Genetic Skin Disorders

OXFORD MONOGRAPHS ON MEDICAL GENETICS

General Editors
ARNO G. MOTULSKY MARTIN BOBROW
PETER S. HARPER CHARLES SCRIVER

Former Editors
J.A. FRASER ROBERTS C.O. CARTER

1. R.B. McConnell: *The genetics of gastrointestinal disorders*
2. A.C. Kopeć: *The distribution of the blood groups in the United Kingdom*
3. E. Slater and V.A. Cowie: *The genetics of mental disorders*
4. C.O. Carter and T.J. Fairbank: *The genetics of locomotor disorders*
5. A.E. Mourant, A.C. Kopeć, and K. Domaniewska-Sobezak: *The distribution of the human blood groups and other polymorphisms*
6. A.E. Mourant, A.C. Kopeć, and K. Domaniewska-Sobezak: *Blood groups and diseases*
7. A.G. Steinbert and C.E. Cook: *The distribution of the human immunoglobulin allotypes*
8. D. Tills, A.C. Kopeć, and R.E. Tills: *The distribution of the human blood groups and other polymorphisms: Supplement I*
10. D.Z. Loesch: *Quantitative dermatoglyphics: classification, genetics, and pathology*
11. D.J. Bond and A.C. Chandley: *Aneuploidy*
12. P.F. Benson and A.H. Fensom: *Genetic biochemical disorders*
13. G.R. Sutherland and F. Hecht: *Fragile sites on human chromosomes*
14. M.d'A Crawfurd: *The genetics of renal tract disorders*
16. C.R. Scriver and B. Childs: *Garrod's inborn factors in disease*
18. M. Baraitser: *The genetics of neurological disorders, second edition*
19. R.J. Gorlin, M.M. Cohen, Jr., and L.S. Levin: *Syndromes of the head and neck, third edition*
20. R.A. King, J.I. Rotter, and A.G. Motulsky: *The genetic basis of common diseases*
21. D. Warburton, J. Byrne, and N. Canki: *Chromosome anomalies and prenatal development: an atlas*
22. J.J. Nora, K. Berg, and A.H. Nora: *Cardiovascular diseases: genetics, epidemiology, and prevention*
24. A.E.H. Emery: *Duchenne muscular dystrophy, second edition*
25. E.G.D. Tuddenham and D.N. Cooper: *The molecular genetics of haemostasis and its inherited disorders*
26. A. Boué: *Fetal medicine*
27. R.E. Stevenson, J.G. Hall, and R.M. Goodman: *Human malformations*
28. R.J. Gorlin, H.V. Toriello, and M.M. Cohen, Jr.: *Hereditary hearing loss and its syndromes*
29. R.J.M. Gardner and G.R. Sutherland: *Chromosome abnormalities and genetic counseling, second edition*
30. A.S. Teebi and T.I. Farag: *Genetic disorders among Arab populations*
31. M. Michael Cohen: *The child with multiple birth defects*
32. W.W. Weber: *Pharmacogenetics*
33. V.P. Sybert: *Genetic skin disorders*

OXFORD MONOGRAPHS ON MEDICAL GENETICS NO. 33

Genetic Skin Disorders

Virginia P. Sybert, M.D.

Professor and Head, Division of Dermatology
Professor, Division of Medicine Genetics,
Department of Pediatrics
Adjunct Professor, Divisions of Dermatology and Medical Genetics,
Department of Medicine
University of Washington School of Medicine and
Children's Hospital and Medical Center
Seattle, Washington

New York Oxford
OXFORD UNIVERSITY PRESS
1997

Oxford University Press

Oxford New York
Athens Auckland Bangkok Bogota
Bombay Buenos Aires Calcutta Cape Town
Dar es Salaam Delhi Florence Hong Kong Istanbul
Karachi Kuala Lumpur Madras Madrid
Melbourne Mexico City Nairobi Paris
Singapore Taipei Tokyo Toronto

and associated companies in
Berlin Ibadan

Published by Oxford University Press, Inc.
198 Madison Avenue, New York, New York 10016

Library of Congress Cataloging-in-Publication Data
Sybert, Virginia P.
Genetic skin disorders / Virginia P. Sybert.
p. cm. (Oxford monographs on medical genetics : no. 33)
Includes bibliographical references and index.
ISBN 0-19-506218-3
1. Skin—Diseases—Genetic aspects. I. Title. II. Series.
[DNLM: 1. Skin Diseases—genetics. WR 218 S981g 1997]
RL793.593 1997
616.5′042—dc21
DNLM/DLC
for Library of Congress 97–2037

1 3 5 7 9 8 6 4 2

Printed in Hong Kong
On acid-free paper

To my mother, Mildred Lerner

Preface

Why another book on inherited skin diseases? At last count there were five in print and one in revision. And really, isn't that enough? Hopefully, no.

This book was born out of my own frustration in finding information quickly and efficiently when dealing with a patient with inherited skin disease in whom there was a question of diagnosis or inheritance or syndromic association.

I modeled this book after David W. Smith's incomparable *Recognizable Patterns of Human Malformation* because it continues to be the one volume turned to most frequently by specialists and generalists when it comes to the visual diagnosis of malformation syndromes. Why? Because the entries are highly formatted and easy to scan, contain pithy information, and provide great photographs for comparison. Most useful is the appendix of differential diagnosis by anomalies; one can quickly scan through the list, thumb through the entries for each entity, eliminate conditions readily from further consideration, and recognize others that one might erroneously not have included. Beyond content, the typeface and formatting of the entries (especially in the third edition) allow for rapid scanning. How material is presented is as important as what material is presented. If you can't find it, it doesn't matter how good it is.

Acknowledgments

I am indebted to many people and many institutions. Maimon Cohen introduced me to clinical genetics at the State University of New York at Buffalo. Judy Hall, Arno Motulsky, and George Stamatoyannopoulos provided a training program nonpareil at Children's Hospital and Medical Center and the University of Washington School of Medicine. Bonnie Pagon has been a colleague of the heart whose opinions have never ceased to help. Karen Stephens made a place, both literally and figuratively, for me without which this book could not have been completed. Ron Scott provided the position that enabled me to stay in Seattle, George Odland allowed me entry into Dermatology and Marvin Scotvold made room for me at Children's. Julie Francis' support has been unflagging. I thank Nancy Esterly for her gracious introduction into the pediatric dermatology community and my colleagues across the country and continents in both genetics and dermatology who have shared their insights and expertise.

I gratefully acknowledge the support of Roche Laboratories and Galderma Laboratories in partially defraying the cost of color printing.

I am grateful for the secretarial assistance of hieroglyphics experts Melanie Kling, Cathy Moore, and Christine Neely-Jones. This book would not have been possible without the expert collaboration of Maxine Covington, whose love of the language and fierce defense of grammar are evident throughout. The availability of the primary resources in the collection of the Health Sciences Library at the University of Washington School of Medicine has been absolutely essential. Unfortunately, funding crises and fashion (financial support for computers seems to overwhelm that for collections) are seriously eroding the ability of my institution to obtain and maintain vital original information. This is to be deplored.

The intellectual rigor and curiosity of the medical students, fellows, and residents in our training programs—pediatrics, family medicine, genetics, and dermatology—are responsible for much of the content in this book. In the eternal quiz show of academic medicine, it is the next generation's "why" that pushes us beyond each answer to the next "I don't know," which in its turn must be answered. They keep laziness at bay.

I am grateful to Oxford University Press for the long leash and patience that they have shown me and most particularly to Jeffrey House, who has been the nicest of principals.

Penultimately, I owe more than can ever be expressed to my patients and their families. I am grateful for their faith, for their generosity, and for their willingness to let me into the most intimate corners of their lives.

Lastly, from Peter and Julia and Ben, my safe harbor, comes the rhythm of my days.

Contents

4. DISORDERS OF PIGMENTATION 262

5. DISORDERS OF THE DERMIS 335

Introduction

This book is not exhaustive or all-inclusive. It is meant to be a readable, handy guide to the diagnosis and differential of inherited skin disorders to which you can refer while the patient is still in your office. The annotated bibliographies contain many review papers and those from readily available journals. Although other sources, including original descriptions and publications in languages other than English, have been used in the writing of each section, I have chosen to emphasize those references that contain interesting additional information that you can easily find if you are interested in further reading. The bibliographies of the cited articles can direct you further to more extensive sources.

Many of the comments reflect my own biases, developed out of 15 years of a highly selective practice of genodermatology. I have tried to make it clear where I differ from dogma.

Descriptions of histopathology, at both the light and electron microscopic levels, are attributed only when the original observations are from articles of general interest. For many descriptions, I depended heavily on several general histopathology texts, including Lever and Schaumburg (1990): *Lever's Histopathology of the Skin,* 7th ed., and Johannessen and Hashimoto (1985): *Electron Microscopy in Human Medicine,* Vol. 11(2): The Skin. For descriptions of the ultrastructure of prenatal skin, Dr. Karen Holbrook was an invaluable resource.

My hope is that the book will be useful to generalists, pediatricians, dermatologists and geneticists. For each disorder I've tried to include the answers to the questions I most often have: What are all the pertinent associated clinical features? What is the differential diagnosis? How is the condition inherited? Where do I or my patient turn now? I strongly urge you to contact medical genetics centers or the various support groups for the most current information regarding treatment, experimental protocols, molecular studies, and prenatal diagnosis. The names and addresses of support groups come from the Directory of National Genetic Voluntary Organizations and Related Resources published by the Alliance of Genetic Support Groups, 35 Wisconsin Circle, Suite 440, Chevy Chase, Maryland 20815-7015, 1-800-336-GENE. 2nd Edition, May 1995. These organizations are an invaluable resource for information and support for you and your patients. They range from kitchen table volunteer groups to highly sophisticated national organizations. NORD—The National Organization for Rare Disorders, P.O. Box 8923, New Fairfield, Connecticut 06812, 1-800-999-6673—is a central clearinghouse for information on rare disorders and can direct you to an appropriate resource if none of those listed seems appropriate.

The medical literature is replete with case reports of recognized syndromes "plus" or recognized syndromes "minus." It is often difficult to tease out those features that are part and parcel of a given disorder and those that are occurring by chance alone and to decide what the minimal diagnostic criteria are. As consistently as possible, the text indicates where I believe that distinct and separate disorders exist and where I believe that the isolated case reports represent variable expressions of a recognized disorder. Every possible combination of anything with something else has been reported at least once and may have occurred only by chance. Almost every nongenetic disease has occurred more than once in at least one family. This book is not meant to be an exhaustive review of every skin finding that has ever been reported to occur in more than one family member nor of every inherited syndrome that has ever shown dermatologic manifestations. For example, the rare occurrence of nevus of Ota in family members did not seem compelling enough to warrant its inclusion as a separate genetic condition. Down syndrome and Noonan syndrome are not included as separate entries because their dermatologic manifestations, while of interest, are irrelevant to their diagnosis.

A few disorders are discussed in this volume (e.g., bathing trunk nevus, Klippel-Trenaunay-Weber syndrome) that do not appear to be inherited but that are traditionally covered by the umbrella of congenital skin disorders. These are included here because it seems natural, appropriate, and useful to do so.

Conditions are grouped arbitrarily into categories reflecting the primary site of the major dermatologic features. Some conditions traditionally have been considered in one group rather than another. For example, bullous congenital ichthyosiform erythroderma is classified as an ichthyosis rather than a bullous disorder. Some conditions defy pigeonholing: Where does incontinentia pigmenti really belong? Is it a disorder of hyperpigmentation, of blistering, or of hyperkerotosis? There is an alphabetical listing of conditions in Appendix C to aid readers in finding them.

The sections on treatment reflect both current recommendations and personal preference. I have tried to avoid dogmatic recommendations, as fashion in medicine changes faster than revisions can be made.

The mode of inheritance given for each entity reflects our current understanding. In some instances, pedigree or molecular proof for a single accepted or presumed mode of inheritance is lacking. Where there is question, I have given the reasons for doubt or listed the evidence for choosing one mode of inheritance over another.

This is not a textbook of genetics. The chapter on practical inheritance sets out guidelines for generating and understanding recurrence risks. Although everyone does not have ready access to a medical genetics center, a referral to a genetics clinic can be of great benefit to families. In very few other medical settings is time set aside for a family to present its agenda of concerns and for a detailed and careful exposition of all the issues surrounding inherited disease.

Appendix B lists diagnoses by dermatologic signs. This list has been designed to serve as a starting point for both dermatologists and geneticists. I have tried to cross-reference physical findings, by both dermatologic nomenclature and medical genetics terminology. By redundancy I hope to cover all of your bases.

These have been arbitrary decisions and have been part of the fun in writing this book. In contrast to refereed journal articles, a book is the unexpurgated result of idiosyncrasy. I have done my best not to lead readers astray. I welcome comments and will appreciate the opportunity to correct errors.

CHAPTER 1

PRACTICAL INHERITANCE

Genetic disorders are unique among diseases in that they affect families and generations, not just individuals. In the diagnosis and discussion of an inherited disorder, the recurrence risk must always be included. Will it happen again? Who is at risk to inherit? What is the magnitude of that risk? How severely will the condition be manifested? The answers to these questions depend on the mode of inheritance and the penetrance and expression of the gene(s) for the disorder.

Inherited disease is usually classified as single gene or Mendelian, chromosomal, or multifactorial or polygenic. Mendelian disorders are further subdivided into autosomal and sex linked, dominant and recessive. In addition to these classic modes of inheritance, we now recognize contiguous gene syndromes, gonadal or somatic mosaicism, imprinting, and mitochrondrial inheritance. Each of these confers its own modification of classic recurrence risks.

If we are to provide accurate genetic counseling, a disorder must be correctly diagnosed, recognized to be or not be genetic, and characterized as to the mode of inheritance. Many genetic conditions are sporadic, occurring only in a single individual in a family. For some disorders, this has resulted in a failure to recognize the genetic nature or a misclassification regarding the mode of inheritance.

The first step in the evaluation of any patient suspected of having a genetic skin disorder is to compile a family history. Often this will clearly delineate the mode of inheritance. More often, the family history will be negative. How can this be explained in the context of a genetic disorder? Perhaps you are mistaken and the family history is not negative. You have asked the wrong question. "Does anyone in your family have neurofibromas" is less likely to elicit a positive response than "Does anyone in your family have lumps or bumps on the skin?" Often the informant simply does not know enough details. Always try to obtain medical records that may be relevant. It is better to be weary than to be wrong.

What if the family history really is negative? Sporadic cases can be the result of new dominant mutations. The gene for the condition has been altered in the formation of the egg or the sperm and is not truly "carried" by either parent. There is no recurrence risk to the parents or siblings in this situation, but the affected individual, who now has one copy of the normal allele and one copy of the mutation, does have a risk of transmitting the condition to offspring. This is the classic 50% risk for autosomal dominant disorders.

Autosomal recessive inheritance often gives a negative family history. With a 1 in 4 risk for each offspring to be affected when both parents are carriers, by chance alone many small sibships will contain only one affected individual. What appears to be sporadic in fact carries a 25% recurrence risk. Autosomal recessive inheritance is often invoked incorrectly when a single child is affected, especially in those disorders where the mode of inheritance is uncertain. Many lethal conditions traditionally thought to be autosomal recessive are the result of new dominant mutations or gonadal mosaicism in the parent, and the recurrence risks are very different (25% vs. 0% vs. indeterminate).

Female carriers of X-linked recessive disorders may not be recognized because they do not express the condition, or there may have been a paucity of males at risk born in the family, giving rise to a negative family history even though multiple female relatives carry the gene.

Nonpaternity plays a role in providing a negative family history. Misattribution of fatherhood occurs in perhaps as many as 10% of all births in the United States. When in doubt, check it out, discreetly.

Phenocopies do exist. There are acquired disorders that can mimic inherited conditions. It is as important to confirm a lack of recurrence as it is to determine the likelihood of it.

More than one mode of inheritance may be responsible for certain disorders. Genocopies, or genetic heterogeneity, have been demonstrated for many conditions. While most cases of epidermolysis bullosa simplex are due to autosomal dominant mutations that result in structurally altered kerating proteins, in a few families autosomal recessive inheritance of null alleles, those that do not make any protein product, is the cause. Recurrence risks are quite different.

Occasionally, a dominant disorder diagnosed in the patient as new will actually be carried by a parent in whom subtle signs are not recognized (minimal expression) or in whom the gene simply results in no detectable phenotypic change (lack of penetrance). It is important to be aware of those genetic conditions in which this phenomenon is common.

How do we establish the likely mode of inheritance for a given disorder? This traditionally has been based on pedigree analysis and biochemical studies. More recently, molecular techniques have been employed to pinpoint specific mutations, and these have established or confirmed the mechanism of inheritance for some genetic disorders.

In autosomal dominant disorders, the pedigree shows generation to generation transmission; males and females are equally at risk. The disorders are often marked by both intrafamilial and interfamilial variability in severity. Occasionally a gene carrier may not express the condition, and so a "skipped" generation appears. The disorder may skip, but the gene does not. The *sine qua non* to prove autosomal dominant rather than X-linked inheritance is the transmission of the disorder from father to son, as fathers do not give their X chromosome to their boy children. Male to male transmission is not required in every family. It need only occur once for a given disorder to confirm autosomal dominant inheritance. The risk to the offspring of an individual with an autosomal dominant disorder to inherit the offending gene is 50%. The risk to express the disorder may be modified by reduced penetrance, variable expressivity, imprinting, and sex-limited expression.

For autosomal recessive disorders, the risk for each pregnancy to carrier parents is 25%. Each unaffected sibling has a 2 in 3 risk to be a carrier, and each healthy parental sibling has a 1 in 2 risk to be a carrier. The likelihood of these individuals having an affected child depends on the carrier frequency of the gene in the general population, which tends to be estimated at 1 in 50 or less except for those very few "common" disorders recognized within certain ethnic groups (e.g., sickle cell anemia, cystic fibrosis). For these conditions the carrier frequency may approach 1 in 10 to 1 in 20 in the at-risk population. The risk for relatives of probands with autosomal recessive diseases, other than the parents, to have affected children is absolutely small, albeit relatively greater than that of the general population. These estimates need to be calculated appropriately for each situation, based on the carrier frequency in the population.

For X-linked recessive conditions, affected fathers will transmit the gene to all of their daughters and to none of their sons, and the risk for disease will devolve upon the grandchildren born to the daughters. Carrier mothers will transmit the gene with a 50% likelihood to each daughter and each son. A son who inherits the gene will express the disorder; a daughter who inherits the gene will be a carrier who may show none, some, or all the signs of the condition. In X-linked dominant disorders, the risk to inherit the gene is the same, but the outcome is different. These conditions are usually lethal in males and result in early embryonic death. Daughters who inherit the gene will usually express the disorder to some degree.

Chromosomal disorders often do not carry a risk for recurrence. Occasionally, a parent may carry his or her chromosomes in a rearranged fashion in which the structure is altered but the genetic content is normal. While this does not have a phenotypic effect, it does put the parent at risk to make chromosomally unbalanced gametes. Thus the pregnancies of such individuals are at risk to inherit unbalanced chromosome rearrangements that have occurred during meiosis. It is rarely necessary to karyotype parents of children with numerical chromosome abnormalities, such as trisomy 21 or trisomy 18, but is almost always required for those children with unbalanced structural alterations.

Multifactorial conditions are believed to result from a combination of genetic and environmental factors, and the recurrence risks are empiric. They are based on what has been observed in population studies. Polygenic conditions are thought to result solely from the interaction of multiple genes, irrespective of the environmental influences. Recurrence risks are again empiric. The risk of recurrence for a multifactorial/polygenic condition decreases as relatedness decreases. First degree relatives (parents, siblings, children) are at higher risk than second (grandparents, grandchildren, aunts, uncles) or third (first cousins) degree relatives. The recurrence risk also increases as the number of affected individuals within a family increases.

There are other factors that alter the magnitude of a recurrence risk and mechanisms that affect genes in ways that can modify risks. *Anticipation,* the observed phenomenon of worsening of certain genetic disorders in subsequent generations, may in some conditions be due to expansion or contraction of regions of the gene referred to as *trinucleotide repeats.* Anticipation has implications for counseling in that it is not only the likelihood of inheriting a disorder but also the likelihood of greater severity that imposes a reproductive burden.

Imprinting refers to the modification of maternal or paternal genes that occurs during the formation of the eggs or sperm so that they are expressed differently in the child if inherited from one parent or the other. For example, a gene may require transmission through a mother to be activated and may not be expressed if inherited from a father. While the risk to transmit the gene remains 50%, this phenomenon results in a different risk to express the disorder depending on the sex of the transmitting parent.

Some pleiotropic syndromes (those involving multiple tissues and organs) result from contiguous gene deletions. The term *contiguous gene deletion* refers to submicroscopic loss of chromosomal material that results in loss of function for several genes. In some instances, these arise de novo; in others they may be inherited. Great variability within contiguous gene syndromes may result from involvement of few or more or specific genes in the same region.

There are genes that reside outside the nuclear chromosome structure, in the cytoplasmic mitochondria. These mitochondrial genes are transmitted exclusively by females to offspring and in variable numbers. Mitochrondrial inheritance results in an unusual pedigree pattern in which transmission is exclusively by females, and the proportion of affected children appears to be random.

Mosaicism for single gene defects and for chromosome abnormalities offers yet another mechanism for occurrence and recurrence of genetic disease. A mutation or chromosomal abnormality arising after fertilization in an early cell of a zygote will be expressed only in the cells derived from the initial target cell. The distribution of those cells will depend on the timing and site of the original error. The gonads of an individual mosaic for such an alteration may or may not contain cells with the abnormality. The risk to have an affected child depends on gonadal involvement and may range from 0% to 50%.

With rapid advances in our ability to diagnose genetic disorders at a clinical and molecular level, to identify carriers, and to provide earlier and earlier prenatal diagnosis, coupled with our increasing understanding of the complexity of control of the expression of genetic disease, it is incumbent upon every practitioner to recognize those disorders with a significant genetic component and to offer to refer individuals and families with these conditions for appropriate genetic diagnosis and counseling.

REFERENCES

Sybert, V.P. (1993). Principles of genetics in the molecular era. A primer for dermatologists. *Arch. Dermatol.* **129,** 1409–1416.

Berg, P., and Singer, M. (1992). *Dealing with genes: the language of heredity.* University Science Books, Mill Valley, CA.
A fine textbook with clear discourse. A palatable refresher for the course you slept through in college.

CHAPTER 2

DISORDERS OF THE EPIDERMIS

Differentiation and Kinetics

ICHTHYOSES

The term *ichthyosis* refers to a group of disorders that have in common scaling of the skin. The term itself has come under criticism; *disorders of keratinization* and *disorders of cornification* have been proposed as more fitting and inclusive labels. The historical and colloquial popularity of *ichthyosis* is likely to keep its usage alive, despite its orthographical complexity (how many "h"s are there?).

These disorders have been classified on the basis of clinical and histologic features and, more recently, biochemical and molecular markers. Prognosis, recurrence risk, and accurate prenatal diagnosis depend on the correct diagnosis. To differentiate ichthyosis vulgaris from sterol sulfatase deficiency has significant implications for families. The recognition of Sjögren-Larsson syndrome in a child with lamellar ichthyosis is critical. It has been the experience of most clinicians dealing with the ichthyoses that a significant proportion of patients appear not quite to fit into a specific recognized category. As with other disorders for which the genetic basis has been elucidated, it is highly likely that even within a single diagnostic category allelic and nonallelic differences will be found (e.g., bullous congenital ichthyosiform erythroderma can result from different mutations in different keratins), and many families will be found to have private mutations.

The reader is referred to the following publications for more detailed reviews of this group of disorders:

Traupe, H. (1989). *The ichthyoses: a guide to clinical diagnosis, genetic counseling, and therapy*. Springer-Verlag, New York.

This is a gem of a book with excellent photographs and a colloquial style that makes hard science and clinical minutiae accessible to a general audience. The author freely presents his own opinions and is clear to indicate what is fact and what is hypothesis.

Williams, M.L., and Elias, P.M. (1987). Genetically transmitted generalized disorders of cornification. The ichthyoses. *Dermatol. Clin.* **5**, 155–178.

This review suggests renaming the ichthyoses as numbered disorders of cornification rather than by eponym. I personally find the classification scheme unworkable, (I just can't remember all those numbers), but the review is excellent.

BULLOUS CONGENITAL ICHTHYOSIFORM ERYTHRODERMA (MIM:113800)

(Epidermolytic Hyperkeratosis; Bullous Erythroderma Ichthyosiform Congenital of Brocq)

DERMATOLOGIC FEATURES

MAJOR. Bullous congenital ichthyosiform erythroderma is rare, occurring in perhaps 1 in 300,000 births. Infants with bullous congenital ichthyosiform erythroderma are born with erythematous, blistering, and denuded skin, with areas of marked hyperkeratosis. In some, only

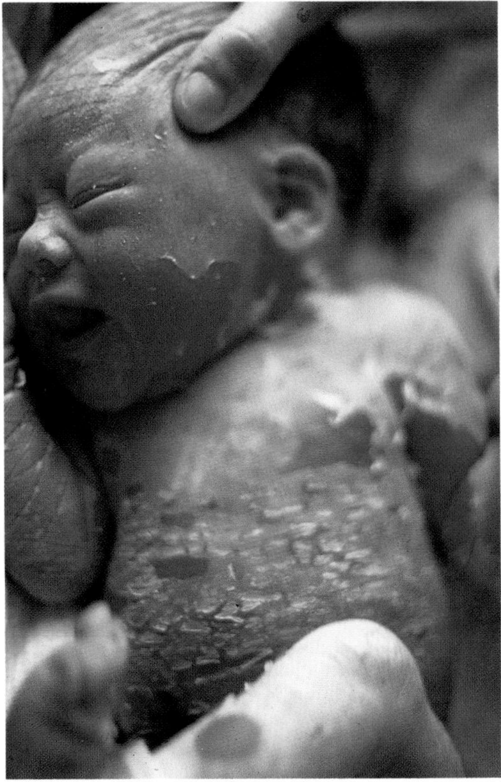

Figure 2.1. Newborn with erythema, scaling, and denuded areas. (From Sybert and Holbrook, 1987.)

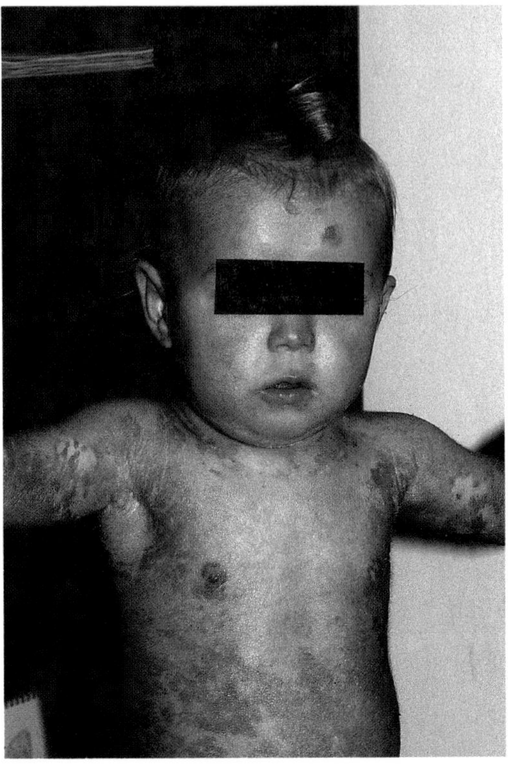

Figure 2.2. Toddler with darker scale; erosions show underlying erythema. (From Sybert and Holbrook, 1987.)

erythroderma and bullae are present at birth, and hyperkeratosis develops later.

Over time there is a gradual decrease in the frequency of blister formation, but an increase in the severity of the ichthyosis. The erythroderma lessens, but persists to some degree throughout life. The skin underlying the ichthyotic plaques is often tender. Skin involvement is generalized in most, with palmar and plantar involvement. There are patients with patchy, inverse, or more limited skin involvement. Significant interfamilial variation in the severity of the ichthyosis is typical of classic bullous congenital ichthyosiform erythroderma. Intrafamilial variation also occurs.

The severity of involvement in adult life cannot be reliably predicted by severity of presentation at birth.

The disorder can be life threatening at birth, with sepsis a not uncommon complication. Cutaneous infection with common pathogens, *Staphylococcus* and *Streptococcus,* is a chronic problem. Patients are often odiferous; the odor is most marked when superinfection is present.

The teeth, hair, and nails are normal, but scalp involvement can be severe, resulting in hair loss because of matted crusts. Heat intolerance is common, presumably because of mechanical inhibition by scale of heat loss from sweating.

Minor. Loss of distal finger pad substance and limited range of motion of the small joints of the hands and feet can occur when palmar and plantar involvement is severe.

One 69-year-old patient with bullous congenital ichthyosiform erythroderma was reported with multiple squamous and basal cell tumors. However, she had previously received two courses of superficial x-ray to treat her ichthyosis. She also developed a breast cancer. No other reports suggested increased occurrence of cutaneous malignancies.

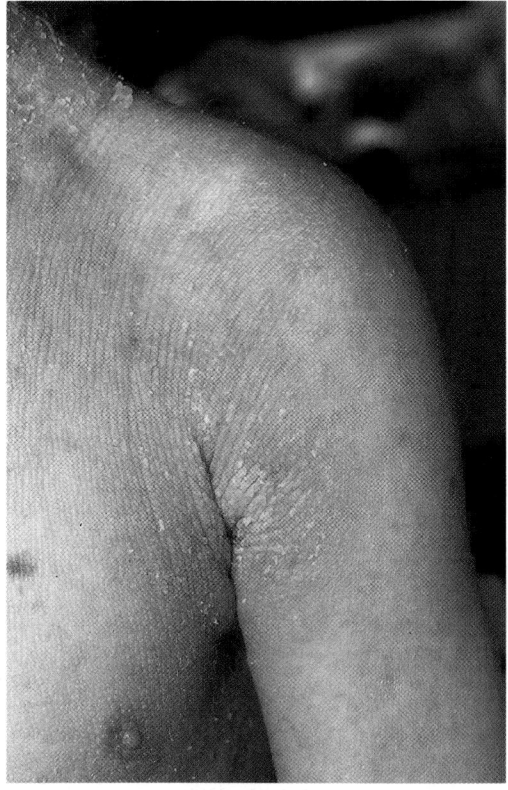

Figure 2.3. Older individual with scale along epidermal skin lines, thickest in axillary folds.

ASSOCIATED ABNORMALITIES

None.

HISTOPATHOLOGY

LIGHT. There is hypergranulosis with orthokeratosis of a compact or basket weave extremely thickened stratum corneum. Cytolysis with blurring of the keratinocyte margins in the upper stratum spinosum and granular layer is typical. The basal layers are usually normal. There may be a minimal inflammatory infiltrate.

EM. Clumping of tonofilaments in the superbasal layers of the epidermis is the hallmark of epidermolytic hyperkeratosis. This feature is not specific to bullous congenital ichthyosiform erythroderma, but can be seen in a number of inherited conditions and in organoid nevi.

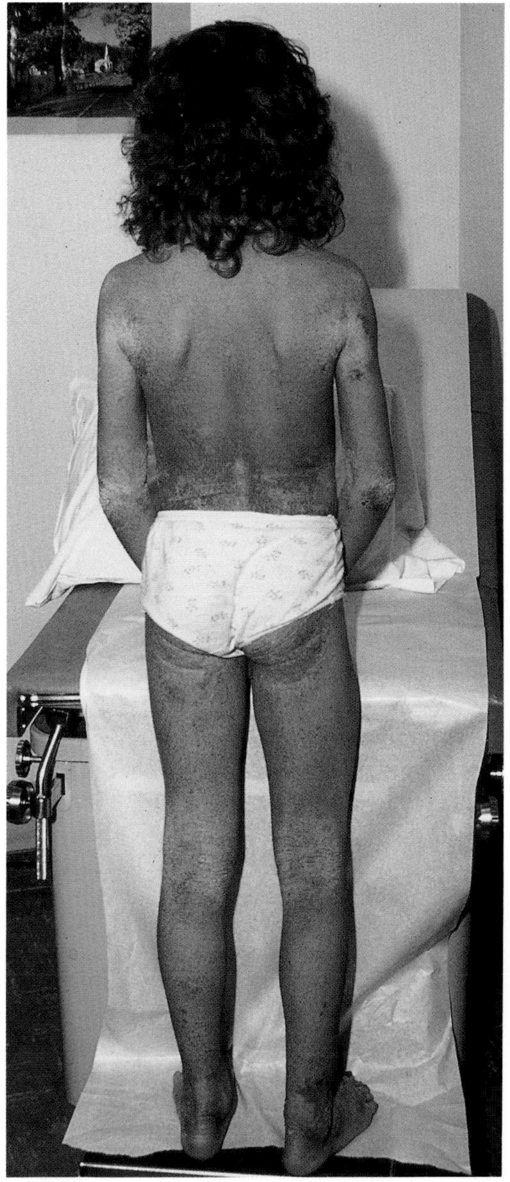

Figure 2.4. Older child with dark, thickened scaling plaques.

BASIC DEFECT

Linkage of bullous congenital ichthyosiform erythroderma to 12p, where the type II keratin gene cluster resides, has been shown, and muta-

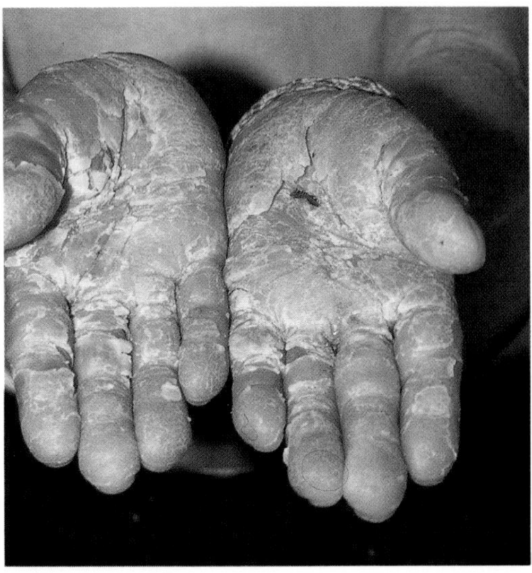

Figure 2.5. Marked palm involvement.

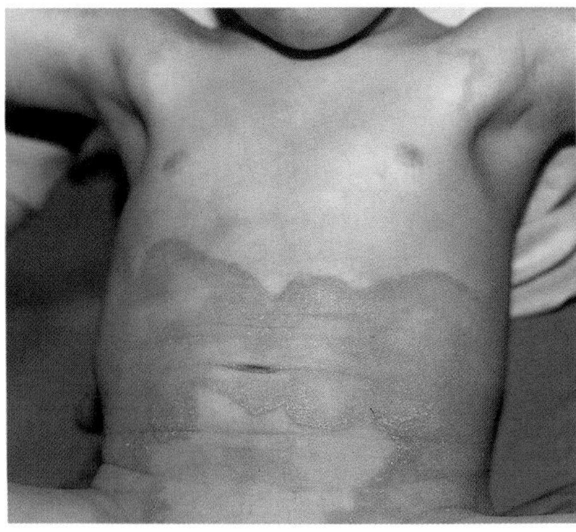

Figure 2.6. Localized involvement. Histologically shows epidermolytic hyperkeratosis. Phenotype reflects allelic heterogenity.

tions in K_1 and K_{10} have been identified in some patients. The introduction of a K_{10} mutation into a transgenic mouse produced animals with a similar phenotype. Abnormal tonofilament aggregates in bullous congenital ichthyosiform erythroderma were composed of K_1 and K_{10} (Yamamoto et al., [J. Invest. Dermatol. 99:19–26, 1992). It is hypothesized that these and other mutations in keratins are responsible for all types of epidermolytic hyperkeratosis.

TREATMENT

Oral retinoids (etretinate, Accutane, and acitretin) have resulted in significant improvement, but must be used with caution because of side effects. Many patients can be titrated to a very low maintenance dose that gives them tolerable, but not maximum, improvement or treat themselves intermittently in efforts to avoid complications.

Fifty percent propylene glycol and water under plastic occlusion for 4–12 hours weekly has been well tolerated by some of my patients with acceptable results.

Lac-Hydrin, 10% urea cream, 10% lactic acid in Eucerin, and glycolic acid lotions can all be somewhat effective. Soaking and gentle debridement of scale, especially of the hands and feet, may be useful to keep mobility intact.

Long-term intermittent use of antibiotics is almost always necessary. Many patients report increased blistering as a sign of impending secondary infection. Low-dose, long-term antibiotic therapy may also decrease the frequency of symptomatic infection. Topical mupirocin (Bactroban) applied to erosions is useful.

In the newborn period, management of increased water loss and increased susceptibility to infection is important.

MODE OF INHERITANCE

Autosomal dominant.

There have been reports of unrelated children with bullous congenital ichthyosiform erythroderma born to parents with extensive linear epidermal nevi distributed along the lines of Blaschko. These nevi demonstrated epidermolytic hyperkeratosis histologically. Somatic mosaicism for mutations in K_{10} have been demonstrated in some of these parents, whose affected children have inherited the abnormal allele and express typical bullous congenital ichthyosiform erythroderma. These cases suggest that the linear epidermal nevus might reflect somatic mosaicism for the gene for bullous congenital ichthyosiform erythroderma. To my knowl-

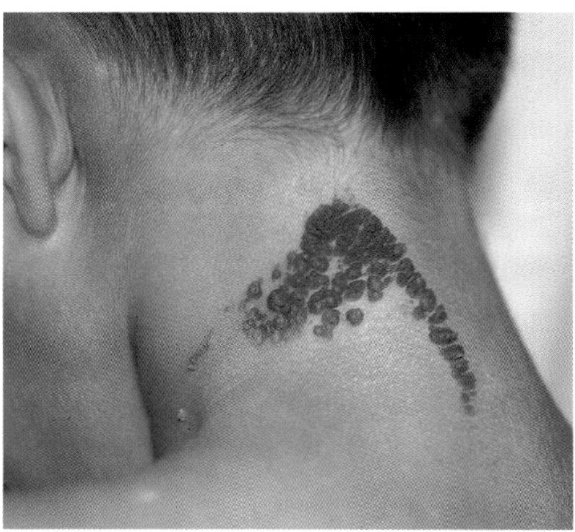

Figure 2.7. Epidermal nevus in distribution along line of Blaschko. Shows epidermolytic hyperkeratosis on biopsy.

edge, there are no reports of individuals with more limited epidermal nevi who have had affected children. There is, however, a single report of a parent with two small areas of nevus comedonicus who had a child with bullous congenital ichthyosiform erythroderma.

PRENATAL DIAGNOSIS

Until recently, fetal skin biopsy has been utilized successfully. With identification of the molecular defects, prenatal diagnosis by direct DNA analysis of CVS or amniotic fluid cells is possible.

DIFFERENTIAL DIAGNOSIS

Infants with nonbullous congenital ichthyosiform erythroderma/lamellar ichthyosis (MIM: 242100) have similar erythroderma and scaling at birth, but have no blistering. Later in childhood, the ichthyosis of nonbullous congenital ichthyosiform erythroderma tends to be marked by flat or plate-like scales, whereas in bullous congenital ichthyosiform erythroderma the scale tends to be thickened and more verruciform. Biopsy will discriminate easily between the two conditions.

The epidermolysis bullosa syndromes, including epidermolysis bullosa letalis (MIM:226650, 226700, 226730), epidermolysis bullosa simplex—Dowling-Meara (MIM: 131760), and epidermolysis bullosa dystrophica (MIM:226200), are marked by blistering and erosions at birth, but generally there is no hyperkeratosis and the infants are rarely erythrodermic. Electron microscopy will distinguish among these conditions.

In incontinentia pigmenti (MIM:308300), the distribution and grouping of small vesicles along the lines of Blaschko is different from the more generalized and random erosions and blisters in bullous congenital ichthyosiform erythroderma. Hyperkeratosis is usually more marked in bullous congenital ichthyosiform erythroderma. Biopsy will differentiate between the conditions.

At birth, infants with the AEC syndrome (Hay-Wells, MIM:106260) can mimic bullous congenital ichthyosiform erythroderma by presenting with erosions and shedding of a collodion membrane. There are no ankyloblepharon in bullous congenital ichthyosiform erythroderma, and cleft lip and cleft palate are absent.

Staphylococcal scalded skin and bullous impetigo in the newborn period can be confused with bullous congenital ichthyosiform erythroderma. Both of these conditions are marked by red, denuded skin, but neither has hyperkeratosis. Appropriate cultures will help discriminate.

Ichthyosis hystrix can be very similar clinically and histologically, but electron microscopy shows difference in tonofilament aggregation. The distribution of lesions in the nevoid form of ichthyosis hystrix is typically along the lines of Blaschko, and this condition may represent somatic mosaicism for bullous congenital ichthyosiform erythroderma. Ichthyosis hystrix of Curth-Macklin (MIM:146590) is more generalized in distribution and is marked by spiny hyperkeratosis rather than verrucous crusting lesions.

Support Group: F.I.R.S.T.
P.O. Box 20921
Raleigh, NC 27619
1-800-545-3286

SELECTED BIBLIOGRAPHY

Cheng, J., Syder, A.J., Yu, Q.-C., Letai, A., Paller, A.S., and Fuchs, E. (1992). The genetic basis of epidermolytic hyperkeratosis: a disorder of differentiation-specific epidermal keratin genes. *Cell* **70,** 811–819.

The authors demonstrate a mutation in codon 156 of K_{10} in affected members in two of six pedigrees studied.

Chipev, C.C., Korge, B.P., Markova, N., Bale, S.J., DiGiovanna, J.J., Compton, J.G., and Steinert, P.M. (1992). A leucine-proline mutation in the H1 subdomain of keratin 1 causes epidermolytic hyperkeratosis. *Cell* **70,** 821–828.

All affected and no unaffected members of a pedigree with bullous congenital ichthyosiform erythroderma had a mutation in K_1.

Nazzaro, V., Ermacora, E., Santucci, B., and Caputo, R. (1990). Epidermolytic hyperkeratosis: generalized form in children from parents with systematized linear form. *Br. J. Dermatol.* **122,** 417–422.

A daughter with generalized bullous congenital ichthyosiform erythroderma was born to a mother whose skin lesions were distributed along the lines of Blaschko. A son with generalized bullous congenital ichthyosiform erythroderma was born to a father with skin lesions also distributed along the lines of Blaschko.

Paller, A.S., Syder, A.J., Chan, Y.M., Yu, Q.C., Hutton, E., Tadini, G., Fuchs, E. (1994). Genetic and clinical mosaicism in a type of epidermal nevus. *N. Engl. J. Med.* **331,** 1408–1415.

Parents of three probands with bullous congenital ichthyosiform erythroderma had epidermal nevi. Lesional skin from the parents showed mutations in 50% of the K_{10} alleles; nonlesional skin had only normal alleles. The affected children showed the same mutations as their parents.

Rothnagel, J.A., Dominey, A.M., Dempsey, L.D., Longley, M.A., Greenhalgh, D.A., Gagne, T.A., Huber, M., Frenk, E., Hohl, D., and Roop, D.R. (1992). Mutations in the rod domains of keratins 1 and 10 in epidermolytic hyperkeratosis. *Science* **257,** 1128–1130.

Three families with epidermolytic hyperkeratosis were studied. One had mild patchy involvement with little blistering, one had widespread involvement and blistering in childhood, and a third sporadic case demonstrated persistent blistering and widespread hyperkeratosis. The family with rare blistering had a defect in K_1; the others had defects in the keratin 10 rod domain. Whether a clinical phenotype: molecular defect correlation will hold up remains to be shown.

Traupe, H. (1989). *The ichthyoses: a guide to clinical diagnosis, genetic counseling, and therapy.* Springer-Verlag, New York, pp. 139–153.

Traupe gives a very nice discourse distinguishing among bullous congenital ichthyosiform erythroderma of Brocq, ichthyosis bullosa of Siemens, and ichthyosis hystrix of Curth-Macklin.

CONTINUAL PEELING SKIN (MIM:270300)

(Keratolysis Exfoliativa Congenita; Deciduous Skin)

DERMATOLOGIC FEATURES

MAJOR. The term, continuous or continual peeling skin, has been used to describe what appear to be two clinically distinct conditions, both rare. In one, onset of asymptomatic peeling of the superficial layers of the epidermis can occur at birth, during childhood, and (as in one reported individual) in adult life. Involvement is usually diffuse, may be patchy or generalized, and palms and soles are usually spared. Seasonal variation has been described. In some, clearing or improvement occurs in summer, in others, in winter. There is no red-

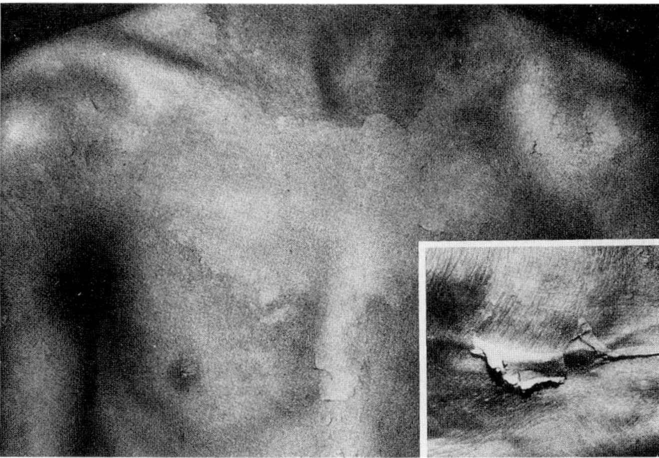

Figure 2.8. Chest of affected individual; inset shows margin of peeling skin. (From Abdel-Hafez et al., 1983.)

ness and no itching, and the lesions are entirely asymptomatic. Traupe refers to this as *type A*.

In the second disorder (*type B,* Traupe), erythema is a primary constant component, and pruritus is part of the disease complex as well. In three unrelated individuals with these findings, serum tryptophan levels were low.

MINOR. In one family with type A, normal-appearing hairs showed light and dark bands with a polarizing microscope.

Hyperpigmentation ranging from slight and brown to more marked gray-brown and dirty-appearing is an inconstant finding.

ASSOCIATED ABNORMALITIES

Short stature has been described in several patients with the red itchy variant of continual peeling skin (type B), but it is not clear that it is actually part of the syndrome. One sporadic patient came from a family with short stature, another had hypogonadotrophic hypogonadism and anosmia, and her sister, purportedly with similar skin findings, had normal stature and no endocrinologic abnormalities.

HISTOPATHOLOGY

LIGHT. Type A: Mild orthohyperkeratosis occurs, with separation of the stratum corneum from the stratum granulosum.

Type B: Parakeratosis and acanthosis are present.

EM. Type A: The plasma membrane of the "peeled" corneocyte remains with the unshed surface cell, suggesting that there is an intracellular cleavage that occurs within the stratum corneum one or more cell layers above the stratum granulosum. Electron-dense lipid-like globular deposits were found between the cells of the stratum corneum.

Type B: Separation appears to occur between the cells of the stratum corneum and stratum granulosum.

BASIC DEFECT

Autoradiography and electron microscopy findings in one patient suggested an increase in the proliferation rate of the epidermis, but the basic defect remains unknown.

TREATMENT

None. The retinoids do not appear to be helpful. Mild emollients may provide some relief.

MODE OF INHERITANCE

Autosomal recessive. Both recurrences within sibships and a high frequency of consanguinity among parents have been noted in both types of continuous peeling skin.

PRENATAL DIAGNOSIS

None.

DIFFERENTIAL DIAGNOSIS

Self-limited desquamation of the stratum corneum (keratosis exfoliativa) can be seen after viral infection, with scarlet fever, Kawasaki disease, and so forth. These are easily distinguished by the associated symptoms. Peeling of the feet is not unusual in chronic foot dermatitis. Peeling can occur with blistering in epidermolysis bullosa simplex (MIM:131800, 131900–131960). Bullae are not part of continual peeling skin. Peeling of the hands and feet is common in hand and foot eczemas as well; these conditions can be distinguished by associated findings.

Variants of lamellar ichthyosis (MIM: 242100) can be marked by peeling of the skin. The collodion membrane present at birth in some ichthyoses can mimic peeling skin, but, once shed, it does not recur. Similarly, some newborns with ectodermal dysplasia may present initially with scaling sheets of skin that do not subsequently recur, but shed to reveal the underlying disorder.

In the Netherton syndrome (MIM:256500), marked by ichthyosis linearis circumflexa, the scales are not easily stripped, and hairs usually show trichorrhexis invaginata. The hair is normal in continual peeling skin. Traupe suggested that type B peeling skin might be allelic to the Netherton syndrome; I believe there may be enough clinical overlap to have resulted in misdiagnosis of some cases of Netherton syndrome as peeling skin, but do not believe the diseases are the same.

Support Group: N.O.R.D.
P.O. Box 8923
New Fairfield, CT
06812
1-800-999-6673

SELECTED BIBLIOGRAPHY

Abdel-Hafez, K., Safer, A.M., Selim, M.M., and Rehak, A. (1983). Familial continual peeling skin. *Dermatologica* **166,** 23–31.

Six cases from two families are presented. There are beautiful photographs and a clear clinical description. In one family, all individuals showed mild hyperpigmentation; in the other, none did.

Behçet, P.E. (1938). Deciduous skin. *Arch. Dermatol. Syphilol.* **37,** 267–271.

This article reviews Fox's original description and describes a 28-year-old male with peeling skin since birth.

Hachem-Zadeh, S., and Holuban, K. (1985). Skin peeling in a Kurdish family. *Arch. Dermatol.* **121,** 545–546.

A brother and sister, born to first cousins who were Kurdish Jews, had itchy red peeling skin present from a few days of life. It improved with age and in summertime.

Kurban, A.K., and Azar, H.A. (1969). Familial continual skin peeling. *Br. J. Dermatol.* **81,** 191–195.

Four of nine siblings, products of a first cousin marriage, had continuous peeling, mild hyperpigmentation, and no erythema.

Traupe, H. (1989). *The ichthyoses: a guide to clinical diagnosis, genetic counseling, and therapy.* New York, Springer-Verlag.

A detailed book on the ichthyoses. Pages 207–210 contain a clear description of peeling skin.

HARLEQUIN FETUS (MIM:242500)

(Harlequin infant; Ichthyosis Congenita Gravior)

DERMATOLOGIC FEATURES

MAJOR. The newborn is covered with thick, armor-like plates of scale that fissure and crack. Eversion of the eyelids (ectropion) and the lips (*eclabium* in English, *eclabion* in French) gives a grotesque "frog-like" appearance to the face. The ears are crumpled and flattened; the nasal tip is flattened with anteversion of the nares. The extremities are swollen and appear edematous due to the tight sausage-like encasement by the thickened stratum corneum. In contrast to the thick yellow scales, the fissures are red and oozing.

MINOR. Eyebrows and eyelashes are usually absent. Scalp hair may or may not be present.

ASSOCIATED ABNORMALITIES

Premature delivery is typical, although some infants are carried to term. Peripartum death is common. Liveborn infants usually die within a few days to weeks due to complications of prematurity, respiratory compromise due to mechanical limitation of ribcage excursion, sepsis, hypothermia, and/or dehydration.

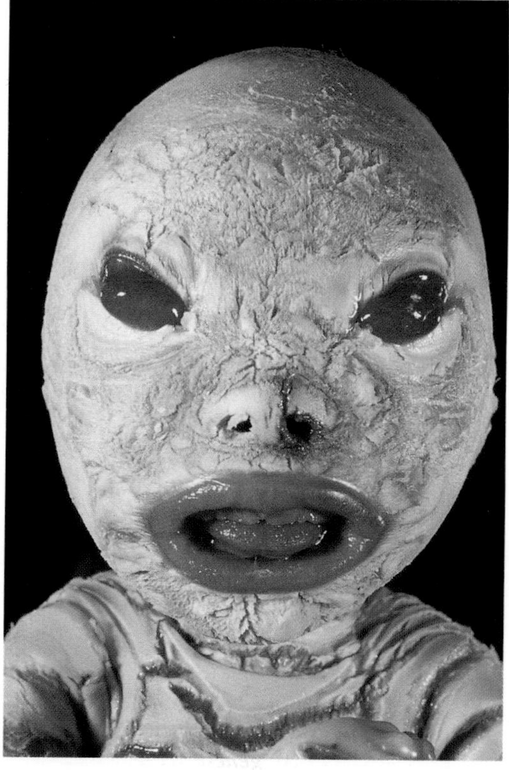

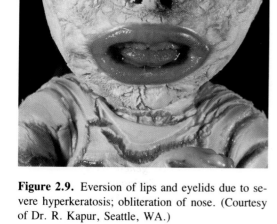

Figure 2.9. Eversion of lips and eyelids due to severe hyperkeratosis; obliteration of nose. (Courtesy of Dr. R. Kapur, Seattle, WA.)

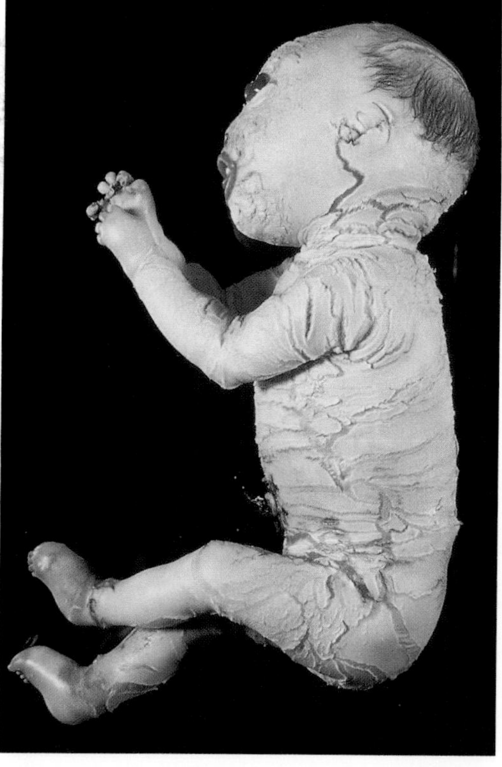

Figure 2.10. Deep cracks and fissures, deformation of ears, sausage-like encasement of hands and feet. (From Dale et al., 1990.)

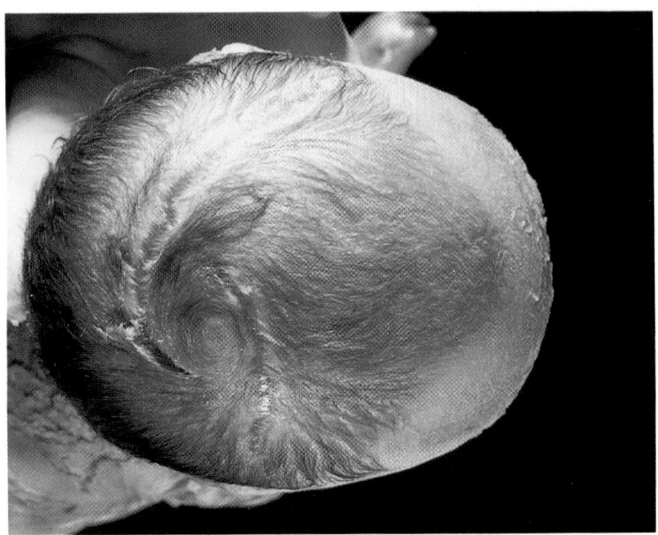

Figure 2.11. Fissures on scalp. Hairs are limited in distribution, but hair shafts appear normal. (Courtesy of Dr. R. Kapur, Seattle, WA.)

Neurologic outcome among survivors is variable, and it is unclear if neurologic impairment is a primary feature of the disorder or a consequence of prematurity and neonatal complications or of drug therapy. Short stature and failure to thrive are typical.

There have been anecdotal reports of a variety of abnormalities, including nonspecific renal tubular defects, alterations in thymic structure, and pulmonary hypoplasia.

HISTOPATHOLOGY

LIGHT. Extraordinary compact orthohyperkeratosis with elongation of rete ridges is seen. In some reports, parakeratosis is described. There are keratin plugs in hair follicles and sweat ducts.

EM. Features include absence of lamellar bodies and presence of vesicles in both the stratum granulosum and stratum corneum. Keratohyaline granules are present but smaller than normal. There is a decrease in tonofilaments. The cell membranes are thickened. Cholesterol crystals have been described. Giant mitochondria have also been noted.

BASIC DEFECT

Unknown. An abnormal cross-beta pattern rather than an alpha pattern of keratin proteins was described in one case. Increased cholesterol and triglyceride with lipid deposits in the stratum corneum have been described in another. There are differences among affected individuals in the presence or absence of hyperproliferative keratins and in profilaggrin. The condition appears to be heterogeneous.

TREATMENT

Survival has now been reported in some of a handful of patients who have received etretinate (approximately 1 mg/kg/day) or 13-*cis*-retinoic acid treatment within a few days of birth. In these infants, the thick plates have shed over a period of weeks, and a severe congenital ichthyosiform erythroderma (CIE) picture has emerged. This phenotype appears to persist once therapy has been stopped.

Careful eye hygiene is mandatory until the ectropion resolves. Management of fluid and electrolytes is complicated because of the extreme water loss, and there are problems with temperature control in these infants. It is often difficult to establish feeding until the eclabium resolves. Scrupulous hygiene and maintenance of humidified atmosphere are important. It is important to recognize that even infants treated with retinoids may succumb during the newborn period.

Harlequin ichthyosis is a severe disorder in which treatment with a medication, which has its own set of significant side effects, results in amelioration of a lethal disease to a severe one with questionable neurologic outcome. The decision to treat or not with retinoids needs to be made on an individual basis with the family. I do not personally support a wholesale recommendation for treatment. Efforts are underway to establish a prospective study to monitor outcome.

MODE OF INHERITANCE

Autosomal recessive. In the literature there is one report that suggests that inheritance may be X-linked recessive. This is based on one sibship in which no females were affected, two of three males had harlequin ichthyosis, and a third was born with a congenital scar on his scalp. There is no compelling evidence to suggest other than autosomal recessive inheritance.

PRENATAL DIAGNOSIS

Skin biopsy at 20–22 weeks gestation will reveal premature keratinization. Multiple reports of prenatal diagnosis by ultrasound that demonstrates decreased movement, swollen limbs, and abnormal facies have all been performed after 24 weeks. Keratinocyte cell clumps, composed of cells containing lipid droplets and amorphous electron dense material, are found in the amniotic fluid. These appear to be a reliable prenatal marker for harlequin ichthyosis, but the earliest time in gestation at which these clumps appear has not been confirmed.

DIFFERENTIAL DIAGNOSIS

The harlequin fetus gives a striking clinical picture, which is not easily confused with any other condition. The thick plates of scale are much more marked than a collodion membrane, although the encasing of the distal extremities may be somewhat similar. A few infants with the Neu-Laxova (MIM:256520) syndrome have had an ichthyosis that appears similar to that of the harlequin fetus. Structural brain abnormalities are a feature of Neu-Laxova and not of harlequin ichthyosis.

Support Group: F.I.R.S.T.
P.O. Box 20921
Raleigh, NC 27619
1-800-545-3286

SELECTED BIBLIOGRAPHY

Dale, B.A., Holbrook, K.A., Fleckman, P., Kimball, J.R., Brumbaugh, S., and Sybert, V.P. (1990). Heterogeneity in harlequin ichthyosis, an inborn error of epidermal keratinization: variable morphology and structural protein expression and a defect in lamellar granules. *J. Invest. Dermatol.* **94,** 6–18.

Ten subjects with harlequin ichthyosis reveal differences in the presence of hyperproliferative keratins and profilaggrin. There is a very preliminary and tentative classification of heterogeneity based on these features. In each of two sets of siblings, findings were concordant.

Hashimoto, K., and Khan, S. (1992). Harlequin fetus with abnormal lamellar granules and giant mitochondria. *J. Cutan. Pathol.* **19,** 247–252.

Extensive electron micrographs from one patient are presented. Report describes two organelles—dense-cored granules and particles containing cored granules. The authors posit that these are abortive lamellar granules and suggest that this is additional evidence in favor of a lipid abnormality in harlequin ichthyosis.

Roberts, L.J. (1989). Long-term survival of a harlequin fetus. *J. Am. Acad. Dermatol.* **21,** 335–339.

A now 9-year-old girl treated initially with 13-

cis-retinoic acid is described. There is a good review of the literature.

Rogers, M., and Scarf, C. (1989). Harlequin baby treated with etretinate. *Pediatr. Dermatol.* **6,** 216–221.

This infant survived to 6 weeks when etretinate was begun. It developed a CIE picture. Of particular importance are the descriptions of neurologic development. At six months the infant could not sit without support; at 1 year the baby was described as normal in intellectual and fine motor functions but delayed by 3 months in gross motor. At 2 years there was a 6-month delay in language and fine motor skills and a greater delay in gross motor skills. Any statement about neurologic normality in an infant or young toddler based on gross screening must be interpreted with caution. We cannot be assured about the intellectual outcome of these treated infants for some time to come.

ICHTHYOSIS BULLOSA OF SIEMENS (MIM:146800)

DERMATOLOGIC FEATURES

Major. The skin appears to be normal at birth. Blistering in response to minor trauma develops in infancy. It is usually localized to hands and feet and the extensor surfaces of the arms and legs. Blisters tend to be small.

Hyperkeratosis develops over time and occurs primarily over the knees, on the elbows, the tops of the wrists and hands, and ankles and feet. It can be more extensive on the extremities. About one-half of affected individuals have periumbilical hyperkeratosis. The involved areas are dark brown and thickened without true scale.

Superficial peeling of the skin is typical. The terms *moulting* and *mauserung* have been used to describe this feature.

There is no underlying erythroderma.

Minor. Recurrent pustules, indistinguishable from those of Sneddon-Wilkinson disease (subcorneal pustular dermatosis), have been described in some families.

ASSOCIATED ABNORMALITIES

None.

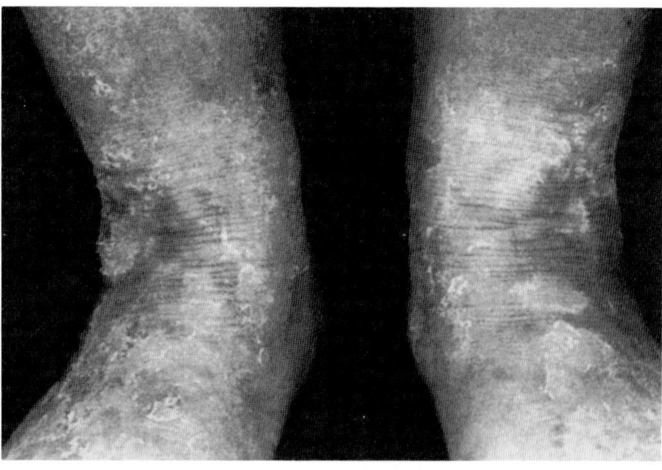

Figure 2.12. Typical hyperkeratosis and collarette scale. (From Steijlen et al., 1991.)

HISTOPATHOLOGY

LIGHT. Orthohyperkeratosis and acanthosis are typical. There is vacuolization of the granular layer cells, which contain irregular clumps in the cytoplasm. When separation within the epidermis occurs, it occurs at this more superficial level.
EM. Clumping of tonofilaments in the granular cells is typical. Occasionally, clumping of tonofilaments in the upper spinous layers can be seen.

BASIC DEFECT

Mutations in the rod domain of keratin 2e presumably result in keratin molecules that disrupt normal filament assembly.

TREATMENT

Emollients and keratolytics, similar to those used for the ichthyoses, may have modest benefit. Acitretin and etretinate treatment was reported successful in one family.

MODE OF INHERITANCE

Autosomal dominant with interfamilial variability of expression. The gene is a member of the type II keratin cluster located at 12q11–13.

PRENATAL DIAGNOSIS

Presumably possible by mutational analysis or by linkage using CVS or amniotic fluid cells.

DIFFERENTIAL DIAGNOSIS

Bullous congenital ichthyosiform erythroderma (MIM:113800) is marked by underlying erythroderma, a feature that is absent in ichthyosis bullosa of Siemens. The superficial shedding of skin in ichthyosis bullosa of Siemens and the localized hyperkeratosis are markedly different. In bullous congenital ichthyosiform erythroderma, the hyperkeratosis tends to be much more scaly, and palms and soles are typically involved, whereas in ichthyosis bullosa of Siemens they are spared. I believe, however, that there is some overlap, and occasionally it may be difficult to determine into which category a given patient falls if the specific molecular defects cannot be identified.

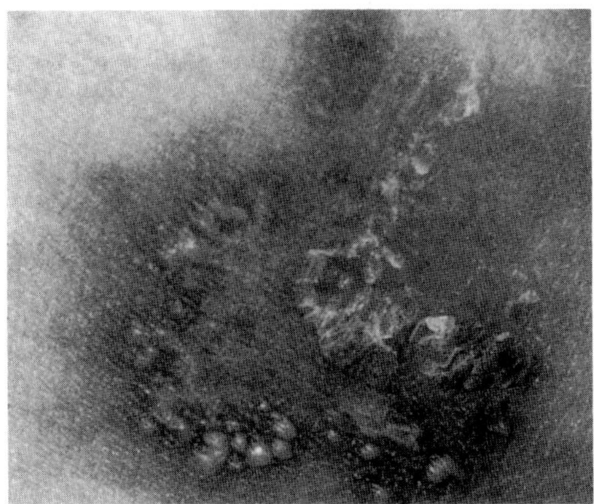

Figure 2.13. Grouped pustules and scaling. (From Steijlen et al., 1990.)

Blistering on the extremities in infancy is a feature of many of the epidermolysis bullosa syndromes. The epidermolysis bullosa simplex disorders (MIM:Many) might be initially considered in the differential diagnosis. Hyperkeratosis is absent in these disorders in young children; it is usually a feature that is limited to palms and soles and develops at a much later age. Skin biopsy will demonstrate a more superficial intraepidermal separation and clumping of tonofilaments in a higher layer in ichthyosis bullosa of Siemens than is seen in epidermolysis bullosa simplex.

Support Group: F.I.R.S.T.
P.O. Box 20921
Raleigh, NC 27619
1-800-545-3286

SELECTED BIBLIOGRAPHY

McLean, W.H.I., Morley, S.M., Lane, E.B., Eady, R.A.J., Griffiths, W.A.D., Paige, D.G.,

Harper, J.I., Higgins, C., and Leigh, I.M. (1994). Ichthyosis bullosa of Siemens—a disease involving keratin 2e. *J. Invest. Dermatol.* **103,** 277–281.

Clearly written with case descriptions and mutation identification in two unrelated British families.

Rothnagel, J.A., Traupe, H., Wojcik, S., Huber, M., Hohl, D., Pittelkow, M.R., Saeki, H., Ishibashi, Y., and Roop, D.R. (1994). Mutations in the rod domain of keratin 2e in patients with ichthyosis bullosa of Siemens. *Nat. Genet.* **7,** 485–489.

This paper succinctly discusses the identification of mutations in ichthyosis bullosa of Siemens and suggests that there is a hot spot, as six unrelated mutational events occurred in the same codon. Although they mention that erythroderma *is* a feature of ichthyosis bullosa of Siemens, this clinical finding is specifically noted as absent in case descriptions.

Steijlen, P.M., Perret, C.M., Stekhoven, J.H.S., Ruiter, D.J., and Happle, R. (1990). Ichthyosis bullosa of Siemens: further delineation of the phenotype. *Arch. Dermatol. Res.* **282,** 1–5.

This paper describes clinical and histopathologic findings in a family.

ICHTHYOSIS HYSTRIX (MIM:146590,146600)

(Porcupine Man; Ichthyosis Hystrix Curth-Macklin; Ichthyosis Hystrix Gravior [Lambert]; Systematized Verrucous Nevus)

Includes Hystrix-Like Ichthyosis with Deafness

DERMATOLOGIC FEATURES

MAJOR. *Hystrix* is the genus name for porcupines and a form of spiky grasses. The term thus evokes an image of the clinical appearance of this disorder, which is marked by plaques of spiny hyperkeratosis. In both the gravior and the Curth-Macklin forms, involvement ranges from patchy to generalized and severe. The palms, soles, and face are generally spared. Involvement of the penis and scrotum may or may not occur. Erythroderma may be present at birth, but is not a feature of the disorder later in life. Seasonal improvement has been described in both forms (Curth-Macklin and Lambert). The distinction between the two disorders may not be real.

Affected infants usually show skin changes within the first few weeks of life, and involvement appears to be progressive. Within affected families, patchy involvement does not distribute along the lines of Blaschko. This is in contrast to the pattern of generalized epidermal nevi, which do track along these lines.

MINOR. Nail involvement with fissuring and splitting of the nail plate has been described in one patient with ichthyosis hystrix Curth-Macklin.

ASSOCIATED ABNORMALITIES

None.

HISTOPATHOLOGY

LIGHT. Orthohyperkeratosis, acanthosis, and papillomatosis with perinuclear vacuolization in the upper spinous and granular layers. Ten to 30% of the keratinocytes are binuclear.

EM. Unbroken concentric shells of tonofibrils encase the nucleus. The lamellar bodies are abnormal. The tonofilament desmosomal attachments are intact. In the *gravior* form, rudimentary tonofilaments are seen. There is no tonofilament clumping.

BASIC DEFECT

Unknown.

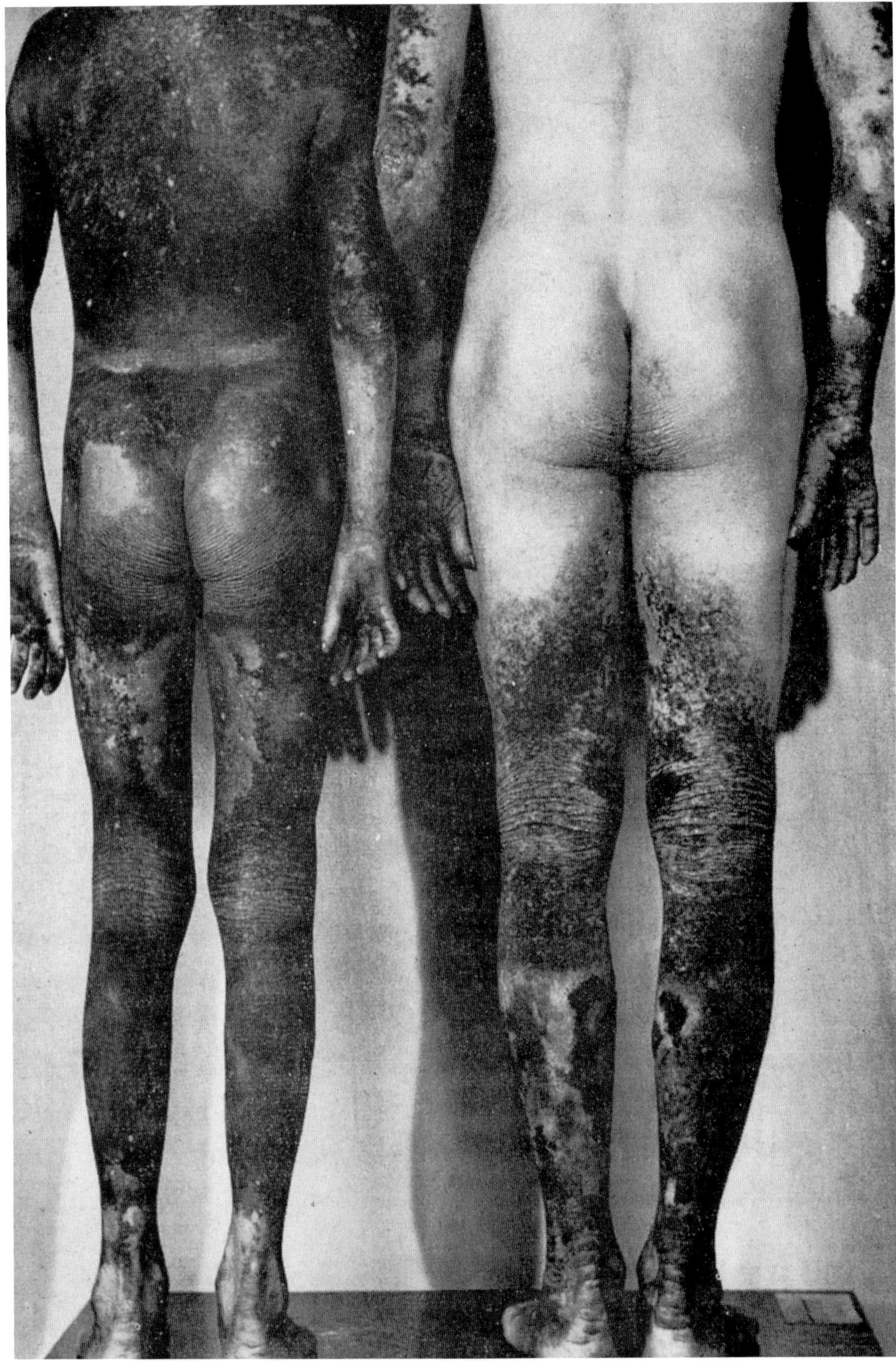

Figure 2.14. Brothers with ichthyosis hystrix with differing degrees of involvement. (From Curth and Macklin, 1954.)

TREATMENT

Oral retinoids may be of some value. Topical humectants (urea, lactic acid, propylene glycol) may be of limited use. One patient reported successful removal of scale by application of a commercial detergent. No details were given.

MODE OF INHERITANCE

Autosomal dominant. The long-held belief that this was a Y-linked disease was based on deliberately misleading pedigree information supplied by the Lambert family.

PRENATAL DIAGNOSIS

None.

DIFFERENTIAL DIAGNOSIS

Ichthyosis hystrix most closely resembles bullous congenital ichthyosiform erythroderma (MIM:113800), but it is distinguished by lack of erythroderma and the absence of blistering. Electron microscopy will differentiate between the two.

Hystrix-like ichthyosis with deafness, or ichthyosis hystrix gravior, type Rheydt, is differentiated by the presence of severe sensorineural hearing loss. Leukoplakia and secondary fungal infections have been described in the Rheydt type. The hearing loss appears to be nonprogressive. Punctate keratitis has been a feature in some individuals. Histopathology is similar to lamellar ichthyosis and distinct from ichthyosis hystrix and bullous congenital ichthyosiform erythroderma.

Organoid nevi can show hystrix-like changes both clinically and histologically. These are usually distributed along the lines of Blaschko and not in the patchy array that ichthyosis hystrix can sometimes demonstrate. The term *systematized epidermal* or *verrucous nevus* might best be dropped or at the least reserved for widespread organoid nevi and not used as one of the synonyms for ichthyosis hystrix.

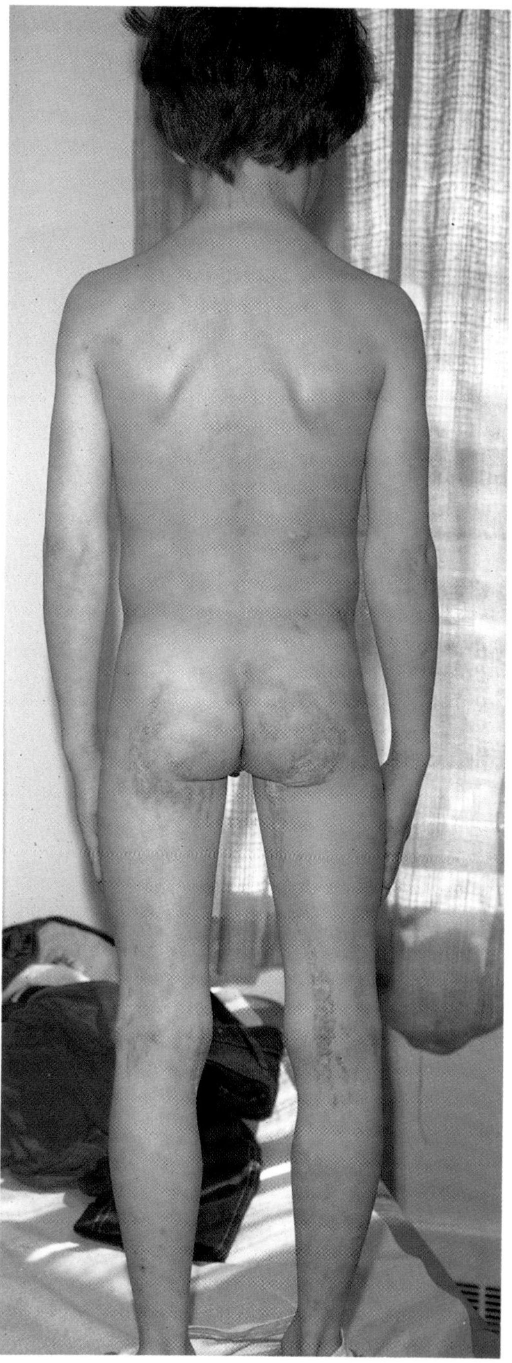

Figure 2.15. In contrast to Fig. 2.14, verrucous lesions are distributed bilaterally along the lines of Blaschko on buttocks and legs in a patient with widespread epidermal nevus.

Support Group: F.I.R.S.T.
P.O. Box 20921
Raleigh, NC 27619
1-800-545-3286

SELECTED BIBLIOGRAPHY

Anton-Lamprecht, I. (1978). Electron microscopy in the early diagnosis of genetic disorders of the skin. *Dermatologica.* **157,** 65–85.

Good electron micrographs of ichthyosis hystrix Curth-Macklin. Also evaluated a patient with ichthyosis hystrix Rheydt.

Bonifas, J.M., Bare, J.W., Chen, M.A., Ranki, A., Neimi, K.-M., and Epstein, E.H. Jr. (1993). Evidence against keratin gene mutations in a family with ichthyosis hystrix Curth-Macklin. *J. Invest. Dermatol.* **101,** 890–891.

Demonstrated absence of linkage to either of the keratin clusters (on 12q and 17q) in one family with ichthyosis hystrix Curth-Macklin.

Curth, H.O., and Macklin, M.T. (1954). The genetic basis of various types of ichthyosis in a family group. *Am. J. Hum. Genet.* **6,** 371–382.

Ollendorff-Curth, H., Allen, F.H. Jr., Schnyder, U.W., and Anton-Lamprecht, I. (1972). Follow-up of a family group suffering from ichthyosis hystrix type Curth-Macklin. *Humangenetik* **17,** 37–48.

Report and revisitation of a single family in which features range from generalized to localized involvement and mild to severe. Ollendorff-Curth, H., is the Curth, H.O. of the 1954 report. There are excellent photos.

Niemi, K.-M., Vortanen, I., Kanerva, L., and Muttilainen, M. (1990). Altered keratin expression in ichthyosis hystrix Curth-Macklin: a light and electron microscopic study. *Arch. Dermatol. Res.* **284,** 198–208.

A proband with short stature, undescended testes, and patchy hyperkeratosis showed abnormal positive staining with antibodies to fetal keratins. The authors state that this disease is clinically distinct from ichthyosis hystrix Curth-Macklin but, because electron microscopic findings were similar, chose to use the same eponym. An unfortunate assumption, as it is clear that the ultrastructural findings are not diagnostically specific.

Penrose, L.S., and Stern, C. (1958). Reconsideration of the Lambert pedigree (ichthyosis hystrix gravior). *Ann. Hum. Genet.* **22,** 258–283.

By historical review of the literature and investigation of parish records, these authors determine that ichthyosis hystrix gravior was autosomal dominant, not Y-linked. There are wonderful illustrations.

ICHTHYOSIS VULGARIS (MIM:146700)

(Ichthyosis Simplex)

DERMATOLOGIC FEATURES

MAJOR. This disorder is characterized by mild to moderate scaling involving primarily extensor surfaces and sparing the flexures and neck. Facial involvement is common. Onset is usually after 6 months of age but may be earlier, and there have been rare reports of infants with ichthyosis vulgaris presenting as collodion babies. Keratosis pilaris is common. The disorder occurs in as many as 1 in 250 individuals and may be underdiagnosed because it can be so mild that affected individuals may not come to medical attention. It improves with age and in warm weather. There is no underlying erythroderma.

MINOR. Hyperlinear palms/soles; pityriasis alba.

ASSOCIATED ABNORMALITIES

Atopic disease occurs in 50% of affected individuals. When atopic dermatitis is severe, it may mask the underlying ichthyosis.

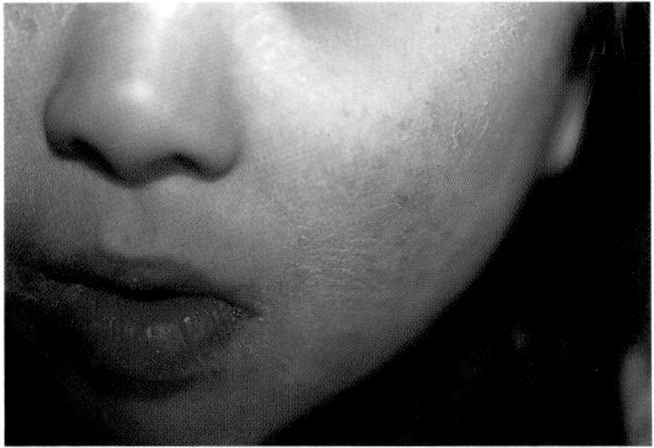

Figure 2.16. Dry, cracked cheeks.

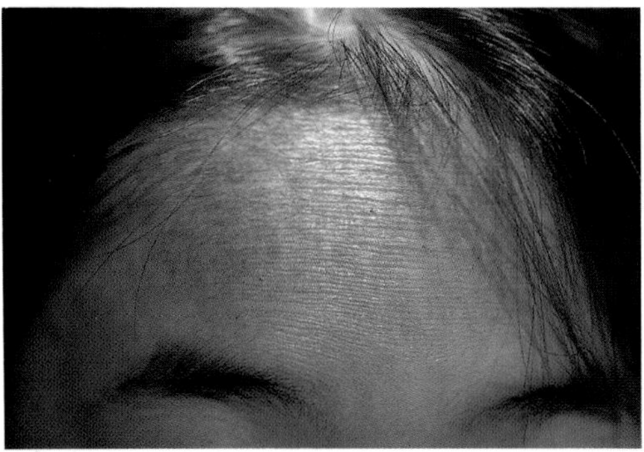

Figure 2.17. Fine, dry furrows on forehead.

HISTOPATHOLOGY

LIGHT. There is a diminished or absent granular layer with orthohyperkeratosis. Occasional follicular plugging and a decrease in the number of sebaceous glands are seen.
EM. There is a decrease to absence of keratohyaline granules. Those present are small and "crumbly."

BASIC DEFECT

Unknown. Cell kinetics, lipids, and keratins are normal. There is a decrease to absence of profilaggrin and filaggrin that correlates with clinical severity of the disorder, suggesting that the basic defect may involve the biosynthesis of these products.

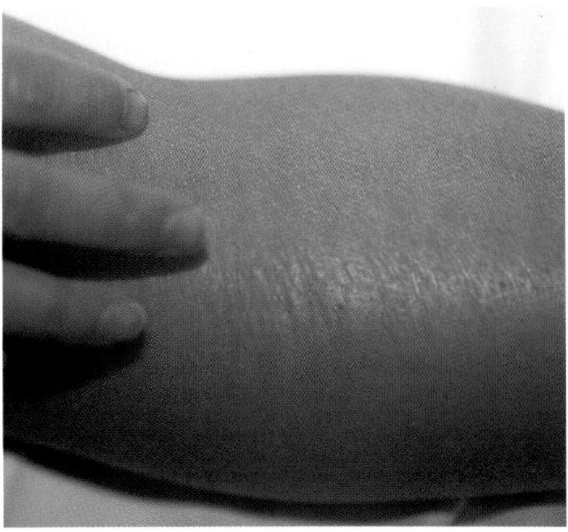

Figure 2.18. Subtle hyperkeratosis of legs with fine, dry wrinkling of skin.

TREATMENT

The skin responds readily to relatively simple treatment, although the ichthyosis can occasionally be refractory. Simple emollients or those containing α-hydroxy acids (e.g., glycolic acid, lactic acid) or urea are beneficial. The associated eczema may be very difficult to treat and in my experience often does not respond until the underlying ichthyosis is brought under control.

MODE OF INHERITANCE

Ichthyosis vulgaris is inherited as an autosomal dominant condition with variable expression and probably reduced penetrance. Males and females are affected equally severely.

PRENATAL DIAGNOSIS

Prenatal diagnosis has not been attempted. It is not known if the ultrastructural defects or biochemical abnormalities are expressed in utero, but it is doubtful, as the disorder usually does not present at birth. The relatively mild nature of the disorder makes the demand for prenatal diagnosis unlikely.

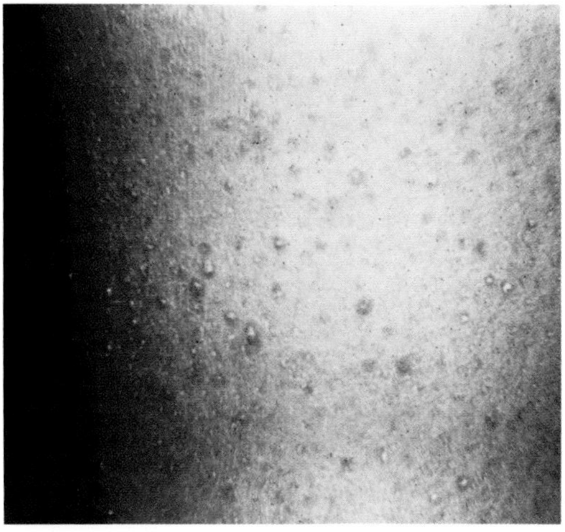

Figure 2.19. Inflammatory papules of keratosis pilaris. (Courtesy of Dr. J. Halloran, Division of Dermatology, University of Washington.)

DIFFERENTIAL DIAGNOSIS

I think it is easy to make the diagnosis of ichthyosis vulgaris but difficult to exclude it. There is a fine line between "normal" xerosis and ichthyosis vulgaris. Many people have isolated keratosis pilaris, and I do not know if this represents minimal expression of ichthyosis vulgaris or a distinct disorder.

X-linked ichthyosis (sterol sulfatase deficiency, MIM:308100) is very similar to ichthyosis vulgaris. Features common to the former and atypical for the latter include involvement of the neck and flexures, sparing of the face, and absence of hyperlinear palms, keratosis pilaris, and atopy. Enzymatic and molecular diagnosis is available for sterol sulfatase deficiency.

Support Group: F.I.R.S.T.
P.O. Box 20921
Raleigh, NC 27619
1-800-545-3286

SELECTED BIBLIOGRAPHY

Anton-Lamprecht, I., and Hofbauer, M. (1972). Ultrastructural distinction of autosomal dominant ichthyosis vulgaris and X-linked ichthyosis. *Humangenetik* **15,** 261–264.

Electron microscopic study of ichthyosis vulgaris contrasted with X-linked ichthyosis (sterol sulfatase deficiency).

Sybert, V.P., Dale, B.A., and Holbrook K.A. (1985). Ichthyosis vulgaris: identification of a defect in synthesis of filaggrin correlated with an absence of keratohyaline granules. *J. Invest. Dermatol.* **84,** 191–194.

A clinical, biochemical, and ultrastructural study of skin from affected and normal individuals from two pedigrees with ichthyosis vulgaris.

Wells, R.S., and Kerr, C.B. (1966). Genetic classification of the ichthyoses. *Arch. Dermatol.* **92,** 1–6.

A study of the major clinical features of X-linked ichthyosis and ichthyosis vulgaris. The authors distinguish the two disorders by a number of clinical criteria.

Williams, M.L. (1983). The ichthyoses—pathogenesis and prenatal diagnosis: a review of recent advances. *Pediatr. Dermatol.* **1,** 1–24.

A review of the ichthyoses, with clinical and biochemical information.

LAMELLAR EXFOLIATION OF THE NEWBORN (MIM:242300)

(Lamellar Ichthyosis of the Newborn; Self-Healing Collodion Baby; Ichthyosis Congenita)

Includes Collodion Baby

DERMATOLOGIC FEATURES

Major. The collodion baby is born covered with a taut, shiny membrane that resembles plastic wrap. The membrane is often fissured and cracked at birth. In lamellar exfoliation of the newborn, it goes on to crack and peel over the course of several weeks to reveal underly-

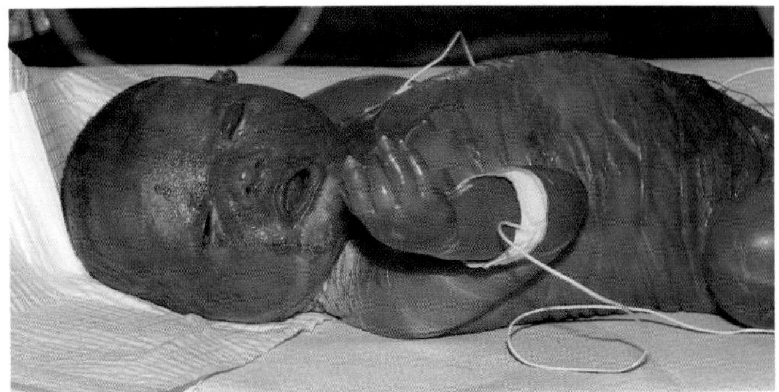

A

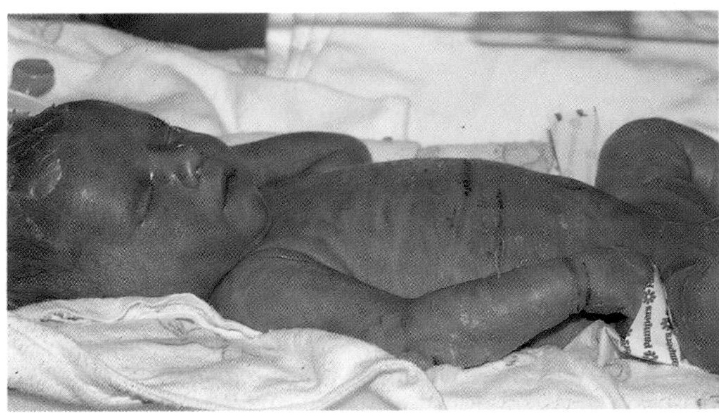

B

Figure 2.20. Infant with lamellar exfoliation of the newborn at 12 hours **(A)** and 8 days **(B)**.

ing normal skin or skin with mild scaling that goes on to resolve. In some children, an underlying, extremely mild ichthyosis may persist.

Ectropion and eclabium (pulling back and eversion of the eyelids and the lips) due to the tautness of the membrane are typical. The pinnae are often crumpled. The tips of the fingers are often tapered, and the hands may be held in partial flexion. These features resolve with shedding of the encasing membrane. There may be underlying redness or ivory color to the skin. Hair and nails are usually normal.

MINOR. Secondary skin infections can develop in the cracks and fissures. Scarring can occur in areas of deep fissuring.

ASSOCIATED ABNORMALITIES

Difficulties with temperature regulation, water loss, and secondary infection and septicemia are complications that can occur in the newborn period. Respiratory difficulty due to restricted chest wall movement can also occur.

HISTOPATHOLOGY

LIGHT. The stratum corneum is thickened and orthokeratotic, and the remainder of the epidermis is normal.

EM. The stratum corneum shows two layers, a normal proximal layer and a distal layer with irregular convoluted horny cells, numerous intercellular Odland bodies (lamellar granules), and nuclear debris with preservation of desmosomes. Small dense granules in the cytoplasm clinging to the cell membrane and desmosomal plate of the horny cells can also be seen (see references Frenk [1980] and de Dobbeleer et al. [1982] for comments).

BASIC DEFECT

Unknown.

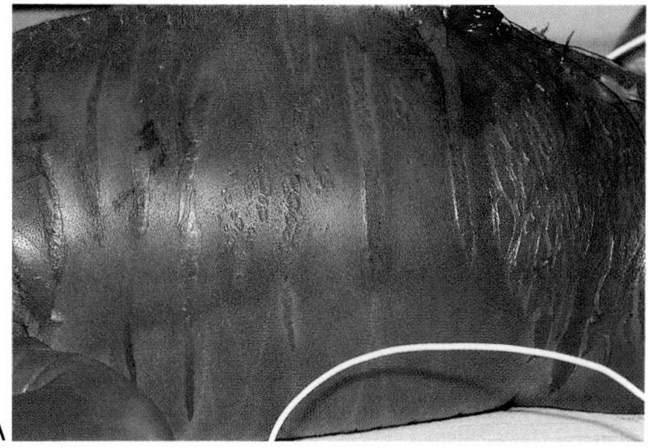

A

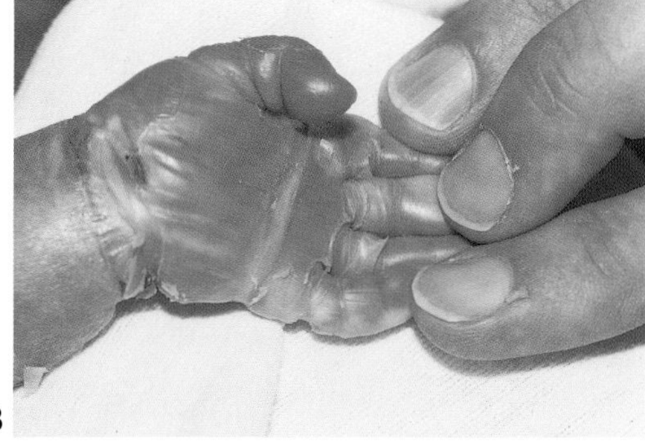

B

Figure 2.21. **(A)** Close-up showing cracks in the collodion membrane. **(B)** Sausage-like encasement of fingers with peeling.

TREATMENT

Use of very light, bland liquid emollients is helpful. Urea and lactic acid containing agents should be avoided because percutaneous absorption can occur. Thicker preparations, creams and greases, tend to delay sloughing and increase the risk of secondary infection.

Maintenance of infection control, scrupulous hygiene, and appropriate neonatal environment are important. Prophylactic antibiotics should not be used. Surveillance skin cultures may be helpful in management. Usually enough of the membrane has shed in 7–10 days to allow for discharge from hospital.

Use of artificial tears until the ectropion resolves helps to prevent corneal damage.

MODE OF INHERITANCE

Autosomal recessive for lamellar exfoliation of the newborn.

PRENATAL DIAGNOSIS

None.

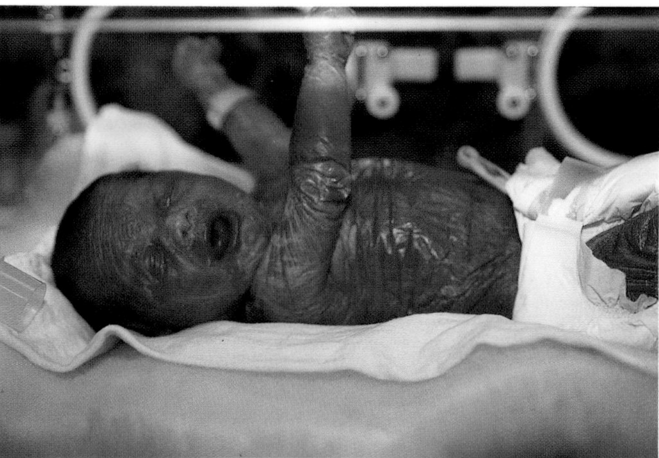

Figure 2.22. Newborn with collodion membrane; after peeling, has mild lamellar ichthyosis with residual ectropion and eclabium.

DIFFERENTIAL DIAGNOSIS

The term *collodion baby* is not diagnostic. A collodion membrane in itself is not specific and has been described with a number of ichthyoses, including lamellar (nonbullous congenital ichthyosiform erythroderma, MIM: 242100), ichthyosis vulgaris (MIM:146700), Netherton syndrome (MIM:256500), Conradi-Hunermann syndrome (MIM:302950, 302960), and the ectodermal dysplasias, especially hypohidrotic ectodermal dysplasia (MIM:305100) and the Hay-Wells (AEC) syndrome (MIM: 106260). Collodion membrane has also been reported in three newborns with type 2 Gaucher disease (MIM:230900). In these infants, the membrane peeled to reveal normal skin.

There is disagreement as to whether sterol sulfatase deficiency (X-linked ichthyosis, MIM:308100) ever presents with a collodion membrane. I am not convinced that it never occurs and would not exclude the possibility of X-linked ichthyosis from the differential diagnosis in a male infant with a collodion membrane.

Biopsy of the membrane is not helpful to discriminate among these possibilities. Diagnostic skin biopsy should be deferred until the membrane has shed to avoid the need for a repeat procedure because the initial biopsy was uninformative.

Support Group: F.I.R.S.T.
P.O. Box 20921
Raleigh, NC 27619
1-800-545-3286

SELECTED BIBLIOGRAPHY

de Dobbeleer, G., Heenen, M., Song, M., and Achten, G. (1982). Collodion baby skin. Ultrastructural and autoradiographic study. *J. Cutan. Pathol.* **9,** 196–202.

Biopsies, at day 2 and month 16 of life, from a female who presented with a collodion membrane and who went on to have apparently normal skin, were evaluated by light and electron microscopy. At 2 days an abnormal distal stratum corneum was seen. At 16 months, despite clinically and ultrastructurally normal skin, her cells showed a higher than normal mitotic index, suggesting that she continued to have a perturbation in cornification.

Frenk, E. (1980). A spontaneously healing collodion baby: a light and electron microscopic study. *Acta Dermatol. Venereol. (Stockh.)* **61,** 168–171.

In contrast to de Dobbeleer et al. (1982), Frenk found no alterations other than a thickened stratum corneum in biopsies on days 1 and 15 in a male infant with this condition. He did find electron microscopic changes in two female infants, similar to those described by de Dobbeleer et al., who then went on to develop lamellar ichthyosis. It seems that skin biopsy in the newborn with collodion membrane is not predictive and should be deferred until the membrane has been shed.

Frenk, E., and de Techtermann, F. (1992). Self-healing collodion baby: evidence for autosomal recessive inheritance. *Pediatr. Dermatol.* **9,** 95–97.

Five affected individuals from an inbred Swiss pedigree are presented, along with a concise review of the literature.

Larrègue, M., Ottavy, N., Bressieux, J.-M., and Lorette, J. (1986). Bèbè collodion. Trente-deux nouvelles observations. *Ann. Dermatol. Venereol.* **113,** 773–785.

The authors review findings from 32 patients of their own and 37 in the literature. Over one-third of the affected infants developed cutaneous bacterial or candidal infections. Four of these became septic, and one developed osteomyelitis. There are useful tables of the differential and of complications. Thirty-eight references.

Reed, W.B., Herwick, R.P. Harville, D., Porter, P.S., and Conant, M. (1972). Lamellar ichthyosis of the newborn. A distinct clinical entity: its comparison to other ichthyosiform erythrodermas. *Arch. Dermatol.* **105,** 394–399.

Beautiful color photographs are presented.

LAMELLAR ICHTHYOSIS (MIM:242100)

(Nonbullous Congenital Ichthyosiform Erythroderma; Autosomal Recessive Ichthyosis; Erythrodermic Autosomal Recessive Lamellar Ichthyosis [EARLI]; Non-erythrodermic Autosomal Recessive Lamellar Ichthyosis [NEARLI])

DERMATOLOGIC FEATURES

MAJOR. This is a heterogenous group of disorders that remains to be classified on a basis that is generally accepted. The conditions share in common presentation at birth of an erythrodermic, scaling infant. Ectropion and eclabium are typical. A collodion membrane is also common.

Over time, the erythroderma tends to fade, but this may vary. The scales may be fine, white and diffuse, or thick, dark, and more plate-like. These clinical features have been the basis for one classification scheme (*lamellar,* dark scale, less erythema; *NCIE,* fine scale, more erythema), but many patients straddle the two descriptions.

All forms of lamellar ichthyosis/nonbullous congenital ichthyosiform erythroderma share in common congenital presentation, persistence of scaling, and absence of blistering.

MINOR. Nails, teeth, and hair are normal, although the hairs may appear thin or sparse because of entrapment by thick scale. Secondary fungal infection is not rare and may go unrecognized. Decreased heat tolerance because of decreased ability to sweat is a complaint in some patients with thicker scales.

ASSOCIATED ABNORMALITIES

Ectropion can persist, resulting in conjunctiva sicca and corneal irritation. Intelligence is normal.

HISTOPATHOLOGY

LIGHT. The granular layer is increased in thickness or normal. There is a mild perivascular lymphocytic infiltrate and mild to moderate hyperkeratosis.

EM. Multiple nonspecific changes. A proposed classification scheme based on electron microscopic features does not correlate with or predict clinical features.

BASIC DEFECT

Heterogeneous. Elevations of *N*-alkanes previously found in a subset of patients with lamellar ichthyosis were probably due to artifact. Recently, different mutations in transglutaminase 1 *(TGM1)* were demonstrated in some, but not all, families with lamellar ichthyosis. The altered enzyme is important in formation of the cornified cell envelope.

TREATMENT

Lactic acid, urea acid, and glycolic acid preparations are all effective to some degree. In severe cases, the oral retinoids may be warranted. See the entry for collodion baby for management in the newborn period.

There have been several case reports of improvement in this condition with hypnosis. I have not attempted to use hypnosis in my patients, although I am intrigued by the idea.

MODE OF INHERITANCE

Autosomal recessive in almost all instances. Several pedigrees with autosomal dominant inheritance of nonbullous congenital ichthyosiform erythroderma have been described. The gene for *TGM1* maps to 14q11.

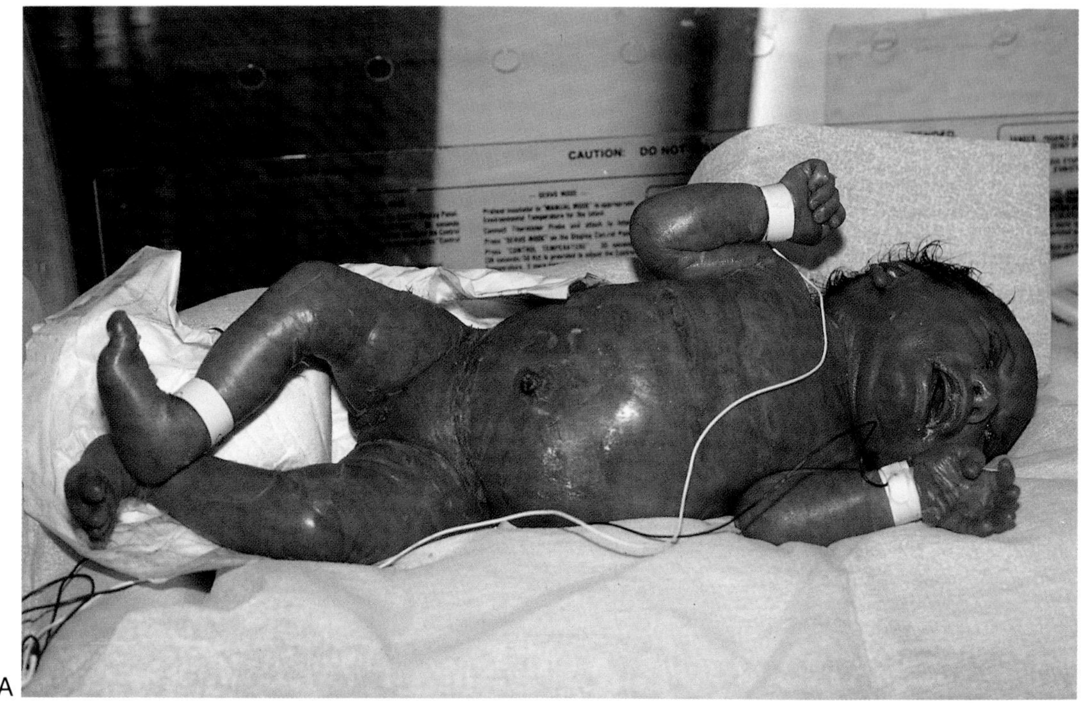
A

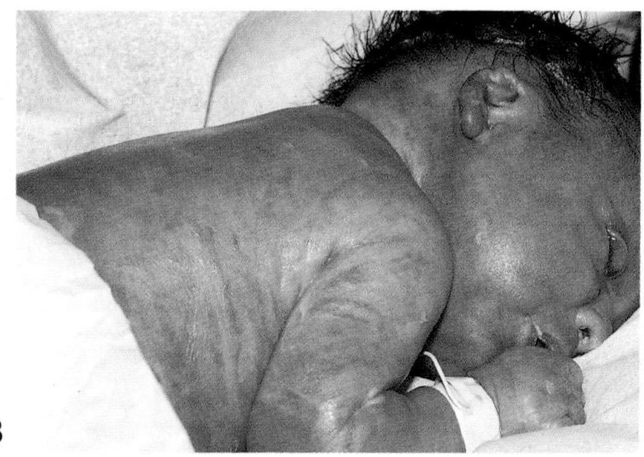
B

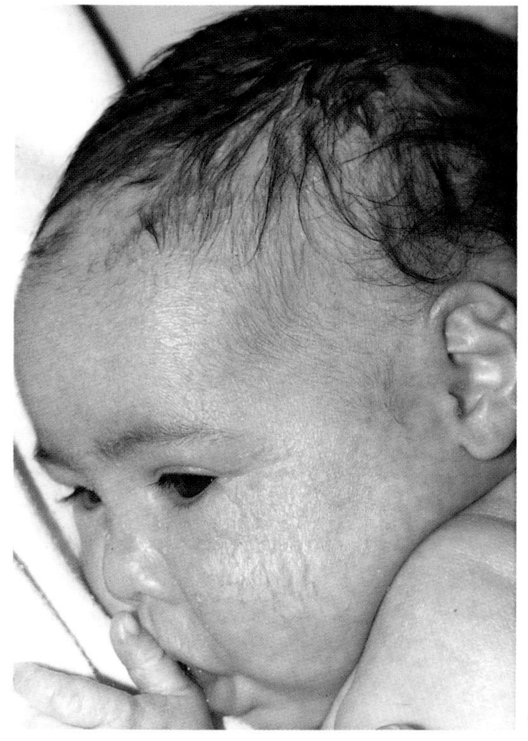
C

Figure 2.23. **(A)** Collodion membrane in newborn with lamellar ichthyosis/nonbullous congenital ichthyosiform erythroderma. Marked ectropion. **(B)** At day 8 still with marked ectropion. Pinna is deformed by the membrane. **(C)** Same infant at 2 months, ectropion resolved. Fine cracking of skin with mild erythroderma.

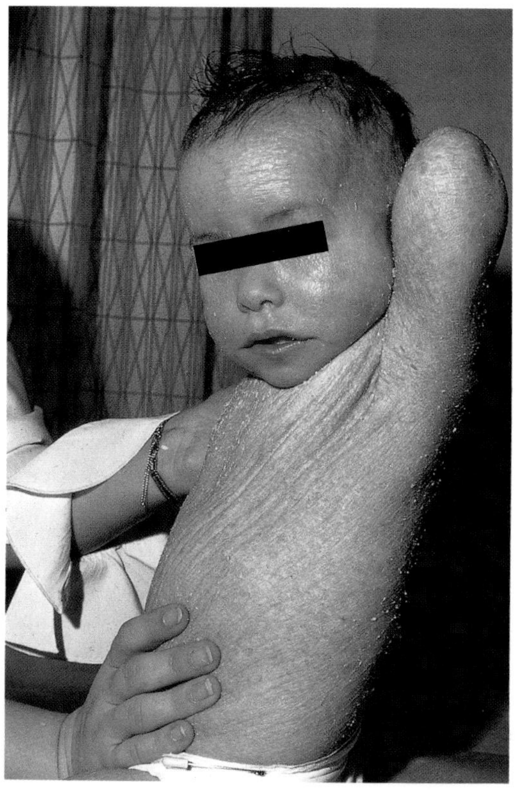

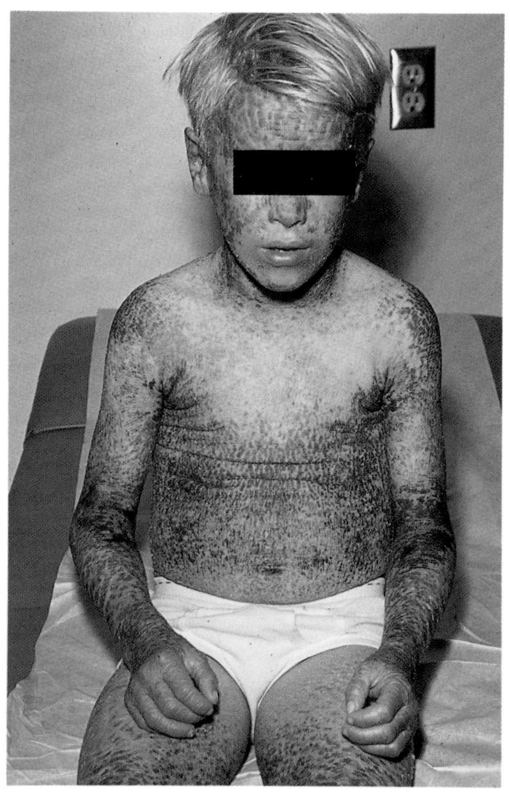

Figure 2.24. **(A)** Finer white scale with erythroderma typical of NCIE. **(B)** The darker adherent plate-like scales and less erythroderma of lamellar ichthyosis.

PRENATAL DIAGNOSIS

Unreliable by fetoscopy and fetal skin biopsy. Although both a correct prenatal diagnosis and exclusion have been performed in two pregnancies, one false-negative diagnosis occurred in a third pregnancy in the same family. Presumably now possible by molecular techniques in families where the mutation has been identified.

DIFFERENTIAL DIAGNOSIS

Many congenital ichthyoses have identical presentations and cannot be distinguished early on from lamellar ichthyosis/nonbullous congenital ichthyosiform erythroderma. Sjögren-Larsson syndrome (MIM:270200), Netherton syndrome (MIM:256500), Rud syndrome (MIM:312770), lamellar exfoliation of the newborn (MIM: 242300), and the trichothiodystrophies (MIM: 234050; 242170, 278730, 275550) can all present with similar clinical findings at birth. Appropriate laboratory tests, skin biopsy, and time may help to differentiate among these.

Tentative classification schema include those based on cell kinetics (NCIE and lamellar ichthyosis); on the ratio of butyrase to glucosidase (NEARLI vs. EARLI), clinical differences (lamellar ichthyosis vs. NCIE and NEARLI vs. EARLI), and ultrastructural alterations (recessive ichthyosis congenita types I through V). None is particularly useful or predictive, as clinical overlap remains significant and inheritance appears to be the same. The concept of heterogeneity is important, but specific diagnostic categories await biochemical findings that are reproducible and distinct and/or identification of specific mutations.

In autosomal dominant lamellar ichthyosis,

A

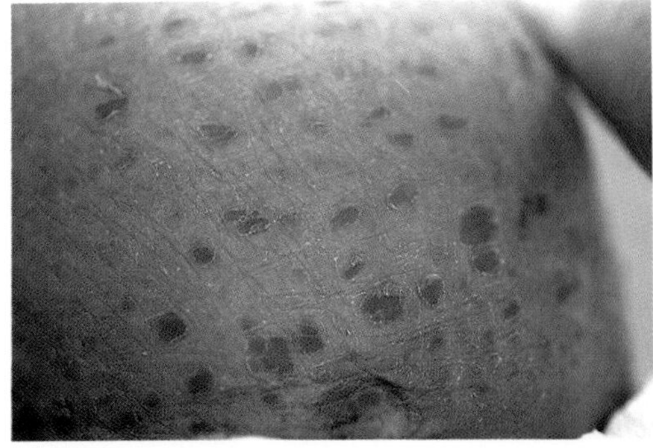

B

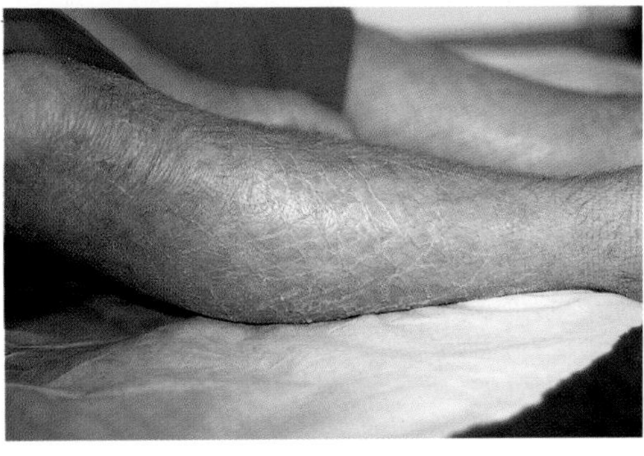

Figure 2.25. **(A)** Plate-like scale of lamellar ichthyosis. **(B)** Intermediate phenotype.

the presence of a distinctive transforming zone between the stratum granulosum and the stratum corneum and elevated triglycerides and fatty acids in scale may distinguish it from autosomal recessive lamellar ichthyosis.

Support Group: F.I.R.S.T.
P.O. Box 20921
Raleigh, NC 27619
1-800-545-3286

SELECTED BIBLIOGRAPHY

Bernhardt, M., and Baden, H.P. (1986). Report of a family with an unusual expression of recessive ichthyosis. *Arch. Dermatol.* **122,** 428–433.

Reviews their records of 42 patients with autosomal recessive lamellar ichthyosis, detailing the clinical heterogeneity of this group.

Kolde, G., Happle, R., and Traupe, H. (1985). Autosomal dominant lamellar ichthyosis: ultrastructural characteristics of a new type of congenital ichthyosis. *Arch. Dermatol. Res.* **278,** 1–5.

Melnik, B., Kuster, W., Hollmann, J., Plewig, G., and Traupe, H. (1989). Autosomal dominant lamellar ichthyosis exhibits an abnormal scale lipid pattern. *Clin. Genet.* **35,** 152–156.

Kolde et al. (1985) and Melnick et al. (1989) provide two reports of the same mother and daughter pair demonstrating differences from autosomal recessive lamellar ichthyosis both in lipids extracted from scale and in electron microscopic findings. Whether these differences will be found in other families is unknown.

Neimi, K.-M., Kanerva, L., and Kuokkanen, K. (1991). Recessive ichthyosis congenita type II. *Arch. Dermatol. Res.* **283,** 211–218.

Findings in a group of patients with lamellar ichthyosis, all of whom had severe scale, but only some of whom had erythroderma. All were found to have cholesterol clefts on electron microscopy. Other electron microscopic findings were variable.

Russell, L.J., DiGiovanna, J.J., Rogers, G.R., Steinert, P.M., Hashem, N., Compton, J.G., and Bale, S.J. (1995). Mutations in the gene for transgluatminase 1 in autosomal recessive lamellar ichthyosis. *Nat. Genet.* **9,** 279–283.

Mutations in *TGM1* found in three ethnically distinct families.

Williams, M.L., and Elias, P.M. (1985). Heterogeneity in autosomal recessive ichthyosis. Clinical and biochemical differentiation of lamellar ichthyosis and nonbullous congenital ichthyosiform erythroderma. *Arch. Dermatol.* **121,** 477–488.

These authors recognized the clinical distinctions among this group. The finding of elevated *N*-alkanes in lamellar ichthyosis has not held up. Authors chose to assign one of two terms—*lamellar ichthyosis and nonbullous congenital ichthyosiform erythroderma*—(which had been previously used synonymously), to each group. This only added to confusion in nomenclature. Until the biochemical and genetic bases have been elucidated, using the terms interchangeably is consistent with historical precedent.

NETHERTON SYNDROME (MIM:256500)

(Comèl-Netherton; Ichthyosis Linearis Circumflexa)

DERMATOLOGIC FEATURES

Confusion about the defining clinical characteristics of Netherton syndrome has several roots: (1) the ichthyosis of the syndrome undergoes evolution and change; (2) not all case reports adequately describe features over time; and (3) it is most likely a heterogeneous condition.

MAJOR. At birth, or within a few days of life, the classic presentation is of an infant with generalized erythroderma and scaling, similar to nonbullous congenital ichthyosiform erythroderma or lamellar ichthyosis. Collodion membrane is rare, but continuous sheets of peeling skin can occur and persist. This initial presentation gradually evolves into the typical pattern of ichthyosis linearis circumflexa, which is marked by migratory serpiginous, circinate plaques of scaling erythema. There is a peculiar double-edged scale along the red peripheral margins of these lesions. The ichthyosis linearis circumflexa may wax and wane, improve with warmth, and is often pruritic. Lichenification of the popliteal and antecubital fossae is common and appears to be independent of atopic disease. The scalp is usually involved with thick, seborrheic-like scaling.

In a minority of patients, the diffuse ichthyosis persists. In a second subset, ichthyosis linearis circumflexa is the first presenting feature, and there is no antecedent generalized involvement.

Hair changes typically are not recognized until the end of the first year of life, and not all hairs are necessarily affected. The hair is thin, fragile, slow growing, and may be sparse. The hairs exhibit trichorrhexis invaginata or bamboo hairs. They give a ball and socket appearance on magnification. Trichorrhexis nodosa and pili torti have also been described. These changes may disappear as childhood progresses. Eyelashes and eyebrows may be affected, as are secondary sexual hairs. While not all patients with ichthyosis linearis circumflexa have been described to have trichorrhexis invaginata, the presence of both features is pathognomonic for Netherton syndrome.

MINOR. Atopic disease has been mentioned in numerous case reports, but critical analysis of family history has not been pursued. The lichenification of the flexures, the pruritis, and the eczematous-like patches of ichthyosis lin-

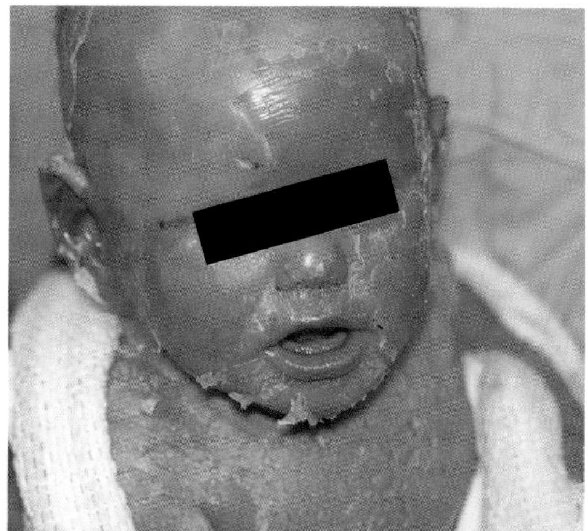
A

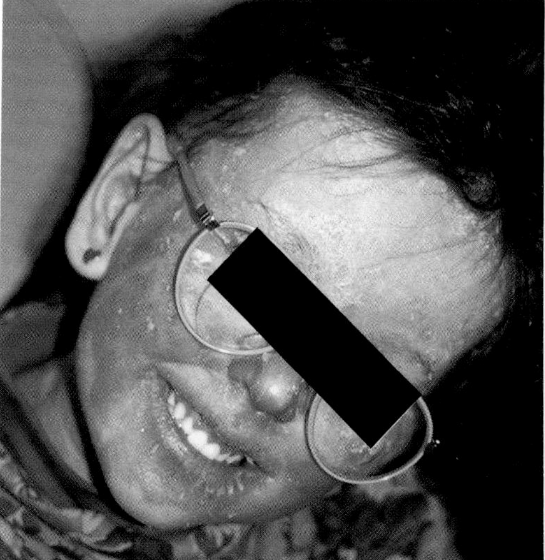
B

Figure 2.26. (A) Continuous sheets of peeling skin with underlying erythroderma. **(B)** Older patient with sparse fragile hair, continued redness and peeling, especially on cheeks and around mouth.

earis circumflexa may lead to a misdiagnosis of severe atopic dermatitis. Urticaria, especially in response to ingestion of nuts, and/or asthma have been noted in about one-fourth to one-third of case reports.

ASSOCIATED ABNORMALITIES

From 10% to 15% of patients in the literature have had mental retardation. Among affected sibships, at least one pair was discordant for mental retardation. The sibling with mental retardation had generalized aminoaciduria. The other did not. The range of reported intellectual impairment has been from mild to severe.

Short stature and failure to thrive are described in almost one-third of cases. A primary defect in intestinal absorption has been suggested but not documented. Eosinophilia and elevated levels of IgE are often seen. IgE levels range from slightly elevated to extraordinarily high (greater than 10,000 IU/ml).

Recurrent infections, both bacterial and candidal, cutaneous and bronchopulmonary, are common and a cause for mortality in a subset of infants. Hypernatremic dehydration in the newborn period has occurred in more than 10% of case reports with Netherton syndrome. A generalized aminoaciduria without obvious cause has been noted in some patients.

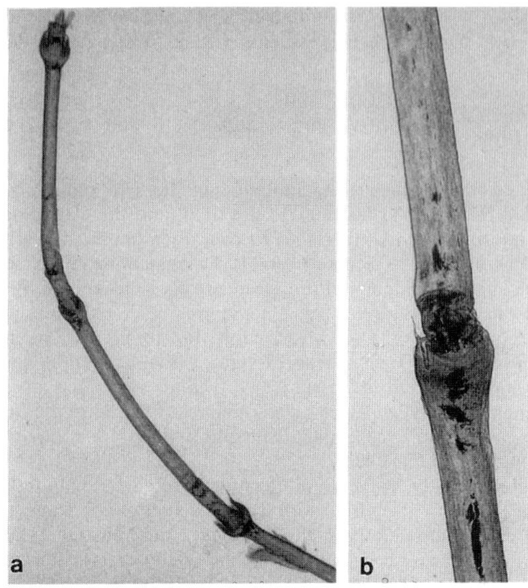

Figure 2.27. Light microscopic appearance of trichorrhexis invaginata. (From Traupe, 1989.)

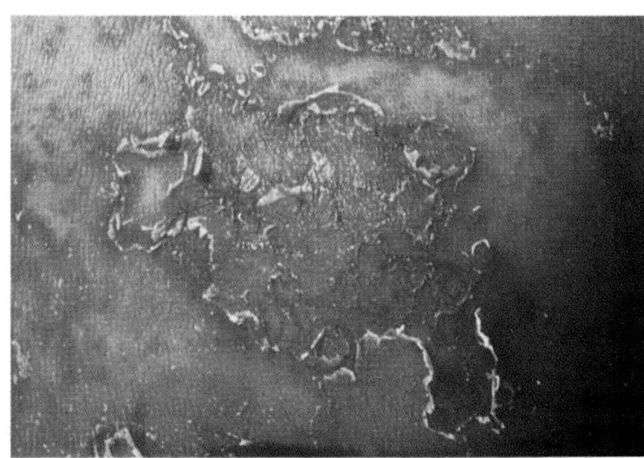

Figure 2.28. Typical double-edged scale of ichthyosis linearis circumflexa. (From Judge, 1994.)

HISTOPATHOLOGY

LIGHT. Acanthosis with orthokeratosis and parakeratosis is typical. Isolated case reports have suggested that features of psoriasis (e.g., Munro microabscesses, elongation of rete ridges) can be seen. There may be a mixed histiolymphocytic infiltrate. Most diagnostic changes are found at the internal border of the double-edged margin of lesions; biopsy material should include the edge and both sides. Under the dissecting microscope the hairs show a typical ball and socket appearance, with the distal hair shaft intussuscepted into a cup formed by the proximal shaft.

EM. There are conflicting reports in the literature that may reflect the heterogeneity of the condition or its variable nature. In a number of reports round or oval bodies containing finely granular material are present in the spinous cells. These are also seen in atopic dermatitis. In the areas around the intussuscepted hair shaft, there is disorganized keratinization.

BASIC DEFECT

Unknown.

TREATMENT

Fluid and electrolyte support during the neonatal period to avoid hypernatremic dehydration secondary to transepidermal water loss is important. Use of light emollients may be helpful. Lac-Hydrin has been reported to be impressively effective in several case reports. I have not had similar success with my two patients with Netherton syndrome. Etretinate treatment has met with mixed success, and it may exacerbate the disease in some individuals. Cyclophosphamide (50 mg p.o./q3d) therapy was reported to be successful in one patient. PUVA (psoralen plus ultraviolet light of the A wavelength) has been used successfully in two patients.

MODE OF INHERITANCE

Autosomal recessive. Consanguinity has been reported in 10% of families.

PRENATAL DIAGNOSIS

None.

DIFFERENTIAL DIAGNOSIS

Traupe believes that continual peeling skin type B (MIM:270300) is the same entity as Netherton syndrome with congenital ichthyosiform erythroderma. I believe that more severe skin findings, failure to thrive, trichorrhexis invaginata, and elevated IgE levels distinguish Netherton from continual peeling skin.

Congenital nonbullous ichthyosiform erythroderma or lamellar ichthyosis (MIM:242100) needs to be excluded. Examination of multiple hairs on more than one occasion may be necessary to detect trichorrhexis invaginata.

Acrodermatitis enteropathica (MIM:201100) can appear quite similar, and careful examination of hairs for trichorrhexis invaginata should be done. Periorificial and distal distribution of skin findings is more typical of acrodermatitis enteropathica. Zinc levels are notoriously inaccurate and may not be reliably discriminatory. An empiric trial of zinc is harmless and may be appropriate during initial evaluation of the patient with Netherton syndrome.

Ichthyosis linearis circumflexa can be confused with autosomal dominant erythrokeratodermia variabilis (MIM:133200). In the latter, the scaling lesions are fixed, not migratory, and onset is usually after the first year of life. Hairs are normal in erythrokeratodermia variabilis. In autosomal dominant erythrokeratodermia *en cocardes,* individual lesions are transient, and hyperkeratosis of the knees and desquamation of the palms and soles occur. Hairs are also normal.

The existence of Leiner disease (MIM: 227100)—explosive seborrheic dermatitis—has been hotly debated. It is a diagnosis that has been applied to some infants who are later found to have Netherton syndrome. Repeated examination of hairs may be required to confirm the diagnosis of Netherton syndrome.

In my experience, there is an association of severe eczematous dermatitis, seborrheic dermatitis, or ichthyotic-like skin changes with severe immune defects that is not diagnostically specific. Infants with severe ichthyosiform erythroderma, severe widespread atopic skin changes, or explosive seborrheic dermatitis may also show poor hair growth, lymphadenopathy (often ascribed to reactive changes secondary to widespread impetiginization), and failure to thrive. Identified syndromes with this constellation include Wiskott-Aldrich syndrome (MIM:301100), Netherton syndrome, and Dubowitz syndrome (MIM:223370). I have seen a number of patients with a variety of real but not diagnostic alterations in lymph node architecture, T- or B-cell defects, and immunoglobulin abnormalities, who present with failure to thrive and severe dermatitis that is unresponsive to conventional therapy. It is likely that some of the infants with Leiner disease fall into this category. To me, the tip-off to suspect one of these conditions is the paucity of hair, which, while striking, could be written off as the far end of normal sparse baby fuzz if one does not recognize its significance.

Skin changes may not be present at birth but evolve over weeks to months. Outcome has been uniformly dismal. I suggest that a full immunologic work-up be undertaken in infants presenting with growth failure, poor hair growth, and generalized eczematous or ichthyosiform skin changes.

Support Group: F.I.R.S.T.
P.O. Box 20921
Raleigh, NC 27619
1-800-545-3286

SELECTED BIBLIOGRAPHY

Netherton, E.W. (1958). A unique case of trichorrhexis nodosa—"bamboo hairs." *A.M.A. Arch. Dermatol.* **78,** 483–487.

This is a lovingly detailed case report with a lucid description of the classic features of the disease. Despite the title, Netherton did not believe the hair changes were true trichorrhexis nodosa. Subsequent reports describe Netherton's patient as having an ichthyosis similar to lamellar ichthyosis, but photos and description clearly indicate that she had generalized erythroderma that progressed to ichthyosis linearis circumflexa.

Shield, J.P.H., Judge, M.R., Reardon, W., Baraitser, M., Nohria, M., Malone, M., and Harper, J.I. (1992). Lethal congenital erythroderma: a newly recognized genetic disorder. *Clin. Genet.* **41,** 273–277.

This paper reviews four families with numerous infants who died with generalized skin changes, nonspecific immune defects and failure to thrive. Although they state no hair defects were found, the one photo of one infant shows no hairs. I believe this presentation is nonspecific and can be seen in a multitude of immune disorders.

Zina, A.M., and Bundino, S. (1979). Ichthyosis linearis circumflexa, Comel and Netherton syndrome: an ultrastructural study. *Dermatologica* **158,** 404–412.

Three patients were evaluated. There is a good discussion of the inconstancy of specific ultrastructural features. The authors argue that, while no feature is diagnostic, taken together a suggestive pattern can confirm the clinical diagnosis.

RESTRICTIVE DERMOPATHY (MIM:275210)

(Tight Skin Contracture Syndrome, Lethal)

DERMATOLOGIC FEATURES

MAJOR. At birth, the skin of these infants is tight and rigid, shiny and red. There may be scaling and areas of marked erosion, especially at the folds (e.g., neck, groin). In those few infants who have survived beyond a few weeks, these changes appear to progress, and the skin becomes more severely tight.

The facies are expressionless, with minimal creases and furrows in the skin.

MINOR. None.

ASSOCIATED ABNORMALITIES

Polyhydramnios and premature rupture of membranes with premature birth are typical. The umbilical cord is often short, and the placenta may be hydropic.

The facies are marked by thin, pinched nares, open small mouth, micrognathia, and crumpled, flattened, or low-set pinnae. These are all secondary to the cutaneous constraint. Choanal atresia or stenosis has been reported in a significant number of affected infants.

Natal teeth have been reported in approximately one-half of the babies with this condition.

Flexion contractures of the joints, presumably secondary to constraint of movement in utero, is a constant finding.

Bony changes have included hypoplasia of the clavicle, radius, ulna, and distal phalanges, overtubulation of the long bones, and wide sutures with large fontanelles. All of these changes have been ascribed to decreased movement in utero.

A

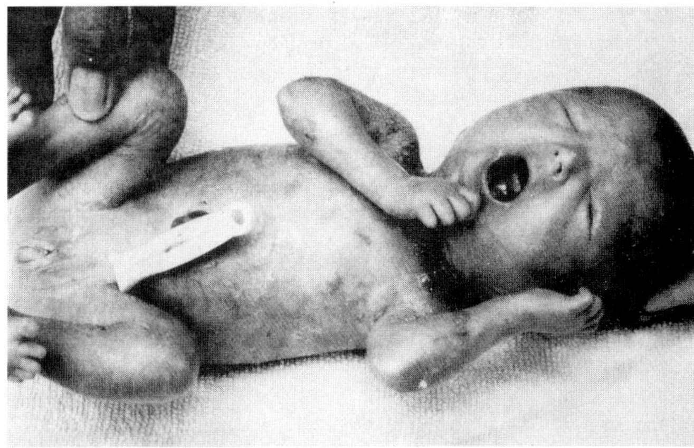

B

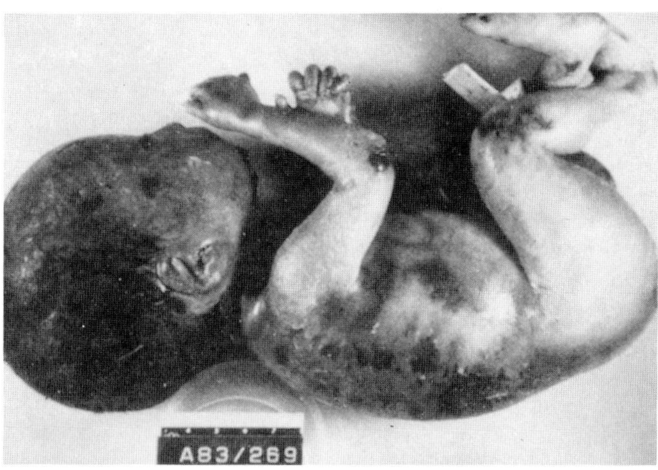

Figure 2.29. **(A)** Typical facies with opened mouth and pinched nares. (From Holbrook et al., 1986.) **(B)** Joints fixed, taunt skin with eroded areas, constricted pinna. (From Witt et al., 1986.)

Pulmonary hypoplasia and respiratory insufficiency or septicemia are the usual causes of death.

In one patient, muscle development was deemed immature on histopathology, consistent with 20–22 weeks rather than 34 weeks of fetal development. A muscle biopsy specimen from an affected sibling was normal.

HISTOPATHOLOGY

Light. Epidermal hyperkeratosis with or without parakeratosis, plus thinning of the dermis and abnormal alignment of the collagen bundles, are typical features. Epidermal appendages are reported as abnormal in most cases. There is an absence of the normal rete ridge pattern and a flattening of the dermo-epidermal junction.

EM. Small collagen fibrils with extremely small or absent elastin fibers are the typical findings. Keratohyaline granules can be abnormal and may fail to aggregate with keratin filaments. These are not consistent features.

BASIC DEFECT

Unknown. Keratin studies have shown increased hyperproliferative keratins but no other abnormalities.

TREATMENT

There is no effective treatment for this condition. To date there have been no long-term survivors.

MODE OF INHERITANCE

Autosomal recessive. There have been multiple recurrences in sibships, and consanguinity between parents is typical.

PRENATAL DIAGNOSIS

None. Fetal skin biopsy at 19 weeks in a pregnancy at risk showed no ultrastructural alterations; the affected infant was subsequently born at 29 weeks after sudden development of polyhydramnios. Whether abnormal suprabasal staining of the epidermis with the monoclonal antibody AE1, which was demonstrated in an affected infant at birth, is present in fetal skin early enough to allow for prenatal diagnosis is unknown.

DIFFERENTIAL DIAGNOSIS

Some cases of restrictive dermopathy have been reported as aplasia cutis congenita, arthrogryposis without specific diagnosis, or as unknowns. Restrictive dermopathy bears great resemblance to the Neu-Laxova syndrome (MIM:256500). The main difference is the presence of structural brain malformations in Neu-Laxova.

In sclerema neonatorum, there is progressive hardening and binding down of previously normal skin, most often occurring in ill premature infants. This can be readily distinguished from restrictive dermopathy.

Infants born with a collodion membrane may appear similar initially, but the membrane cracks, fissures, and begins to peel within a few days to weeks, while the skin in restrictive dermopathy persists in its abnormal appearance. Newborns with a collodion membrane rarely, if ever, have significant large joint fixation. Histologically the collodion membrane can be distinguished by the absence of the dermal alterations seen in restrictive dermopathy and the presence of a normal rete ridge pattern.

Infants with the fetal akinesia sequence and/or arthrogryposes such as Pena-Shokeir (MIM:208150) or COFS (MIM:214150) may show similar joint and facial changes, but the skin in these two conditions is normal, and structural brain malformations are typical.

Epidermolysis bullosa dystrophica and junctional-letalis (MIM:132000, 226600, 226700, 226730), in which absence of the skin can occur, have been confused with both aplasia cutis congenita and restrictive dermopathy. While there may be some joint involvement of the lower limbs where skin has been denuded in congenital epidermolysis bullosa, generalized contractures are not seen and the facies are not abnormal. Microstomia is not part of the epidermolysis bullosa syndromes. Histology and electron microscopy should allow for correct diagnosis.

The Mennonite patients with autosomal recessive arthrogryposis, edema, and taut eroding skin described by Lowry et al. (1985) probably had restrictive dermopathy.

Support Group: F.I.R.S.T.
P.O. Box 20921
Raleigh, NC 27619
1-800-545-3286

SELECTED BIBLIOGRAPHY

Holbrook, K.A., Dale, B.A., Witt, D.R., Hayden, M.R., and Toriello, H.V. (1987). Arrested epidermal morphogenesis in three newborn infants with a fatal genetic disorder (restrictive dermopathy). *J. Invest. Dermatol.* **88,** 330–339.

Witt, D.R., Hayden, M.R., Holbrook, K.A., Dale, B.A., Baldwin, V.J., and Taylor, G.P. (1986). Restrictive dermopathy: a newly recognized autosomal recessive skin dysplasia. *Am. J. Med. Genet.* **24,** 631–648.

The authors coined the term "restrictive dermopathy" and described two sibships and in a subsequent paper a third patient (sibling to others previously reported by Toriello). Electron microscopic and keratin studies are described.

Lowry, R.B., Machin, G.A., Morgan, K., Mayock, D., Marx, L. (1985). Congenital contractures, edema, hyperkeratosis, and intrauterine growth retardation: a fatal syndrome in Hutterite and Mennonite kindreds. *Am. J. Med. Genet.* **22,** 531–43.

Two Hutterite and one Mennonite families.

Pierard-Franchimont, C., Pierard, G.E., Hermanns-Le, T., Arrese-Estrada, J., Verloes, A., and Mulliez, N. (1992). Dermatopathological aspects of restrictive dermopathy. *J. Pathol.* **167,** 223–228.

Verloes, A., Mulliez, N., Gonzalez, M., Laloux, F., Hermanns-Le, T., Pierard, G.E., and Koulischer, L. (1992). Restrictive dermopathy, a lethal form of arthrogryposis multiplex with skin and bone dysplasias: three new cases and review of the literature. *Am. J. Med. Genet.* **43,** 539–547.

Histologic and clinical descriptions of two (Pierard-Franchimont, et al.), and a third (Verloes, et al.), unrelated infants with restrictive dermopathy. Abnormal decreased dendritic staining with factor XIIIa and/or aberrant expression of L1 antigen led authors to suggest that the condition results from maturational delay in all components of skin development. The Verloes, et al. paper gives a detailed description of the clinical features.

X-LINKED RECESSIVE ICHTHYOSIS (MIM:308100)

(Sterol Sulfatase Deficiency; X-linked Ichthyosis Vulgaris; Ichthyosis Nigricans)

DERMATOLOGIC FEATURES

MAJOR. Estimates of incidence range from 1 in 2,000 to 1 in 9,500 male births. All the body surfaces are involved, with the exception of the face, palms, and soles, with large yellow-brown scales. This is not invariable; finer white scaling or grayish scaling can predominate in some individuals. The color and distribution of the scales has given rise to the description "dirty neck disease."

Although frank scaling is usually not recognized until 3–6 months of age, a retrospective study suggested that significant skin peeling does occur within a few days of life, after which the skin appears to be relatively normal until scaling becomes obvious within the first year.

MINOR. None.

ASSOCIATED ABNORMALITIES

Asymptomatic diffuse corneal opacities are seen on slit-lamp examination. These are situated deep in the corneal stroma. From 25% to 50% of males and some carrier females have these findings.

The absence of placental sterol sulfatase activity results in low to absent estriol levels in maternal urine and in amniotic fluid. Spontaneous initiation of labor may not occur, and post-term delivery is seen in approximately one-

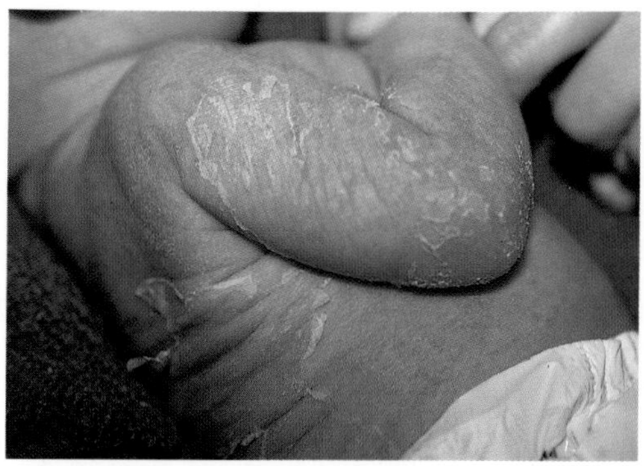

Figure 2.30. Peeling membrane and erythroderma in male with X-linked ichthyosis.

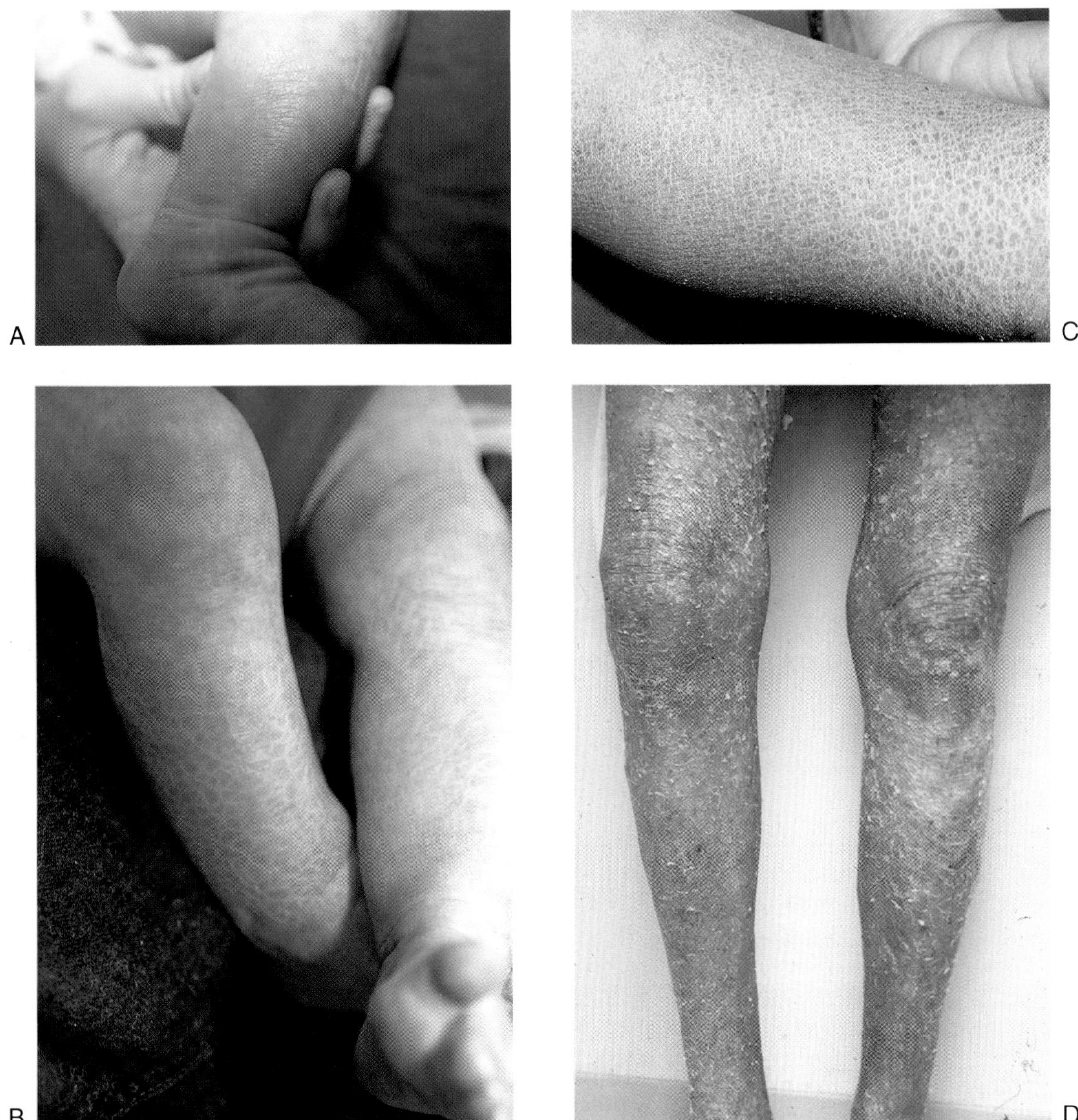

Figure 2.31. Varying degrees of scale in four individuals **(A–D)** with X-linked ichthyosis.

third of patients. Birth weight appears to be below the 50% for normal males.

Cryptorchidism occurs in about one-fifth of affected males. Testicular carcinoma, independent of a history of cryptorchidism, has been reported in four patients. Two had seminomas, one an embryonal carcinoma in one testis and a seminoma in the other. In the fourth, the tumor type was not described. We have also had one patient with X-linked recessive ichthyosis present with testicular malignancy. Testicular self-examination should be taught to all boys with this condition.

HISTOPATHOLOGY

Light. Orthohyperkeratosis with occasional minimal parakeratosis and an increased granular layer. These findings are not invariable.
EM. No diagnostic changes.

BASIC DEFECT

Deficiency of sterol sulfatase results in inability to cleave cholesterol sulfate. In over 80% of individuals there is a gene deletion at the STS locus on the short arm of the X chromosome.

TREATMENT

Twice daily application of topical keratolytics, including urea and lactic acid creams, or propylene glycol 50–50 with water under plastic occlusion overnight once a week is effective. I have not had a patient require oral retinoids for adequate control.

MODE OF INHERITANCE

X-linked. Most female carriers do not express skin changes, and, in those who do, changes are minimal and rarely exceed mild dryness. Female carriers may have corneal abnormalities.

The sterol sulfatase locus escapes inactivation; thus normal females have an almost twofold level of activity compared with normal males. Female carriers of X-linked recessive ichthyosis have sterol sulfatase levels at or below the mean for normal males. The locus is Xp22.3, and the gene has been cloned.

PRENATAL DIAGNOSIS

Prenatal diagnosis is possible by molecular detection of deletions at the STS locus and also by evaluation of closely linked DNA markers in those families in whom there is not a deletion. Measurement of sterol sulfatase activity in cells obtained during chorionic villus sampling or in amniocytes is also possible, as is measurement of amniotic fluid and maternal urine estriol levels. A number of authors state that prenatal diagnosis is not warranted because of the relative mildness of this condition. In my practice, prior to the time that prenatal diagnosis became available, I encountered several families in whom the genetic risk resulted in a decision not to reproduce, suggesting that prenatal diagnosis may be desired by some families.

DIFFERENTIAL DIAGNOSIS

The skin changes are similar to those of ichthyosis vulgaris (MIM:146700) but distinguished by flexural distribution, absence of hyperlinear palms and keratosis pilaris, sparing of the face except for the preauricular areas, involvement of the neck, lack of improvement with age, and no association with atopy.

Some patients described as having the Rud syndrome (MIM:312770)—comprised of ichthyosis similar to X-linked recessive ichthyosis, hypogonadism and cryptorchidism, and with or without mental retardation, polyneuropathy, short stature, or anosmia—had sterol sulfatase deficiency. Although severe X-linked recessive ichthyosis can mimic mild lamellar/nonbullous congenital ichthyosiform erythroderma (MIM: 242100), the latter condition always presents at birth, the former almost never. Enzymatic assay and/molecular studies will discriminate.

Support Group: F.I.R.S.T.
P.O. Box 20921
Raleigh, NC 27619
1-800-545-3286

SELECTED BIBLIOGRAPHY

Basler, E., Grompe, M., Parenti, G., Yates, J., and Ballabio, A. (1992). Identification of point mutations in the steroid sulfatase gene of three patients with X-linked ichthyosis. *Am. J. Hum. Genet.* **50,** 483–491.

Reviews molecular studies and reports three different point mutations in patients without deletions.

Mevorah, B., Frenk, E., Muller, C.R., and Ropers, H.H. (1981). X-linked recessive ichthyosis in three sisters and evidence for homozygosity. *Br. J. Dermatol.* **105,** 711–717.

This is a fascinating pedigree in which a carrier female and her affected first cousin husband had three affected homozygous and one carrier heterozygous daughters who again transmitted the disorder appropriately for an X-linked condition. Diagnosis was confirmed by sterol sulfatase levels.

Shackleton, C., Williams, M.L., and Epstein, E.H., Jr. (1988). Diagnostic tests for recessive X-linked ichthyosis. *Pediatr. Dermatol.* **5**, 211–212.

Lipoprotein electrophoresis is unreliable (I share these authors' experience). Authors give instructions for obtaining cholesterol sulfate levels, which will be elevated in X-linked recessive ichthyosis.

Shapiro, L.J., Weiss, R., Webster, D., and France, J.T. (1978). X-linked ichthyosis due to steroid sulfatase deficiency. *Lancet* **i**, 70–72.

Shapiro, L.J., Weiss, R., Buxman, M.M., Vidgoff, J., and Dimond, R.L. (1978). Enzymatic basis of typical X-linked ichthyosis. *Lancet* **ii**, 756–757.

Recognition and confirmation of the enzymatic basis of the disease initially in two pedigrees and then in 25 unrelated patients from around the world.

Wells, R.S., and Kerr, C.B. (1966). Clinical features of autosomal dominant and sex-linked ichthyosis in an English population. *Br. Med. J.* **1**, 947–950.

This is my all-time favorite study in which careful observation of clinical features and pedigree data allowed for determination of distinguishing diagnostic features between these disorders. Nary a microscope, test tube, or reagent was used.

ERYTHROKERATODERMAS

ERYTHROKERATODERMIA VARIABILIS (MIM:133200)

(Mendes da Costa Disease; Keratosis Rubra Figurata; Erythrokeratoderma Figurata Variabilis)

Includes Erythrokeratodermia Variabilis *en Cocarde*, Giroux-Barbeau Syndrome

---

DERMATOLOGIC FEATURES

Major. This condition is marked by two types of skin changes. There are migratory patches of erythema that may be circinate, targetoid, or geographic and last for minutes to days to months. These may gradually become hyperkeratotic, erythematous, and fixed. There may be a thin circumferential white margin of vasoconstriction surrounding the lesions.

The second skin change is a hyperkeratotic plaque with yellow-brown-gray scale. These areas are sharply demarcated with geographic borders and are usually fixed. These develop independent of the fleeting erythema. Some affected individuals have both stable and transient plaques. In one large pedigree, some family members had only stable lesions and others had only transient.

The face, extensor surfaces of the extremities, trunk, and buttocks are usually involved. Onset is typically in infancy, and there is progression through childhood with stabilization at puberty. Improvement and regression with age and warmth have been described, as has complete but transient clearing after febrile illness. In the *en cocarde* variant, rosette or target-like erythematous patches predominate, but it is not clear that the disorder is genetically or clinically distinct from classic erythrokeratodermia variabilis.

Minor. Involvement of the palms and soles with keratoderma can also occur. Itching is an occasional complaint.

ASSOCIATED ABNORMALITIES

None.

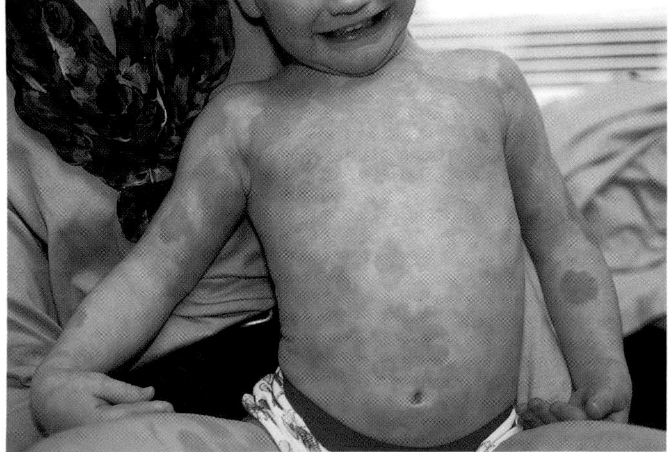

A

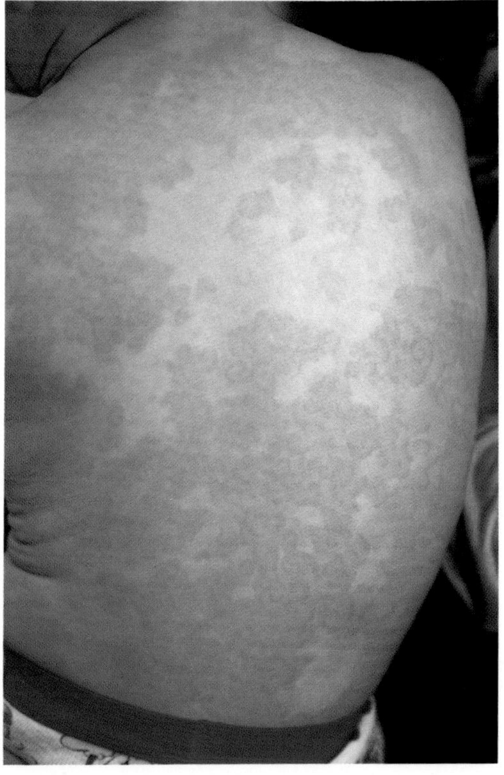

B

Figure 2.32. (A,B) Widespread involvement of trunk with skip areas.

HISTOPATHOLOGY

LIGHT. Orthohyperkeratosis with thickened granular layer, irregular acanthosis, and papillomatosis. There is a mild superficial perivascular lymphocytic infiltrate.

EM. Decreased number of lamellar bodies. There is one report of reduction in Langerhans cells. This has not been confirmed by others.

BASIC DEFECT

Unknown. The cell proliferation rate is reportedly normal.

TREATMENT

Treatment with isotretinoin has resulted in complete clearing. Treatment with etretinate and Acitretin has also resulted in improvement or clearing.

MODE OF INHERITANCE

Autosomal dominant. Linkage has been established to the Rh locus on the short arm of chromosome 1 at 1p31.3–p33. There are two reports of two sets of affected sisters with normal parents.

PRENATAL DIAGNOSIS

None.

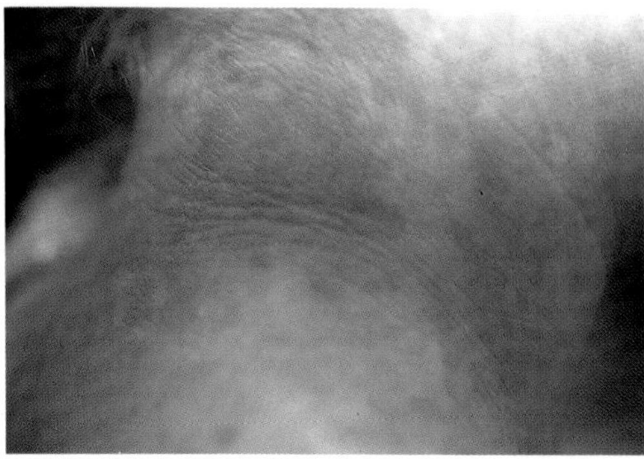

Figure 2.33. Close-up of neck showing thickening of epidermis and accentuation of skin lines.

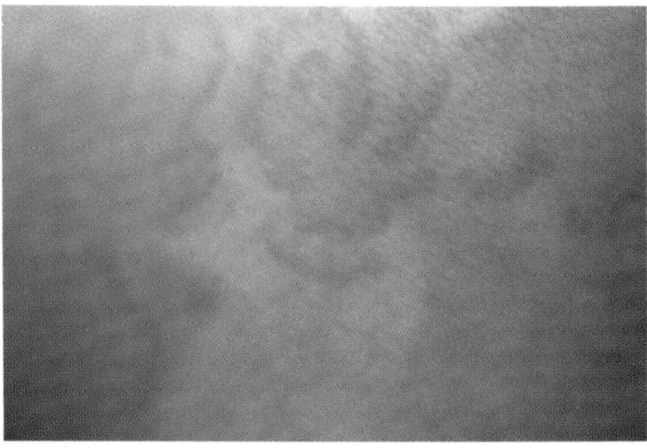

Figure 2.34. Arcuate margins of concentric erythema resembling Chinese silk embroidery.

DIFFERENTIAL DIAGNOSIS

In progressive systemic erythrokeratoderma, the trunk is usually spared; in erythrokeratodermia variabilis it is usually involved. Palmar and plantar involvement is more typical of progressive systemic erythrokeratoderma. There is a considerable overlap between the two disorders, and some case reports span the two.

Psoriasis can usually be differentiated by its silvery, micaceous scale and by the distribution of plaques. Skin biopsy will differentiate.

In Giroux-Barbeau syndrome (ichthyosis and ataxia, MIM:133190) the skin changes are somewhat similar. Patients have progressive ataxia beginning in the fourth to fifth decades. Linkage to the same region on chromosome 1p has been shown.

The ichthyosis of Netherton syndrome (MIM:256500)—ichthyosis linearis circumflexa—can be distinguished from erythrokeratodermia variabilis by its doubled-edged scale.

Support Group: F.I.R.S.T.
P.O. Box 20921
Raleigh, NC 27619
1-800-545-3286

SELECTED BIBLIOGRAPHY

Giroux, J.-M., and Barbeau, A. (1972). Erythrokeratodermia with ataxia. *Arch. Dermatol.* **106,** 183–188.

This is a huge French-Canadian kindred that presented with skin changes of patchy scaling erythema, primarily on the distal extremities. Skin changes can improve in adult life and may disappear. There is also improvement with warm weather. The ataxia is progressive and develops in the fourth to fifth decades, just as the skin involvement appears to subside. Nystagmus and loss of deep tendon reflexes is typical. Inheritance is autosomal dominant. Histopathologic changes are common to both ichthyosis vulgaris and erythrokeratodermia variabilis.

McFadden, N., Oppedal, B.R., Ree, K., and Brandtzaeg, P. (1987). Erythrokeratoderma variabilis: immunohistochemical and ultrastructural studies of the epidermis. *Acta Dermatol. Venereol. (Stockh.)* **67,** 284–288.

One patient showed abnormal staining for cytokeratin PKK2 in the stratum corneum. PKK2 is usually confined to the basal epidermal and follicular epithelial cells. This abnormal staining disappeared, and clinical clearing occurred, when the patient was treated with etretinate.

Mendes da Costa, S. (1925). Erythro-et keratodermia variabilis in a mother and daughter. *Acta Dermatol. Venereol.* **6,** 255–261.

A beautiful description of the clinical features. Argues for the return of the lovingly detailed case report to our current publishable papers. Mendes da Costa's name is also given to a disorder of blistering, and this may cause some confusion.

Schnyder, U.W., and Sommacal-Schopf, D. (1957). Fourteen cases of erythrokeratodermia figurata variabilis within one family. *Acta Genet.* **7,** 204–206.

Remarkably varied clinical descriptions among affected family members.

vander Schroeff, J.G., van Leeuwen-Cornelisse, I., van Haeringen, A., and Weent, L.N. (1988). Further evidence for localization of the gene of erythrokeratodermia variabilis. *Hum. Genet.* **80,** 97–98.

Cumulative maximum lod score of 9.93 (theta = 0.03) for linkage between erythrokeratodermia variabilis and Rh. There were two recombinants. These numbers are based on two distinct pedigrees, but the authors believe both probably had a common ancestor because they both come from the same geographically isolated area.

PITYRIASIS RUBRA PILARIS (MIM:173200)

(Keratosis Circumscripta)

DERMATOLOGIC FEATURES

MAJOR. Palmar-plantar hyperkeratosis with a smooth thickened appearance and a peculiar yellow-orange or salmon hue, with sharp demarcation of the borders, is classic for pityriasis rubra pilaris. There is a generalized, patchy perifollicular erythema and fine powdery scaling. The perifollicular papules have a central hyperkeratotic plug surrounded by a yellow-orange ring. The individual lesions coalesce into the salmon-colored plaques typical of the disorder.

The elbows, knees, backs of the hands and feet, and ankles are preferred sites of involvement. The hands and feet may become edematous.

The scalp is involved in almost one-half of reported patients. The typical salmon-hued rash is present with thick, adherent scale.

The entire skin surface can be involved. Islands of sparing are typical.

Classification of pityriasis rubra pilaris into distinct clinical subtypes has been complicated by significant overlap among them (see Table 2.1).

MINOR. Nail dystrophy with thickening, pitted yellow lines, opacities of the nail plate, hyperkeratosis of the nail bed, and punctate subungual hemorrhages can occur.

Ectropion has been described.

ASSOCIATED ABNORMALITIES

None.

Table 2.1. Classification of Pityriasis Rubra Pilaris Based on Clinical Manifestations and Prognosis

Subgroup	*Skin*	*% Remission by 3 Years*	*% of Patients with Pityriasis Rubra Pilaris*
Type I: classic adult	Diffuse involvement, erythroderma, islands of clear skin	80	55
Type II: atypical adult	Ichthyosiform scaling, sparse hair	20	5
Type III: classic juvenile	Same as type I, with onset in first few years of life	16–60	10
Type IV: circumscribed juvenile	Follicular hyperkeratosis of knees and elbows, onset prior to puberty	32–60	25
Type V: atypical juvenile	Onset in first few years, chronic course	0	5

Modified from Griffiths (1980)

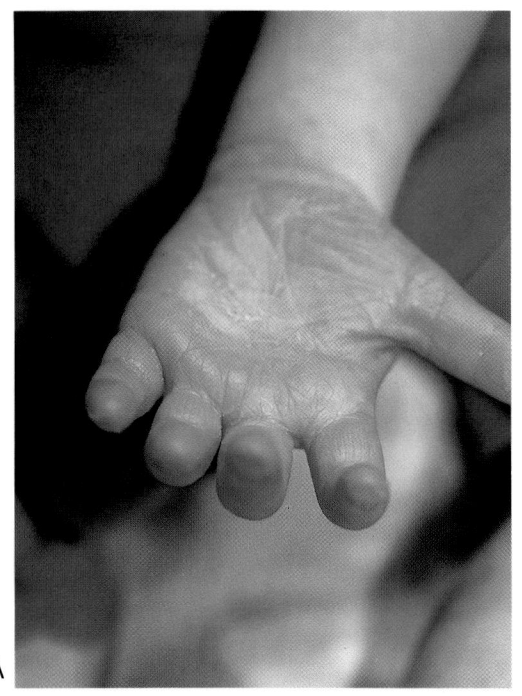

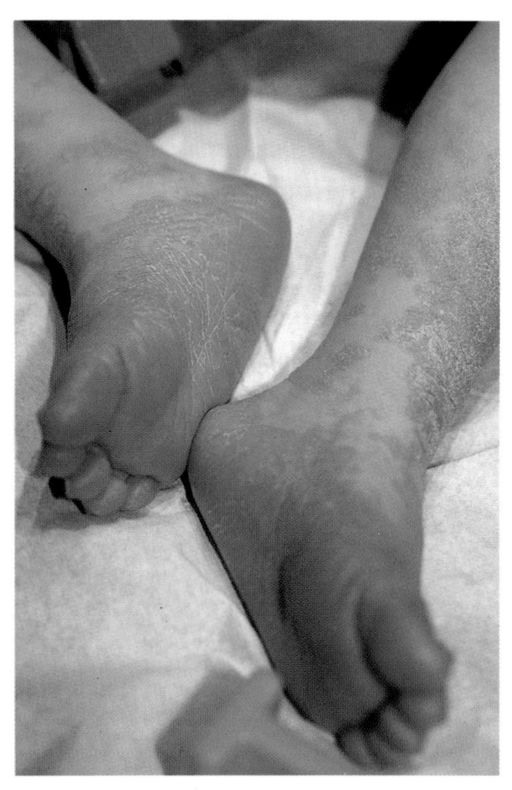

Figure 2.35. Palmar (**A**) and plantar (**B**) erythema and scale with orange hue.

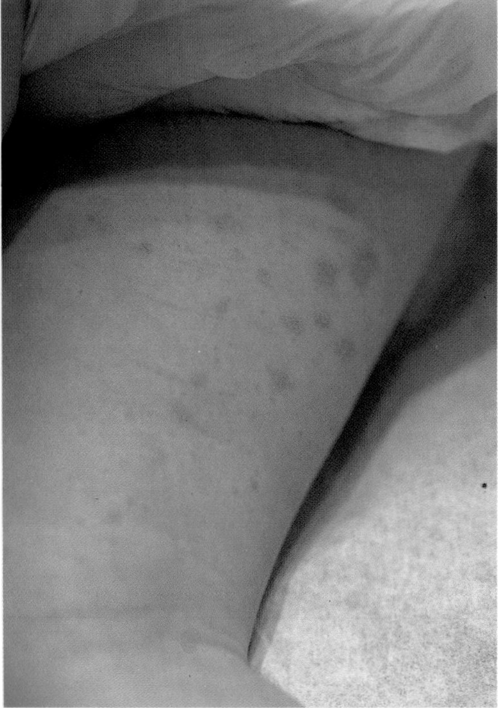

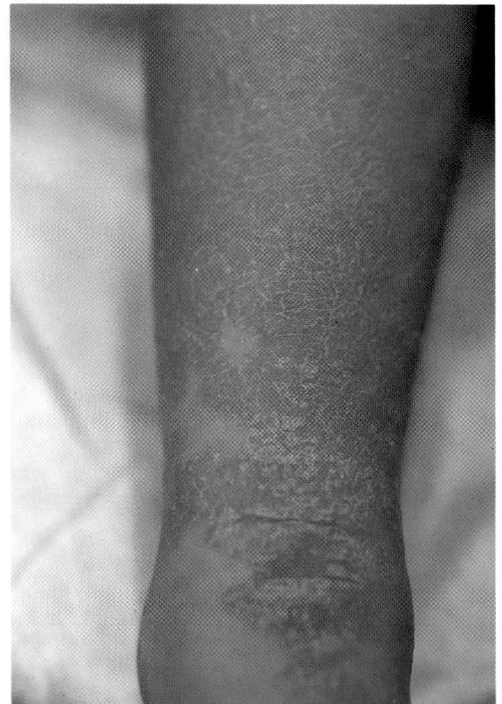

Figure 2.36. (**A**) Individual papules. (**B**) Coalescence into plaques with island of sparing.

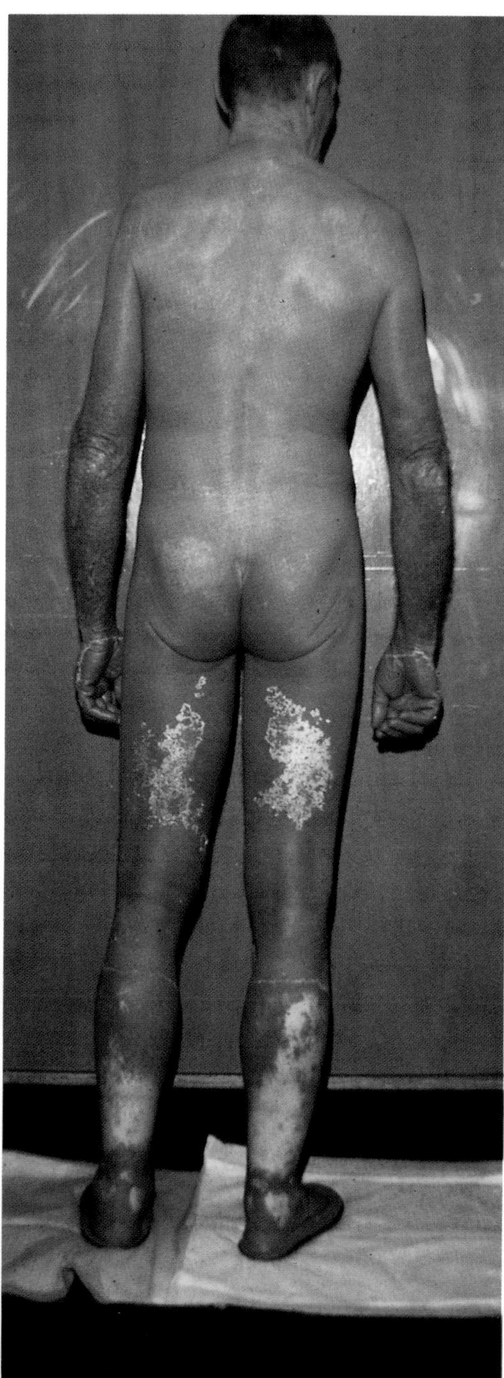

Figure 2.37. Marked areas of normal skin in generalized disease. (Courtesy of Division of Dermatology, University of Washington.)

HISTOPATHOLOGY

LIGHT. There is compact acanthosis of the epidermis with hyperkeratosis and patchy parakeratosis. The suprapapillary plates are thickened. The hair follicles are filled with keratotic plugs, and there may be perifollicular parakeratosis. There are patchy foci of basal liquefaction and spongiosis.

EM. Decreased tonofilaments and desmosomes and increased lamellar granules occur. Basal lamina at the dermo-epidermal junction shows focal splits.

BASIC DEFECT

Unknown. It has been suggested that there may be a defect in transport or delivery of retinoids to tissue, but serum retinol-binding protein levels are normal.

TREATMENT

Vitamin A 150,000–300,000 IU daily is effective in about one-third of patients. Vitamin A toxicity rarely occurs in patients with pityriasis rubra pilaris even when these high doses are used.

Etretinate and 13-*cis*-retinoic acid are also effective and may result in remission in a greater proportion of patients. With its longer half-life and therefore high potential for teratogenicity, etretinate is less desirable than isotretinoin.

Methotrexate, azathiaprine (Imuran), and stanozolol are not uniformly effective and represent second-line drugs for patients who fail vitamin A or retinoid treatment.

PUVA and UVB are not useful.

Many other drugs have been tried with limited success.

MODE OF INHERITANCE

Autosomal dominant when inherited. Most cases have been sporadic. It is impossible to distinguish clinically between genetic and acquired pityriasis rubra pilaris in the absence of a family history. Arguments have been made by several authors that, when inherited, pityriasis rubra pilaris actually represents atypical ichthyosis or psoriasis because of the small proportion of patients with pityriasis rubra pilaris with a positive family history.

PRENATAL DIAGNOSIS

None.

DIFFERENTIAL DIAGNOSIS

Palmoplantar keratodermas (MIM:148400, 140600, 144200, 148350) do not usually have scalp involvement, although they can share in common with pityriasis rubra pilaris involvement of other areas in addition to palms and soles and, similar to pityriasis rubra pilaris, may not present at birth.

Plaques of psoriasis (MIM:177900) have a silvery scale, and the erythema is red, not the salmon hue of pityriasis rubra pilaris. The follicular plugging of pityriasis rubra pilaris is distinctive. The Koebner phenomenon and itching are rare in pityriasis rubra pilaris, common in psoriasis.

Seborrheic dermatitis usually does not involve the palms and soles.

Vitamin A deficiency can be distinguished by history and differs histologically from pityriasis rubra pilaris. Patchy parakeratosis and an inflammatory infiltrate in the upper dermis are found in pityriasis rubra pilaris but not in vitamin A deficiency.

Support Group: F.I.R.S.T.
P.O. Box 20921
Raleigh, NC 27619
1-800-545-3286

SELECTED BIBLIOGRAPHY

Cohen, P.R., and Prystowsky, J.H. (1989). Pityriasis rubra pilaris: a review of diagnosis and treatment. *J. Am. Acad. Dermatol.* **20,** 801–807.

Review article summarizing approach to treatment.

Dicken, C.H. (1994). Treatment of classic pityriasis rubra pilaris. *J. Am. Acad. Dermatol.* **31,** 997–999.

Reviews treatment outcomes in 75 patients at the Mayo Clinic. Patients were aged 16–81 years.

Gelmetti, C., Schiuma, A.A., Cerri, D.C., and Gianotti, F. (1986). Pityriasis rubra pilaris in childhood: a long-term study of 29 cases. *Pediatr. Dermatol.* **3,** 446–451.

Describes course of disease in 29 children and makes a case for not treating children because they tend to have self-limited disease that resolves within a year. I am not sure I agree with this position, as the disease can be devastating while active, and, in my experience, problems with vitamin A toxicity are rare.

Griffiths, W.A.D. (1976). Pityriasis rubra pilaris—an historical approach. *Clin. Exp. Dermatol.* **1,** 37–50.

A detailed review of the literature and of 90 cases at St. John's Hospital.

Griffiths, W.A.D. (1980). Pityriasis rubra pilaris. *Clin. Exp. Dermatol.* **5,** 105–112.

An attempt-to classify pityriasis rubra pilaris into five subtypes with regard to clinical presentation and prognosis.

PROGRESSIVE SYMMETRIC ERYTHROKERATODERMA (MIM:None)

(Darier-Gottron Disease)

DERMATOLOGIC FEATURES

Major. Symmetric red scaling plaques on the buttocks, groin, and knees appear soon after birth, progress, then stabilize, and may improve after puberty. The face may also be involved. Palmar and plantar involvement occurs in approximately one-half of patients. The trunk is usually spared.

Minor. None.

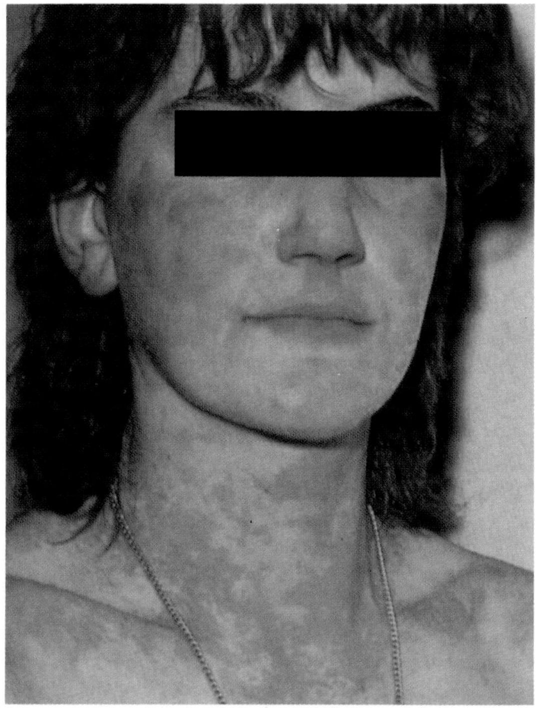

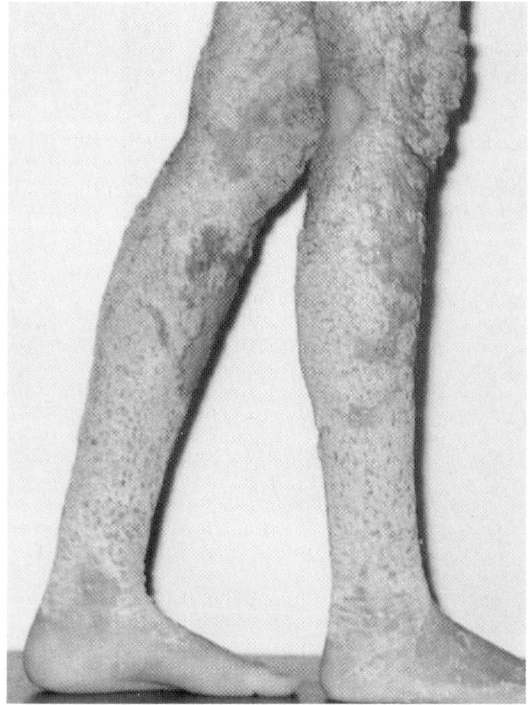

Figure 2.38. **(A)** Symmetric erythematous plaques on face and neck of mother. **(B)** More marked hyperkeratosis on legs with some islands of sparing. (From Dupertuis, 1991.)

ASSOCIATED ABNORMALITIES

None.

HISTOPATHOLOGY

LIGHT. Acanthosis with basket-weave hyperkeratosis and a normal granular layer with occasional parakeratosis. Granular cells show perinuclear vacuolization.

EM. Essentially normal. Granular cells show increased numbers of swollen mitochondria; not all cells and not all mitochondria within the same cell are abnormal. There are increased numbers of lipid vacuoles in the stratum corneum.

BASIC DEFECT

Unknown. An increase in cell proliferation has been demonstrated.

TREATMENT

Standard keratolytics—lactic acid, glycolic acid, and urea formulations—usually are minimally effective. Oral retinoids may be useful. Benefits and risks of treatment in light of severity of disease need to be weighed on an individual basis.

MODE OF INHERITANCE

Autosomal dominant.

PRENATAL DIAGNOSIS

None.

DIFFERENTIAL DIAGNOSIS

Among the palmoplantar keratodermas, buttocks and extremity involvement is not rare.

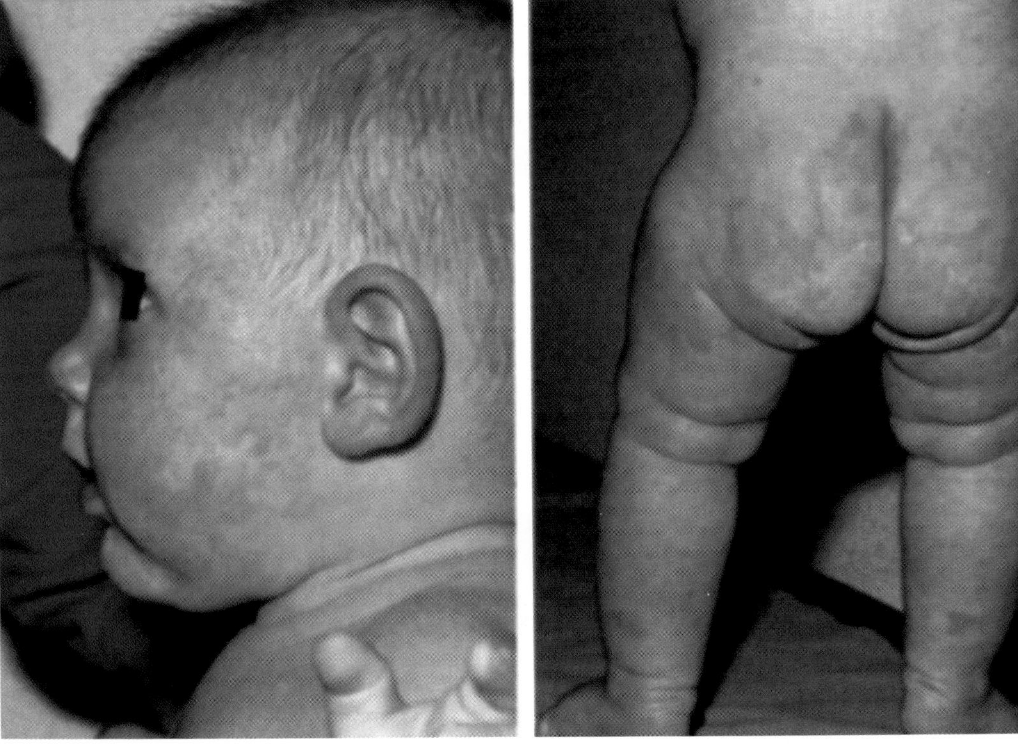

Figure 2.39. Lesions on cheeks **(A)** and buttocks and legs **(B)** in son. (From Dupertuis, 1991.)

Differentiating among these and from progressive symmetric erythrokeratoderma with accuracy is not always possible. All of the conditions appear to be autosomal dominant. Localized pityriasis rubra pilaris (MIM:173200) is marked by perifollicular erythema and hyperkeratosis. Biopsy should help discriminate. Progressive symmetric erythrokeratodermia usually lacks the classic fleeting erythema of erythrokeratodermia variabilis (MIM:133200), and the distribution of hyperkeratosis spares the trunk in progressive symmetric erythrokeratoderma and involves it in erythrokeratodermia variabilis. However, in at least one family, a child with erythrokeratodermia variabilis had a mother and a grandfather with clinically typical progressive symmetric erythrokeratoderma. Both conditions are autosomal dominant with abnormalities limited to the skin.

Support Group: F.I.R.S.T.
P.O. Box 20921
Raleigh, NC 27619
1-800-545-3286

SELECTED BIBLIOGRAPHY

Darier, J. (1911). Erythrokératodermie verruqueuse en nappes symétrique et progressive. *Bull. Soc. Fr. Dermatol. Syphiligr.* **22,** 252–264.

In this case report of a boy with onset of progressive keratodermia at 1 year, Darier argues forcibly that the condition is different from verrucous congenital nevus. However, the photographs and the histopathology are strikingly similar to the latter and far more severe and verrucoid than most subsequent case reports of progressive symmetric erythrokeratoderma.

Hopsu-Havu, V.K., and Tuohimaa, P. (1971). Erythrokeratodermia congenitalis progressiva symmetrica (Gottron). II. An analysis of epidermal cell proliferation. *Dermatologica* **142,** 137–144.

Autoradiographic studies of one patient show a threefold increase in the mitotic index of lesional skin. This was in contrast to the normal cell kinetics in erythrokeratodermia variabilis reported in a German study. However, other case reports of erythrokeratodermia variabilis have described an increased cell turnover rate. Caution must be exercised in giving credence to this as a differentiating feature.

Nazzaro, V., and Blanchet-Bardon, C. (1986). Progressive symmetric erythrokeratodermia. Histological and ultrastructural study of a patient before and after etretinate. *Arch. Dermatol.* **122,** 434–440.
Detailed electron microscopic study with good color photographs of the patient.

ACROKERATODERMA

ACROKERATOELASTOIDOSIS (MIM:101850)

(Costa Disease)

Includes Hereditary Papulotranslucent Acrokeratoderma

DERMATOLOGIC FEATURES

Major. Asymptomatic firm thickened skin of the palms and soles is dotted with individual papules that are yellow-gray in color and typically shiny. They may achieve confluence. The backs and sides of the fingers are involved. In some descriptions, involvement continues up the shins. Onset is in late childhood and early adult life.
Minor. Occasional hyperhidrosis. Knuckle pads are reported in some.

ASSOCIATED ABNORMALITIES

None.

HISTOPATHOLOGY

Light. Orthohyperkeratosis with fragmentation and thinning and disaggregation of elastic fibers in the dermis. The dermal collagen may show homogenization.
EM. Decreased fibroblasts and extracellular elastic fibers.

BASIC DEFECT

Unknown.

TREATMENT

None.

MODE OF INHERITANCE

Autosomal dominant.

PRENATAL DIAGNOSIS

None.

DIFFERENTIAL DIAGNOSIS

Xanthomas can mimic acrokeratoelastoidosis in appearance. Serum lipids are normal in Costa

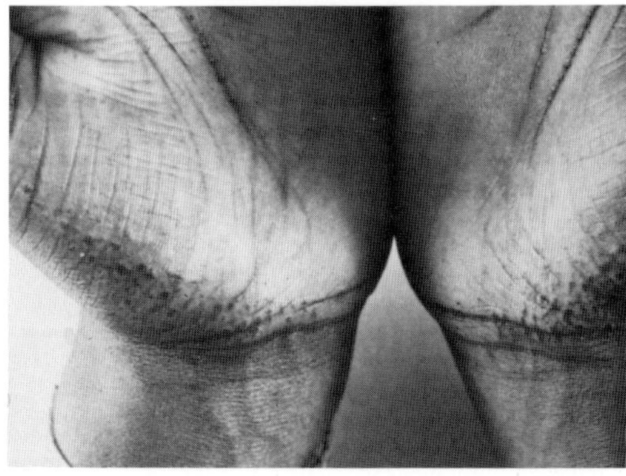

Figure 2.40. Tiny crater-like lesions at edges of palms. (From Dowd et al., 1983.)

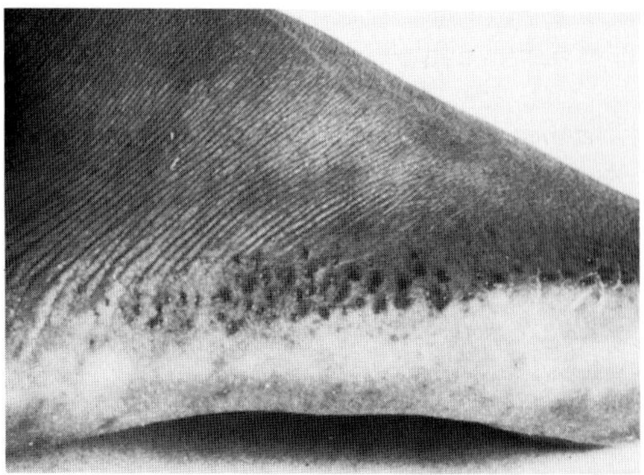

Figure 2.41. Similar changes on foot. (From Dowd et al., 1983.)

disease. Focal acral hyperkeratosis (Dowd) is clinically similar. No alterations in elastic fibers are found with light microscopy.

In hereditary autosomal dominant papulotranslucent acrokeratoderma (MIM:101840), yellowish-white translucent papules develop in similar distribution after puberty. These are histologically differentiated by hyperkeratosis and normal elastic fibers. Similar changes can occur in the elderly due to trauma and actinic damage. These are termed *degenerative collagenous plaques* and are easily differentiated by history. Plane warts can appear similar, and some patients with acrokeratoelastoidosis were mistakenly treated for warts for years.

Support Group: F.I.R.S.T.
P.O. Box 20921
Raleigh, NC 27619
1-800-545-3286

SELECTED BIBLIOGRAPHY

Costa, O.G. (1954). Acrokeratoelastoidosis. *A.M.A. Arch. Dermatol.* **70,** 228–231.

Only description by Costa in English. (This was a sporadic case.)

Dowd, P.M., Horman, R.R.M., and Black, M.M. (1983). Focal acral hyperkeratosis. *Br. J. Dermatol.* **109,** 97–103.

Fifteen patients (seven from three families) with clinical features identical to acrokeratoelastoidosis. Elastic fiber changes were absent in biopsy specimens. Is this a disorder genetically distinct from acrokeratoelastoidosis? I am not sure it is important from a patient care standpoint—same prognosis, same inheritance.

Greiner, J., Kruger, J., Palden, L., Jung, E.G., and Vogel, F. (1983). A linkage study of acrokeratoelastoidosis. Possible mapping to chromosome 2. *Hum. Genet.* **63,** 222–227.

Very provisional linkage to several markers on 2. This is a large family originally reported by Jung.

Johansson, E.A., Kariniemi, A.-L., and Niemi, K.-M. (1980). Palmoplantar keratoderma of punctate type: acrokeratoelastoidosis Costa. *Acta Dermatol. Venereol.* **60,** 149–153.

Ten patients in six families showed no changes in elastin with light microscopy, but variable disaggregation of elastic fibers in the reticular dermis was found with electron microscopy. This raises the possibility that Costa disease and focal acrokeratosis may be identical.

Jung, E.G., and Beil, F.U. (1973). Acrokeratoelastoidosis mimicking palmoplantar xanthomata. *Nutr. Metab.* **15,** 124–127.

A report of the disease in a German patient. The authors suggest that the distribution of papules in acrokeratoelastoidosis is between the dermal ridges, whereas xanthomas occur on the ridges.

ACROKERATOSIS VERRUCIFORMIS (HOPF) (MIM:101900)

DERMATOLOGIC FEATURES

Major. Flat-topped, flesh-colored to tan, polygonal papules, similar in appearance to plane warts, develop on the backs of the hands and the tops of the feet and may extend up along the wrists and ankles. The hands are usually more involved than the feet. Involvement

A
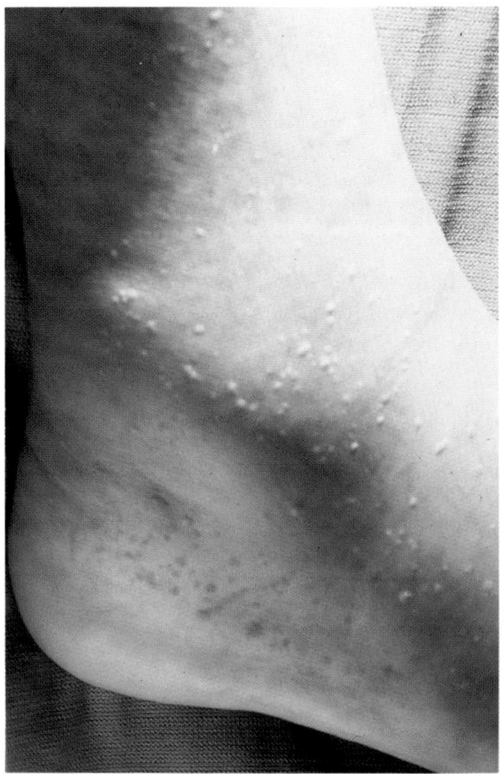

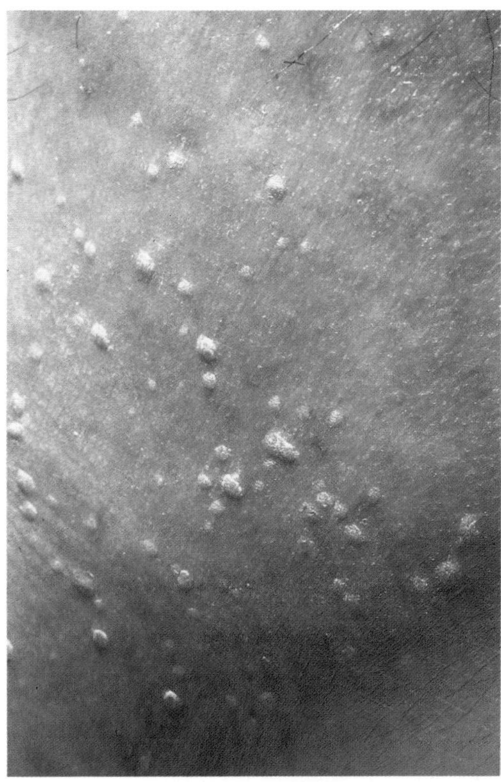
B

Figure 2.42. **(A)** Horny papules over ankle, punctate lesions at margin of sole. **(B)** Close-up showing resemblance to warts. (Courtesy of Division of Dermatology, University of Washington.)

of the neck has been reported. Onset is usually in late childhood, but has occurred at ages 6 months to 40 years.

Punctate hyperkeratoses of the palms, often described as "better felt than seen," occur. These lesions can be embedded and result in dropout of the dermal ridge pattern if palm prints are taken. The term *horny pearls* has been used to describe them. Diffuse palmar thickening has also been noted.

The nails are usually abnormal; fingernails are more involved than toenails. The findings are nonspecific and include whitening, thinning, longitudinal striations, friability, and brittleness. One of Hopf's two original patients had normal nails.

Minor. There may be an increased tendency for blistering with trauma.

Generalized mild ichthyosis has been described in a few patients.

There have been two reports of malignant degeneration in acrokeratosis verruciformis.

ASSOCIATED ABNORMALITIES

None. There is a brief clinical description of two brothers with mental retardation, choroideremia, nystagmus, hypohidrosis, and an "acrokeratosis verruciformis-like" eruption that was offered by van den Bosch as a new form of ectodermal dysplasia. None of these features has been reported in other patients with acrokeratosis verruciformis.

HISTOPATHOLOGY

Light. Hyperkeratosis without parakeratosis, mild to moderate acanthosis, and a conspicuous granular layer with no vacuolization are the classic features.

EM. No information.

BASIC DEFECT

Unknown.

TREATMENT

None.

MODE OF INHERITANCE

Autosomal dominant.

PRENATAL DIAGNOSIS

None.

DIFFERENTIAL DIAGNOSIS

The acral lesions of Darier-White disease (MIM:124200) are indistinguishable clinically and histologically from acrokeratosis verruciformis. This, along with the occurrence of acrokeratosis verruciformis with or without Darier-White in several pedigrees, has led many to claim that the two disorders reflect the variable expression of a single gene. Others maintain that there is a distinct entity, acrokeratosis verruciformis of Hopf, that does not carry with it a risk for more widespread cutaneous involvement typical of Darier-White.

The lesions of epidermodysplasia verruciformis (MIM:226400,305350) are clinically similar to the papules of acrokeratosis verruciformis. Pityriasis versicolor-like changes of epidermodysplasia verruciformis are not described in acrokeratosis verruciformis. The histology is different, and viral particles are not found in acrokeratosis verruciformis.

The flat-topped papules of lichen planus can mimic acrokeratosis verruciformis. They are usually more violaceous and have Wickham's striae, which are not seen in the papules of acrokeratosis verruciformis. Unlike lichen planus, there is no lymphocytic infiltrate in acrokeratosis verruciformis.

Support Group: N.O.R.D.
P.O. Box 8923
New Fairfield, CT
06812
1-800-999-6673

SELECTED BIBLIOGRAPHY

Herndon, J.H., and Wilson, J.D. (1966). Acrodermatosis verruciformis (Hopf) and Darier's disease. Genetic evidence for unitary origin. *Arch. Dermatol.* **93,** 305–310.

This is a kindred with 12 affected individuals. Features range from white nails with subungual keratoses only, to palmar pits only, to acrokeratosis verruciformis, to acrokeratosis verruciformis with palmar and plantar keratoderma, to two patients with lesions on their neck and body, one of which appeared more typical of Darier-White disease. This individual had dyskeratotic changes on biopsy from a lesion from the back, but acrokeratosis verruciformis-like changes in a lesion from the foot. This is quite typical of Darier-White disease in which the acral lesions show a different histology than those on the trunk. The authors of this paper are uncertain whether there are one, two, or three diseases segregating in this family.

Niedelman, M.L. (1947). Acrokeratosis verruciformis (Hopf): report of 14 cases in one family with four generations with a review of the literature. *Arch. Dermatol. Syphilol.* **56,** 48–63.

Niedelman, M.L., and McKusick, V.A. (1962). Acrokeratosis verruciformis (Hopf). A follow-up study. *Arch. Dermatol.* **86,** 779–782.

These are the initial report and a follow-up report 15 years later with addition of 10 affected individuals, for a total of 24 family members with acrokeratosis verruciformis. Onset occurred within the first year of life; males and females were equally affected. In this family, ichthyotic skin is described, but details are not given. Verrucae plana-like lesions, discrete and confluent, occurred on the backs of the hands and the feet and on the palms. Niedelman reviews the literature and cites three case reports of acrokeratosis verruciformis prior to Hopf.

Niordson, A.M., and Sylvest, B. (1965). Bullous dyskeratosis follicularis and acrokeratosis verruciformis. *Arch. Dermatol.* **92,** 166–168.

This is a report of a family in whom acrokeratosis verruciformis of Hopf is transmitted through three generations. One of the affected individuals had lesions of acrokeratosis verruciformis, Darier-White, and a question of Hailey-Hailey disease. This individual had two children, one of whom had Darier-White and one of whom had both Darier-White and acrokeratosis verruciformis. It is difficult to sort this family out, as, in the biopsy material from the one patient with all three diseases, parakeratosis was seen in all lesions, a finding not typical of acrokeratosis verruciformis.

Panja, R.K. (1977). Acrokeratosis verruciformis (Hopf). A clinical entity? *Br. J. Dermatol.* **96,** 643–652.

This author argues that Darier-White disease and acrokeratosis verruciformis are distinct entities. The major distinguishing features are the greasy scale of Darier-White, absence of malignant change, and difference in histopathology, even in the acral lesions. He describes one patient with acrokeratosis verucciformis who developed malignant changes on the palm at age 62.

Waisman, M. (1960). Verruciform manifestation of keratosis follicularis, including a reappraisal of hard nevi (Unna). *A.M.A. Arch. Dermatol.* **81,** 1–19.

This author argues that Darier-White and acrokeratosis verucciformis are the same disease, the latter being a mild expression of the former. He presents clinical and histologic data to support his hypothesis and notes that one of Hopf's original patients went on to develop typical lesions of Darier-White disease.

HEREDITARY PALMOPLANTAR KERATODERMAS

The hereditary palmoplantar keratodermas (HPPKs) or hyperkeratoses are a group of conditions characterized by abnormal thickening of the palms and soles. They are distinguished one from the next by severity (mutilating vs. nonmutilating), distribution (punctate vs. generalized, limitation to palms and soles or involving other areas [transgradiens]), associated abnormalities (periodontitis, esophageal carcinoma, ichthyosis), histopathology (epidermolytic vs. nonepidermolytic), and mode of inheritance. As with most groups of genetic disorders, clinical overlap is typical, distinguishing features often do not, private syndromes abound, and definitive classification may not always be possible.

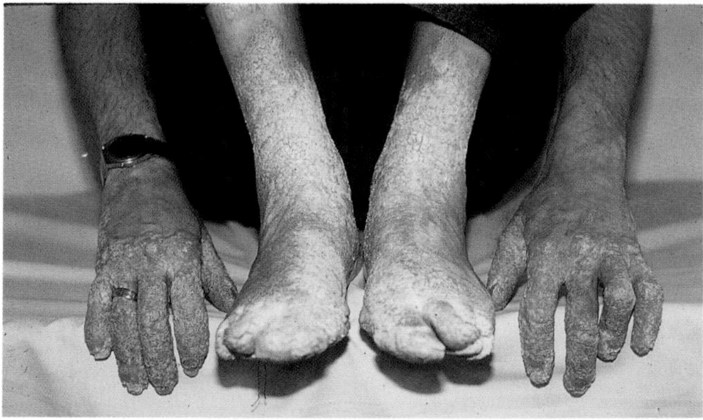

Figure 2.43. Severe palmar and plantar hyperkeratosis with progression onto legs and tops of hand. This patient does not fit into a recognized category. (From Sybert et al., 1988.)

For the purpose of pursuing our understanding of the underlying mechanisms of these disorders, the ability to distinguish among them clearly is of paramount importance. However, for clinical management, the ability to separate those with autosomal recessive inheritance from those with autosomal dominant transmission, and those at risk for associated complications from those who are not, may be all that is necessary. The patient who comes to me for treatment for severe HPPK, which has been present in her family for three generations with limited variability in severity, does not need to know if she has Greither, Unna-Thost, or Vörner syndrome, as inheritance, treatment, and limitation of disease to the skin are common to all three. However, if I wished to use her family for molecular studies, definitive diagnosis would be required before trying to add the lod score from her family to those of any other.

Treatment for these disorders in basically the same, and histopathology is often not distinctive.

Prenatal diagnosis, in general, is not available. As specific mutations are identified, this will change.

SELECTED BIBLIOGRAPHY

Itin, P.H. (1992). Classification of autosomal dominant palmoplantar keratoderma. Past, present, future. *Dermatology* **185,** 163–165.

Presents scheme for classification that recognizes overlap and confusion.

Lucker, G.P.H., Van de Kerkhof, P.C.M., and Steijlen, P.M. (1994). The hereditary palmoplantar keratoses: an updated review and classification. *Br. J. Dermatol.* **131,** 1–14.

Another good review. Table lists Sybert syndrome, referring to a family we reported. I would prefer to describe it as HPPK dominant extensive, as we remain ignorant of the basic defect to date.

HEREDITARY PALMOPLANTAR KERATODERMA WITH DEAFNESS (MIM:124500)

DERMATOLOGIC FEATURES

Major. This is probably not a single disorder but an association common to several HPPKs. Palmoplantar hyperkeratosis develops in mid-childhood and may or may not spare the arch of the foot. In one family, onset of skin changes was in the late teens. Constriction bands have been described in some affected individuals.

Minor. Nail dystrophy with koilonychia was reported in one family. Keratoderma of the elbows and knees was described in another.

ASSOCIATED ABNORMALITIES

Progressive sensorineural hearing loss with onset in infancy may lead to total deafness. Hearing loss can be present at birth.

In one family with HPPK and deafness, hereditary sensorimotor neuropathy was also described.

HISTOPATHOLOGY

Light. Hyperkeratosis with nonspecific changes.

EM. No information.

BASIC DEFECT

Unknown.

TREATMENT

Topical therapies for the hyperkeratosis include soaking in supersaturated saline solutions and

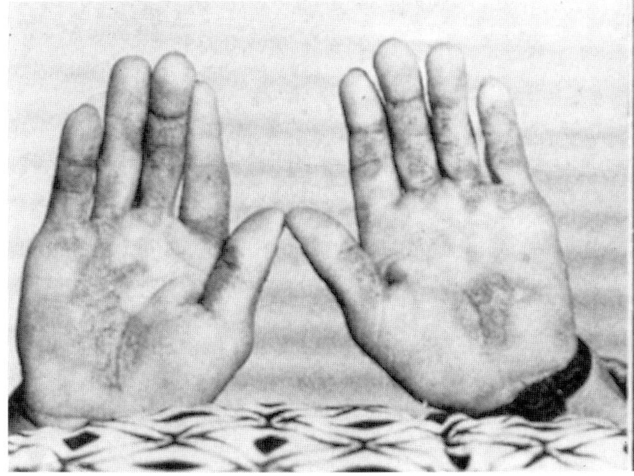
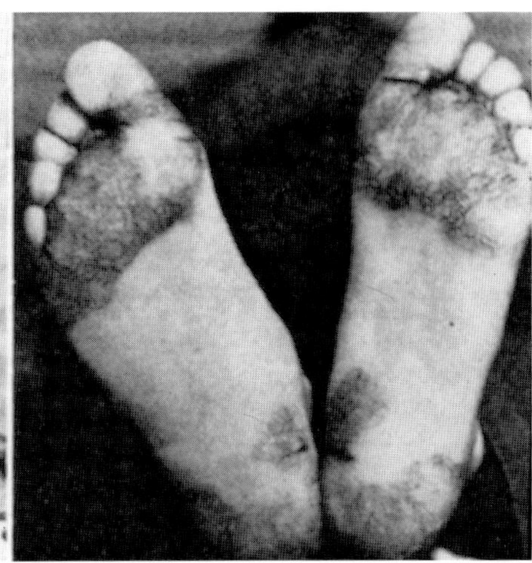

Figure 2.44. Palms and soles with thickening primarily over areas of pressure. (From Bititci, 1975.)

then gentle debridement and 50% propylene glycol in water under plastic occlusion overnight weekly. The use of mechanical debulkers such as dental drill with a sanding bit, paring down of the hyperkeratoses, and so forth can be successful for some patients.

Therapy with oral retinoids, including etretinate, isotretinoin, and acitretin, has been attempted with variable success.

MODE OF INHERITANCE

Autosomal dominant.

PRENATAL DIAGNOSIS

None.

DIFFERENTIAL DIAGNOSIS

Hypertrophic nail changes distinguish pachyonychia congenita (MIM:167200) from disorders that share in common with it HPPK and hearing loss. Congenital deafness has also been reported in the Papillon-Lefèvre syndrome (MIM: 245000); progressive deafness has been described in HPPK with leukonychia and knuckle pads (MIM:149200) and in Vohwinkel syndrome (which McKusick lists as synonymous with HPPK and deafness).

Support Group: F.I.R.S.T.
P.O. Box 20921
Raleigh, NC 27619
1-800-545-3286

SELECTED BIBLIOGRAPHY

Blanchet-Bardon, C., Nazzaro, V., and Puissant, A. (1987). Clinically specific type of focal palmoplantar keratoderma with sensorineural deafness: an entity. *Dermatologica* **175,** 148–151.

A sporadic case with clinical features similar to the report of Hatamochi et al.

Hatamochi, A., Nakagawa, S., Ueki, H., Miyoshi, K, and Iuchi, I. (1982). Diffuse palmoplantar keratoderma with deafness. *Arch. Dermatol.* **118,** 605–607.

A consanguineous pedigree in which many individuals have deafness without HPPK is described. No individual with both transmitted HPPK alone, but individuals with only deafness transmitted either deafness or deafness and HPPK. It is a hard pedigree to sort out.

Sharland, M., Bleach, N.R., Goberdhan, P.D., and Patton, M.A. (1992). Autosomal dominant palmoplantar hyperkeratosis and sensorineural deafness in three generations. *J. Med. Genet.* **29,** 50–52.

Male-to-male transmission is demonstrated.

HEREDITARY PALMOPLANTAR KERATODERMA EPIDERMOLYTIC HYPERKERATOSIS (MIM:144200)

(Vörner Syndrome; Epidermolytic Palmoplantar Keratoderma [EPPK]; Localized Epidermolytic Hyperkeratosis)

DERMATOLOGIC FEATURES

Major. Diffuse yellow palmoplantar hyperkeratosis on an erythematous base with erythematous margins involving the surface of the palms and soles. It is clinically identical to Unna-Thost disease (MIM:148400). Onset is at birth or soon after.

Minor. Occasional reports of blistering of the hands and feet, especially in early childhood. Unclear if secondary to dermatophyte infection, increased sweating, or the underlying inherited disease.

ASSOCIATED ABNORMALITIES

One family has been reported with early onset breast and ovarian cancer. There is an early onset breast cancer gene that has been mapped to the same region as epidermolytic palmoplantar keratoderma. The genetic relationship between the skin findings and malignancy is uncertain.

Hereditary sensorimotor neuropathy has been described in several families. In one, disuse atrophy and pes cavus secondary to restriction of feet by hyperkeratosis mimicked Charcot-Marie-Tooth. Nerve conduction velocities were normal.

HISTOPATHOLOGY

Light. The features of epidermolytic hyperkeratosis are present with perinuclear vacuolization of the keratinocytes in the granular and spinous layers and large irregular keratohyalin granules. These changes may be patchy in distribution.

EM. Abnormal clumps of tonofilaments and keratohyaline granules. Tonotubular keratin filaments were described in a single individual from a large pedigree.

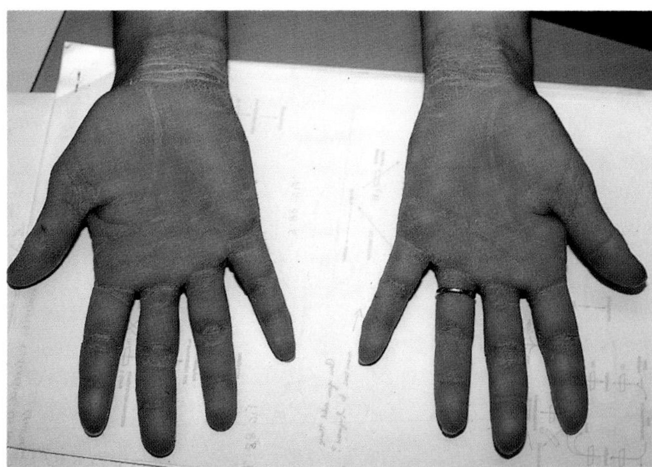

Figure 2.45. The underlying erythema extends up onto the volar surface of the wrists. The hyperkeratosis is less marked at sites of movement.

BASIC DEFECT

Linkage to acidic keratin cluster at 17q12–q21 in some families and allelic mutations in K_9 have been found.

TREATMENT

Topical therapies for hyperkeratosis include soaking in supersaturated saline solutions and then gentle debridement and 50% propylene glycol in water under plastic occlusion overnight weekly. The use of mechanical debulkers such as dental drill with a sanding bit, paring down of the hyperkeratoses, and so forth can be successful for some patients.

Therapy with oral retinoids, including etretinate, isotretinoin, and acitretin, has been attempted with variable success.

MODE OF INHERITANCE

Autosomal dominant.

PRENATAL DIAGNOSIS

None.

DIFFERENTIAL DIAGNOSIS

Epidermolytic hyperkeratosis is also a feature of many dermatologic conditions that are clinically distinct from epidermolytic palmoplantar keratoderma. It is not a specific diagnostic finding. Epidermolytic hyperkeratosis has been demonstrated in a presumed autosomal recessive form of palmoplantar keratoderma characterized by eczematous patches and periorbital involvement. Epidermolytic hyperkeratosis has been described in hereditary painful callosities (MIM:114140). These occur later in life and are limited in distribution to pressure points. Epidermolytic hyperkeratosis was also described in a single patient with Richner-Hanhart syndrome (MIM:276600). Clinically identical findings without epidermolytic hyperkeratosis are typical of the autosomal dominant HPPK reported in Sweden, Unna-Thost (MIM: 148400). It and Vörner syndrome may be identical.

Support Group: F.I.R.S.T.
P.O. Box 20921
Raleigh, NC 27619
1-800-545-3286

SELECTED BIBLIOGRAPHY

Blanchet-Bardon, C., Nazzaro, V., Chevrant-Breton, J., Espie, M., Kerbrat, P., and le Marec, B. (1989). Hereditary epidermolytic palmoplantar keratoderma associated with breast and ovarian cancer in a large kindred. *Br. J. Dermatol.* **117,** 363–370.

Early onset adenocarcinoma of the breast and/or ovaries developed in 8 of 10 females of age of risk with hereditary palmoplantar keratoderma; one woman had breast cancer without palmoplantar keratoderma. She developed breast cancer at age 67, much later than other family members. One male with palmoplantar keratoderma died of adenocarcinoma of the colon. A subsequent study of this family demonstrated a point mutation in K9 segregating with the skin findings (*Nat. Genet.* **6,** 106–109, 1994).

Bonifas, J.M., Matsumura, K., Chen, M.A., Berth-Jones, J., Hutchinson, P.E., Zloczower, M., Fritsch, P.O., and Epstein, E.H., Jr. (1994). Mutations of keratin 9 in two families with palmoplantar epidermolytic hyperkeratosis. *J. Invest. Dermatol.* **103,** 474–477.

Navsaria, H.A., Swensson, O., Ratnavel, R.C., Shamsher, M., McLean, W.H.I., Lane, E.B., Griffiths, W.A.D., Eady, R.A.J., and Leigh, I.M. (1995). Ultrastructural changes resulting from keratin-9 gene mutations in two families with epidermolytic palmoplantar keratoderma. *J. Invest. Dermatol.* **104,** 425–429.

Reis, A., Hennies, H.-C., Langbein, L., Digweed, M., Mischke, D., Drechsler, M., Schröck, E., Royer-Pokora, B., Franke, W.W., Sperling, K., and Küster, W. (1994). Keratin 9 gene mutations in epidermolytic palmoplantar keratoderma (EPPK). *Nat. Genet.* **6,** 174–179.

Two different point mutations in *KRT9*. In some families, no mutations in *KRT9* have been identified. Locus heterogeneity is a possibility.

Küster, W., and Becker, A. (1992). Indication for the identity of palmoplantar keratoderma type Unna-Thost with type Vörner. Thost's family revisited 110 years later. *Acta Dermatol Venereol. (Stockh.)* **72,** 120–127.

The authors were able to trace the origins of these patients back to Thost's original family. They note the patchy distribution of epidermolytic hyperkeratosis and propose to rename in favor of Vörner. I'd prefer HPPK with or without EH or EPPK.

Reis, A., Küster, W., Eckardt, R., and Sperling, K. (1992). Mapping of a gene for epidermolytic palmoplantar keratoderma to the region of the acidic keratin gene cluster at 17q12-q21. *Hum. Genet.* **90,** 113–116.

Suggest *KRT9* as candidate gene. It is mapped to the region of linkage and is strongly expressed only in palmar and plantar epidermal cells.

Requena, L., Schoendorff, C., and Sanchez Yus, E. (1991). Hereditary epidermolytic palmoplantar keratoderma (Vörner type)—report of a family and review of the literature. *Clin. Exp. Dermatol.* **16,** 383–388.

Large Spanish pedigree. Good table of disorders with epidermolytic hyperkeratosis and listing of previously published papers. Fifty-one references.

Tropet, Y., Zultak, M., Blanc, D., Laurent, R., and Vichard, Ph. (1989). Surgical treatment of epidermolytic hereditary palmo-plantar keratoderma. *J. Hand Surg. (Am.)* **14A,** 143–149.

Reviews surgical experience in the literature and discusses merits of different approaches to grafting.

HEREDITARY PALMOPLANTAR KERATODERMA HOWEL-EVANS (MIM:148500)

(Tylosis with Esophageal Carcinoma)

DERMATOLOGIC FEATURES

MAJOR. Onset of hyperkeratosis of the palms and soles usually occurs after age 10 years. The soles are more severely involved than the palms. Rough skin is a feature in young children and was recognized by family members to presage development of palm and sole involvement.

Leukoplakia is common.

MINOR. Widespread keratosis pilaris.

Epidermal inclusion cysts in the axillae were described in one family.

ASSOCIATED ABNORMALITIES

Esophageal carcinoma, usually involving the lower two-thirds of the esophagus, develops in adult life, at a mean age of 45 years. It has been estimated that 95% of patients will develop malignancy by age 65 years, but this is based on actuarial prediction and not on actual numbers.

HISTOPATHOLOGY

LIGHT. Changes of leukoplakia in the oral mucosa occur with keratosis, spongiosis, and acanthosis.

EM. Abnormal keratohyaline granules, cytoplasmic vacuoles, and intranuclear particles are found in oral mucosa.

BASIC DEFECT

Unknown.

TREATMENT

Prompt attention should be given to complaints of dysphagia. It is unclear if routine screening

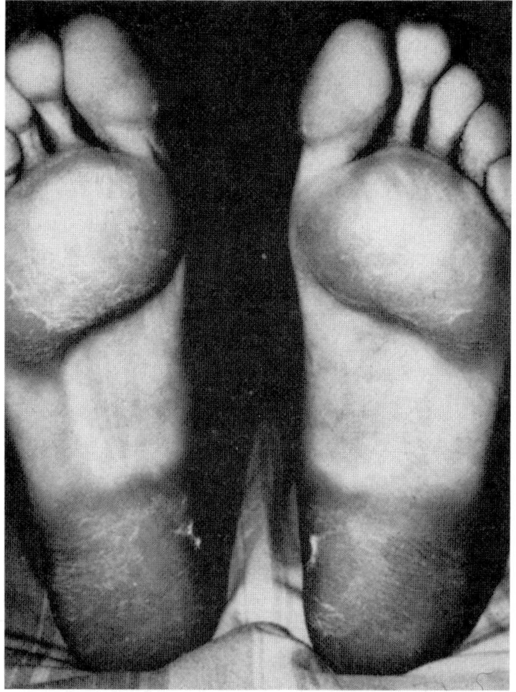

Figure 2.46. Grossly thickened plaques on the balls of feet and heels. (From O'Mahony et al., 1984.)

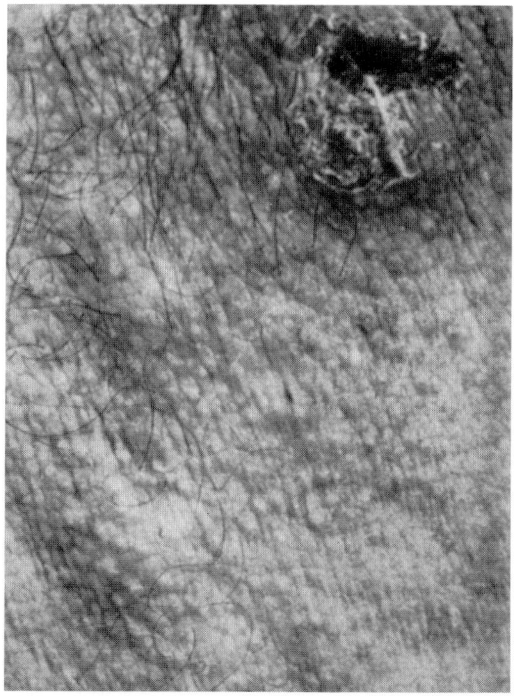

Figure 2.47. Follicular hyperkeratosis and cysts in axilla. (From O'Mahony et al., 1984.)

for esophageal changes is useful, as tumors can grow very quickly and the changes of dysplasia may be widespread and the prediction of which areas will become malignant is difficult.

Topical therapies for the hyperkeratosis include soaking in supersaturated saline solutions and then gentle debridement and 50% propylene glycol in water under plastic occlusion overnight weekly. The use of mechanical debulkers such as dental drill with a sanding bit, paring down of the hyperkeratoses, and so forth can be successful for some patients.

Therapy with oral retinoids, including etretinate, isotretinoin, and acitretin, has been attempted with variable success.

MODE OF INHERITANCE

Autosomal dominant.

PRENATAL DIAGNOSIS

None.

DIFFERENTIAL DIAGNOSIS

Onset of signs is later than in most of the other HPPKs and involvement appears more mild; otherwise it is impossible to differentiate Howel-Evans from other HPPKs unless there is a family history of carcinoma of the esophagus.

Support Group: F.I.R.S.T.
P.O. Box 20921
Raleigh, NC 27619
1-800-545-3286

SELECTED BIBLIOGRAPHY

Ashworth, M.T., Nash, J.R.G., Ellis, A., and Day, D.W. (1991). Abnormalities of differentiation and maturation in the oesophageal squamous epithelium of patients with tylosis: morphologic features. *Histopathology* **19,** 303–310.

Annual esophagoscopies in 29 members of a

pedigree with Howel-Evans syndrome revealed changes ranging from nonspecific alteration to dysplasia. Changes in severity occurred over months. Esophagitis was common. Dysplasia developed in three patients while on oral retinoids. Malignant change in one individual was multifocal.

Harper, P.S., Harper, R.M.J., and Howel-Evans, A.W. (1970). Carcinoma of the oesophagus with tylosis. *Q.J. Med.* **39,** 317–333.

Howel-Evans, W., McConnell, R.B., Clarke, C.A., and Sheppard, D.M. (1958). Carcinoma of the oesophagus with keratosis palmaris et plantaris (tylosis). A study of two families. *Q. J. Med.* **27,** 413–429.

Elegant study and follow-up 12 years later of two large pedigrees. Worth reading for the thinking that the physicians displayed in their approach to the family vis-à-vis their perceptions of the risks versus the benefits of genetic counseling.

HEREDITARY PALMOPLANTAR KERATODERMA OLMSTED (MIM:None)

(Mutilating Palmoplantar Keratoderma with Periorificial Keratotic Plaques)

DERMATOLOGIC FEATURES

MAJOR. This is an extremely rare disorder with onset of painful progressive thickening of the palms and soles in the first few years of life. These begin as discrete lesions and gradually achieve confluence. The borders are erythematous. Constriction of fingers leading to autoamputation is typical.

Perioral, perinasal, periumbilical, and pericrural involvement with hyperkeratotic fissured plaques is typical and progressive. Its onset is usually later than involvement of the palms and the feet. Areas of hyperkeratosis have developed in response to pressure or trauma.

MINOR. Oral leukokeratosis has been described in two of four reported cases.

The nails of one affected individual were tiny and yellow; in another they were thickened.

Hyperhidrosis of the palms can occur.

Alopecia was noted in two patients.

ASSOCIATED ABNORMALITIES

Joint hypermobility was described in one patient.

One case report of a boy with similar distribution of skin lesions without ainhum had corneal dyskeratosis.

Intellectual slowness is reported in some and normal intelligence in others, with some question of psychosocial neglect playing a role in the former.

HISTOPATHOLOGY

LIGHT. Massive hyperkeratosis with both ortho- and parakeratosis. The granular layer may be reduced.

EM. No information.

BASIC DEFECT

Unknown.

TREATMENT

There has been marginal success in reducing pain with skin grafting.

Topical therapies for hyperkeratosis include soaking in supersaturated saline solutions and then gentle debridement and 50% propylene glycol in water under plastic occlusion over-

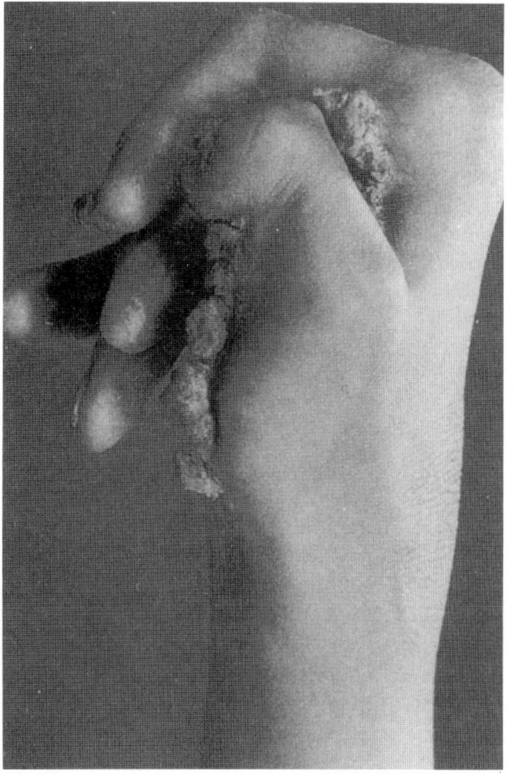

A

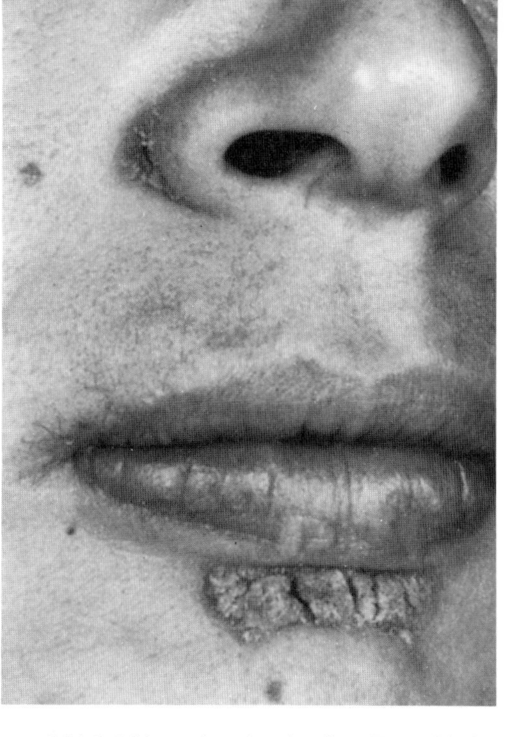

B

Figure 2.48. **(A)** Severe contractures of fingers with hyperkeratosis. **(B)** Hyperkeratotic plaques at nasolabial folds and under the lip. (From Lucker and Steijlen, 1994.)

night weekly. The use of mechanical debulkers such as dental drill with a sanding bit, paring down of the hyperkeratoses, and so forth can be successful for some patients.

Therapy with oral retinoids, including etretinate, isotretinoin, and acitretin has been attempted with variable success.

MODE OF INHERITANCE

Autosomal dominant versus X-linked. Only one mother–son affected pair was reported; all other cases were sporadic. The boy had more widespread and more severe disease than his mother.

PRENATAL DIAGNOSIS

None.

DIFFERENTIAL DIAGNOSIS

Acrodermatitis enteropathica (MIM:201100) can have a similar distribution of skin lesions and alopecia. Nonresponsiveness to zinc therapy will discriminate between the two. The skin lesions in acrodermatitis enteropathica are usually more eczematous and less hyperkeratotic.

Constriction bands also occur in the Vohwinkel syndrome (MIM:124500), which is distinguished by starfish-shaped hyperkeratoses on the dorsal hands and lack of periorificial involvement. Mal de Meleda (MIM:248300) is similar, although perioral involvement seems more severe in the Olmsted syndrome.

Support Group: F.I.R.S.T.
P.O. Box 20921
Raleigh, NC 27619
1-800-545-3286

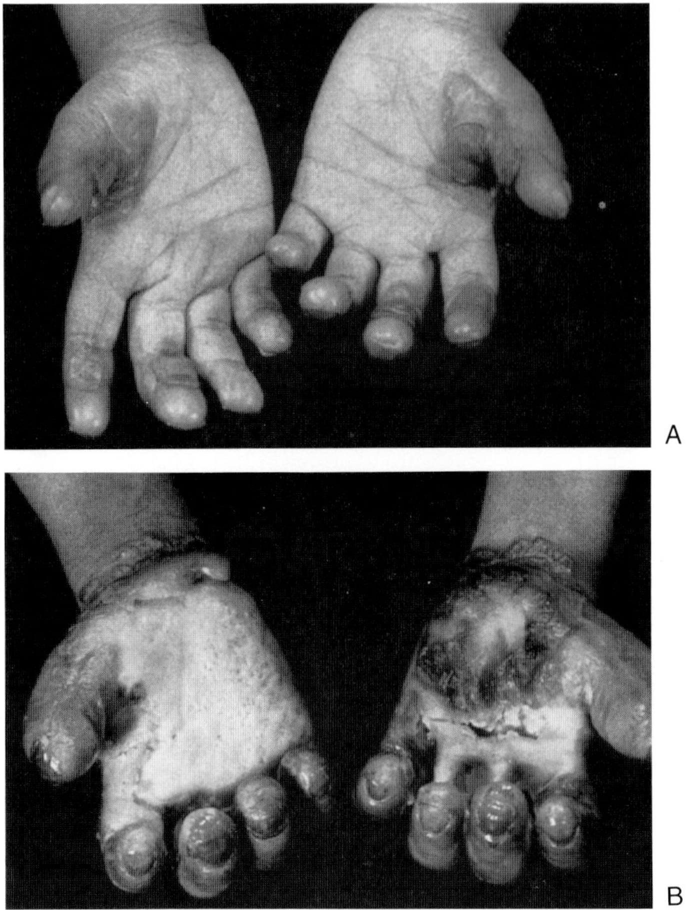

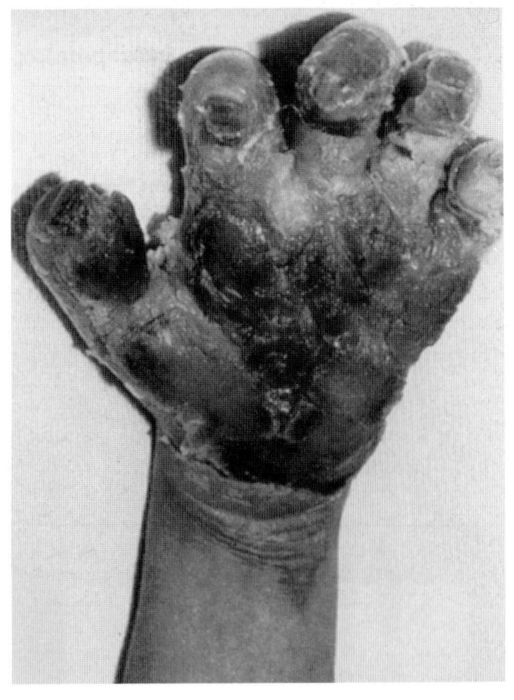

Figure 2.49. Hands at ages 25 months **(A),** 40 months **(B),** and 51 months **(C)** showing progressive involvement. (From Atherton et al., 1990.)

SELECTED BIBLIOGRAPHY

Atherton, D.J., Sutton, C., and Jones, B.M. (1990). Mutilating palmoplantar keratoderma with periorificial keratotic plaques (Olmsted's syndrome). *Br. J. Dermatol.* **122,** 245–252.
Case report of an affected mother and son. Mother much more mildly involved, with lesions limited to the palms and soles.

Lucker, G.P.H., and Steijlen, P.M. (1994). The Olmsted syndrome: mutilating palmoplantar and periorificial keratoderma. *J. Am. Acad. Dermatol.* **31,** 508–509.
A 33-year-old male had been treated for years as acrodermatitis enteropathica. Surgical excision led to pain relief, without improvement in contractures or return of function.

Olmsted, H.C. (1927). Keratodermia palmaris et plantaris congenitalis. Report of a case showing associated lesions of unusual location. *Am. J. Dis. Child.* **33,** 757–764.
A detailed case report.

HEREDITARY PALMOPLANTAR KERATODERMA PUNCTATE (MIM:148600)

(Keratoderma Punctata Punctatum; Keratodermia Palmoplantaris Papulosa; Buschke-Fisher-Brauer Disease; Keratodermia Palmoplantare Papuloverrucoides Progressiva)
Includes Porokeratosis Punctata Palmaris et Plantaris

DERMATOLOGIC FEATURES

MAJOR. This is probably a heterogeneous group of disorders. Onset of discrete islands of hyperkeratosis on the palms and soles is usually in late childhood through middle age. Lesions are discrete and diffuse, may be symmetrical, and may be few or many in number. Although changes are usually limited to the palms and soles, other body sites may be affected. Papules range in size from 2 to greater than 10 mm. Some affected individuals have many, many small lesions; others have a few large verrucoid lesions. Although some families tend to have multiple tiny excrescences and others have fewer larger lesions, there is also intrafamilial variation in these features. Usually the lesions are asymptomatic; occasionally pain is a complaint.

Removal of the thickened crust often leaves a depression with a surrounding keratotic rim. It is stated that manual labor causes worsening of the disorder.

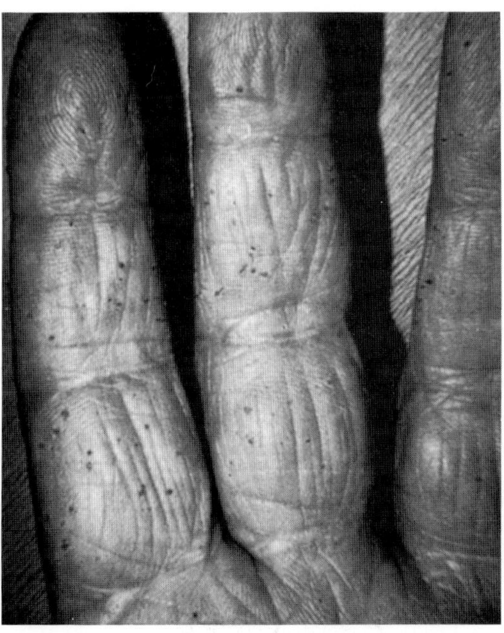

Figure 2.50. Spiny projections on fingers. (From Osman et al., 1992.)

MINOR. Nail changes including fissures, onychogryphosis, and loosening of the nail plate are sometimes described. Not all nails are affected in the same individual. In one reported family, the keratosis was associated with diffuse macular hypopigmentation, which was noted in infancy.

ASSOCIATED ABNORMALITIES

In one family, superficial corneal opacities were described.

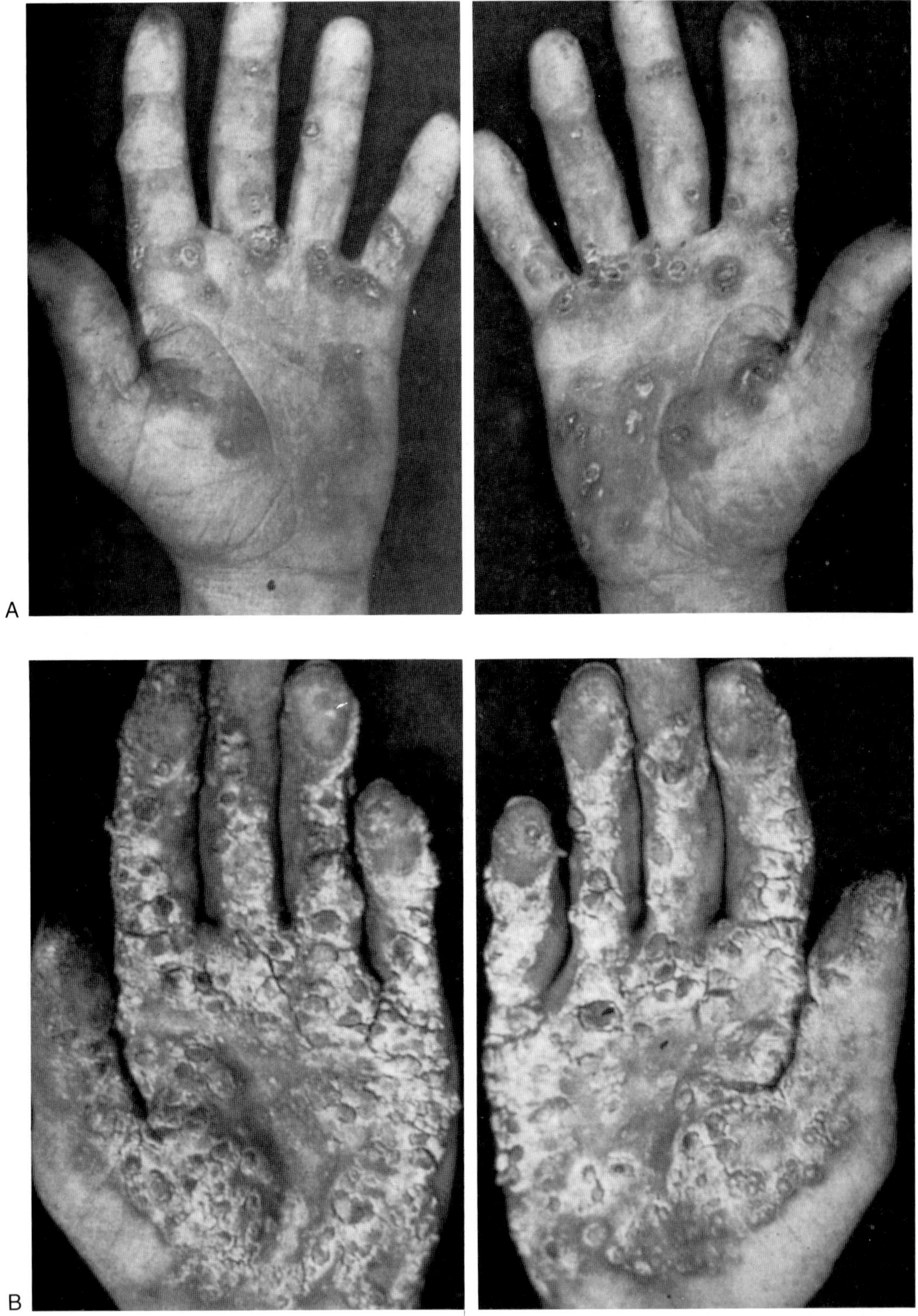

Figure 2.51. Fifty-one-year old **(A)** and 60-year-old **(B)** brothers showing progression of involvement with age. (From Žmegač and Sarajlič, 1964.)

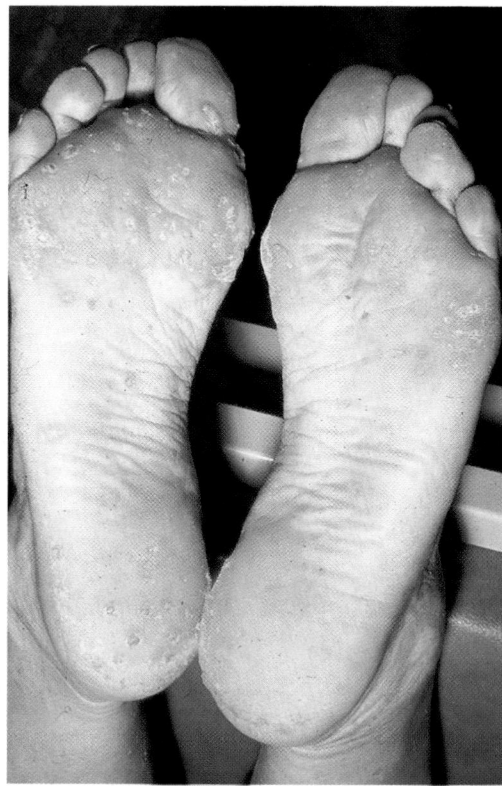

Figure 2.52. Soles with punctate lesions. (Courtesy of Division of Dermatology, University of Washington.)

HISTOPATHOLOGY

LIGHT. Orthohyperkeratosis with a thinned or thickened granular layer.
EM. A decreased absence of keratohyaline granules in some, irregular keratohyaline granules in others.

BASIC DEFECT

Unknown.

TREATMENT

Topical therapies for the hyperkeratosis include soaking in supersaturated saline solutions and then gentle debridement and 50% propylene glycol in water under plastic occlusion overnight weekly. The use of mechanical debulkers such as dental drill with a sanding bit, paring down of the hyperkeratoses, and so forth can be successful for some patients.

Therapy with oral retinoids, including etretinate, isotretinoin, and acitretin, has been attempted with variable success.

MODE OF INHERITANCE

Autosomal dominant.

PRENATAL DIAGNOSIS

None.

DIFFERENTIAL DIAGNOSIS

A supposedly acquired form of spiny palmar hyperkeratosis has been described and labeled *punctate porokeratotic keratoderma.* The lesions in this disorder are tiny and exhibit parakeratotic plugs. One pedigree has been described. The males in this family with autosomal dominant inheritance of spiny hyperkeratoses (MIM:175860) also had sebaceous hyperplasia of the face and neck.

In acrokeratoelastoidosis (MIM:101850) and hereditary papulotranslucent keratoderma (MIM:101840), the hyperkeratotic papules cannot be unroofed, and histology is different.

Support Group: F.I.R.S.T.
P.O. Box 20921
Raleigh, NC 27619
1-800-545-3286

SELECTED BIBLIOGRAPHY

Buchanan, R.N., Jr. (1963). Keratosis punctata palmaris et plantaris. *Arch. Dermatol.* **88,** 644–650.
"To the family . . . the defect is known as 'HalliBurton' marks. [In this] family of first rate ability and recognized integrity . . . the HalliBurton mark is one proudly borne." The discussion and following comments to this paper

that were presented at the American Dermatologic Association meeting provide a fascinating time warp (e.g., "intelligent and white race," "Crick's codon").

Osman, Y., Daly, T.J., and Don, P.C. (1992). Spiny keratoderma of the palms and soles. *J. Am. Acad. Dermatol.* **26,** 879–881.

Reviews the literature and nomenclature problems with punctate keratoderma and punctate porokeratosis.

Žmegač, Z.J., and Sarajlić, M. V. (1965). A rare form of an inheritable palmar and plantar keratosis. *Dermatologica* **130,** 40–52.

Three generation family. Marked variability in skin changes. Describes eye findings in detail.

HEREDITARY PALMOPLANTAR KERATODERMA STRIATA (MIM:148700)

(Brunauer-Fuhs-Siemens)

DERMATOLOGIC FEATURES

Major. Onset of linear brown-grayish hyperkeratotic streaks on the palms, more diffuse involvement on the feet, is in the first to second decades. Suspicious changes may be present earlier in childhood, but go unrecognized. These changes may be exacerbated by trauma.

Minor. In two families, curly hair was described; not all individuals demonstrated this finding.

ASSOCIATED ABNORMALITIES

None.

HISTOPATHOLOGY

Light. Acanthosis and papillomatosis with an increase in the granular layer.

EM. Tightly packed tonofibrils and abnormal large masses of keratohyaline granules.

BASIC DEFECT

Unknown.

TREATMENT

Topical therapies for hyperkeratosis include soaking in supersaturated saline solutions and then gentle debridement and 50% propylene glycol in water under plastic occlusion overnight weekly. The use of mechanical debulkers such as dental drill with a sanding bit, paring down of the hyperkeratoses, and so forth can be successful for some patients.

Therapy with oral retinoids, including etretinate, isotretinoin, and acitretin has been attempted with variable success.

MODE OF INHERITANCE

Autosomal dominant. Linkage to 18q12 has been suggested. The desmosomal cadherin gene resides in this region and may be a candidate gene.

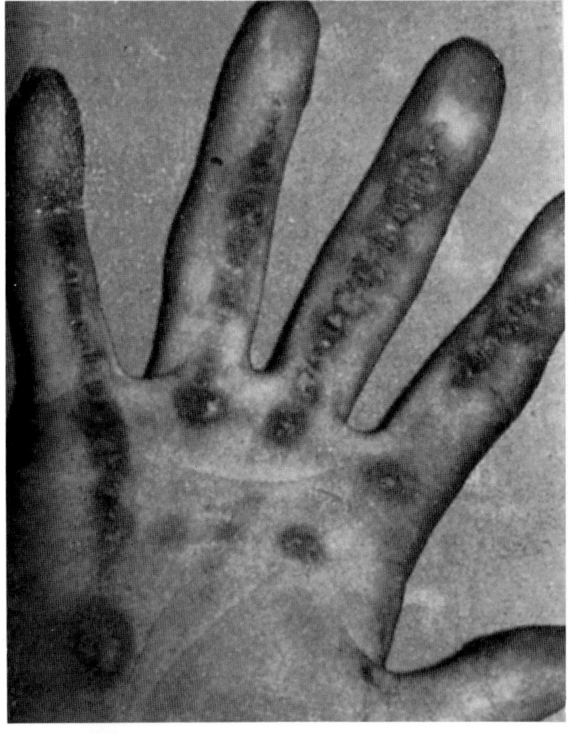
A

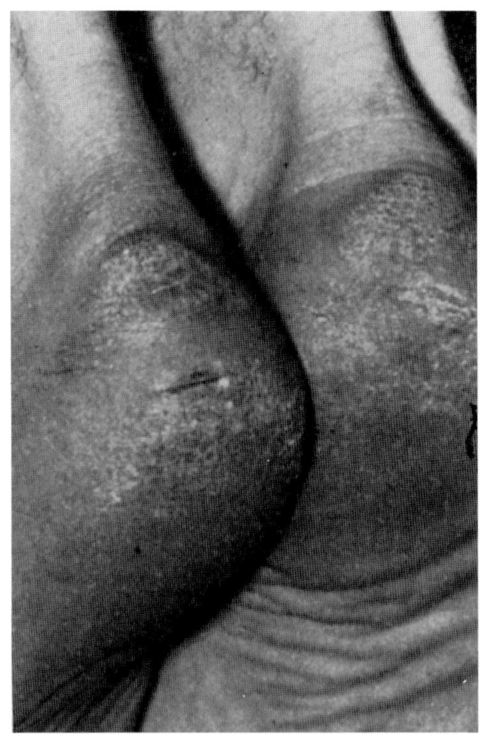
B

Figure 2.53. **(A)** Linear hyperkeratoses on fingers and palm. **(B)** Thickening of heels with sparing of arch. (From Baes et al., 1969.)

PRENATAL DIAGNOSIS

None.

DIFFERENTIAL DIAGNOSIS

There may be overlap with HPPK punctata (MIM:148600); round islands of hyperkeratosis were described in some family members of a pedigree with striata. Epidermal nevi are unlikely to be as symmetric or in such limited distribution, and they are usually present at birth or soon thereafter.

Support Group: F.I.R.S.T.
P.O. Box 20921
Raleigh, NC 27619
1-800-545-3286

SELECTED BIBLIOGRAPHY

Baes, H., de Beukelaar, L., and Wachters, D. (1969). Kératodermie palmo-plantaire variante. *Ann. Dermatol. Syphiligr. (Paris)* **96,** 45–50.

Beautifully detailed evaluation of a four-generation pedigree with remarkable clinical variation.

Fartasch, M., Vigneswaran, N., Diepgen, T.L., and Hornstein, O.P. (1990). Abnormalities of keratinocyte maturation and differentiation in keratosis palmoplantaris striata. Immunohistochemical and ultrastructural study before and during etretinate therapy. *Am. J. Dermatopathol.* **12,** 275–282.

This is a single case report with abnormal staining for involucrin and profillaggrin. Good electron micrographs.

HEREDITARY PALMOPLANTAR KERATODERMA UNNA-THOST (MIM:148400)

(Tylosis; Hereditary Palmoplantar Keratoderma)

Includes Greither Syndrome

DERMATOLOGIC FEATURES

MAJOR. The palms and soles are initially red. This is noted at or soon after birth. There is gradual thickening of the skin with diffuse hyperkeratosis. The margins often remain red and may expand up along the lateral aspects of the hands and feet, up onto the volar wrists and dorsal heels. The hyperkeratosis may be smooth and waxy or irregular and verrucous. Constriction and tapering of the soft tissue of the distal fingertips and contractures of the hand, all due to the hyperkeratosis, are common.

The hyperkeratoses may be limited to pressure-bearing areas or cover the entire surface. The degree and pattern of involvement can vary between the hands and feet of the same individual, within families, and among families.

In Greither syndrome (transgrediens form), involvement of knees, elbows, shins, and forearms is a variable finding, as is progression of involvement. Onset is typically a bit later than in classic Unna-Thost, but not invariably so. These features also show marked intra- and interfamily variability and may not indicate genetically distinct conditions.

MINOR. Dermatophyte infection is reported in about one-third of patients. It is often difficult to treat, but successful treatment often results in clinical improvement of the hyperkeratosis.

Acrocyanosis of the distal one-third of the extremities, which clears with elevation, has been described in one pedigree.

I have seen patients (in different families) with perianal and pericrural involvement, the presence of which was not described voluntarily but found only upon complete examination. Whether this feature is more common in Unna-Thost than is generally appreciated or whether it delineates a genetically distinct condition is unclear to me.

ASSOCIATED ABNORMALITIES

Clinodactyly of the fifth fingers has been reported in several pedigrees. It is not invariably present among affected family members. Photographs of the hands suggest that these patients may have a generalized brachydactyly.

HISTOPATHOLOGY

LIGHT. Hyperkeratosis with a decrease in the granular layer. The features of epidermolytic hyperkeratosis are present in some individuals in some families.

EM. Normal and abnormal keratohyaline granules are seen. The latter are round and less electron dense and are present in the lower stratum granulosum.

BASIC DEFECT

A mutation in keratin 1 has been demonstrated in one family.

TREATMENT

Dermatophyte infections are refractory to most treatments. Topical 1% econazole nitrate in 50% propylene glycol with water resulted in negative cultures and some improvement in scaling and fissuring.

Topical therapies for hyperkeratosis include soaking in supersaturated saline solutions and then gentle debridement and 50% propylene glycol in water under plastic occlusion overnight weekly. The use of mechanical debulkers such as dental drill with a sanding bit, paring down of the hyperkeratoses, and so forth can be successful for some patients.

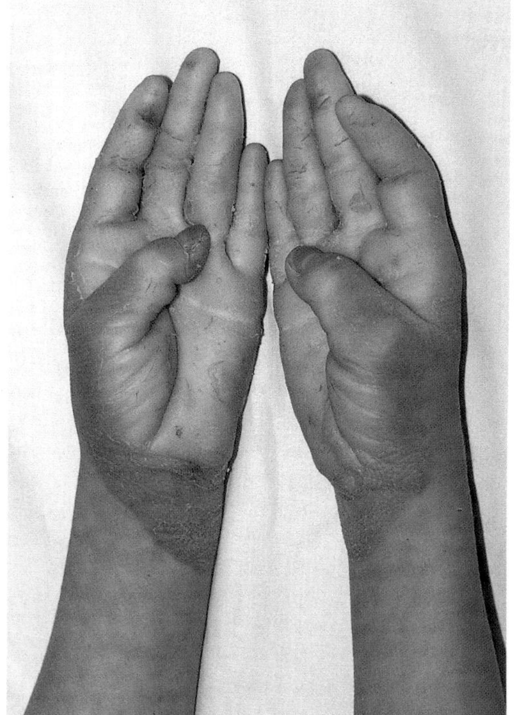

A

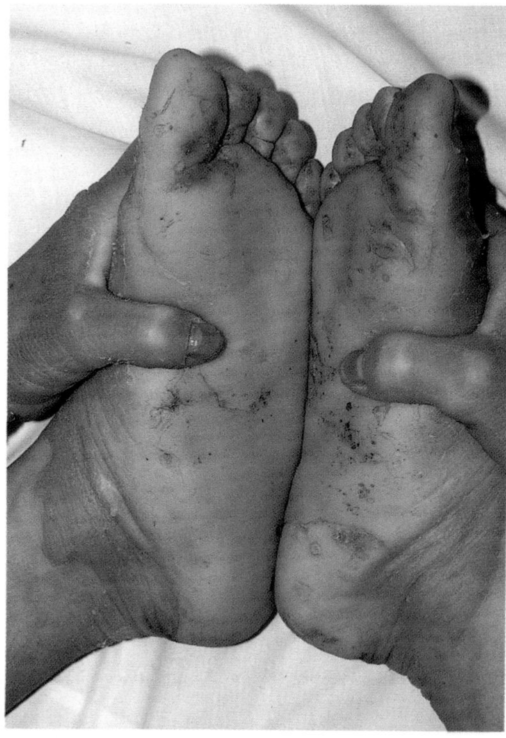

B

Figure 2.54. Palms **(A)** and soles **(B)** in 10 year old. The erythema extends beyond the hyperkeratosis.

Therapy with oral retinoids, including etretinate, isotretinoin, and acitretin, has been attempted with variable success.

Both split thickness and full thickness grafting have been successful in some cases.

MODE OF INHERITANCE

Autosomal dominant. The variability of clinical expression may reflect genetic heterogeneity or extrinsic factors affecting expression of the same mutant allele. The gene for K1 maps to 12q11–q13, where the type II keratins reside.

PRENATAL DIAGNOSIS

None.

DIFFERENTIAL DIAGNOSIS

Other forms of HPPK may be difficult to distinguish reliably.

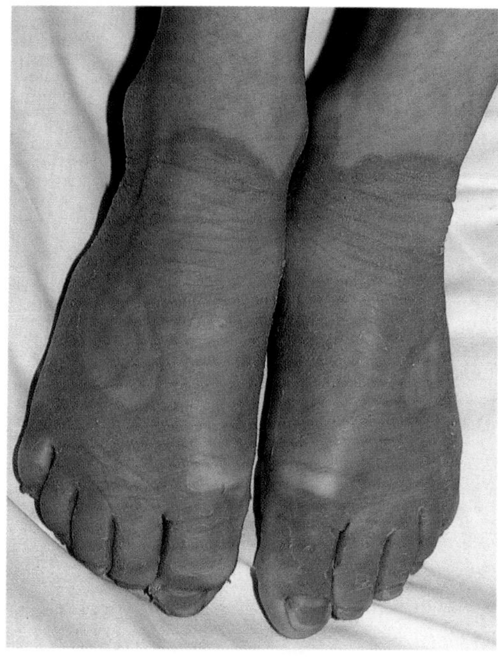

Figure 2.55. Erythema of the top of feet in same patient as in Fig. 2.54 with sharply demarcated borders.

In Vörner disease (epidermolytic palmoplantar keratoderma, MIM:144200), the clinical features are identical. Historically, the histologic features of epidermolytic hyperkeratosis separated Vörner disease from Unna-Thost. However, a recent reevaluation of one of the descendants of the Thost family demonstrated epidermolytic hyperkeratosis on biopsy. It is likely that the historical distinctions of Unna-Thost and Vörner will fall into disuse, and the disorders will be identified by their mutations.

HPPK and clinodactyly (MIM:148520) may not be a different syndrome.

Several pedigrees with suspected autosomal recessive inheritance of HPPK clinically identical to Unna-Thost have been described.

Concern for development of esophageal carcinoma in all sporadic cases, in which a family history of benign HPPK is not available, is probably appropriate. Onset of palmoplantar hyperkeratosis in the Howel-Evans variant of HPPK (MIM:148500) is usually later than that of Unna-Thost. Most individuals with Howel-Evans have oral mucosal changes. Careful dental evaluation may be helpful to differentiate this disorder.

In scleroatrophic and keratotic dermatosis of the limbs (Huriez syndrome, MIM:181590), there are atrophic and sclerodermatous-like changes of the dorsal hands and hypoplasia of the nails. Inheritance is autosomal dominant.

Pachyonychia congenita (MIM:167200) and Clouston syndrome (MIM:129500) can present with palmar and plantar hyperkeratosis. The associated features of each will differentiate them from Unna-Thost disease.

Support Group: F.I.R.S.T.
P.O. Box 20921
Raleigh, NC 27619
1-800-545-3286

SELECTED BIBLIOGRAPHY

Kansky, A., and Arzensek, J. (1979). Is palmoplantar keratoderma of Greither's type a separate nosologic entity? *Dermatologica* **158,** 244–248.

A family with some members having both HPPK and hyperkeratosis of the knees, others with one or the other finding.

Kimonis, V., DiGiovanna, J.J., Yang, J.-M., Doyle, S.Z., Bale, S.J., and Compton, J.G. (1994). A mutation in the V1 end domain of keratin 1 in non-epidermolytic palmar-plantar keratoderma. *J. Invest. Dermatol.* **103,** 764–769.

Despite lack of epidermolytic hyperkeratosis, mutation in K1 demonstrated. The variable region of the keratin 1 molecule was altered; this is different from the structural change in K1 seen in bullous congenital ichthyosiform erythroderma.

Klintworth, G.K., and Anderson, I.F. (1961). Tylosis palmaris et plantaris familiaris associated with clinodactyly. *S. Afr. Med. J.* **35,** 170–175.

Some family members with both clinodactyly and HPPK, others with only one or the other. Photographs of clinodactyly in this and other reports suggest brachydactyly with short palms. This impression of short hands is supported by description of simian creases in the Mexican families in other reports. Perhaps two unrelated disorders together?

Nielsen, G. (1985). Two different clinical and genetic forms of hereditary palmoplantar keratoderma in the northernmost county of Sweden. *Clin. Genet.* **28,** 361–366.

This is a follow-up study of one performed 20 years earlier. Among 18 offspring born to couples in which both parents were affected with HPPK, none had unusually severe disease or other findings suggestive of homozygosity.

HEREDITARY PALMOPLANTAR KERATODERMA VOHWINKEL (MIM:124500)

(Keratodermia Hereditaria Mutilans)

DERMATOLOGIC FEATURES

MAJOR. There are characteristic honeycombed diffuse hyperkeratoses of the palms and soles and starfish-like keratoses on the backs of the hands, fingers, and toes. These appear to be specific to Vohwinkel syndrome but are not always present. Linear hyperkeratoses of the knees and elbows can also occur. Constriction bands (pseudo-ainhum) that form deep furrows around digits and can result in autoamputation are common. The hyperkeratoses appear soon after birth; constriction bands develop at around age 5 years or thereafter. The constriction bands appear to be distinct from the hyperkeratosis. The latter can result in decreased range of motion of the hands.

MINOR. Progressive alopecia or sparse or fuzzy hair has been described in some patients, but is not universally found. Ridging of the nails with thickening of the nail plates and onychogryphosis are occasionally seen. Mild ichthyosis similar to ichthyosis vulgaris has been described in one pedigree.

ASSOCIATED ABNORMALITIES

Hearing loss has occasionally been described. Whether these individuals fit into one of the HPPK syndromes with hearing loss or whether deafness is a nonspecific finding for many HPPKs, including Vohwinkel, is unclear.

HISTOPATHOLOGY

LIGHT. Hyperkeratosis, acanthosis, and a thickened granular layer.

EM. Swollen mitochondria within the spinous and granular cells. Increased numbers of membrane coating granules with lipid-like vacuoles in the stratum corneum. Increased numbers of normal desmosomes in the spinous layer.

BASIC DEFECT

A mutation in loricrin, a protein involved in the structure of the cornified cell envelope, has been identified in one family.

TREATMENT

Topical therapies for the hyperkeratosis include soaking in supersaturated saline solutions and then gentle debridement and 50% propylene glycol in water under plastic occlusion overnight weekly. The use of mechanical debulkers such as dental drill with a sanding bit, paring down of the hyperkeratoses, and so forth can be successful for some patients.

Therapy with oral retinoids, including etretinate, isotretinoin, and acitretin, has been attempted with variable success.

MODE OF INHERITANCE

Autosomal dominant with documented male-to-male transmission. Linkage to 1q21 has been demonstrated. This is the location of a group of genes known as the epidermal differentiation complex and includes, among others, the genes for loricrin, involucrin, trichohyalin and profilaggrin.

PRENATAL DIAGNOSIS

None.

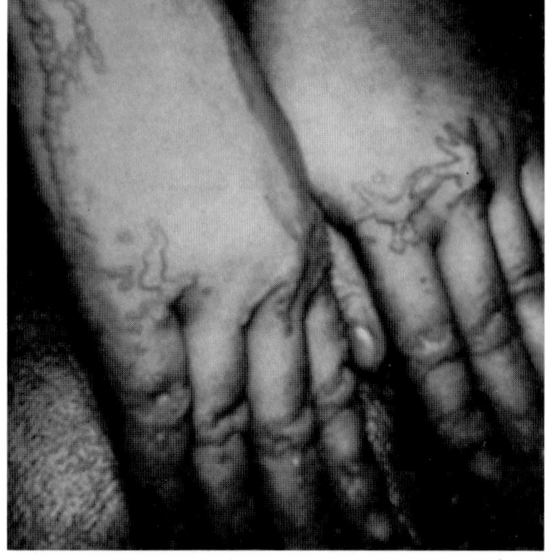

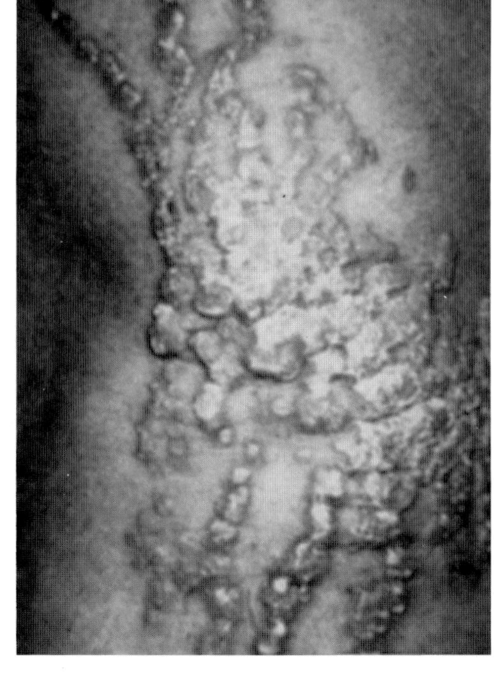

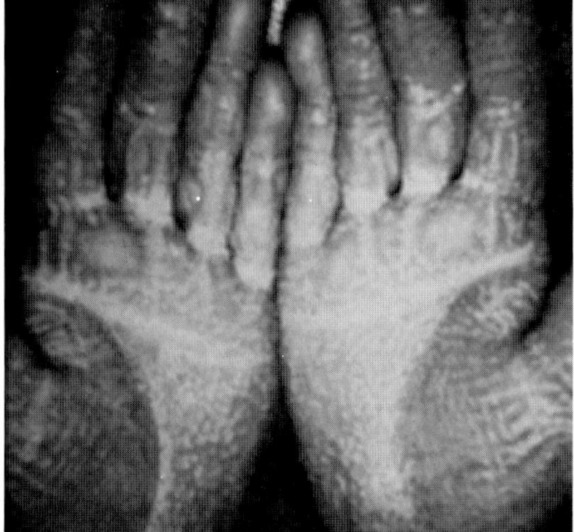

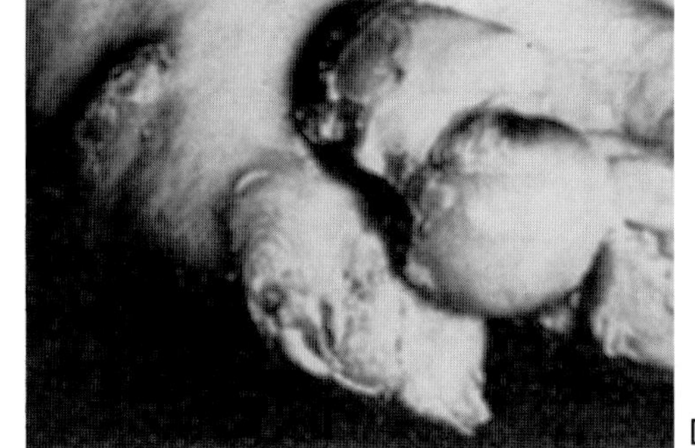

Figure 2.56. **(A)** Starfish hyperkeratoses of hands. **(B)** Hyperkeratoses over knees. **(C)** Honeycombed keratoses of the palms. **(D)** Ainhum-like bands around the toes. (From Gibbs and Frank, 1966.)

DIFFERENTIAL DIAGNOSIS

All other forms of HPPK, especially the Olmsted syndrome, which is distinguished by periorificial involvement, are in the differential diagnosis of the Vohwinkel syndrome. One family has been described with possible autosomal recessive inheritance of generalized ichthyosis and palmoplantar changes similar to that of Vohwinkel, but with more extensive linear keratotic papules arranged in cords vertically across flexures. Pseudo-ainhum was present in some affected family members.

Support Group: F.I.R.S.T.
P.O. Box 20921
Raleigh, NC 27619
1-800-545-3286

SELECTED BIBLIOGRAPHY

Gibbs, R.C., and Frank, S.B. (1966). Keratoderma hereditaria mutilans (Vohwinkel). *Arch. Dermatol.* **94,** 619–625.

Case report. Beautiful photos. Clear discussion of the differential diagnosis of constriction bands.

Pujol, R.M., Moreno, A., Alomar, A., and de Moragas, J.M. (1989). Congenital ichthyosiform dermatosis with linear keratotic flexural papules and sclerosing palmoplantar keratoderma. *Arch. Dermatol.* **125,** 103–106.

Affected siblings born to consanguineous parents.

Vohwinkel, K.H. (1929). Keratoma hereditarium mutilans. *Arch. f. Dermat. u. Syph.* **158,** 354–364.

Photographs of his original patient are striking, showing involvement of palms, volar wrists, and discrete polygonal papules over the dorsi of the hands. Constriction bands are remarkable. There is a cribriform appearance to the soles and discrete lesions over the knees. Vohwinkel's article was received April 2, 1929, and published in August.

Wigley, J.E.M. (1928). A case of hyperkeratosis palmaris et plantaris associated with ainhum-like constriction of the fingers. *Proc. R. Soc. Med.* **21,** 1715–1716.

Clinically identical case to Vohwinkel's, presented in May 1928 at the Royal Society of Medicine. Perhaps Wigley-Vohwinkel for the eponymists?

MAL DE MELEDA (MIM:248300)

(Mal de Mljet)

DERMATOLOGIC FEATURES

Major. Diffuse palmar and plantar thickening appears soon after birth. The hyperkeratosis is usually yellow and smooth, but may become thickened, irregular, and gray-brown. The finger webs may be involved. Restriction of extension of the fingers and hands is common.

Hyperhidrosis with odor is typical, as is

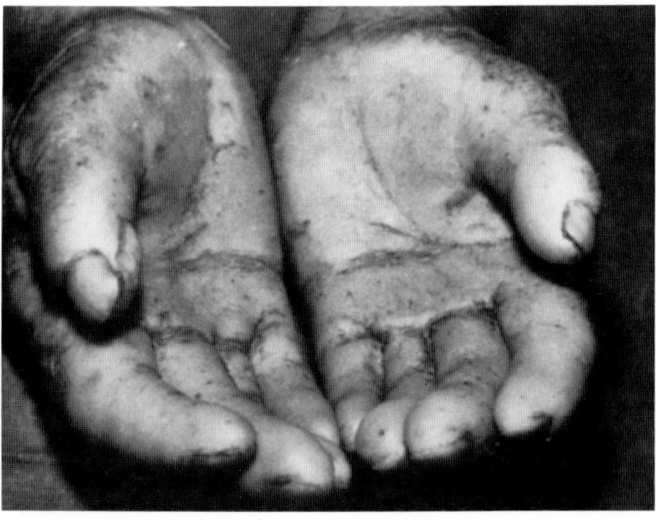

Figure 2.57. Palms showing diffuse hyperkeratosis. (From Franceschetti et al., 1972.)

onychogryphosis and loss of soft tissue of the fingerpads. Extension up onto the volar wrists and dorsal heels is seen in about half of patients, and patches of hyperkeratosis on the knees, elbows, and the axillae are not uncommon. Perioral erythema giving a cheleitis-like picture similar to Olmsted syndrome occurs in about half of patients.

Minor. Ainhum (constricting tissue bands) are reported in a minority of patients.

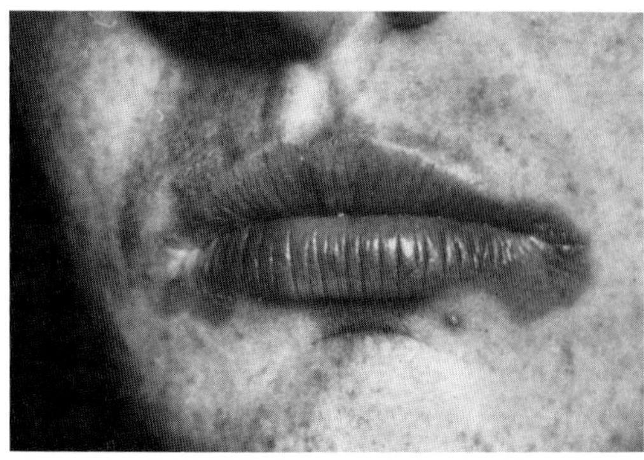

Figure 2.58. Perioral involvement. (From Franceschetti et al., 1972.)

ASSOCIATED ABNORMALITIES

The distal phalanges are described as short, but it is not clear if this is secondary to longstanding constriction of the fingertips by hyperkeratosis or if it is a primary bony alteration.

HISTOPATHOLOGY

Light. Orthohyperkeratosis with a normal granular layer.

EM. No information.

BASIC DEFECT

Unknown.

TREATMENT

See Unna-Thost disease.

MODE OF INHERITANCE

Autosomal recessive. The disease was reported initially in inhabitants of Mljet, but subsequently has been described in other European ethnic groups.

PRENATAL DIAGNOSIS

None.

DIFFERENTIAL DIAGNOSIS

All of the palmoplantar keratodermas need to be considered in the diagnosis of Mal de Meleda syndrome. If the ethnic origin of the patient is Dalmatian, Mal de Meleda is most likely. Recognition of onset in infancy may be more typical of Mal de Meleda. In an isolated case, it may not be possible to differentiate autosomal recessive from autosomal dominant disease. Four families from the Greek island of Naxos had skin changes consistent with Mal de Meleda. In addition, they had very curly hair (also described in HPPK striata, MIM:148700), cardiac conduction abnormalities, cardiomegaly, and right ventricular abnormalities. These patients may represent a distinct autosomal recessive disorder.

Support Group: F.I.R.S.T.
P.O. Box 20921
Raleigh, NC 27619
1-800-545-3286

SELECTED BIBLIOGRAPHY

Franceschetti, A.Th., Reinhart, V., and Schnyder, U.W. (1972). La Maladie de Meleda. *J. Genet. Hum.* **20,** 267–296.

Spectacular pedigree with individuals in five affected generations, most the result of consanguineous matings within the same family. The pedigree supports autosomal recessive inheritance, but could be autosomal dominant with reduced penetrance. Table of features of different HPPK syndromes underscores the overlap among them.

Niles, H.D., and Klumpp, M.M. (1939). Mal de Meleda. Review of the literature and report of four cases. *Arch. Dermatol. Syphilol.* **39,** 409–421.

Interesting approach to genetics. Four case reports, one from a consanguineous mating, who also had an affected brother. Another patient had an affected father, paternal uncle, paternal grandfather, and granduncle, yet the authors incorrectly state "data on family background not sufficient . . . [to] determine if the trait was dominant or recessive." Based on the pedigree, this individual had an autosomal dominant disorder, raising questions about the appropriateness of diagnosis of Mal de Meleda.

Protonotarios, N., Tsatsopoulou, A., Patsourakos, P., Alexopoulos, D., Gezerlis, P., Simitsis, S., and Scampardonis, G. (1986). Cardiac abnormalities in familial palmoplantar keratosis. *Br. Heart J.* **56,** 321–326.

Two of nine individuals from four families had skin involvement without cardiac involvement. All nine individuals had curly rough hair. Skin changes were identical to Mal de Meleda but limited to palms and soles. Forty relatives without skin changes were examined also, and had no cardiac defects.

PAPILLON-LEFÈVRE (MIM:245000)

(Keratosis Palmoplantaris with Periodontopathia)

Includes Focal Palmoplantar and Gingival Hyperkeratosis

DERMATOLOGIC FEATURES

MAJOR. Beginning in infancy, the palms and soles become reddened and then progressively hyperkeratotic. The margin of erythema is often "transgredient," i.e., over onto the dorsal finger webs, up onto the volar wrists, and onto the achilles tendon.

Other skin surfaces, including the backs of the hands and feet, knees, elbows, forearms, and shins, may also be affected. This generally occurs later in childhood.

MINOR. Onychodystrophy with pitting, streaking, and grooving is nondiagnostic and occasional.

Relapsing pyodermas occur in about one-fifth of patients.

ASSOCIATED ABNORMALITIES

Juvenile periodontitis with inflammation of the gums and loss of teeth occurs in all patients. Both primary and secondary dentition are involved. Onset of gingivitis is usually about age 2–3 years. After all the primary teeth are shed, gingivitis resolves until secondary teeth erupt and the process begins anew, again to resolve after all permanent teeth are shed. There is swelling and pyorrhea of the alveolar gum ridges, and alveolar bone resorption results in loss of teeth.

Calcifications of the falx cerebri and choroid plexus are described in a minority of patients.

Acroosteolysis was reported in one woman.

There are rare occurrences of infection of internal organs (liver, lung, kidney, and abdominal cavity). There is a questionable defect in polymorphonuclear chemotaxis and impaired B- and T-cell reactivities.

In a few pedigrees, arachnodactyly has been described. Although the term *Marfan syndrome* has been used to describe some of these patients, they have no other findings of Marfan syndrome. The eponym Haim-Munk has been appended to these families.

Although mental retardation is alluded to in review papers, the case reports do not suggest an increased incidence.

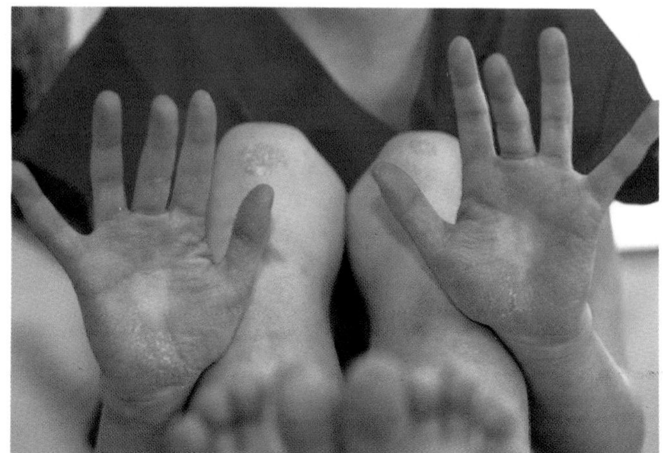

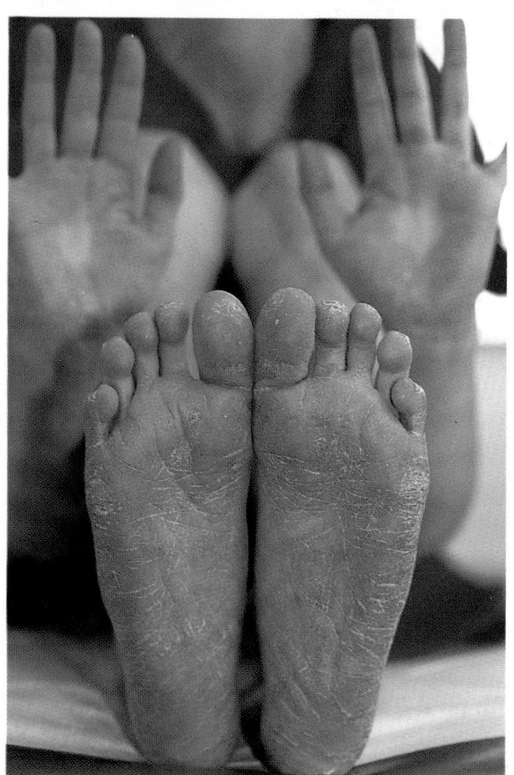

Figure 2.59. Hands (**A**) and feet (**B**) with marked erythema and mild hyperkeratosis in an 8-year-old.

HISTOPATHOLOGY

LIGHT. Hyperkeratosis with mild perivascular infiltrate in the dermis. There is occasional parakeratosis. The gums show severe inflammation.

EM. Lipid-like vacuoles in the granular cells and reduced tonofilaments with rectangular or globular keratohyalin. Similar vacuoles are seen in the stratum corneum cells. This is based on a report of one family.

BASIC DEFECT

Unknown. As periodontosis occurs in leukocyte adhesion deficiency and, given inconstant laboratory indicators of immune deficiency and in-

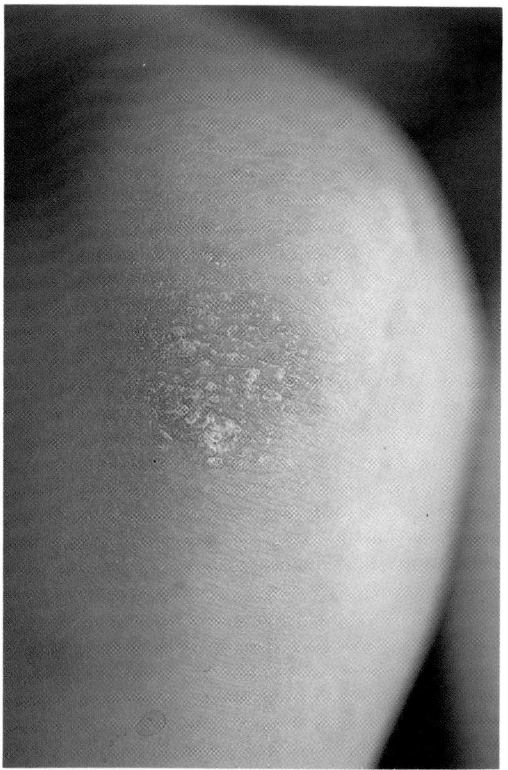

Figure 2.60. Red, scaling patch on knee.

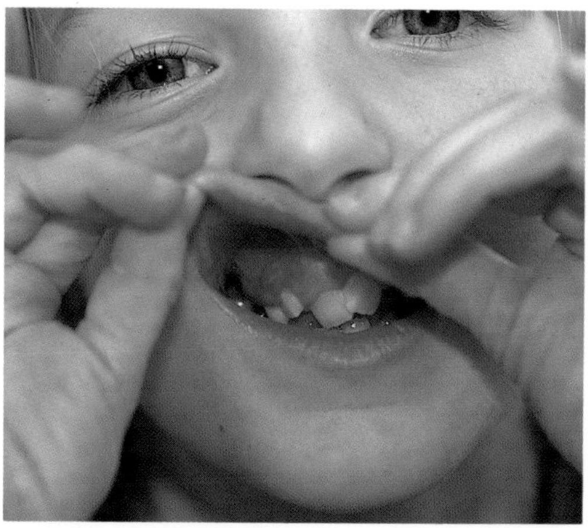

Figure 2.61. Boggy gums with aphthous ulcer and erythema.

creased frequency of skin infections in Papillon-Lefèvre, it is tempting to posit an underlying defect in immunocompetency.

An increase in collagen production by gingival fibroblasts has been reported once.

TREATMENT

Use of etretinate or acitretin has resulted in improvement in skin findings and in preservation of teeth. Although the skin lesions recurred after cessation of treatment, gum disease did not. In another study, etretinate therapy resulted in cessation of bouts of pyoderma in three affected individuals. In a third case report, a patient without a history of prior infections developed two bacterial liver abscesses while on etretinate.

One report of successful autologous split thickness grafting with an 18-month follow-up. Photographs are not impressive.

Aggressive dental management with tooth extraction is currently conventional therapy aimed at preservation of alveolar bone.

MODE OF INHERITANCE

Autosomal recessive.

PRENATAL DIAGNOSIS

None.

DIFFERENTIAL DIAGNOSIS

Biopsy will differentiate the gum changes of hyperkeratosis from inflammatory gingivitis. Psoriasis can give a similar cutaneous appearance, but age of onset and presence of gum disease, as well as histopathology, will differentiate.

Other forms of palmoplantar hyperkeratosis may show identical skin changes, but they do not share gum disease.

Early onset periodontitis can be a feature of immune defects as can eczematous and seborrhea-like skin changes. These cutaneous findings are usually more diffuse than the skin changes of Papillon-Lefèvre.

An autosomal dominant disorder, focal palmoplantar and gingival keratosis (MIM: 148730) is marked by development of hyperkeratosis on the palms and soles, primarily at pressure points, and hyperkeratosis of the margins of the gums and the palate without tooth loss. The buccal mucosa is usually spared. Onset of skin changes and gum changes is in midchildhood to puberty. Subungual hyperkeratosis is typical.

Support Group: F.I.R.S.T.
P.O. Box 20921
Raleigh, NC 27619
1-800-545-3286

REFERENCES

Baer, P.N. (1989). Preventing loss of teeth in patients with Papillon-Lefèvre syndrome. *J. Pedod.* **13,** 182–183.

Proposes that removal of primary teeth, followed by a regimen of tetracycline, can result in preservation of secondary teeth. Cites three instances.

Gorlin, R.J., Sedano, H., and Anderson, V.E. (1964). The syndrome of palmar–plantar hyperkeratosis and premature periodontal destruction of the teeth. A clinical and genetic analysis of the Papillon-Lefèvre syndrome. *J. Pediatr.* **65,** 895–908.

A single case report with an excellent literature review. Ninety-two references.

Haneke, E. (1979). The Papillon-Lefèvre syndrome: keratosis palmoplantaris with periodontopathy. *Hum. Genet.* **51,** 1–35.

Review article of 150 cases in the literature. One hundred fifty-nine references.

Hart, T.C., and Shapira, L. (1994). Papillon-Lefèvre syndrome. *Periodontol. 2000* **6,** 88–100.

Somewhat redundant, but quite complete review. Detailed description of excruciatingly meticulous oral hygiene protocols with relatively limited success in retaining teeth. Ninety-eight references.

Nazzaro, V., Blanchet-Bardon, C., Mimoz, C., Revuz, J., and Puissant, A. (1981). Papillon-Lefèvre syndrome. Ultrastructural study and successful treatment with acitretin. *Arch. Dermatol.* **124,** 533–539.

One family with three affected children. Better response to acitretin than etretinate in one.

Papillon, Lefèvre, P. (1924). Deux cas de kératodermie palmaire et plantaire symétrique familiale (Maladie de Meleda) chez le frère et la soeur. Coexistence dans deux cas d'alterations dentaires graves. *Bull. Soc. Fr. Dermatol. Syphiligr.* **31,** 82–87.

Described changes as indistinguishable from mal de Meleda in a brother and a sister, noting the dental abnormalities. Many citations give Monsieur Papillon the initials M.M., which stood for "Messieurs" in the original publications. Despite my efforts I have been unable to find his first name and would be grateful for information.

Young, W.G., Newcomb, G.M., and Daley, T.J. (1982). Focal palmoplantar and gingival hyperkeratosis syndrome. Report of a family with cytologic, ultrastructural and histochemical findings. *Oral Surg. Oral Med. Oral Pathol.* **53,** 473–482.

Clear discussion and extensive histopathology for this autosomal dominant disorder. Thirty references.

SCLEROATROPHIC AND KERATOTIC DERMATOSIS OF THE LIMBS (MIM:181590)

(Sclerotylosis; Huriez Syndrome)

DERMATOLOGIC FEATURES

Major. At birth, atrophic red skin is present on the hands and feet, more pronounced on the hands. The skin is thin and parchment-like over the backs of the hands, feet, and fingers. At birth, the palms and soles are hyperkeratotic, again the hands more so than the feet. The fingertips may appear mummified. Raynaud phenomenon is absent, and there are no

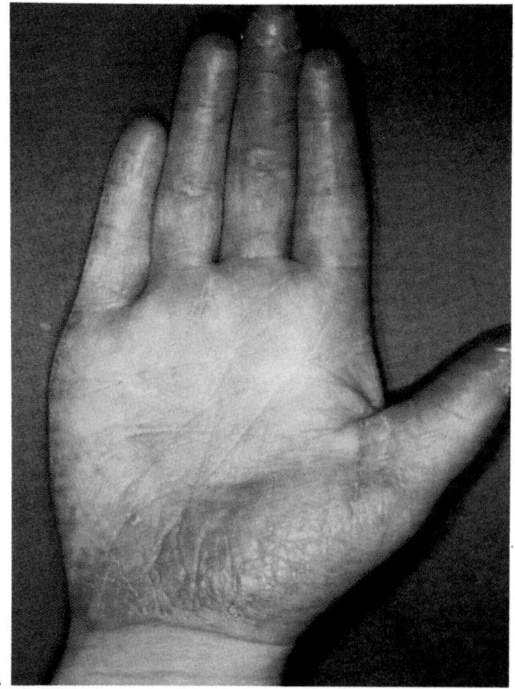

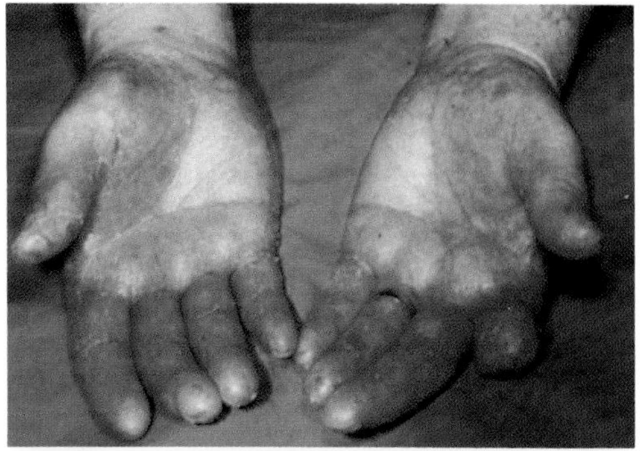

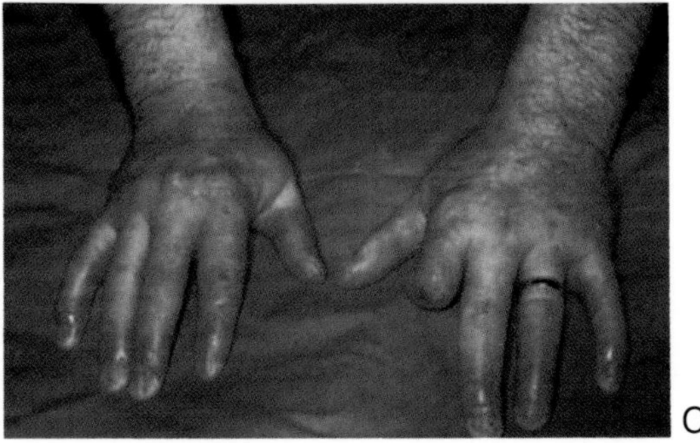

Figure 2.62. **(A)** Absence of dermatoglyphics, short distal phalanges; hyperkeratosis stops at the edge of the palm. **(B)** Severe involvement; squamous cell carcinoma of the index finger resulted in amputation. **(C)** Spindling of fingers and nail atrophy. (From Delaporte et al., 1995.)

capillary changes of scleroderma. These changes progress in early childhood and then stabilize.

The nails are often hypoplastic, spoon shaped, or fissured.

MINOR. Eleven of 86 affected individuals in eight families developed squamous cell carcinoma in involved skin as adults.

ASSOCIATED ABNORMALITIES

None.

HISTOPATHOLOGY

LIGHT. The hyperkeratotic areas show orthokeratosis with occasional parakeratosis. Features of thinning of the epidermis and dermis are inconsistently seen. The granular layer is increased. There is a minimal perivascular lymphocytic infiltrate in some. There are similar changes in the atrophic areas.

EM. Hyperkeratotic lesions show dense bundles of tonofilaments and abundant keratohyaline clumps. Atrophic areas share these features. In addition, the dermis of the atrophic areas is marked by irregularly bordered, nonhomogeneous elastic fibers.

BASIC DEFECT

Unknown. Provisional linkage to the MNS blood group.

TREATMENT

Monitoring for malignant changes. One successful outcome with long-term oral retinoid treatment.

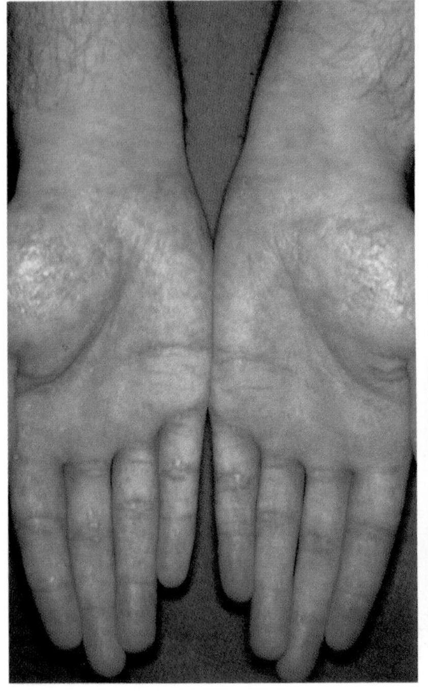

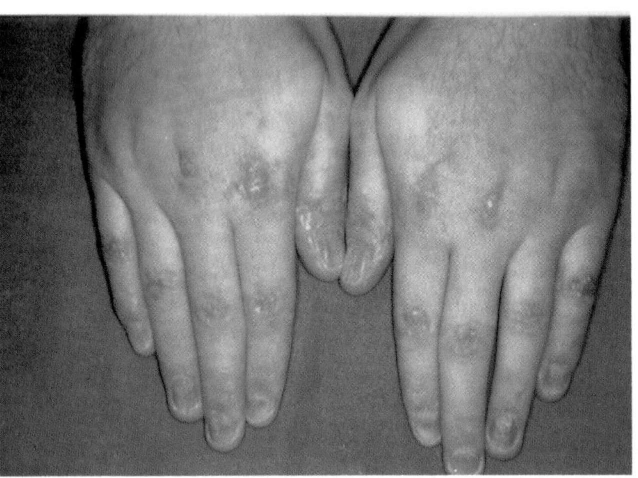

Figure 2.63. **(A)** Hands of younger patient with punctate porokeratotic appearance to palms. **(B)** Atrophy of nails with atrophic areas over the knuckles. (From Delaporte et al., 1995.)

MODE OF INHERITANCE

Autosomal dominant. Male-to-male transmission is documented.

PRENATAL DIAGNOSIS

None.

DIFFERENTIAL DIAGNOSIS

Scleroderma does not present at birth or with hyperkeratosis of the palms. Other HPPKs do not have the sclerodactyly of Huriez syndrome.

Support Group: N.O.R.D.
P.O. Box 8923
New Fairfield, CT 06812
1-800-999-6673

SELECTED BIBLIOGRAPHY

Delaporte, E., N'Guyen-Mailfer, C., Janin, A., Savary, J.B., Vasseur, F., Feingold, N., Piette, F., and Bergoend, H. (1995). Keratoderma with scleroatrophy of the extremities or sclerotylosis (Huriez syndrome): a reappraisal. *Br. J. Dermatol.* **133,** 409–416.

Reevaluation of one of Huriez's original families, with 27 of 114 members affected. Microscopic and ultrastructural features reported for three. They describe hypohidrosis (presumably of the palms and soles) in half of affected individuals.

Huriez, Cl., Deminati, M., Agache, P., Delmas-Marsalet, Y., and Mennecier, M. (1969). Génodermatose scléro-atrophiante et kératodermique des extrémités. *Ann. Dermatol. Syphilligr. (Paris)* **96,** 135–146.

Detailed review of two large pedigrees.

POROKERATOSES

POROKERATOSIS OF MIBELLI (MIM:175800, 175850, 175900)

Includes Porokeratosis Palmaris Plantaris et Disseminata (PPPD); Disseminated Superficial Actinic Porokeratosis (DSAP); Linear Porokeratosis; Porokeratosis Palmaris et Plantaris (PPP); and Degos Disease

---

DERMATOLOGIC FEATURES

MAJOR. Common to all forms of porokeratosis are round, mildly erythematous to brown, hyperkeratotic, slightly depressed lesions, with a surrounding, raised, hyperkeratotic border. Lesions are typically small, a few millimeters in diameter (DSAP, PPP, PPPD), or plaque-like and annular (Mibelli) or mixed. Distribution may be generalized (Mibelli, DSAP), linear (linear porokeratosis), limited to palms and soles (PPP), or any combination of these (PPPD). There may be a predilection for sun-exposed areas (DSAP) or for acral distribution (Mibelli). On the palms and soles, lesions tend to have a punched-out appearance. Hand and foot involvement usually, but not always, precedes involvement elsewhere. Some patients report exacerbation with sunlight exposure; some complain of pruritis.

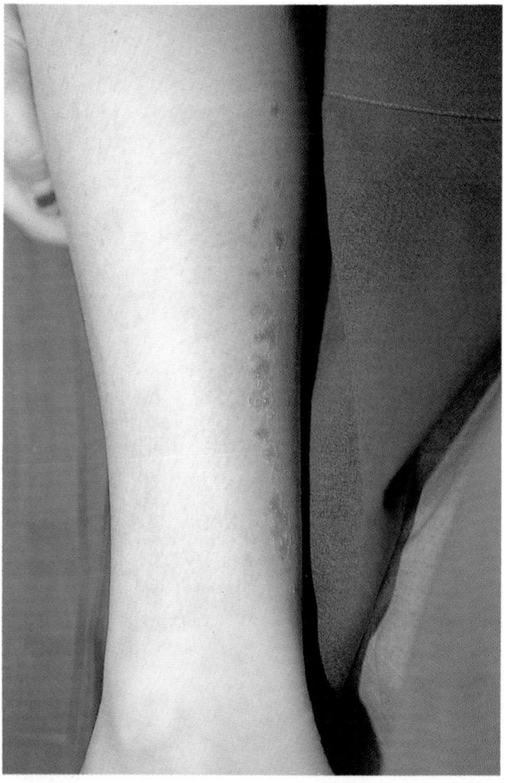

Figure 2.64. Linear lesions on leg of child, with erythema and surrounding raised border.

Onset tends to be in childhood (linear, Mibelli) or in later teens or early adult life (DSAP, PPPD). The existence of several families with expression of more than one type of porokeratosis among members, and individuals expressing more than one phenotype of porokeratosis, suggest that the distinctions among these conditions may be artificial.

MINOR. It is unclear if an increased risk for squamous cell carcinomas developing within porokeratotic lesions exists. Lesions on the oral mucosa have been described in PPPD.

ASSOCIATED ABNORMALITIES

None.

HISTOPATHOLOGY

LIGHT. The hallmark is a circumferential cornoid lamella—a horn of parakeratotic cells arising from a dell in the epidermis. Dyskeratosis with vacuolization of keratinocytes and a chronic lymphohistiocytic infiltrate in the dermis are common to all forms of porokeratosis. **EM.** Intraepidermal edema with intracellular perinuclear edema of keratinocytes is typical. An increase in the number of Langerhans cells has been described. Duplication of the basal lamina of the dermal–epidermal junction has also been noted.

BASIC DEFECT

Unknown.

TREATMENT

PPPD and Mibelli respond to retinoids, but the discomfort of treatment may exceed the discomfort of the disease. Freezing with liquid nitrogen gives varying response. I have treated one patient with porokeratosis of Mibelli with liquid nitrogen with questionable success; she was pleased with the results, but I was not.

MODE OF INHERITANCE

Autosomal dominant. In several pedigrees where only siblings were affected, the parents were normal by history only and not examined. Many pedigrees show male-to-male transmission. Heterogeneity of phenotype within families is common.

PRENATAL DIAGNOSIS

None.

DIFFERENTIAL DIAGNOSIS

Linear porokeratosis occurs sporadically, and actinic damage and immunosuppression can also cause porokeratosis. Biopsy will distinguish porokeratosis from other clinical entities if uncertainty exists. Conditions in which cornoid lamella have been occasionally found (rarely is the lamella circumferential as it is in porokeratosis) are clinically distinct and will not be confused.

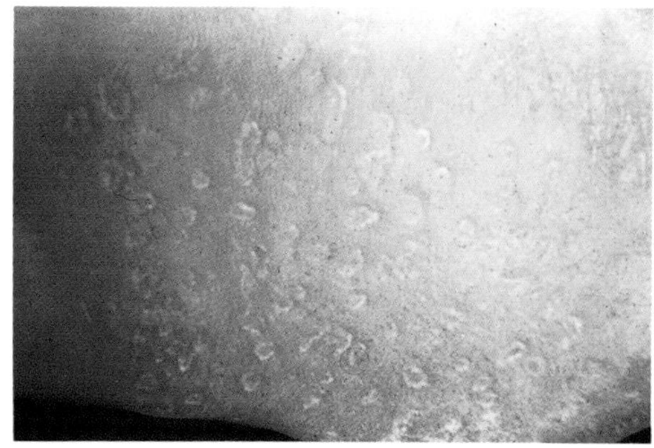

Figure 2.65. Multiple depressed lesions without erythema on the sole. (Courtesy of Division of Dermatology, University of Washington.)

The lesions of Degos disease (malignant atrophic papulosis) may appear somewhat similar. In malignant atrophic papulosis, asymptomatic pea-sized pink lesions that develop atrophic white centers and surrounding pink telangiectatic borders appear on any skin surface. Biopsy shows atrophy with hyperkeratosis and mucin in the dermis with endothelial proliferation within deep dermal vessels. Internal organs may or may not be involved.

Support Group: N.O.R.D.
P.O. Box 8923
New Fairfield, CT
06812
1-800-999-6673

SELECTED BIBLIOGRAPHY

Anderson, D.E., and Chernosky, M.E. (1969). Disseminated superficial actinic porokeratosis. Genetic aspects. *Arch. Dermatol.* **99,** 408–412.
Ten pedigrees are described.

Commens, C.A., and Shumack, S.P. (1987). Linear porokeratosis in two families with disseminated superficial actinic porokeratosis. *Pediatr. Dermatol.* **4,** 209–214.
A nice table with familial occurrence of linear porokeratosis in association with other forms.

Guss, S.B., Osbourn, R.A., and Lutzner, M.A. (1971). Porokeratosis plantaris palmaris et disseminata. A third type of porokeratosis. *Arch. Dermatol.* **104,** 366–373.

A table differentiating among porokeratosis of Mibelli, DSAP, and PPPD is given. This is perhaps moot. One affected family member developed melanoma in a site not affected by porokeratosis. Another patient developed two squamous cell carcinomas.

Kisch, L.S., and Bruynzeel, D.P. (1984). Six cases of malignant atrophic papulosis (Degos' disease) occurring in one family. *Br. J. Dermatol.* **111,** 469–471.

Two generations affected. Equal number of males and females, but no male-to-male transmission.

Shaw, J.C., and White, C.R., Jr. (1984). Porokeratosis plantaris palmaris et disseminata. *J. Am. Acad. Dermatol.* **11,** 454–460.

A clear review with good photos of histopathology and clinical lesions.

OTHER DISORDERS OF THE EPIDERMIS

ABSENCE OF DERMATOGLYPHICS (MIM:125540, 136000)

(Absence of Fingerprints; Baird Syndrome; Reed Syndrome)

DERMATOLOGIC FEATURES

MAJOR. This condition is marked by absence of fingertip ridge patterns, absence of sweating on palms and soles, and ridged, thinned nails with attachment to the hyponychium. There are two subtypes that are distinguished by additional clinical features. There is palmoplantar thickening in the Baird subtype, in which transient congenital milia have also been described. Congenital blistering of fingers and soles occurs in the Reed subtype.

MINOR. Cutaneous syndactyly of the toes and/or fingers.

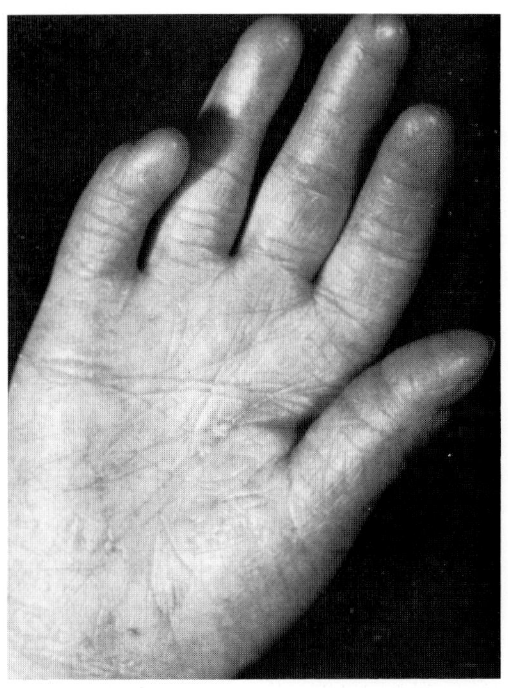

Figure 2.66. Contractures and absence of normal dermal ridge pattern. (From Baird, 1964.)

ASSOCIATED ABNORMALITIES

Camptodactyly of the fingers and/or toes was a feature in 12 of 13 affected individuals in Baird's family.

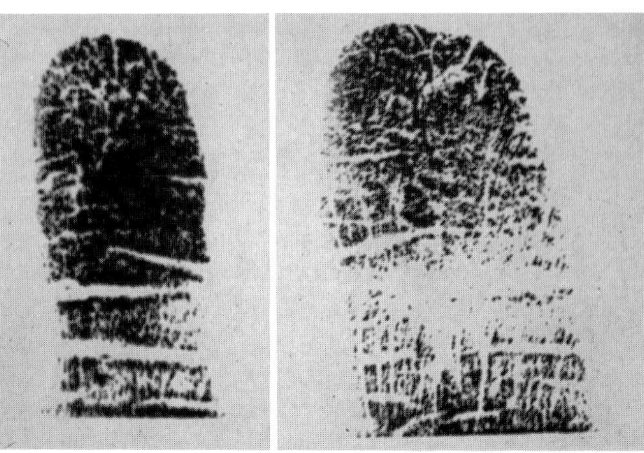

Figure 2.67. Fingerprints of an affected individual. (From Baird, 1964.)

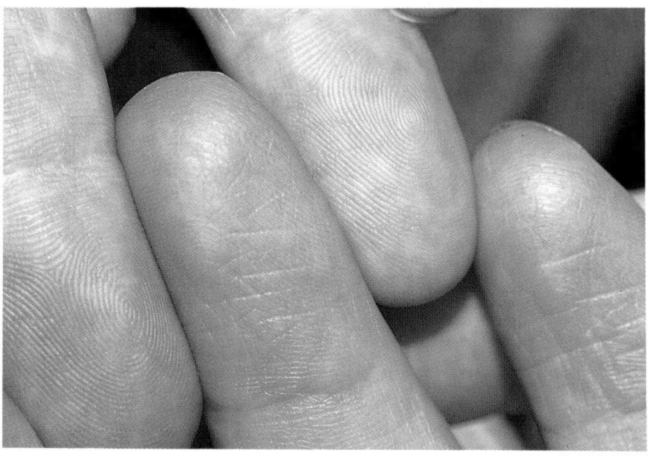

Figure 2.68. Second and fourth fingers from the left belong to an individual with hypohidrotic ectodermal dysplasia showing absence of normal dermatoglyphic pattern.

HISTOPATHOLOGY

Unknown.

BASIC DEFECT

Unknown.

TREATMENT

None.

MODE OF INHERITANCE

Autosomal dominant.

PRENATAL DIAGNOSIS

Not applicable.

DIFFERENTIAL DIAGNOSIS

Although effacement of epidermal ridges can accompany chronic hand dermatitis, this is easily differentiated from absence of dermatoglyphics. Males with hypohidrotic ectodermal dysplasia (HED) (MIM:305100) often have no fingerprint patterns. The associated features of HED preclude confusion with absence of dermatoglyphics. In epidermolysis bullosa junctional-progressiva (MIM:226500), there is gradual loss of the fingerprint pattern. Nail dystrophy and blistering are persistent.

Support Group: N.O.R.D.
P.O. Box 8923
New Fairfield, CT
06812
1-800-999-6673

SELECTED BIBLIOGRAPHY

Baird, H.W. III (1964). Kindred showing congenital absence of the dermal ridges (fingerprints) and associated anomalies. *J. Pediatr.* **64,** 621–631.

Baird, H.W. III (1968). Absence of fingerprints in four generations. Letter to the Editor. *Lancet* **ii,** 1250.

The letter adds three new affected members to the pedigree reported by the author in 1964. There are good photographs in the 1964 article.

Reed, T., and Schreiner, R.L. (1983). Absence of dermal ridge patterns: genetic heterogeneity. *Am. J. Med. Genet.* **16,** 81–88.

Report of a pedigree with male-to-male transmission.

Cirillo-Hyland, V.A., Zackai, E.H., Honig, P.J., Grace, K.R., Schnur, R.E. (1995). Reevaluation of a kindred with congenital absence of dermal ridges, syndactyly, and facial milia. *J. Am. Acad. Dermatol.* **32:**315–318.

Examined a newborn member of Baird's original pedigree. Baby had two vesicles—one on hand, one on foot. Authors argue that Baird and Reed "subtypes" are the same disorder.

ACANTHOSIS NIGRICANS (MIM:100600)

(Keratosis Nigricans)

DERMATOLOGIC FEATURES

Major. The brown to black velvety thickening of the skin of acanthosis nigricans can occur anywhere on the body, but has a predilection for flexures of the neck, axillae, and antecubital and popliteal fossae. Its appearance differs from hyperpigmentation alone in that the skin markings are also accentuated and thickened. Initially, there may be only a light brown discoloration, which progresses to the classic deep brown thick plaques. In longstanding disease, papillomas and warty excrescences may occur. There are no clinical features of the skin changes that distinguish isolated acanthosis nigricans from that associated with systemic or syndromic abnormalities.

Minor. Mucosal involvement may occur. Soft fleshy papules may develop on the hands, forearms, legs, and face. One family reported with absence of eyebrows and eyelashes.

ASSOCIATED ABNORMALITIES

Acanthosis nigricans can be isolated or associated with malignancy, obesity, insulin resistance, and a number of genetic and/or dysmorphic syndromes. In some of the syndromic associations the underlying cause for the acanthosis nigricans may be altered glucose metabolism and increased insulin levels. In others, it is unknown.

In association with obesity, it is often termed *pseudoacanthosis nigricans*. In my opinion, the term serves no useful purpose and should be dropped.

Syndromic associations include: *Crouzon craniofacial dysostosis (MIM:123500):* This is an autosomal dominant syndrome of craniosynostosis, hypertelorism, hypoplastic maxilla, and parrot-beaked nose. I have seen one patient with this syndrome who had very extensive acanthosis nigricans. She had normal insulin and glucose levels and was slender. Suslak et al. (1985) reported a parent and child, both of whom had Crouzon syndrome and acanthosis nigricans.

Seip syndrome (lipodystrophy [Berardinelli syndrome] MIM:269700): This condition is marked by generalized lipodystrophy, hyperlipemia, hepatomegaly, nonketotic insulin-resistant diabetes mellitus, and acanthosis nigricans. Polycystic ovaries, muscular hypertrophy, and mental retardation have been reported in some patients.

Rabson-Mendenhall syndrome (MIM: 262190): This is an autosomal recessive disorder of pineal hyperplasia, insulin-resistant diabetes mellitus, coarse facies, and hirsuitism. There appears to be a decrease in insulin receptors in this condition.

Prader-Willi syndrome (MIM:176270): The acanthosis nigricans reported in some patients with Prader-Willi syndrome may be in association with obesity and diabetes and not a primary feature of the syndrome.

Bloom syndrome (MIM:210900): The occurrence of acanthosis nigricans in one patient with Bloom syndrome may have been secondary to malignancy and not a primary feature of the syndrome.

Familial insulin resistance with acanthosis nigricans, acral hypertrophy, and muscle cramps (MIM:200170): This is a presumed autosomal recessive disorder reported in one kindred.

Stein-Leventhal (MIM:184700): This autosomal dominant disorder of polycystic ovaries and hirsutism can have associated acanthosis nigricans.

Rud syndrome (MIM:312770): A possibly X-linked recessive form of ichthyosis, epilepsy, retardation, and retinitis pigmentosa. Acanthosis nigricans may be associated with an underlying endocrinopathy and not a primary feature.

HISTOPATHOLOGY

Light. Hyperkeratosis and papillomatosis, mild acanthosis, and little hyperpigmentation are seen in involved skin.
EM. No information.

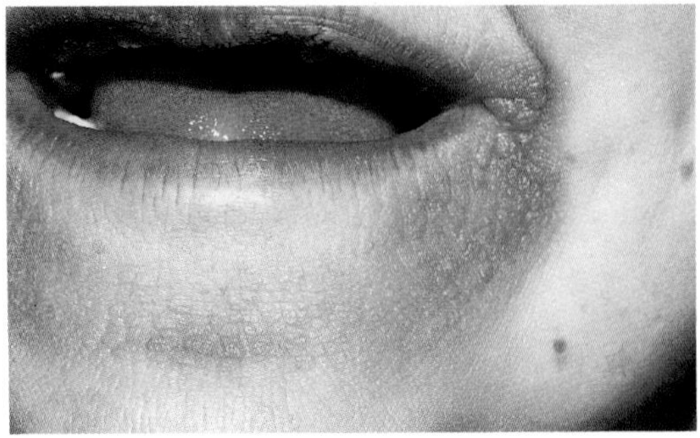

Figure 2.69. Early changes of slightly thickened brown plaques around mouth in patient with Crouzon syndrome.

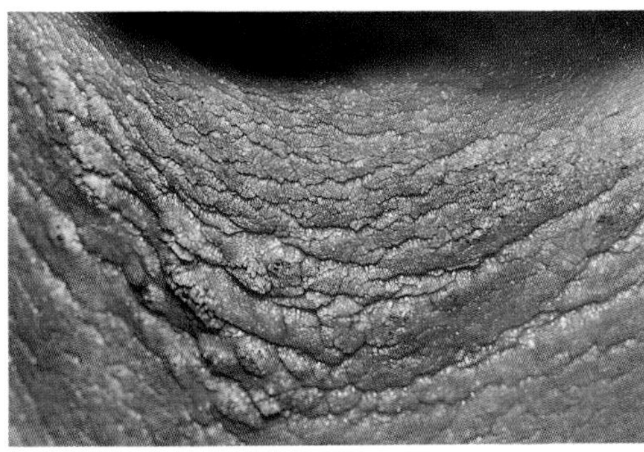

Figure 2.70. More advanced disease with deep furrows and excrescences.

BASIC DEFECT

It has been suggested that the unifying pathway for the association of acanthosis nigricans with a variety of insulin-resistant conditions is local tissue resistance to insulin. This results in a general hyperinsulinemia, with increased binding of insulin to insulin-like growth factor receptors and consequent stimulation of dermal fibroblasts or epidermal keratinocytes. A similar role of growth stimulation by tumor products has been posited for acanthosis nigricans associated with malignancy.

TREATMENT

None effective. Keratolytics are of minimal help. Treatment of underlying disease, when present, may result in remission of acanthosis nigricans. There has been one report of response to 10–20 g/day of ω-3 fatty-acid-rich fish oil in a patient with lipodystrophic diabetes. She stopped the medication for other reasons, and follow-up is not available. I have tried this in one patient with Crouzon syndrome and acanthosis nigricans, and she has had a moderate response with improvement, but not clearing, of her acanthosis nigricans.

MODE OF INHERITANCE

Isolated acanthosis nigricans can be autosomal dominant or sporadic. I am not certain that true, isolated acanthosis nigricans outside of syndromes such as Stein-Leventhal syndrome or disorders of insulin resistance has been shown to be inherited in a regular pattern. In acanthosis nigricans associated with a syndrome, the mode of inheritance depends on the syndrome.

PRENATAL DIAGNOSIS

None.

DIFFERENTIAL DIAGNOSIS

Lichenification and hyperpigmentation secondary to dermatitis might be confused with acanthosis nigricans at first glance but is easily distinguished clinically. Epidermal nevi (MIM:163200) may be brown and verrucous. They tend to be distributed along the lines of Blaschko and not localized to neck and axillae. The histologic findings are different.

Support Group: N.O.R.D.
P.O. Box 8923
New Fairfield, CT 06812
1-800-999-6673

SELECTED BIBLIOGRAPHY

Curth, H.O., and Aschner, B.M. (1959). Genetic studies on acanthosis nigricans. *Arch. Dermatol.* **79,** 55–66.

Nine pedigrees of benign acanthosis nigricans in which multiple family members were affected, at least one of which was a family with Stein-Leventhal with variable expression of acanthosis nigricans and polycystic ovaries.

Flier, J.S. (1985). Metabolic importance of acanthosis nigricans. *Arch. Dermatol.* **121,** 193–194.

Discussion of the role of insulin resistance in causation of acanthosis nigricans.

Rendon, M.I., Cruz, P.D., Sontheimer, R.D., and Bergstresser, P.R. (1989). Acanthosis nigricans: a cutaneous marker of tissue resistance to insulin. *J. Am. Acad. Dermatol.* **21,** 461–469.

Case report of two patients with acanthosis nigricans. They present an algorithm for assessment of patients with acanthosis nigricans and an overview of the mechanism of the disease.

Sheretz, E.F. (1988). Improved acanthosis nigricans with lipodystrophic diabetes during dietary fish oil supplementation. *Arch. Dermatol.* **124,** 1094–1096.

Case report of improvement in acanthosis nigricans with ω-3 fatty-acid-rich dietary fish oil.

Stuart, C.A., Pate, C.J., and Peters, E.J. (1989). Prevalence of acanthosis nigricans in an unselected population. *Am. J. Med.* **87,** 269–272.

A survey of 1,400 children in the sixth and eighth grades. Acanthosis nigricans was found in 13.1% blacks, 5.5% Hispanics, and 0.04% whites. There was a clear association with racial background and obesity. The authors evaluated 12 of the 102 children with acanthosis nigricans further for elevations in insulin. Their data are, however, presented in a way that cannot be interpreted. The results in these 12 patients were reported in a histogram that included 127 other individuals' test results. I do not believe any inference can be drawn from their data other than that there is a clear predilection of the disorder for specific ethnic groups and that the prevalence (7%) of acanthosis nigricans is higher than previously believed and much higher than frank insulin resistance or diabetes in a teenage population.

Suslak, L., Glista, B., Gertzman, G.B., Lieberman, L., Schwartz, R.A., and Desposito, F. (1985). Crouzon syndrome with periapical cemental dysplasia and acanthosis nigricans: the pleiotropic effect of a single gene? *Birth Defects* **XXI(2),** 127–134.

Report of mother and son with both disorders. Acanthosis nigricans had developed by age 2 years in the son.

DARIER-WHITE DISEASE (MIM:124200)

(Darier Disease; Keratosis Follicularis; Psorospermose Folliculaire Vegetante)

DERMATOLOGIC FEATURES

Major. Yellow, tan, or brown rough, firm papules that often have a greasy scale or crust are distributed in a seborrheic pattern on the face, at the hair margins, the middle and upper chest, intertriginous areas, ears, and back. They may become confluent, forming plaques. When the crust is removed, a central pore can often be seen. Onset of skin changes is typically in the late first through fourth decades, most commonly around puberty. Lesions first appear on the middle-chest or upper shoulders and neck in half of patients. The condition is usually itchy, and blistering is common. These symptoms are exacerbated with heat, exercise, and sunlight. Occasionally hemorrhage into the lesions occurs. Hemorrhagic lesions were found in 6% of patients in one series.

Warty, hypertrophic plaques may develop. These are often odiferous. Large dilated follicular openings mimicking giant comedones can be seen.

Flat-topped, skin-colored to brown papules without the greasy scale are distributed acrally on the tops of the hands and feet and are similar to acrokeratosis verruciformis of Hopf in appearance and pattern. These lesions may be the earliest sign of the disorder.

Punctate keratoses, both pits and papules, of the palms and soles are seen in approximately 85% of patients.

Ninety to 100% of patients will have nail changes. These include longitudinal red or white subungual streaks that may traverse the length of the nail. Where the streak meets the free nail margin, V-shaped notches or clefts occur. The combination of red and white bands with notching is pathognomonic for Darier-White. Keratoses can develop on any part of the nail apparatus. Longitudinal ridging and friability of the nail plate are common. Not all nails are necessarily involved; fingernails are usually more affected than toenails.

Whitish umbilicated or cobblestone papules can be found on all oral mucosal surfaces, larynx, esophagus, and rectum. The palate is most commonly affected. Oral involvement tends to be a later manifestation than cutaneous involvement. Recurrent parotid gland swelling can be a problem. This is thought to be due to squamous metaplasia of the ductal lining, which results in obstruction.

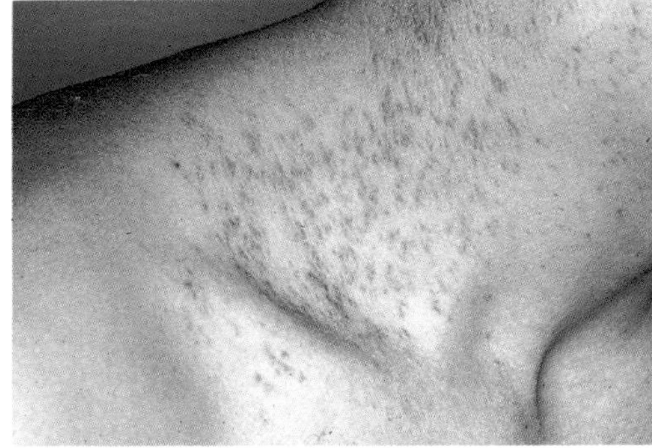

Figure 2.71. Brown, rough papules over the neck and upper chest.

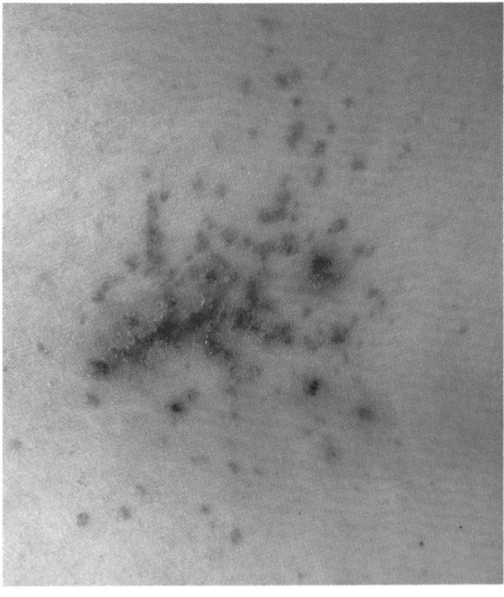

Figure 2.72. Hemorrhagic crusted lesions.

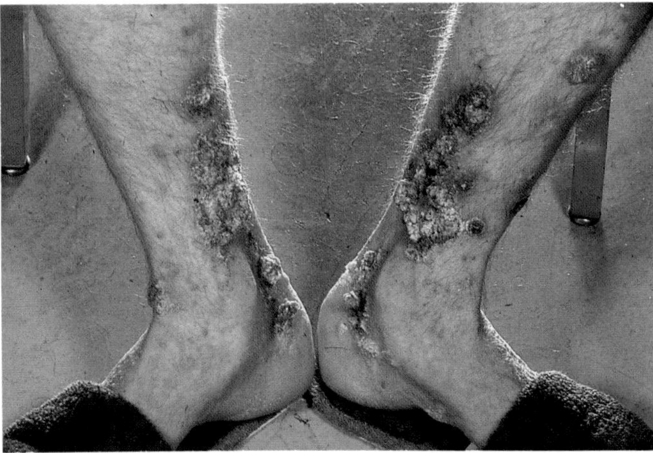

Figure 2.73. Vegetative plaques.

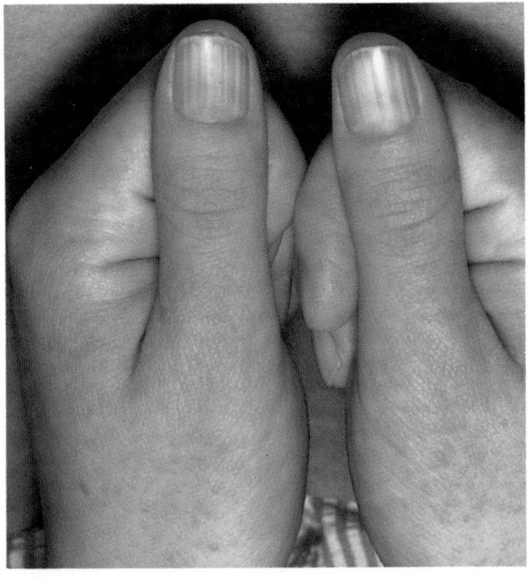

Figure 2.74. White streaks in nails, subtle hyperkeratotic papules over thumbs and hands.

Each of the manifestations of Darier-White can occur individually and at different times. Onset of the classic nail and skin changes may be preceded by other findings for many years, often obscuring the correct diagnosis. Although there may be fluctuation in severity, spontaneous remission has not been reported.

MINOR. Rarely, Darier-White can present solely as hemorrhagic macules and blisters, usually palmar and plantar, often in the setting of diffuse palmoplantar hyperkeratosis.

Single lesions of warty dyskeratoma have been reported in three patients with Darier-White disease.

Although the disorder is usually generalized, a zosteriform or nevoid distribution has been described, perhaps the result of somatic mosaicism.

In some patients, the distribution of lesions is flexural, rather than seborrheic.

Odor is a complaint common to almost half of affected individuals, and secondary bacterial infection often contributes to this.

Eczema herpeticum, from both herpes simplex and vaccinia, has been reported at least 20 times, often occurring after sun exposure. In two cases, there were no lesions of Darier-White present at the time eczema herpeticum developed.

ASSOCIATED ABNORMALITIES

Eye: Asymptomatic opacities in the periphery of the cornea have been described in some patients. Two brothers with retinitis pigmentosa and Darier-White disease have been reported. This probably reflects a stochastic rather than causal association.

Bone: Cystic changes in the bones were reported in four patients, but may be due to factors other than the skin disease. After seeing an individual with Darier-White disease who had bone cysts secondary to dietary osteomalacia with secondary hyperparathyroidism, Crisp et al. (1992) surveyed 30 additional patients with Darier disease and found no bone cysts. They argue against an association.

Malignancy: There is a question of increased risk for skin cancer in Darier-White; very few cases have been reported.

Immune system: A variety of immune defects have been suggested in Darier-White disease, but none has been confirmed. Secondary infection in the crusted and warty plaques is common, and this has led to the idea that an immune defect might play a role in the disorder. It seems more likely that the hyperkeratoses provide an environment seductive to skin pathogens, while at the same time interfering with the mechanical integrity required for the skin's defenses. The same phenomenon may play a role in bullous congenital ichthyosiform erythroderma and in other conditions in which a thickened erose crust occurs.

Psychiatric: It has been stated that mental retardation is more common in Darier-White disease. This is difficult to critique from the literature. One survey from Denmark stated that 5 of 51 patients were mentally defective; it was the authors' impression that others, particularly those they termed destitute, were also intellectually handicapped, but no details are given, and family histories were not reviewed for the possibility of unrelated causes of mental retardation. A retrospective study of five patients ascertained through dermatologic records of hospital inpatients demonstrated psychological or intellectual deficits in all. However, as all hospitalizations had been for neurologic problems, not for dermatologic complications, ascertainment bias is obvious. It has been suggested that suicidal ideation is more common among patients with Darier-White disease than among patients with other disfiguring skin disorders, but the number of patients studied was small.

HISTOPATHOLOGY

LIGHT. Skin: features of dyskeratosis with classic corps ronds and grains believed to represent dead or dying keratinocytes, acantholysis, and suprabasal clefting or lacunae are typical. Uninvolved skin is normal histologically.

Nail features include no suprabasal clefts, but there is presence of multinucleated giant cells and absence of inflammatory infiltrate in the nail bed.

EM. There is a decrease in the number of desmosomes with loss of tonofilament–desmosomal association in the epidermal cells. The corps ronds are composed of dense keratohyaline masses and tonofilaments. The grains are nuclear remnants surrounded by dyskeratotic elements.

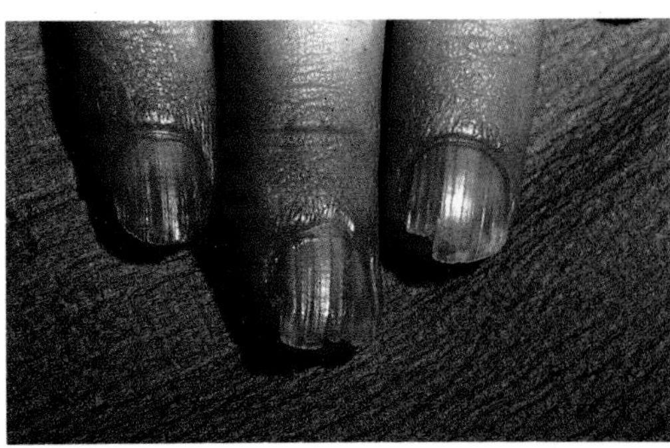

Figure 2.75. Red and white streaks with notching of free nail margin. (Courtesy of Division of Dermatology, University of Washington.)

BASIC DEFECT

Unknown. Abnormalities in tonofilament formation, in various aspects of the immune system, and a primary abnormality in desmosomes have been posited but not confirmed.

TREATMENT

Etretinate and acitretin, the latter in doses of 10–30 mg/day, may be beneficial clinically. When it becomes generally available, the latter may be preferrable because of its shorter half-life. Topical 13-*cis*-retinoic acid has also been effective, although it is not available commercially. Dermabrasion gives temporary cosmetic relief.

MODE OF INHERITANCE

Autosomal dominant with intrafamilial and interfamilial variability in severity. Penetrance appears to be 100% by late adult life. The condition has been mapped to 12q23–24, distal to the keratin gene cluster.

PRENATAL DIAGNOSIS

None.

DIFFERENTIAL DIAGNOSIS

In the early stages, patients may be misdiagnosed with eczema or seborrhea. Lack of response to standard therapy should lead to biopsy and correct diagnosis.

The lesions of acrokeratosis verruciformis of Hopf (MIM:101900) are identical to the acral lesions of Darier-White, and, if this is the first presenting sign in an individual with Darier-White disease, the correct diagnosis may be delayed until the more typical greasy lesions appear.

Epidermodysplasia verruciformis (MIM: 226400, 305350) is also clinically similar to acral Darier-White disease, but can be distinguished histologically by the presence of viral particles.

Hailey-Hailey disease (benign familial pemphigus) (MIM:169600) can mimic bullous Darier-White, but blistering erosive changes are far more typical and keratotic papules are less common in Hailey-Hailey disease. Although the nails in Hailey-Hailey disease may show broad white bands, they are not friable or notched, and red bands are absent. Electron microscopy may help to differentiate between the two conditions.

Support Group: F.I.R.S.T.
P.O. Box 20921
Raleigh, NC 27619
1-800-545-3286

SELECTED BIBLIOGRAPHY

Blackman, H.J., Rodrigues, M.M., and Peck, G.L. (1980). Corneal epithelial lesions in keratosis follicularis (Darier's disease). *Ophthalmology* **87,** 931–943.

Sixteen of 21 patients ascertained by skin disease had asymptomatic peripheral opacities of the cornea with central corneal epithelial irregularity. The opacities varied in size and shape and were similar in degree but not in distribution in the two eyes. There was no correlation with age or severity of skin involvement. One patient had central changes without peripheral opacities. Ten patients were examined prior to retinoid treatment, 11 patients after. Other findings unique to individual patients are detailed.

Burge, S.M. (1989). Darier's disease, keratins and proteases: a review. *J. R. Soc. Med.* **82,** 673–676.

Reviews what is known or hypothesized about the basic defect in Darier-White.

Burge, S.M., and Wilkinson, J.D. (1992). Darier-White disease: a review of the clinical features in 163 patients. *J. Am. Acad. Dermatol.* **127,** 40–50.

This is an excellent review of the range of the dermatologic findings. One hundred twenty-three patients from a total of 163 records were examined by Dr. Burge. An additional 18 were interviewed by telephone. Of particular interest was the abandonment of oral retinoid therapy by a fourth of treated patients despite its efficacy because of what might be considered minor but discomfiting side effects.

Caulfield, J.B., and Wilgram, G.F. (1963). An electron microscope study of dyskeratosis and acantholysis in Darier's disease. *J. Invest. Dermatol.* **41,** 57–65.

Biopsies from five patients, four with a positive family history, were evaluated by electron microscopy. The authors believe the primary defect in Darier-White disease may be in tonofilament formation. They underscore the differences in the pathology of Hailey-Hailey, in which, while tonofilaments are increased in number, they do not aggregate into clumps and are not associated with keratohyaline granules.

Crisp, A.J., Roland Payne, C.M.E., Adams, J., Brenton, D.P., Meyrick Thomas, R.H., Black, M.M., Pope, F.M., Wilkinson, J. D., and MacDonald, L.M. (1992). The prevalence of bone cysts in Darier's disease: a survey of 31 cases. *Clin. Exp. Dermatol.* **19,** 78–83.

Authors argue against a causal relationship between the concurrent diseases.

King, D.F. (1982). A footnote to "the tale of the psorosperm." *Am. J. Dermatopathol* **4,** 313–314.

This historical footnote contains the following quote from White regarding his second patient with Darier-White disease: "After the examination . . . had been completed, the surprising discovery was made that the person described in my former article, whom she then accidentally met in the waiting room, was her father . . . It was found . . . that the daughter had been adopted by another family in infancy and that her father had not seen her since she was a year old." Once again, we must learn to mistrust the negative family history.

Macleod, R.I., and Munro, C.S. (1991). The incidence and distribution of oral lesions in patients with Darier's disease. *Br. Dent. J.* **171,** 133–136.

Twenty-four (19 with a positive family history) of 50 patients with Darier disease contacted agreed to be examined. Twelve of these had oral involvement, which occurred in both familial and sporadic cases. None of five subjects less than 35 years old had oral involvement. Thirty percent of the 24 had recurrent parotid gland swelling. Includes excellent pictures of the oral mucosal changes.

Medansky, R.S., and Woloshin, A.A. (1961). Darier's disease. An evaluation of its neuropsychiatric component. *Arch. Dermatol.* **84,** 482–484.

Psychiatric investigation of five patients with Darier-White disease and review of the literature regarding intellectual problems, which is helpful in delineating how uncertain the occurrence and significance of intellectual deficit and psychiatric disease are.

Oxholm, A., Oxholm, P., da Cunha Bang, F., and Horrobin, D.F. (1990). Abnormal essential fatty acid metabolism in Darier disease. *Arch. Dermatol.* **126,** 1308–1311.

Because essential fatty acid deficiency shares several features in common with Darier-White disease, these authors studied 13 unrelated adults with Darier-White disease, four of whom were on low-dose retinoid therapy. They found significantly reduced levels of the δ-6-desaturase metabolites of linolenic and α-linolenic acids, suggesting a defect in the δ-6-desaturase enzyme. These findings have not been confirmed to date.

HEREDITARY PAINFUL CALLOSITIES (MIM:114140)

(Keratosis Palmoplantaris Nummularis)

DERMATOLOGIC FEATURES

MAJOR. This disorder is rare and possibly heterogeneous. The major feature is development of thick, painful calluses on pressure points of feet in early childhood after walking has been established. These can also develop on the hands if manual labor is performed. Calluses can interfere with function. They are typically not erythematous. I have seen one family in whom the callosities were not painful.

MINOR. Two families reported with blistering at the edge of the calluses. One family had periungual and subungual hyperkeratoses. One child had involvement of the shins, perhaps secondary to crawling. One older patient developed calluses below the knees, associated with frequent kneeling.

ASSOCIATED ABNORMALITIES

None.

HISTOPATHOLOGY

LIGHT. Massive hyperkeratosis. In only the family with blistering were cytolysis and dyskeratosis reported.

EM. Variable. Clumping of tonofilaments has been described in one family.

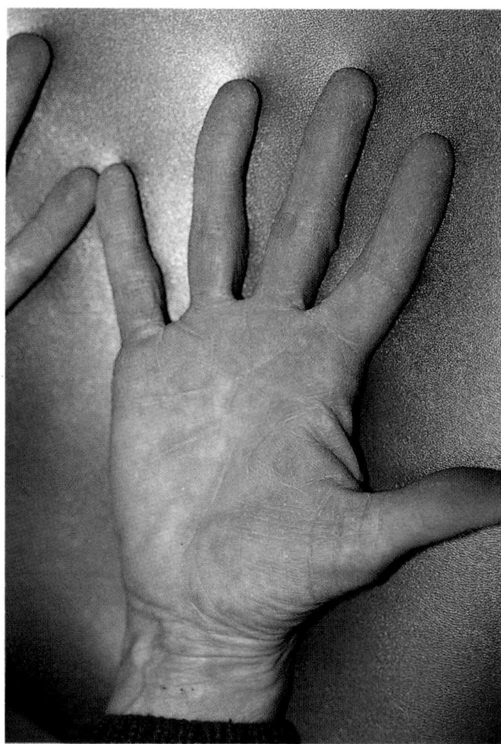

Figure 2.76. Calluses along palmar creases where pressure occurs.

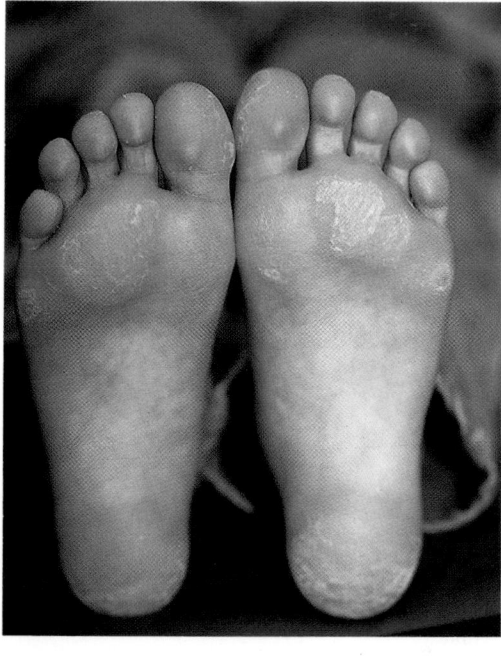

Figure 2.77. Involvement of weight-bearing surfaces of feet.

BASIC DEFECT

Unknown.

TREATMENT

Mechanical debridement and use of orthopedic shoes. There is poor response to retinoids.

MODE OF INHERITANCE

Autosomal dominant.

PRENATAL DIAGNOSIS

None.

DIFFERENTIAL DIAGNOSIS

Other palmoplantar hyperkeratoses (MIM: many) need to be considered. In both the one family and one sporadic case I have seen, the lesions were true calluses with marked accentuation of normal skin lines in contrast to the verrucous or shiny hyperkeratosis of palmoplantar keratoderma. Some cases in the literature described as HPPK papulosa (Buschke-Fischer or Brauer) may have been confused with hereditary painful callosities. Underlying erythema or erythema at the margins is typical of HPPK and not of hereditary painful callosities.

Support Group: F.I.R.S.T.
P.O. Box 20921
Raleigh, NC 27619
1-800-545-3286

SELECTED BIBLIOGRAPHY

Dupre, A., Bonafe, J.-L., and Cristol, B. (1979). Treatment of hereditary painful callosities with tretinoin (Letter). *Arch. Dermatol.* **115,** 638–639.
This letter incorrectly assumed that hereditary

painful callosities were equivalent to HPPK Buschke-Fischer, and this misconception has been perpetuated in McKusick's catalog and subsequent reports. HPPK Buschke-Fischer does respond to retinoids; hereditary painful callosities do not.

Roth, W., Penneys, N.S., and Fawcett, N. (1978). Hereditary painful callosities. *Arch. Dermatol.* **114,** 591–592.

Baden, H.P., Bronstein, B.R., and Rand, R.E. (1984). Hereditary callosities with blisters. Report of a family and review. *J. Am. Acad. Dermatol.* **11,** 409–415.

Case reports of families with microscopy findings.

Wachters, D.H., Frensdorf, E.L., Hausman, R., and van Dijk, E. (1983). Keratosis palmoplantaris nummularis ("hereditary painful callosities"). Clinical and histopathologic aspects. *J. Am. Acad. Dermatol.* **9,** 204–209.

Three families with somewhat differing features are presented.

KERATOSIS FOLLICULARIS SPINULOSA DECALVANS (MIM:308800)

DERMATOLOGIC FEATURES

MAJOR. Flesh-colored, spiny hyperkeratotic papules develop on the face, trunk, and extremities, usually in infancy and early childhood. Elbows, knees, and extensor surfaces are involved. There may be some improvement at puberty. Absence of the eyebrows almost invariably occurs, with absence of the eyelashes less frequent. Scarring alopecia of the scalp is typical.

MINOR. Nail changes of "high cuticles," where the free margin of the cuticle extends up to the middle of the nail plate, have been described.

ASSOCIATED ABNORMALITIES

Photophobia is common and is moderate to severe. It tends to improve in adult life. Affected individuals have a corneal dystrophy characterized by punctate subcorneal opacities. The photophobia may be caused by these corneal opacities, which refract light abnormally. Of six female carriers examined, only one showed corneal changes, which were mild. None of these obligate carriers had photophobia.

HISTOPATHOLOGY

LIGHT. Focal parakeratosis and mild follicular hyperkeratosis are found in the epidermis of the hyperkeratotic papules; there is mild dermal perifollicular fibrosis and a minimal lymphocytic infiltrate.

EM. No information.

BASIC DEFECT

Unknown.

TREATMENT

Photoprotection for the eyes. There is no effective treatment for the skin lesions; keratolytics may give minimal relief. Retinoids have not been tried.

MODE OF INHERITANCE

X-linked recessive. The term *X-linked dominant* has also been applied. This may be a semantic argument. It is clear that not all female carriers show any manifestations, and the range of severity in females is typical for carriers

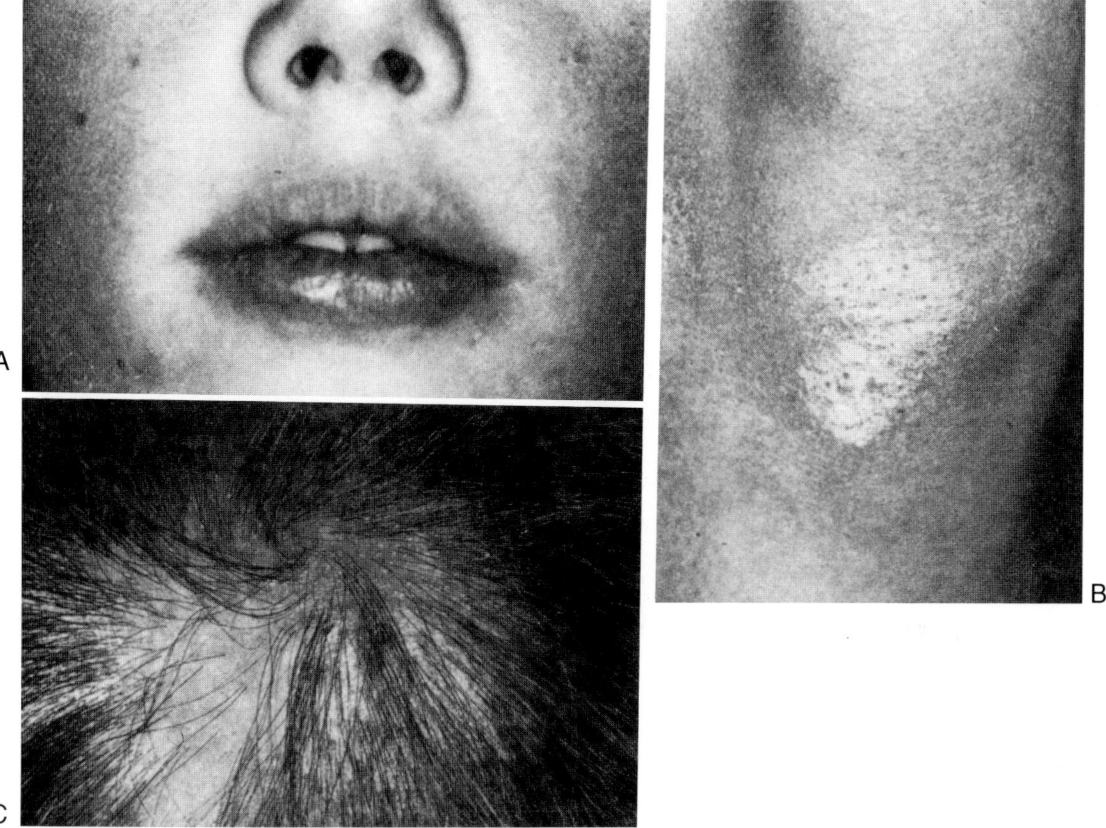

Figure 2.78. **(A)** Follicular hyperkeratosis over the face with sparing around the nose. **(B)** Marked involvement over the knee. **(C)** Scarring alopecia. (From van Osch et al., 1992.)

for X-linked recessive traits. The absence of clinical findings in a female does not ensure her a noncarrier status.

Linkage to Xp22.13–p22.2 has been established in a large Dutch pedigree.

PRENATAL DIAGNOSIS

None.

DIFFERENTIAL DIAGNOSIS

In ulerythema ophryogenes and inflammatory keratosis pilaris, the papules are erythematous, in contrast to the most often flesh-colored papules of keratosis follicularis spinulosa decalvans.

Atrichia congenita with papular lesions (MIM:209500) is similar to keratosis follicularis spinulosa decalvans, but involvement of the scalp is more severe. Histology of the papules shows epithelial cysts, not the plugged follicles of keratosis follicularis spinulosa decalvans. Atrichia congenita is most likely autosomal recessive.

In lichen spinulosis, an acquired self-limited condition typically occurring in childhood, spiny papules occur in discrete patches that favor the elbows, knees, abdomen, buttocks, thighs, and neck and may be quite widespread. It usually responds to local therapy with keratolytics. Histologically there are dilated hair follicles with keratin plugs. I think this condition is much more common than appreciated and is usually not brought to the physician's attention because it is asymptomatic.

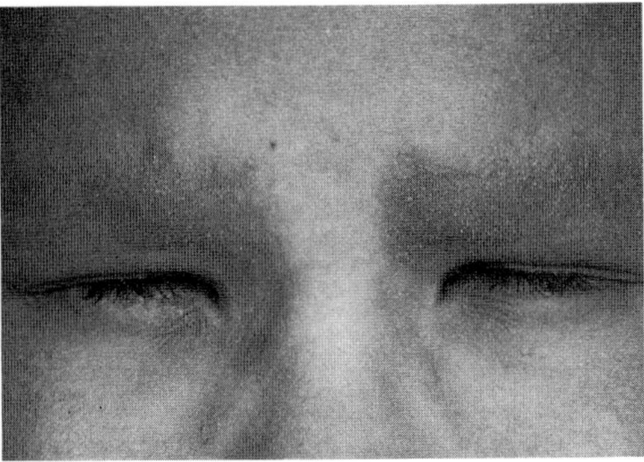

Figure 2.79. Follicular plugging and erythema with loss of hairs in eyebrows, similar to ulerythema ophryogenes. (From van Osch et al., 1992.)

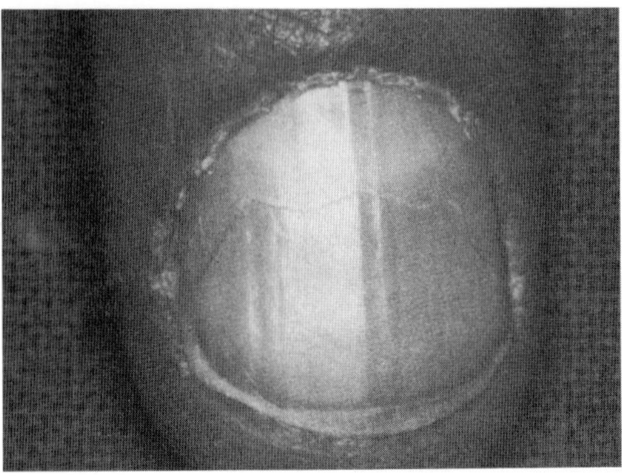

Figure 2.80. Very high cuticle on the fingernail. (From van Osch et al., 1992.)

Britton et al. (1978) described a patient with onset at birth of skin changes consisting of generalized thickening and hyperkeratosis, spiny filiform projections over all the skin surface, most pronounced on the scalp, perinasal region and ear lobes. He had conjunctivitis and decreased tearing with no evidence of corneal changes. He also had hypoplastic nails, deafness, failure to thrive, a question of developmental delay, and no scalp or body hair. This patient may have had the KID (keratitis-ichthyosis-deafness) syndrome (MIM:148120) in which skin changes may appear similar to keratosis follicularis spinulosa decalvans, but corneal changes and hearing deficits, as well as mode of inheritance, are distinctive.

Cantu et al. (1974) reported an X-linked pedigree in which affected individuals had keratosis follicularis, cerebral atrophy, severe mental retardation, and proportionate short stature with delayed bone age, alopecia, and absence of the hair, eyebrows, and eyelashes.

Marks (1967) reported a family with an X-linked skeletal dysplasia (epiphyseal dysplasia), cataracts, subepithelial corneal dystrophy, plantar hyperkeratosis, and diffuse horny follicular spines and small red follicular papules. Intelligence was normal.

The term *ichthyosis follicularis* has been applied to a group of disorders. These diverse case reports share in common generalized scaling of the skin, which is not a feature of keratosis follicularis spinulosa decalvans.

Many case reports in the literature in which the authors use the term *keratosis follicularis spinulosa decalvans* are better described as involving widespread ichthyotic changes with horny prominence, often with diffuse erythema as well as thickening of the skin. These case reports result in a spectrum of clinical features, a wide range of skin findings, and uncertain mode of inheritance being erroneously attributed to the single-gene disorder of keratosis follicularis spinulosa decalvans. To add a final fillip of confusion, Darier-White disease (MIM:124200) is also called *keratosis follicularis*. The greasy papules and patches of Darier-White are clinically distinctive.

Support Group: F.I.R.S.T.
P.O. Box 20921
Raleigh, NC 27619
1-800-545-3286

BIBLIOGRAPHY

Britton, H., Lustig, J., Thompson, B.J., Meyer, S., Esterly, N.B. (1978). Keratosis follicularis spinulosa decalvans. An infant with failure to thrive, deafness, and recurrent infections. *Arch. Dermatol.* **114,** 761–764.

Cantu, J.M., Hernandez, A., Larracilla, J., Trejo, A., Macotela-Ruiz, E., (1974). A new X-linked recessive disorder with dwarfism, cerebral atrophy, and generalized keratosis follicularis. *J. Pediatr.* **84,** 564–567.

Marks, R. (1967). Follicular hyperkaratosis and ocular abnormalities associated with Fairbanks syndrome. *Brit J. Dermatol.* **79,** 168–169.

Case reports of keratosis follicularis spinulosa decalvans-like skin changes in individuals and families along with unusual findings. These may very well be distinct disorders.

Kuokkanen, K. (1971). Keratosis follicularis spinulosa decalvans in a family from Northern Finland. *Acta Dermatol Venereol. (Stockh.)* **51,** 146–150.

A most interesting family in whom palmoplantar hyperkeratosis and keratosis follicularis spinulosa decalvans were independently segregating. Two putative carrier females had a seborrheic/eczematous disorder as well. Six of eight obligate carriers showed no manifestations. Onset was later in life than usual with keratosis follicularis spinulosa decalvans, and the photographs are strongly suggestive of atrophoderma vermiculatum on the face.

Rand, R., and Baden, H.P. (1983). Keratosis follicularis spinulosa decalvans. Report of two cases and literature review. *Arch. Dermatol.* **119,** 22–26.

These authors coin the term "keratosis pilaris atrophicans" for those disorders of keratosis pilaris with inflammation followed by atrophy. They would put ulerythema ophryogenes, keratosis pilaris, and keratosis follicularis spinulosa decalvans in the same basket. One of their patients had a mother with ichthyosis vulgaris and keratosis pilaris and a sister with keratosis pilaris only. Their other patient was a female with progressive alopecia and inflammatory keratosis pilaris. Neither of these cases fits with classic descriptions of keratosis follicularis spinulosa decalvans. Inflammation has not played a significant role in keratosis follicularis spinulosa decalvans. The X-linked inheritance of keratosis follicularis spinulosa decalvans has been well established, and it deserves splitting from ulerythema ophryogenes and keratosis pilaris.

van Osch, L.D.M., Oranje, A.P., Keukens, F.M., van Voorst Vader, P.C., and Veldman, E. (1992). Keratosis follicularis spinulosa decalvans: a family study of seven male cases and six female carriers. *J. Med. Genet.* **29,** 36–40.

Follow-up study of first family described by Siemens in 1926 and Waardenburg in 1961. There were 34 affected males and two obligate female carriers.

KNUCKLE PADS (MIM:149100, 126900)

(Pachydermodactyly)

Includes Bart-Pumphrey Syndrome

DERMATOLOGIC FEATURES

Major. There appear to be two distinct conditions described by the term *knuckle pads.* One is marked by hyperkeratotic thickened lesions and the other by subcutaneous thickening or nodules with an overlying epidermis that has lost normal markings.

The first form is typically associated with palmoplantar keratoderma; the latter is seen in individuals with Dupuytren contracture and/or Peyronie disease (MIM:126900). Both types of knuckle pads can occur with other findings as well.

The proximal interphalangeal joints are most commonly affected. Distal interphalangeal and metacarpal phalangeal joints may also be involved. The toes rarely show changes. Any or all of the digits may affected. The lesions are usually asymptomatic, although they can occasionally itch or be mechanically bothersome. In type II, the knuckle pads usually precede development of contractures.

Minor. None.

ASSOCIATED ABNORMALITIES

None.

HISTOPATHOLOGY

LIGHT. In type I, there is marked thickening of the epidermis and the stratum corneum. In type II, there is thickening of the dermis with irregular collagen bundles and an increase in collagen, with hyperkeratosis of the overlying stratum corneum.
EM. Increased numbers of fibroblast-like and myofibroblast-like cells and macrophages and fine collagen fibers in type II.

BASIC DEFECT

Unknown.

TREATMENT

Mixed results with application of potent corticosteroids.

MODE OF INHERITANCE

Autosomal dominant. Most cases have been sporadic.

PRENATAL DIAGNOSIS

None.

DIFFERENTIAL DIAGNOSIS

Trauma, especially occupational, can result in callosities that mimic knuckle pads. These calluses retain normal skin line markings, which knuckle pads do not. Knuckle pads can be seen in association with leukonychia, deafness, and palmoplantar hyperkeratosis (Bart-Pumphrey syndrome, MIM: 149200). They are also described in a number of other palmoplantar keratodermas and in acrokeratoelastoidosis (MIM: 101850). Patients with Ehlers-Danlos syndrome type I can occasionally have knuckle pads. Subcutaneous granuloma annulare can mimic knuckle pads; in granuloma annulare there are likely to be lesions elsewhere as well. Biopsy may be required if question remains.

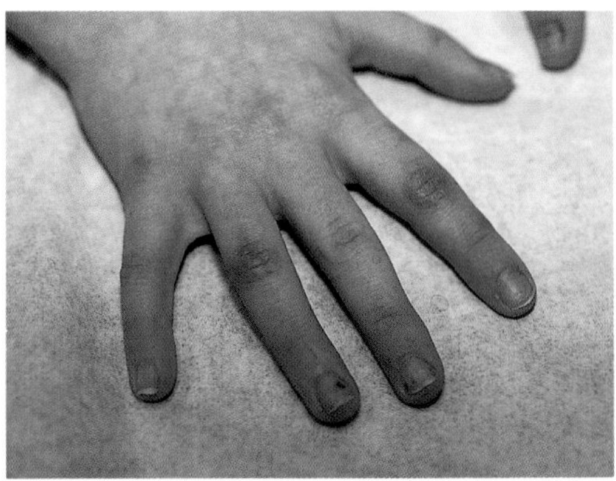

Figure 2.81. Early changes of thickening and erythema over PIP joints. Most obvious on the index finger.

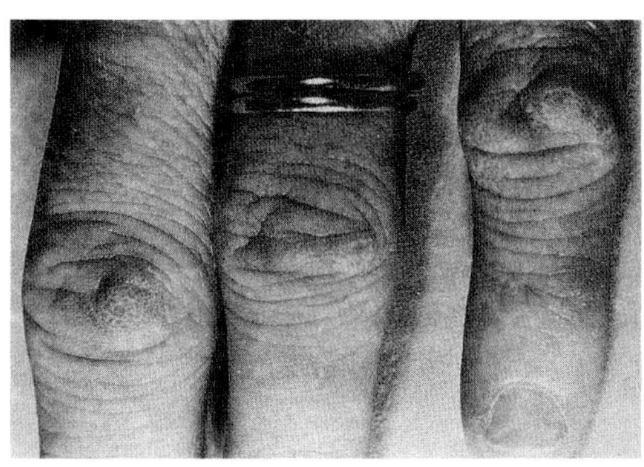

Figure 2.82. Knuckle pads in patient with Bart-Pumphrey syndrome. (From Ramer et al., 1994.)

Support Group: N.O.R.D.
P.O. Box 8923
New Fairfield, CT
06812
1-800-999-6673

SELECTED BIBLIOGRAPHY

Garrod, A.E. (1893). On an unusual form of nodule upon the joints of the fingers. *St. Bartholomew's Hosp. Rep.* **29,** 157–161.

Garrod, A.E. (1904). Concerning pads upon the finger joints and their clinical relationships. *Br. J. Med.* **2,** 8.

Initial report of three patients, one of whose brothers were also affected and whose father has Dupuytren's. The subsequent paper described 12 cases, of which nine had a personal or family history of Dupuytren's with knuckle pads.

Hueston, J.T., and Wilson, W.F. (1973). Knuckle pads. *Aust. N.Z.J. Surg.* **42,** 274–277.

Reviews subcutaneous knuckle pads.

Morginson, W.J. (1955). Discrete keratodermas over the knuckle and finger articulations. *A.M.A. Arch. Dermatol.* **71,** 349–353.

Reviews hyperkeratotic knuckle pads.

Paller, A.S., and Hebert, A.A. (1986). Knuckle pads in children. *Am. J. Dis. Child.* **140,** 915–917.

The authors present four cases, two with palmoplantar keratoderma. There is a review of the literature.

Ramos Silva, J. (1956). Coussinets des phalanges ("Pulvillus digiti"). *Ann. Dermatol. Syphiligr. (Paris)* **83,** 22–33.

Beautiful photographs of knuckle pads in Renaissance art.

Richards, T.B., Gamble, J.F., Castellan, R.M., and Matthias, T. (1987). Knuckle pads in live-chicken hangers. *Contact Dermatitis* **17,** 13–16.

Vegetarianism does not protect; knuckle pads have also been described in gardeners.

KYRLE/FLEGEL DISEASE (MIM:149500,144150)

(Hyperkeratosis Follicularis et Parafollicularis in Cutem Penetrans; Hyperkeratosis Lenticularis Perstans)

DERMATOLOGIC FEATURES

MAJOR. Kyrle disease and Flegel disease are both extraordinarily rare and share in common many features. Debate has raged as to the relationship between the two, and the major differentiating feature has been histopathology. Reports of the presence of typical microscopic findings of both diseases in each of two individuals has put question to the separate identity of the disorders.

Both are characterized by the development in middle age of a generalized eruption of small (Flegel) to medium (Kyrle) sized flattish scaly red-brown lesions that may develop a hyperkeratotic plug. Legs are the primary site of involvement. Palms, soles, and mucous membranes are spared. Old lesions may resolve a new ones develop. Coalescence into plaques (Kyrle) has been described. Koebnerization is more typical of Flegel but has been described for Kyrle disease also.

MINOR. In one family with Flegel disease, squamous cell carcinoma developed in uninvolved sites in four of six affected family members; one relative had squamous cell carcinoma without Flegel disease.

ASSOCIATED ABNORMALITIES

An association with diabetes mellitus and/or glucose tolerance test abnormalities has been noted for both disorders. Chronic renal disease is often associated, especially in nonfamilial cases. It has been estimated that 10% of patients on renal dialysis will develop Kyrle disease.

In one pedigree with Kyrle disease, 3 of 13 affected individuals had anterior stromal corneal opacities; two of these had posterior subcapsular cataracts.

HISTOPATHOLOGY

LIGHT. In Kyrle disease, a keratotic plug with patchy parakeratosis fills an epithelial invagination. There is basophilic debris in the base of the plug. Perforation is variable. In Flegel

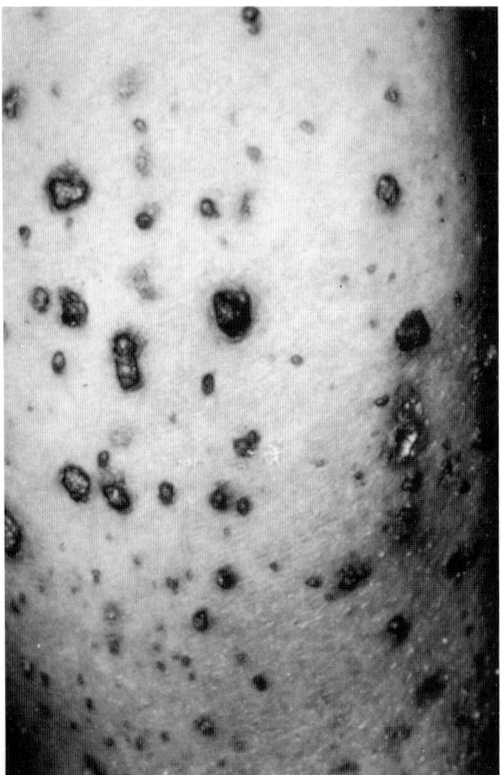

Figure 2.83. Keratotic plugs and fine scale in Kyrle disease. (From Cunningham et al., 1987.)

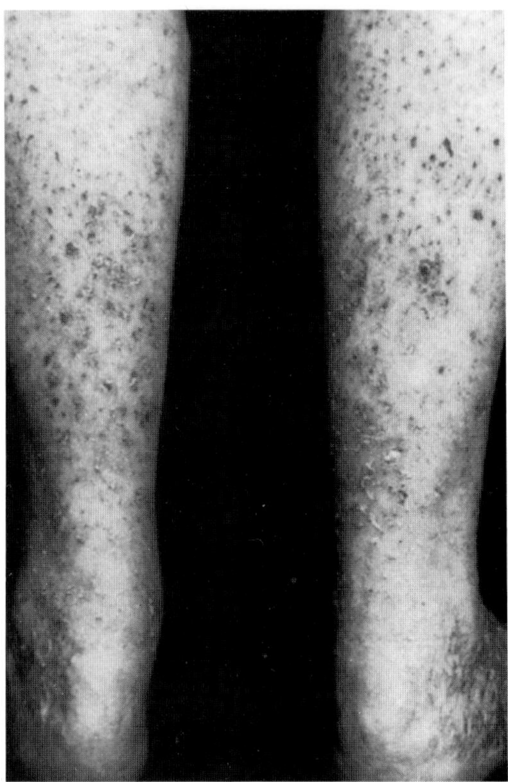

Figure 2.84. Hyperkeratotic lesions scattered over legs. (From Tidman et al., 1987.)

disease, there is compact hyperkeratosis with occasional parakeratosis with decrease to absence of the granular layer. There is a bandlike lymphohistiocytic infiltrate in the papillary dermis.

EM. In Flegel disease, there is reduction in keratohyaline granules with intracytoplasmic inclusions in the dermal infiltrate. Absence of lamellar bodies been described in some but not all patients.

BASIC DEFECT

Unknown.

TREATMENT

5-Fluorouracil is reported to be effective, and there has been mixed success with tretinoin.

MODE OF INHERITANCE

Unclear. Most cases are sporadic. Some pedigrees have involved sibships only; one pedigree demonstrates pseudodominance. Flegel disease has been described in three generations in one pedigree; in two in another.

PRENATAL DIAGNOSIS

None.

DIFFERENTIAL DIAGNOSIS

In perforating folliculitis only the follicles are involved, the papules are smaller, and coalescence does not occur. Lesions usually contain a curled hair. In reactive perforating collagenosis (MIM:216700) onset is in childhood. Individual lesions may be shorter lived. Involvement of the face and upper extremities is more common, and histopathology shows necrotic changes in collagen. Lesions often developed in sites of trauma. There is a significant clinical overlap with Kyrle disease. Inheritance is probably autosomal recessive. Response to topical tretinoin has been reported.

Elastosis perforans serpiginosa (MIM: 130100) is usually more circinate and more localized. The histopathology will differentiate elastosis perforans serpiginosa from other conditions. Although elastosis perforans serpiginosa is listed in the dominant catalog, recurrences in three sibships (one consanguineous) have also been described in the literature. The lesions of Darier-White disease (MIM: 124200) tend to have a greasier-appearing scale, and the distribution tends to be in the upper extremities. Biopsy will differentiate.

Support Group: N.O.R.D.
P.O. Box 8923
New Fairfield, CT
06812
1-800-999-6673

SELECTED BIBLIOGRAPHY

Ayala, F., and Donofrio, P. (1983). Elastosis perforans serpiginosa. Report of a family. *Dermatologica* **166,** 32–37.

Two brothers born to first cousins once removed. Onset began in the second year of life.

Bean, S.F. (1969). Hyperkeratosis lenticularis perstans. A clinical, histopathologic, and genetic study. *Arch. Dermarol.* **99,** 705–709.

Bean, S.F. (1972). The genetics of hyperkeratosis lenticularis perstans. *Arch. Dermatol.* **106,** 72.

Three generation pedigree initially described in 1969. Onset in late adult life may hamper recognition of the inheritance of the disorder.

Beveridge, G.W., and Langlands, A.V. (1973). Familial hyperkeratosis lenticularis perstans associated with tumours of the skin. *Br. J. Dermatol.* **88,** 453–458.

Unclear if malignancy is segregating independently in this family. All skin tumors except one arose in skin sites unaffected by hyperkeratosis lenticularis perstans. In addition to squamous cell carcinoma, one patient had anaplastic carcinoma of the lung.

Ford, T.C., Mirarchi, J.A., and Castillo, J. (1990). Kyrle's disease. A rare case report and surgical treatment. *J. Am. Podiatr. Med. Assoc.* **80,** 151–155.

No mention of genetics but a good review of clinical features and the literature.

Langeveld-Wildschut, E.G., Toonstra, J., van Vloten, W.A., and Beemer, F.A. (1993). Familial elastosis perforans serpiginosa. *Arch. Dermatol.* **129,** 205–207.

Presents two generation family with male-to-male transmission and reviews previous familial reports which suggest either genetic heterogeneity or incomplete penetrance.

Patterson, J.W. (1984). The perforating disorders. *J. Am. Acad. Dermatol.* **10,** 561–581.

Reviews perforating disorders. Suggests that Kyrle disease always is acquired and is not genetic.

Pearson, L.H., Smith, J.G. Jr., and Chalker, D.K. (1987). Hyperkeratosis lenticularis perstans (Flegel's disease). Case report and literature review. *J. Am. Acad. Dermatol.* **16,** 190–195.

Isolated report with color photographs.

Tidman, M.J., Price, M.L., and MacDonald, D.M. (1987). Lamellar bodies in hyperkeratosis lenticularis perstans. *J. Cutan. Pathol.* **14,** 207–211.

In contrast to others, these authors found no alterations in lamellar bodies in four individuals studied.

ULERYTHEMA OPHRYOGENES (MIM:209700)

(Keratosis Pilaris Atrophicans Faciei; Folliculitis Rubra; Atrophoderma Vermiculata)

Includes Erythromelanosis Follicularis Faciei et Colli

DERMATOLOGIC FEATURES

Major. Small, horny, rough follicular papules develop in the eyebrows and on the cheeks in infancy or early childhood. They are usually on an erythematous base. As resolution occurs, pitted scars and eyebrow loss may result.

In atrophoderma vermiculata, which may be the same disorder or genetically distinct, the onset of the lesions occurs later in childhood, and the preauricular and cheek areas are most frequently involved. The follicular plugs leave honeycomb scarring when they are shed.

Minor. None.

ASSOCIATED ABNORMALITIES

Ulerythema ophryogenes has been noted in association with Noonan syndrome (MIM: 163950). The causal relationship between the two conditions is not known.

HISTOPATHOLOGY

Light. Early in the process there is hyperkeratosis of pilosebaceous units with a mild, nonspecific inflammatory infiltrate. Cheek lesions may show cystic dilation and dense subepidermal aggregation of apparently normal elastic fibers. Late stages are marked by atrophy of sebaceous glands and hair follicles and dermal fibrosis.

EM. No information.

BASIC DEFECT

Unknown.

TREATMENT

Keratolytics such as urea or the α-hydroxy acids (α-glycolic acid, lactic acid) may be beneficial. A few of my patients with atrophoderma vermiculata have responded well to topical retinoids.

MODE OF INHERITANCE

Autosomal dominant. It is not clear why McKusick lists atrophoderma vermiculata as a possi-

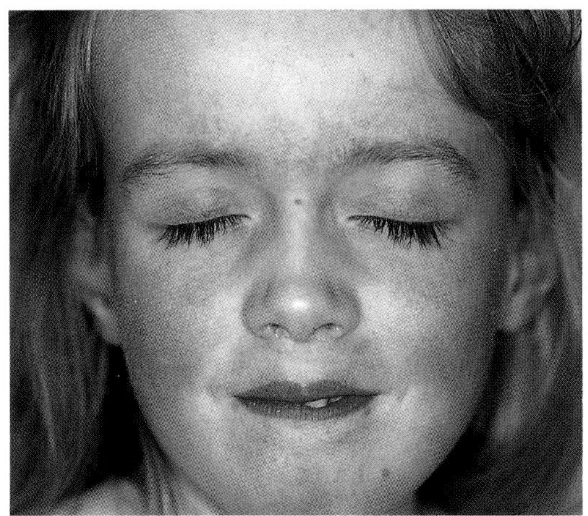

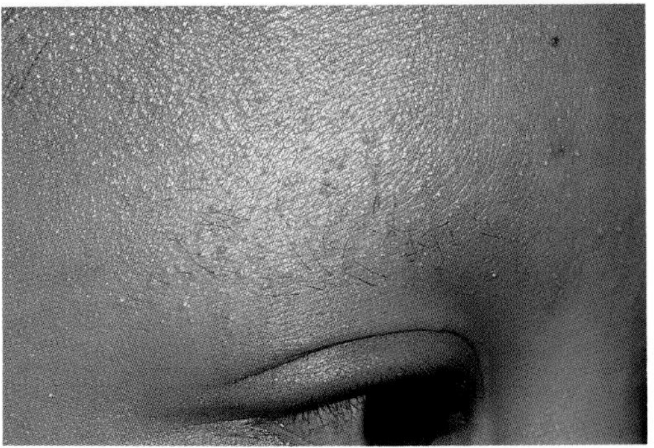

Figure 2.85. **(A)** Involvement of eyebrows without loss of hairs. **(B)** Involvement of eyebrows with hair loss.

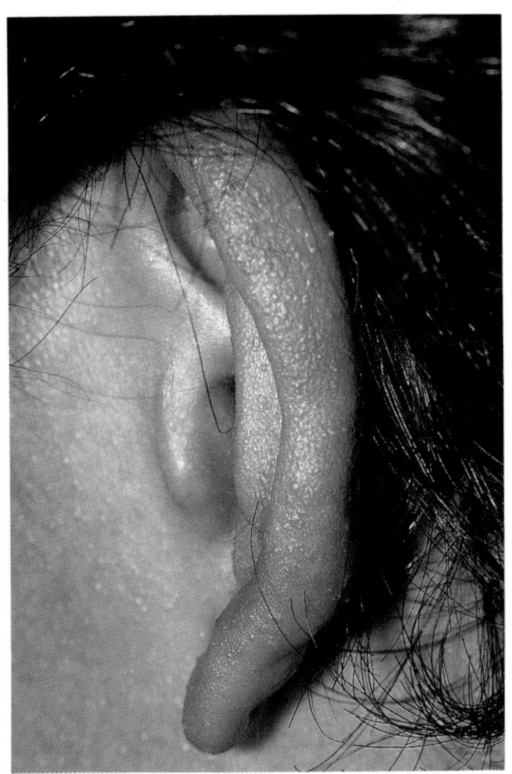

Figure 2.86. Involvement of pinna.

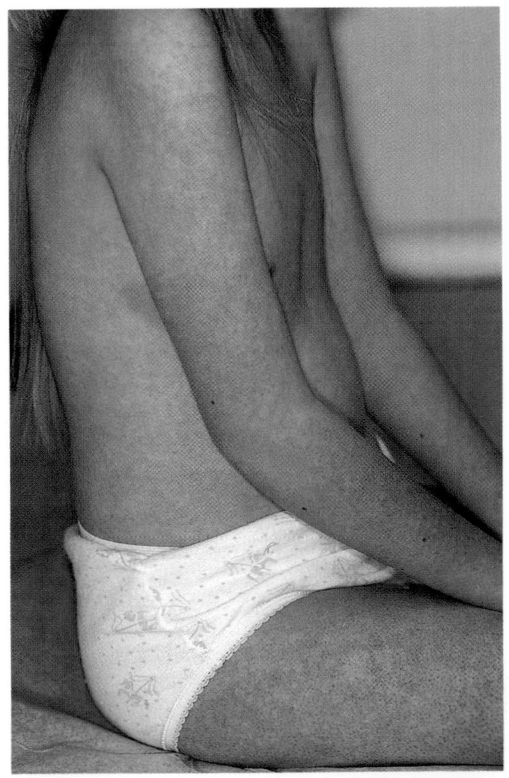

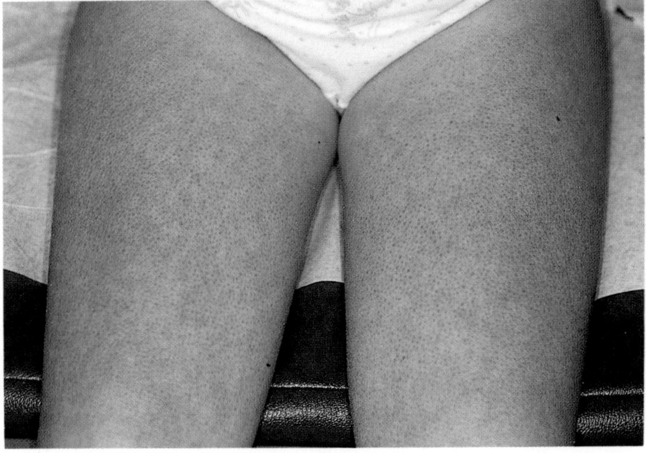

Figure 2.87. **(A)** Arms and legs. **(B)** Close-up of involvement of the thighs.

ble autosomal recessive condition, as the evidence cited for autosomal recessive inheritance is one pedigree of an affected mother with two affected children. An affected father and daughter have been reported in the literature, and we have seen an affected father and daughter.

PRENATAL DIAGNOSIS

None.

DIFFERENTIAL DIAGNOSIS

The individual lesions of isolated keratosis pilaris or keratosis pilaris in association with ichthyosis vulgaris (MIM:146700) may be difficult to distinguish clinically from ulerythema ophryogenes. Distribution of lesions in the former is usually on the outer aspects of the upper arms and tops of the thighs, although the cheeks may be involved. The erythema is usually less, the eyebrows are usually not involved, and resolving lesions do not leave scars in keratosis pilaris. The red, perifollicular hyperkeratoses of keratosis follicularis spinulosa decalvans (MIM:308800) can appear similar, and loss of eyebrows also occurs. Photophobia, with corneal dystrophy and scarring alopecia of the scalp, are features of keratosis follicularis spinulosa decalvans not seen in ulerythema. The horny papules of Darier-White disease (MIM:124200) are greasier in appearance, and involvement is more widespread.

Cardiofaciocutaneous syndrome is the name given to individuals with features of Noonan syndrome (MIM:163950) plus curly hair with a high frontal and temporal hairline, koilonychia, and ulerythema ophryogenes. In my opinion, it represents a subset of Noonan syndrome.

Erythromelanosis follicularis faciei et colli (MIM:None) is marked by asymptomatic brown follicular keratotic papules that develop in adolescence on the face, eyebrows, ears, neck, and upper arms. There is both erythema and hyperpigmentation. The lack of scarring and sparing of eyebrow hairs plus the hyperpigmentation differentiate this from ulerythema ophryogenes, but the disorders are very similar. There have been three familial reports; most cases are sporadic.

Support Group: F.I.R.S.T.
P.O. Box 20921
Raleigh, NC 27619
1-800-545-3286

SELECTED BIBLIOGRAPHY

Davenport, D.D. (1904). Ulerythema ophryogenes. *Arch. Dermatol.* **89,** 74–80.

A single case report of an affected male whose condition did not respond to vitamin A given intramuscularly.

Frosch, P.J., Brumage, M.R., Schuster-Pavlovic, C., et al. (1988). Atrophoderma vermiculatum. *J. Am. Acad. Dermatol.* **18,** 538–542.

Case report of a father and daughter with atrophoderma vermiculatum. There is an excellent discussion of differential diagnosis and overlap with ulerythema ophryogenes.

Pierini, D.D., and Pierini, A.M. (1979). Keratosis pilaris atrophicans faciei (ulerythema ophryogenes): a cutaneous marker in the Noonan syndrome. *Br. J. Dermatol.* **100,** 409–416.

Discusses the association of ulerythema ophryogenes and Noonan syndrome.

Ward, K.A., Moss, C., and McKeown, C. (1994). *Br. J. Dermatol.* **131,** 270–274.

Presents family and reviews literature, arguing against cardio-facio-cutaneous syndrome representing a distinct disorder.

Yanez, S., Velasco, J.A., and Gonzalez, M.P. (1993). Familial erythromelanosis follicularis faciei et colli—an autosomal recessive mode of inheritance. *Clin. Exp. Dermatol.* **18,** 283–285.

Acay, M.C. (1993). Erythromelanosis follicularis faciei et colli: A genetic disorder? Letter. *Int. J. Dermatol.* **32,** 542.

Acay reported a sister–brother pair and an affected son, mother, and maternal grandmother. Yanez et al. (1993) described two affected siblings, offspring of a third cousin mating.

SYNDROMIC DISORDERS

CHILD SYNDROME (MIM:308050)

(Ichthyosiform Erythroderma, Unilateral, with Ipsilateral Malformations, Especially Absence Deformity of Limbs)

DERMATOLOGIC FEATURES

MAJOR. The skin changes may be present at birth but can develop weeks after birth. The involved areas are red, thickened, with a greasy adherent yellow scale. Areas of involvement can change over time, and spontaneous regression has been reported, as well as late occurrence in previously uninvolved skin.

Clinically, the lesions are very similar to an inflammatory linear verrucous epidermal nevus. Some have proposed the term *psoriasiform epidermal nevus* to refer to both of these lesions.

Classically, the entire right or entire left half of the body is involved, but there are some reports of lesions confined to smaller areas defined by the lines of Blaschko. Islands of unaffected skin on the involved side, also following the lines of Blaschko, have been noted.

MINOR. Involved nails can be grossly deformed, hyperkeratotic, and dysplastic.

ASSOCIATED ABNORMALITIES

Skeletal: The skeletal changes are usually, but not always, ipsilateral with the skin findings. Unilateral defects of the long bones range from

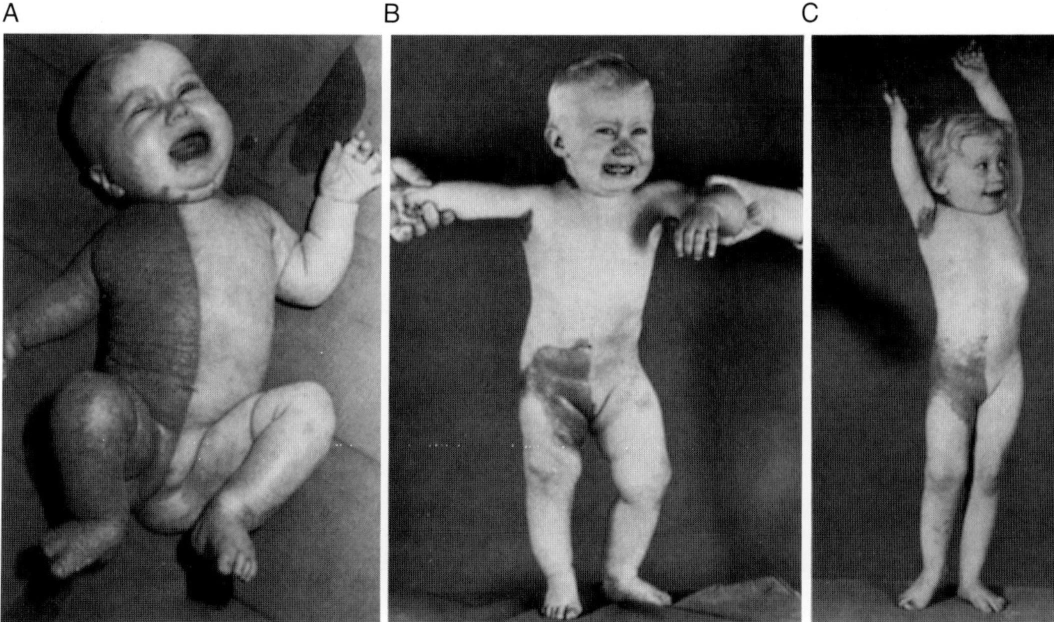

Figure 2.88. (A–C). Skin involvement sharply demarcated at the midline, with changes over time. There is ipsilateral limb hypoplasia. (From Happle et al., 1980.)

minimal to terminal transverse defects of phalanges to complete absence of the long bones. Unilateral vertebral anomalies can result in scoliosis. Unilateral pelvic, calvarial, mandibular, clavicular, scapular, and rib hypoplasia have all been reported. Unilateral stippling of the epiphyses has been found.

Neurologic: Ipsilateral hypoplasia of the brain, cranial nerves, and/or spinal cord has been described. Some patients have normal intellect.

Other: Cardiac and renal malformations are frequent. At autopsy, one patient was found to have hypoplasia of multiple organs, including the thyroid, adrenals, ovaries, and fallopian tubes.

HISTOPATHOLOGY

LIGHT. The epidermis is acanthotic and spongiotic with parakeratotic and orthokeratotic stratum corneum. The granular layer can be increased or absent. There is a lymphohistiocytic infiltrate present in the dermis.

EM. There is a reduction in keratin filaments and keratohyalin and an increase in mitochondria. Malformation of cementsomes is described. Keratohyalin is globular rather than stellate; there is unidentified abnormal material in the intracellular spaces. There are some differences in findings among case reports.

BASIC DEFECT

Unknown. Fibroblasts cultured from the involved skin of a CHILD patient had a lower proliferative rate, generated PGE_2 prior to confluence, and produced greater amounts of PGE_2 when stimulated with indomethacin than did cultured cells from the uninvolved skin of the same individual. The authors interpreted these findings to indicate that the ichthyosis in CHILD syndrome may be the result of dermal, rather than epidermal, factors. Tissue from a second patient demonstrated continued production of K_5 and K_{14}, basal cell keratins, throughout the upper cell layers of the epidermis and decreased suprabasal production of K_1 and K_{10}, the keratins of differentiation. Cells in culture did not differ from normal in the keratins produced, but did appear morphologically altered.

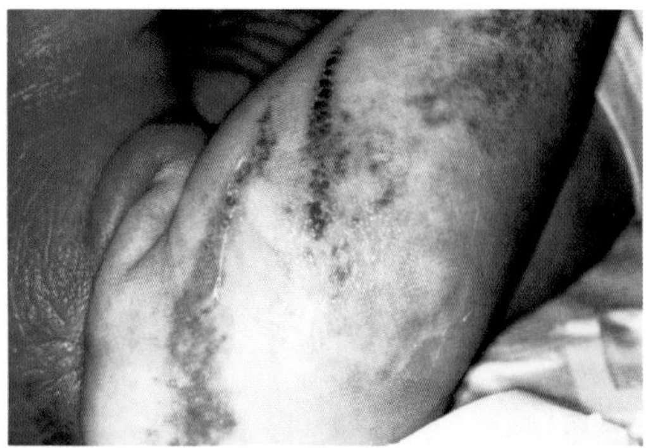

Figure 2.89. Upper thigh and abdomen with thickened leather-like changes; hyperkeratotic streaks on other leg. (From Hashimoto et al., 1995.)

Epiphyseal stippling is characteristic of the peroxisomal diseases. Its presence in CHILD syndrome suggests that investigation into defects in long chain fatty acid degradation may be fruitful.

TREATMENT

Usual treatment for ichthyosis, including urea or α-hydroxy acid–based emollients, is not particularly helpful.

Orthopedic management of the limb defects and appropriate treatment of the visceral abnormalities must be individualized.

MODE OF INHERITANCE

Unknown. Almost all cases have been sporadic. Happle et al. (1980) have proposed that CHILD is an X-linked lethal dominant trait. Most reported patients are female.

There has been one report of two affected sisters born to healthy parents, which could be explained by gonadal mosaicism in a parent, with extreme lyonization in each of the offspring.

One report described psoriasis in the mother and grandmother and possible psoriasis in a maternal aunt of a proband. This report has been inappropriately cited as a documented familial occurrence of CHILD. A third report stated that a maternal aunt of the proband died in infancy of congenital heart disease, and "it was noted the left side of her body was smaller than the right." A maternal first cousin once removed died at 3 months of age with a "similar problem, and, in addition, had skin lesions." What the skin lesions were and whether limb malformations were present are not stated. This seems rather weak support for familial occurrence.

PRENATAL DIAGNOSIS

None.

DIFFERENTIAL DIAGNOSIS

Moss and Burn suggested (1990) that the isolated linear inflammatory verrucous epidermal nevus (ILVEN) was at one end of a continuum shared by CHILD, perhaps reflecting a postzygotic somatic mutation for the same defect. When the mutation occurs very early it results in diffuse unilateral involvement; when it occurs later in embryogenesis, involvement is much more limited. Others believe ILVEN is distinguished from CHILD by intense pruritus and by its failure to show female predominance.

Epidermal nevus syndrome (MIM:163200) is a sporadic condition that encompasses a heterogeneous group of disorders including sebaceous nevus syndrome. Some cases of CHILD syndrome have been described as having epidermal nevus. The skin lesions of CHILD tend to be more ichthyosiform with erythroderma and those of the epidermal nevus syndrome more verrucous, usually without erythroderma.

Conradi-Hunermann syndrome (chondrodysplasia punctata, MIM:302960) shares in common with CHILD syndrome limb defects, unilateral or asymmetric involvement, and stippling of the epiphyses. Follicular atrophoderma is not a feature of CHILD syndrome, and widespread, bilateral patchy skin involvement with ichthyosiform erythroderma is far more typical of Conradi-Hunermann. The "feather edge" scaling of Conradi-Hunermann is distinctive.

Support Group: F.I.R.S.T.
P.O. Box 20921
Raleigh, NC 27619
1-800-545-3286

SELECTED BIBLIOGRAPHY

Dale, B.A., Kimball, J.R., Fleckman, P., Hebert, A.A., and Holbrook, K.A. (1992). CHILD syndrome: lack of expression of epidermal differentiation markers in lesional ichthyotic skin. *J. Invest. Dermatol.* **98,** 442–449.

Investigation of keratin production and epithelial cell culture characteristics in one patient with CHILD.

Falek, A., Heath, C.W. Jr., Ebbin, A.J., and McLean, W.R. (1968). Unilateral limb and skin deformities with congenital heart disease in two siblings: a lethal syndrome. *Pediatrics* **73,** 910–913.

Two sisters born to unrelated healthy parents. A third pregnancy ended in a spontaneous loss.

Goldyne, M.E., and Williams M. (1989). CHILD syndrome. Phenotypic dichotomy in eicosanoid metabolism and proliferative rates among cultured dermal fibroblasts. *Clin. Invest.* **84,** 357–360.

Cells cultured from involved and uninvolved skin demonstrated differences in proliferation and PGE_2 production from one patient with CHILD syndrome.

Happle, R., Koch, H., and Lenz, W. (1980). The CHILD syndrome. Congenital hemidysplasia with ichthyosiform erythroderma and limb defects. *Eur. J. Pediatr.* **134,** 27–33.

Detailed review of 18 cases with two new of their own. Propose the acronym CHILD and argue that the disorder is X-linked lethal dominant.

Hashimoto, K., Topper, S., Sharata, H., and Edwards, M. (1995). CHILD syndrome: analysis of abnormal keratinization and ultrastructure. *Pediatr. Dermatol.* **12,** 116–129.

Detailed electron micrograph study of a single patient.

Moss, C., and Burn, J. (1990). CHILD +

ILVEN = PEN or PENCIL. *J. Med. Genet.* **27**, 390–391.

The authors propose that CHILD and ILVEN represent distal ends of a continuum that results from postzygotic mutation, the expression of which is dependent on the stage in embryogenesis at which the mutation occurs.

Shear, C.S., Nyhan W.L., Frost, P., and Weinstein, G. (1971). Syndrome of unilateral ectromelia, psoriasis and central nervous system anomalies. *Birth Defects* **7(8)**, 197–203.

The proposita with a family history of psoriasis had been reported previously by Cullen et al. (*Arch. Dermatol.* **99**, 724–729, 1969). Autoradiographic studies demonstrated increased cell proliferation in cells cultured from the involved side. Her skin findings improved during a short course of methotrexate.

CHONDRODYSPLASIA PUNCTATA (MIM:118650, 215100, 302950, 302960)

(Chondrodystrophica Calcificans Congenita; Conradi-Hunermann Disease; Happle Syndrome)

The term *chondrodysplasia punctata* is not disease specific, and stippling of the epiphyses is a feature of many disorders. However, the term has been selectively applied to several conditions marked by ichthyosis and bone changes. The eponym Conradi-Hunermann syndrome has also been used for several of these conditions.

DERMATOLOGIC FEATURES

MAJOR. The skin findings in both the X-linked dominant form and the autosomal recessive or rhizomelic form of chondrodysplasia punctata are similar. Skin changes are seen in almost all individuals with the X-linked dominant form and reported in about 25% of patients with the autosomal recessive form.

At birth there is often a thick cheesy tenacious quality to the vernix with underlying adherent scale and erythroderma. Remnants of a collodion membrane, particularly on the extremities and around the hands and feet, may be present.

The scaling has a feather-like edge. It has been described as horny or spikey, but it looks more like the edging on lace to me. In the X-linked recessive form of chondrodysplasia punctata, which is part of a contiguous gene syndrome, the ichthyosis is more similar to that of sterol sulfatase deficiency.

Follicular atrophoderma is the second major skin finding. The term refers to dells or icepick-like scars and/or dilated follicular orifices. While the follicular atrophoderma is usually distributed along the lines of Blaschko, the ichthyosis may be patchy, diffuse, along the lines of Blaschko, or without obvious pattern.

MINOR. Patchy scarring alopecia is typical. The hairs that are present may be coarse, wiry, lusterless, or sparse. *Pseudopelade* is a term that has been used in the literature to describe the alopecia. There may be thinning to absence of the eyebrows and eyelashes.

ASSOCIATED ABNORMALITIES

Stippling of the epiphyses represents premature calcification. The pattern of distribution of stippling differs among the chondrodysplasia punctata syndromes but may not be distinctive enough to allow for diagnostic certainty. As bone maturation proceeds and the epiphyses begin to calcify further, the stippled appearance is lost. Coronal clefting of the vertebrae is common. The skeletal changes are typically asymmetric with variable shortening of the limbs in the X-linked dominant form, severe and symmetric in the rhizomelic form. Mild short stature and limb length discrepancy is frequently seen in the X-linked dominant form.

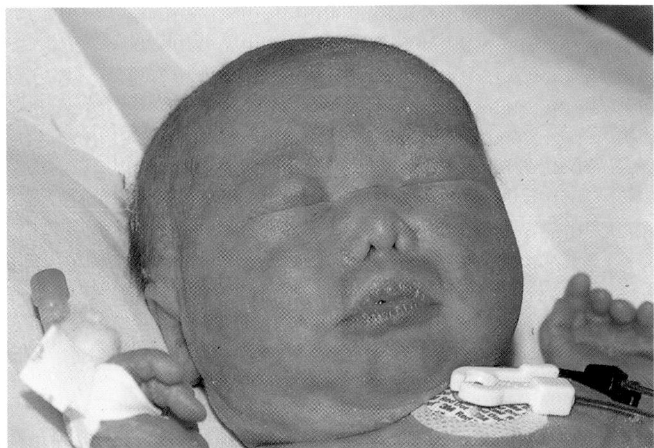

A

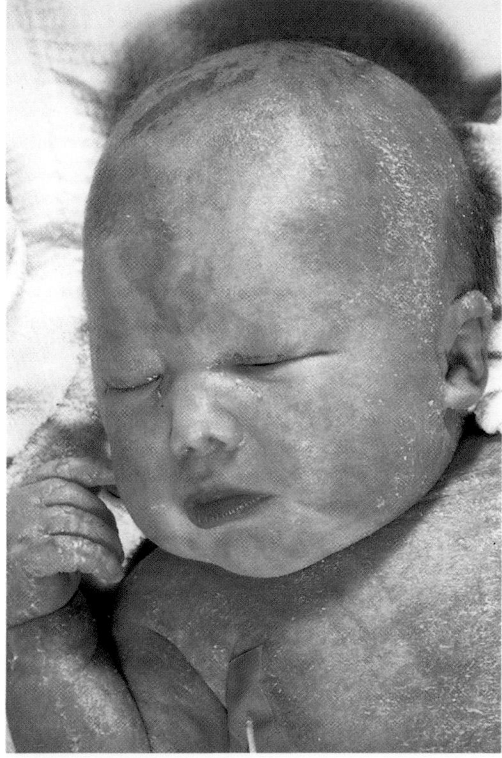

B

Figure 2.90. **(A,B)** Two newborns. The nostrils are pinched, philtrum and lips are full, and there is a rim of fine scalp hairs with baldness over the pate.

In the autosomal recessive form, dwarfing is severe and constant.

Eye findings are also common. Changes are seen in 70% of patients with the autosomal recessive form and are usually bilateral and symmetric. They are less frequently seen in the X-linked dominant form and tend to be asymmetric or unilateral. Cataracts are the typical feature, but microcornea and microophthalmia are also described.

The facial appearance associated with chondrodysplasia punctata is shared by all forms—a flattened nasal tip with a very short columella, and often deep vertical grooving between the nasal tip and the nostrils is typical.

Intelligence in the X-linked dominant form was normal in 13 of 15 cases in which intellectual development was mentioned.

HISTOPATHOLOGY

Light. The changes are nonspecific. There is thickening of the stratum corneum with focal hyperparakeratosis, a decreased granular layer, and marked follicular plugging, which may stain positively for calcium.

EM. Small vacuoles, some of which contain needle-like calcium inclusions, are seen in the keratinocytes in the granular layer.

BASIC DEFECT

Unknown. In the autosomal recessive form there is an increase in red blood cell plasmalogen with a deficiency of DHAP-AT, suggesting that it may be a peroxisomal disorder.

The X-linked dominant form appears to be homologous to the bare patches locus in the mouse. A candidate gene, *BGN,* has been pro-

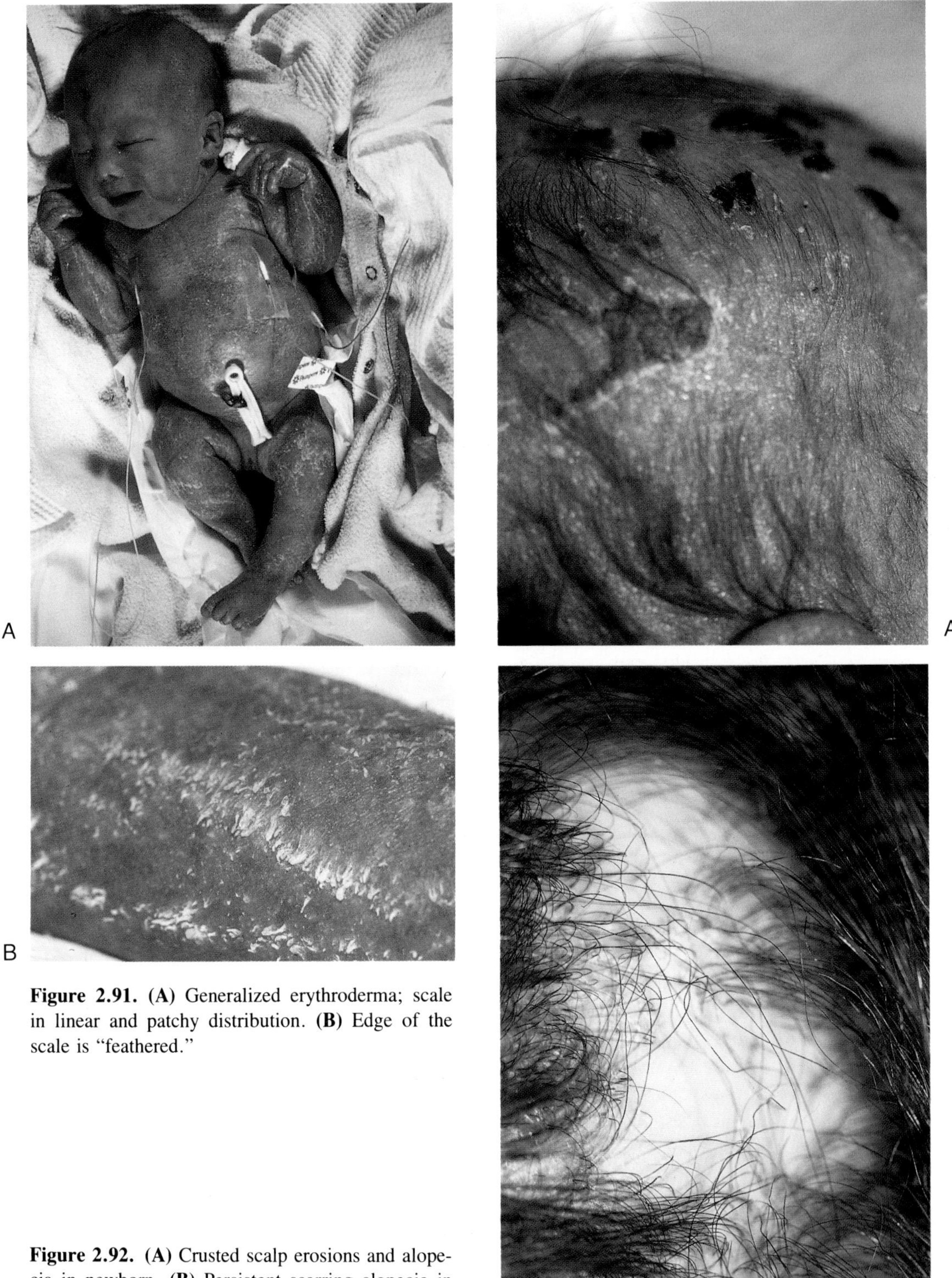

Figure 2.91. **(A)** Generalized erythroderma; scale in linear and patchy distribution. **(B)** Edge of the scale is "feathered."

Figure 2.92. **(A)** Crusted scalp erosions and alopecia in newborn. **(B)** Persistent scarring alopecia in adult.

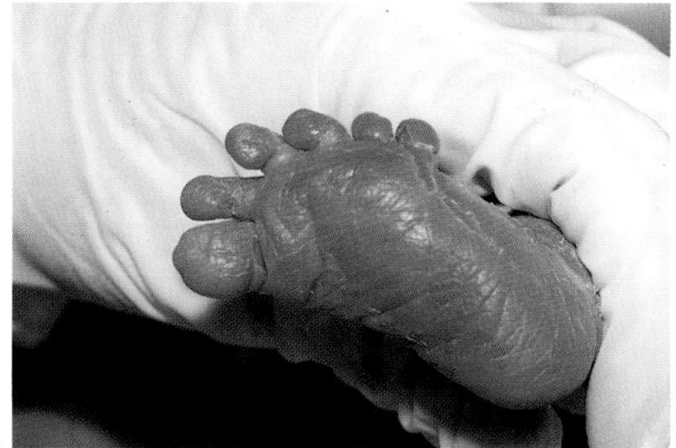

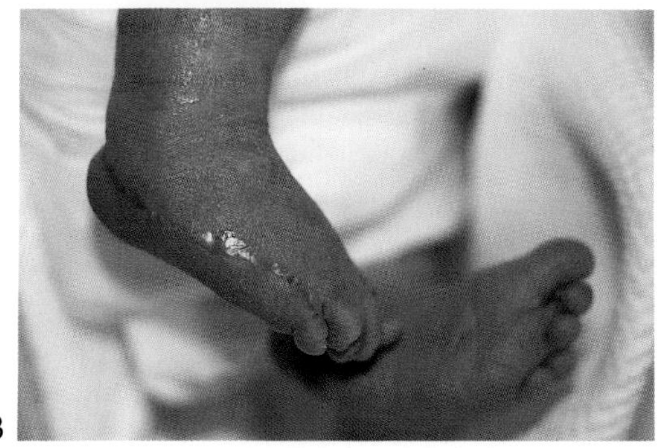

Figure 2.93. **(A)** Foot showing polydactyly and remnants of collodion membrane. **(B)** Different infant with linear remnant of membrane and scaling on foot.

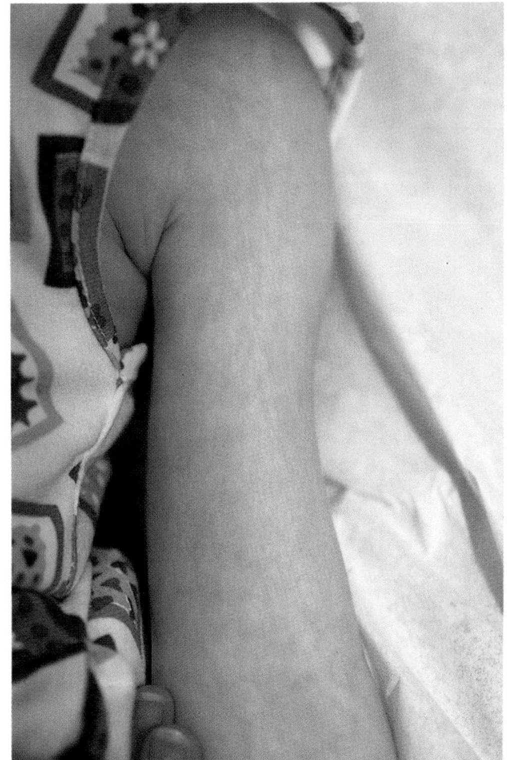

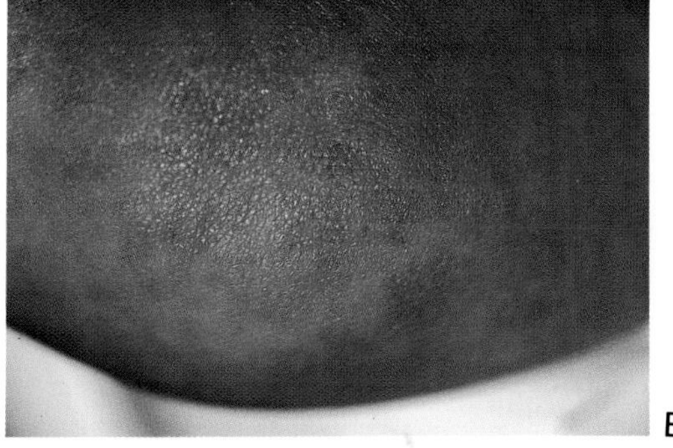

Figure 2.94. **(A)** Linear hypopigmented streaks in a now 6 year old. **(B)** Follicular atrophoderma (coarse follicular pores) in adult.

posed, but linkage studies do not support a relationship with the disease.

TREATMENT

The ichthyotic skin changes resolve fairly rapidly over several months to a year. In my experience, less treatment is more. Light liquid emollients will help to speed up shedding of any collodion membrane remnants; use of thick creams and ointments usually retards this process. The erythroderma fades on its own, and the scaling is usually relatively asymptomatic. If topical urea or lactic acid containing agents do not result in improvement, I am inclined to stick with simple emollients and let nature do its job. Orthopedic management is important, as is careful ophthalmologic follow-up.

MODE OF INHERITANCE

X-linked dominant: This is the most common form of chondrodysplasia punctata that I have seen. This may be ascertainment bias, as the dermatologic findings usually far overshadow the skeletal abnormalities in the X-linked dominant form compared with the autosomal recessive rhizomelic form. The condition may map to Xq27–28.

Autosomal recessive: Marked by severe symmetric rhizomelic shortening of the limbs. By complementation studies, this disorder is biochemically and genetically heterogeneous.

Autosomal dominant: I am unconvinced that any case of chondrodysplasia punctata that might be autosomal dominant in inheritance has skin findings. Almost all of the reports with skin findings claimed to represent autosomal dominant inheritance are of sporadic cases with no family history.

X-linked recessive: These may all be the result of submicroscopic deletions of the sterol sulfatase locus (Xp22.3–Xpter), with deletion of contiguous genes resulting in other features including stippled epiphyses. The gene for chondrodysplasia punctata appears to be distal to the STS locus.

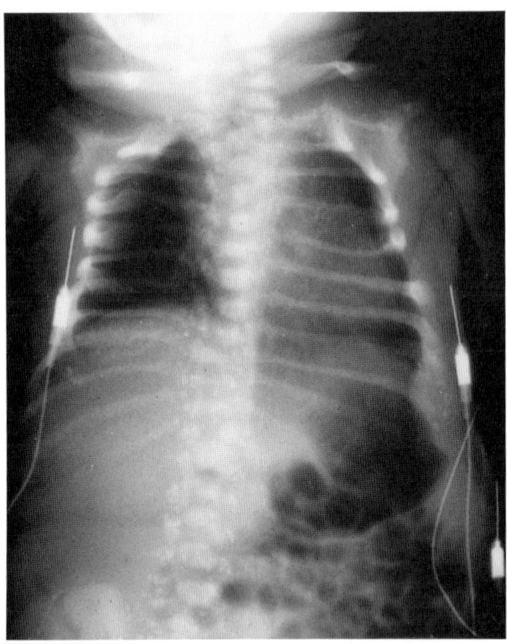

Figure 2.95. Multiple areas of stippling.

PRENATAL DIAGNOSIS

Unreliable.

DIFFERENTIAL DIAGNOSIS

The skin changes of chondrodysplasia punctata can appear somewhat similar to those of Netherton syndrome (MIM:256500). In ichthyosis linearis circumflexa, the ichthyosis may also be serpiginous, but it lacks the feathery border of chondrodysplasia punctata. Trichorrhexis invaginata is not a feature of chondrodysplasia punctata, and follicular atrophoderma is not a feature of Netherton syndrome. CHILD syndrome (MIM:308050) is marked by segmental ichthyosis. Unilateral skeletal involvement with stippling of the epiphyses and limb reduction defects has been reported. In contrast to chondrodysplasia punctata, the skin changes are not generalized, but limited to one half or less of the body. Although chondrodysplasia punctata is marked by congenital erythroderma, in my experience it is readily distinguished from bullous congenital ichthyosiform erythroderma (MIM:113800), in which skin changes are usually much more diffuse. Infants with chondrodysplasia punctata can present with remnants of a collodion membrane similar to nonbullous congenital ichthyosiform erythroderma (MIM:242300, 242100, 146750). Underlying differences in the distribution of the erythroderma and the ichthyosis, along with the typical facial and skeletal features, will make the diagnosis clear. The feathery edge of the scale of chondrodysplasia punctata is quite distinctive and, once seen, becomes an easily recognized feature. None of the other congenital erythrodermas are marked by stippling of the epiphyses. Some babies with chondrodysplasia punctata have mistakenly been labeled as incontinentia pigmenti (MIM:308300) in the literature. While the distribution of skin lesions in the two disorders is similar, the nature of the skin changes is not, and the conditions are difficult to confuse clinically.

Stippling of the epiphyses is a feature of many conditions, most notably Zellweger syndrome (MIM:214100), infantile Refsum syndrome (MIM:266510) and Coumadin/warfarin syndrome. These and other types of chondrodysplasia punctata (MIM:Many) have no skin changes.

Support Group: F.I.R.S.T.
P.O. Box 20921
Raleigh, NC 27619
1-800-545-3286

SELECTED BIBLIOGRAPHY

Bennett, C.P., Berry, A.C., Maxwell, D.J., and Seller, M.J. (1992). Chondrodysplasia punctata: another possible X-linked recessive case. *Am. J. Med. Genet.* **44,** 795–799.

Useful table of disorders of which chondrodysplasia punctata is a feature, with references.

Happle, R., Matthiass, H.H., and Micher, E. (1977). Sex-linked chondrodysplasia punctata? *Clin. Genet.* **11,** 73–76.

First argument for what in retrospect was obvious, the likelihood that at least one form of chondrodysplasia punctata was X-linked dominant. Previous descriptions of families failed to recognize that only females were involved. The term *dominant,* without adjectival adjunct, was used in most of these earlier reports.

Kolde, G., and Happle, R. (1984). Histologic and ultrastructural features of the ichthyotic skin in X-linked dominant chondrodysplasia punctata. *Acta Dermatol. Venereol. (Stockh.)* **64,** 389–394.

Light and electron microscopy of two children with X-linked dominant chondrodysplasia punctata. The authors state that the changes are different from other ichthyoses, but they do not compare their findings to skin changes in the rhizomelic form. Thus I do not know if biopsy can be helpful to distinguish between the two chondrodysplasia punctata/ichthyosis syndromes.

Manzke, H., Christopher, E., and Wiedemann, H.-R. (1980). Dominant sex-linked inherited chondrodysplasia punctata: a distinct type of chondrodysplasia punctata. *Clin. Genet.* **17,** 97–107.

Intrigued by a case report of Happle et al. (1977), these authors reviewed several of their own patients with chondrodysplasia punctata and found two families with an affected mother and daughter.

Sheffield, L.J., Danks, D.M., Mayne, V., and Hutchinson, L.A. (1976). Chondrodysplasia punctata—23 cases of a mild and relatively common variety. *J. Pediatr.* **89,** 916–923.

Twenty-three of 44 patients with stippling of the epiphyses are discussed in detail. All had stippling of the calcaneus. None had cataracts, some had intellectual impairment that was mild, and one-sixth died. One set of dizygotic twins and one sibship of three, all of whom were exposed to phenytoin and phenobarbital in utero, were affected. I am convinced they represent a teratogenic entity, and this report serves only to expand the conditions in which stippling is a feature. All other patients had a negative family history. None had skin changes.

Traupe, H., Muller, D., Atherton, D., Kalter, D.C., Cremers, F.P.M., van Oost, B.A., and Ropers, H.-H. (1992). Exclusion mapping of the X-linked dominant chondrodysplasia punctata/ichthyosis/cataract/short stature (Happle) syndrome: possible involvement of an unstable premutation. *Hum. Genet.* **89,** 659–665.

The authors failed to find linkage with any of 26 informative markers along the X chromosome, including those in the Xq28 region. The authors present several explanations and favor the idea of an unstable premutation that is silent in males.

Traupe, H., van den Ouweland, A.M.W., van Oost, B.A., Vogel, W., Vetter, U., Warren, S.T., Rocchi, M., Darlis, M.M.G., and Ropers, H.-H. (1992). Fine mapping of the human biglycan (BGN) gene within the Xq28 region employing a hybrid cell panel. *Genomics* **13,** 481–483.

The authors endow X-linked dominant chondrodysplasia punctata with Happle's name, which serves, in my opinion, no useful or distinguishing purpose and only adds to the list of terms under which one must search in computer databases for references. Dr. Happle deserves full marks for his recognition of the X-linked dominant nature of the disorder and for pointing out the homology between the condition of bare patches in the mouse and this disorder. Rather than to continue to muddy the eponymous waters, it seems reasonable to me to continue with the interchangeable use of *X-linked dominant Conradi-Hunermann* or *X-linked dominant chondrodysplasia punctata* until the disorder can be identified by its molecular or biochemical defect.

ICHTHYOSIS WITH HYPOGONADISM (MIM:312770)

(Rud Syndrome)

DERMATOLOGIC FEATURES

MAJOR. Although there are compelling arguments that Rud syndrome does not exist, enough cases of ichthyosis with hypogonadism have been described to warrant an entry here, recognizing that each patient may represent a distinct disorder, some of which may have resulted from contiguous gene syndromes involving the sterol sulfatase locus on the X chromosome.

The ichthyosis is congenital or presents soon after birth. It is generalized and ranges from mild to severe, most similar to X-linked recessive ichthyosis or ichthyosis vulgaris.

MINOR. None.

ASSOCIATED ABORMALITIES

Hypogonadism is reported in both males and females but more easily recognized in the former. It may be primary or hypogonadotrophic in origin. Affected males are often eunuchoid in appearance.

Anosmia has been reported. Affected individuals with hypogonadism and anosmia most likely have Kallman syndrome and X-linked recessive ichthyosis as a result of a contiguous gene deletion.

Short stature is an inconstant finding.

Mental retardation and epilepsy have been termed cardinal features of the disorder, but are also inconstant findings.

Hypertrophic polyneuropathy has been described in two patients.

Retinitis pigmentosa has been reported twice.

HISTOPATHOLOGY

LIGHT. Nonspecific changes.

EM. Nonspecific changes.

BASIC DEFECT

Unknown. There are probably submicroscopic deletions of the sterol sulfatase and Kallman loci in some individuals.

TREATMENT

Emollients for the ichthyosis, including lactic acid, urea, and glycolic acid. All patients with Rud syndrome need high resolution karyotyping to detect X;Y translocations or X-chromosome deletions, testing for sterol sulfatase deficiency biochemically and/or with molecular probes, and testing for anosmia and appropriate endocrinologic evaluation.

MODE OF INHERITANCE

Autosomal recessive and X-linked recessive.

PRENATAL DIAGNOSIS

None.

DIFFERENTIAL DIAGNOSIS

In DeSanctis-Caccione syndrome (MIM: 278800), short stature and hypogonadism are associated with photosensitivity and changes of xeroderma pigmentosa, not ichthyosis. The trichothiodystrophies types C and D (MIM: 234050, 275550) overlap with Rud syndrome. Hair abnormalities are not reported in Rud syndrome, but to my knowledge polarized light microscopic evaluation of hairs has not been attempted.

Support Group: F.I.R.S.T.
P.O. Box 20921
Raleigh, NC 27619
1-800-545-3286

SELECTED BIBLIOGRAPHY

Perrin, J.C.S., Idemoto, J.Y., Sotos, J.F., Maurer, W.F., and Steinberg, A.G. (1976). X-linked syndrome of congenital ichthyosis, hypogonadism, mental retardation and anosmia. *Birth Defects* **12(5),** 267–274.

Describes individuals with hypogonadotrophic hypogonadism. No karyotyping or evaluation for sterol sulfatase levels. These individuals might have had submicroscopic X chromosome deletions.

York-Moore, M.E., and Rundle, A.T. (1962). Rud's syndrome. *J. Ment. Defic. Res.* **6,** 108–118.

Case report with good review of the heterogeneous group of patients to whom the eponym has been applied.

Young, I.D., and Hughes, H.E. (1982). Sex-linked mental retardation, short stature, obesity and hypogonadism: report of a family. *J. Ment. Defic. Res.* **26,** 153–162.

Four males in a large pedigree with short stature, mental retardation, obesity, and hypogonadism. Sterol sulfatase levels, karyotyping, and fragile X testing were normal in the one male evaluated. Only one of the brothers had ichthyosis, one had atopic dermatitis, one had freckling, and one had a "chronic" skin condition that was not further described.

KID SYNDROME (MIM:148120)

(Keratitis-Ichthyosis-Deafness; Senter Syndrome; Atypical Ichthyosis with Deafness and Keratitis)
Includes Autosomal Recessive KID Syndrome (Desmons Syndrome)

DERMATOLOGIC FEATURES

Major. There is generalized thickening of the skin marked by confluent, discrete, small, horny papules. The skin has been described as leather-like and grainy. Changes are present at birth or soon thereafter and progressive. Severity ranges from marked to overwhelmingly severe. Hyperkeratotic plaques on the face, ears, elbows, knees, and backs of the hands and feet may have an erythematous base. These plaques may be more widespread in more severely affected individuals.

The palms and soles are involved, and the dermal ridge pattern on the fingertips is typically interrupted by numerous horny papules.

Scalp hairs are usually sparse or absent, and eyelashes, eyebrows, and secondary sexual hairs are also sparse or absent.

Recurrent pyoderma and fungal infections of the skin are common, and scarring may result.

Minor. Decreased sweating due to occlusion of sweat ducts by scale has been reported. Sweat glands themselves are normal.

Squamous cell carcinoma of the tongue has been reported in two children and of the skin in four adults; in two, involvement was multifocal. Leukokeratosis and scrotal tongue have also been described.

ASSOCIATED ABNORMALITIES

Neurosensory deafness is probably congenital and nonprogressive. Hearing loss ranges from mild to profound; most individuals have severe hearing loss. Cochlear abnormalities have been described.

Four-fifths of patients develop a vascularizing keratitis during infancy and childhood, preceded by recurrent blepharoconjunctivitis. Corneal ulcerations and pannus ultimately lead to blindness. Although one case was affected at birth, usually changes do not appear until 2–4 years of age. Rarely onset of eye involvement has occurred in adult life. Approximately one-third of patients have photophobia as well.

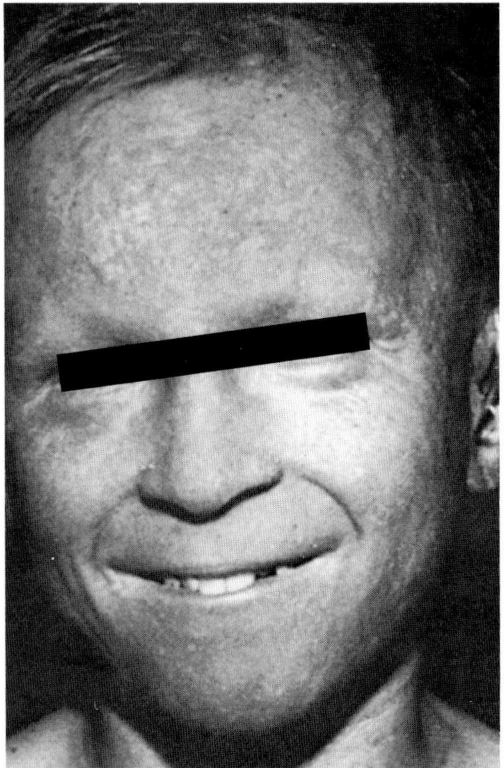

Figure 2.96. Moderately involved child with scarring alopecia and hyperkeratotic lesions. Hearing aid in place for deafness. (From Langer et al., 1990.)

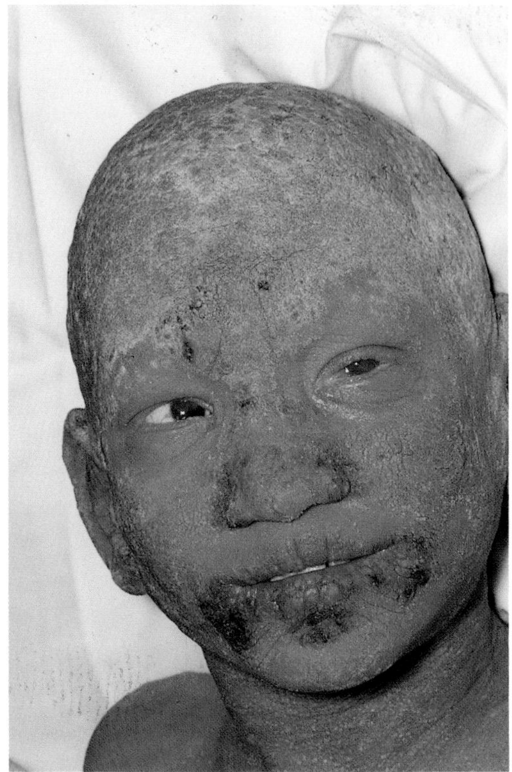

Figure 2.97. Severely involved child with complete alopecia and keratitis.

Intelligence is normal.

Teeth may be malformed or small.

Shortening of the achilles tendon has been reported in four patients. Progressive restriction of joint movement due to the skin changes is not rare.

Cerebellar hypoplasia was reported in one patient who had normal intelligence.

Acroosteolysis and severe arthritis have been reported in one patient.

HISTOPATHOLOGY

LIGHT. Nonspecific acanthosis with basketweave orthohyperkeratosis.

EM. Lamellar granules are normal. Keratohyaline bundles may be thickened and clumped.

BASIC DEFECT

Unknown.

TREATMENT

None specific for the skin. The oral retinoids have been disappointing. Surveillance for development of skin and mucosal malignancy is important. Fungal infections appear to respond to oral ketoconazole or fluconazole.

Corneal grafts revascularize rapidly with subsequent loss of vision. Careful ophthalmological evaluation and follow-up are necessary.

Hearing aids and appropriate school placement are part of management.

A

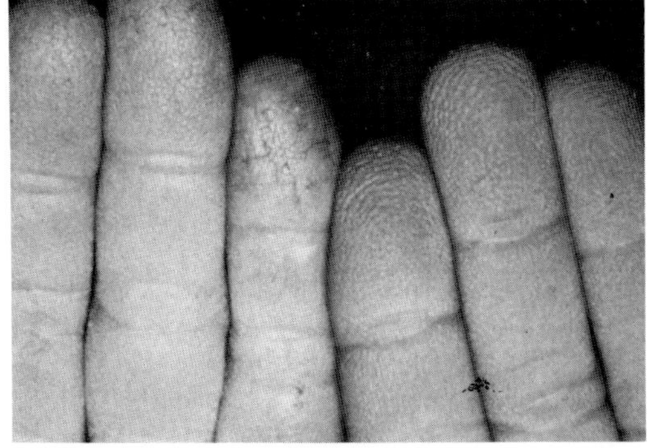

B

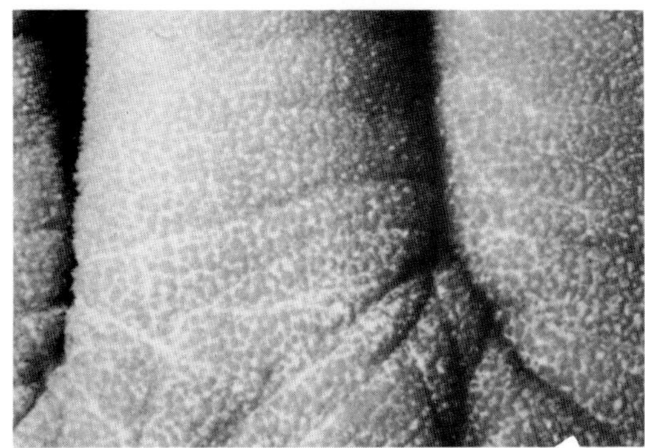

Figure 2.98. **(A)** Hands of daughter (right) and mother (left). **(B)** Close-up shows spicules of hyperkeratosis. (From Nazzaro et al., 1990.)

MODE OF INHERITANCE

Autosomal dominant. Male-to-male transmission has occurred. As expected in this severe disease, most cases are sporadic.

PRENATAL DIAGNOSIS

None to date.

DIFFERENTIAL DIAGNOSIS

The KID-recessive form (Desmons syndrome, MIM:242150) shares with KID its skin changes and deafness. Affected individuals usually have no eye findings. In addition they develop progressive hepatic cirrhosis and apparent glycogen storage in midlife. Mental retardation was reported in one patient. The skin of infants with ichthyosis and immune defects may appear similar to that of children with KID. Although recurrent skin infection is common in KID, death from systemic infection in infancy and early childhood is rare. Deafness and progressive keratitis may help to differentiate KID. I think there is considerable overlap with this group of ichthyoses with immune defects and the KID syndrome and that heterogeneity within the KID syndrome is likely.

The ichthyosis in Sjögren-Larsson syndrome (MIM:270200) is more dry and scaly and less spiny. Ataxia is not part of KID, and the eye findings in Sjögren-Larsson are different. Skin changes in keratosis follicularis spinulosa decalvans (MIM:308800) are very similar, but there are no hearing abnormalities in keratosis follicularis spinulosa decalvans.

Support Group: F.I.R.S.T.
P.O. Box 20921
Raleigh, NC 27619
1-800-545-3286

SELECTED BIBLIOGRAPHY

Desmons, F., Bar, J., and Chevillard, Y. (1971). Érythrodermie ichthyosiforme congénitale sèche surdi-mutité, hepatomégalie, de transmission récessive autosomique. Étude d'une famille. *Bull. Soc. Fr. Dermatol. Syphiligr.* **78,** 585–591.

None of three affected siblings born to first cousins had significant eye findings. Intelligence was normal.

Hazen, P.G., Walker, A.E., Stewart, J.J., Carney, J.F., Engstrom, C.W., and Turgeon, K.L. (1992). Keratitis, ichthyosis and deafness (KID) syndrome. Management with oral ketoconazole therapy. *Int. J. Dermatol.* **31,** 58–59.

Hazen, P.G., Carney, P., and Lynch, W.S. (1989). *Int. J. Dermatol.* **28,** 190–191.

Two reports of this 48-year-old woman for whom treatment with oral ketoconazole resulted in improvement in skin changes and unmasking of multiple squamous cell carcinomas that had previously been obscured by hyperkeratosis. The authors believe treatment has slowed the development of new tumors and slowed the progression of neovascularization of the patient's corneal transplants.

Nazzaro, V., Blanchet-Bardon, C., Lorette, G., and Civatte, J. (1990). Familial occurrence of KID (keratitis, ichthyosis, deafness) syndrome. Case reports of a mother and daughter. *J. Am. Acad. Dermatol.* **23,** 385–388.

Clear review of clinical features.

Skinner, B.A., Greist, M.C., and Norins, A.L. (1981). The keratitis, ichthyosis and deafness (KID) syndrome. *Arch. Dermatol.* **117,** 285–289.

Case report and literature review giving name to the disorder. Tabular review of case reports.

Tuppurainen, K., Fräki, J., Karjalainen, S., Paljärvi, L., Suhonen, R., and Ryynänen, M. (1988). The KID syndrome in Finland. A report of four cases. *Acta Ophthalmol. (Copenh.)* **68,** 692–698.

Father and two sons and one sporadic case are described.

Wilson, G.N., Squires, R.H., Jr., and Weinberg, A.G. (1991). Keratitis, hepatitis, ichthyosis and deafness. Report and review of KID syndrome. *Am. J. Med. Genet.* **40,** 255–259.

Report of a patient with Desmons syndrome (KID-AR) and review of KID.

NEU-LAXOVA SYNDROME (MIM:256520)

DERMATOLOGIC FEATURES

Major. This syndrome is probably heterogeneous, and there is considerable intrafamilial and interfamilial variation in clinical features. The descriptions of skin changes, as given by nondermatologists, range from lemon-colored thin scaly skin to tight scaly skin to harlequin-fetus-like changes. The term *ichthyosis* has probably been used inappropriately in this disorder. Most photographs suggest that the skin is taut, shiny, with limited scaling, resembling restrictive dermopathy. Tissue edema is almost always present and may be extreme on the hands and feet.

The eyelids are often hypoplastic and retracted.

Minor. Scalp hair may be absent.

ASSOCIATED ABNORMALITIES

Microcephaly is a constant finding, with structural brain malformations including, but not limited to, lissencephaly and agyria, absence of the corpus callosum, calcifications, and atrophy. Affected siblings may have different central nervous system malformations.

Severe intrauterine growth retardation, prematurity, and stillbirth are typical, as is a short umbilical cord.

The facies are marked by hypertelorism, sloping forehead, and retracted lids with exposed globes, but these features are not univer-

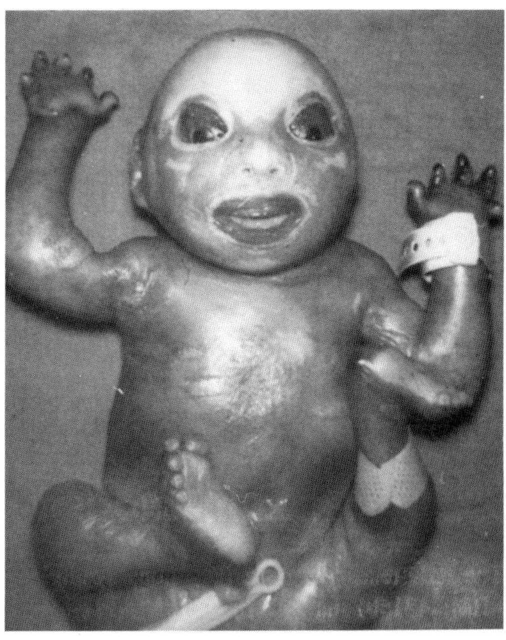

Figure 2.99. Swollen puffy hands, deficient eyelids, eclabium, and taut encasement by skin. (From Ejeckam et al., 1986.)

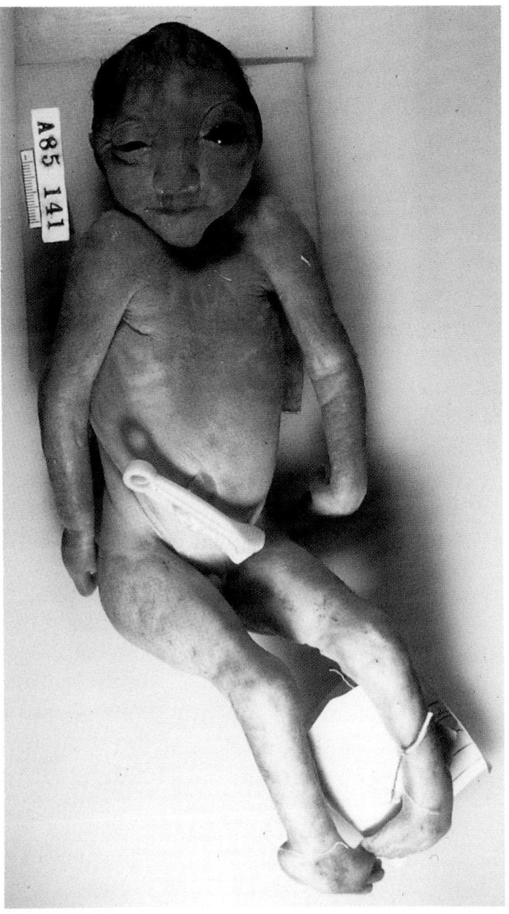

Figure 2.100. Fixed joints and abnormal facies. (Courtesy of Dr. R.A. Pagon, Seattle, Washington.)

sal. Cataracts have occasionally been described.

The limbs are held in flexion. Neu-Laxova is believed to be one of the syndromes resulting in the fetal akinesia sequence.

Siblings discordant for cleft lip and cleft palate have been reported.

HISTOPATHOLOGY

LIGHT. A questionable increase in subcutaneous tissue and edema of the dermis have been described. Orthohyperkeratosis with a normal granular layer.

EM. No information.

BASIC DEFECT

Unknown.

TREATMENT

None. The condition is uniformly lethal.

MODE OF INHERITANCE

Autosomal recessive.

PRENATAL DIAGNOSIS

Currently unreliable. Decrease in fetal movement and edema with abnormal head configuration and intrauterine growth retardation have all been reported in affected fetuses, but late in the second trimester. Intrauterine retardation appears to develop in the midsecond trimester. Whether any of these features are present before 24 weeks of fetal development is unknown.

DIFFERENTIAL DIAGNOSIS

The facies in some cases of Neu-Laxova syndrome resemble those of restrictive dermopathy (MIM:275210), as do the skin changes. The structural brain malformations differentiate between the two.

Infants with harlequin ichthyosis (MIM: 242500) have everted lips rather than a mouth fixed in open position, and the plate-like scales are far more marked. The eyelids in harlequin ichthyosis are everted and the globes often obscured by the exposed inner lids. In Neu-Laxova syndrome, the lids are hypoplastic and pulled away, exposing the globes. In only one report labeled as Neu-Laxova were skin changes clinically similar to harlequin ichthyosis, and this report was unconvincing. The presence of microcephaly and structural brain abnormalities in a stillborn with severe scaling would push one to a diagnosis of Neu-Laxova syndrome.

Infants with COFS Syndrome (Pena-Shokeir

II, MIM:214150) can resemble Neu-Laxova. In the original report (Neu et al., 1971), one of the affected siblings could easily have been diagnosed as COFS. In general, infants with COFS do not have skin changes.

Support Group: F.I.R.S.T.
P.O. Box 20921
Raleigh, NC 27619
1-800-545-3286

The Compassionate Friends (TCF)
P.O. Box 3696
Oak Brook, IL 60522-3696
1-708-990-0010

SELECTED BIBLIOGRAPHY

Curry, C.J. (1982). Letter to the Editor: further comments on the Neu-Laxova syndrome. *Am. J. Med. Genet.* **13,** 441–444.

An attempt to classify subtypes of Neu-Laxova syndrome. This classification has not been accepted but accurately reflects the heterogeneity within this phenotype.

Ejeckam, G.G., Wadhwa, J.K., Williams, J.P., and Lacson, A.G. (1986). Neu-Laxova syndrome: report of two cases. *Pediatr. Pathol.* **5,** 295–306.

Good clinical photographs and excellent photomicrographs.

Neu, R.L., Kajii, T., Gardner, L.I., Nagyfy, S.F., and King, S. (1971). A lethal syndrome of microcephaly with multiple congenital anomalies in three siblings. *Pediatrics* **47,** 610–612.

These three affected siblings were as dissimilar as they were similar.

Seemanova, E., and Rudolf, R. (1985). The Neu-Laxova syndrome. *Am. J. Med. Genet.* **20,** 13–15.

Perfect example of the reason for confusion in diagnosis. Retrospective diagnosis based on descriptions and photographs of a patient born nine years earlier. Photographs show harlequin-like ichthyosis, but no abnormalities were noted at postmortem examination (it was unclear if the brain was examined or not). No histopathology of the skin was available, and yet the authors elected to diagnose the patient as Neu-Laxova syndrome because of edema of the hands and feet. Chromosome studies were not done. There was severe intrauterine growth retardation, but a head circumference measurement was not obtained. As far as I can tell, this baby does not have a diagnosis, and labeling it as Neu-Laxova is not warranted.

NEUTRAL LIPID STORAGE DISEASE WITH ICHTHYOSIS (MIM:275630)

(Chanarin-Dorfman Syndrome; Triglyceride Storage Disease with Impaired Long Chain Fatty Oxidation)

DERMATOLOGIC FEATURES

MAJOR. The ichthyosis is present at birth, and at least one infant was born with a collodion membrane. There may be mild erythroderma, ectropion, and eclabium. The scale is fine, white to gray in color, and involves all skin surfaces. The disorder is most clinically similar to nonbullous congenital ichthyosiform erythroderma.

MINOR. None.

ASSOCIATED ABNORMALITIES

As might be expected in a storage disease, with the exception of the ichthyosis, all other findings are of later onset and progressive.

Neurologic status may be normal. Developmental delay or mental retardation was described in 4 of 13 patients. It is unclear whether this is related to the disorder or to polygenic effects of consanguinity. In one family, mental

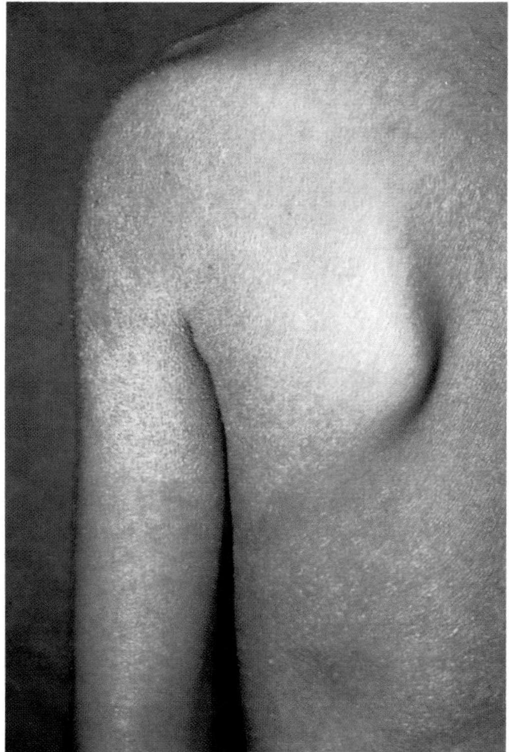

Figure 2.101. Fine, white scale with underlying erythroderma. (From Venencie et al., 1993.)

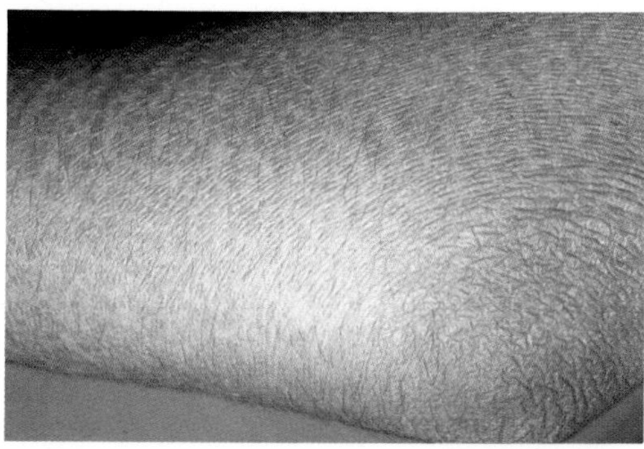

Figure 2.102. Close-up of dark wrinkled skin with brown scale in affected sister. (From Venencie et al., 1993.)

retardation was clearly segregating independently. Nystagmus and ataxia were described in 2 of 11 patients reported as of 1985.

Some affected individuals develop a progressive mild myopathy. Cataracts and electroretinogram alterations are reported in more than half. Progressive neurosensory deafness also occurs in more than half of affected individuals. Hepatosplenomegaly without liver dysfunction is typical. Fatty degeneration is present on liver biopsy.

HISTOPATHOLOGY

LIGHT. Lipid droplets are seen in many tissues and cell types. Not all cells are affected to the same degree in the same individual. Heterozygotes show lipid inclusions in eosinophils. The ichthyotic skin is hyperkeratotic with patchy parakeratosis and focal spongiosis. There may be a mild perivascular inflammatory infiltrate in the upper dermis.

EM. Demonstrates that lipid is stored within the cytoplasm in droplets, not within organelles.

BASIC DEFECT

Storage of triglycerides but not cholesterol or cholesterol esters. The basic defect remains unknown.

TREATMENT

Keratolytics, including urea, lactic acid or glycolic acid based emollients, for the ichthyosis. There is no treatment available for the metabolic defect.

MODE OF INHERITANCE

Autosomal recessive.

PRENATAL DIAGNOSIS

Not performed. Potentially feasible by fetal skin biopsy if lipid accumulation is present in utero.

DIFFERENTIAL DIAGNOSIS

Intracellular triglyceride storage is not unique to neutral lipid storage disease with ichthyosis, but the combination of this feature with ichthyosis is specific. The ichthyosis is similar to that of nonbullous congenital ichthyosiform erythroderma (MIM:242100), and affected infants may present with a collodion membrane (MIM: 242300). Microscopic analysis of white blood cells will demonstrate typical inclusions diagnostic for neutral lipid storage disease with ichthyosis. Refsum syndrome (MIM:266500) is differentiated by later onset of ichthyosis, absence of lipid droplets on smear, and accumulation of phytanic acid.

Support Group: F.I.R.S.T.
P.O. Box 20921
Raleigh, NC 27619
1-800-545-3286

SELECTED BIBLIOGRAPHY

DiDonato, S., Garavaglia, B., Strisciuglo, P., Barrone, C., and Andria, G. (1988). Multisystem triglyceride storage disease due to a specific defect in degradation of endocellularly synthesized triglycerides. *Neurology* **38,** 1107–1110.

Evaluation of two unrelated patients demonstrating that, except for degradation of endogenous triglycerides, fibroblasts appear to have normal lipid metabolism and are able to degrade exogenous triglyceride. The nature of the specific defect remains elusive.

Williams, M.L., Koch, T.K., O'Donnell, J.J., Frost, P.H., Epstein, L.B., Grizzard, W.S., and Epstein, C.J. (1985). Ichthyosis and neutral lipid storage disease. *Am. J. Med. Genet.* **20,** 711–726.

Inbred Palestinian Christian family demonstrating pseudodominance. Affected father, product of a first cousin mating, had three affected children by his first cousin spouse. Both his wife and mother (obligate heterozygotes) had lipids droplets in eosinophils. This is a nice review with helpful tables.

REFSUM DISEASE (MIM:266500)

(Heredopathica Atactica Polyneuritiformis; Phytanic Acid Oxidase Deficiency)

DERMATOLOGIC FEATURES

MAJOR. Onset of mild generalized scaling may occur in childhood but is usually delayed until adolescence. The skin changes are clinically similar to ichthyosis vulgaris, including hyperlinear palms. Skin changes often develop long after other symptoms and may revert to normal with lowering of phytanic acid levels. Over one-half of reported patients have had skin changes.

MINOR. None.

ASSOCIATED ABNORMALITIES

Progressive ataxia, progressive peripheral neuropathy, loss of deep tendon reflexes, and elevation of cerebrospinal fluid protein are classic features of the disorder.

Progressive visual loss with retinal changes of retinitis pigmentosa has its onset usually in the second decade. Miosis is also a common feature, and lenticular opacities have been described. Anosmia is an almost universal finding and usually precedes the visual symptoms. Progressive sensorineural hearing loss is typical. Cardiac arrhythmias with atrioventricular conduction impairment and bundle branch block are common and may precipitate sudden death.

Shortening of the tubular bones of the hands and feet and a conical terminal phalanx of the thumb are seen in approximately one-third of the patients. Flattening of the epiphyses of the knees and elbows is also common.

HISTOPATHOLOGY

LIGHT. There is a decrease in the granular layer with mild orthohyperkeratosis and an increase in lipid droplets in keratinocytes and dermal nevus cells.

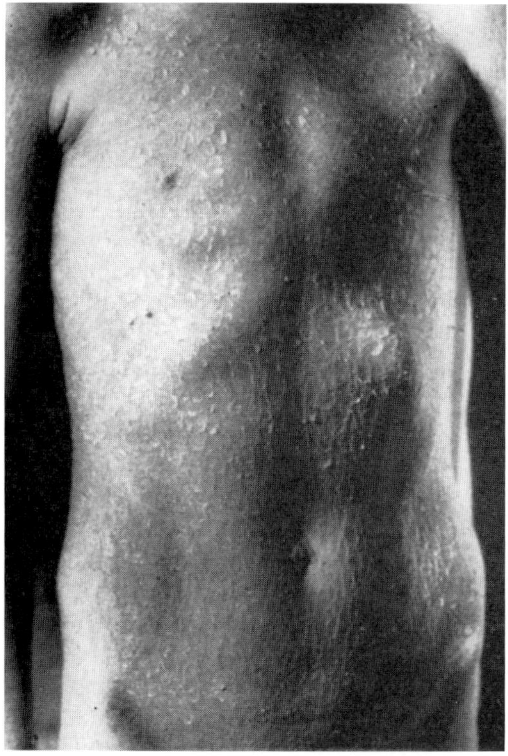

Figure 2.103. Eight-year-old female. (From Refsum et al., 1949.)

EM. Giant degenerated mitochondria with accumulation of lipid droplets in basal keratinocytes.

BASIC DEFECT

Defect in the α-oxidation of phytanic acid.

TREATMENT

Dietary restriction of phytanic acid (no dairy products and no green vegetables) will reverse many of the changes. Plasmapheresis during initiation of dietary restriction to manage mobilization of tissue stores of phytanic acid is often necessary. Plasmapheresis may also be used as an adjunct to continued diet therapy. The skin changes, neuropathy, and cardiac arrhythmias reverse or improve with lowering of phytanic acid levels. The retinitis pigmentosa and hearing loss do not, suggesting that these latter are consequences of long-term storage rather than reflecting current levels of phytanic acid.

A

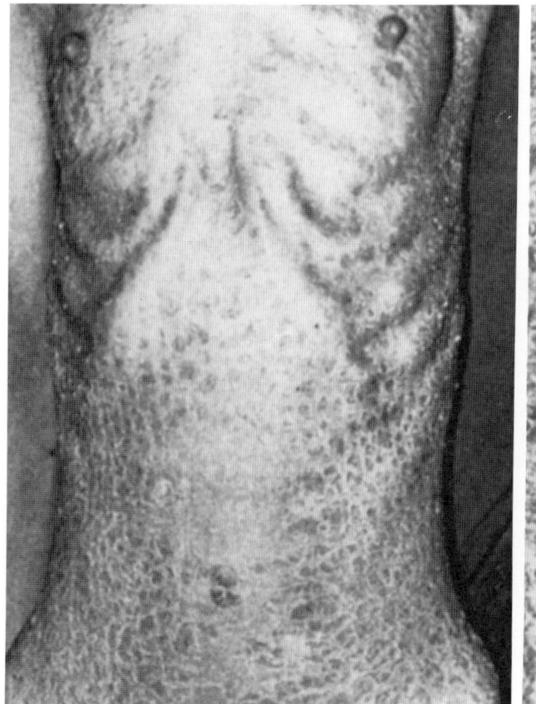

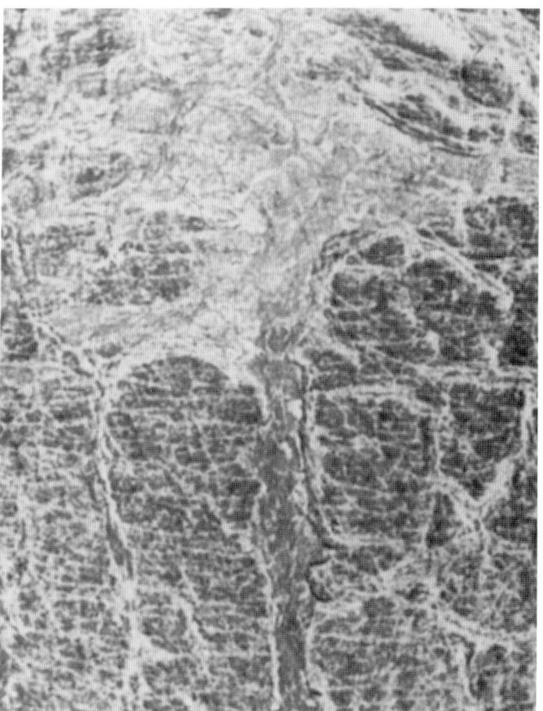

B

Figure 2.104. **(A)** Thirty-seven-year old female. **(B)** Close-up of scale. (From Davies et al., 1977.)

MODE OF INHERITANCE

Autosomal recessive.

PRENATAL DIAGNOSIS

To my knowledge this has not been performed but theoretically should be possible. It has been performed for infantile Refsum disease, which is a different disorder.

DIFFERENTIAL DIAGNOSIS

Patients with Usher syndrome (MIM:276900) share in common with Refsum syndrome retinitis pigmentosa and deafness, but lack skin changes and ataxia. Phytanic acid levels are normal. In Sjögren-Larsson syndrome (MIM: 270200), onset of ataxia is in the first few years of life, and the ichthyosis is congenital.

The diagnosis of Refsum disease should be considered in any patient with retinitis pigmentosa and hearing loss or in individuals with progressive ataxia. The skin changes are often absent, and thus the diagnosis may not be brought to mind.

Support Group: National Ataxia Foundation (NAF)
15500 Wayzata Blvd., #750
Wayzata, MN 55391
1-612-473-7666

F.I.R.S.T.
PO Box 20921
Raleigh, NC 27619
1-800-545-3286

The Foundation Fighting Blindness
1401 Mount Royal Ave, 4th Floor
Baltimore, MD 21217-4245
1-800-683-5555

SELECTED BIBLIOGRAPHY

Gibberd, F.B., Billimoria, J.D., Goldman, J.M., Clemens, M.E., Evans, R., Whitelaw, M.N., Retsas, S., and Sherratt, R.M. (1985). Heredopathia atactica polyneuritiformis: Refsum's disease. *Acta Neurol. Scand.* **72,** 1–17.
A fascinating read. Case reports detail the impact of disease and treatment. Extensive specific dietary recommendations given. Thirty-nine references.

Watkins, P.A., and Mihalik, S.J. (1990). Mitochondrial oxidation of phytanic acid in human and monkey liver: implication that Refsum's disease is not a peroxisomal disorder. *Biochem. Biophys. Res. Commun.* **167,** 580–586.
Argues that defect in oxidation is mitochondrial, not peroxisomal, in origin.

RICHNER-HANHART SYNDROME (MIM:276600)

(Type II Tyrosinemia; Tyrosinosis Oculocutaneous Type)

DERMATOLOGIC FEATURES

MAJOR. Blisters appear on the palms, soles, and tips of the fingers and then progress to hyperkeratosis with fissuring. These linear verrucous papules and plaques are surrounded by erythema and are painful. Onset may be within the first years of life or as late as the teen years. Skin lesions are not invariably present, even among siblings.

MINOR. Occasional hyperhidrosis of the palms and soles.

ASSOCIATED ABNORMALITIES

Mental retardation to varying degrees is described in less than half of the reported patients. There is no correlation with the presence or

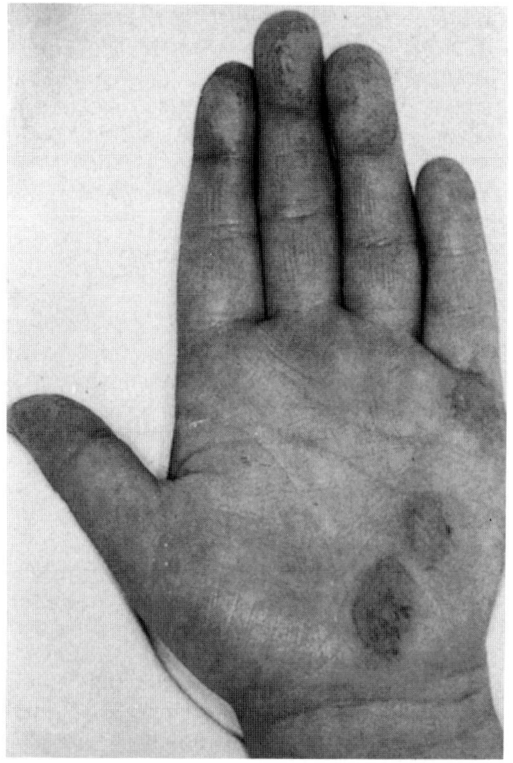

Figure 2.105. Thickened plaques on palm and fingertips. (From Fraser et al., 1987.)

severity of the eye and/or skin findings and mental retardation.

Dendritic corneal ulcers can develop in the first months of life, presaged by photophobia and increased tearing, or not occur until middle age. Eye changes are not invariable, even among siblings. Eye changes may precede or develop after skin findings. Nystagmus and strabismus are occasionally described.

HISTOPATHOLOGY

LIGHT. Changes of epidermolytic hyperkeratosis with papillomatosis and acanthosis. Bullae are present in the upper epidermis.

EM. Abnormal needle-shaped "crystal ghosts," presumably tyrosine crystals, can be seen in the cytoplasm of keratinocytes, along with aggregation of tonofilaments. There is some variability in the findings described.

BASIC DEFECT

Deficiency of hepatic tyrosine aminotransferase. Ranch minks have the same autosomal recessive disease, and similar clinical features develop in rats fed low tyrosine diets.

TREATMENT

Dietary management with decreased phenylalanine and tyrosine will clear skin lesions and keratitis. One report of success with etretinate (authors feared poor compliance with diet in a patient who only had skin lesions). One report of skin grafting to a lesion on the heel stated that there was no recurrence.

Of 12 liveborn children of 5 affected mothers, 2 had microcephaly and mental retardation. Dietary management during pregnancy may or may not be appropriate or helpful.

MODE OF INHERITANCE

Autosomal recessive. One-half of cases are of Italian origin. The gene maps to 16q22.1–22.3.

PRENATAL DIAGNOSIS

Potentially possible by linkage or direct mutational analysis if mutations are known.

DIFFERENTIAL DIAGNOSIS

Easily differentiated from other hereditary palmoplantar keratodermas by elevated levels of serum and urinary tyrosine. The same is true for other bullous disorders such as epidermolysis bullosa simplex Weber-Cockayne (MIM: 131800) and transient bullous dermolysis of the newborn (MIM:131705).

Support Group: N.O.R.D.
P.O. Box 8923
New Fairfield, CT
06812
1-800-999-6673

SELECTED BIBLIOGRAPHY

Goldsmith, L.A., and Laberge, C. (1989). Tyrosinemia and related disorders. In *The Metabolic and Molecular Bases of Inherited Disease*. Scriver, C.R., Beaudet, A.L., Sly, W.S., and Valle, D. (eds.). McGraw-Hill, New York, 6th ed., pp. 547–554.
Excellent review

Natt, E., Kida, K., Odievre, M., DiRocco, M., and Scherer, G. (1992). Point mutations in the tyrosine aminotransferase gene in tyrosinemia type II. *Proc. Natl. Acad. Sci. U.S.A.* **89,** 9297–9301.
Compound heterozygosity for mutant alleles demonstrated in two of three patients analyzed. In the third, offspring of a consanguineous mating, two different mutations were found on one allele, and homozygosity was suspected.

SJÖGREN-LARSSON SYNDROME (MIM:270200)

DERMATOLOGIC FEATURES

MAJOR. This is a relatively rare form of ichthyosis. I have made the diagnosis in one patient. The ichthyosis of Sjögren-Larsson syndrome is diffuse, with dark hyperkeratosis and mild to moderate scaling. The scale is itchy, and the linear grayish marks that scratching leaves on the skin are a classic feature. Although all surfaces are involved, the greatest thickening is seen on the lower trunk. Erythema is a minimal and occasional feature and when present does not persist beyond infancy. At birth, the skin changes are indistinguishable from lamellar ichthyosis. A collodion membrane has never been described. Although skin changes are usually present at birth, onset may occur as late as several months, and the ichthyosis may worsen during the first year, after which severity is not significantly altered by age. It may, as do most ichthyoses, improve mildly with warm climate.

Nails and hair are normal. Scalp involvement is typical, but the central face is generally spared. Palms and soles may be thickened.

MINOR. There may be a mild reduction in sweating, and relative heat intolerance is an infrequent complaint.

ASSOCIATED ABNORMALITIES

The typical neurologic feature of Sjögren-Larsson syndrome is a marked spastic diplegia or tetraplegia, more severe in the lower limbs. Many patients become wheelchair-bound by adolescence. Progression of neurologic disability seems to cease after puberty. Although neurologic symptoms may not develop until middle to late childhood, they are present by 30 months of age in most patients. Nonprogressive mental retardation is an invariable feature of classic Sjögren-Larsson syndrome and can range from mild to severe. Epilepsy occurs in about one-third of patients.

Reported skeletal findings include mild short stature (one-third) and thoracic kyphosis. The short stature may be secondary to contractures and/or to scoliosis rather than representing primary growth failure.

The classic eye findings are glistening white dots in the fundus that cluster about the macula and may number as few as 5 or as many as 50 or more. There is no correlation between the number of dots and the severity of spasticity, mental retardation, or ichthyosis, and there does not appear to be a significant increase in the number of dots with age. These are present in 100% of typical patients. Macular degeneration is seen in 10%–30% of patients. Superficial corneal opacities are described in approximately one-half of affected individuals. Complaints of photophobia are typical.

Defective enamel of the secondary teeth is a minor finding.

Although mortality is increased, early death due to infection is thought to have been secondary to poor care or a consequence of complications of severe mental retardation rather than to endogenous immune dysfunction.

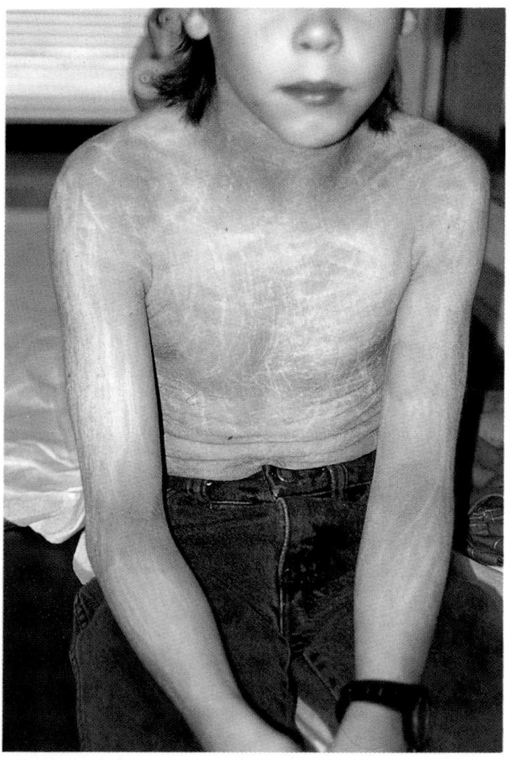

Figure 2.106. Generalized severe xerosis with multiple scratch marks visible. This is a pruritic ichthyosis.

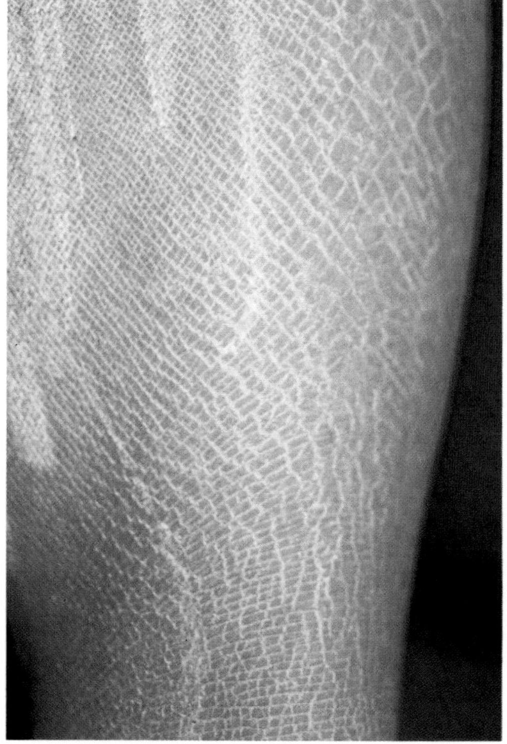

Figure 2.107. Close-up of brown adherent scale and fine white powdery scratch trails.

HISTOPATHOLOGY

Light. Slight generalized parakeratosis with moderate to marked hyperkeratosis and thickened granular layer, acanthosis, and papillomatosis are typical. A mild perivascular infiltrate with round cells and slight irregularities in pigmentation are also described.
EM. Increased number of mitochondria and prominent Golgi apparatus in the keratinocytes. Abnormal lamellar inclusions in the cytoplasm of stratum corneum cells are seen in both ichthyotic and uninvolved skin.

BASIC DEFECT

An accumulation of long chain fatty alcohol due to a reduction in the activity of the enzyme fatty alcohol:nicotinamine adenine dinucleotide oxidoreductase (FAO). This enzyme's activity is dependent in part on fatty aldehyde dehydrogenase, which is deficient in Sjögren-Larsson Syndrome.

TREATMENT

Keratolytics may be helpful for the skin. Etretinate has also been successful. Justification for its use must be made on a patient by patient basis. Dietary restriction of fats with medium chain fatty acid supplementation is currently being evaluated for both neurologic and dermatologic effects in controlled studies. Improvement on such a diet has been reported anecdotally.

MODE OF INHERITANCE

Autosomal recessive. The gene *FALDH* has been identified and maps to 17p11.2.

PRENATAL DIAGNOSIS

Electron microscopy of fetal skin at 23 or 24 weeks gestation shows hyperkeratosis, but enzymatic assay of cultured amniocytes appears to be more accurate with less risk. Molecular methods utilizing chorionic villus samples should be possible.

DIFFERENTIAL DIAGNOSIS

Among the ichthyoses, severe ichthyosis vulgaris (MIM:146700), NCIE/lamellar ichthyosis (MIM:242100), and sterol sulfatase deficiency (MIM:308100) are similar, the last most so. Although individuals with both sterol sulfatase deficiency and Sjögren-Larsson syndrome have corneal opacities, they are superficial in Sjögren-Larsson syndrome, deep in X-linked ichthyosis. Retinal changes are absent in X-linked ichthyosis. Appropriate metabolic testing, measurement of alcohol dehydrogenase activity in cultured fibroblasts or leukocytes, or histochemical staining of skin biopsy for hexanol dehydrogenase for Sjögren-Larsson syndrome and blood cholesterol sulfate levels for X-linked ichthyosis will differentiate between the two.

Support Group: F.I.R.S.T.
P.O. Box 20921
Raleigh, NC 27619
1-800-545-3286

SELECTED BIBLIOGRAPHY

Jagell, S. (1981). *Sjögren-Larsson Syndrome in Sweden. An Epidemiological, Genetic, Clinical, and Biochemical Study*. Medical Dissertation, University of Umea.

Jagell, S., Gustavson, K.-H., and Holmgren, G. (1981). Sjögren-Larsson syndrome in Sweden. A clinical, genetic, and epidemiological study. *Clin. Genet.* **19,** 233–256.

Excellent in-depth description of Sjögren-Larrson syndrome. Jagell's dissertation (1981) contains several published papers and much greater detail, but is less easily accessed. Jagell found two-thirds of 35 patients in Sweden to have IQs less than 50. Other parts of the dissertation appear in other publications.

Kelson, T.L., Craft, D.A., and Rizzo, W.B. (1992). Carrier detection for Sjögren-Larsson syndrome. *J. Inherit. Metab. Dis.* **15,** 105–111.

All of 11 obligate heterozygotes had FAO activity or FALDH (fatty aldehyde dehydrogenase) activities that were below normal range when an 18-carbon substrate was used. Authors recommend testing for both enzymes for greater accuracy.

Rizzo, W.B., Dammann, A.L., Craft, D.A., Black, S.H., Tilton, A.H., Africk, D., Chaves-Carballo, E., Holmgren, G., and Jagell, S. (1989). Sjögren-Larsson syndrome: inherited defect in the fatty alcohol cycle. *J. Pediatr.* **115,** 228–234.

Eight patients (four Swedish, one American black, two American whites, and one Chilean) were evaluated. All eight had decreased FAO activity (approximately 18%) in fibroblasts. Three of three tested had decreased activity (22%) in leukocytes also. Heterozygotes showed partial deficiency.

Tabsh, K., Rizzo, W.B., Holbrook, K.H., and Theroux, N. (1993). Sjögren-Larsson syndrome: technique and timing of prenatal diagnosis. *Obstet. Gynecol.* **82,** 700–703.

Fetal skin biopsy at 19 weeks showed no abnormal features, although cultured amniocytes demonstrated reduced FAO activity. Rebiopsy at 23 1/2 weeks showed hyperkeratosis. Authors recommend biochemical diagnosis.

Cohesion

EPIDERMOLYSIS BULLOSA

The epidermolysis bullosa syndromes share in common easy fragility of the skin, manifested by blistering with little or no trauma. They are differentiated into three major categories by the level in the skin at which blisters form:

Simplex: Separation occurs above the plasma membrane of the basal keratinocyte, in the basal or suprabasal layer of the epidermis (nonscarring).

Junctional: Separation occurs above the basement membrane of the dermis, within the lamina lucida of the dermo-epidermal junction (nonscarring). As atrophy may develop over time, the term *atrophicans* has been applied to this group by the Europeans.

Dystrophic: The blister forms below the basement membrane, and the basement membrane is attached to the blister roof (scarring).

The epidermolysis bullosa syndromes are further delineated on the basis of distribution of lesions (localized or generalized), mode of inheritance, associated clinical features, and ultrastructural alterations. Distinct mutations in the keratin genes have been found in epidermolysis bullosa simplex. Alterations in the type VII collagen gene *(COL7A1)* have been demonstrated in most forms of dystrophic epidermolysis bullosa. Defects in subunits of laminin 5 (also called nicein, kallinin, and epiligrin) *(LAMC2, LAMB3)* and in other components of hemidesmosomes *(BPAG2, LAD1, ITGβ4)* appear likely to be causal in junctional epidermolysis bullosa. Within the next few years, molecular diagnosis for many types of epidermolysis bullosa will become available.

While there is agreement as to diagnostic criteria for some forms of epidermolysis bullosa, controversy exists regarding the validity of more rare subtypes and the criteria for further subdiagnoses. Gedde-Dahl's monograph on epidermolysis bullosa (1971) remains an excellent review of the disorders, although for discussion of more recent biochemical and molecular work one must look to the current literature.

I have included only those subtypes of epidermolysis bullosa that have met with general acceptance. Within the discussion of the differential diagnoses for these I have included some of the less well-characterized subtypes. Even within these subcategories, further genetic heterogeneity is likely to exist.

Bart syndrome (MIM:132000) is an autosomal dominant form of epidermolysis bullosa, initially thought to be a simplex form. It is characterized by congenital absence of the skin on the lower legs and feet, nonscarring blistering of the skin and oral mucosa, and nail abnormalities. Electron microscopy was not originally performed in this family. Subsequently, it was recognized that many types of epidermolysis bullosa—dystrophic, junctional, and perhaps simplex—can present with congenital absence of the skin. Reevaluation of this family has demonstrated a decrease in anchoring fibrils and linkage to type VII collagen *(COL7A1)*. Thus, this family has epidermolysis bullosa dystrophica. Whether the family described has a unique subtype of epidermolysis bullosa dystrophica remains uncertain.

Epidermolysis bullosa acquisita is an acquired form of epidermolysis bullosa dystrophica thought to result from the development of autoantibodies to type VII collagen. It will not be discussed further.

Clinical diagnosis is often problematic in the more severe types of epidermolysis bullosa. A positive Nikolsky sign (blistering of uninvolved skin after rubbing) is common to all; mucosal and nail involvement and the presence or absence of milia may not be helpful discriminators. It is often easy to mistake postinflammatory changes for those of scarring.

With the exception of the diagnosis of

Weber-Cockayne syndrome, which can be made clinically in the presence of a positive family history, transmission electron microscopy is the *sine qua non* for the diagnosis of epidermolysis bullosa. Light microscopy is inadequate and unacceptable for the accurate diagnosis of epidermolysis bullosa. Immunofluorescent antibody/antigen mapping is used primarily as an adjunct to electron microscopic diagnosis, as a rapid method of prenatal diagnosis, and as a research tool. For those without access to electron microscopy, immunofluorescence studies may be more easily obtained and can help to distinguish among, and in some instances within, the major diagnostic groups. It may prove valuable in the future for specific subtype diagnosis.

The leading edge of a fresh (less than 12 hours old) or mechanically induced blister with some normal adjacent skin should be biopsied. Older blisters undergo change that may obscure the diagnostic morphology. There is argument about using a punch biopsy versus an elliptical or shave excision, with some believing that the punch can introduce confusing artifact. In our hands, careful use of the punch to avoid loss of the epidermis has been successful.

A national registry for individuals with epidermolysis bullosa was established in the United States by the National Institutes of Health in 1986. There are four regional centers. They can be contacted most easily through D.E.B.R.A.

The care of a patient with epidermolysis bullosa may be straightforward or complicated and frustrating. The lists of bandages, dressings, antibiotics, medications, and so forth are legion, and I refer you to Lin and Carter (1992) or to D.E.B.R.A. for specifics regarding treatment.

SELECTED BIBLIOGRAPHY

Bruckner-Tuderman, L., Schnyder, U.W., and Baran, R. (1995). Nail changes in epidermolysis bullosa: clinical and pathogenetic considerations. *Br. J. Dermatol.* **132,** 339–344.

Nice review with good photographs and discussion of nail changes in all three types of epidermolysis bullosa.

Eady, R.A.J., and Dunnill, M.G.S. (1994). Epidermolysis bullosa: hereditary skin fragility diseases as paradigms in cell biology. *Arch. Dermatol. Res.* **287,** 2–9.

Review of current state of knowledge regarding molecular defects in the three major groups of epidermolysis bullosa.

Fine, J.-D., Bauer, E.A., Briggaman, R.A., Carter, D.M., Eady, R.A.J., Esterly, N.B., Holbrook, K.A., Hurwitz, S., Johnson, L., Lin, A., Pearson, R., and Sybert, V.P. (1991). Revised clinical and laboratory criteria for subtypes of inherited epidermolysis bullosa. A consensus report by the Subcommittee on Diagnosis and Classification of the National Epidermolysis Bullosa Registry. *J. Am. Acad. Dermatol.* **24,** 119–135.

An epic review of the diagnostic features of epidermolysis bullosa in an attempt to devise a unified scheme for classification. It is important to recognize that consensus does not equal unanimity.

Gedde-Dahl, T. Jr. (1971). *Epidermolysis Bullosa. A Clinical, Genetic, and Epidemiological Study.* Johns Hopkins Press, Baltimore.

Although Gedde-Dahl has a more recent review (*Acta Dermatol. Venereol. Suppl.* **95,** 74–87, 1981), I find the 1971 monograph more readable and interesting.

Haber, R.M., Hanna, W., Ramsay, C.A., and Boxall, L.B.H. (1985). Hereditary epidermolysis bullosa. *J. Am. Acad. Dermatol.* **13,** 252–278.

A compact, readable clinical review of the epidermolysis bullosa syndromes.

Lin, A., and Cartin, D.M. (eds.) (1992). *Epidermolysis Bullosa. Basic and Clinical Aspects.* Springer-Verlag, New York.

Excellent chapters on noncutaneous involvement and management. The chapter on prenatal diagnosis is exceptionally well written, but already outdated.

EPIDERMOLYSIS BULLOSA SIMPLEX DOWLING-MEARA (MIM:131760)

(Epidermolysis Bullosa Simplex Herpetiformis)

Includes Epidermolysis Bullosa Simplex with Mottled Hyperpigmentation; Epidermolysis Bullosa Simplex with Muscular Dystrophy

DERMATOLOGIC FEATURES

MAJOR. Widespread and severe blistering and/or multiple grouped clumps of small blisters (whose resemblance to the blisters of juvenile dermatitis herpetiformis gave the disorder one of its names) are typical. Hemorrhagic blisters are common. Onset is usually at birth, and severity varies greatly, both within and between families. Skin involvement can be severe enough to result in neonatal infant death. During middle to late childhood, improvement occurs and blistering may be a minimal component of the disorder in adult life. Unlike other forms of epidermolysis bullosa, the Dowling-Meara variant appears to improve with heat or warmth in some individuals. Spontaneous prolonged clearing with fevers has been reported.

Progressive hyperkeratosis, punctate or diffuse, of the palms and soles begins in childhood. It may be the major complaint of patients in adult life.

The mucosa can be involved; this usually resolves with age.

MINOR. Nail dystrophy and milia, typically thought to be features limited to dystrophic disease, are common.

Both hyperpigmentation and hypopigmentation can occur.

ASSOCIATED ABNORMALITIES

None.

A

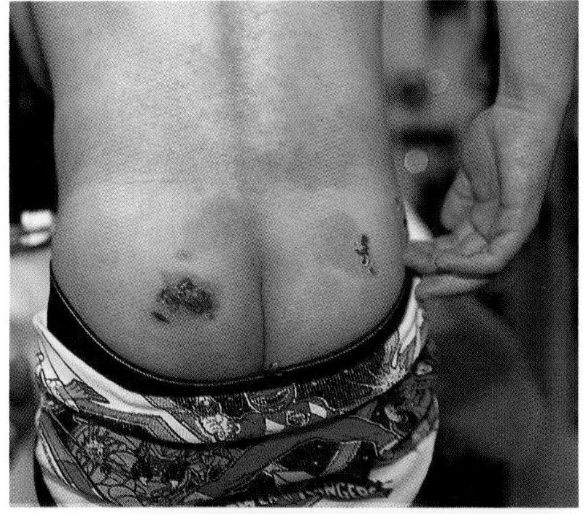

B

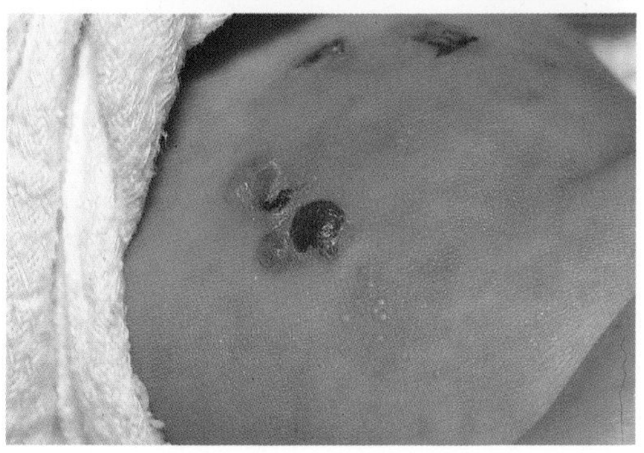

Figure 2.108. (A) Grouped blisters. Healing areas are red without scarring. Hyperpigmentation. **(B)** Hemorrhagic grouped blisters. Milia are present without evidence of scarring.

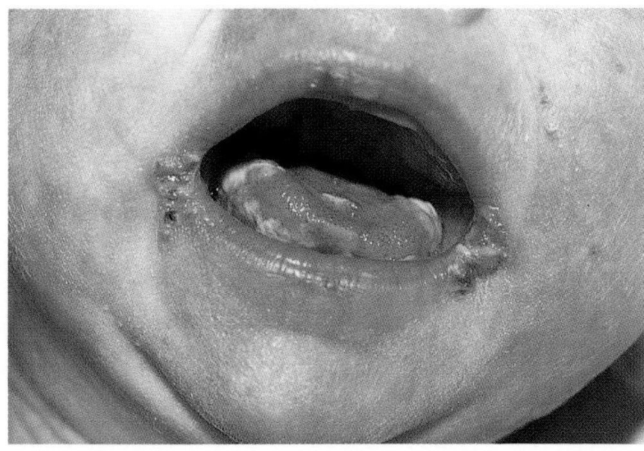

Figure 2.109. Oral involvement. This infant died of sepsis.

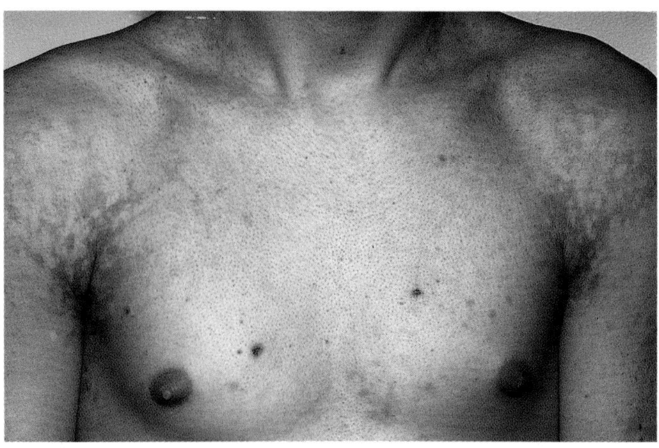

Figure 2.110. Marked lacy reticular hyperpigmentation. Few small erosions on chest.

HISTOPATHOLOGY

Light. The blister occurs within the basal keratinocytes. Eosinophils occasionally are present.

EM. Clumping of tonofilaments in the basal keratinocytes is the distinguishing hallmark of the disorder. One study noted two distinct types of changes: round clumping and whisk-type clumping, and suggests that these may be specific to specific mutations.

BASIC DEFECT

Defects in the basic keratin 5 *(KRT5)* on chromosome 12 and the acidic keratin 14 *(KRT14)* on chromosome 17 have been demonstrated. The abnormal proteins exert a dominant negative effect on keratin filament assembly.

TREATMENT

Standard dressing care for blisters, skin protection, and attention to secondary infection are necessary. Lancing of blisters before they can spread by the pressure of their own fluid may be helpful.

Use of keratolytics and softening agents for the palmoplantar hyperkeratosis in adulthood has some limited benefit. I have had one patient treated with Accutane (13-*cis*-retinoic acid) who noted an improvement in hyperkeratosis and a decrease in blisters.

Cyproheptadine (Periactin) in standard doses has been reported to reduce blistering in two anecdotal reports. In a small clinical trial we performed, it clearly was beneficial in some patients and, in my opinion, deserves a trial in all.

In infants and children with more severe involvement, failure to thrive may be a problem. Nutritional support may be required.

MODE OF INHERITANCE

Autosomal dominant, with many sporadic cases.

PRENATAL DIAGNOSIS

Possible by direct mutational analysis, linkage, or fetoscopy and fetal skin biopsy.

DIFFERENTIAL DIAGNOSIS

Epidermolysis bullosa superficialis is similar in clinical appearance. Milia and atrophic scarring can occur. Patients may have oral and ocular involvement. The nails may or may not be

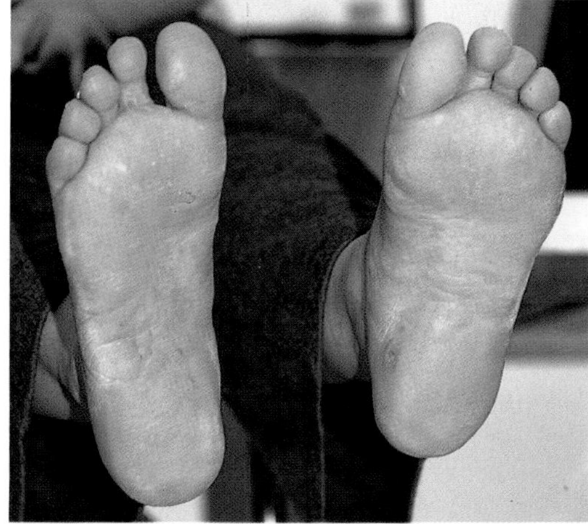
A

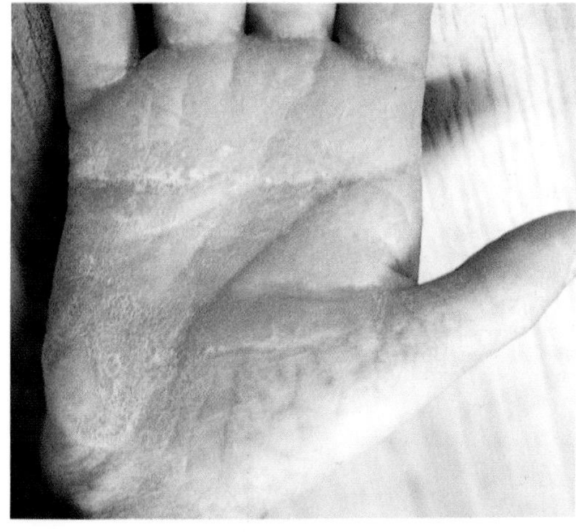
B

Figure 2.111. Plantar (**A**) and palmar (**B**) hyperkeratosis in older patients.

affected. This condition is also autosomal dominant. Electron microscopy shows a split just below the stratum corneum, rarely in the lower two-thirds of the epidermis. This condition is extremely rare and I have never seen it.

Epidermolysis bullosa simplex (EBS) occurs with muscular dystrophy (MIM:226670). There are a number of case reports of EBS with marked skin changes: atrophy, scarring, and associated with muscle disease, with or without nail dystrophy. The forms of muscular dystrophy have included limb–girdle muscular dystrophy,"congenital muscular dystrophy," myasthenia gravis, and facioscapulohumeral muscular dystrophy. The specific relationship between the skin and the muscle diseases is unclear. Recent work has demonstrated alterations in plectin, an intermediate filament present in both skin and muscle, in some individuals with epidermolysis bullosa and a slowly progressive muscular dystrophy. Inheritance in most cases has been consistent with autosomal recessive transmission. Severe widespread blistering in the presence of atrophy and scarring, coupled with blistering within the epidermis, should raise the possibility of one of these entities, rather than EBS Dowling-Meara.

In EBS with mottled hyperpigmentation (MIM:131960) the blisters are not grouped and pigment is more distinctive in a lentigo or freckle-like distribution. There is both hyperpigmentation and hypopigmentation, which can also be seen in EBS Dowling-Meara. Atrophy of the skin of the hands and feet is common in EBS mottled hyperpigmentation and is not part of EBS Dowling-Meara. EBS mottled hyperpigmentation worsens with heat. Caries are common in EBS mottled hyperpigmentation, perhaps due to poor dental hygiene. Clumping of tonofilaments is an ultrastructural feature common to both, but in EBS mottled hyperpigmentation it is claimed that there is a specific discontinuity of the basement membrane zone. I believe EBS mottled hyperpigmentation is clinically very similar to Kindler-Weary syndrome (MIM:173650) and may not be genetically distinct.

Incontinentia pigmenti (MIM:318310 might be confused in the newborn period. The blisters in EBS Dowling-Meara do not distribute along the lines of Blaschko but tend to be grouped in clusters. Verrucous changes on the trunk and extremities are not part of EBS Dowling-Meara. A biopsy will differentiate.

Epidermolysis bullosa junctional (EBJ) (MIM:226610, 226700, 226730) and recessive epidermolysis bullosa dystrophica (EBD) (MIM:226600) can look similar to severe EBS Dowling-Meara at birth. Electron microscopy will allow for correct diagnosis.

Support Group: D.E.B.R.A.
40 Rector Street, 8th Floor
New York, NY 10006
1-212-693-6610

SELECTED BIBLIOGRAPHY

Buchbinder, L.H., Lucky, A.W., Ballard, E., Stanley, J.R., Stolar, E., Tabas, M., Bauer, E.A., and Paller, A.S. (1986). Severe infantile EBS: Dowling-Meara type. *Arch. Dermatol.* **122,** 190–198.

Demonstrates how severe EBS Dowling-Meara can be. Clinical confusion with EBD occurred, misdiagnoses were made when based on light microscopy alone, and one infant died.

Coleman, R., Harper, J.I., and Lake, B.D. (1993). Epidermolysis bullosa simplex with mottled hyperpigmentation. *Br. J. Dermatol.* **128,** 679–685.

Two members of a four generation pedigree with male-to-male transmission were studied. The pigmentation occurred slowly, in areas that never had blistered. Keratoderma was also a feature, similar to EBS Dowling-Meara. They found no tonofilament clumping.

Dowling, G.B., and Meara, R.H. (1954). Epidermolysis bullosa resembling juvenile dermatitis herpetiformis. *Br. J. Dermatol.* **66,** 139–143.

Four children; in one onset of blisters did not begin until 3 months of age. None had a positive family history, and the authors incorrectly inferred autosomal recessive inheritance. A lesson to remember.

Fine, J.-D., Johnson, L., and Wright, T. (1989). Epidermolysis bullosa simplex superficialis. *Arch. Dermatol.* **125,** 633–638.

A large pedigree with many generations and male-to-male transmission. Despite the superficial level of the split, many cutaneous findings, including atrophic scarring, nail changes, and oral involvement.

Holbrook, K.A., Wapner, R., Jackson, L., and Zaeri, N. (1992). Diagnosis and prenatal diagnosis of epidermolysis bullosa herpetiformis (Dowling-Meara) in a mother, two affected children, and an affected fetus. *Prenat. Diagn.* **12,** 725–739.

More interesting for the subtext than for the prenatal diagnosis. A woman, who claimed to have no history of blistering, had two affected children by two different fathers. Each child was diagnosed as having EBJ or EBD. Skin biopsy material from a fetus fathered by a third male showed clumping of tonofilaments. The mother was requestioned and found to have had blisters in childhood. On examination she was then noted to have hyperkeratotic palms and soles. Biopsy specimens from the two previously affected children were reviewed and found to have features typical of EBS Dowling-Meara.

Salih, M.A.M., Lake, B.D., El Hag, M.A., and Atherton, D.J. (1985). Lethal epidermolytic epidermolysis bullosa: a new autosomal recessive type of epidermolysis bullosa. *Br. J. Dermatol.* **113,** 135–143.

An inbred kinship with numerous affected sibships. Lethal in some in infancy. Clinically similar to EBS Dowling-Meara, but worsens with heat. Electron microscopy is described as showing split within the basal keratinocytes, "poorly organized," "disorganized and fragmented" tonofilaments; cannot be evaluated from the photographs.

Stephens, K., Sybert, V.P., Wijsman, E.M., Ehrlich, P., and Spencer, A. (1993). A keratin 14 mutational hot spot for epidermolysis bullosa simplex, Dowling-Meara: implications for diagnosis. *J. Invest. Dermatol.* **101,** 240–243.

Of 10 individuals and/or families with EBS Dowling-Meara, six had a G–A or C–T substitution in codon 125 of the gene for K14, suggesting a "hot spot" for mutations.

Tadini, G., Ermacora, E., Cambiaghi, S., Brusasco, A., and Cavalli, R. (1993). Positive response to 5HT-2 antagonists in a family affected by epidermolysis bullosa Dowling-Meara type [Letter]. *Dermatology* **186,** 80.

Oral pipamperone at 20 mg/day in an infant and 180 mg/day in a mother resulted in complete clearing of blisters. Side effects included developmental delay in the infant and drowsiness in the mother. Cyproheptadine was tried at 4 and 8 mg/day, respectively, with marked improvement and no side effects.

Vassar, R., Coulombe, P.A., Degenstein, L., Albers, K., and Fuchs, E. (1991). Mutant keratin expression in transgenic mice causes marked abnormalities resulting in a human genetic skin disease. *Cell* **64,** 365–380.

A beautiful study in which mice transgenic for a partially deleted human *K14* gene showed blistering, intraepidermal separation, and clumping of tonofilaments.

EPIDERMOLYSIS BULLOSA SIMPLEX GENERALIZED (MIM:131900)

(EBS Koebner)

DERMATOLOGIC FEATURES

Major. The clinical features that help to distinguish dominant EBS Koebner from other simplex forms of epidermolysis bullosa include

1. Generalized distribution without clustering of blisters
2. Occasional oral involvement
3. Occasional vaginal involvement
4. Occasional nail involvement

Minor. Milia (keratin and sebum retained within pilosebaceous units) are said not to occur in nonscarring epidermolysis bullosa; in my experience they can be seen in any rapidly healing tissue. While milia are less common in dominant EBS Koebner than in dominant EBS Dowling-Meara, they do occur.

Occasionally, hyperkeratosis of the palms and soles can develop. This feature can be seen in all three major forms of EBS, but is most common in EBS Dowling-Meara.

ASSOCIATED ABNORMALITIES

There are infrequent descriptions of corneal abnormalities in generalized EBS. Most individuals do not have eye problems.

Muscular dystrophies of various types (spinal muscular atrophy, progressive muscular dystrophy, congenital hypotonia) have been described in a few families with EBS and presumed autosomal recessive inheritance. The clinical appearance of the epidermolysis bullosa is more typical of EBD or epidermolysis bullosa atrophicans, although biopsy specimens show an intraepidermal split. Most reports do not describe ultrastructure evaluation. Recent work suggests that the hemidesmosomes lack normal connections to keratin intermediate filaments. A risk to develop muscular dystrophy is not a realistic concern for families with typical EBS Koebner.

HISTOPATHOLOGY

Light. Multiloculated blisters in the basal layer are typical, usually developing below the cell nuclei. Bits of basal cell cytoplasm may remain attached to the dermis after separation.

EM. The split occurs within or just above the basal cells. There is cytolysis of the cytoplasm below the nuclei. Tonofilaments are not clumped, but may be destroyed.

BASIC DEFECT

Molecular defects in the genes for keratin 5 *(KRT5)* on chromosome 12q and keratin 14 *(KRT14)* on chromosome 17q have been demonstrated in many families. Alterations in the plectin gene or the hemidesmosomal gene *HD1* may be causal in EBS with muscular dystrophy.

TREATMENT

Mechanical protection of the skin. Topical mupirocin (Bactroban) for erosions. As with all forms of epidermolysis bullosa, there appears to be some improvement with age. Lancing of blisters to decompress them is beneficial in most patients; in some it is not helpful.

MODE OF INHERITANCE

Autosomal dominant with 100% penetrance; marked intrafamilial variability in severity. Rare reports of consanguineous pedigrees consistent with autosomal recessive inheritance. Recessive inheritance appears to be associated with homozygosity for null alleles; dominant with heterozygosity for mutations causing structural alterations, consistent with a dominant negative effect.

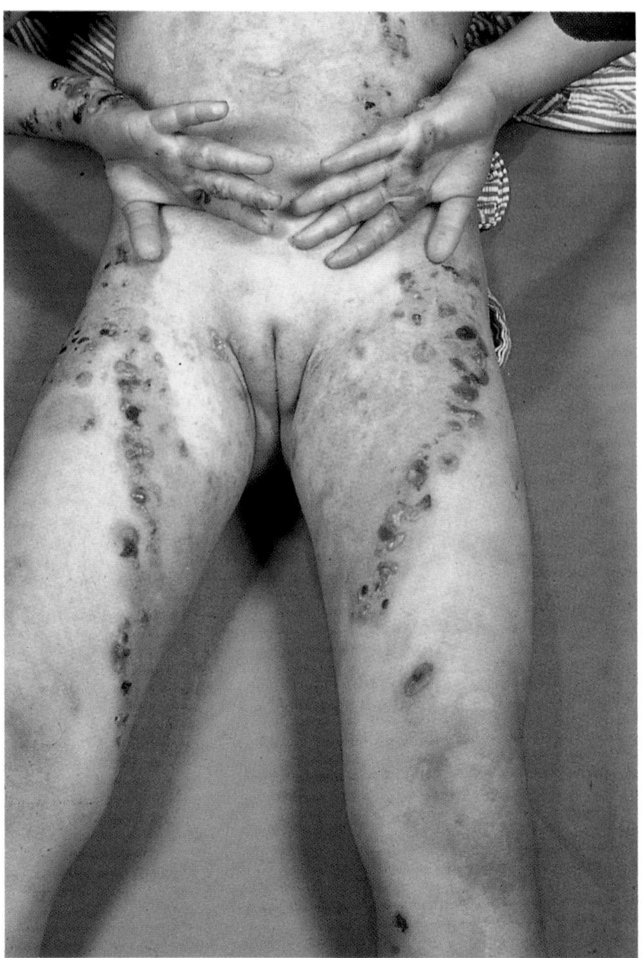

Figure 2.112. Widespread blistering, both hemorrhagic and serous.

PRENATAL DIAGNOSIS

Prenatal diagnosis by fetoscopy and fetal skin biopsy for electron microscopy and/or immunofluorescence studies is possible for dominant EBS Koebner. To my knowledge it has not been done. Linkage or mutation analysis for keratin 14 or keratin 5 using chorionic villous samples or amniotic fluid cells is now feasible.

DIFFERENTIAL DIAGNOSIS

All the blistering diseases of infancy need to be considered in the differential diagnosis. Most can be ruled out clinically. Other forms of generalized epidermolysis bullosa such as EBS Dowling-Meara (MIM:131760), EBJ (MIM:226610, 226700, 226730), and EBD (MIM:131700, 131800, 226600) can be differentiated by electron microscopy. There is significant clinical overlap with EBS Weber-Cockayne (MIM:131800). In many EBS Weber-Cockayne families there will be some individuals with more generalized involvement typical of EBS Koebner. Conversely, Koebner's original patient developed blisters only on her hands and feet and under her corset. The disorders are allelic; either phenotype can result from mutations in K_5 or K_{14}. Perhaps mutation analysis will allow for more specific prediction of severity within families.

Bullous impetigo and staphylococcal scalded skin can be ruled out by appropriate bacterial cultures. Transient bullous disease of infancy (MIM:131705) may be difficult to distinguish clinically. Electron microscopy will demonstrate a subepidermal separation in transient bullous disease. Transient acropustulosis of infancy occurs primarily in black infants and is characterized more by pustules than blisters, which develop without trauma. In incontinentia pigmenti (MIM:308310) blisters tend to be grouped, and rapid progression to verrucous lesions is typical. Biopsy will show eosinophils in incontinentia pigmenti. These are not present in significant numbers in EBS Koebner.

There are a few consanguineous pedigrees reported with severe epidermolysis bullosa simplex in siblings. It is striking that in all, while electron microscopic findings demonstrate an intraepidermal split, the clinical picture is characterized by atrophy, scarring, mucosal involvement, and a phenotype more similar to EBD or EBJ atrophicans.

Infants with bullous mastocytosis (MIM: 154800) can present with widespread blisters; the presence of purple nodules or typical mast cell lesions is usually a clue to the correct diagnosis. Biopsy will differentiate between the two conditions.

Support Group: D.E.B.R.A.
40 Rector Street, 8th Floor
New York, NY 10006
1-212-693-6610

SELECTED BIBLIOGRAPHY

Bonifas, J.M., Rothman, A.L., and Epstein, E.H. Jr. (1991). Epidermolysis bullosa simplex: evidence in two families for keratin gene abnormalities. *Science* **254,** 1202–1205.

In one family with generalized skin fragility but blisters primarily on the hands and the feet, a T–C change in exon 6 of the keratin 14 gene was demonstrated. In a family with only acral blistering, linkage was shown to the region of chromosome 12 encoding keratin 5.

Humphries, M.M., Sheils, D.M., Ferrar, G.J., Kumar-Singh, R., Kenna, P.F., Mansergh, F.C., Jordan, S.A., Young, M., and Humphries, P. (1993). A mutation (Met–Arg) in the type 1 keratin (K14) gene responsible for autosomal dominant epidermolysis bullosa simplex. *Hum. Mutat.* **2,** 37–42.

A different point mutation in a different exon of K14 described in a separate family.

Rugg, E.L., McLean, W.H.I., Lane, E.B., Pitera, R., McMillan, J.R., Dopping-Hepenstal, P.J.C., Navsaria, H.A., Leigh, I.M., and Eady, R.A.J. (1994). A functional "knockout" of human keratin 14. *Genes Dev.* **8,** 2563–2573.

Chan, Y., Anton-Lamprecht, I., Yu, Q.-C., Jackel, A., Zabel, B., Ernst, J.P., and Fuchs, E. (1994). A human keratin 14 "knockout": the absence of K14 leads to severe epidermolysis bullosa simplex and a function for an intermediate filament protein. *Genes Dev.* **8,** 2574–2587.

Two different probands, products of consanguineous matings, both homozygous for different mutations leading to effective null alleles of K_{14}.

Stephens, K., Zlotogorski, A., Smith, L., Ehrlich, P., Wijsman, E., Livingston, R.J., and Sybert, V.P. (1995). Epidermolysis bullosa simplex: a keratin 5 mutation is a fully dominant allele in epidermal cytoskeletal function. *Am. J. Hum. Genet.* **56,** 577–585.

In a consanguineous family with EBS Koebner, one individual was homozygous for the causal mutation in K_5. Her clinical features were not significantly worse than those of her heterozygous relatives, demonstrating the true dominant negative effect of the mutation.

EPIDERMOLYSIS BULLOSA SIMPLEX LOCALIZED (MIM:131800)

(EBS Weber-Cockayne)

Includes Kallin Syndrome; EBS Ogna

DERMATOLOGIC FEATURES

MAJOR. Blisters are usually confined to the hands and feet, although they can occur anywhere, given adequate trauma. I have seen patients develop blisters on the buttocks after horseback riding and around the waist after wearing a tight belt. The palms and soles are usually more involved than the backs of the hands and the tops of the feet. Symptoms are worse in warm weather (as is true for all forms of epidermolysis bullosa except dominant EBS Dowling-Meara) and worsen with sweating. Blisters are rarely present at birth. The first episodes may occur on the knees and shins with crawling or on the feet at about 18 months after walking is firmly established. Some affected individuals do not manifest the disease until adolescence or early adult life, and the classic story is that of the army recruit with Weber-Cockayne who blisters severely after his first enforced march.

MINOR. Occasionally, a nail may be shed if a large blister occurs in the nail bed. Hyperkeratosis of the palms and soles can develop in later childhood and adult life.

ASSOCIATED ABNORMALITIES

None.

HISTOPATHOLOGY

LIGHT. Intraepidermal cell lysis and separation.

EM. The split often occurs above the basal cells in the upper stratum Malpighii, below the granular layer. This is a higher split than that of dominant EBS Koebner, but the level of splitting may reflect the degree of trauma rather than the specific gene defect, and splitting in the basal layer is also described in Weber-Cockayne.

BASIC DEFECT

Molecular defects in the gene for keratin 5 (*KRT5*) on chromosome 12q and in the gene for keratin 14 (*KRT14*) on chromosome 17q have been demonstrated in many families with EBS Weber-Cockayne.

TREATMENT

Drysol or Peri-dri (20% aluminum chloride) or topical glutaraldehyde applied to the soles and palms to decrease sweating may be helpful. Lancing of blisters speeds healing and prevents lateral spread by the pressure of blister fluid. Avoidance of trauma and protection are primary.

MODE OF INHERITANCE

Autosomal dominant with 100% penetrance. Only one pedigree suggestive of autosomal recessive inheritance has been reported.

PRENATAL DIAGNOSIS

Potentially possible by molecular analysis of chorionic villi or amniotic fluid cells.

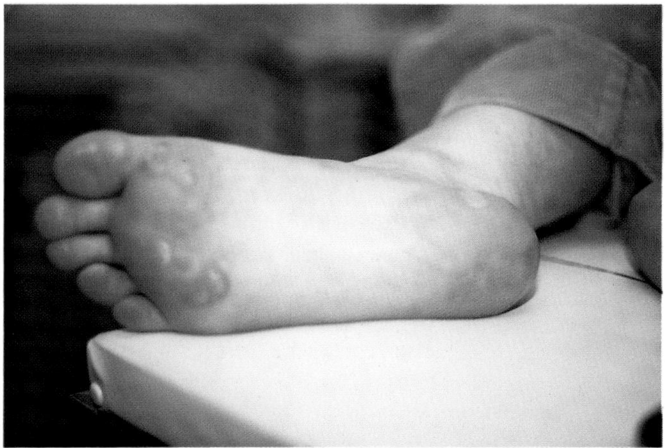

Figure 2.113. Blisters on foot.

DIFFERENTIAL DIAGNOSIS

EBD, EBJ, and EBS Dowling-Meara can be differentiated by electron microscopy. It is sometimes difficult to distinguish between EBS Weber-Cockayne and EBS Koebner (MIM: 131900) clinically, and there are no reliable ultrastructural indicators. In some families, involvement is clearly limited to hands and feet, and a diagnosis of Weber-Cockayne fits best; in some, generalized blistering as in EBS Koebner is the rule; but in many, involvement is somewhere in between. It is clear from molecular studies that the distinction between the two is arbitrary and clinical in that they are allelic disorders with considerable overlap in phenotype.

Transient acropustulosis of infancy occurs primarily in black infants and is characterized more by pustules than blisters. Normal blistering with trauma is usually a one-time episode; in EBS Weber-Cockayne, chronicity is the key. Sweaty foot dermatitis or dyshidrotic eczema with peeling can be confused with EBS Weber-Cockayne; erythema, chapping, and eczematous changes are absent in EBS Weber-Cockayne. The Ogna variant (MIM:131950) of EBS has been reported only in one kindred in Norway. These individuals had blisters primarily on the hands and feet coupled with bruising. This disorder has been linked to glutamate pyruvate transaminase, which maps to chromosome 8.

Support Group: D.E.B.R.A.
40 Rector Street, 8th Floor
New York, NY 10006
1-212-693-6610

SELECTED BIBLIOGRAPHY

Fine, J.D., Johnson, L., Wright, T., and Horiguchi, Y. (1989). Epidermolysis bullosa simplex: identification of a kindred with autosomal recessive transmission of the Weber-Cockayne variety. *Pediatr. Dermatol.* **6,** 1–5.

Three of five individuals in two sets of double third cousins (coefficient of inbreeding 1/64) were affected with typical Weber-Cockayne; palms and soles were the only sites of blistering. A second cousin of one of these sibships (coefficient of inbreeding 1/32) was also affected, but had more severe, widespread involvement with scars, milia, hypopigmentation, dystrophic nails, and mucosal involvement. Could this be due to compound heterozygosity?

Gamborg-Nielsen, P., and Sjolund, E. (1985). Epidermolysis bullosa simplex localisata associated with anodontia, hair and nail disorders: a new syndrome. *Acta Dermatol. Venereol.* **65,** 526–530.

The sisters Kallin, for whom the disorder is named, shared in common hypodontia and blisters of the feet. Sister A had transient alopecia that resolved and mild onychogryphosis of the toenails. Biopsy of a blister showed subcorneal cleavage. Sister B had blisters on the hands, mildly curved fingernails and toenails, thinned brittle hair, and unilateral deafness. With hematoxylin and eosin stain, the blisters were seen in the midepidermis. Electron microscopy was not performed on either sister.

Niemi, K.-M., Sommer, H., Kero, M., Kanerva, L., and Haltia, M. (1988). Epidermolysis bullosa simplex associated with muscular dystrophy and recessive inheritance. *Arch. Dermatol.* **124,** 551–554.

A sister and brother with blisters, atrophic changes, nail dystrophy, mild scarring, and tooth loss had progressive weakness. Muscular dystrophy of different types have been reported with epidermolysis bullosa of uncertain types. Usually, information about ultrastructural features is lacking. The reasons for all of these associations remain unclear. In some, mutations in the plectin gene are believed to be causal.

EPIDERMOLYSIS BULLOSA JUNCTIONAL GENERALIZED (MIM:226700, 226730)

(EBJ Herlitz; EBJ Herlitz-Pearson; EBJ Letalis; EBJ Gravis)

Includes EBJ with Pyloric Atresia

DERMATOLOGIC FEATURES

MAJOR. Blistering is generalized, severe, and almost invariably present at birth. Blisters may be hemorrhagic. Hands, feet, buttocks and perineum, abdomen, and face may all be involved. All mucosal surfaces—oral, respiratory, gastrointestinal, and genitourinary—may be affected.

Death in infancy is typical but not invariable. Sepsis is a common complication leading to death. Sloughing of the respiratory mucosa with obstruction and sudden death is also a major cause of mortality. Hoarseness of the cry indicates respiratory involvement and is an ominous augury.

Among survivors, a common feature is exuberant granulation tissue, which develops around the nose and mouth and can occur at fingertips.

MINOR. Nails are commonly shed and may not regrow. Balanitis is reported in uncircumcised males.

ASSOCIATED ABNORMALITIES

Pyloric atresia has been reported in a subset of fetuses and infants with EBJ. This association is likely specific to one form of EBJ rather than a feature common to a genetically heterogeneous group.

Hydronephrosis and interstitial nephritis have been mentioned in individual case reports.

Chronic anemia is a secondary complication, probably due to nutritional inadequacy, anemia of chronic disease, and blood loss from erosions.

Corneal erosions and scarring and blistering of the eyelids with blepharitis were described in 50% of patients in one series.

Dysplastic teeth and cobblestoning of the enamel have been noted. Severe dental problems with caries may result from poor dental toilet because of fragile gums as well as from the primary enamel dysplasia.

HISTOPATHOLOGY

LIGHT. Immunofluorescent labeling with GB3 (which recognizes nicein) or 19-DEJ-1 is diminished or absent.

EM. The split occurs within the lamina lucida, below the plasma membrane of the epidermal keratinocyte. There is a paucity to absence of hemidesmosomes, and the hemidesmosomes that are present are usually hypoplastic.

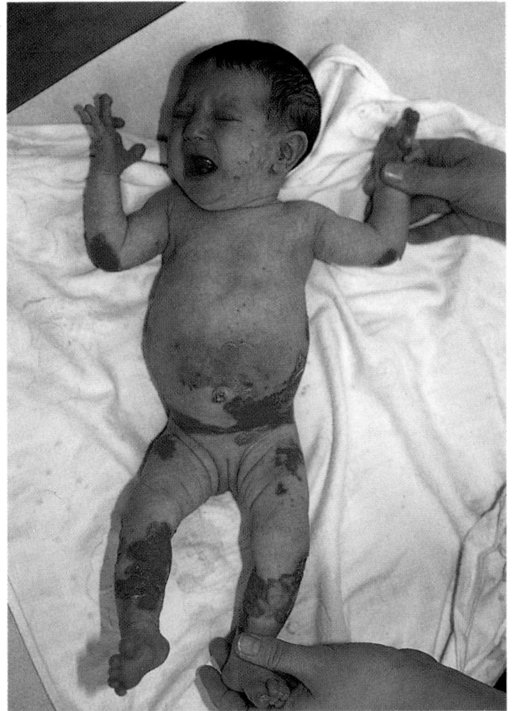
A

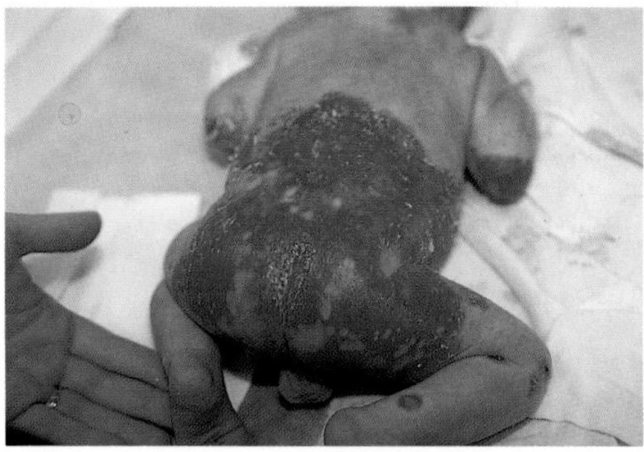
B

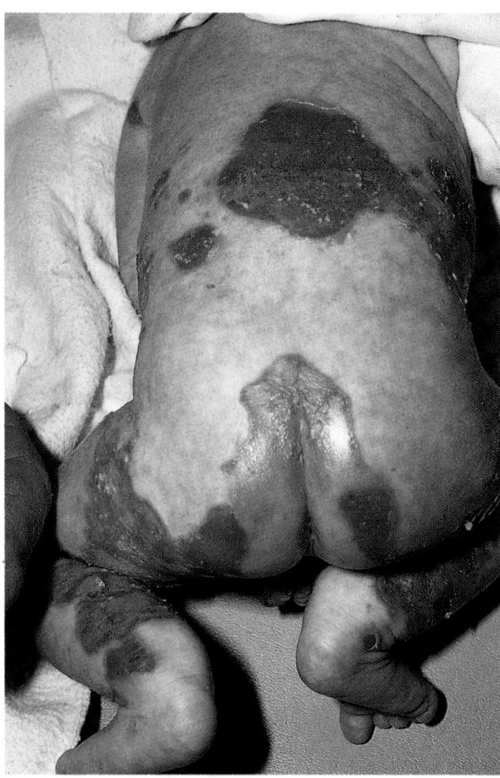
C

Figure 2.114. (A–C) Infants with severe lethal disease showing widespread and superficial erosions.

BASIC DEFECT

Defects in subunits of laminin 5 (nicein/kalinin) appear to be causal. In one patient with EBJ and pyloric atresia, compound heterozygosity for mutations in the β_4-integrin gene *(ITGβ4)* was found.

TREATMENT

Standard wound treatment with appropriate dressings and vigilance against secondary infection are basic. Treatment is tedious and complicated and must be individualized.

Use of tracheostomy when respiratory involvement occurs is arguable. Outcome of tracheostomies have ranged from death to inability to decannulate to successful extubation. Decisions regarding major intervention need to be made on a case by case and family by family basis.

Appropriate nutritional supplementation, use of occupational and physical therapy, and appropriate dental support are mainstays of care. Placement of a gastrostomy tube may be desirable for some infants whose survival is threatened by inanition rather than by respiratory compromise. In a small number of infants with EBJ and repaired pyloric atresia, persistent malabsorption and protein-losing enteropathy defied medical management.

Circumcision is probably warranted to prevent balanitis in males.

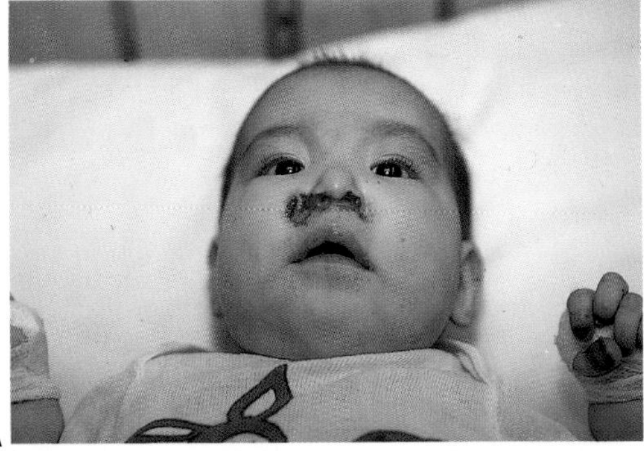
A

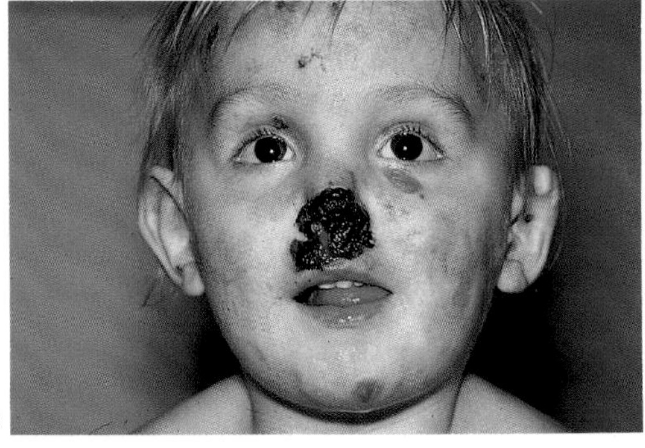
B

Figure 2.115. Typical perinasal involvement with granulation tissue. Older child **(B)** survived and lost to follow-up at age 8 years. Younger one **(A)** died of sepsis at age 13 months.

DIFFERENTIAL DIAGNOSIS

The mitis or generalized benign atrophic form of junctional epidermolysis bullosa (MIM: 226650) is indistinguishable clinically and morphologically. The diagnostic discriminator is time. Survival beyond infancy is limited almost entirely to the atrophic group. Infants with recessive EBD (MIM:226600) and severe epidermolysis bullosa simplex-Koebner (MIM: 131900) or epidermolysis bullosa simplex-Dowling-Meara (MIM:131760) can appear with identical clinical features at birth. Electron microscopy will distinguish among these entities.

Nongenetic causes of blistering (e.g., infection, toxic epidermal necrolysis, staphylococcal scalded skin) must always be excluded. Infants with bullous mastocytosis may present with widespread blistering; there are usually accompanying nodules and plaques composed of mast cell infiltrates. Biopsy will distinguish.

Support Group: D.E.B.R.A.
40 Rector Street, 8th Floor
New York, NY 10006
1-212-693-6610

MODE OF INHERITANCE

Autosomal recessive. Genes map to 1q51 *(LAMC2)*, 1q32 *(LAMB3)*, 18q11.2 *(LAMA3)*, and 17q11-qter *(ITGβ4)*.

PRENATAL DIAGNOSIS

Fetoscopy and fetal skin biopsy using both electron microscopy and fluorescent antibody probes has been successful. Monoclonal antibody staining of amniocytes has also proven reliable. α-Fetoprotein appears to be elevated in EBJ with pyloric atresia but is not necessarily elevated in other forms of EBJ. In EBJ with pyloric atresia, ultrasound examination may reveal a positive "snowflake sign" or evidence of gastric obstruction. Molecular diagnosis is likely to be widely available by the time this is published.

SELECTED BIBLIOGRAPHY

Dolan, C.R., Smith, L.T., and Sybert, V.P. (1993). Prenatal detection of epidermolysis bullosa letalis with pyloric atresia in a fetus with abnormal ultrasound and elevated alpha-fetoprotein. *Am. J. Med. Genet.* **47,** 395–400.

The diagnosis of EBJ with pyloric atresia was made unexpectedly by the presence of an elevated maternal serum α-fetoprotein level, elevated amniotic fluid levels of α-fetoprotein and acetylcholinesterase, and gastric dilation and a snowflake sign—echogenic particles in the amniotic fluid—at 20 weeks of pregnancy. The diagnosis was confirmed postmortem. There is a review of the literature. Fetoscopy and fetal skin biopsy remain the gold standard for prenatal diagnosis, pending identification of the gene defects involved.

Gil, S.G., Brown, T.A., Ryan, M.C., and Carter, W.G. (1994). Juntional epidermolysis bullosis: defects in expression of epiligrin/nicein/kalinin and integrin B4 that inhibit hemidesmosome formation. *J. Invest. Dermatol.* **103,** 31S–38S.

Vidal, F., Aberdam, D., Miquel, C., Christiano, A.M., Pulkkinen, L., Uitto, J., Ortonne, J.P., and Meneguzzi, G. (1995). Integrin beta 4 mutations associated with junctional epidermolysis bullosa with pyloric atresia. *Nat. Genet.* **10,** 229–234.

A patient with EBJ pyloric atresia had reduced expression of integrin $\beta 4$. The Vidal et al. (1995) paper demonstrates a single patient with EBJ and pyloric atresia with compound heterozygosity for mutations in this integrin.

Tidman, M.J., and Eady, R.A.J. (1986). Hemidesmosome heterogeneity in junctional epidermolysis bullosa revealed by morphometric analysis. *J. Invest. Dermatol.* **86,** 51–56.

Skin biopsies from five infants with lethal EBJ, three children with "indeterminate" disease, and three adults with "non-lethal" disease were studied. Although there were differences in the number and size of hemidesmosomes between patients, there were no consistent differences between the groups. Thus, electron microscopic findings do not reliably predict outcome.

Vailly, J., Pulkkinen, L., Christiano, A.M., Tryggvason, K., Uitto, J., Ortonne, J.-P., and Meneguzzi, G. (1995). Identification of a homozygous exon-skipping mutation in the *LAMC2* gene in a patient with Herlitz's junctional epidermolysis bullosa. *J. Invest. Dermatol.* **104,** 434–437.

Vailly, J., Pulkkinen, L., Miquel, C., Christiano, A.M., Gerecke, D., Burgeson, R.E., Uitto, J., Ortonne, J.-P., and Meneguzzi, G. (1995). Identification of a homozygous one-basepair deletion in exon 14 of the *LAMB3* gene in a patient with Herlitz junctional epidermolysis bullosa and prenatal diagnosis in a family at risk for recurrence. *J. Invest. Dermatol.* **104,** 462–466.

Baudoin, C., Miquel, C., Blanchet-Bardon, C., Gambini, C., Meneguzzi, G., and Ortonne, J.-P. (1995). Herlitz juntional EB keratinocytes display heterogeneous defects of nicein/kalinin gene expression. *J. Clin. Invest.* **93,** 862–869.

Three reports of different mutations and alterations in different components of laminin 5 (nicein/kalinin) and prenatal exclusion of the disorder by mutational analysis in a fetus at risk.

EPIDERMOLYSIS BULLOSA JUNCTIONAL GENERALIZED ATROPHIC BENIGN (MIM:226650)

(Mitis; Disentis; GABEB)

Includes EBJ Localisata; EBJ Progressiva; EBJ Inversa; EBJ Cicatricial; LOGIC

DERMATOLOGIC FEATURES

MAJOR. The term *benign* is legitimately applied to this group only in perspective to the lethality of the Herlitz form. Despite the high likelihood of survival beyond infancy, the burden of this disorder is significant. Blisters are present at birth but decrease in frequency with age. Healing with atrophy and shiny cigarette paper-like changes, rather than scarring, is the rule. Milia are stated not to occur. Nail dystrophy with thickening, fracturing, and loss of nail plates is common, as is scarring alopecia, which can involve the scalp, pubic and axillary hairs, eyebrows, and eyelashes.

Blistering of the mucosa and esophageal and laryngeal involvement with stenosis can occur, as can urethral involvement.

MINOR. Hyperkeratosis of the palms and soles is described in a number of case reports. The significance of hyperpigmented lesions or nevocytic nevi reported in a few patients is unclear.

ASSOCIATED ABNORMALITIES

Corneal ulcers occur rarely. Tooth abnormalities include "abraded enamel," "defects in enamel," "caries," and tooth loss, presumably secondary to caries. One 26-year-old patient was described with EBJ and wasting muscle disease of unclear type.

HISTOPATHOLOGY

LIGHT. The basement membrane remains with the blister floor.
EM. Cleavage occurs within the lamina lucida. Hemidesmosomes may be degenerated, decreased in number, or absent. The anchoring fibrils are normal.

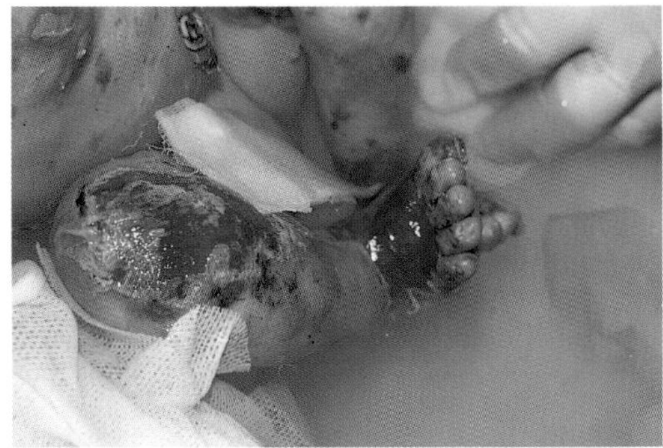

Figure 2.116. Erosions and blisters in a newborn with "mitis" junctional epidermolysis bullosa.

BASIC DEFECT

Mutations in *LAMB3*—the β 3 chain of laminin 5—and a deficiency of the bullous pemphigoid antigen have been demonstrated in one and three patients, respectively.

TREATMENT

Dilantin treatment has enjoyed anecdotal success. The usual need for skin protection, wound dressing, management of infection, nutrition, and dental care applies.

MODE OF INHERITANCE

Autosomal recessive. *LAMB3* maps to 1q32, *BPAG2* to 10q24.3. Likely to have locus and allelic heterogeneity.

PRENATAL DIAGNOSIS

Should be possible by molecular techniques.

DIFFERENTIAL DIAGNOSIS

Mild forms of EBJ have been described individually but may or may not represent allelic, nonallelic, or identical disorders. The specific diagnostic categories are not clear cut, and individual patients may fit better between rather than within categories.

In localized EBJ (EBJ localisata), newborns present with absence of nails. Blistering ensues in childhood and then may improve in adult life. Teeth are carious. Partial alopecia has been described. Blisters can occur anywhere, but are most frequently on the shins. This may not be a causally distinct variant of EBJ.

In EBJ progressiva (MIM:226500), skin and nail involvement begin in childhood. Loss of dermatoglyphics and mild finger contractures ensue. Palmar hyperkeratosis and oral involvement also develop over time. Electron microscopy showed separation between the lamina lucida with amorphous material deposited in the lamina rara in some. Unlike in other forms of EBJ, hemidesmosomes appear normal.

Individuals with inverse EBJ can present with generalized blistering at birth, which, within months, becomes limited primarily to the groin and axillae, although the recurrence of truncal involvement in childhood is described. The anus can also be involved. The oral mucosa and the cornea may be affected; teeth and nails may also be abnormal. White spots (albostriate) appear on the trunk and extremities. These can be raised or flat and atrophic.

Cicatricial EBJ is extremely rare. The clinical appearance is similar to recessive EBD. Blisters heal with scarring and with pseudoamputation of the digits, but electron microscopy shows a split in the lamina lucida with sparse, small hemidesmosomes. The LOGIC syndrome

A

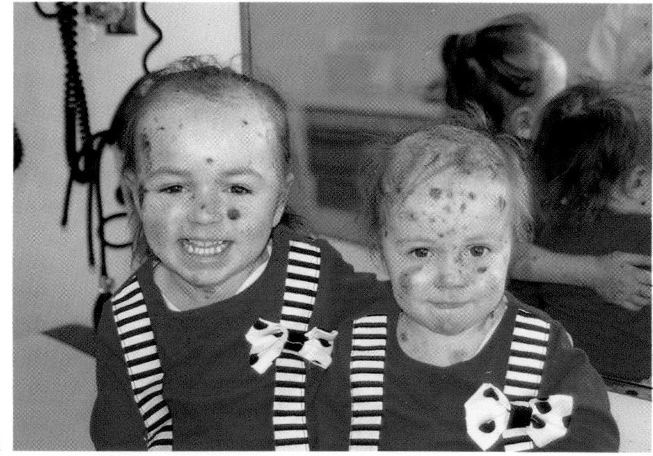

B

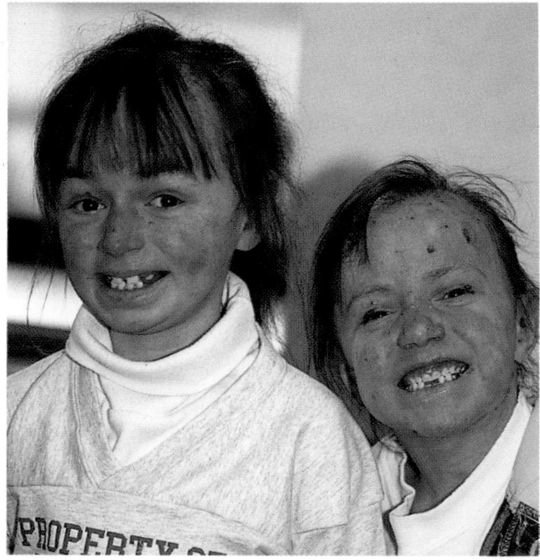

Figure 2.117. **(A)** Same patient as in Fig. 2.116 now at age 4 with her 2-year-old sister. **(B)** At ages 9 and 7. Both have sparse hair and scarring alopecia.

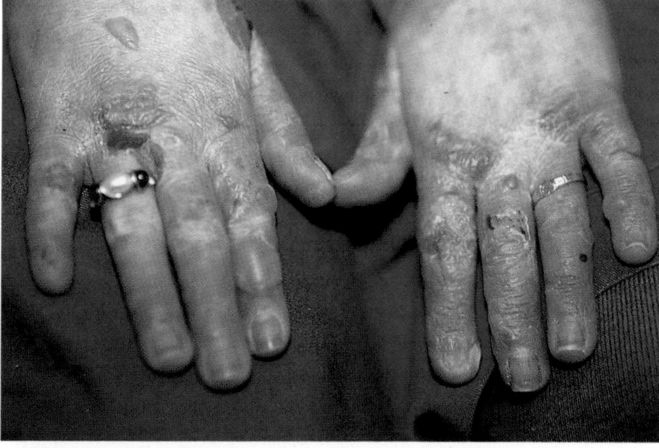

Figure 2.118. Hands showing serous and hemorrhagic blisters. Nail dystrophy, atrophic scarring, but no cutaneous fusion.

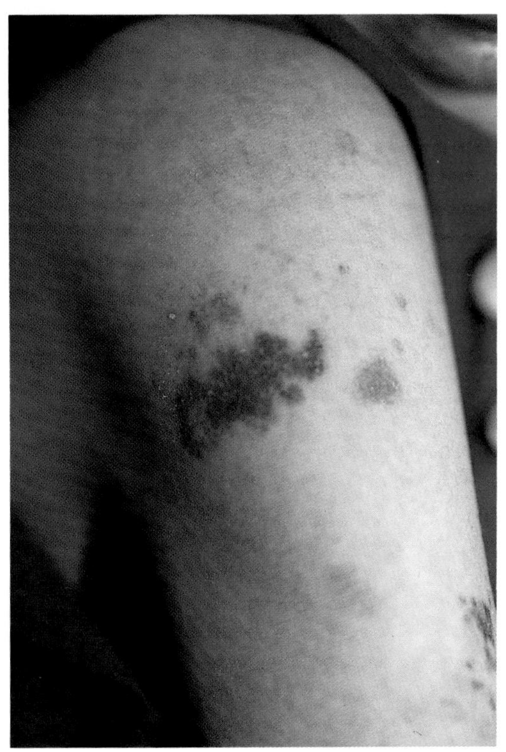

Figure 2.119. Peculiar hyperpigmentation and atrophic scars.

Figure 2.120. (A) Mild disease; hypopigmented scars. **(B)** Feet with nail changes; hypopigmented healed sites.

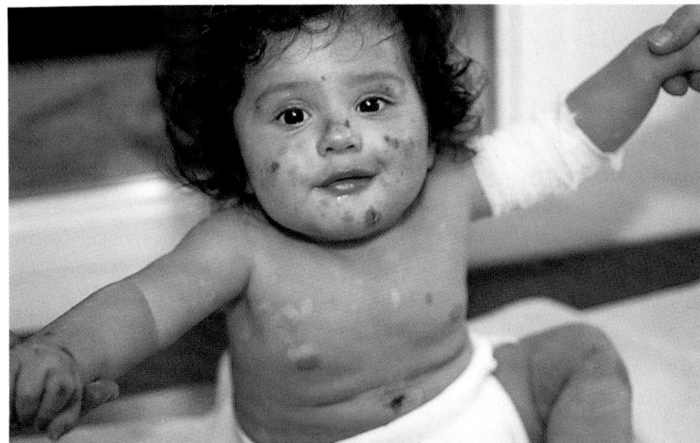

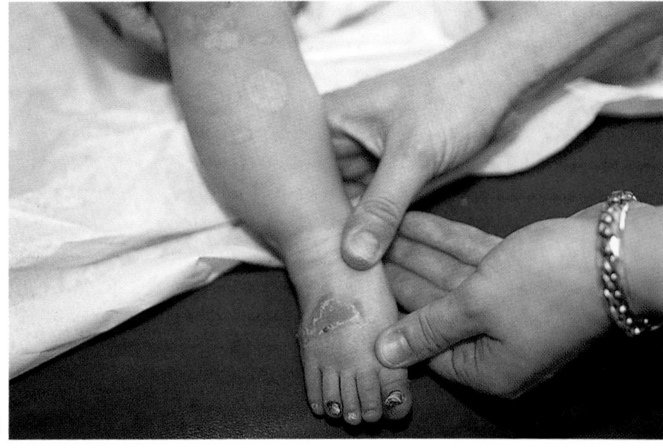

is a disorder described in Muslim Punjabis. Progressive *l*aryngeal and *o*cular *g*ranulation in *I*ndian *c*hildren is the major clinical finding. Skin erosions, nail dystrophy, and tooth abnormalities are also features. Blistering does not occur. Purportedly there are no electron microscopic changes of EBJ, but one sentence in a review noted that an abnormality in hemidesmosomes was found in one patient.

The clinical picture of EBJ letalis (MIM:226700) is identical at birth. In survivors the presence of granulation tissue around the nose may serve to distinguish EBJ letalis from generalized atrophic benign EBJ.

Support Group: D.E.B.R.A.
40 Rector Street, 8th Floor
New York, NY 10006
1-212-693-6610

SELECTED BIBLIOGRAPHY

Bircher, A.J., Lang-Muritano, M., Pfaltz, M., and Bruckner-Tuderman, L. (1993). Epidermolysis bullosa junctional progressiva in three siblings. *Br. J. Dermatol.* **128,** 429–435.

Fully evaluated three affected sibships. Good photographs and review of the literature.

Haber, R.M., and Hanna, W. (1987). Epidermolysis bullosa progressiva. *J. Am. Acad. Dermatol.* **16,** 195–200.

Case report. Patient presented with nail dystrophy at age 8 that progressed to permanent shedding of all nails. Blisters developed in the teen years. There was oral involvement with blisters without dental caries. Patient had palmar and plantar hyperkeratosis and loss of dermatoglyphics. Electron microscopic studies of a blister showed the level of separation to be within the lamina lucida and the presence of normal anchoring fibrils. In nonblistered skin, hemidesmosomes were normal. The authors suggested that EBD progressiva, described by Gedde-Dahl, is actually this junctional disorder.

Haber, R.M., Hanna, W., Ramsey, C.A., and Boxall, L.B.H. (1985). Cicatricial junctional epidermolysis bullosa. *J. Am. Acad. Dermatol.* **12,** 836–844.

Progressive nasal scarring resulting in obstruction was typical. A sporadic case and 4 affected siblings of a 10 member sibship are described. Two of the affected brothers died in their twenties from renal problems of an unknown nature. Electron microscopy of the skin showed separation within the lamina lucida, normal anchoring fibrils, and rudimentary hemidesmosomes.

Hintner, H., and Wolff, K. (1982). Generalized atrophic benign epidermolysis bullosa. *Arch. Dermatol.* **118,** 375–384.

Eight cases, four from one family. Detailed clinical description and excellent photos and photomicrographs.

Jonkman, M.F., de Jong, M.C., Heeres, K., Pas, H.H., van der Meer, J.B., Owaribe, K., Martinez-de-Velasco, A.M., Niessen, C.M., and Sonnenberg, A. (1995). 180-kD bullous pemphigoid antigen (BP180) is deficient in generalized atrophic benign epidermolysis bullosa. *J. Clin. Invest.* **95,** 1345–1352.

Skin from three unrelated patients with EBJ generalized atrophic benign showed negative staining with antibodies to bullous pemphigoid antigen. Staining was normal in skin from four individuals with EBJ Herlitz, one with "pretibial EBJ" and one with cicatricial EBJ.

McGrath, J.A., Pulkkinen, L., Christiano, A.M., Leigh, I.M., Eady, R.A.J., and Uitto, J. (1995). Altered laminin 5 expression due to mutations in the gene encoding the $\beta 3$ chain *(LAMB3)* in generalized atrophic benign epidermolysis bullosa. *J. Invest. Dermatol.* **104,** 467–474.

Three affected family members share compound heterozygosity for recessive mutations in the *LAMB3* gene. This family had normal staining to bullous pemphigoid antigen. Obviously, EBJ generalized atrophic benign is heterogeneous both clinically and causally.

EPIDERMOLYSIS BULLOSA DYSTROPHICA COCKAYNE-TOURAINE (MIM:131800, 131750, 132000)

(Dominant Epidermolysis Bullosa Dystrophica)

Includes Pasini, Bart, and Neurotrophica

DERMATOLOGIC FEATURES

MAJOR. Blisters can appear in the newborn period or as late as several years of age. In the Cockayne-Touraine variant of EBD, blisters tend to occur on the extremities, elbows, knees, and the digits. However, widespread blistering can also occur. In EBD Pasini, blisters tend to be more widespread. In both, blisters can occur in oral mucosa. Blisters heal with scarring. Scars may be thickened or atrophic. Mitten deformities do not occur. Milia are typically seen. All types of dominant EBD can have dystrophic nails.

The albupapuloid lesions characteristic of the Pasini variant are small whitish papules resembling scars or grouped milia. They can occur in areas without preceding blisters, and in a Koebner distribution (at sites of trauma). They predominate on the lower back, but can develop anywhere. They can coalesce into plaques. I am not convinced that they are specific to the Pasini variant.

In "Bart syndrome," congenital absence of skin over the tibias is a common finding. Scarring is variable.

As with most, if not all, forms of epidermolysis bullosa, blistering tends to decrease as patients age.

MINOR. Squamous cell carcinoma has been reported in some patients.

ASSOCIATED ABNORMALITIES

None.

HISTOPATHOLOGY

LIGHT. The albupapuloid lesions show variable and nonspecific changes.

EM. Separation occurs below the basement membrane. Anchoring fibrils are absent or hypoplastic and/or decreased in number. Attempts at correlation of ultrastructural features with clinical phenotype have not been uniformly successful.

BASIC DEFECT

Defects in type VII collagen have been demonstrated in both autosomal dominant and autosomal recessive epidermolysis bullosa dystrophica. Linkage to the *COL7A1* locus on chromosome 3 has been confirmed, and specific molecular defects have been found in some individuals.

TREATMENT

Standard blister management with lancing of blisters and atraumatic dressings. Protection of the skin is important.

MODE OF INHERITANCE

Autosomal dominant.

PRENATAL DIAGNOSIS

Fetal skin biopsy for electron microscopic evaluation. Linkage studies and direct mutational analyis are rapidly becoming methods of choice.

DIFFERENTIAL DIAGNOSIS

Localized recessive EBD, or mild recessive EBD Hallopeau-Siemens (MIM:226600) can be

A

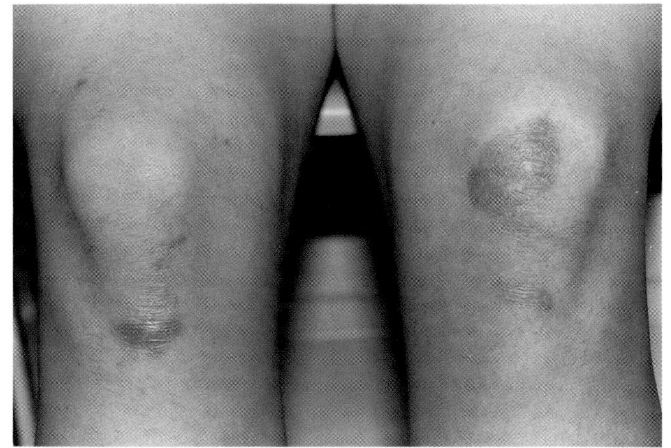

B

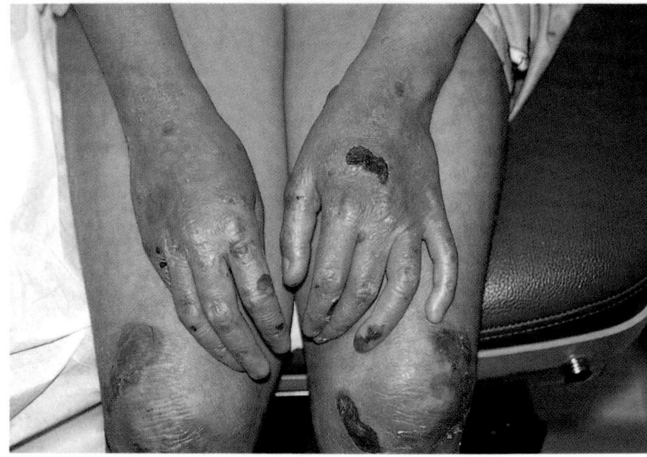

Figure 2.121. **(A)** Mild scarring over knees. **(B)** More severe involvement.

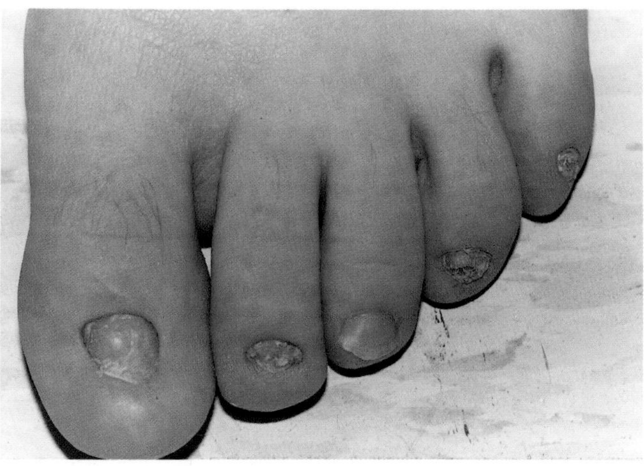

Figure 2.122. Nail changes.

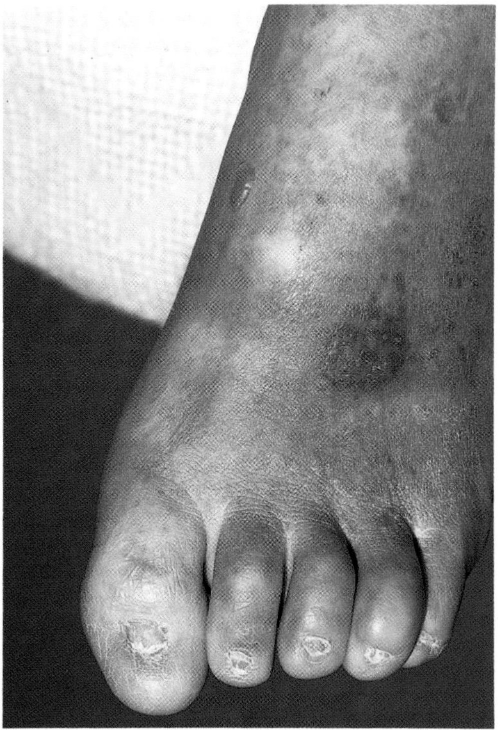

Figure 2.123. Patient from Bart's original family, with nail changes, scarring, pigment changes, and blister.

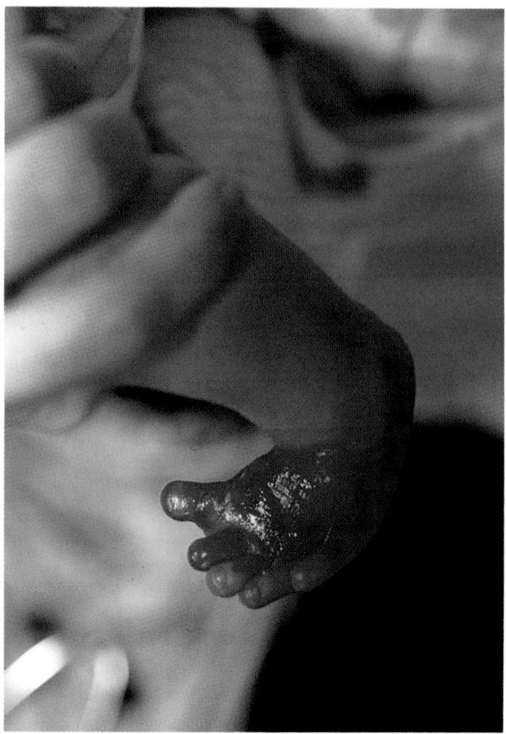

Figure 2.124. Aplasia cutis congenita of the lower leg and foot in localized dystrophic epidermolysis bullosa.

difficult to distinguish from dominant EBD. In sporadic cases, it may not be possible to differentiate autosomal dominant from autosomal recessive recurrence risks if a specific mutation cannot be identified in the affected individual.

A form of EBD with localized involvement and onset in late childhood (EBD neurotrophica, MIM:226500) has been described in a few families in Norway. Initially it was thought to be associated with progressive deafness, but this proved not to be true; the two disorders segregated independently. In EBD inversa (MIM:226450), sites of blistering are the genitalia, trunk, axillae, neck, and upper legs, and esophageal involvement is typical.

Support Group: D.E.B.R.A.
40 Rector Street, 8th Floor
New York, NY 10006
1-212-693-6610

SELECTED BIBLIOGRAPHY

Bouwes Bavinck J.N., van Haeringen, A., Ruiter, D., and van der Schroeff, J.G. (1987). Autosomal dominant epidermolysis bullosa dystrophica: are the Cockayne-Touraine, the Pasini and the Bart-types different expressions of the same mutant gene? *Clin. Genet.* **31,** 416–424.

A large pedigree with 25 affected members. Five were born with congenital absence of the skin. The authors also discuss a previously reported family in whom some members had albupapuloid lesions, others not, and one of whom had absence of the skin overlying the tibias. Authors argue for locus homogeneity, i.e., both Pasini and Cockayne-Touraine result from mutations in type VII collagen, and allelic heterogeneity.

Uitto, J., and Christiano, A.M. (1994). Molecular basis for the dystrophic forms of epidermolysis bullosa: mutations in the type VII collagen gene. *Arch. Dermatol. Res.* **287,** 16–22.

Clearly written review of mutations and mechanism.

Zelickson, B., Matsumura K., Kist, D., Epstein, E.H. Jr., and Bart, B. J. (1995). Bart's syndrome: ultrastructure and genetic linkage. *Arch. Dermatol.* **131,** 663–668.

Reevaluation of Bart's original pedigree. Ultrastructural features include poorly formed anchoring fibrils and a split below the lamina densa. Linkage to *COL7A1* on 3p with a lod score of 3.26 at 5% recombination. Ten of 37 affected members did not have congenital localized absence of the skin.

EPIDERMOLYSIS BULLOSA DYSTROPHICA, HALLOPEAU-SIEMENS (MIM:226600)

(Recessive Epidermolysis Bullosa Dystrophica Generalized Gravis; REBD Mutilans)

Includes Inversa, Mitis, and Localized Recessive

DERMATOLOGIC FEATURES

MAJOR. Blisters are present at birth or within the first few days of life. They may be serous or hemorrhagic. Blistering around nail plates is common, as is oral involvement. Blisters spread and enlarge under their own tension. Classically the blisters are tense with thick blister roof. This is not always readily clinically appreciated; thus its use as a diagnostic clue is limited.

Ulcerations and erosions are typical and may take long periods of time to heal. Milia are common within the healing sites. Itching is a frequent complaint.

Scars may be superficial and atrophic, or deeper and thickened. Pseudoamputation of digits due to scarring and fusion between the fingers and between the toes resulting in mitten deformities is the hallmark of the disorder. Early loss of nail plates with scarring is typical. Patchy scarring alopecia is a frequent finding.

The oral, gastrointestinal, and ocular mucous membranes are typically involved, and scarring may lead to gastrointestinal obstruction, ankyloglossia and microstomia, and eye problems.

Squamous cell carcinoma of the skin and mucosa develop in adult life between the ages of 20 and 40. These may be due to chronic injury (similar to the risk for cutaneous malignancy in burn scars) rather than being a direct result of the gene defect(s). It is unclear whether the risk for melanoma is increased.

MINOR. Congenital absence of the skin can occur and usually involves the lower extremities.

ASSOCIATED ABNORMALITIES

Blisters of the lids and conjunctivae are typical. Ectropion and occlusion of tear ducts with scar tissue can occur. Corneal involvement is less common. Mucosal involvement is the rule; esophageal strictures develop in many, as does anal stenosis. Nutrition is complicated by increased protein and caloric requirements and limited ability to eat solids and roughage. Constipation is a common problem.

Affected individuals often have a very *maigre* appearance to the face with small pinched nares and small pointed chin. Dental caries appear to be secondary to involvement of the gums and poor dental hygiene rather than due to primary enamel defects.

Growth retardation, anemia, and hypoalbuminemia are typical and mortality from inanition, cardiac failure, chronic infection and metastatic cutaneous and mucosal malignancy is a major feature of young adult life.

A

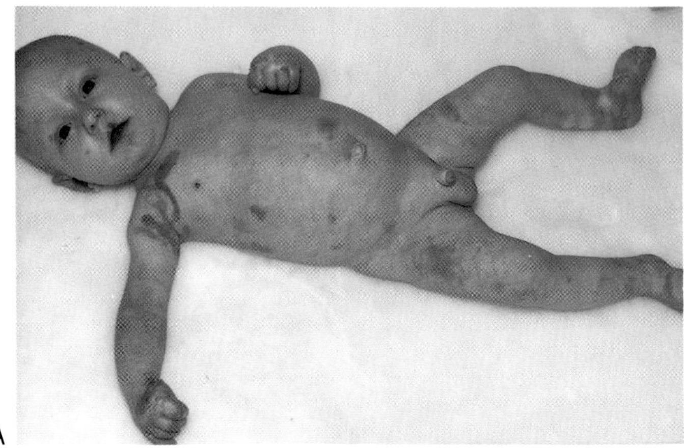

B

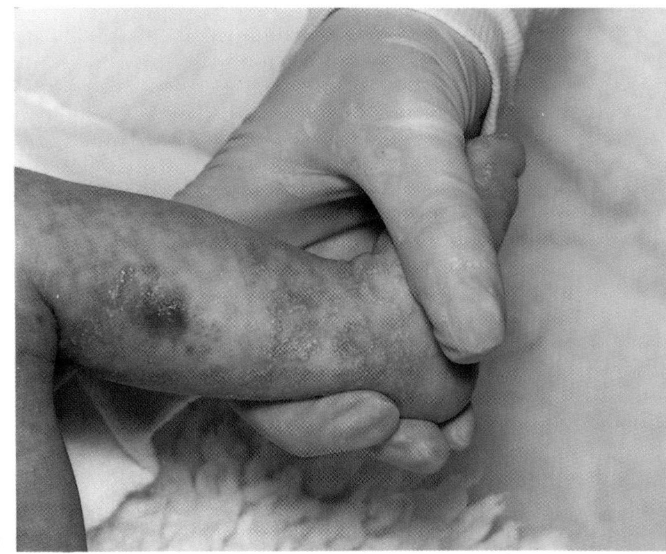

Figure 2.125. (A,B) Infant with multiple erosions, milia, and hemorrhagic blisters.

HISTOPATHOLOGY

LIGHT. Monoclonal antibodies to basement membrane proteins (19-DEJ-1 and GB3) will stain the blister roof; abnormal, patchy, or no staining of the blister floor with LH7:2 (antibody to type VII collagen).

EM. Separation occurs within the dermis below the basement membrane. There is a decrease to absence of anchoring fibrils in both normal and blistered skin. Storage of type VII collagen demonstrated in one patient.

BASIC DEFECT

Defects in type VII collagen. Many mutations are being reported. Compound heterozygosity for mutations is likely. Correlation of clinical severity with molecular defect is yet to be established.

TREATMENT

Standard and meticulous blister care is paramount. Lancing of blisters is almost always

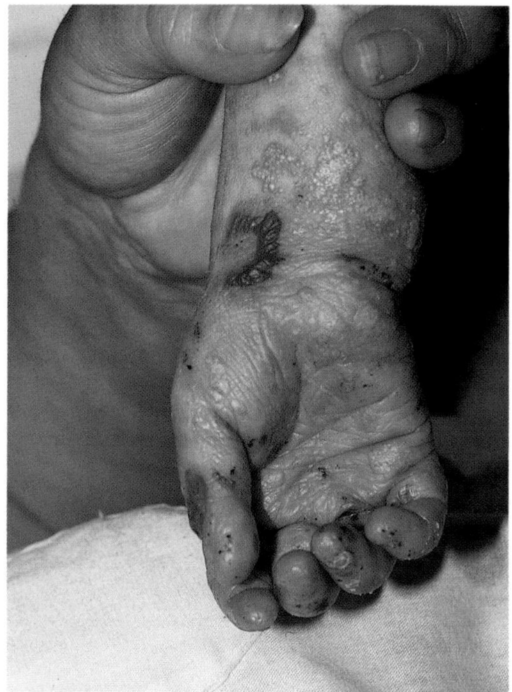

A

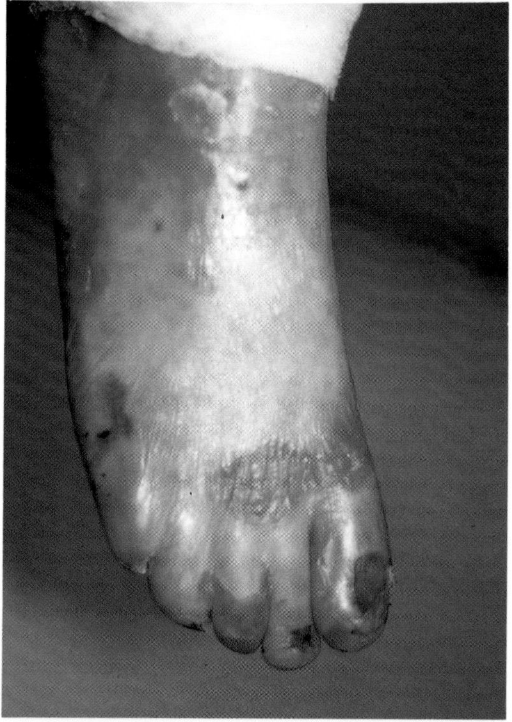

B

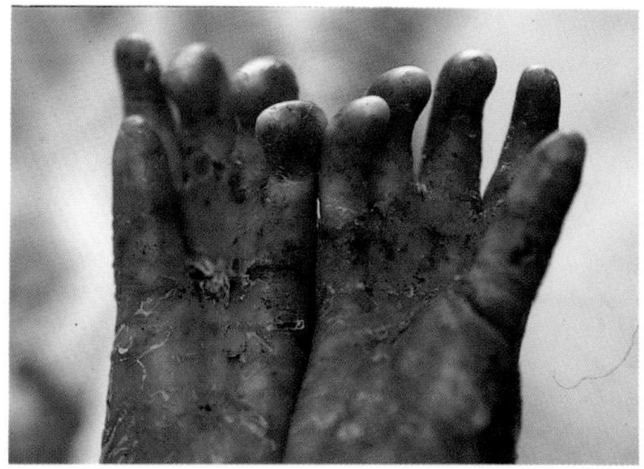

C

Figure 2.126. **(A)** Hemorrhagic blisters, erosions, nail dystrophy, and milia. **(B)** Foot of the same patient showing early fusion of toes and loss of nails. **(C)** Pseudoamputation of distal phalanges in hands of same patient 5 1/2 years later.

beneficial, as they will enlarge from the pressure of the blister fluid if left alone. Dressing care is complicated, and careful separation of healing digits is important. A host of nonadherent bandages (e.g., N-terface, Vigilon, vaseline impregnated gauze) is available, and care needs to be individualized. Surgical stripping of the fused fingers and toes may be indicated in some instances. Infection is a common complicating factor, and careful surveillance is mandatory. Mupirocin (Bactroban) applied to erosions may speed healing and reduce infection. Nutritional support, treatment of anemia, and occupational and physical therapy become increasingly important with age. Hydantoin has limited utility; it may be beneficial in reducing blister formation in a few individuals. In the only controlled study performed to date, there was no significant benefit seen. Management of nutrition may require steps as extreme as colonic interposition for esophageal stenosis if esophageal stenosis does not respond to dilatation or gastrostomy placement.

Particular attention to surveillance examinations for malignancy becomes more important with age.

MODE OF INHERITANCE

Autosomal recessive. The gene *COL7A1* maps to 3p21.1–p21.3.

PRENATAL DIAGNOSIS

Fetal skin biopsy obtained under ultrasound guidance for ultrastructural evaluation has been

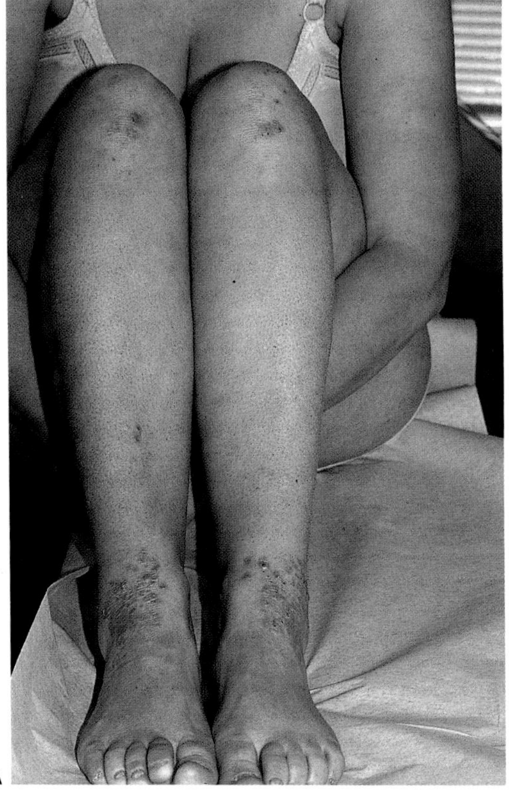

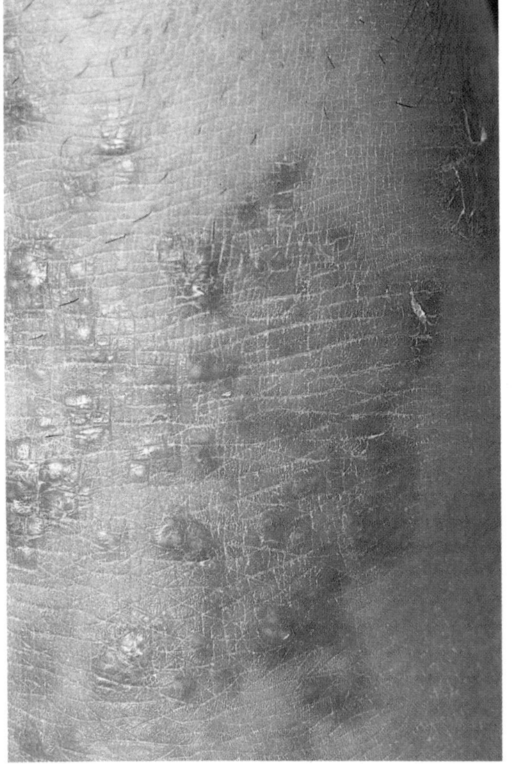

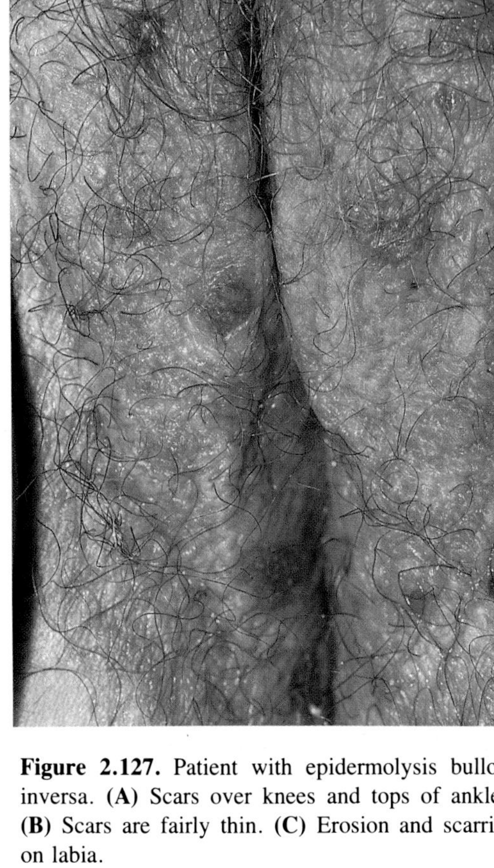

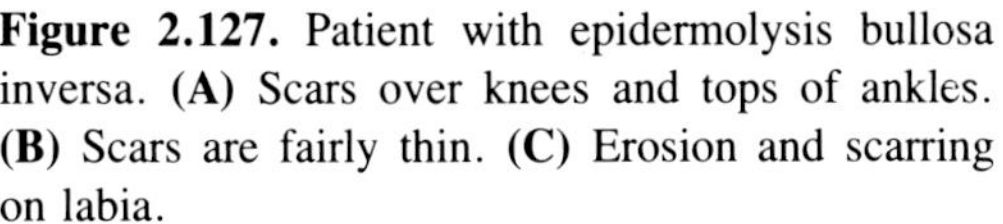

Figure 2.127. Patient with epidermolysis bullosa inversa. **(A)** Scars over knees and tops of ankles. **(B)** Scars are fairly thin. **(C)** Erosion and scarring on labia.

utilized in the past. Molecular diagnosis by linkage analysis and direct mutational probes for *COL7A1* is now possible in informative families.

DIFFERENTIAL DIAGNOSIS

There are many milder forms of recessive epidermolysis bullosa dystrophica (REBD) that must be considered in the differential diagnosis of REBD Hallopeau-Siemens. These include REBD mitis, which is only distinguished by more mild involvement. The scalp is usually spared, and mitten deformities do not occur, although mild syndactyly may develop. Mucosal lesions tend to be less severe. There are no ultrastructural or molecular discriminators between this form of REBD and the Hallopeau-

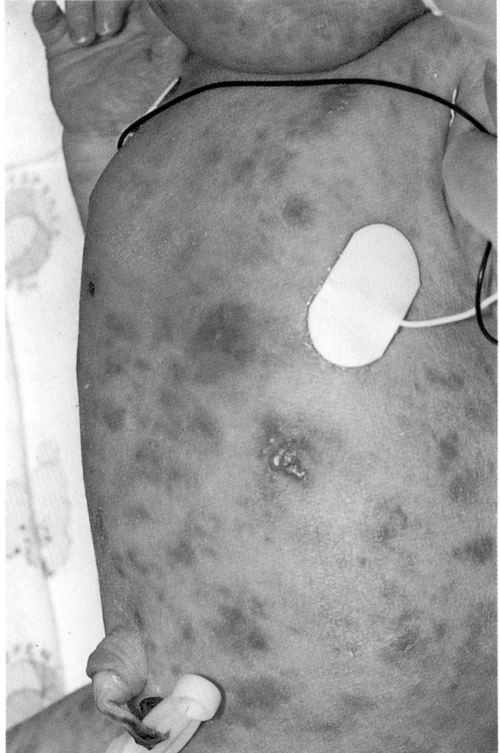

Figure 2.128. Infant with bullous mastocytosis; infiltrated purple lesions and marked blistering.

Siemens form of REBD. Localized REBD (MIM:None) begins in infancy, and blisters are limited to the extremities. Loss of nails is typical. I am unconvinced that this condition really exists. In Gedde-Dahl's monograph, most cases were sporadic, and families with "recessive localized EB" were distantly related to a pedigree with autosomal dominant EBD. Dominant EBD (MIM:131750, 131800) can be clinically similar to REBD mitis and, rarely, can be as severe as REBD Hallopeau-Siemens. In sporadic cases, the mode of inheritance cannot always be determined with certainty on clinical grounds alone. Molecular analysis should ultimately provide accurate recurrence risk information.

Transient bullous dermatolysis of the newborn (MIM:131705) is clinically and ultrastructurally similar. Healing occurs without significant scarring, and this autosomal dominant disorder resolves in the first few years of life. Storage of type VII collagen in keratinocytes is a constant feature of transient bullous dermatolysis; it has also been seen in an infant with REBD Hallopeau-Siemens.

In REBD inversa (MIM:226450), blistering is generalized during infancy, but tends to become limited to the flexures, groin, and trunk with age. Severe oral involvement is the rule, and esophageal stenosis is common. Some patients have corneal erosions. Microstomia, ankyloglossia, and loss of the separation between the lips and gums are frequent features, as they are in REBD Hallopeau-Siemens. EBS Dowling-Meara (MIM:131760), EBS Koebner (MIM:131900), and EBJ (MIM:226700) can be clinically indistinguishable at birth unless a positive family history is available. Electron microscopy will allow for correct diagnosis.

Bullous mastocytosis (MIM:154800), AEC syndrome (MIM:106260), and rarely, hypohidrotic ectodermal dysplasia (MIM:305100) can present with blistering or peeling, denuded skin. The associated features should allow for ready exclusion of these conditions.

Support Group: D.E.B.R.A.
40 Rector Street, 8th Floor
New York, NY 10006
1-212-693-6610

SELECTED BIBLIOGRAPHY

Bruckner-Tuderman, L., Niemi, K.-M., Kero, M., Schnyder, U.W., and Reunala, T. (1990). Type VII collagen is expressed but anchoring fibrils are defective in dystrophic epidermolysis bullosa inversa. *Br. J. Dermatol.* **122,** 383–390.

Case report with good clinical description. Authors hypothesize that REBD inversa might be heterogeneous and that, although type VII collagen molecules are made, they cannot be properly assembled into anchoring fibrils.

Christiano, A.M., Greenspan, D.S., Hoffman, G.G., Zhang, X., Tamai, Y., Lin, A.N., Dietz, H.C., Hovnanian, A., and Uitto, J. (1993). A missense mutation in type VII collagen in two affected siblings with recessive dystrophic epidermolysis bullosa. *Nat. Genet.* **4,** 62–66.

Homozygosity for methionine to lysine mutation in two siblings and heterozygosity in their mother and maternal half-brother. Numerous other mutations have been reported at meetings. While homozygosity for mutant type VII collagen genes has been shown in some affected individuals, for many affected individuals only one mutant allele, shared by one heterozygote parent, has been identified, raising the possibility that some individuals may have their second mutant allele as the result of new mutation.

Dunnill, M.G.S., Richards, A.J., Milana, G., Mollica, F., Atherton, D., Winship, I., Farrall, M., Al-Imara, L., Eady, R.A.J., and Pope, F.M. (1994). Genetic linkage to the type VII collagen gene (COL7A1) in 26 families with generalised recessive dystrophic epidermolysis bullosa and anchoring fibril abnormalities. *J. Med. Genet.* **31,** 745–748.

Sixteen of 26 families informative for one marker. Twenty-four of 25 informative for another. Noted marked interfamilial variability in severity. Did not comment about intrafamilial homogeneity.

Hovnanian, A., Hilal, L., Blanchet-Bardon, C., Bodemer, C., de Prost, Y., Stark, C.A., Christiano, A.M., Dommergues, M., Terwilliger, J.D., Izquierdo, L., Conteville, P., Dumez, Y., Uitto, J., and Goossens, M. (1995). DNA-based prenatal diagnosis of generalized recessive dystrophic epidermolysis bullosa in six pregnancies at risk for recurrence. *J. Invest. Dermatol.* **104,** 456–461.

Linkage studies in four families, direct mutational analysis in two. All six fetuses had at least one normal allele. Diagnosis of REBD excluded.

EPIDERMOLYSIS BULLOSA DYSTROPHICA PRETIBIAL (MIM:131850)

DERMATOLOGIC FEATURES

Major. The blisters are confined primarily but not exclusively to the pretibial area. Blistering may begin in infancy, childhood, or adult life. Healing occurs with scarring and milia. Nail dystrophy is typical. Itching is a common complaint.

Minor. Albupapuloid lesion—raised, small, whitish papules—have been described in a few patients.

ASSOCIATED ABNORMALITIES

None.

HISTOPATHOLOGY

Light. Basement membrane attached to blister roof.

EM. At the sites of predilection, there is a decrease in anchoring fibrils or fibrils that are normal in structure but irregularly spaced. At sites where blistering does not usually occur, anchoring fibrils may be normal in number or somewhat reduced.

BASIC DEFECT

Linkage to *COL7A1* demonstrated.

TREATMENT

Usual blister care, including lancing of blisters to prevent lateral spread and nonirritating dressings. Cyproheptadine may help to reduce itching.

MODE OF INHERITANCE

Autosomal dominant.

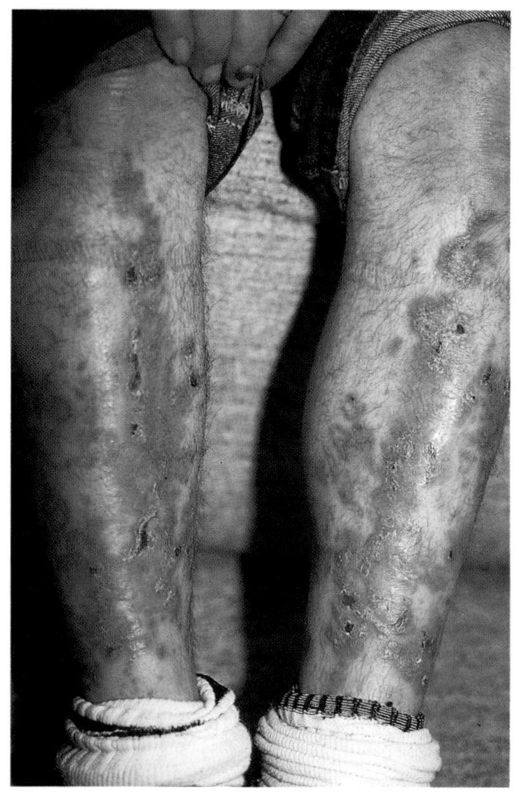
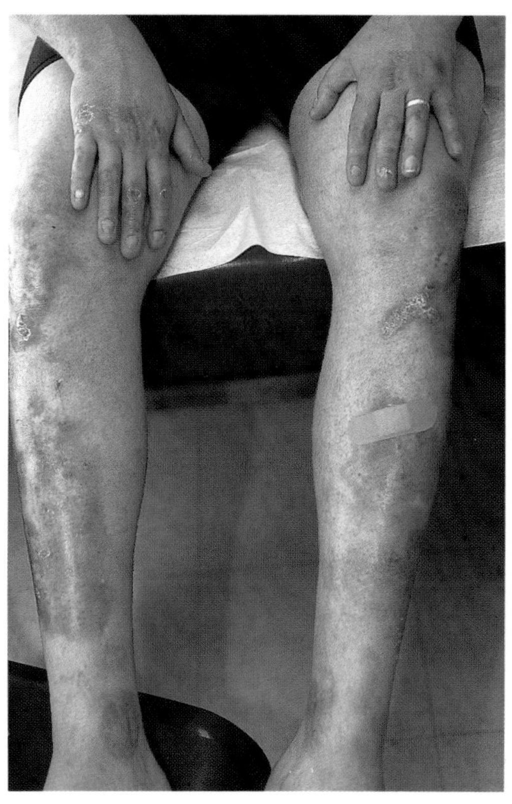

Figure 2.129. **(A)** Marked inflammatory changes, erosions, excoriations, hemosiderin deposition, and atrophic thick epidermis. **(B)** In addition to shins, hands are involved with dystrophic nails and scarring.

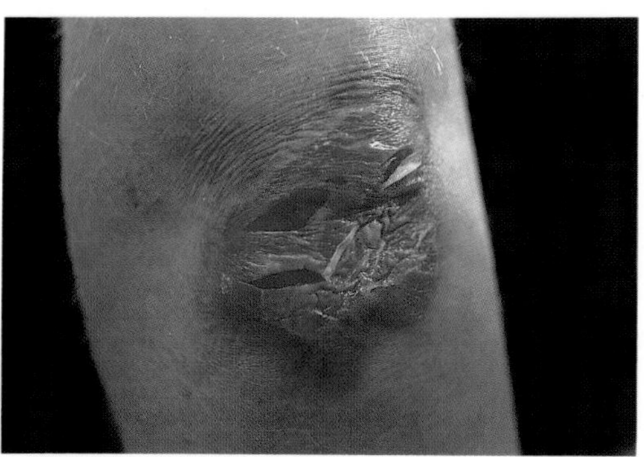

Figure 2.130. Blister on elbows overlying older scar.

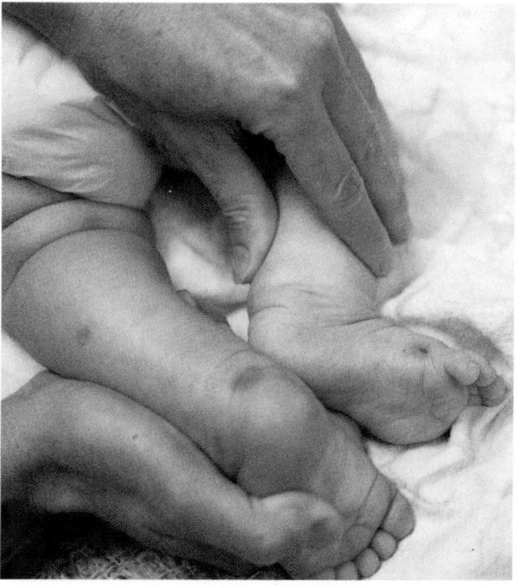

Figure 2.131. Daughter of patient in Fig. 2.129. She has few scattered blisters and no pretibial involvement at this age.

PRENATAL DIAGNOSIS

Possible by linkage studies.

DIFFERENTIAL DIAGNOSIS

When onset of blistering and itching is delayed until late in childhood or adult life, a misdiagnosis of prurigo nodularis or dermatitis artifactua is possible. Nail changes and/or positive family history should help to distinguish EBD pretibial.

It is argued that EBD pretibial is not a distinct entity, but a variation in expression of other forms of epidermolysis bullosa. Families with pretibial involvement and clinical overlap with both dominant EBD Cockayne-Touraine (MIM:131800) and Pasini (MIM:131750) have been described. EBD pretibial does not appear to be the same as forms of EBD with congenital absence of pretibial skin, in which blistering is usually more widespread.

Support Group: D.E.B.R.A.
40 Rector Street, 8th Floor
New York, NY 10006
1-212-693-6610

SELECTED BIBLIOGRAPHY

Lee, J.Y.-Y., Chen, H.-C., and Lin, S.-J. (1993). Pretibial epidermolysis bullosa: a clinicopathologic study. *J. Am. Acad. Dermatol.* **29:**974–981.

This is a very interesting paper in which overlap among the dominant dystrophic epidermolysis bullosa syndromes is well laid out. In 2 of 13 families, only siblings were affected, arguing for autosomal recessive inheritance in some cases of pretibial epidermolysis bullosa. However, in one of these, the proband later developed esophageal involvement, and the possibility of REBD inversa or REBD Hallopeau-Siemens rather than EBD pretibial seems more likely.

Naeyaert, J.M., Nuytinck, L., De Bie, S., Beele, H., Kint, A., and De Paepe, A. (1995). Genetic linkage between the collagen type VII gene *COL7A1* and pretibial epidermolysis bullosa with lichenoid features. *J. Invest. Dermatol.* **104,** 803–805.

Family interesting in marked variability, severity, and delayed onset of signs until after 10 years of age.

TRANSIENT BULLOUS DERMATOLYSIS OF THE NEWBORN (MIM:131705)

(Epidermolysis Bullosa Dystrophica Dominant Neonatal Form)

DERMATOLOGIC FEATURES

MAJOR. Extensive blistering is present at birth, but resolves within the first 1–2 years. Healing occurs with little or no scarring. Milia may be present.

Nails may be lost, and the oral mucosa may be involved.

MINOR. None.

ASSOCIATED ABNORMALITIES

None.

HISTOPATHOLOGY

LIGHT. Intracytoplasmic deposits that stain with LH7:2 (a monoclonal antibody to type VII collagen) are seen in the keratinocytes.

EM. On immunoelectron microscopy, perinuclear staining with LH7:2 is seen in the basal keratinocytes. In one patient, storage of this material within vacuoles was demonstrated.

BASIC DEFECT

A defect in type VII collagen is suspected.

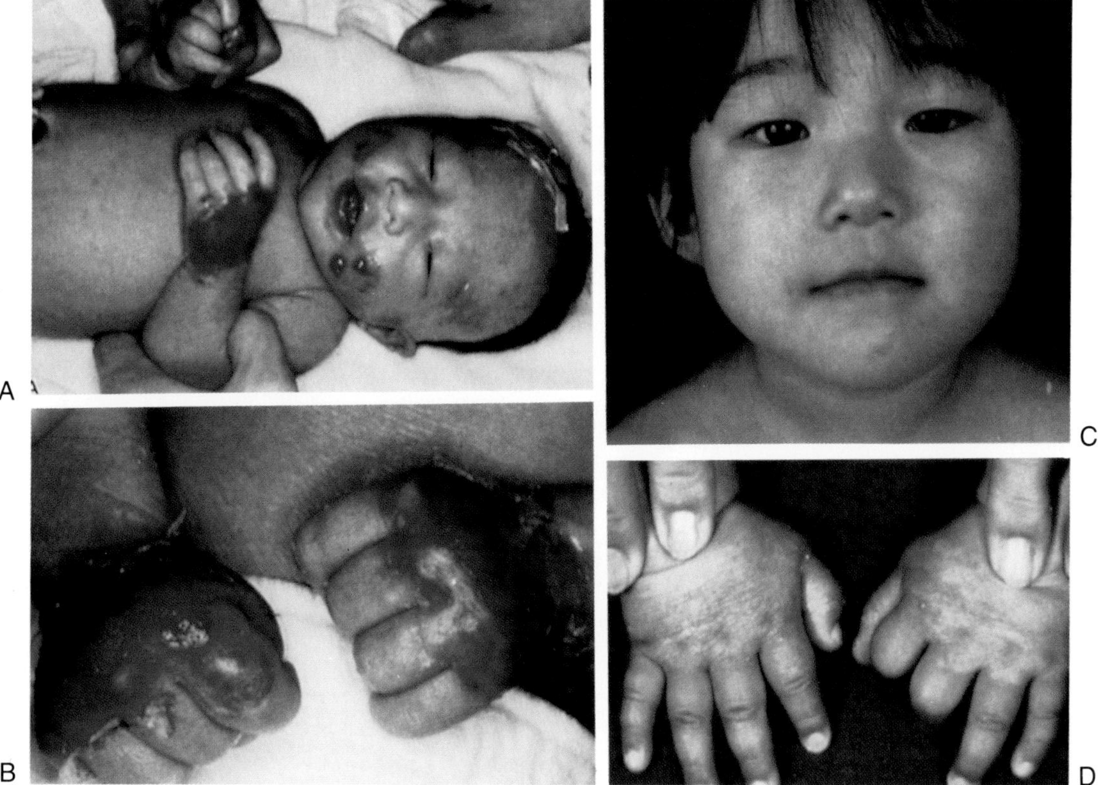

Figure 2.132. **(A,B)** Affected infant at 2 days of age. **(C)** Age 3 1/2 years. **(D)** Age 1 1/2 years. Milia on backs of hands are the only residua. (From Hashimoto et al., 1989.)

TREATMENT

Standard care, as for epidermolysis bullosa, with lancing of blisters to prevent lateral spread, nonadherent and nonirritative dressings and topical mupirocin for erosions.

MODE OF INHERITANCE

Autosomal dominant.

PRENATAL DIAGNOSIS

None.

DIFFERENTIAL DIAGNOSIS

Transient bullous dermatolysis of the newborn is indistinguishable clinically from all of the epidermolysis bullosa syndromes (MIM:Many) that present at birth. The electron microscopic feature of intrakeratinocytic storage of material that stains with LH7:2 will eliminate most from further consideration. However, some patients with other forms of dystrophic epidermolysis bullosa can show similar storage of type VII collagen. It may not be possible, therefore, to distinguish severe recessive epidermolysis bullosa dystrophica (MIM:226600) from the more benign transient dermatolysis of the newborn until the clinical course becomes evident.

Acropustulosis of infancy is an acquired disorder in which tiny vesicles and pustules occur primarily on the extremities. It resembles transient bullous dermatolysis only in its temporary nature and is readily distinguished clinically. Bullous dermatosis of childhood or linear IgA disease usually does not present in the neonatal period and is marked by greater inflammatory changes and rosettes of large blisters. It often masquerades as severe bullous impetigo. Immunofluorescence studies will show deposition of IgA along the basement membrane.

Support Group: D.E.B.R.A.
40 Rector Street, 8th Floor
New York, NY 10006
1-212-693-6610

SELECTED BIBLIOGRAPHY

Fine, J.-D., Horiguchi, Y., Stein, D.H., Esterly, N.B., and Leigh, I.M. (1990). Intraepidermal type VII collagen. *J. Am. Acad. Dermatol.* **22,** 188–195.

Four patients, two from dominant pedigrees, showed positive staining for LH7:2 in epidermal cells, around the nuclei within the cytoplasm. Anchoring fibrils were decreased in number.

Hashimoto, K., Matsumoto, M., and Iacobelli, D. (1985). Transient bullous dermatolysis of the newborn. *Arch. Dermatol.* **121,** 1429–1438.

These authors were the first to describe this condition. They found stellate bodies within the rough endoplasmic reticulum in cells of the lower epidermis. One patient was subsequently restudied by Fine et al. (1990).

Phillips, R.J., Harper, J.I., and Lake, B.D. (1992). Intraepidermal collagen type VII in dystrophic epidermolysis bullosa: report of five new cases. *Br. J. Dermatol.* **126,** 222–230.

Of five patients with intraepidermal storage of type VII collagen, one fit best with transient bullous dermatolysis, one with mild REBD, one with EBD pretibial, and one with mild REBD with anal involvement. One fetus was diagnosed prenatally. The authors caution against the prognostic value of the finding of intracytoplasmic storage of type VII collagen. They also note changes in electron microscopic findings over time.

Smith, L.T., and Sybert, V.P. (1990). Intraepidermal retention of type VII collagen in a patient with recessive dystrophic epidermolysis bullosa. *J. Invest. Dermatol.* **94,** 261–264.

This infant, born to consanguineous parents in whose family other consanguineous matings had also resulted in infants with lethal epidermolysis bullosa, had type VII collagen stored in large vesicles in the basal and suprabasal keratinocytes. Storage cannot be used as a specific feature for transient bullous dermatolysis.

HAILEY-HAILEY DISEASE (MIM:169600)

(Benign Familial Pemphigus)

DERMATOLOGIC FEATURES

MAJOR. Vesicles and subsequent superficial craters and erosions develop on the neck and in the axillae, groins, and perineum. Blistering can also occur in the antecubital fossae, on the scalp and extremities, below the breasts, and on the trunk, but these areas tend to be involved less frequently. Onset is usually after puberty during the third and fourth decades of life. Clinical severity may improve, remain static, or worsen over time. Many affected individuals will have a positive Nikolsky sign.

Friction, heat, and injury can result in blister formation at any site. Over time, involved areas may show chronic maceration with vegetations, or fine scaling and erythema. Secondary impetigenization and/or candidiasis is common. Pain, itching, and odor are frequent complaints.

Lesions may be crusted plaques with raised, fissured margins, wet erosive plaques, and plaques with soft vegetations. These changes reflect chronic long-standing disease.

MINOR. One patient with Hailey-Hailey disease had seborrheic dermatitis-like changes on the scalp that on biopsy showed histologic features of benign familial pemphigus.

Longitudinal white bands on the nails are reported. This was noted by one author in 50% of his patients, based on personal experience, and there is no other documentation for this feature in the literature.

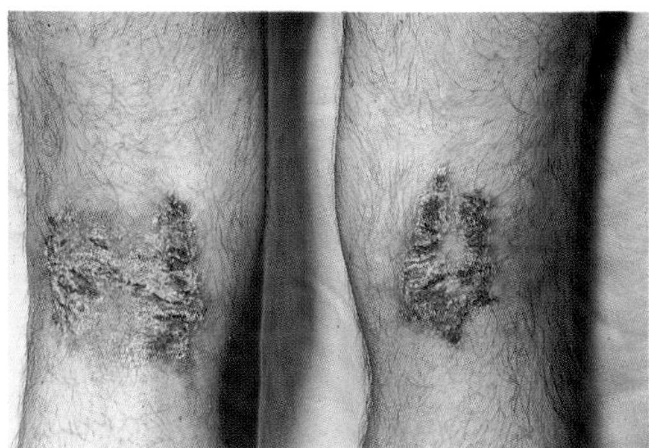

Figure 2.133. Superficial erosions and crusting on an erythematous base. Small blisters are visible. (Courtesy of Dr. J. Halloran, Division of Dermatology, University of Washington.)

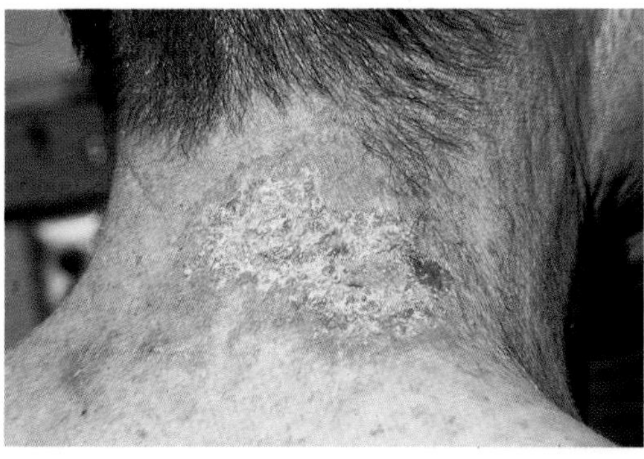

Figure 2.134. Thicker, more vegetative plaques in the popliteal fossae. (Courtesy of Dr. J. Halloran, Division of Dermatology, University of Washington.)

ASSOCIATED ABNORMALITIES

None.

HISTOPATHOLOGY

LIGHT. Acantholysis is present in the lower midepidermis with the occasional appearance of corps ronds and grains. Immunofluorescent staining for bullous pemphigus antigen is negative.

EM. At first there is a dissociation of tonofilaments and desmosomes and then clumping of tonofilaments and disappearance of desmosomes. Separation occurs above the basement membrane with partial adherence of the basal cells to the base of the blister. Alterations in the microvilli in the prickle cell layer were described in one study.

BASIC DEFECT

Unknown.

TREATMENT

Excision of and split thickness grafts to involved areas has moderate success. Blistering often recurs along graft margins but may be more tolerable than if the entire area were left untreated. Twenty percent aluminum chloride (Drysol, Peridri) to decrease sweating may decrease blistering. Dermabrasion may be successful. A host of other therapeutic modalities, including Clobetasol, antibiotics, electrodessication, cryotherapy, CO_2 laser, and cyclosporine, have been mentioned. Success with each was anecdotal.

MODE OF INHERITANCE

Autosomal dominant. Family studies are inadequate to address penetrance. The gene has been mapped to 3q21–q24.

PRENATAL DIAGNOSIS

None.

DIFFERENTIAL DIAGNOSIS

Hailey-Hailey disease is distinguished from other blistering disorders by limitation of blisters to inverse sites, absence of extracutaneous manifestations, and negative immunofluorescence studies. Pemphigus vulgaris is marked by blistering at any cutaneous site. There is positive immunofluorescence with IgG and C3. Familial cases of all variants of pemphigus have been reported, but they constitute a minute fraction of individuals with these diseases. Hidradenitis suppurative (MIM:142690) involves the axilla and the groin; typical lesions are cysts, sinus tracts, and inflammatory pustules, not erosions or vegetative plaques. Darier-White disease (MIM:124200) has a similar histologic picture, although corps ronds and grains are more common in Darier-White. Greasy scale is not part of Hailey-Hailey disease, and typical distribution of lesions is different. Some have argued that the two disorders are the same, but linkage mapping of Darier-White to 12q excludes this. EBD inversa (MIM:226450) can be differentiated from Hailey-Hailey disease by nasopharyngeal involvement, scarring, and ultrastructural features of decreased numbers and/or abnormal anchoring fibrils. Clumping of tonofilaments is a feature of EBS Dowling-Meara (MIM:148066). The location of blisters and age of onset of Hailey-Hailey disease should easily differentiate the two conditions.

Because erosions and vegetations on an erythematous base rather than blisters may predominate in the clinical picture of Hailey-Hailey, bacterial and fungal infections, eczema, seborrheic dermatitis, psoriasis, intertrigo, and condyloma acuminata must be excluded. Conversely, individuals with Hailey-Hailey disease may be misdiagnosed as one of these entities.

Support Group: D.E.B.R.A.
40 Rector Street, 8th Floor
New York, NY 10006
1-212-693-6610

SELECTED BIBLIOGRAPHY

Burge, S.M. (1992). Hailey-Hailey disease: the clinical features, response to treatment and prognosis. *Br. J. Dermatol.* **126,** 275–282.

Thirty-four individuals were examined, 20 were interviewed by telephone. Medical records of an additional four were reviewed. Gives a nice overview of the disorder.

Crotty, C.P., Scheen, R. III, Masson, J.K., and Winkelmann, R.K. (1981). Surgical treatment of familial benign chronic pemphigus. *Arch. Dermatol.* **117,** 540–542.

Five patients were treated by excision and grafting with fair to good results in four, death by pulmonary embolus in one. It is important to remember that death can be a consequence of surgery and that this mode of treatment has risks beyond therapeutic failure.

Hailey, H., and Hailey, H. (1939). Familial benign chronic pemphigus. *Arch. Dermatol. Syphilol.* **39,**679–685 and *Arch. Dermatol.* **118,** 774–780.

The brothers Hailey described two sets of brothers with this disease. They stated that the disease was familial. Subsequent reports confirmed vertical and male-to-male transmission. The Haileys were sons of a doctor, showing the autosomal dominant male-limited transmission often seen in the medical profession.

Hamm, H., Metze, D., and Broker, E.-V. (1994). Hailey-Hailey disease: eradication by dermabrasion. *Arch. Dermatol.* **130,** 1143–1149.

Ten patients, 46 sites, median follow-up time 42 months (3–72 months). Eighty-three percent of treated areas remained disease free.

Michel, B. (1982). Commentary: Hailey-Hailey disease. *Arch. Dermatol.* **118,** 781–783.

A nice summary of the literature, clearly written, with succinct descriptions. Thirty-one references.

CHAPTER 3

DISORDERS OF EPIDERMAL APPENDAGES

Hair

There are a host of genetic conditions that affect hair growth, structure, and distribution either in isolation or as part of more generalized syndromes. Little is understood about genetic control of body hair distribution in humans. Unusual hair patterns can be seen in many pleiotropic syndromes associated with mental retardation and have been the subject of innumerable case reports. These patterns include a generalized increase in numbers of pigmented body hairs, increased length of hairs, and unusual hair whorls. Reviews and general references about normal hair growth and hair abnormalities are given in the Bibliography.

This section includes entries of isolated and syndromic structural hair abnormalities, hereditary alopecias, and hypertrichoses. I have not included alopecia areata/totalis/universalis (MIM: 104000). The genetics of this relatively common cause of hair loss are unclear and fit best with either autosomal dominant inheritance with reduced penetrance or with a polygenic model; a positive family history is elicited in 10%–20% of patients, and a 6% risk to first degree relatives has been estimated.

Hair abnormalities as part of ectodermal dysplasia syndromes can be found in the section on ectodermal dysplasias. There are many case reports and reports of pedigrees with structural hair abnormalities and other dysmorphic and developmental abnormalities that are far too numerous to discuss individually. The specific hair defects may differ within a family, and often a variety of structural defects are found in hairs from a single individual.

SELECTED BIBLIOGRAPHY

Birnbaum, P.S., and Baden, I.H. (1987). Heritable disorders of hair. *Dermatol. Clin.* **5,** 137–153.

Mitchell, A.J., and Krall, E.A. (eds.) (1987). Hair disorders. *Dermatol. Clin.* **5,** 467–640.

Rook, A. (1991). *Diseases of the hair and scalp.* Blackwell Scientific, Oxford.

Whiting, D.A. (1987). Structural abnormalities of the hair shaft. *J. Am. Acad. Dermatol.* **16,** 1–25.

ALOPECIAS

LOOSE ANAGEN HAIR (MIM:None)

(Pluckable Hair; Short Anagen Hair)

DERMATOLOGIC FEATURES

MAJOR. The presenting complaint is usually "the hair doesn't grow" or "she's never needed a haircut." These changes are noted in early childhood. The hair is easily shed or pulled from the scalp, but is not fragile. The hair may be sparse or appear normally distributed but

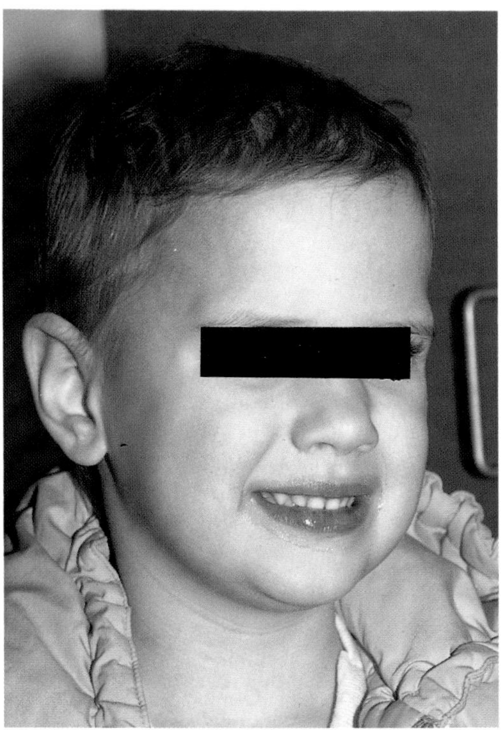

Figure 3.1. Five-year-old with short hair that has never been cut. Normal eyebrows, eyelashes, and teeth.

short. Eyebrows, eyelashes, nails, teeth, and skin are normal. Hair color may be lighter than normal for family. The hairs appear to improve with age, becoming thicker, longer, and more dense, although they are still easily pulled out.
MINOR. None.

ASSOCIATED ABNORMALITIES

None.

HISTOPATHOLOGY

LIGHT. There is distortion of the anagen hair bulbs with absence of the inner and outer root sheaths.
EM. EM shows changes similar to light microscopy. The cuticle is absent from the hair bulb.

BASIC DEFECT

Unknown.

TREATMENT

Reassurance that the problem is likely to ameliorate with age.

MODE OF INHERITANCE

Possibly autosomal dominant with variable clinical expression. As the condition improves with age, it may go unrecognized in parents.

PRENATAL DIAGNOSIS

None.

DIFFERENTIAL DIAGNOSIS

All structural malformations of the hair should be excluded by a microscopic evaluation of the hair shaft and root. Alopecia areata is distinguished by patchy rather than diffuse thinning, and the patches in alopecia areata are usually completely devoid of hair. In telogen effluvium the pulled hairs are in telogen, not anagen. In trichotillomania, the presence of broken hairs and normal anagen bulbs should allow for easy exclusion of loose anagen hair.

Support Group: National Alopecia Areata Foundation
P.O. Box 150760
San Rafael, CA 94915-0760
415-456-4644

SELECTED BIBLIOGRAPHY

Baden, H.P., Kvedar, J.C., and Magro, C.M. (1992). Loose anagen hair is a cause of hereditary hair loss in children. *Arch. Dermatol.* **128,** 1349–1353.
Of 14 patients reviewed, one had a mother with

no symptoms but abnormal anagen hairs on microscopic evaluation. A second patient had a clinically normal mother and sister; hairs from both showed typical microscopic changes. The paper details the histopathologic and electron microscopic changes in hair bulbs.

Price, V.H., and Gummer, C.L. (1989). Loose anagen syndrome. *J. Am. Acad. Dermatol.* **20,** 249–256.

Report of 27 cases from 24 families. All had light-colored hair.

MALE PATTERN BALDNESS (MIM:109200)

(Androgenetic Hair Loss)

DERMATOLOGIC FEATURES

MAJOR. Gradual thinning and ultimate loss of hair over the vertex of the scalp with general sparing of the parietal and occipital regions is typical for male pattern baldness. Different patterns are recognized; all show progression with age. By age 70, only one-third of human males have no evidence of significant balding.

Hairs in the affected areas gradually convert from pigmented terminal hairs to vellus hairs. In affected females, the hairs generally do not completely miniaturize, and the density of follicles may decrease.

MINOR. Some argue that males with male pattern baldness have increased body hair on the chest. This is disputed by others.

ASSOCIATED ABNORMALITIES

Male pattern alopecia in genetically susceptible females may occur with exposure to exogenous or endogenous androgens; thus a source of excess androgen production should always be sought in a female with male pattern baldness.

HISTOPATHOLOGY

LIGHT. The hair follicles in the involved scalp have been "transformed" to vellus hairs with short follicles; there are clumps of elastic fibers within the remnants of the fibrous root sheath and long thin blood vessels coursing up to the base of the miniaturized follicle.

EM. No information.

BASIC DEFECT

A diminution in the size of the hair follicle occurs in progressive cycles, going from terminal to vellus hairs; the anagen phase becomes shorter. The process requires (1) aging, (2) genetic susceptibility and, (3) androgens.

TREATMENT

The treatments for male pattern baldness are legion. Currently, popular choices include topical Rogaine (minoxidil), scalp reduction, and hair transplants.

MODE OF INHERITANCE

Possibly autosomal dominant with partial sex-limited expression. There are surprisingly few and modest published studies attempting to define the inheritance of male pattern baldness. Females who exhibit thinning of the hair prior to middle age are believed to be homozygotes for male pattern baldness. The gene frequency appears to be most common in Caucasians, less so in Africans, and least frequent in Amerindians, Asians, Inuits, and Yupiks.

PRENATAL DIAGNOSIS

None.

DIFFERENTIAL DIAGNOSIS

In telogen effluvium, there is a rapid generalized thinning of hair that involves the entire scalp. The rapidity of onset and the history of precipitating factors should easily differentiate this process from male pattern baldness. Trichotillomania might rarely present as a confounder—broken hairs and history should exclude male pattern baldness. In females, the possibility of an exogenous androgen source should always be excluded by history, clinical examination and/or appropriate laboratory testing.

Senescent baldness refers to the thinning of the hair that occurs in both sexes after age 50, is a "normal" function of aging, and is not genetically dependent.

Support Group: None

SELECTED BIBLIOGRAPHY

Harris, H. (1946). The inheritance of premature baldness in men. *Ann. Eugen.* **13,** 172–181.

Found 13% of 900 males were prematurely bald. Sixty-six percent of the brothers were bald if the father of the proband was also bald, and 46% of the brothers were bald if the father was not. Fifty-six percent of bald men had bald fathers. The authors concluded that this was consistent with an autosomal dominant gene and that premature baldness was genetically distinct from senescent baldness.

Kuster, W., and Happle, R. (1984). The inheritance of common baldness: two B or not two B? *J. Am. Acad. Dermatol.* **11,** 921–926.

They argue against a two-allele system and for polygenic inheritance. They state that "careful family studies . . . are lacking and we admit that we have not embarked on such studies either." Their arguments are not compelling, and they fail to recognize the contribution of occult carrier mothers to the risk to offspring.

Montagna, W. (1973). Baldness: a disease? *J. Am. Med. Wom. Assoc.* **28,** 447–450, 458.

Perhaps the genetic basis of baldness remains elusive because of what Montagna describes: "man [is] a difficult, largely unsuitable, and often unpleasant subject for study." Montagna argues, as a balding biologist, that male pattern baldness is but an alternative step in the dance of life.

Osborn, D. (1916). Inheritance of baldness. *J. Hered.* **7,** 347–355.

The author sets out to debunk the theory that pressure from hats is a cause for hair loss. He states that it is a sex-limited autosomal dominant trait, similar to the inheritance of horns in sheep. He distinguishes between pattern baldness and congenital alopecia and alopecia of illness.

Sălomon, T. (1968). Genetic factors in male pattern alopecia. In *Biopathology of Pattern Alopecia.* Baccaredda-Boy, A., Moretti, G., and Frey, J.R. (eds.). Karger, New York. pp 39–49.

One hundred nineteen males. The author examined living family members, reviewed photos, and took histories. Sixteen patients had no family history, 65 had two generations, 24 three generations, and 3 had four generations of involvement. Eleven probands had two-generation families with both parents affected. There was an association of increasing amounts of chest hair, but not back hair, in affected individuals. The author's interpretation of homozygosity versus heterozygosity in males and females is based on incorrect assumptions, evident by examining the published pedigrees.

Smith, M.A., and Wells, R.S. (1964). Male-type alopecia, alopecia areata, and normal hair in females. Family histories. *Arch. Dermatol.* **89,** 95–98.

Fifty-six females with thinning of the hair were compared with two control groups: females with alopecia areata and females with no hair problems. Fifty-four percent of first degree male relatives over 30 and 20% of all female relatives were bald in the group with male pattern baldness. In the alopecia areata families, 23% of first degree male relatives and 7% of all female relatives were bald. There was no greater likelihood of having affected relatives in the females with severe male pattern hair loss than in those with less severe loss.

Snyder, L.H., and Yingling, H.C. (1935).

Studies in human inheritance XII. The application of the gene-frequency method of analysis to sex-influenced factors, with especial reference to baldness. *Hum. Biol.* **7**, 608–615.

Examined over 4,000 inmates of a state hospital for the insane who were older than 35 years of age. Forty-three percent of the males were bald, as were 8% of the females. They propose a sex-limited autosomal dominant condition, with females expressing only if homozygous.

MARIE UNNA SYNDROME (MIM:146550)

(Hereditary Hypotrichosis; Hypotrichosis Congenita Hereditaria)

Includes Atrichia; Hypotrichosis Simplex; Hypotrichosis with Light-Colored Hair and Facial Milia; Hypotrichosis Jeanselme and Rime; IFAP

DERMATOLOGIC FEATURES

MAJOR. At birth, some affected individuals have little or no hair. Others are reported to have normal neonatal hair. Bald infants go on to develop sparse, coarse, wiry, twisted hair in childhood. In those with normal hair at birth, the hairs become abnormal in early childhood. There may be early and progressive alopecia in adult life. The eyebrows, eyelashes, and body hair are involved, as are beard, axillary, and pubic hairs.

MINOR. None.

ASSOCIATED ABNORMALITIES

None.

HISTOPATHOLOGY

LIGHT. The hairs are twisted, coarse, and irregular. There is marked longitudinal ridging. Individual hairs from the same individual may appear normal or demonstrate these findings.

Scalp biopsy specimens have shown a decrease in the number of pilosebaceous units and some perifollicular scarring.

EM. Same as light microscopy. Patchy loss of the normal cuticular scale of the hair shaft has been described.

BASIC DEFECT

Unknown.

TREATMENT

None.

MODE OF INHERITANCE

Autosomal dominant.

PRENATAL DIAGNOSIS

None.

DIFFERENTIAL DIAGNOSIS

In *hypotrichosis simplex (MIM:146520)* the scalp hair is normal at birth and is lost in childhood. The hypotrichosis of Marie Unna syndrome is usually congenital, although not always. In hypotrichosis simplex, the hairs are normal until their loss occurs. In Marie Unna syndrome, the hairs are coarse and twisted. All hairs except those of the scalp are normal in hypotrichosis simplex, in contrast to the facial and body hair involvement of Marie Unna syndrome.

Hypotrichosis with light-colored hair and facial milia (MIM:146530): Based on one pedigree, congenital sparseness of scalp hair that improves at puberty is the only consistent abnormality. The facial milia may not be present. The hair of affected individuals was lighter than that of unaffected individuals, but still normal by visual and microscopic inspection. Tensile strength, growth rates, sulfur amino acid contents, and the x-ray diffraction pattern of hair from affected individuals were normal.

Hypotrichosis Jeanselme and Rime: This is an autosomal dominant hypotrichosis syndrome with onset in late infancy and involvement of scalp, facial, and body hairs. Mild keratosis pilaris and fragile nails were described in the proband. The skin of her scalp felt mildly thickened and irregular. It is not clear to me that this syndrome is distinct from Marie Unna disease.

Atrichia (MIM:209500, 209501, 241900): There may be several distinct forms of atrichia congenita. In one form, absence of scalp hair may be partial or complete; eyebrows, eyelashes, and body hair are diminished or absent, scalp biopsy material shows absence of follicles, and any hairs present are fine and hypopigmented. In another form, the neonatal hairs of infants with autosomal recessive atrichia are lost and not replaced. The hair follicles show cystic malformations. The skin is covered with flesh-colored follicular papules, which develop in late childhood and increase in number over the years. The papules represent epithelial cysts filled with keratin. Eyebrows and eyelashes may be involved. Body hair is absent. When coupled with photophobia, this constellation is referred to as IFAP—*i*chthyosis *f*ollicularis, *a*trichia, and *p*hotophobia. Its inheritance is either autosomal recessive or X-linked recessive. There are reports of an autosomal recessive disorder termed *hypotrichosis* that is clinically similar to atrichia. It is not at all clear to me where atrichia stops and hypotrichosis begins.

There are numerous case reports of individuals with atrichia and mental retardation, with or without microcephaly, with or without other features. For each of these, occasional recurrences in siblings have suggested either autosomal recessive or X-linked recessive inheritance. In isolated cases, accurate recurrence risks are not possible to calculate.

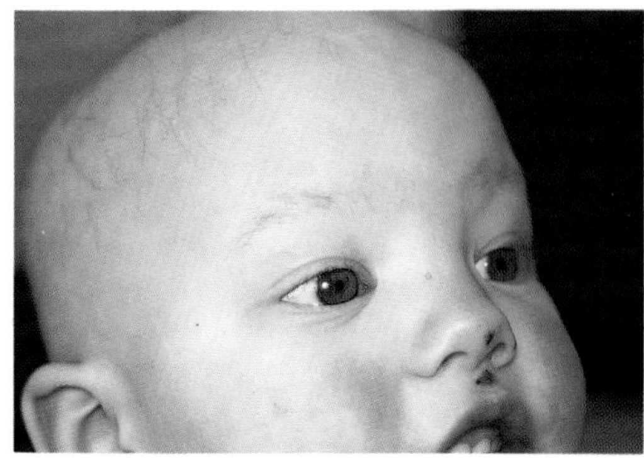

Figure 3.2. Fine, sparse hair. Sparse eyebrows and eyelashes.

Support Group: N.O.R.D.
P.O. Box 8923
New Fairfield, CT 06812
1-800-999-6673

SELECTED BIBLIOGRAPHY

Damste, Th.J., and Prakken, J.R. (1954). Atrichia with papular lesions, a variant of congenital ectodermal dysplasia. *Dermatology.* **108,** 114–122.

Report of three cases of atrichia. One patient, whose grandparents were first cousins, had two of her six siblings affected and two affected maternal second cousins.

Hamm, H., Meinecke, P., and Traupe, H. (1991). Further delineation of the ichthyosis follicularis, atrichia, and photophobia syndrome. *Eur. J. Pediatr.* **150,** 627–629.

Case report. Review of literature showed eight affected males in six families, no affected females. The authors note the marked variability in the presence and severity of nondiagnostic features (e.g., epilepsy), suggesting that they may not be truly associated with the disorder itself.

Jeanselme, E., and Rime (1924). Un cas d'alopécie congénitale familiale. *Bull. Soc. Fr. Dermatol. Syphiligr.* **31,** 79–82.

Description of a single family with multiple

generations. Affected individuals had normal hair at birth that fell out at 8–9 months, to be replaced by hairs that fractured, grew slowly, or not at all. The skin of the scalp was described as thickened and irregular. There was no keratosis pilaris. The hairs that were present were normal in appearance and caliber.

Parrish, J.A., Baden, H.P., Goldsmith, L.A., and Matz, M.H. (1979). Studies of the density and the properties of the hair in a new inherited syndrome of hypotrichosis. *Br. J. Dermatol.* **101,** 331–339.

Biochemical and clinical studies of a family with a hypotrichosis characterized by congenitally sparse, but otherwise normal, scalp hair that improved at puberty. Most affected individuals had multiple facial milia.

Peachey, R.D.G., and Wells, R.S. (1971). Hereditary hypotrichosis (Marie Unna type). *Trans. St. Johns Hosp. Dermatol. Soc.* **57,** 157–166.

Three extensive pedigrees are described in detail, and histologic features of hairs and scalp biopsies are presented.

Stevanovic, D.V. (1970). Hereditary hypotrichosis congenita: Marie Unna type. *Br. J. Dermatol.* **83,** 331–337.

Detailed description of the histology of the hair follicles in a patient with Marie Unna hypotrichosis. The author hypothesized that unilateral bulges of the external root sheath, that they observed in one hair, might compress the inner root sheath and mechanically result in distortion of the keratinization pattern of the hair shaft.

Toribio, J., and Quinones, P.A. (1974). Hereditary hypotrichosis simplex of the scalp. Evidence for autosomal dominant inheritance. *Br. J. Dermatol.* **91,** 687–696.

An eight generation pedigree demonstrating autosomal dominant inheritance of progressive hair loss beginning in middle to late childhood and reaching greatest severity in the early twenties. Eyebrows, eyelashes, body hair, and secondary sexual hairs were all normal. Histologic samples showed miniature hair follicles very similar to alopecia areata, but without the inflammatory infiltrate of alopecia areata. Clinical photos resemble the picture of diffuse alopecia areata.

Unna, M. (1925). Uber hypotrichosis congenital hereditaria. *Dermatol. Wochenschr.* **81,** 1167–1178.

Why Marie Unna has her first and last names appended to the syndrome she described is a mystery to me. Affirmative action?

HIRSUTISM

GINGIVAL FIBROMATOSIS AND HYPERTRICHOSIS (MIM:135400)

DERMATOLOGIC FEATURES

MAJOR. Excessive body and facial hair in a distribution identical to hypertrichosis lanuginosa occurs. Some reports describe the hair as coarser and darker than in hypertrichosis lanuginosa, but I have seen one affected individual with fine long vellous hairs. The hair may be abnormal at birth or become obvious within the first few years of life, or not develop until puberty. Gingival hyperplasia develops in the first few years of life and will engulf the teeth. The gums are pink, extremely firm, and pebbly or nodular in appearance. They completely obscure the teeth, and the patient appears edentulous.

MINOR. None.

ASSOCIATED ABNORMALITIES

One report in the Chinese medical literature described benign virginal hypertrophy of the

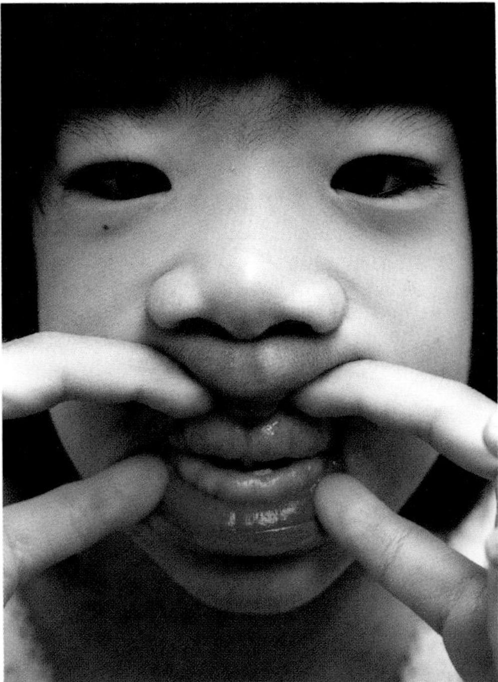

Figure 3.3. Overgrowth of gums. Distal tip of lower central incisor barely visible. Marked synophrys and low frontal hair line.

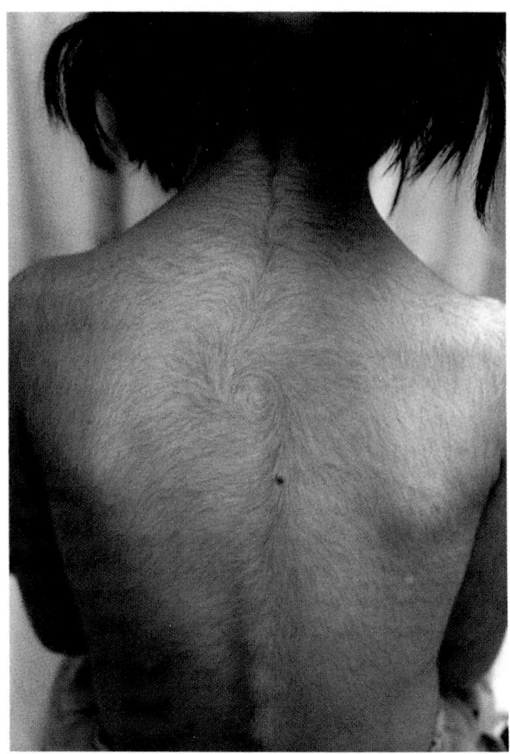

Figure 3.4. Hirsutism of back.

breasts in a patient with sporadic classic gingival fibromatosis and hypertrichosis. She also had aortic insufficiency and mitral stenosis. She may have had the Byars-Jurkiewicz syndrome or Cowden syndrome rather than this disorder.

Most patients with this condition have been mentally normal. In two reports, two patients with gingival fibromatosis who were labeled as having hypertrichosis also had mental retardation and epilepsy. These two appear minimally hirsute with mild synophrys in the clinical photographs.

HISTOPATHOLOGY

LIGHT. The gingiva show remarkably elongated rete ridges overlying dense fibrous connective tissue with increased amounts of mucopolysaccharides.

EM. Two populations of fibroblasts, one of thick cells associated with areas rich in ground substance but poor in fibrous collagen, and one with thin cells in collagen-rich areas, have been described.

BASIC DEFECT

Unknown. Collagens have been normal. Cell culture characteristics of fibroblasts have differed from normal, demonstrating a shorter lifespan and increased fragility and producing reduced amounts of collagen.

TREATMENT

Surgical debulking of the gums is necessary to preserve teeth and function, but recurrence is inevitable and repeat procedures will be necessary. In reports from Argentina and Britain, total tooth extraction resulted in normal gum remodeling. Follow-up periods range from 5 to 14 years. This procedure coupled with the use of dentures resulted in remarkably improved oral function.

MODE OF INHERITANCE

Autosomal dominant.

PRENATAL DIAGNOSIS

None.

DIFFERENTIAL DIAGNOSIS

Gingival hypertrophy is a feature of many nondermatologic conditions and is rarely the reason for presentation to a dermatologist. However, it can be seen in a few inherited skin disorders.

In the Cross syndrome (MIM:257800), gingival fibromatosis can occur in association with hypopigmentation, seizures, and severe mental retardation. One of the reported patients had recurrent periodontitis, perhaps causing gum thickening.

Hypertrichosis, fibroadenomas of the breast, and gingival fibromatosis occur in the Byars-Jurkiewicz syndrome, which may be a subset of the Cowden syndrome (MIM:158350). In the Rutherfurd syndrome (MIM:180900), gingival hypertrophy occurs in association with corneal dystrophy. In the Laband syndrome (Zimmerman-Laband, MIM:135500), hypertrichosis, aplasia, or dysplasia of the fingernails overlying "whittled" terminal phalanges, hypertrophy of the nasal tip and ears, and hypermobility accompany the gum changes. Hepatosplenomegaly has also been described.

Gingival hypertrophy can also occur in isolation (MIM:135300).

Cherubism (Ramon syndrome, MIM: 266270) is an autosomal recessive condition marked by progressive bony enlargement of the mandible and maxilla, mild mental retardation, and seizures. Hypertrichosis of the face and pubic region was reported in one of two affected brothers. This is not to be confused with autosomal dominant cherubism (MIM: 118400), which is manifested by bony changes alone.

Juvenile hyaline fibromatosis (Murray-Puretic-Drescher syndrome, MIM:265700) is a presumably autosomal recessive disorder marked by hyaline deposits in the skin, progressive joint contractures, recurrent infections, and the appearance of calcified subcutaneous nodules and superficial white papules, atrophoderma, and scleroderma in infancy or early childhood with progressive skeletal deformities. Hypertrichosis is not a feature, although gingival enlargement may be.

Isolated hypertrichosis lanuginosa congenita (MIM:145700, 307150) is not associated with gingival fibromatosis.

Support Group: N.O.R.D.
P.O. Box 8923
New Fairfield, CT
06812
1-800-999-6673

SELECTED BIBLIOGRAPHY

Cuestas-Carnero, R., and Bornancini, C.A. (1988). Hereditary generalized gingival fibromatosis associated with hypertrichosis: report of five cases in one family. *J. Oral Maxillofac. Surg.* **46,** 415–420.

Five members of a family with male-to-male transmission are described. The hypertrichosis involved the face and arms in all affected individuals; in one, the back was also involved. Treatment by dental extraction and debulking resulted in normal gum formation with a 14-year follow-up.

Johnson, B.D., El Guindy, M., Ammons, W., Narayanan, A.S., and Page, R.C. (1986). A defect in fibroblasts from an unidentified syndrome with gingival hyperplasia as the predominant feature. *J. Periodontal Res.* **21,** 403–413.

Cell culture studies were performed in one patient with gingival hyperplasia who was described as hirsute. I suspect this patient had gingival fibromatosis and hypertrichosis.

Witkop, C.J. Jr. (1971). Heterogeneity in gingival fibromatosis. *Birth Defects* **VII(7),** 210–221.

Excellent detailed review with 134 references. Little regarding pathogenesis has been learned since this article appeared.

HYPERTRICHOSIS LANUGINOSA CONGENITA (MIM:145700, 307150)

(Hypertrichosis Universalis)

Includes Ambras Syndrome; CAMHR Syndrome; Barber-Say Syndrome

DERMATOLOGIC FEATURES

MAJOR. The entire body surface except the mucosa, palms, soles, prepuce, glans penis, and labia minora is covered with fine, long hairs that may be blonde to black in color. They may be present at birth, or progressive development of hairiness may occur in infancy. In some, the hairs are lost in childhood; in others, they persist into adult life. Within the same family different patterns of hair development and resolution have occurred.

MINOR. None.

ASSOCIATED ABNORMALITIES

One patient with congenital glaucoma has been described.

A sibship with hypertrichosis, cataracts and mental retardation (CAMHR) has been reported. Photographs suggest that these infants were hirsute and did not have true hypertrichosis.

One infant presented with a neonatal tooth, as had her unaffected father and multiple paternal relatives. Statements are made that missing teeth is a common feature in this condition, but this is not documented in other case reports of hypertrichosis lanuginosa.

A brother and sister, along with two additional sporadic cases, with hypertrichosis, cardiomegaly, and skeletal abnormalities, including a narrow thorax, platyspondyly, Erlenmeyer flask changes to the long bones, and generalized osteopenia have been described.

HISTOPATHOLOGY

LIGHT. An increase in the number of hair follicles that extended into the subcutaneous tissue was found in tissue from one patient.

EM. No information.

BASIC DEFECT

Unknown.

TREATMENT

Depilation, shaving, and other methods of hair removal.

MODE OF INHERITANCE

1. Autosomal dominant.
2. X-linked dominant (Macias-Flores et al., 1984)

PRENATAL DIAGNOSIS

None.

DIFFERENTIAL DIAGNOSIS

Hirsutism refers to increased hair growth in females and children in a male pattern distribution (beard, arms, legs, chest) and may result from many endocrinologic, pharmacologic, and genetic causes. These causes should be sought in any child with acquired hair growth.

Generalized hypertrichosis is a feature of congenital erythropoietic porphyria (Gunther disease, MIM:263700), but its onset is gradual and not congenital.

Infants with leprechaunism (Donohue syndrome, MIM:246200) have increased facial hair. Their abnormal facies, failure to thrive, and insulin resistance are not features of hypertrichosis lanuginosa.

In Stein-Leventhal syndrome (polycystic ovaries, obesity, hirsutism; MIM:184700), hirsutism is acquired and distributed in the pattern

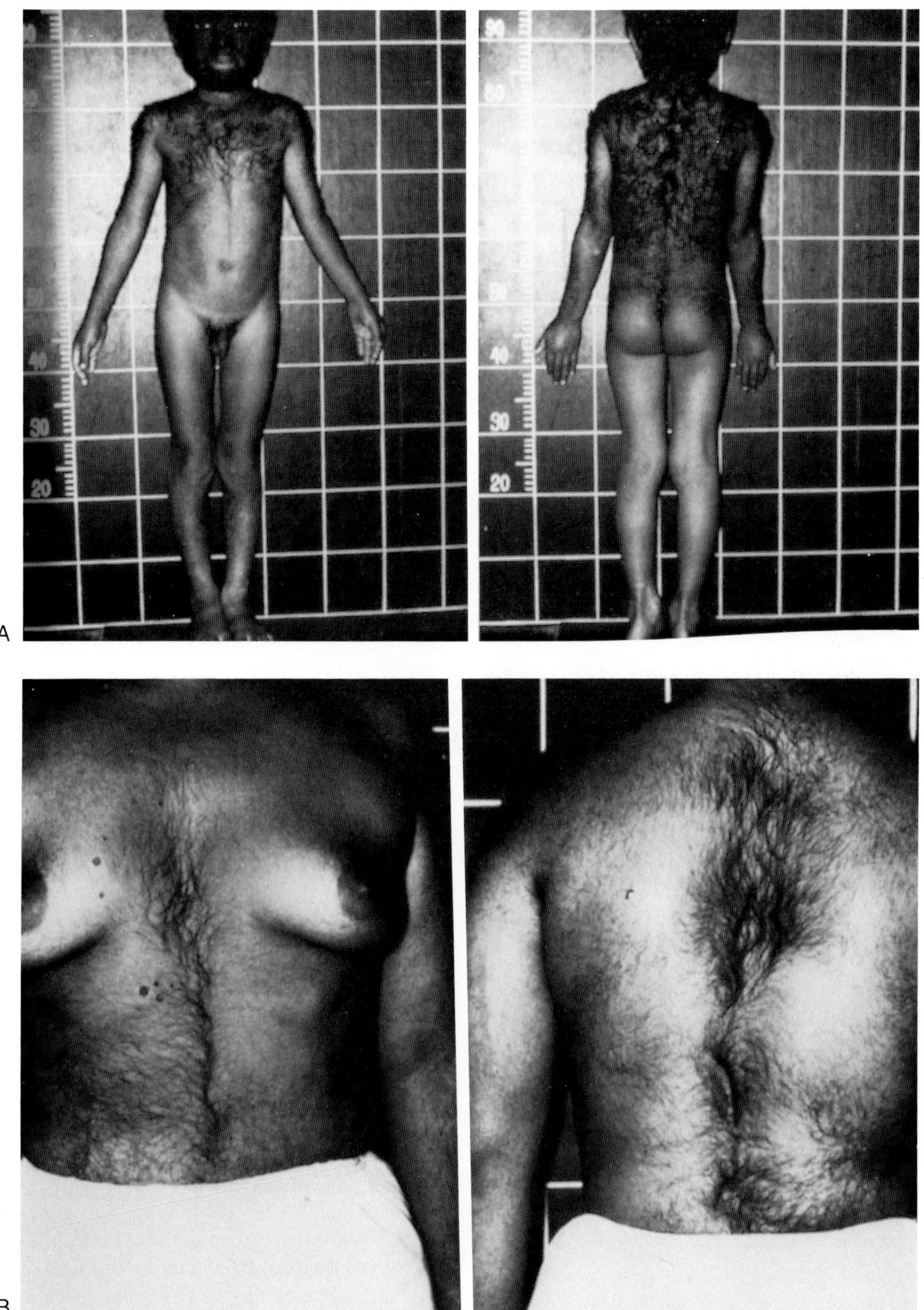

Figure 3.5. Son **(A)** and mother **(B)** with X-linked hypertrichosis lanuginosa. (From Macias-Flores et al., 1984.)

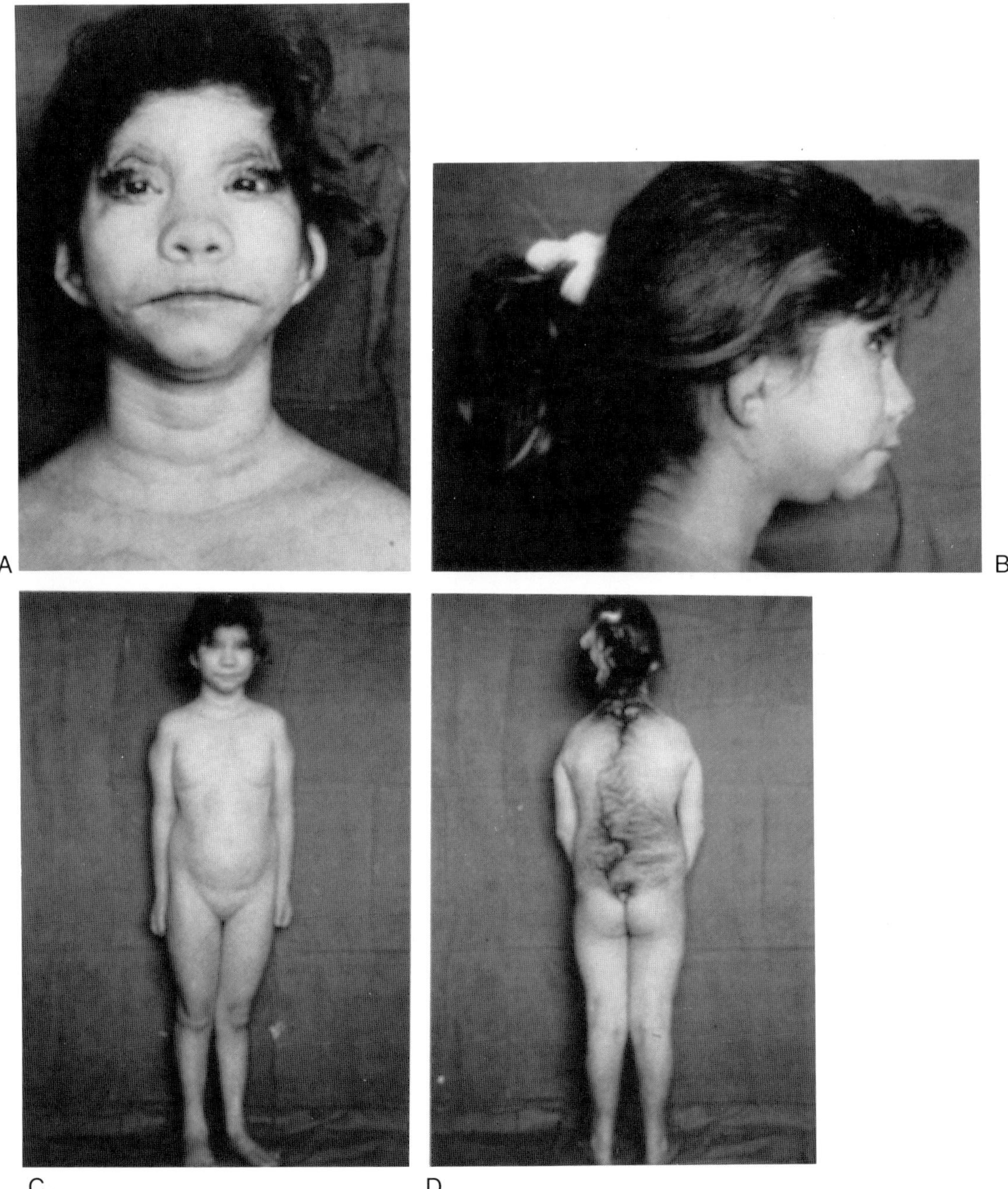

Figure 3.6. (A–D) Patient with Barber-Say syndrome: abnormal facies with macrostomia, abnormal eyebrows and eyelashes, abnormal ears, and hirsutism of the back. (From Santana et al., 1993.)

of normal male secondary sexual hairs (beard, mustache, body hair).

Nevoid hypertrichosis is marked by congenital or postnatal appearance of circumscribed areas of coarse hair growth on a background of normal pigment. Becker's nevi and congenital hairy melanocytic nevi can also be hypertrichotic, as can smooth muscle hamartomas and plexiform neurofibromas. All these lesions can be distinguished by clinical differences (e.g., pigmentation, coarse nature of hair, localized involvement) and by histopathology.

Localized facial and digital hypertrichosis was described in the Schinzel-Gideon syndrome (MIM:269150), and facial hirsutism is a feature of Cornelia de Lange syndrome (MIM:122470), both of which can be distinguished from hypertrichosis universalis by their clinical features.

Hypertrichosis is also associated with gingival fibromatosis (MIM:135400).

Children with Barber-Say syndrome have marked hypertrichosis of the back and neck, bushy lateral eyebrows, and long eyelashes. Facies are notable for a large mouth and abnormal external ears. The skin is wrinkled, lax, and atrophic, with a prominent vascular pattern. Intelligence and growth are normal. Inheritance is uncertain. All cases have been sporadic.

Support Group: N.O.R.D.
P.O. Box 8923
New Fairfield, CT
06812
1-800-999-6673

SELECTED BIBLIOGRAPHY

Baumeister, F.A.M., Egger, J., Schildhauer, M.T., and Stengel-Rutkowski, S. (1993). Ambras syndrome: delineation of a unique hypertrichosis universalis congenita and association with a balanced pericentric inversion (8) (p11.2;q22). *Clin. Genet.* **44,** 121–128.

Authors suggest the eponym Ambras after the first documented case in the family of Ambras Castle. The affected woman had six accessory nipples, and her hairs were vellus. Extensive discussion of types of hairs.

Beighton, P. (1970). Congenital hypertrichosis lanuginosa. *Arch. Dermatol.* **101,** 669–672.

Report of an affected male whose father had a history of hairiness in infancy with persistence of luxuriant eyebrows and eyelashes in adult life.

Cantú, J.M., García-Cruz, D., Sanchez-Corona, J., Hernandez, A., and Nazara, Z. (1982). A distinct osteochondrodysplasia with hypertrichosis—Individualization of a probable autosomal recessive entity. *Hum. Genet.* **60,** 36–41.

Two siblings and two isolated cases with hypertrichosis that improved with age but remained clinically obvious, who had unusual skeletal features and cardiomegaly. Intelligence was normal.

Felgenhauer, W.-R. (1969). Hypertrichosis lanuginosa universalis. *J. Genet. Hum.* **17,** 1–44.

Written in French, this article describes a mother and her two children with hypertrichosis lanuginosa universalis. There are several tables categorizing the different types of hypertrichosis and hirsutism and an exhaustive review of the European and historical literature. Plates from early references are included, along with clinical photos of Felgenhauer's patients.

Figuera, E., Pandolfo, M., Dunne, P.W., Cantú, J.M., and Patel, P.E. (1995). Mapping the congenital generalized hypertrichosis locus to chromosome Xq24–q27.1. *Nat. Genet.* **10,** 202–207.

Follow-up of the original family of Macías-Flores et al. (1984).

Macías-Flores, M.A., García-Cruz, D., Rivera, H., Escobar-Luján, M., Melendrez-Vega, A., Rivas-Campos, D., Rodríguez-Collazo, F., Moreno-Arellano, J., and Cantú, J.M. (1984). A new form of hypertrichosis inherited as an X-linked dominant trait. *Hum. Genet.* **66,** 66–70.

Nine authors describe 25 affected individuals in five generations with no male-to-male transmission and more severe expression in males than in females. The photographs are striking. Hypertrichosis is present at birth, worsens through childhood, and, in females, improves somewhat after puberty. The lower extremities are the least involved. The hair distribution in females, while described as "patchy" by the authors, did not distribute along the lines of Blaschko but appeared to concentrate along the midline trunk and face.

LEPRECHAUNISM (MIM:246200)

(Donohue Syndrome)

Includes Rabson-Mendenhall Syndrome

DERMATOLOGIC FEATURES

Major. At birth, hirsutism is a prominent feature, with fine, downy hairs particularly prominent over the face. The skin appears loose because of loss of subcutaneous tissue, and excessive wrinkling can be marked. The skin turgor is normal. The term *pachyderma* has been used to describe the redundant wrinkled skin, but it is not truly thickened except around the genitalia and lips.

Minor. Rugations around the anus, lips, and vulva are often described. Premature breast and nipple enlargement are common features.

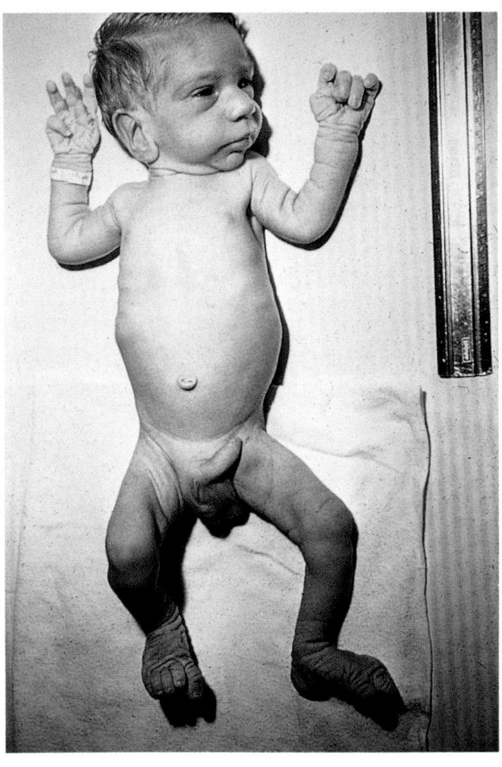

Figure 3.7. Redundant skin of hands and feet, large phallus, lack of adipose tissue. (Courtesy of Dr. J.G. Hall, Vancouver, British Columbia.)

ASSOCIATED ABNORMALITIES

Severe intrauterine growth retardation is an invariable finding. This growth deficiency persists postnatally, and failure to thrive results in death, usually within the first year of life. A few long-term survivors have been described in the literature.

The facies are marked by large, posteriorly rotated ears, prominent eyes with shallow orbits, and micrognathia. There is a simian, wizened appearance to the visage.

Abdominal protruberance with hepatomegaly contrasts sharply with the emaciated appearance of the face and limbs.

The penis and clitoris may be oversized. Polycystic ovaries are a common finding in females.

Severe hyperinsulinemia is the rule, with insulin levels reaching to greater than 100 times normal.

It is unclear if intelligence is affected; most case reports are of extremely sick infants who die.

HISTOPATHOLOGY

Light. No information.

EM. No information.

BASIC DEFECT

Homozygosity or compound heterozygosity for abnormalities in the insulin receptor gene has been demonstrated. It has been suggested that these mutations may also affect other cell surface receptors, such as those for epidermal growth factor.

TREATMENT

None effective.

MODE OF INHERITANCE

Autosomal recessive.

PRENATAL DIAGNOSIS

Successful prenatal exclusion of leprechaunism by measuring insulin receptor function of cultured amniocytes has been done. Theoretically it is now possible to diagnose leprechaunism prenatally by use of molecular techniques if the mutation(s) are known.

DIFFERENTIAL DIAGNOSIS

In congenital generalized lipodystrophy, emaciation is not present at birth, and muscle hypertrophy is. The severity of leprechaunism distinguishes it from the more benign generalized lipodystrophy. Insulin receptors are normal in congenital generalized lipodystrophy. Rabson-Mendenhall syndrome (MIM:262190) is marked by premature eruption of teeth, genital and ovarian hypertrophy, insulin-resistant diabetes mellitus, generalized hirsutism, acanthosis nigricans, and acromegalic facial features that develop in childhood. The patients are also reported to have thickened nails. Hyperplasia of the pineal gland was demonstrated on postmortem examination. In one patient with Rabson-Mendenhall syndrome, compound heterozygosity for mutations in the insulin receptor gene was demonstrated. Thus it is not clear that the condition deserves its own eponym.

Support Group: N.O.R.D.
P.O. Box 8923
New Fairfield, CT
06812
1-800-999-6673

SELECTED BIBLIOGRAPHY

Donohue, W.L., and Uchida, I. (1954). Leprechaunism. A euphuism for a rare familial disorder. *J. Pediatr.* **45,** 505–519.

Great photographs and a must-read justification of the use of the term *leprechaunism.* A *euphuism* involves the use of a highfaluting or hoity-toity term; a *euphemism* is the substitution of a gentler, kinder one. I think the authors must have meant the latter.

Kadowaki, T., Kadowaki, H., Rechler, M.M., Serrano-Rios, M., Roth, J., Gorden, P., and Taylor, S.I. (1990). Five mutant alleles of the insulin receptor gene in patients with genetic forms of insulin resistance. *J. Clin. Invest.* **86,** 254–264.

Homozygosity for a missense mutation in the insulin receptor gene in a patient with leprechaunism, compound heterozygosity for a different missense, and nonsense mutation in a patient with Rabson-Mendenhall and a patient with type A insulin resistance.

Longo, N., Langley, S.D., Griffin, L.D., and Elsas, L.J. II (1992). Reduced m-RNA and a nonsense mutation in the insulin-receptor gene produce heritable severe insulin resistance. *Am. J. Hum. Genet.* **50,** 998–1007.

An infant with classic leprechaunism who died at 7 months of age was heterozygous for a paternal mutation that resulted in a premature stop codon. The maternally inherited allele was normal in the protein coding region. Authors suggest that the second mutation affected a region of the gene involving control of expression. The paper is very difficult to read, and no information is given regarding glucose homeostasis in either parent, although the mother's cells behaved abnormally in culture.

LOCALIZED HYPERTRICHOSIS (MIM:139600, 239840)

(Hairy Elbows; Hairy Neck; Hypertrichosis Cubiti; Cervical Hypertrichosis)

DERMATOLOGIC FEATURES

MAJOR. Conditions in which inherited, site-specific abnormal hair growth have been reported are hypertrichosis cubiti and both anterior and posterior cervical hypertrichosis.

In hairy elbows, lanugo hairs, present at birth or developing soon thereafter, occur on the extensor surfaces of the elbows extending from midhumerus to midforearm. Involvement is bilateral. One male with this condition had a sister with generalized hypertrichosis.

In anterior cervical hypertrichosis, the patch of hair is at the sternal notch; in posterior, it is over the cervical vertebrae. In both conditions, the abnormal hair is present at birth.

MINOR. None.

ASSOCIATED ABNORMALITIES

In two pedigrees with hypertrichosis cubiti, short stature has been associated, as it has been in some sporadic cases. It is not clear whether the short stature and increased hair growth are inherited independently or result from the effects of a single gene. The type of short stature appears to differ between families; it was proportionate in one family, disproportionate in another.

In one family with posterior cervical hypertrichosis, kyphoscoliosis was associated. In another with anterior cervical hypertrichosis, the three affected individuals also had a peripheral neuropathy.

HISTOPATHOLOGY

LIGHT. There is a questionably increased number of normal hair follicles without structural alteration.

EM. No information.

BASIC DEFECT

Unknown.

TREATMENT

None.

MODE OF INHERITANCE

Hypertrichosis cubiti: unknown. An affected mother and daughter were cited in one report; affected siblings were reported among the Amish. McKusick cites this condition as a probable autosomal dominant, but it may be genetically heterogeneous.

Posterior cervical hypertrichosis: X-linked recessive or autosomal dominant. Although a multigeneration family was reported, there was no opportunity for male-to-male transmission in the pedigree.

Anterior cervical hypertrichosis: questionable autosomal rescessive. This was a highly inbred kindred with an affected mother, son, and paternal aunt, who was also first cousin to the mother.

PRENATAL DIAGNOSIS

None.

DIFFERENTIAL DIAGNOSIS

Localized patches of hair growth are most often sporadic, can be associated with congenital melanocytic nevi, smooth muscle hamartomas, Becker's nevi, or plexiform neurofibromas. Biopsy and histopathology will differentiate among these different conditions. A ring of hypertrichosis surrounding a scarred or hairless

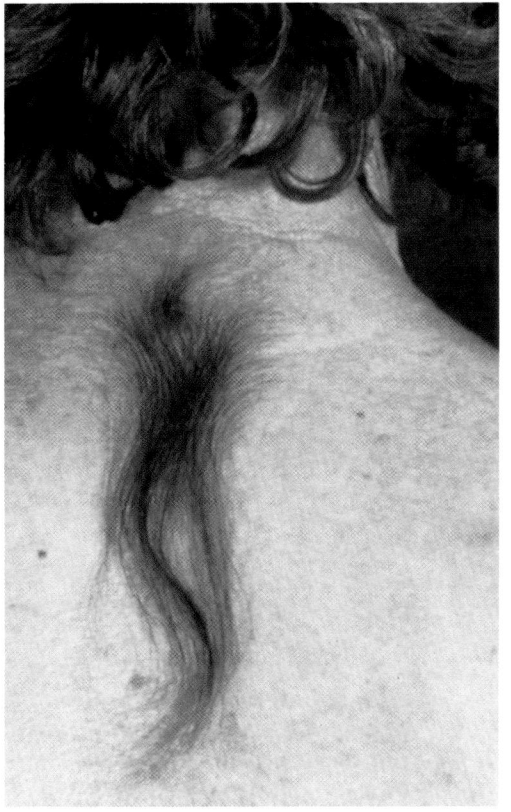

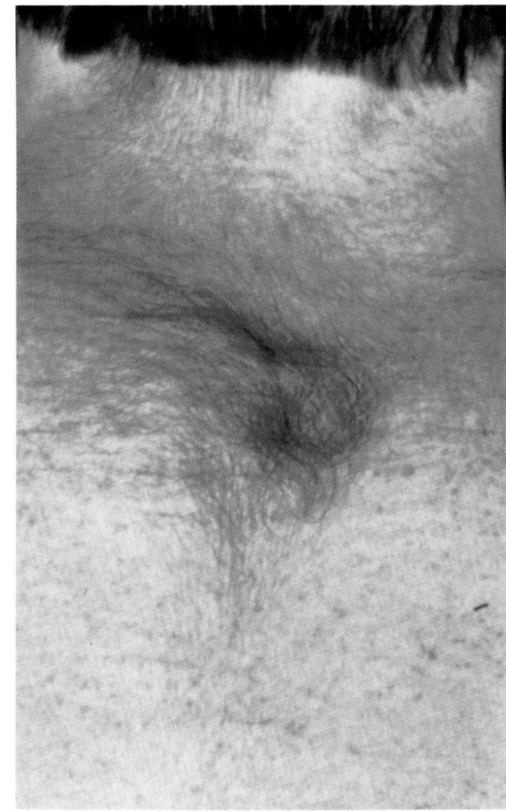

Figure 3.8. (A,B) Patches of hair on neck. (From Reed, 1989.)

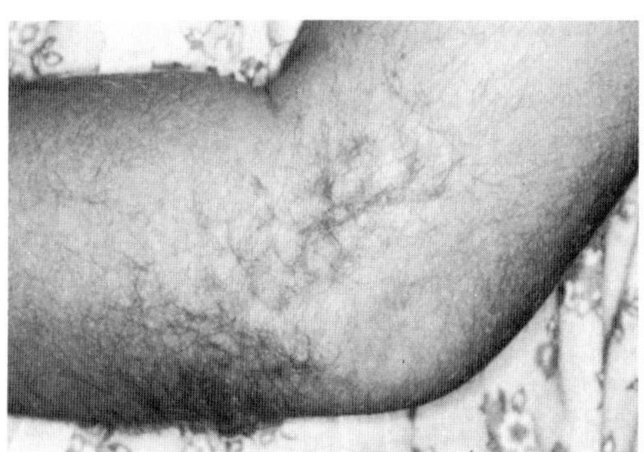

Figure 3.9. Thick, curly hair on lateral aspect of the elbow. (From Rudolph, 1985.)

area on the scalp warrants evaluation for a neuroectodermal rest or encephalocele. Infants with localized patches of hair growth over the midline back should have evaluation for vertebral bony abnormalities and occult meningoceles.

Support Group: N.O.R.D.
P.O. Box 8923
New Fairfield, CT
06812
1-800-999-6673

SELECTED BIBLIOGRAPHY

Edwards, M.J., Crawford, A.E., Jammu, V., and Wise, G. (1994). Hypertrichosis "cubiti" with facial asymmetry. *Am. J. Med. Genet.* **53,** 56–58.

Title is misleading. Patient had hypertrichosis of the right zygoma, right upper lip, on the trunk along the lines of Blaschko (right greater than left), and on the right thigh; suggestive of the X-linked form of hypertrichosis lanuginosa.

MacDermot, K.D., Patton, M.A., Williams, M.J.H., and Winter, R.M. (1989). Hypertrichosis cubiti (hairy elbows) and short stature: a recognisable association. *J. Med. Genet.* **26,** 382–385.

A mother and daughter with rhizomelic short stature, mild skeletal changes, and hairy elbows are reported. Two affected sporadic males with proportionate short stature and normal skeletal surveys are also described.

Reed, O.M., Mellette, J.R., Jr., and Fitzpatrick, J.E. (1989). Familial cervical hypertrichosis with underlying kyphoscoliosis. *J. Am. Acad. Dermatol.* **20,** 1069–1072.

Kyphoscoliosis and scoliosis were clinically evident and confirmed by x-rays. There were no vertebral body abnormalities noted. The patch of hair was posterior.

Trattner, A., Hodak, E., Sagie-Lerman, T., David, M., Nitzan, M., and Garty, B.Z. (1991). Familial congenital anterior cervical hypertrichosis associated with peripheral, sensory, and motor neuropathy—a new syndrome? *J. Am. Acad. Dermatol.* **25,** 767–770.

An inbred kindred in which ocular albinism and thalassemia minor were also segregating. The authors state that no individual had neuropathy without a patch of cervical hair, but do not detail how careful the examination of other family members was.

POLYCYSTIC OVARIAN DISEASE (MIM:184700)

(Stein-Leventhal Syndrome; Polycystic Ovary Syndrome; Polycystic Ovarian Syndrome)

DERMATOLOGIC FEATURES

MAJOR. Hirsutism, excessive growth of hair in females at sites usually associated with male secondary sexual changes, is a common presenting sign of Stein-Leventhal syndrome. The fine vellus hairs of the body and face differentiate into pigmented coarse terminal hairs. Onset is usually around menarche, and the rate of progression is slow. Seventy percent of affected females have objective hirsutism.

Almost all women with "idiopathic hirsutism" will have an underlying ovarian source for increased androgen production.

MINOR. Acanthosis nigricans, velvety brown thickening of the skin of the axillae, neck, and midchest, occurs in those with insulin resistance. It is more common in those individuals with Stein-Leventhal syndrome who are obese. A small proportion of affected females will develop male pattern baldness, and perhaps 10% will have significant problems with acne.

There is some suggestion that males who carry the gene for Stein-Leventhal syndrome have premature balding. In one report, males had an increased amount of body hair evident at birth. Oligospermia was described in one case report.

ASSOCIATED ABNORMALITIES

Elevated luteinizing hormone levels, menstrual irregularities, anovulatory cycles, and polycystic ovaries are classic features. Not all patients have demonstrably enlarged ovaries. Even when the ovaries are normal in size, there will be thecal cell hyperplasia and follicular cysts. Infertility occurs in almost three-fourths of affected females.

Forty percent of patients are obese.

Insulin resistance and diabetes are common. In one study, 20% of obese females with polycystic ovary disease developed diabetes or abnormal glucose tolerance tests before age 30.

HISTOPATHOLOGY

LIGHT. The hairs are pigmented terminal hairs that appear to be normal in number.

EM. No information.

BASIC DEFECT

Unknown. Peripheral conversion of androgens to dihydrotestosterone is increased either because of tissue factors or because of increased substrate.

TREATMENT

A variety of hormonal therapies have been used, including birth control pills, estrogens, and cyproteroneacetate. Spironolactone may be effective. Weight loss may result in improvement in ovarian function in some patients.

Clomiphene has been used to induce fertility; ovarian wedge resection used to be the treatment of choice, but is now used in a minority of patients.

MODE OF INHERITANCE

Probably autosomal dominant with sex-limited expression. Delineation of the mode of inheritance is hampered by the lack of clear diagnostic criteria.

PRENATAL DIAGNOSIS

None.

DIFFERENTIAL DIAGNOSIS

The congenital hypertrichoses include congenital hypertrichosis lanuginosa (MIM:145700), congenital generalized hypertrichosis (MIM: 307150), and hypertrichosis with gingival fibromatosis (MIM:135400). In these disorders, hair growth is present at birth or soon after. Endocrine abnormalities and polycystic ovaries are not typical features. Both males and females are affected. Isolated or idiopathic hirsutism, without other features of Stein-Levinthal syndrome, can occur in the absence of other signs of virilization or androgen excess. It is probably caused by increased overall activity of endogenous androgens, either by local conversion or by increased production.

In the congenital adrenal hyperplasias (partial 21-hydroxylase deficiency, 3-β-hydroxy-δ-5-steroid dehydrogenase deficiency, and 11-β-hydroxylase deficiency), patients may occasionally present with acquired hirsutism. Appropriate laboratory evaluation will help to distinguish among these possibilities.

Other sources of androgens such as ovarian tumors, adrenal tumors, Cushing syndrome, and medications can result in hirsutism as a presenting complaint.

The degree of "normal" hairiness differs among ethnic groups. Thus, there is a sliding definition of hirsutism. In some individuals it may be difficult to distinguish that which is indicative of underlying polycystic ovarian disease.

Support Group: N.O.R.D.
P.O. Box 8923
New Fairfield, CT
06812
1-800-999-6673

SELECTED BIBLIOGRAPHY

Ferriman, D., and Gallwey, J.D. (1961). Clinical assessment of body hair growth in women. *J. Clin. Endocrinol. Metab.* **21,** 1440–1447.

The authors devised a scoring system for "semi-quantitative assessment" of hairiness in females. This scale is used extensively in the literature. They use a composite score devised from a 5-point grading system for each of 11 body sites.

Jahanfar, S., and Eden, J.A. (1993). Idiopathic hirsutism or polycystic ovary syndrome. *Aust. N.Z. J. Obstet. Gynaecol.* **33,** 414–416.

The authors screened 173 women with hirsutism. Eighty-six percent of 96 with normal menstrual cycles, 97% of 44 with oligomenorrhea, and 94% of 33 with amenorrhea had ultrasound evidence of polycystic ovaries. The authors suggest that there is no true "idiopathic" hirsutism.

Legro, R.S. (1995). The genetics of polycystic ovary syndrome. *Am. J. Med.* **98,** 9S–16S.

Very nice review of the factors confounding classic pedigree analysis in polycystic ovarian syndrome. There is a lack of clear distinction between affected and unaffected individuals in many instances. They review all the studies to date and discuss linkage as a powerful tool to elucidate the inheritance of polycystic ovary syndrome. However, given the difficulty of assigning family members, especially males, to affected or unaffected categories (a *sine qua non* for linkage studies), this seems a problematic approach to me.

Lunde, O., Magnus, P., Sandvik, L., and Hoglo, S. (1989). Familial clustering in the polycystic ovarian syndrome. *Gynecol. Obstet. Invest.* **28,** 23–30.

A cohort of 132 females with polycystic ovaries and two or more of menstrual irregularities, hirsutism, infertility, obesity. A control group of 71 females with no gynecologic disease (all were fertile). In response to a questionnaire, 19% of group 1 patients had fathers with early baldness and/or excessive hairiness. This occurred in 10% of the control group. Twenty percent of the brothers had similar findings compared with 2% of brothers in the control group. Thirty-one percent of mothers had signs of polycystic ovarian disease compared with 3% in the control group, and 31% of sisters were similarly affected compared with 7% in the control group. This study is subject to all of the errors of self-administered questionnaires.

Robinson, S., Rodin, R.A., Deacon, A., Wheeler, M.J., and Clayton, R.N. (1992). Which hormone tests for the diagnosis of polycystic ovaries syndrome? *Br. J. Obstet. Gynaecol.* **99,** 132–238.

Total testosterone is the best single indicator. Coupled with androstenedione and luteinizing hormone, these authors claim it provides definitive testing.

Shelly, D.R., and Dundif, A. (1990). Polycystic ovary syndrome. *Compr. Ther.* **16,** 26–34.

Very nice, clearly written review, with recommendations for diagnosis, workup, and management.

HAIR SHAFT ABNORMALITIES, ISOLATED

MONILETHRIX (MIM:158000, 177750, 252700)

(Beaded Hair)

DERMATOLOGIC FEATURES

Major. In monilethrix the hairs appear beaded, with wide (normal) and narrow (abnormal) regularly distributed nodes. The hairs are fragile at the constricted sites and break easily. There may be partial to total alopecia. The hairs usually become more normal at puberty. Eyelashes, eyebrows, and body hair, both vellus and terminal, are uninvolved. Not all the scalp hairs are abnormal, and in some individuals only a patch or two are involved. Intrafamilial variation in severity is common.

Pseudomonilethrix, characterized by irregular spacing of nodes, is also autosomal dominant and clinically appears the same.

Minor. Some affected individuals have keratosis pilaris.

ASSOCIATED ABNORMALITIES

None.

HISTOPATHOLOGY

Light. The hairs are not twisted. There are evenly spaced, wide nodes 0.7 to 1 mm apart, separated by narrow internodes.

EM. On cross section, the nodes are normal. The cuticle and the cortex are abnormal in the internodes, with alterations in cortical cells and their tonofibrils and abnormal deposits of cystine positive material. Ito et al. (1990) described cytoplasmic vacuoles in the cortical and cuticular cells.

A

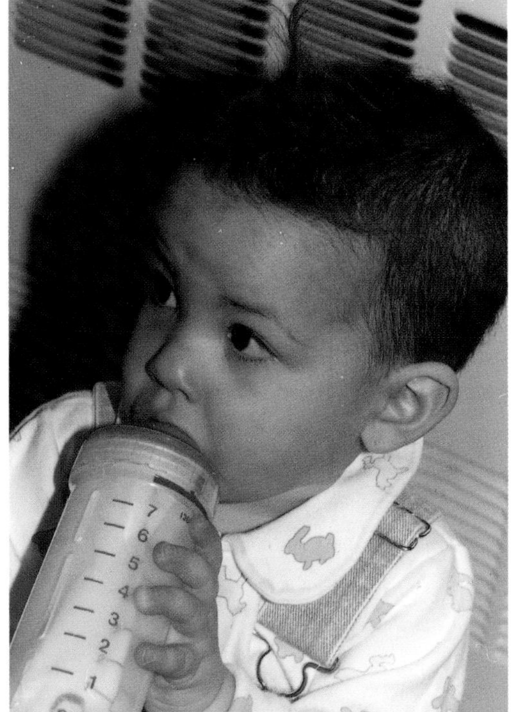

B

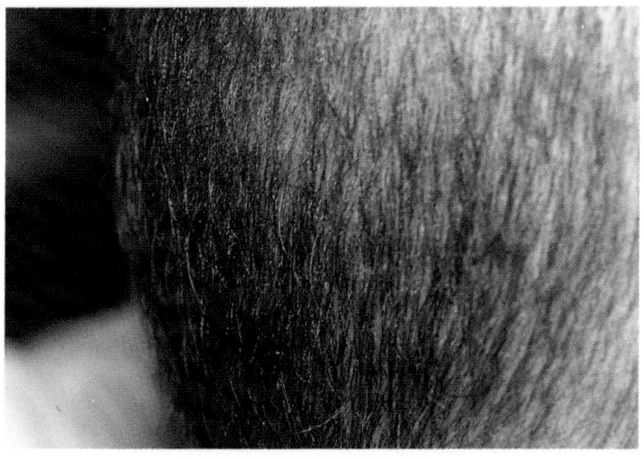

Figure 3.10. **(A)** Hairs are normal in number but short. **(B)** Close-up shows beaded appearance of hairs.

BASIC DEFECT

Unknown.

TREATMENT

Gentle handling of hair to minimize breakage.

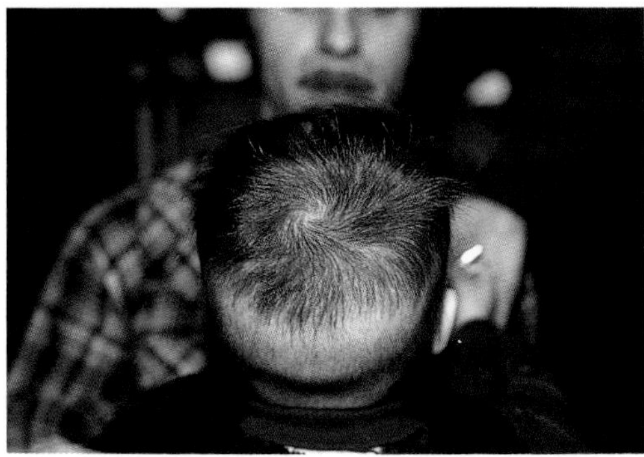

Figure 3.11. Hairs are worn off around occiput due to fragility.

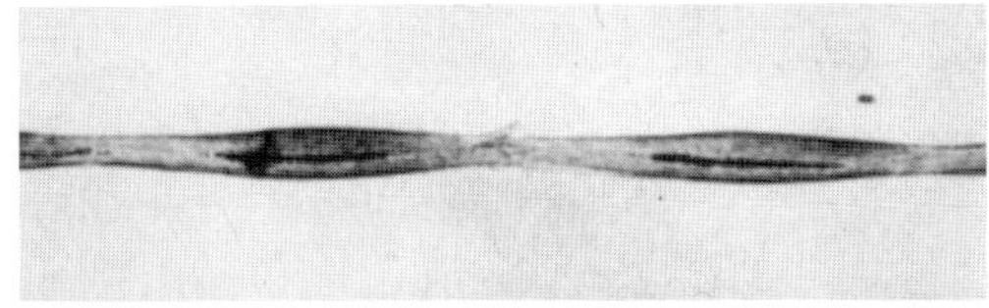

Figure 3.12. Hairs under light microscope with broad and narrow regions. (From Price, 1975.)

MODE OF INHERITANCE

Autosomal dominant inheritance with variable expression is demonstrated in most pedigrees. Solomon and Green (1963) noted a 2:1 ratio of affected females to males; Schaap et al. (1982), just the reverse. Although autosomal recessive inheritance has been suggested for some families with monilethrix, the published pedigrees interpreted as suggesting autosomal recessive inheritance are also consistent with autosomal dominant inheritance. Linkage to the type II keratin cluster on 12q has been demonstrated in two families.

PRENATAL DIAGNOSIS

None.

DIFFERENTIAL DIAGNOSIS

Other structural hair shaft abnormalities are in the differential diagnosis of monilethrix. In pili torti (MIM:261900), the twists of the hair shaft can make it appear as if there are wide and narrow areas. The twists require refocusing up and down the hair shaft with the light or dissecting microscope, whereas the length of the hair with monilethrix remains in the same plane of focus.

Support Group: N.O.R.D.
P.O. Box 8923
New Fairfield, CT
06812
1-800-999-6673

BIBLIOGRAPHY

Baker, H. (1962). An investigation of monilethrix. *Br. J. Dermatol.* **74,** 24–30.

Report of a family with monilethrix and the lack of significant clinical response to treatment by protection from light, intradermal and subcutaneous injections of hydrocortisone acetate, and Grenz rays. Baker noted that the hairs grew at the rate of one node–internode complex per day.

Bentley-Phillips, B., Bayles, M.A.H., and Grace, H.J. (1974). Pseudo-monilethrix. Further family studies. *Humangenetik* **25,** 331–337.

This is a follow-up study of the authors' original pedigree and two new families. Affected individuals have dry, coarse, unruly, thin, or "difficult to manage" hair. These changes are usually of late childhood onset and occur in the context of overbrushing and overmanipulation of the hairs. The irregularly spaced nodes are actually depressions, demonstrated by scanning electron microscopy. The authors believe pseudomonilethrix is a distinct and real genetic entity. I am unconvinced. The changes described, which include twists in the hair and trichorrhexis nodosa-like changes, as well as the nodes, could be the result of mechanical damage. These families may have a condition predisposing to fragile hairs, which then show these secondary structural changes.

Gummer, C.L., Dawber, R.P.R., and Swift, J.A. (1981). Monilethrix: an electron microscopic and electron histochemical study. *Br. J. Dermatol.* **105,** 529–541.

A detailed study of the ultrastructural changes in monilethrix with an extended discussion regarding possible biochemical mechanisms.

Ito, M., Hashimoto, K., Katsuumi, K., and Sato, Y. (1990). Pathogenesis of monilethrix: computer stereography and electron microscopy. *J. Invest. Dermatol.* **95,** 186–194.

This is a detailed report of scanning and transmission electron microscopy of hairs and a scalp biopsy from a single patient with monilethrix. In contrast to others, the authors believe that the nodes and internodes of monilethrix are not regularly spaced, as they demonstrated irregular involvement in the hairs of this patient and in another patient published previously. However, the literature they cite is the family of Bentley-Phillips et al. (1974), which did not have monilethrix.

Schaap, T., Even-Paz, Z., Hodes, M.E., Cohen, M.M., and Hachem-Zadeh, S. (1982). The genetic analysis of monilethrix in a large inbred kindred. *Am. J. Med. Genet.* **11,** 469–474.

The authors posit autosomal dominant inheritance with great intrafamilial variability and penetrance of 100%. While some of the affected family members could have been homozygous for the monilethrix gene because of consanguinity, there was no difference in severity of the hair findings between them and presumed heterozygotes.

Solomon, I.L., and Green, O.C. (1963). Monilethrix. Its occurrence in seven generations, with one case that responded to endocrine therapy. *N. Engl. J. Med.* **269,** 1279–1282.

Report of a large pedigree ascertained through several probands. They note the improvement with age and the intrafamilial variability.

Summerly, R., and Donaldson, E.M. (1962). Monilethrix. A family study. *Br. J. Dermatol.* **74,** 387–391.

Five of nine affected members of a five generation pedigree are described.

PILI ANNULATI (MIM:180600)

(Ringed Hair; Spangled Hair)

DERMATOLOGIC FEATURES

MAJOR. The "ringed" hairs show alternating light and dark bands, visible to the eye. When viewed in the light microscope, these bands are reversed. The hairs grow at a normal rate. There is disagreement as to whether the cavities in the hairs are sites of easy breakage. Many reports claim normal strength and length of the hairs.

Only scalp hairs are affected.

MINOR. None.

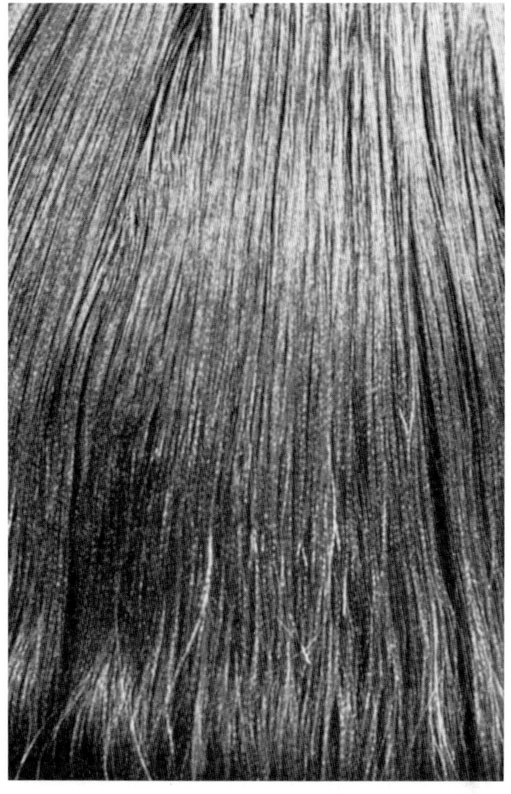

Figure 3.13. Clinical appearance of hair. (From Juon, 1942.)

ASSOCIATED ABNORMALITIES

None.

HISTOPATHOLOGY

LIGHT. The cortical fibers of the abnormal bands contain air-filled spaces, as do the cortical cells. These spaces appear bright with reflected light, but do not permit transmitted light to pass through and appear dark under light microscopy.

EM. The cuticle of involved bands shows undulations on the surface and in longitudinal sections. Cross sections of the cortex demonstrate increased intracellular spaces among the macrofibrils.

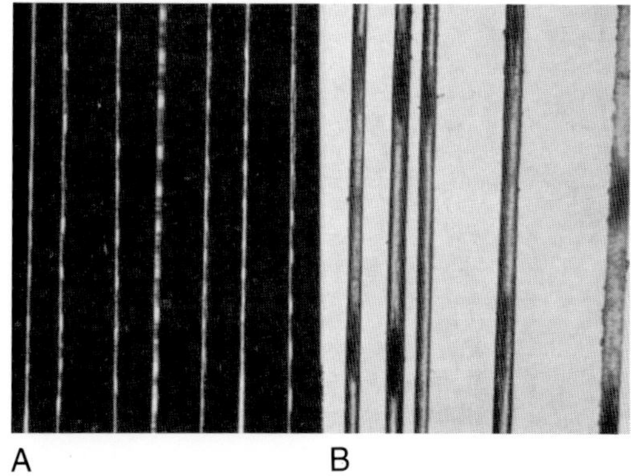

Figure 3.14. **(A)** Hairs with reflected light. **(B)** Hairs with transmitted light showing reversal of banding. (From Juon, 1942.)

BASIC DEFECT

There may be an abnormality in the formation of the microfibril matrix complex.

TREATMENT

None.

MODE OF INHERITANCE

Autosomal dominant.

PRENATAL DIAGNOSIS

None.

DIFFERENTIAL DIAGNOSIS

At first glance, monilethrix (MIM:158000, 252200) or beaded hairs might appear similar to pili annulati. It is clearly different on closer inspection.

Support Group: N.O.R.D.
P.O. Box 8923
New Fairfield, CT
06812
1-800-999-6673

SELECTED BIBLIOGRAPHY

Ashley, L.M., and Jacques, R.S. (1950). Four generations of ringed hair. *J. Hered.* **41,** 82–84.

Report of a family and review of the literature substantiating autosomal dominant inheritance.

Gummer, C.L., and Dawber, R.P.R. (1981). Pili annulati: electron histochemical studies on affected hair. *Br. J. Dermatol.* **105,** 303–309.

A detailed discussion of electron microscopic findings in pili annulati.

Price, V.H., Thomas, R.S., and Jones, F.T. (1968). Pili annulati: optical and electron microscopic studies. *Arch. Dermatol.* **98,** 640–647.

Study of hairs from one affected female. The authors proved that the areas that were bright with reflected light were air-filled cavities by demonstrating that they filled with a variety of liquids. Good electron micrographs and interesting discussion.

PILI TORTI (MIM:261900)

(Twisted Hair; Kinky Hair)

Includes Bjornstad Syndrome

DERMATOLOGIC FEATURES

MAJOR. The scalp hairs are sparse, break easily, and appear dry and coarse. When examined under the microscope, they show twisting. Typically 180 degree twists are irregularly distributed along the hair shaft and are the weak sites at which fracturing of the hairs occurs. Both scalp and body hair may be involved. In isolated pili torti, the changes may

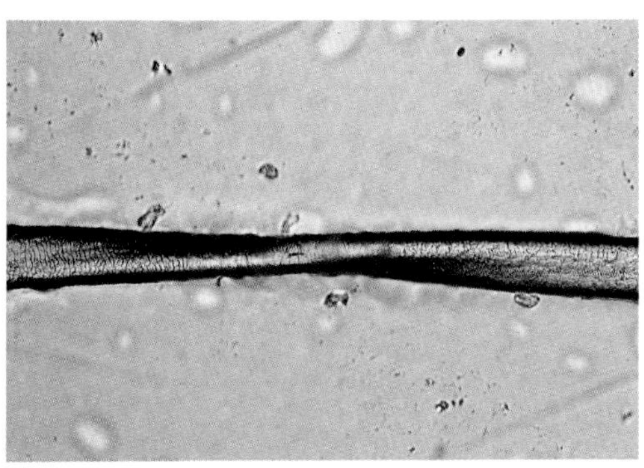

Figure 3.15. Twists in hair shaft. (Courtesy of Dr. D. Benjamin, Seattle, Washington.)

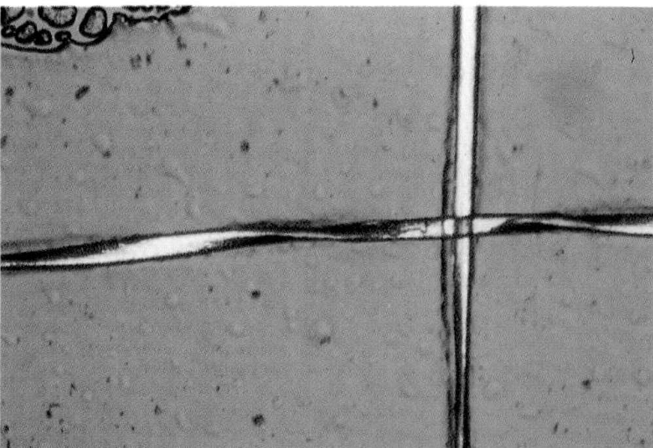

Figure 3.16. Under polarized light. (Courtesy of Dr. D. Benjamin, Seattle, Washington.)

not be congenital, but have onset in early childhood. In some cases of isolated pili torti, the hairs were reported to normalize at puberty.

MINOR. Enamel hypoplasia has been reported in some affected individuals.

ASSOCIATED ABNORMALITIES

Syndromic associations for pili torti include:

Menkes disease (MIM:309400): This is an X-linked disorder of copper uptake in which the pili torti may result from a defect in the formation of disulfide bonds in keratin. Female carriers for Menkes may have patchy distribution of pili torti. Other structural hair abnormalities such as trichorrhexis nodosa and monilethrix can also be found. Neurologic and vascular abnormalities, typical of Menkes disease, are not part of isolated pili torti.

Pili torti and deafness (Bjornstad syndrome, MIM:262000): Several reports of pedigrees with siblings affected with pili torti and progressive sensorineural hearing loss have been reported. Deafness in these families was detected within the first year.

Pili torti, sensorineural deafness, and secondary hypogonadism (MIM:262000): This may be the same disorder as pili torti with deafness. The hypogonadism was of late onset secondary to a deficiency of luteinizing hormone and was present in two of the three affected siblings. The deafness was progressive and severe. Eyebrows, eyelashes, scalp, and body hair were involved.

Pili torti and ichthyosis (MIM:256500): Netherton syndrome can exhibit pili torti in addition to trichorrhexis invaginata.

Pili torti and ectodermal dysplasia: Ocular, tooth, and nail abnormalities have been reported in association with pili torti in a few families.

Pili torti may also be acquired in association with systemic diseases such as lupus erythematosus and may occur in the hairs surrounding the scars of cicatricial alopecia from a variety of causes.

HISTOPATHOLOGY

LIGHT. The hair shafts are flattened and twisted around their axes at irregular intervals. The twists range from 90 to 360 degrees.

EM. The cuticle is normal.

BASIC DEFECT

Unknown.

TREATMENT

None. Careful and gentle hair grooming is essential, as these hairs are fragile.

MODE OF INHERITANCE

Isolated pili torti may be autosomal dominant or autosomal recessive. Menkes is X-linked recessive. Pili torti with deafness appears to be autosomal recessive.

PRENATAL DIAGNOSIS

None for isolated pili torti.

DIFFERENTIAL DIAGNOSIS

Other structural hair shaft abnormalities including monilethrix (MIM:158000, 252200) are in the differential diagnosis of pili torti. Pili torti can be differentiated from monilethrix under the light microscope. The narrow (twisted) and wide (flat) areas of the hair with pili torti are not in the same plane of focus, while the narrow and normal areas in monilethrix are all in the same plane.

Support Group: N.O.R.D.
P.O. Box 8923
New Fairfield, CT
06812
1-800-999-6673

SELECTED BIBLIOGRAPHY

Appel, B., and Messina, S.J. (1942). Pili torti hereditare. *N. Engl. J. Med.* **226,** 912–915.

Report of sibship with two affected sisters and a brother. A paternal aunt and grandmother were reported to be affected. Scalp hair and eyebrows were involved. Severity varied. The enamel of the teeth was defective. The authors suggested that the condition can improve at puberty.

Beare, J.M. (1952). Congenital pilar defect showing features of pili torti. *Br. J. Dermatol.* **64,** 366–372.

A report of a father and four of eight offspring (three female, one male) with isolated pili torti. Onset was late; loss of eyebrows and eyelashes occurred in early childhood, and the scalp hair became involved in the teens. Body and secondary sexual hair were absent or sparse. All affected individuals had psychiatric or neurologic diseases ranging from "severe congenital idiocy" in the 26-year-old son to "low mentality" and "irresponsibility" in others. Trichorrhexis nodosa was also seen.

Crandall, B.F., Samec, L., Sparkes, R.S., and Wright, S.W. (1973). A familial syndrome of deafness, alopecia, and hypogonadism. *J. Pediatr.* **82,** 461–465.

Three male siblings with progressive sensorineural hearing loss, pili torti, and defects in luteinizing hormone are reported.

Petit, A., Dontenwille, M.M., Blanchet-Bardon, C., and Civatte, J. (1993). Pili torti with congenital deafness (Bjornstad's syndrome)—report of three cases in one family, suggesting autosomal dominant transmission. *Clin. Exp. Dermatol.* **18,** 94–95.

Affected mother, son, and daughter. However, father was also deaf. He is described as deaf from infancy, "suspected to be a consequence of meningitis." Nonetheless, caution is warranted in excluding his hearing loss as potentially genetic and contributing to his children's.

Ronchese, F. (1932). Twisted hairs (pili torti). *Arch. Dermatol.* **26,** 98–109.

Isolated case report of an otherwise normal girl with hair abnormalities present since birth. The hairs on the occiput were more severely involved. Subsequently a second sibling was noted to be affected.

PILI TRIANGULI ET CANALICULI (MIM:191480)

(Uncombable Hair; Spun Glass Hair)

DERMATOLOGIC FEATURES

Major. The hairs are coarse, wiry, frizzy, refractile, and "wild" in appearance. They may stand straight up from the scalp. The hair is described as unmanageable. The hairs are usually blond or silvery and may grow normally or at a slower rate. Eyebrows, eyelashes, and body hair appear normal. In one of our patients, neonatal hair was entirely normal. It was replaced by classic uncombable hair by 6 months of age.

The condition may be more common than the medical literature would suggest. Two patients I have seen with this condition were referred for unrelated skin diseases. The parents were aware of the "problem" hair but had not sought medical attention for it, nor had it been commented on in medical records, although it was striking.

Minor. Although nails are reportedly normal in this disorder, one of my patients had chronic, recurrent onychomycosis beginning at age 2 years. Perhaps a subtle defect in nail growth or structure resulted in increased susceptibility to fungal infection.

ASSOCIATED ABNORMALITIES

None.

HISTOPATHOLOGY

Light. Longitudinal canals can sometimes be appreciated. More useful is examination of

A

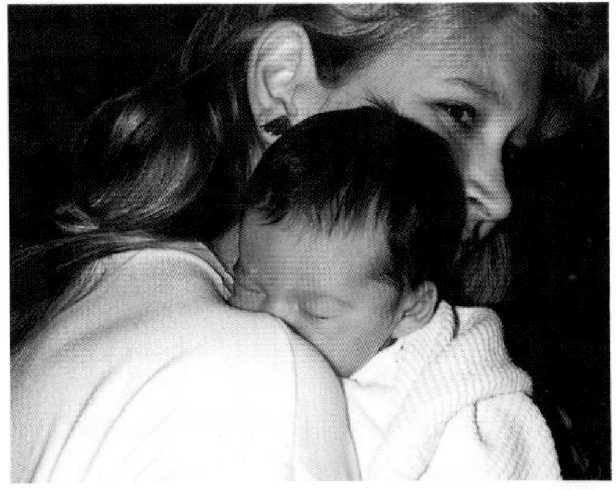

B

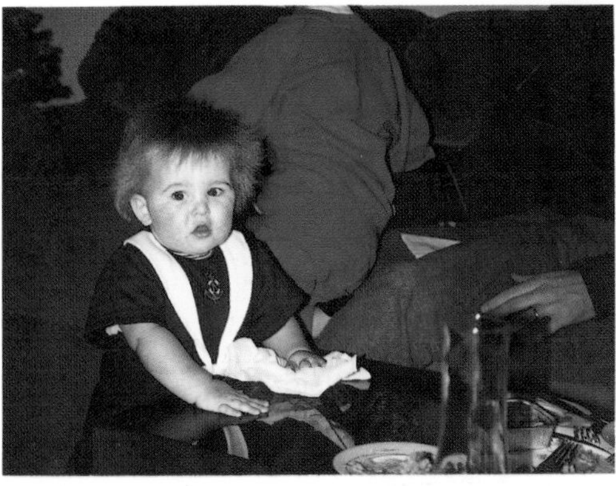

Figure 3.17. **(A)** At 2 weeks of age, newborn hairs are normal. **(B)** By 13 1/2 months, wild mop of spangled hairs has developed.

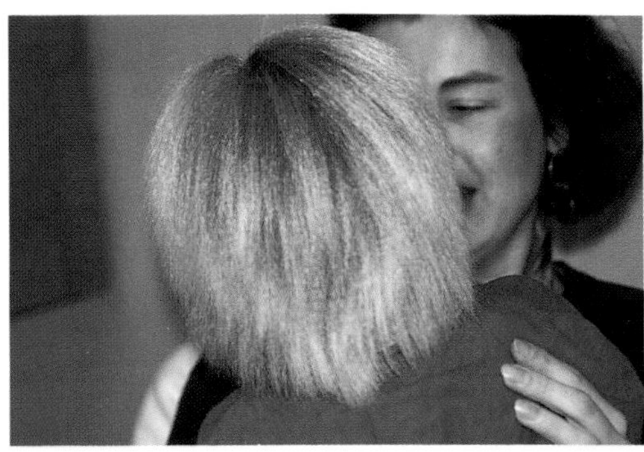

Figure 3.18. Spangling is obvious, along with the light color of the hair.

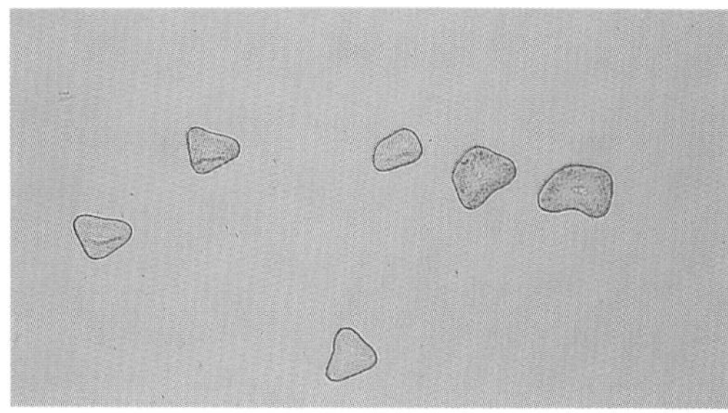

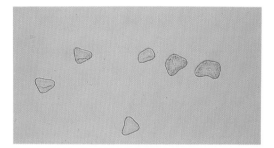

Figure 3.19. On cross section of paraffin-imbedded hairs, triangular and odd shapes easily identified. (Courtesy of Dr. D. Benjamin, Seattle, Washington.)

hairs embedded in paraffin and cut in cross section, which show a kidney bean or triangular shape. (I am indebted to Dr. Denis Benjamin for this inexpensive method.)

EM. The cuticle scales are densely packed, and a median broad canal or groove runs down the shaft of the hairs, which are oval or kidney-bean in shape rather than round.

BASIC DEFECT

Unknown.

TREATMENT

Gentle handling of the hair and creative styling are the only treatments. The condition may improve with puberty.

MODE OF INHERITANCE

Autosomal dominant.

PRENATAL DIAGNOSIS

None.

DIFFERENTIAL DIAGNOSIS

Other structural hair abnormalities are distinguished by clinical and ultrastructural appearance. Uncombable hair has been reported in one patient with Wilson disease (MIM: 277900). Median grooving of the hairs has been reported in Marie Unna syndrome (MIM: 146550).

Support Group: N.O.R.D.
P.O. Box 8923
New Fairfield, CT
06812
1-800-999-6673

SELECTED BIBLIOGRAPHY

Hebert, A.A., Charvow, J., Esterly, N.B., and Fretzin, D.F. (1987). Uncombable hair (pili trianguli et canaliculi): evidence for dominant inheritance with complete penetrance based on scanning electron microscopy. *Am. J. Med. Genet.* **28,** 185.

Report of an affected brother and sister. Hairs from their clinically normal father showed pili trianguli et canaliculi on scanning electron microscopy.

Mallon, E., Dawber, R.P.R., De Berker, D., and Ferguson, D.J.P. (1994). Cheveaux incoiffables—diagnostic, clinical and hair microscopic findings, and pathogenic studies. *Br. J. Dermatol.* **131,** 608–614.

No major breakthrough in basic understanding. Interestingly, affected hairs appeared to weather less than normal hairs and were equally strong.

TRICHORRHEXIS INVAGINATA (MIM:None)

(Bamboo Hair)

DERMATOLOGIC FEATURES

Major. The hairs in trichorrhexis invaginata are friable, thin, and often broken and short. The hair shafts have an irregular distribution of nodules along their length. These nodules are believed to form from intussuception of a distal keratinized hair cuticle into a proximal soft, nonkeratinized cortex.

Minor. None.

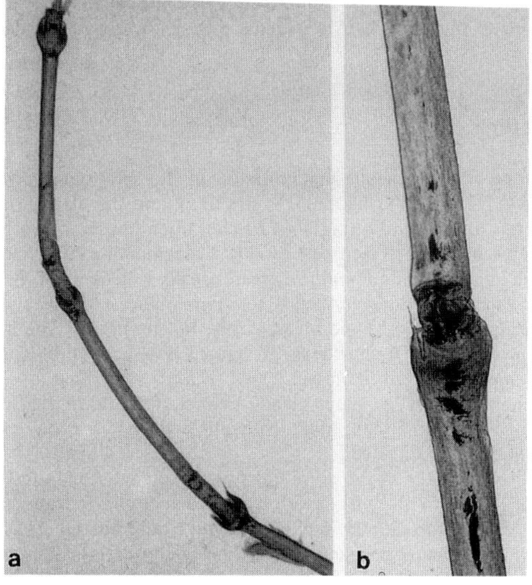

Figure 3.20. Appearance of hair under light microscope. (From Traupe, 1989.)

ASSOCIATED ABNORMALITIES

Trichorrhexis invaginata is the major hair finding in Netherton syndrome (MIM:256500), which is associated with ichthyosis linearis circumflexa. In Netherton syndrome, trichorrhexis invaginata may not be present early on and, when present, may not involve all hairs. Repeat hair examination is mandatory if the diagnosis of Netherton is suspected. Trichorrhexis invaginata has been reported in other ichthyosiform dermatoses as well and can be induced by trauma to normal hair.

HISTOPATHOLOGY

Light. The nodes give a ball-and-socket appearance in which a clubbed distal portion of the hair shaft is compressed into a cupped expansion of the proximal shaft.

EM. Same.

BASIC DEFECT

A partial defect in the conversion of sulfhydryl groups to disulfide bonds in the cortex has been posited.

TREATMENT

Gentle hair care and avoidance of trauma.

MODE OF INHERITANCE

The inheritance pattern is that of the associated syndrome.

PRENATAL DIAGNOSIS

None.

DIFFERENTIAL DIAGNOSIS

Other structural hair abnormalities can be distinguished by light or electron microscopy.

It is important to recognize that trichorrhexis nodosa and trichorrhexis invaginata may be nonspecific markers of increased hair fragility for a variety of reasons and can be seen in hairs of patients with other structural hair abnormalities. Many hairs from several areas must be examined along their lengths, as scalp involvement may be patchy and distribution along the hair shaft irregular.

Support Group: N.O.R.D.
P.O. Box 8923
New Fairfield, CT 06812
1-800-999-6673

SELECTED BIBLIOGRAPHY

Altman, J., and Stroud, J. (1969). Netherton syndrome and ichthyosis linearis circumflexa: psoriasiform ichthyosis. *Arch. Dermatol.* **100,** 550–558.

Report of two patients with Netherton syndrome and ichthyosis linearis circumflexa. The authors suggest that this pattern of scaling skin is typical of Netherton syndrome and propose that psoriasiform ichthyosis be used as a unifying term for the unusual ichthyoses reported in association with trichorrhexis invaginata.

Ito, M., Ito, K., and Hashimoto, K. (1984). Pathogenesis in trichorrhexis invaginata (bamboo hair). *J. Invest. Dermatol.* **83,** 1–6.

Scanning electron microscopy of plucked hairs from three patients with Netherton syndrome showed, in addition to trichorrhexis invaginata, pili torti, trichorrhexis nodosa, and torsion nodules. Based on an increased number of sulfhydryl groups, the authors suggested that incomplete conversion of these to disulfide bonds might be the cause of the hair shaft changes. Good electron and light microscopic micrographs.

TRICHORRHEXIS NODOSA (MIM:NONE)

DERMATOLOGIC FEATURES

Major. In trichorrhexis nodosa, the hair shaft is marked by irregularly spaced swellings where the cuticle has been lost and the fibers of the cortex exposed. The hair fractures at these sites.

Isolated congenital trichorrhexis nodosa is extremely rare. Trichorrhexis nodosa may be a marker of general fragility of hair from a variety of causes rather than a distinct clinical entity. It is a common finding in normal individuals who have chemically or mechanically damaged their hair.

Minor. None.

ASSOCIATED ABNORMALITIES

Hairs from individuals with Menkes syndrome (MIM:309400), argininosuccinic aciduria

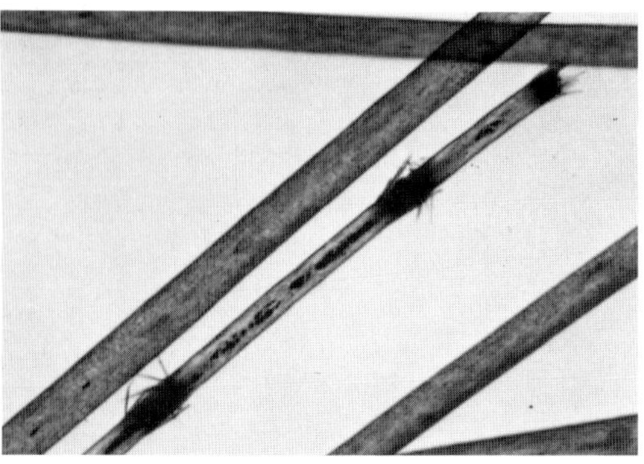

Figure 3.21. Hair with trichorrhexis nodosa under light microscope showing frayed broomstick on end appearance. (From Porter, 1971.)

(MIM:207900), and the trichothiodystrophies (MIM:234050, 242170, 278730) may show trichorrhexis nodosa.

HISPATHOLOGY

LIGHT. The nodes give the appearance of broomsticks head to head, with apposition of the frayed, split cortical fibers.
EM. There is loss of the cuticle with fraying of the cortical fibers at these sites.

BASIC DEFECT

Mechanical or chemical damage to the hair is the major cause of trichorrhexis nodosa in normal individuals. Patients with argininosuccinic aciduria are deficient in arginine and have increased amounts of citrulline, both of which are major constituent amino acids of the hair. This may result in more brittle, weaker hairs that develop trichorrhexis nodosa easily.

TREATMENT

Gentle hair care and avoidance of trauma.

MODE OF INHERITANCE

The inheritance pattern is that of the associated syndrome.

PRENATAL DIAGNOSIS

Specific for associated syndrome.

DIFFERENTIAL DIAGNOSIS

Other structural hair abnormalities can be distinguished by light or electron microscopy.

It is important to recognize that trichorrhexis nodosa and trichorrhexis invaginata may be nonspecific markers of increased hair fragility for a variety of reasons and can be seen in hairs of patients with other structural hair abnormalities such as pili torti or monilethrix. Many hairs must be examined along their lengths, as scalp involvement may be patchy and distribution along the hair shaft irregular.

Support Group: N.O.R.D.
P.O. Box 8923
New Fairfield, CT
06812
1-800-999-6673

SELECTED BIBLIOGRAPHY

Chernosky, M.E., and Owens, D.W. (1966). Trichorrhexis nodosa. Clinical and investigative studies. *Arch. Dermatol.* **94,** 577–585.

Owens, D.W., and Chernosky, M.E. (1966). Trichorrhexis nodosa in vitro reproduction. *Arch. Dermatol.* **94,** 586–588.

Chernosky and Owens (1966) report 49 patients with trichorrhexis nodosa. One patient had a positive family history with an affected mother. Trauma was the single definable cause in most patients. Excellent photographs. Owens and Chernosky (1966) report that they were able to reproduce lesions of trichorrhexis nodosa in samples from 53 normal-appearing scalp hairs by mechanical rubbing.

Ito, M., Ito, K., and Hashimoto, K. (1984). Pathogenesis in trichorrhexis invaginata (bamboo hair). *J. Invest. Dermatol.* **83,** 1–6.

Scanning electron microscopy of plucked hairs from three patients with Netherton syndrome showed, in addition to trichorrhexis invaginata, pili torti, trichorrhexis nodosa, and torsion nodules. Based on an increased number of sulfhydryl groups in the hairs, the authors suggested that incomplete conversion of these to disulfide bonds might be the cause of the hair shaft changes. Good electron microscopy and light micrographs.

WOOLLY HAIR (MIM:194300, 278150, 278200)

Includes CHANDS

DERMATOLOGICAL FEATURES

MAJOR. Woolly hair is a condition that may involve all the scalp hairs or be localized as woolly hair nevi. In generalized woolly hair, the hairs are extremely curly and coarse in texture. The diameter of the curls is about 0.5 cm. In the presumed autosomal recessive form of woolly hair, the hairs are pale and fracture readily. It is said that in autosomal dominant hereditary woolly hair, the hairs usually grow normally, are normally pigmented, and are not fragile. However, many reports of patients with the autosomal dominant form describe pale, blond hairs that demonstrate easy breakage. Woolly hair nevi are congenital lesions, usually localized to a small region in the scalp. I have seen one patient with multiple lesions. They are not genetic and can be associated with other organoid nevi.

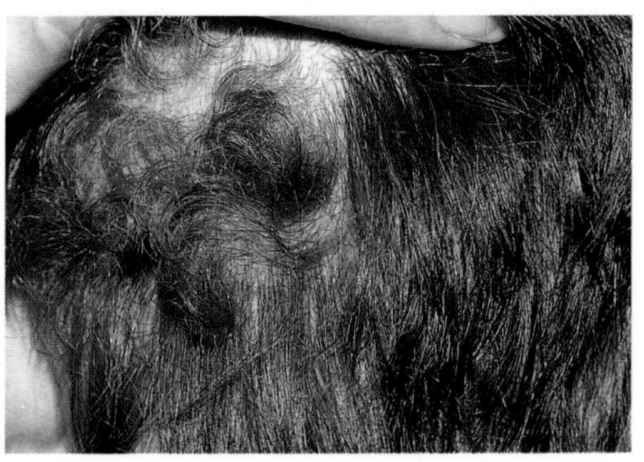

Figure 3.22. Woolly hair nevi at temple.

MINOR. Lesions of trichorrhexis nodosa have been reported in woolly hair but may result from trauma by brushing or combing of the tightly curled hairs rather than reflecting a primary or intrinsic defect.

ASSOCIATED ABNORMALITIES

Woolly hair and ulerythema ophryogenes have been reported in a patient with Noonan syndrome (MIM:163950), an autosomal dominant disorder of short stature, ptosis, mild mental deficiency, webbed neck, and pulmonic stenosis. Both the hair and skin findings may be more common in Noonan syndrome than previously recognized.

Salamon (1963) reported a sibship with woolly hair, generalized hypotrichosis, bat ears, and everted lips. The last two features were inherited separately as unlinked autosomal dominant traits and were not thought to be related to the woolly hair.

HISTOPATHOLOGY

LIGHT. The changes are not pathognomonic. The affected hairs show twisting 180 degrees around their axes, are oval in cross section, and may exhibit trichorrhexis nodosa.

EM. The hairs may show changes of weathering and the findings of trichorrhexis nodosa.

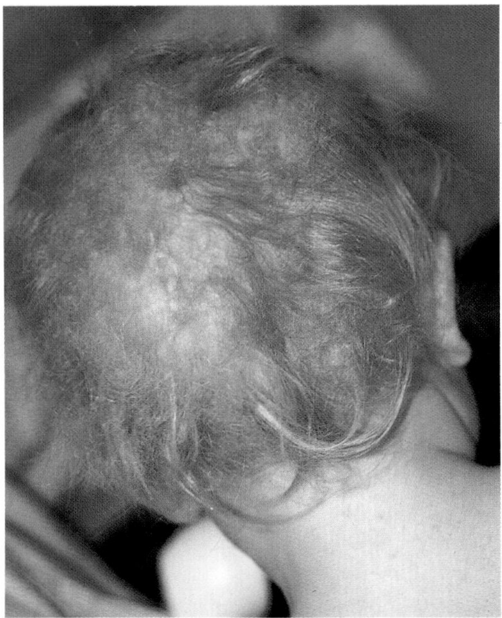

Figure 3.23. More extensive woolly hair nevus.

BASIC DEFECT

Unknown.

TREATMENT

Gentle handling of hair and appropriate styling. The condition may ameliorate with age.

MODE OF INHERITANCE

Autosomal dominant in most instances. With the exception of a report by Hutchinson et al. (1974) of one child who was the offspring of a second cousin mating and the two siblings in Salamon's report (1963), all well-documented cases have been autosomal dominant or sporadic, and there is no compelling evidence for autosomal recessive inheritance.

PRENATAL DIAGNOSIS

None.

DIFFERENTIAL DIAGNOSIS

The hair in CHANDS (*c*urly *h*air, *a*nkyloblepharon, and *n*ail *d*y*s*plasia) (MIM:214350) is similar to woolly hair. The associated features are distinctive. CHANDS has been described in only one kindred (in which ataxia telangiectasia was segregating independently), and the photos of the hair and nail changes are not striking.

Individuals with BIDS (hair–brain syndrome) (MIM:234050) or other trichothiodystrophies have hair that at first glance appears similar. The very fragile, brittle quality of the hair is distinct from woolly hair, as are the associated neurologic, endocrinologic, and skeletal abnormalities.

Patients with woolly hair should be carefully evaluated for features of Noonan syndrome (MIM:163950), which may be quite subtle in its expression.

Support Group: N.O.R.D.
P.O. Box 8923
New Fairfield, CT
06812
1-800-999-6673

SELECTED BIBLIOGRAPHY

Hutchinson, P.E., Cairns, R.J., and Wells, R.S. (1974). Woolly hair. Clinical and general aspects. *Trans. St. Johns Hosp. Dermatol. Soc.* **60,** 160–177.

Two pedigrees with multiple generations, one of which showed male-to-male transmission, are presented. A third, sporadic case was the product of a second cousin mating. Forearm hair was involved in some patients, and trichorrhexis nodosa and pili annulati were noted in some. Hair structure and growth rate were evaluated. The growth rate of the hair appeared normal.

Mohr, O.I. (1932). Woolly hair: a dominant mutant character in man. *J. Hered.* **23,** 345–352.

Schokking, C.Ph. (1934). Another woolly hair mutation in man. *J. Hered.* **25,** 337–340.

Mohr (1932) and Schokking (1934) provide two wonderful clinical portraits of pedigrees with woolly hair. Great family photographs. Both authors felt compelled to argue that the trait did not result from hybridization with African races, but was a true, distinct mutation in Caucasians.

Neild, V.S., Pegum, J.S., and Wells, R.S. (1984). The association of keratosis pilaris atrophicans and woolly hair, with and without Noonan's syndrome. *Br. J. Dermatol.* **110,** 357–362.

The authors describe one pedigree with three affected members in three generations with woolly hair, two of whom also had ulerythema. An unrelated isolated case of a female with Noonan syndrome, woolly hair, and ulerythema ophyrogenes is also described.

Ormerod, A.D., Main, R.A., Ryder, M.L., and Gregory, D.W. (1987). A family with diffuse partial woolly hair. *Br. J. Dermatol.* **116,** 401–405.

A three generation family in which multiple members had two populations of scalp hair, normal and tightly kinked or curled, in approximately a 2:1 ratio. Clinically, the abnormal hairs were similar to woolly hairs. However, on cross section they appeared round, not oval. On electron microscopy, the affected hairs showed frequent kinks that changed the direction of the hair shaft. The hair follicles were normal on light microscopy.

Salamon, T. (1963). Uber Eine familie mit reccessiver Kraushaarigkeit, Hypotrichose und anderen Anomalien. *Hautarzt* **14,** 540–544.

Two consanguineous matings (one of first cousins, one of second cousins in the same family) of individuals normal by history resulted in offspring with woolly hair and hypohidrosis. In German with no English summary.

Verbov, J. (1978). Woolly hair—study of a family. *Dermatologica* **157,** 42–47.

A geneticist's nightmare—a single consanguineous pedigree with apparent autosomal dominant transmission of woolly hair. The proband, product of a first cousin mating, had woolly hair and absence of the lower eyelashes, was deaf (as was her brother with normal hair) and had ichthyosis vulgaris (as did her first cousin with normal hair and hearing). Her father, two other siblings, three first cousins, two paternal aunts, a paternal uncle, and paternal grandmother had isolated woolly hair. Good clinical photographs.

Wyre, H.W., Jr. (1978). Cutaneous manifestations of Noonan's syndrome. *Arch. Dermatol.* **114,** 929–930.

Case report with a table of the dermatologic features of Noonan syndrome.

HAIR SHAFT ABNORMALITIES, SYNDROMIC

MENKES DISEASE (MIM:309400)

(Kinky Hair Disease, Steely Hair Syndrome)

DERMATOLOGIC FEATURES

Major. The hair in Menkes disease is fine, silver or white, and fragile. There is often a paucity of hair at birth, and the eyebrows and eyelashes may remain sparse. The hairs have a kinky or wiry appearance. The hair changes may not be present in newborn hair, and not all hairs are necessarily affected. Neurologically normal carrier females may show pili torti in some of their hairs.

The skin is thin, often mottled, with a cutis marmorata pattern and pale in color. The skin has a doughy, lax quality. Uneven skin pigmentation, along the lines of Blaschko or unilateral, has been described in some carrier females.

Minor. The scalp has been described as scaly in a few case reports. There are occasional descriptions of a seborrheic dermatitis-like or scaling rash on the body.

ASSOCIATED ABNORMALITIES

Affected infants are hypotonic, develop seizures within a few days to months of life, and show profound developmental delays. In some, development may initially appear normal, but loss of milestones occurs within the first year. There have been a few individuals with only mild mental retardation. Feeding difficulties are typical. Death usually ensues within the first year of life, although long-term survival into the early teens has been reported in a few individuals. In these, microcephaly is typical. There is a tortuosity of blood vessels in the central nervous system and elsewhere. These are visible by traditional angiography or, more recently, magnetic resonance angiography (MRA). The intima of the vessels is marked by fragmentation of the internal elastic lamina.

Low birth weight is an inconstant finding; premature birth is common.

Neonatal hypothermia is a typical feature, with core temperatures of 33°–35°C. Its basis is uncertain. Osteoporosis with metaphyseal flaring and wormian bones of the skull are common radiologic findings. The skull changes develop within the first few months, the metaphyseal changes soon after. The ribs and the femurs are common sites for metaphyseal changes.

The typical facial appearance of these patients results from absence of hair, eyebrows, and eyelashes, along with pallor, lack of facial expression, and full cheeks.

Serum ceruloplasmin levels are grossly decreased.

HISTOPATHOLOGY

LIGHT. The hairs show twisting along the longitudinal axis (pili torti). The twisting may not be regular. The hairs have decreased pigment and narrow diameter. As with any fragile hair, trichorrhexis nodosa is common.

EM. The mean dermal collagen fibril diameter is decreased; elastin fibers are very sparse and amorphous.

BASIC DEFECT

Mutations in the Menkes gene (*MNK*) result in increased copper uptake across the brush border of the lumen of the small intestine, but failure to transport copper from these cells into the plasma. This results in total body copper deficiency. Copper-dependent enzymes include tyrosinase (thus the decrease in skin and hair color), lysyl oxidase (thus the defects in elastin and collagen cross-linking), monoamine oxidase (possibly related to the pili torti), cytochrome oxidase (possibly relating to the hypothermia), and ascorbate oxidase (resulting in the skeletal changes).

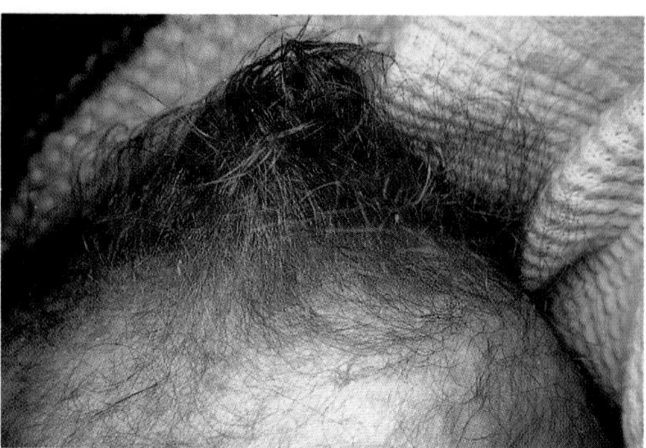

Figure 3.24. Sparse, wiry, refractile hairs, some with silvery sheen. Baby is of mixed African and European descent.

TREATMENT

Subcutaneous copper histidine treatment and intramuscular injection of other copper salts have been reported with varying success. As "mild" forms of the disorder exist, it is difficult to assess the effects of treatment unless the natural course of the disease in untreated siblings is available for comparison.

MODE OF INHERITANCE

X-linked recessive. There are rare reports of manifesting female carriers. The Menkes gene has been isolated and is mapped to Xq13.3

PRENATAL DIAGNOSIS

Now available by mutational analysis. Previously by measuring ^{64}Cu incorporation by

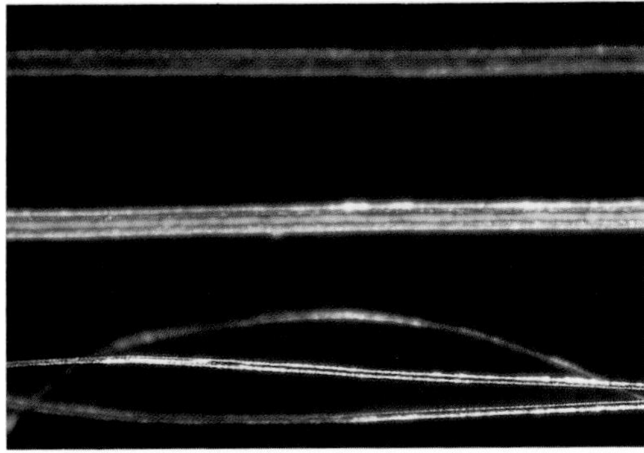

Figure 3.25. Normal pigmented hair (top), normal gray hair (middle), and hairs from infant with Menkes disease (bottom). (From Sybert and Holbrook, 1987.)

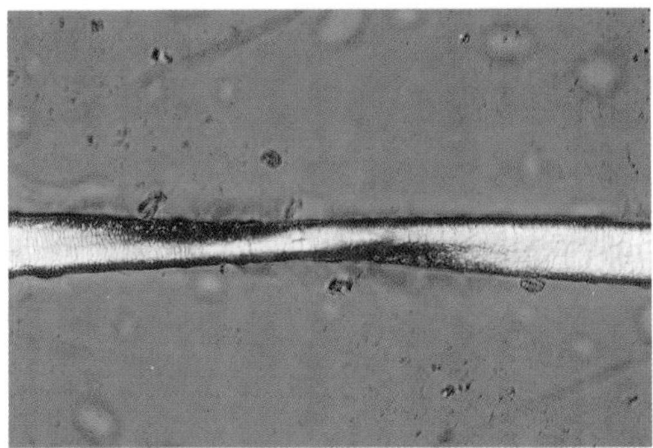

Figure 3.26. Twist in hair nicely highlighted with polarized light. (Courtesy of Dr. D. Benjamin, Seattle, Washington.)

chorionic villus cells or amniotic fluid cells with good, but not complete, reliability.

DIFFERENTIAL DIAGNOSIS

Pili torti is not pathognomonic for Menkes disease. It can be isolated (MIM:261900) or found in association with deafness (Bjornstad syndrome, MIM:262000).

Occipital horn disease (EDS IX, X-linked cutis laxa, MIM:304150) is allelic to Menkes disease. The disorder is clinically different in the greater laxity of skin, the absence of seizures or severe mental retardation, and the presence of exostoses (occipital horns) on the occiput and long bones. In addition, bladder diverticuli are common in EDS IX. Both conditions show a decrease in serum copper, a decrease in serum ceruloplasmin, and an increase in ^{64}CU incorporation.

In the absence of a positive family history, scurvy and rickets might be considered initially based on the bone changes alone in "mild" cases.

The twisting of the hairs creates the illusion of wide and narrow areas along the hair shaft and has led to the misdiagnosis of monilethrix (MIM:158000). In pili torti, the hair shaft shifts in and out of focus as the lens traverses its length. In monilethrix, the wide nodes and narrow internodal areas remain in the same plane of focus.

Wilson disease (MIM:277900) is also characterized by low serum copper and low serum ceruloplasmin levels, but it is easily distinguished by an entirely different clinical course.

Support Group: Corporation for Menkes Disease (CMD)
5720 Buckfield Court
Fort Wayne, IN 46804
1-219-436-0137

SELECTED BIBLIOGRAPHY

Danks, D.M., Campbell, P.E., Stevens, B.J., Mayne, V., and Cartwright, E. (1972). Menkes's kinky hair syndrome. An inherited defect in copper absorption with widespread effects. *Pediatrics* **50,** 188–201.

Danks, D.M., Campbell, P.E., Walker-Smith, J., Stevens, B.J., Gillespie, J.M., Blomfield, J., and Turner, B. (1972). Menkes' kinky-hair syndrome. *Lancet* **i,** 1100–1103.

These authors applied what was known about sheep to humans. Recognizing the similarities between the hair of patients with Menkes and the wool of sheep suffering from nutritional copper deficiency, along with the vascular changes of copper deficiency in other animals (swine, chicks, turkeys, and cattle), Danks and colleagues looked at copper levels in seven affected infants and demonstrated decreased values. The *Pediatrics* article contains more clinical detail. They describe monilethrix in the hairs in the *Lancet* report, but retract this in the *Pediatrics* report.

Gerdes, A.-M., Tønnesen, T., Horn, N., Grisar, T., Marg, W., Muller, A., Reinsch, R., Barton, N.W., Guiraud, P., Joannard, A., Richard, M.J., and Guttler, F. (1990). Clinical expression of Menkes syndrome in females. *Clin. Genet.* **38,** 452–459.

The first patient was a sister of a boy with Menkes. The second had an affected uncle. Her karyotype was 45,X/46,XX. In a third patient, the diagnosis of Menkes was based on neurologic abnormalities, pili torti, and osteoporosis, but her copper uptake studies were normal. All three of these patients were severely affected. These authors review other reports of carriers in the literature.

Harris, E.D. (1993). Menkes' disease: perspective and update on a fatal copper disorder. *Nutr. Rev.* **51,** 235–238.

Succinct review of the possible mechanisms of action of the *MNK* gene.

Sarkar, B., Lingertat-Walsh, K., and Clarke, J.T.R. (1993). Copper histidine therapy for Menkes disease. *J. Pediatr.* **123,** 828–830.

Tümer, Z., Horn, N., Tønnesen, T., Christodoulou, J., Clarke, J. T. R., Sarkar, B. (1996) Early copper-histidine treatment for Menkes disease. *Nat. Genet.* **12,** 11–13.

"Success" with three patients and failure in five. One was 12 years old prior to therapy, suggesting that he had a mild variant to begin with. In the other two "successful patients," treatment was started at 1 month of age. Neurologic status is normal in these two infants, although they have had "major non-neurologic problems attributable to Menkes." In five patients in whom treatment was begun between 2 and 7 months of age, although the serum copper normalized, neurologic deterioration progressed. The authors suggest that very early initiation of treatment might work. There were no sibling controls to determine the natural course of the disease in any of these individuals. In the follow-up letter (Tümer et al., 1996), the mutations in two of the successfully treated patients (born premature and treated within four weeks after birth) were identified and were consistent with an expected to be severe phenotype. The authors thus are encouraged by the potential utility of very early treatment.

Tønnesen, T., Kleijer, W.J., and Horn, N. (1991). Incidence of Menkes disease. *Hum. Genet.* **86,** 408–410.

Based on their experience as a catchment lab for pre- and postnatal diagnosis of Menkes disease, they estimate an incidence of 1 in 254,000 (including those fetuses aborted). Previous estimates started at 1 in 35,000 to 1 in 90,000 to 1 in 114,000. If these authors are correct, Menkes disease is 70 times less common than Duchenne muscular dystrophy.

Wheeler, E.M., and Roberts, P.F. (1976). Menkes's steely hair syndrome. *Arch. Dis. Child.* **51,** 269–274.

Hydronephrosis, hydroureter, and bladder diverticuli are described in three males with typical Menkes disease. Given the allelic relationship to X-linked cutis laxa and the urinary findings of that disorder, it is not surprising that a small subset of patients with Menkes disease will also have urinary tract involvement. It is not a typical feature.

TRICHODENTOOSSEOUS SYNDROME (MIM:190320)

Includes Trichodental Syndrome

DERMATOLOGIC FEATURES

Major. At birth the hair is full and kinky. It may remain coarse, thick, and tightly curled or may become straight by adult life. Fingernails may be thin, striated, and peel in layers. Toenails may be thickened or normal.

Minor. None.

ASSOCIATED ABNORMALITIES

Teeth are small and pitted with hypoplastic enamel. There is taurodontism, and the teeth have large pulp chambers. They are prone to caries. Affected individuals are usually edentulous by age 30 years.

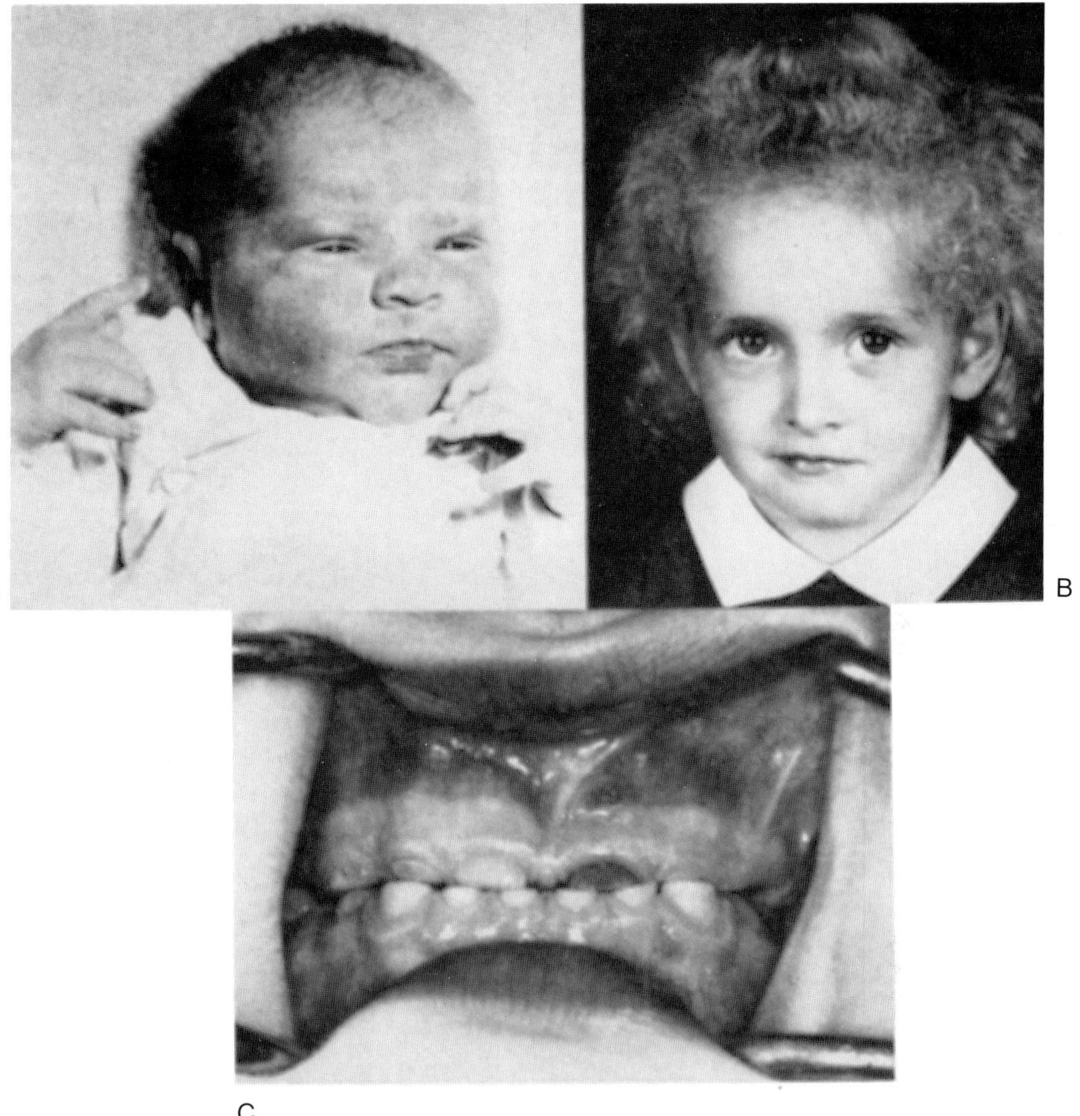

Figure 3.27. **(A)** Kinky hair as newborn. **(B)** Persistence of hair changes at age 5 years. **(C)** Eroded teeth; a cyst is visible above the upper left incisor. (From Lichtenstein et al., 1972.)

The skull is marked by dolichocephaly, frontal bossing, and a square jaw. Premature fusion of the cranial sutures occurred in 70% of the patients evaluated. Increased bone density is typical and asymptomatic, with no increase in fracture rate.

HISTOPATHOLOGY

LIGHT. Hairs appear normal.
EM. No information.

BASIC DEFECT

Unknown.

TREATMENT

Agressive dental care. There is no information regarding the effectiveness of newer techniques such as sealants to prevent decay.

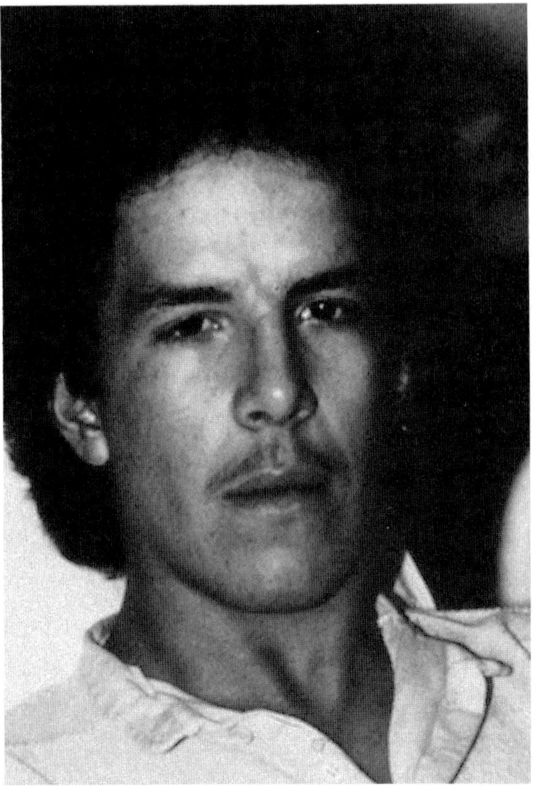
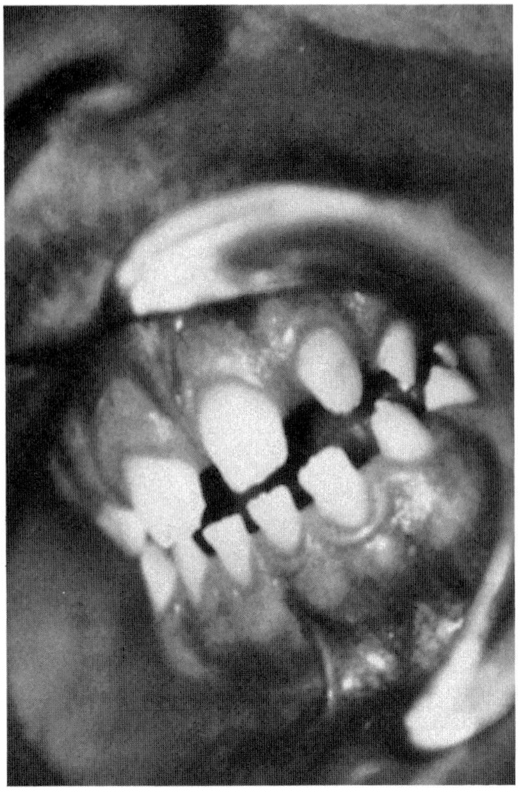

A B

Figure 3.28. **(A)** Frizzy hair. **(B)** Abnormally shaped teeth with pitting. (From Quattromani et al., 1983.)

MODE OF INHERITANCE

Autosomal dominant with male-to-male transmission. Although, genetic heterogeneity has been proposed, functional counseling differences are nil. All types have autosomal dominant inheritance and variable hair, nail, and skeletal findings, with abnormal teeth as a constant finding.

PRENATAL DIAGNOSIS

None.

DIFFERENTIAL DIAGNOSIS

Tooth and nail syndrome (Witkop syndrome, MIM:189500) lacks the hair changes. CHANDS (MIM:214350) shares curly hair and nail changes in common. Teeth are normal in CHANDS; ankyloblepharon filiforme adnatum are typical. Curly hair can be seen in Noonan syndrome (MIM:163950), the cardiofacial cutaneous syndrome (MIM:115150), and woolly hair (MIM:194300), all of which are easily distinguished by absence of tooth findings and presence of other abnormalities. Autosomal dominant trichodental syndrome (MIM:None) is marked by fine short hair with a short anagen phase and hypodontia with peg-shaped teeth. The nails are normal.

Support Group: N.F.E.D.
219 East Main, Box 114
Mascoutah, IL 62258-0114
1-618-566-2020

SELECTED BIBLIOGRAPHY

Lichtenstein, J., Warson, R., Jorgenson, R., Dorst, J.P., and McKusick, V.A. (1972). The Tricho-dento-osseous (TDO) syndrome. *Am. J. Hum. Genet.* **24,** 569–582.

An extensive pedigree from Virginia. The authors were able to fully evaluate 10 affected family members. One of 107 affected individuals had bilateral sensorineural deafness, which is probably unrelated.

Melnick, M., Shields, E.D., and El-Kafrawy, A.H. (1977). Tricho-dento-osseous syndrome: a scanning electron microscopic analysis. *Clin. Genet.* **12,** 17–27.

Thin tooth enamel with pits and depressions, with a mineral content similar to dentin, was found. The authors demonstrated an abnormal collagenous membrane around the apices of the teeth.

Robinson, G.C., Miller, J.R., and Worth, H.M. (1966). Hereditary enamel hypoplasia: its association with characteristic hair structure. *Pediatrics* **37,** 498–502.

A four generation family from British Columbia. Hair appeared normal but tightly curled. If teeth were not abnormal, the hair would probably not have been brought to medical attention. The nails in some were friable and peeling; they were thickened in other affected members.

Quattromani, F., Shapiro, S.D., Young, R.S., Jorgenson, R.J., Parker, J.W., Blumhardt, R., and Reece, R.R. (1983). Clinical heterogeneity in the tricho-dento-osseous syndrome. *Hum. Genet.* **64,** 116–121.

Shapiro, S.D., Quattromani, F.L., Jorgenson, R.J., and Young, R.S. (1983). Tricho-dento-osseous syndrome: heterogeneity or clinical variability. *Am. J. Med. Genet.* **16,** 225–236.

Perhaps duplicate publication of this family was warranted because Quattromani et al. (1983) and Shapiro et al. (1983), could not agree. The Quattromani et al. paper supports genetic unity with clinical heterogeneity; the Shapiro et al. paper favors genetic heterogeneity. In the latter publication, Figure 6 is upside down, but it is correctly oriented in Figure 3b of the Quattromani et al. publication.

In arguing for heterogeneity, Shapiro et al. credit Lichtenstein et al. (1972) with evaluation of 107 patients radiologically. In fact, only 10 affected individuals were so examined.

TRICHO-RHINO-PHALANGEAL SYNDROME (MIM:150230, 190350, 275500)

(Langer-Gideon [Type II]; TRPS-I; TRPS-II)

Includes Type I and Type II

DERMATOLOGIC FEATURES

MAJOR. Scanty, slow-growing, fragile scalp hairs are typical of tricho-rhino-phalangeal syndrome (TRPS-I) and Langer-Gideon syndrome (TRPS-II). There is often a very high frontal hairline with bitemporal regression. Early balding may occur in both males and females.

The eyebrows may be thickened medially and thin and absent laterally in tricho-rhino-phalangeal syndrome type I. This is referred to as *signe de sourcil,* which means "sign of the eyebrow" (a term, perhaps, of limited descriptive utility). In contrast, the eyebrows may be generous in Langer-Gideon syndrome. Eyelashes and secondary sexual hairs may also be scanty.

MINOR. Nails may be thin and slow-growing in both conditions.

Redundant hyperelastic skin has been described in a number of patients with Langer-Gideon syndrome.

ASSOCIATED ABNORMALITIES

Neurologic: Mental retardation and microcephaly are hallmarks of Langer-Gideon syndrome, although Langer et al. (1984) suggest that this is not invariable.

Facies: The facial features in both tricho-rhino-phalangeal syndrome type I and Langer-Gideon syndrome are characterized by a prominent bulbous "pear-shaped" nasal tip and a very long philtrum.

Orthopedic: Multiple exostoses are a primary and distinguishing feature of Langer-Gideon syndrome and make their appearance in early childhood. Cone-shaped epiphyses in the hands and feet, most often involving the middle phalanges, result in dystrophic changes to the fingers and toes. The specific pattern of involvement is referred to as "type 12 coned epiphyses." Abnormal patellae with recurrent dislocation and abnormal femoral heads and necks are shared by both types of tricho-rhino-phalangeal syndrome, as is degenerative joint disease in adulthood and mild to moderate short stature. Avascular necrosis of the hip is a common complication, and bone age is often retarded.

Frequent respiratory infections have been alluded to in descriptions of patients with Langer-Gideon syndrome, but may be secondary to aspiration due to hypotonia and neurologic dysfunction rather than reflecting an underlying immune defect.

HISTOPATHOLOGY

LIGHT. Hair diameters are thinner than normal. The ratio of telogen to anagen hairs is normal. The dermal papillae surrounding the hairs are hypoplastic; the hair matrix is normal. These findings were described in one patient.

EM. The hair cuticle was normal in one patient; in another, irregular spacing between cuticular cells with ragged, broken cuticular margins and exposure of the cortex were demonstrated. Both patients had thin hair shaft diameter.

BASIC DEFECT

Deletions of 8q24.12 have been found in several patients with tricho-rhino-phalangeal syndrome type I; most are normal cytogenetically. Linkage to COL2A1 has been excluded in tricho-rhino-phalangeal syndrome type I.

In Langer-Gideon syndrome, deletions of the long arm of 8 (8q22–8q24), with a critical region of 8q24.1, have been implicated. Involvement of 8q24.13 seems to ensure mental retardation and exostoses.

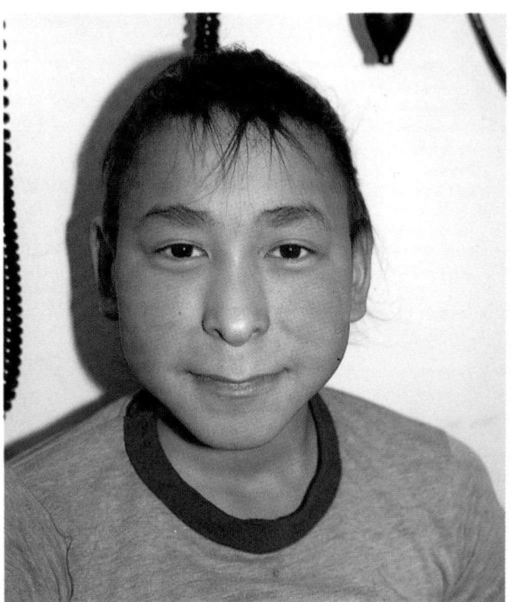

A

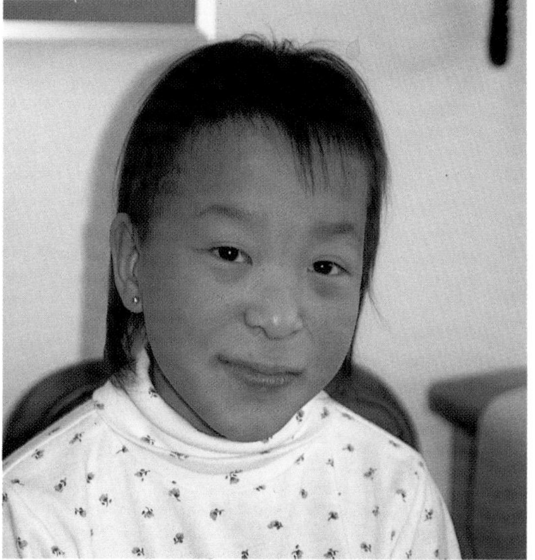

B

Figure 3.29. Sparse hair and typical "pear-shaped" nose. **(A)** Alaskan native. **(B)** Japanese.

A 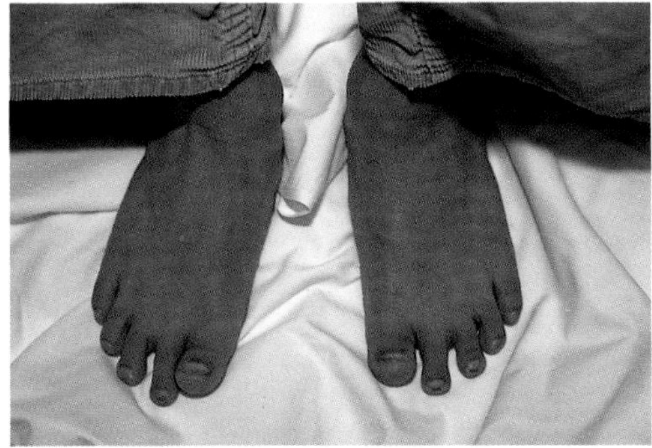

B 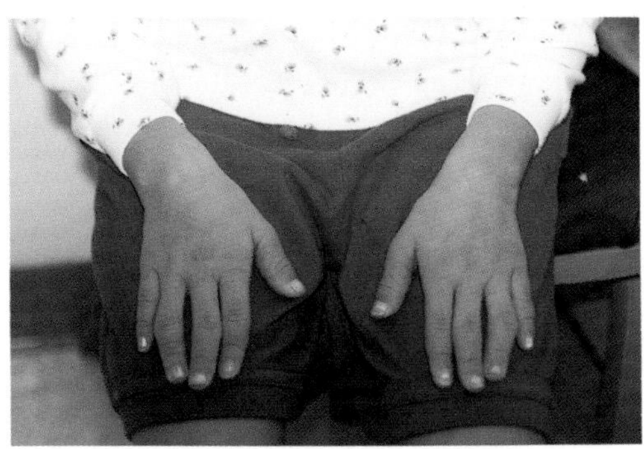

Figure 3.30. Feet **(A)** and hands **(B)** of patient in 3.29B.

TREATMENT

Orthopedic management of progressive hip and knee degenerative arthritis is often required in adult life in tricho-rhino-phalangeal syndrome type I.

MODE OF INHERITANCE

Tricho-rhino-phalangeal syndrome type I: autosomal dominant. There have been a few reports of affected siblings with normal parents and/or consanguinity among parents, raising the possibility of an autosomal recessive genocopy.

Langer-Gideon syndrome: appears to be chromosomal. Most cases have been sporadic.

PRENATAL DIAGNOSIS

There is potential only for the prenatal detection of chromosomal deletions derived from parental translocations.

DIFFERENTIAL DIAGNOSIS

Misdiagnoses of Larsen syndrome (MIM: 150250, 245600) because of joint laxity and Ehlers-Danlos type I syndrome (MIM:130000) due to hyperelastic redundant skin have been made in the medical literature. The associated facies and hair abnormalities of the tricho-rhino-phalangeal syndromes should differentiate them readily, although correct diagnosis in the newborn period may remain problematic.

Much has been written about the variability of tricho-rhino-phalangeal syndrome, but in my reading of the case reports it seems that a great deal of the heterogeneity has been introduced by labeling as "tricho-rhino-phalangeal syndrome" families with unique disorders that share some features in common, but are actually different entities. This appears to reflect the investigators' biases regarding pathognomonic features, e.g., one family is included because of nasal configuration, despite normal epiphyses; another is excluded when the nasal configuration is different, although type 12 coning of the epiphyses is present.

Support Group: Little People of America, Inc. (LPA)
P.O. Box 9897
Washington, D.C. 20016
1-800-243-9273

SELECTED BIBLIOGRAPHY

Buhler, E.M., Buhler, U.K., Beutler, C., and Fessler, R. (1987). A final word on the tricho-rhino-phalangeal syndrome. *Clin. Genet.* **31,** 273–275.

These authors argue that TRPS-I and TRPS-II are not separate entities but reflect a contiguous gene syndrome. I find this an unpalatable way to conceptualize genetic diseases. While it appears true that TRPS-II results from a chromosomal deletion involving several (more than one) genes, it is entirely possible that TRPS-I results from a single gene mutation or deletion. Certainly many families with clear-cut autosomal dominant inheritance of TRPS-I exist, and most patients are cytogenetically normal. This is not to say that they might not also be chromosomally deleted at a submicroscopic level, but the implications for both prognosis and recurrence are significantly different for a diagnosis of TRPS-I versus a diagnosis of TRPS-II. The authors' reasoning seems analogous to claiming that a male with hemophilia A and chronic granulomatous disease has the same disease as a male with chronic granulomatous disease alone because a chromosomal deletion can result in either, depending on its size. Overlap, clinically and/or cytogenetically, does not confer identity. The patient in this report underscored again the difficulty of making a firm clinical diagnosis. The patient lacked the eyebrow sign and had entirely normal hair.

Cope, R., Beals, R.K., and Bennett, R.M. (1986). The tricho-rhino-phalangeal dysplasia syndrome: report of eight kindreds, with emphasis on hip complications, late presentations, and premature osteoarthritis. *J. Pediatr. Orthop.* **6,** 133–138.

This is a good review of orthopedic complications.

Goldblatt, J, and Smart, R.D. (1986). Tricho-rhino-phalangeal syndrome without exostoses, with an interstitial deletion of 8q23. *Clin. Genet.* **29,** 434–438.

This patient with a microdeletion is described as having TRPS-II without exostoses, but the clinical photograph does not show the typical facies of tricho-rhino-phalangeal syndrome. The patient has a normal philtrum and a broad, fleshy nasal tip with well-defined broad alae nasi and shortening of the distal phalanges without involvement of the middle phalanges or metacarpals.

Langer, L.O., Jr., Krassikof, N., Laxova, R., Scheer-Williams, M., Lutter, L.D., Gorlin, R.J., Jennings, C.G., and Day, D.W. (1984). The tricho-rhino-phalangeal syndrome with exostoses (or Langer-Gideon syndrome): four additional patients without mental retardation, and review of the literature. *Am. J. Med. Genet.* **19,** 81–111.

This is an excruciatingly detailed analysis of the literature with five new cases of TRPS-II, which the authors chose to call TRPSE (E = exostoses). They argue for a wider range of intellectual function in TRPS-II, with 29% of patients functioning in the normal to dull–normal range; the remainder are mildly to severely retarded. Three of their five case reports, however, had significant cognitive dysfunction, despite borderline or normal IQ. A fourth patient was frankly retarded, and only one appeared to be entirely within normal limits. This paper is a good source for reported frequency of specific findings in TRPS-II.

Naritomi, K., and Hiroyama, K. (1989). Partial trisomy of distal 8q derived from mother with mosaic 8q23.3–24.13 deletion, and relatively mild expression of tricho-rhino-phalangeal I. *Hum. Genet.* **82,** 199–201.

The authors describe the mother to have a typical TRPS-I face, but the photograph does not demonstrate abnormal eyebrows or a bulbous nasal tip. Her skeletal findings included short stature, short fourth and fifth metacarpals, but no coning of the epiphyses or middle phalangeal involvement. The daughter had normal radiographs at age 17 months, a short upturned nose, and normal hair. I am not convinced that the diagnosis of TRPS-I is justified, and it may have been inspired by the cytogenetic findings rather than the clinical features.

Prens, E.P., Peereboom-Wynia, J.D.R., De-Bruyn, W.C., van Joost, T.H., and Stolz, E. (1984). Clinical and scanning electron microscopic findings in a solitary case of tricho-rhino-phalangeal syndrome type I. *Acta Dermatol. Venereol.* **64,** 249–253.

Van Neste, D., and Dumortier, M. (1982). Tricho-rhino-phalangeal syndrome. Disturbed geometric relationships between hair matrix and dermal papillae in scalp hair bulbs. *Dermatologica* **165,** 16–23.

Evaluation of hairs and scalp biopsy from a 13-year-old girl (Van Neste) and hairs from a 21-year-old female (Prens) with TRPS-I.

TRICHOTHIODYSTROPHY (MIM:SEE BELOW)

(Synonyms: See Below)

DERMATOLOGIC FEATURES

Major. This is a heterogeneous group of disorders, and several attempts have been made to classify them based on associated features.

The unifying clinical finding in the trichothiodystrophies is brittle, fragile, poorly growing hair, which shows a pattern of bright and dark bands on polarization. The scalp hairs, eyebrows, and eyelashes are invariably involved. Body, axillary, and pubic hairs can also be affected.

The nails are usually abnormal. They may be friable and thinned and demonstrate longitudinal ridging, horizontal splitting, and koilonychia. Conversely, they may be thickened distally and yellowed.

Ichthyosis, clinically similar to lamellar ichthyosis, with erythroderma and scaling without blistering, is a major feature distinguishing several subsets of trichothiodystrophy. Some newborns presented as collodion babies.

Minor. Eczema has been noted in some case reports. It does not appear to be a specific finding to any subgroup.

In patients with photosensitivity (PIBIDS), unusual freckling and cutaneous malignancies have not been described. This is in contrast to xeroderma pigmentosum D, with which PIBIDS shares the same defect in DNA repair.

ASSOCIATED ABNORMALITIES

As stated above, it is the associated abnormalities that have allowed for potential classification of trichothiodystrophy. Below is my approach, which varies somewhat from that of others. I do not think eponyms should be used as distinct diagnostic entities, as overlap clearly occurs. Rather, the classification system should be viewed as a way to categorize individuals reasonably for prognosis pending identification of specific mutations.

All types share in common the hair findings.

Type A: hair, with or without nails.

Type B (Sabinas syndrome, MIM:211390): hair, with or without nails, with mental retardation.

Type C (Pollitt syndrome, MIM:275550): hair, with or without nails; with mental retardation, folliculitis, and retarded bone age; with or without caries.

Type D (BIDS: brittle hair with infertility, developmental delay, short stature; hair–brain syndrome, MIM:234050): hair; with or without nails; with mental retardation and short stature; with or without decreased gonadal function.

Type E (IBIDS: ichthyosis with BIDS, Tay syndrome, MIM:242170): hair; with or without nails; with mental retardation and short stature; with or without decreased gonadal function, lenticular opacities/cataracts, and failure to thrive/"progeria" with loss of subcutaneous tissue; with microcephaly; with or without ataxia and calcification of the basal ganglia; with erythroderma and scale. These patients may present as collodion babies.

Type F (PIBIDS: photosensitivity with IBIDS, MIM:278720): All of the features of type E, plus photosensitivity.

Type G (trichothiodystrophy with immune defects, MIM:258360): hair; with or without mental retardation; with chronic neutropenia or immunoglobulin deficiency. The immune defects are usually mild; one patient had transient combined immunodeficiency. The hairs in two of these patients showed trichorrhexis nodosa, and birefringence was not mentioned; one of these patients was intellectually normal.

Although in most discussion sections of many papers on trichothiodystrophy dental caries are commonly noted, they were actually mentioned in only a few cases of various types of trichothiodystrophy. The caries may be a finding more likely associated with mental retardation and poor dental hygiene than a primary feature of the disorders.

HISTOPATHOLOGY

LIGHT. The hairs show a distinctive pattern of light and dark bands under polarizing light. There may be twisting of the hair shaft, and trichorrhexis nodosa-like nodes are found. A skin biopsy from one patient with BIDS showed a decrease in the granular layer and hyperkeratosis.

EM. On scanning electron microscopy of the hair there were abnormal and/or incomplete cuticle formation with irregular twisting and trichoschisis (transverse fracturing of the hairs). Transmission electron microscopy demon-

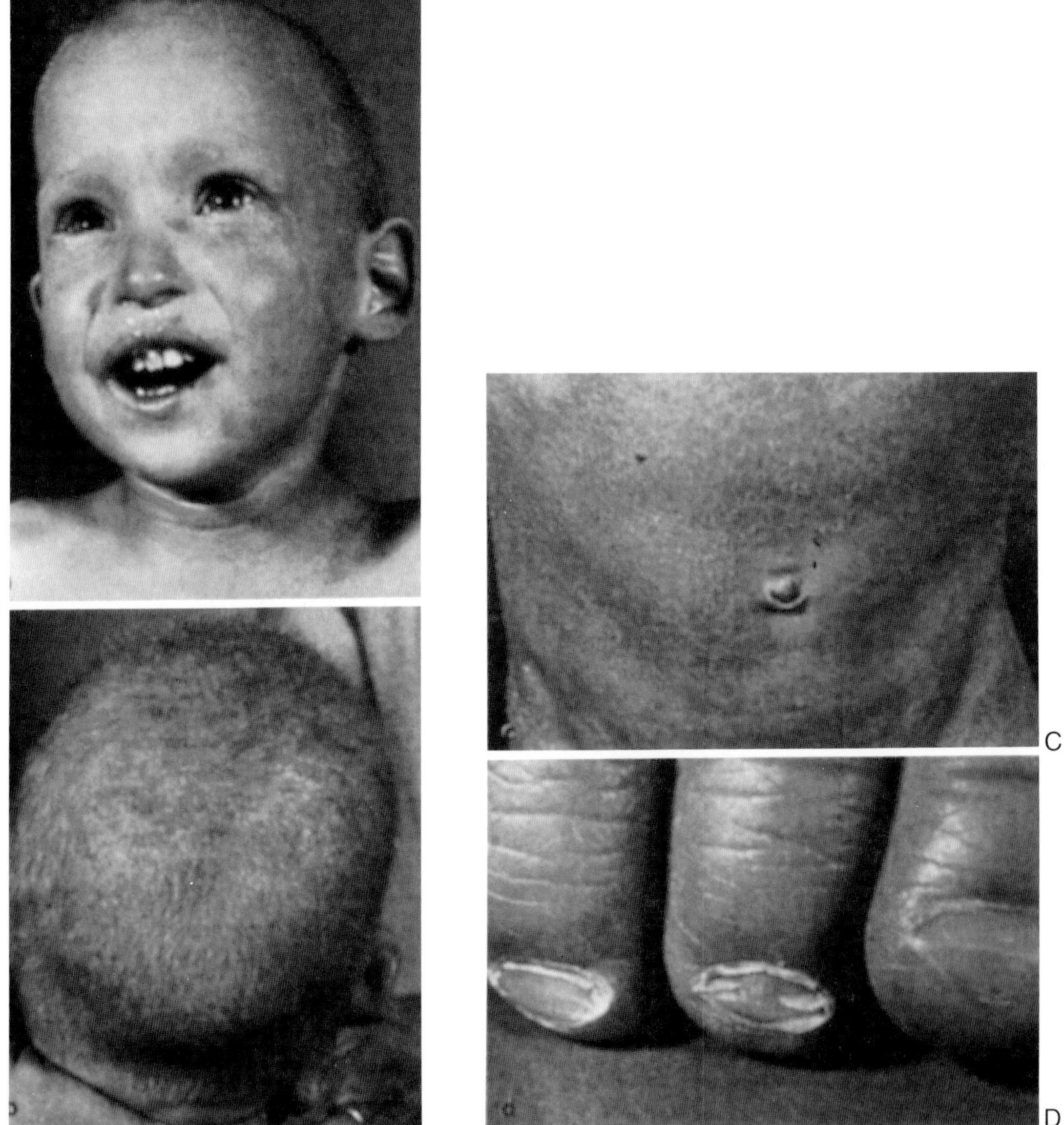

Figure 3.31. (A–D) Sparse broken hair, scaling on trunk, and splitting of nail plates. (From Happle et al., 1984.)

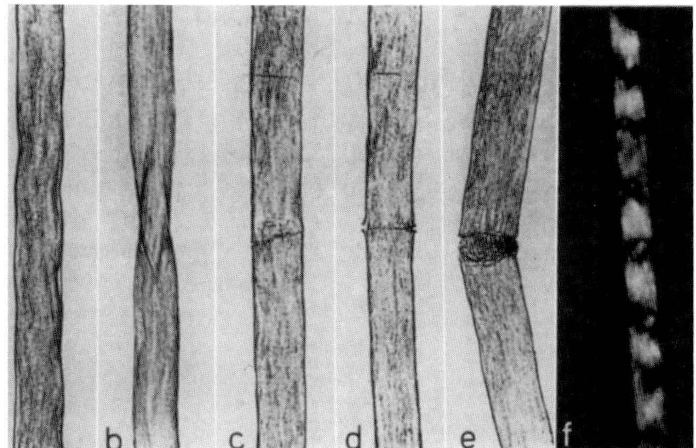

Figure 3.32. **(A–E)** Structural alterations in hair shafts with folding and trichoschisis. **(F)** Alternating dark and light bands under polarizing light. (From Happle et al., 1984.)

strated abnormal whorled and irregular arrangement of microfibrils. Membrane-bound vacuoles filled with granular filamentous material were found in the cytoplasm of the epidermal keratinocytes in one patient with follicular hyperkeratosis and trichothiodystrophy.

BASIC DEFECT

The hairs from all types of trichothiodystrophy show a decrease in cystine to 10%–50% of normal. This reflects a decrease to absence of ultra high sulfur proteins, which are major components of the hair cuticle. The defective cuticle results in a hair that is more readily weathered and develops trichorrhexis nodosa and fractures. The nails also show this deficiency in high sulfur proteins. The assumption is that all forms of trichothiodystrophy result from alterations in the biochemical pathway involved in making these proteins, but a specific defect has not been found.

Cells from patients with PIBIDS do show a defect in excision repair of ultraviolet light–induced DNA damage, which is the same defect as that of xeroderma pigmentosum complementation group D.

The heterogeneity of the trichothiodystrophies makes biochemical characterization difficult. Any series of patients may include different allelic and nonallelic mutations, and attempts to confirm findings in one patient may be foiled by analysis of a second who may not have the same disorder.

TREATMENT

Photoprotection in PIBIDS. There is no other specific treatment for the conditions. Appropriate emollient therapy for those patients with ichthyosis may be helpful.

MODE OF INHERITANCE

Autosomal recessive.

PRENATAL DIAGNOSIS

The PIBIDS syndrome has been diagnosed prenatally in several pregnancies at risk by measurement of repair to ultraviolet light–induced DNA damage in chorionic villus cells, cultured amniocytes, or fetal skin biopsy tissue. With identification of mutations in *ERCC2,* molecular diagnosis may be possible in some families.

DIFFERENTIAL DIAGNOSIS

The trichothiodystrophies can be differentiated from other simple hypotrichoses on the basis of the hair findings. The hairs in Netherton syndrome (MIM:256500) show trichorrhexis invaginata, not the dark and light bands of trichothiodystrophy. Although the ichthyosis in both conditions can be similar, the more typical ichthyosis of Netherton is ichthyosis lineara circumflexa.

Infants with Menkes disease (MIM:309400) can appear clinically similar to trichothiodystrophies without ichthyosis. Microscopic analysis of hairs will show the typical pili torti in infants with Menkes disease. It is reasonable to measure copper and ceruloplasmin levels in patients with suspected trichothiodystrophy to rule out Menkes disease.

The ichthyosis of trichothiodystrophy is similar to that of the Sjögren-Larsson syndrome (MIM:270200), as are the ataxia and short stature. Patients with Sjögren-Larsson syndrome have normal hair and nails, and about one-half of the patients will show glistening dots in the retina. The defect in FAO activity in Sjögren-Larsson syndrome differentiates between the two conditions biochemically.

Individuals with xeroderma pigmentosa D (MIM:278730) share in common with PIBIDS only photosensitivity; they show no other cutaneous features of PIBIDS. They have early malignant skin changes in contrast to PIBIDS. McKusick includes PIBIDS under the xeroderma pigmentosum group D entry.

I do not know if hairs from a person affected with these other conditions have been analyzed for cystine, so I cannot conclude that biochemical analysis of hair will differentiate trichothiodystrophy from all other conditions. Light and scanning electron microscopic findings do appear to be specific and thus are useful to discriminate among all these disorders.

Support Group: N.O.R.D.
P.O. Box 8923
New Fairfield, CT 06812
1-800-999-6673

SELECTED BIBLIOGRAPHY

Broughton, B.C., Steingrimsdottir, H., Weber, C.A., and Lehmann, A.R. (1994). Mutations in the xeroderma pigmentosum group D DNA repair/transcription gene in patients with trichothiodystrophy. *Nat. Genet.* **7,** 189–193.

Identified mutations in xeroderma pigmentosum group D (*ERCC2*). Four patients with trichothiodystrophy (all from cell lines, no clinical information given) are described; all were compound heterozygotes. Hypothesize how hair abnormalities might occur, based on mutations, but cannot explain lack of malignant skin changes.

Gillespie, J.M., Marshall, R.C., and Rogers, M. (1988). Trichothiodystrophy—biochemical and clinical studies. *Australas. J. Dermatol.* **29,** 85–93.

Analysis of hairs from three unrelated individuals with trichothiodystrophy. All showed typical structural alterations; each showed decrease in high sulfur and absence of ultra high sulfur compounds, but differed from each other in electrophoretic pattern of the high sulfur proteins, supporting the concept of heterogeneity within trichothiodystrophy.

Itin, P.H. and Pittelkow, M.R. (1990). Trichothiodystrophy: review of sulfur-deficient brittle hair syndromes and association with the ectodermal dysplasias. *J. Am. Acad. Dermatol.* **22,** 705–717.

Complete review of trichothiodystrophy. Table of features is all-inclusive from literature reports. Eighty-eight references.

Price, V.H., Odom, R.B., Ward, W.H., and Jones, F.T. (1980). Trichothiodystrophy. Sulfur-deficient brittle hair as a marker for a neuroectodermal symptom complex. *Arch. Dermatol.* **116,** 1375–1384.

Very lucid description of the theoretical basis for the hair abnormalities.

Van Neste, D. (1989). Dysplasies pilaires congénitales; conduite a tenir et intérêt de diverses méthodes de diagnostic. *Ann. Dermatol. Venereol.* **116,** 251–263.

Van Neste has written extensively on hair abnormalities, mostly in French. This review of hair dystrophies includes his diagnostic framework for trichothiodystrophy and has very good photographs of a variety of hair shaft abnormalities.

Nails

While the nails are primarily involved in many ectodermal dysplasia syndromes and may show secondary changes in a multitude of other genetic conditions, there are very few inherited "pure" nail disorders.

Included in this section are those disorders traditionally identified through nail changes, including one form of ectodermal dysplasia. Conditions in which nail changes may occur, but are not major or diagnostic features, are discussed in other sections or have not been included in this volume if dermatologic findings are not major hallmarks (e.g., Turner syndrome [hyperconvex or concave nails]).

Absence and hypoplasia of the nails usually reflect alterations in the underlying phalanges, as does fusion of the nail plate. The anonychia described in association with aplasia cutis congenita, Coffin-Siris, ectrodactyly, and a host of skeletal dysplasias reflects the underlying bony alterations rather than being primary. The term *racquet nails* describes the short broad nail associated with the short distal phalanx of the thumb in brachydactyly D and is not a distinct entity of nail dystrophy alone. Fused or bifid nails overlie fused or bifid terminal phalanges.

Chromosomal disorders may also demonstrate alterations in nail development. Teratogens such as hydantoin and phenobarbital may also cause nail hypoplasia. Loss of nails is common in the epidermolysis bullosa syndromes; thickening is typical of palmoplantar keratodermas. It is rare that the nail change will be the major key to diagnosis in these conditions.

Some of the nail changes that have been claimed to be syndromic are, in fact, nonspecific and may be seen in a variety of conditions. These changes include yellow nails, which can be associated with malignancy, edema, lymphedema of any cause, nephrotic syndrome, chronic lung disease, and koilonychia, which can occur in many metabolic disturbances, result from environmental insult, and be seen in association with monilethrix. Although isolated koilonychia has also been reported with autosomal dominant inheritance, not all nails are necessarily involved. Therefore I have chosen not to include koilonychia or yellow nails as distinct inherited entities.

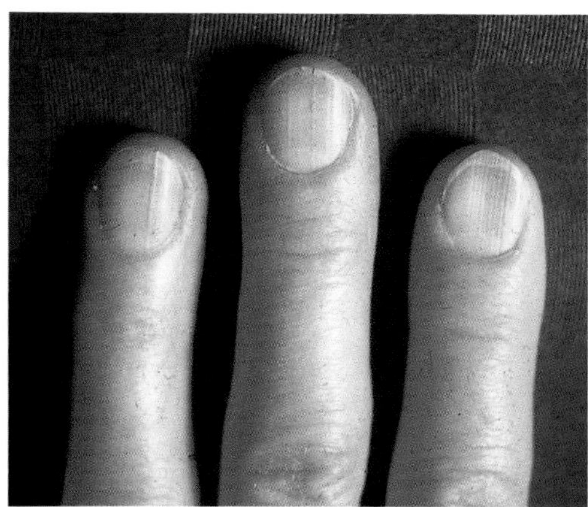

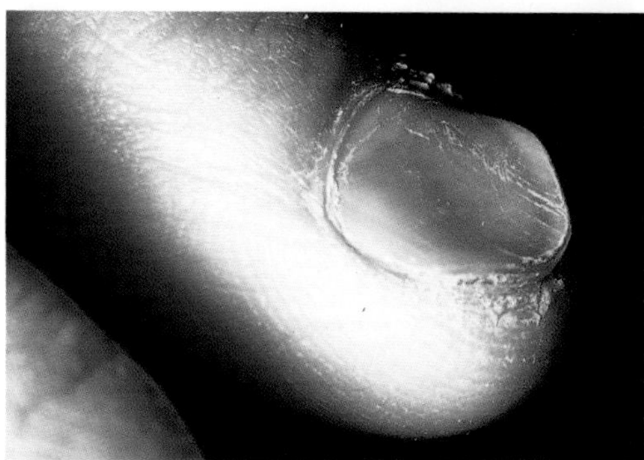

Figure 3.33. **(A)** Mild koilonychia of varying degree. **(B)** Severe spooning. (Courtesy of Division of Dermatology, University of Washington.)

Among the more intriguing, to me, of nail anomalies is the ectopic nail. Reported rarely, and never familial, these are foci of nail development in the volar or lateral aspect of the finger, separate and distinct from the normal nail plate. These are considered hamartomatous by most authors. However, we have seen one patient with bilaterally symmetric involvement, suggesting that a genetic factor rather than a stochastic developmental abnormality might be involved.

NAIL DISORDERS, ISOLATED

CONGENITAL MALALIGNMENT OF THE GREAT TOENAILS (MIM: None)

DERMATOLOGIC FEATURES

MAJOR. There is lateral deviation of one or both great toenails present at birth. This results in recurrent paronychia secondary to ingrown toenails. Both medial and lateral deviation have been reported. Onychogryphosis of the involved nails has also been described.
MINOR. None.

ASSOCIATED ABNORMALITIES

None.

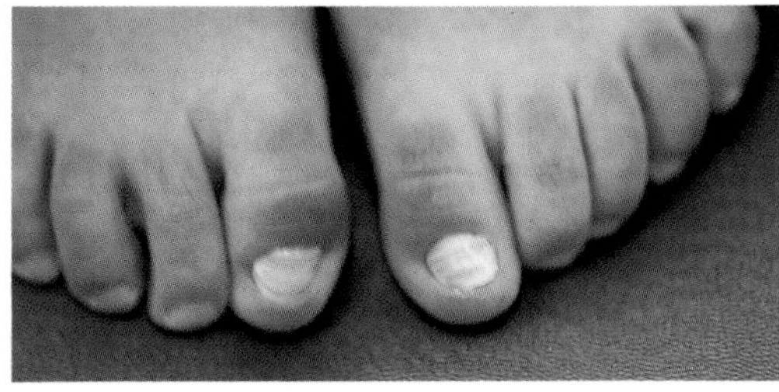

Figure 3.34. Deviated great toenails; lamellated appearance to plate.

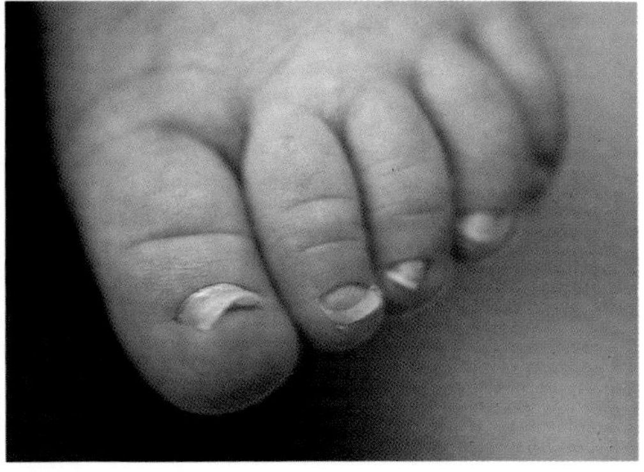

Figure 3.35. Thickening of nail plate; third nail is also deviated.

HISTOPATHOLOGY

LIGHT. No information.
EM. No information.

BASIC DEFECT

Unknown.

TREATMENT

Spontaneous resolution may occur. If repeated paronychia become unmanageable, removal of the nail plate and ablation of the nail matrix is the only effective treatment.

MODE OF INHERITANCE

Autosomal dominant. Most cases have been sporadic.

PRENATAL DIAGNOSIS

Not applicable.

DIFFERENTIAL DIAGNOSIS

A mistaken diagnosis of onychomycosis is readily avoided by a careful history.

Support Group: Not applicable.

SELECTED BIBLIOGRAPHY

Baran, R., and Bureau, H. (1983). Congenital malalignment of the big toenail as a cause of ingrowing toenail in infancy. Pathology and treatment (a study of thirty cases). *Clin. Exp. Dermatol.* **8,** 619–623.

This series includes monozygous twins, one with one toenail affected, the other with both toenails involved.

Dawson, T.A.J. (1979). An inherited nail dystrophy principally affecting the great toenails. *Clin. Exp. Dermatol.* **4,** 309–313

Dawson, T.A.J. (1982). An inherited nail dystrophy principally affecting the great toenails: further observations: Letter to the Editor. *Clin. Exp. Dermatol.* **7,** 455–456.

A three-generation family with male-to-male transmission is described. Although the great toenails were most severely involved, others were too. Subungual debris and green-yellow color changes were also present. Bacterial and fungal cultures were not reported, so onychomycosis or pseudomonas infection could not be excluded. Fungal infections of the toenails are uncommon in children; in my experience, when a child presents with onychomycosis, invariably one or both parents are also affected. Five years after his initial presentation, Dawson reported almost complete resolution in one family member who had been treated with topical tetracycline and nystatin. Nonetheless, he does not suggest in his article that infection played a role in the nail changes.

Harper, K.J., and Beer, W.E. (1986). Congenital malalignment of the great toenails—an inherited condition. *Clin. Exp. Dermatol.* **11,** 514–516.

Affected identical twin girls of a set of triplets; the third child was an unaffected boy.

FAMILIAL DYSTROPHIC SHEDDING OF THE NAILS (MIM: None)

DERMATOLOGIC FEATURES

Major. Loss of nails begins in childhood. The toenails appear to be more involved than the fingernails. After shedding, which is usually painless, regrowth may be normal or a dystrophic nail plate may grow in. Loss can be permanent. As one nail regrows, the neighbor may loosen and be shed.

In reports of nail shedding without epidermolysis bullosa, shedding preceded development of nail dystrophy. In the reports of nail

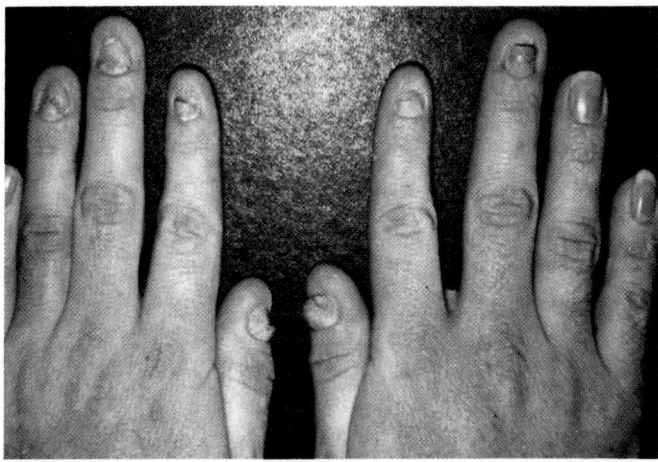

Figure 3.36. Nails in various stages of involvement; the fourth and fifth on the right and the fifth on the left are currently well formed, although hyperpigmented. (From Martin and Rudolph, 1980.)

shedding associated with epidermolysis bullosa, dystrophy of the nails preceded shedding.
MINOR. None.

ASSOCIATED ABNORMALITIES

None.

HISTOPATHOLOGY

LIGHT. In one patient, biopsy tissues of the nail matrix and the nail were normal.
EM. No information.

BASIC DEFECT

Unknown.

TREATMENT

None.

MODE OF INHERITANCE

Autosomal dominant.

PRENATAL DIAGNOSIS

None.

DIFFERENTIAL DIAGNOSIS

Nails can be lost in all forms of epidermolysis bullosa (MIM:Many), recurrently or permanently. A history of cutaneous blistering differentiates these diseases from isolated periodic nail shedding. Shedding of the nail plate can occur after trauma or after severe illness. Appropriate historical information should be sought.

One family has been described in whom progressive dystrophy and periodic shedding of only the great toenails began after puberty. Multiple epidermal inclusion cysts appear to be segregating as a second, unrelated autosomal dominant condition in the same family.

Support Group: N.O.R.D.
P.O. Box 8923
New Fairfield, CT 06812
1-800-999-6673

SELECTED BIBLIOGRAPHY

Main, R.A. (1973). Periodic shedding of the nails. *Br. J. Dermatol.* **88,** 497–498.

Report of a family with epidermolysis bullosa in which the proband had only shedding of the nails. Other family members with mild blistering of the hands and feet had also lost nails.

Martin, S., and Rudolph A.H. (1980). Familial dystrophic periodic shedding of the nails. *Cutis* **25,** 622–625.

Case report of a multigenerational family.

Oliver, W.J. (1927). Recurrent onychoptosis occurring as a family disorder. *Br. J. Dermatol.* **39,** 297.

Oliver described a healthy 12-year-old boy with recurrent periodic shedding of the nails whose mother shed her nails in a similar manner, losing one or two nails every 7–8 months. Two maternal uncles were also reported to be affected. The nail that was involved at the time that Oliver saw the patient showed blackening with a broad white transverse line at the base. This is suggestive of loss due to trauma, but does not explain the positive family history.

Samman, P.D., and Fenton, D.A. (1986). *The Nails in Disease.* William Heinemann Medical Books, London, 4th ed., pp. 183–184.

Periodic shedding of the nails must be exceedingly rare. In the 27 years spanned by the first and fourth editions of this excellent book, no new case reports or further details have been added to the original description of the disorder.

LEUKONYCHIA (MIM:151600)

(White Nails; Albugo)

DERMATOLOGIC FEATURES

MAJOR. The white color of the nails may be stippled (leukonychia punctata), streaky (leukonychia striata) or complete (leukonychia totalis). In at least one report, a mother with leukonychia totalis had two daughters with only the distal portion of the nail plate involved (leukonychia partialis).
MINOR. None.

ASSOCIATED ABNORMALITIES

Deafness has been reported in several syndromes in association with partial or total leukonychia.

Duodenal ulcer disease and gallstones were reported in two pedigrees with leukonychia. Some individuals had either one or the other manifestation. It could not be proved that the two features were segregating independently.

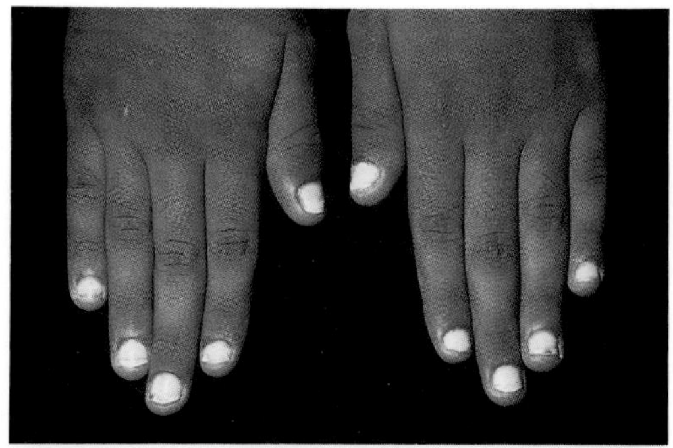

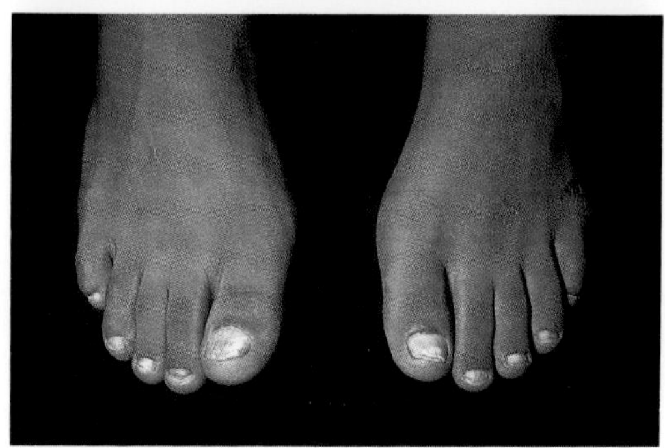

Figure 3.37. **(A)** Fingernails. **(B)** Toenails with congenital leukonychia totalis.

HISTOPATHOLOGY

LIGHT. An abnormal band in the middle of the nail plate comprised of larger than normal cells with large nuclei was described in a case of congenital leukonychia striata. A stratum granulosum with keratohyaline granules was seen in some areas overlying the stripe.
EM. No information.

BASIC DEFECT

Unknown.

TREATMENT

None.

MODE OF INHERITANCE

Autosomal dominant.

PRENATAL DIAGNOSIS

None.

DIFFERENTIAL DIAGNOSIS

Leukonychia, sebaceous cysts, and renal calculi (MIM:151600): Involved nails may show koilonychia in addition to the color change. Epidermal inclusion cysts are typical and widespread. The chemical composition of the renal calculi is not stated. Inheritance is autosomal dominant. McKusick does not differentiate this condition from isolated leukonychia.

Leukonychia, palmoplantar hyperkeratosis, knuckle pads, and deafness (MIM:149200): Can be distinguished from leukonychia alone by the presence of the associated abnormalities. I think it is appropriate to exclude hearing abnormalities in any individual with total leukonychia.

Enamel hypoplasia, progressive sensorineural hearing loss, and punctuate leukonychia (MIM:234580): Reported in a brother and sister pair. Only the secondary teeth were affected with hypoplasia of the enamel. Hearing was normal in the first year of life.

Trauma is by far the most common cause of Beau's lines and white spots in the nails. Leukonychia secondary to trauma can be excluded both by history and by nicking the nail and following the white lines and dots as the nail grows out. McKusick reports that he has seen one family with autosomal dominant inheritance of white spots, which he has termed *leukonychia maculata* (MIM:151550).

Acquired leukonychia has been associated with a host of *infectious diseases* and with *occupational exposures*.

Support Group: N.O.R.D.
P.O. Box 8923
New Fairfield, CT
06812
1-800-999-6673

SELECTED BIBLIOGRAPHY

Albright, S.D., III, and Wheeler, C.E. (1964). Leukonychia. Total and partial leukonychia in a single family with a review of the literature. *Arch. Dermatol.* **90,** 392–399.

A mother with total involvement and two daughters with proximal leukonychia. A very nice review of the known associations with leukonychia.

Bart, R.S., and Pumphrey, R.E. (1967). Knuckle pads, leukonychia and deafness—a dominantly inherited syndrome. *N. Engl. J. Med.* **276,** 202–207.

In this pedigree, hearing loss detected in infancy or early childhood was progressive, and the degree of loss was variable. Knuckle pads, when present, appeared in the first few years of life. Leukonychia was found in all examined affected members and had not been remarked upon by the family members but was pointed out to them by the authors.

Kruse, W.T., Cawley, E.P., and Cotterman, C.W. (1951). Hereditary leukonychia totalis. *J. Invest. Dermatol.* **17,** 135–140.

The authors state that in Bavaria white spots in the nails indicate the number of years to live. This is a very well written report of a family with a review of the literature.

Medansky, R.S., and Fox, J.M. (1960). Hereditary leukonychia totalis. *Arch. Dermatol.* **82,** 412–414.

Fourteen affected members in a five generation family with male-to-male transmission are reported.

TWENTY NAIL DYSTROPHY (MIM:161050)

(Onychodystrophy Totalis)

DERMATOLOGIC FEATURES

MAJOR. Flattening, thinning, pitting, and longitudinal striations of the nail plate may be seen at birth and worsen with age. There are no other skin findings, and health is unaffected.

MINOR. None.

ASSOCIATED ABNORMALITIES

None.

HISTOPATHOLOGY

LIGHT. Thickening and acanthosis of the nail bed with a mild mononuclear infiltrate at the

A
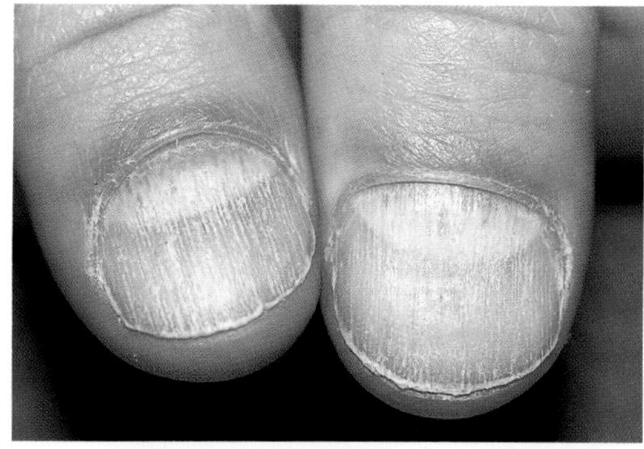

B
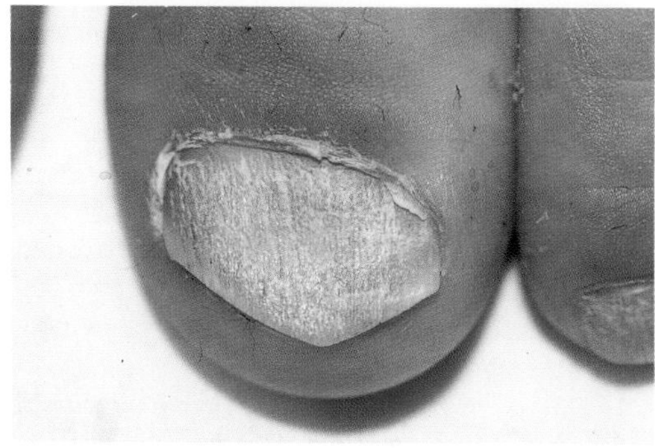

Figure 3.38. **(A)** Thumbnails. **(B)** Toenail.

dermis was reported in one patient. No features were thought to be remarkably abnormal.
EM. No information.

BASIC DEFECT

Unknown.

TREATMENT

None.

MODE OF INHERITANCE

Autosomal dominant.

PRENATAL DIAGNOSIS

None.

DIFFERENTIAL DIAGNOSIS

Twenty nail dystrophy can be a feature of lichen planus, alopecia areata, vitiligo, and psoriasis. Isolated, acquired twenty nail dystrophy in the absence of other disease has also been reported. Onset is in early to late childhood, and all twenty nails are involved. The thumb nails and great toenails may be yellowed and thickened, while other nails are thin and friable. This condition, in contrast to the inherited disorder, shows gradual improvement and resolution by adulthood.

In nail-patella syndrome (MIM:161200), although the described changes of the nails can be similar, usually not all nails are involved, and nail-patella is distinguished by its other features—iliac horns, abnormal elbows and patellae, and renal disease.

Support Group: N.O.R.D.
P.O. Box 8923
New Fairfield, CT
06812
1-800-999-6673

SELECTED BIBILIOGRAPHY

Arias, A.M., Yung, C.W., Rendler, S., Soltani, K., and Lorincz, A.L. (1982). Familial severe twenty nail dystrophy. *J. Am. Acad. Dermatol.* **7,** 349–352.

A 37-member pedigree with 21 affected individuals in five generations with male-to-male transmission. Four individuals were examined by the authors. One individual had only 18 nails involved, another had anonychia at birth with appearance of dystrophic nails at age 3.

Commens, C.A. (1988). Twenty nail dystrophy in identical twins. *Pediatr. Dermatol.* **5,** 117–119.

Identical twin sisters with classic nail changes that had been stable since birth. No clinical response to high dose vitamin A treatment or topical steroids under occlusion occurred.

Hazelrigg, D.E., Duncan, C., and Jaratt, M. (1977). Twenty nail dystrophy of childhood. *Arch. Dermatol.* **113,** 73–75.

Six case reports of children who developed twenty nail dystrophy with no other cutaneous abnormalities and no family history. In one child with onset at age 7, gradual improvement was apparent by age 12.

Pavone, L., LiVolti, S., Guaneri, B., LaRosa, M., Sorge, G., Incorpora, G., and Mollica, F. (1982). Hereditary twenty nail dystrophy in a Sicilian family. *J. Med. Genet.* **19,** 337–340.
This is a report of a three-generation family with male-to-male transmission of nail changes present at birth and worsening with age. There was no evidence for any other skin abnormalities.

NAIL DISORDERS, SYNDROMIC

NAIL-PATELLA SYNDROME (MIM:161200)

(Hereditary Onycho-Osteodysplasia [HOOD]; Turner-Keiser Syndrome; Fong Disease; Oesterricher-Turner Syndrome)

Includes COIF, Congenital Anonychia, Anonychia with Limb Defects, Anonychia with Flexural Pigmentation, Anonychia of the Thumbnails, Onychodystrophy with Deafness.

DERMATOLOGIC FEATURES

MAJOR. The nail dystrophy in nail-patella syndrome can be quite variable. Nail changes are almost always congenital but can be progressive. They are usually symmetric, with the thumbnails most consistently and most severely involved. Slight longitudinal ridging may be the mildest manifestation. Longitudinal clefting and splitting of the nail plate; abnormally shaped, triangular, or absent lunulae; and slow growth of the nail may occur. Absence of the lateral half of the thumbnails alone can be seen, as can shortening and narrowing of the thumbnails. Koilonychia has been described. Anonychia of one, several, or all fingers can occur. Severity seems to decrease from the radial to the ulnar side. Ninety-eight percent of patients have nail changes; one-third involve the thumb only, one-third involve the thumb and index finger, one-third have involvement of all of the nails. Toenails are involved in approximately one-seventh of affected individuals.

MINOR. None.

ASSOCIATED ABNORMALITIES

Bony abnormalities of the elbows with elongation and deformation of the radial neck, hypoplasia of the capitellum and lateral epicondyle of the humerus occur. Bowing of the radial shaft is also found. Subluxation of the radial head is a common occurrence, and there is limited range of motion at the elbows with sparing of flexion. More than 90% of affected individuals have changes at the elbow.

Iliac horns, which are pathognomonic and asymptomatic, arise from the external iliac fossa, are bilateral, and can be palpable. They are reported in approximately 80% of patients in the literature.

Hypoplasia to absence of the patellae with hypoplasia of the lateral femoral condyles and fibular head and dysplasia of the tibial plateau occur in 90% of patients. Patellar subluxation and dislocation are common.

Scapular changes are reported in about 40% of patients. These include thickening of the lateral border and hypoplasia of the glenoid. Madelung deformity has also been documented,

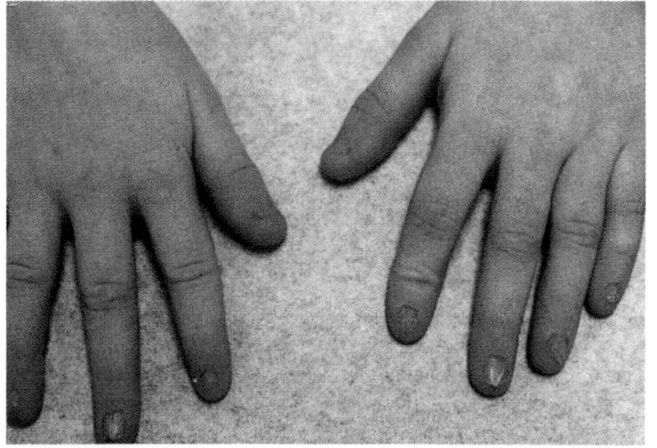

A

C

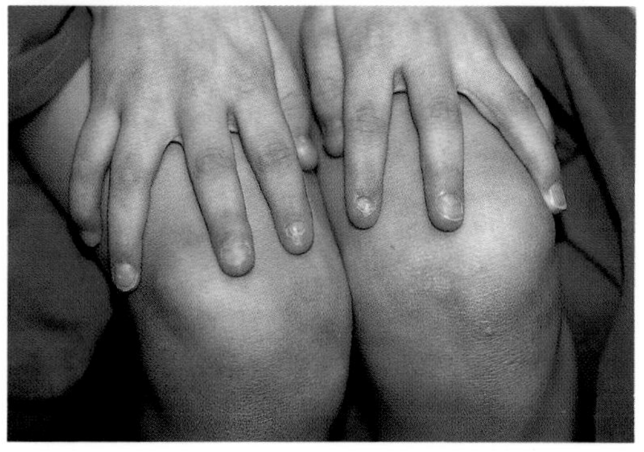

B

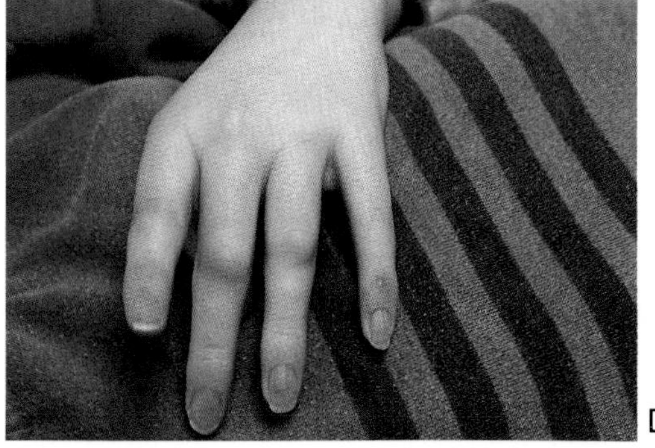

D

Figure 3.39. **(A)** Absent nails on thumbs. Abnormal nails on index fingers; all nails are affected. **(B)** Anonychia of the thumbs; longitudinal clefting, triangular lunulae; no kneecaps. **(C)** Micronychia on the index finger, koilonychia on the third finger, dystrophic fourth fingernail. **(D)** Absent lunulae.

and clubfoot has been reported as an incidental finding in a few patients.

The renal changes in nail-patella syndrome can range from relatively benign glomerulonephritis to nephrosis to need for renal transplantation. The first renal manifestation is usually proteinuria; hematuria can also occur. It has been suggested that structural renal malformations including duplication of the ureters may also be a feature of nail-patella syndrome. On electron microscopy there are defects in the renal basement membrane.

A clover-leaf distribution of dark pigment around the central area of the iris has been described in some patients.

HISTOPATHOLOGY

Light. One report has shown changes in elastin fibers with fragmentation and an increase in numbers throughout the dermis except in the papillae, where the fibers were thin. A second report from another patient showed no changes in elastin.

EM. Thickening of the basement membrane at the dermo-epidermal junction with reduplication of the lamina densa is a major feature. Multilaminated basement membranes surround most dermal vessels.

BASIC DEFECT

Unknown.

TREATMENT

The nail changes usually do not require any treatment. Recurrent dislocation of the elbows and kneecaps may require orthopedic intervention. Treatment for renal complications may be required.

It is reasonable to screen individuals with nail-patella syndrome for structural renal malformations and to follow them for the development of significant renal complications.

MODE OF INHERITANCE

Autosomal dominant. It has been suggested that there are two allelic (based on linkage to ABO) forms of the disorder, one with and one without nephropathy. Recurrence risk for nephropathy may be as high as 25% in families with a history of renal disease (a 50% risk for transmission of the gene and a 50% risk for the development of renal disease in individuals with nail-patella syndrome with a positive family history of kidney involvement). The risk for renal disease may be less than 5% if there is no renal disease in the family. The gene has been mapped to 9q34.

PRENATAL DIAGNOSIS

To my knowledge, prenatal diagnosis for nail-patella syndrome has not been performed. The recombination fraction with ABO is approximately 10%.

DIFFERENTIAL DIAGNOSIS

The triad of nail, bone, and kidney changes of nail-patella syndrome readily distinguishes it from other nail dystrophies. However, the nail changes alone are not pathognomonic and can be part of a number of other syndromes.

Congenital onychodysplasia (COIF): This condition is characterized by nail changes limited to the hands and usually involving only the index fingers. Nails may be absent, small, or comprised of two rudimentary small nail plates. The distal third of the underlying phalanges may be hypoplastic with irregularities or bifurcation of the tips. In one report, one case had Poland anomaly as well. Similar nail changes can be seen in association with structural bony alterations such as syndactyly and brachydactyly. While most reports of COIF have been sporadic, recurrence in siblings has been described. Recurrence risk in isolated COIF without an underlying bony disorder such as brachydactyly is probably low.

Congenital anonychia (MIM:107000, 206800): Pedigrees consistent with both autosomal dominant and autosomal recessive inheritance of anonychia are in the literature. The nails are absent, and the underlying nail beds appear to be normal. Rudimentary nail plates occasionally are present. There are no underlying skeletal abnormalities. Mixed anonychia and onychodystrophy has also been reported in families.

Anonychia with limb defects (MIM:106900, 106990): Any alteration in phalangeal structure such as brachydactyly, terminal transverse defects, and absence deformities will alter the overlying nail plate with changes ranging from complete absence of the nail to mild shortening alone. The nail changes are not specific, and the diagnosis depends on recognizing the underlying bony dysplasia.

Anonychia with flexural pigmentation (MIM: 106750): Affected individuals have thin, peeling skin of the palms and soles, congenital absence or hypoplasia of the nails, and slow-growing, coarse but thin hair. In addition, hyperpigmentation and hypopigmentation of the groin, axillae, natal cleft, and areolae develop. Dermatoglyphics may be poorly formed. This condition is also in the differential of absence of dermatoglyphics (MIM:125540).

Anonychia of the thumbnails (MIM:188200): One patient reported with anonychia of the thumbnail subsequently proved to have nail-patella syndrome. A second report gave no x-ray information, so the possibility of nail changes secondary to an underlying bony abnormality of the thumbs could not be excluded. I am not convinced that this is a distinct entity.

Onychodystrophy with deafness (MIM: 124480, 220500): This is a heterogeneous category. Sensorineural hearing loss and alteration in nail development are associated in several syndromes. In one family with vertical transmission of sensorineural hearing loss and anonychia, terminal hypoplasia of the distal phalanges, triphalangeal thumbs, and absence of the distal phalanges of the fifth fingers were also found. In the family reported with autosomal recessive transmission, nails were dystrophic, not absent. Affected individuals in a third family with deafness and nail changes similar to those of nail-patella syndrome had oligodontia and peg-shaped teeth. Although several generations were involved, there was no male-to-male transmission.

Support Group: N.O.R.D.
P.O. Box 8923
New Fairfield, CT
06812
1-800-999-6673

SELECTED BIBLIOGRAPHY

NAIL-PATELLA SYNDROME

Burkhart, C.G., Bhumbra, R., and Iannone, A.M. (1980). Nail-patella syndrome. A distinctive clinical and electron microscopic presentation. *J. Am. Acad. Dermatol.* **3,** 251–256.

This is a case report with electron microscopy of the skin.

Campeau, E., Watkins, D., Rouleau, G.A., Babul, R., Buchanan, J.A., Meschino, W., and Der Kaloustian, V.M. (1995). Linkage analysis of the nail-patella syndrome. *Am. J. Hum. Genet.* **56,** 243–247.

Further mapping of nail-patella syndrome to 9q34.1. Authors think *COL5A1* unlikely to be the causal gene, as it maps to 9q34.3.

Carbonara, P., and Alpert, M. (1964) Hereditary osteo-onychodysplasia (HOOD). *Am. J. Med. Sci.* **248,** 139–151.

Review of the literature with extensive photos and tables. Carbonara and Alpert point out that the diagnosis of nail-patella syndrome usually is made in patients presenting for other reasons, during which evaluation recognition of the syndrome occurs and a family history is elicited.

Duncan, J.G., and Souter, W.A. (1963). Hereditary onycho-osteodystrophy. The nail-patella syndrome. *J. Bone Joint Surg. Br.* **45B,** 242–258.

Review of the literature with extensive photos and tables.

Gibbs, R.C., Berczeller, P.H., and Hyman, A.B. (1964). Nail-patella-elbow syndrome. *Arch. Dermatol.* **89,** 196–199.

Case report of an affected female with histopathology of the skin showing fragmentation of the elastin fibers.

Lommen, E.J.P., Hamel, B.C.J., and Te Slaa, R.L. (1987). Nephropathy in hereditary osteoonychodysplasia (HOOD); variable expression or genetic heterogeneity. *Prog. Clin. Biol. Res.* **305,** 157–160.

Two distinct pedigrees with HOOD, one with and one without renal disease. The authors suggest a risk of 50% for renal involvement and 10% risk for renal failure in families with a positive history of renal disease. They calculated that there was a less than 5% risk for renal involvement in affected individuals from families with HOOD without renal disease.

Lucas, G.L., and Opitz J.M. (1966). The nail-patella syndrome. Clinical and genetic aspects of five kindreds with 38 affected family members. *J. Pediatr.* **68,** 273–288.

Review of the literature with extensive photos and tables.

OTHER DISORDERS

Feinmesser, M., and Zelig, S. (1961). Congenital deafness associated with onychodystrophy. *Arch. Otolaryngol.* **74,** 507–508.

Affected siblings, offspring of double first cousins, are described. There were no bony changes in the hands. The nails appeared dystrophic, short, and thickened.

Hopsu-Havu, V.K., and Jansen, C.T. (1973). Anonychia congenita. *Arch. Dermatol.* **107,** 752–753.

Four of 10 siblings born to parents who were consanguineous by three separate routes were affected. The proband was ascertained at a "social occasion." She had not sought medical advice for her nail abnormalities.

Kitayama, Y., and Tsukada, S. (1983). Congenital onychodysplasia. Report of 11 cases. *Arch. Dermatol.* **119,** 8–12.

Good clinical descriptions and x-rays of affected patients with a review of the literature. The authors suggest that vascular insult may be the cause of the onychodysplasia based on similar nail findings in a girl who suffered traumatic ischemia to a digit on days 3–5 of life.

Millman, A.J., and Strier, R.P. (1982). Congenital onychodysplasia of the index finger.

Report of a family. *J. Am. Acad. Dermatol.* **7,** 57–65.

Nine affected individuals in five generations with male-to-male transmission are described. Micronychia and polynychia of the index fingers with underlying bifid terminal phalanges was found in one of two patients examined radiologically. Thickening and curving of the small nail plate was noted and the term *rolled micronychia* was suggested.

Verbov, J. (1975). Anonychia with bizarre flexural pigmentation—an autosomal dominant dermatosis. *Br. J. Dermatol.* **92,** 469–474.

Two generations affected with anonychia and flexural pigmentation with no male-to-male transmission.

ONYCHOTRICHODYSPLASIA AND NEUTROPENIA (MIM:258360)

Includes Cartilage Hair Hypoplasia

DERMATOLOGIC FEATURES

MAJOR. Alopecia is present at birth and is followed by slow growth of fine, sparse hairs. The eyebrows and eyelashes are sparse and short. There is an absence of body hairs and development of sparse pubic hair with absence of axillary hair. The nails are hypoplastic with ridging, splitting, and koilonychia.

MINOR. Mild keratosis pilaris is described in some patients. Conjunctivitis secondary to irritation from short in-turning eyelashes is common.

ASSOCIATED ABNORMALITIES

Recurrent bacterial infections including tonsillitis, sinusitis, otitis, and cystitis are common. Chronic neutropenia with absolute neutrophil counts of 1,000–2,500 per milliliter is a defining feature of the disorder. Mild mental retardation is typical. Of seven patients described, one had normal intelligence.

HISTOPATHOLOGY

LIGHT. The hairs show trichorrhexis nodosa, possibly secondary to trauma to thin, weak shafts.

EM. Hairs show loss of cuticle.

BASIC DEFECT

Unknown.

TREATMENT

Appropriate antibiotic therapy for infections; careful eyelid care with plucking of the irritating lashes.

MODE OF INHERITANCE

Autosomal recessive, based on occurrence in siblings of consanguineous parents.

PRENATAL DIAGNOSIS

None.

DIFFERENTIAL DIAGNOSIS

Other forms of atrichia and hypotrichosis (MIM:Many) must be differentiated from this disorder. It is the only condition in which hypotrichosis is associated with neutropenia. Cartilage-hair hypoplasia (metaphyseal chondrodysplasia, McKusick type, MIM:250250) is

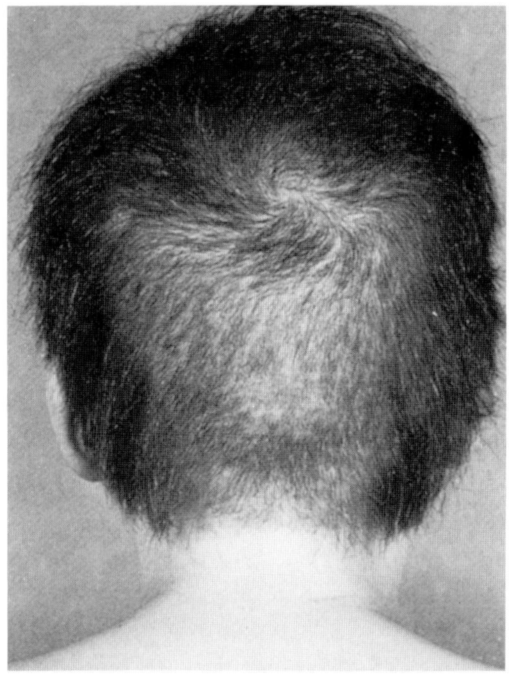

Figure 3.40. Short hairs, broken due to fragility. (From Verhage et al., 1987.)

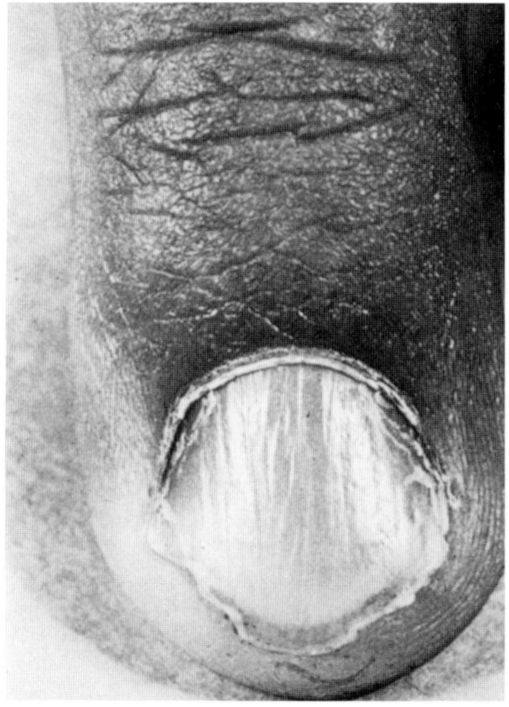

Figure 3.41. Brittle, flaking nail with longitudinal striae. (From Verhage et al., 1987.)

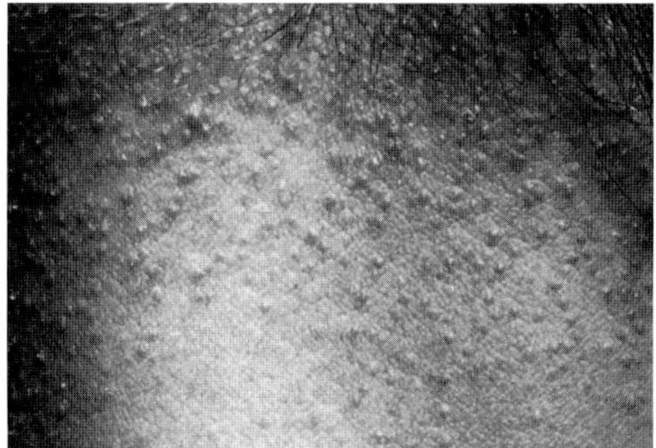

Figure 3.42. Perifollicular hyperkeratosis at the nape. (From Verhage et al., 1987.)

characterized by short stature, normal intelligence, and no nail changes. In cartilage-hair hypoplasia, lymphopenia is the more typical hematologic finding.

Individuals with cyclic neutropenia do not have hair abnormalities.

Support Group: N.O.R.D.
P.O. Box 8923
New Fairfield, CT
06812
1-800-999-6673

SELECTED BIBLIOGRAPHY

Hernandez, A., Olivares, F., and Cantu, J.-M. (1979). Autosomal recessive onychotrichodysplasia, chronic neutropenia and mild mental retardation. Delineation of the syndrome. *Clin. Genet.* **15,** 147–152.

Two siblings. The authors describe the hairs as showing trichorrhexis (splitting), but offer no further description.

Itin, P.H., and Pittelkow, M.R. (1991). Trichothiodystrophy with chronic neutropenia and mild mental retardation. *J. Am. Acad. Dermatol.* **24,** 356–358.

On scanning electron micrographs, the hairs showed cuticular loss. There was a decreased sulfur content in the hairs, suggesting that onychotrichodysplasia with neutropenia may be categorized among the trichothiodystrophies.

PACHYONYCHIA CONGENITA (MIM:167200, 167210)

Includes Jadassohn-Lewandowsky; Jackson-Lawler; Onychogryposis

Samman and Fenton (1986) proposed four types of pachyonychia congenita: classic type I (Jadassohn-Lewandowsky type); type II, (Riehl), which is similar to type I but more mild and with chronic oral leukoplakia; type III (Jackson-Lawler), which is characterized by natal teeth, multiple epidermal inclusion cysts, with or without other abnormalities; and type IV, in which affected individuals have widespread macular pigmentation in the neck and axillae with moderate nail and skin changes. Other classifications distinguish a type III in which all the classic features are present and in addition there is corneal dystrophy (Schafer-Brunauer syndrome). Yet another scheme was suggested by Feinstein et al. (1988) in which the type IV form of pachyonychia congenita was characterized by mental retardation, laryngeal involvement, and alopecia. More recently with discovery of specific mutations, Jadassohn-Lewandowsky is referred to as PC-1; Jackson-Lawler as PC-2.

Among the many classification schemes, the major similarities appear to be in the diagnostic significance of (1) corneal dystrophy, (2) presence of natal teeth and multiple cysts (either steatocystoma multiplex or epidermal inclusion cysts), and (3) absence of oral leukoplakia.

I agree with Schonfeld's (1980) position that not all these distinctions may be warranted, overlap within families does occur, and one cannot accurately predict in many families whether an individual at risk for pachyonychia congenita will be spared a specific finding. I am also convinced that any inherited disorder with thickened nails in association with a second dermatologic feature has been labeled as pachyonychia congenita in case reports, further muddying the diagnostic waters.

DERMATOLOGIC FEATURES

MAJOR. The fingernails and toenails are thickened, friable, and darkened. Distal involvement may be greater than proximal involvement. Nail changes can be seen at birth and usually present within the first year of life. Although involvement is often symmetric, not all nails are necessarily involved. The toenails and fingernails of

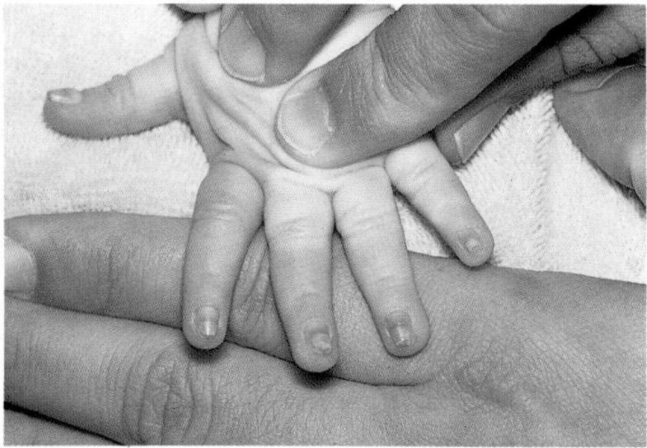

A

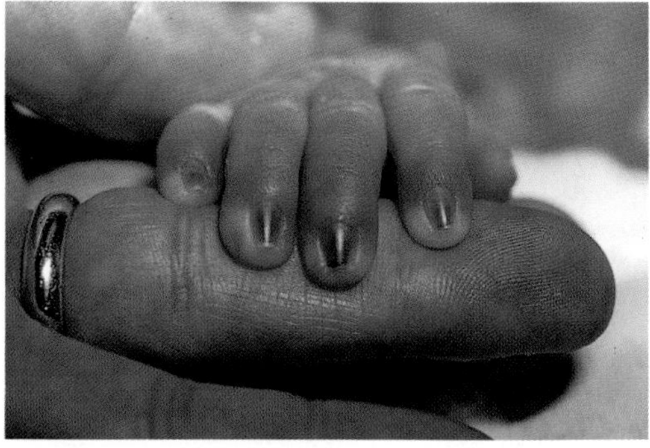

B

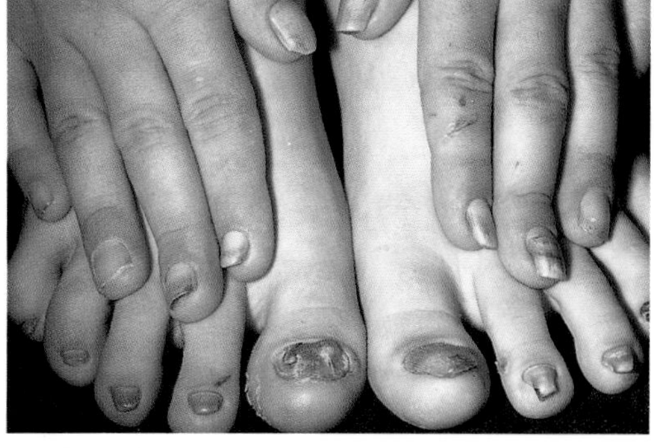

C

Figure 3.43. (A–C) Varying nail changes in individuals with pachyonychia congenita. (C, courtesy of Dr. P. Fleckman, Seattle, Washington.)

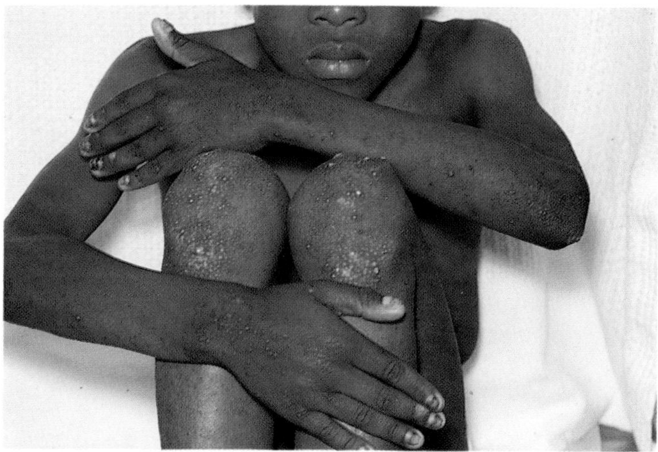

Figure 3.44. Nail changes and typical follicular hyperkeratosis over knees and arms.

the thumbs and index fingers tend to be more severely involved. The distal nail bed, as well as the nail plate, is also thickened. Nails may be shed; new nails are also dystrophic.

Hyperkeratosis and hyperhidrosis of the palms and soles are common.

Follicular hyperkeratosis, primarily of the elbows and knees, develops. More widespread distribution of these skin lesions can also occur.

MINOR. There are occasional reports of blistering of the soles.

Epidermal inclusion cysts, steatocystoma multiplex, and cylindromas have been reported. There is some confusion about the histopathology of these lesions in pachyonychia congenita, and there may be overlap. These skin changes occur later in childhood and adult life and are typical of Jackson-Lawler (PC-2).

Alopecia, which may be congenital or occur later, and/or thinning and loss of sheen of the hair are described in some patients, typically in those with Jackson-Lawler (PC-2). Coarseness of eyebrows and body hair, with pili torti of the hair shafts, has been described as well in this group.

Reticulated hyperpigmentation of the neck and axillae can occur and may represent a distinct subtype.

Hidradenitis suppurativa was described in one family.

ASSOCIATED ABNORMALITIES

Oral leukoplakia of the mucosa of the mouth and on the tongue is histologically similar to white sponge nevus. Malignant degeneration has not been reported. This feature is primarily seen in the Jadassohn-Lewandowsky form (PC-1) and is absent in the Jackson-Lawler variant (PC-2).

Natal teeth are occasionally present, as are malformed teeth, primarily in the Jackson-Lawler variant (PC-2).

The evidence for association with mental retardation in the literature is not compelling, and I suspect that this is not a true feature of pachyonychia congenita.

HISTOPATHOLOGY

LIGHT. The nail plate and proximal nail matrix are normal. The nail bed shows marked hyperkeratosis. The distal nail matrix is hypertrophic. There is some disagreement about microscopic features.

Oral mucosa: Acanthosis, parakeratosis, and intracellular vacuolization are seen.

Hyperkeratoses: Hyperkeratosis, parakeratosis, acanthosis, and a moderate increase in

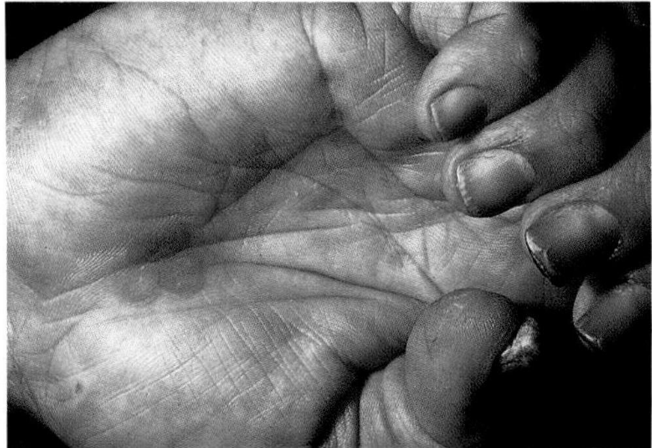

Figure 3.45. Nail changes and focal hyperkeratosis of palm and thumb. (Courtesy of Dr. P. Fleckman, Seattle, Washington.)

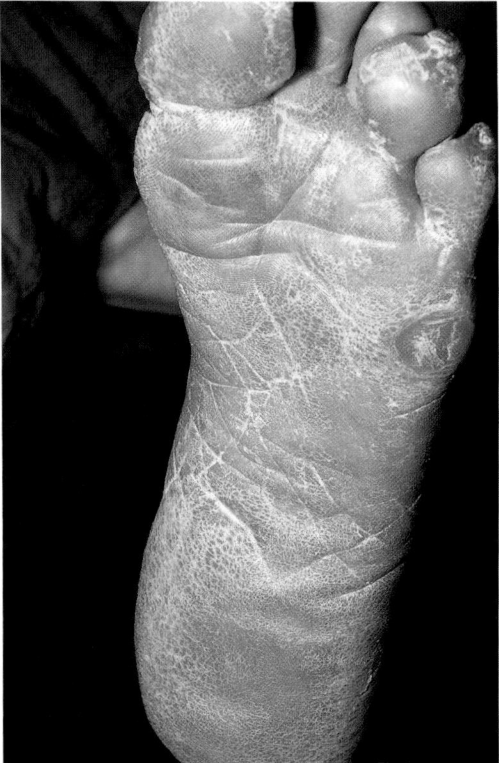

Figure 3.46. Hyperkeratosis of the sole. (Courtesy of Dr. P. Fleckman, Seattle, Washington.)

the granular layer with a minimal lymphocytic infiltrate in the upper dermis are reported in some biopsy specimens, orthohyperkeratosis and a decreased granular layer in others. It is unclear if these findings are site or patient specific.

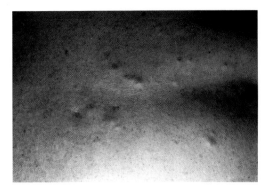

Figure 3.47. Epidermal inclusion cysts.

EM. Dense aggregation of tonofilaments at the periphery of the basal keratinocytes and abnormal keratohyalin have been described. These changes are not specific.

BASIC DEFECT

A mutation in K17 has been demonstrated in one family with Jackson-Lawler (PC-2). Heterozygosity for a nonsense mutation in K16 has been found in one pedigree with Jadassohn-Lewandowsky (PC-1); heterozygosity for a deletion in K6a in another.

TREATMENT

Treatment is primarily symptomatic. Emollients and keratolytics (e.g., Lac-Hydrin, glycolic acid, salicylic acid) can be used for the hyperkeratoses. Routine grinding of the nail plates can keep their interference with function at a minimum, but the nails remain cosmetically dystrophic. If limitation of hand function becomes unacceptable, ablation of the nail matrix is the only permanent effective therapy for the dystrophic nails. There has been mixed success with treatment with oral retinoids.

MODE OF INHERITANCE

Autosomal dominant. Both Jackson-Lawler (PC-2) and Jadassohn-Lewandowsky (PC-1) types have been mapped to the type I keratin cluster on 17q. *KRT6* resides on 12q.

PRENATAL DIAGNOSIS

Possible in some instances by mutation or linkage analysis.

DIFFERENTIAL DIAGNOSIS

The involvement of the nails in pachyonychia congenita can often be distal and may be clinically indistinguishable from fungal infection on the basis of nail changes alone. KOH and fungal cultures are always appropriate.

The nail changes of dyskeratosis congenita (MIM:305000) are quite different from those of pachyonychia congenita, more similar to those of lichen planus, with hypoplasia and pterygia of the nails rather than thickening.

Onychogryphosis, the development of claw or talon nails, is usually acquired. One family with claw-like nail changes and plantar hyperkeratoses is described by McKusick (MIM: 164680). One individual had dry, coarse hair. Although five generations were involved, no male-to-male transmission occurred.

Support Group: N.O.R.D.
P.O. Box 8923
New Fairfield, CT 06812
1-800-999-6673

SELECTED BIBLIOGRAPHY

Feinstein, A., Friedman, J., and Schewach-Millet, M. (1988). Pachyonychia congenita. *J. Am. Acad. Dermatol.* **19,** 705–711.

Schonfeld, P.H.R. (1980). The pachyonychia congenita syndrome. *Acta Dermatol. Venereol.* (Stockh.) **60,** 45–49.

Sivasundram, A., Rajagopalan, K, and Sarojini, T. (1985). Pachyonychia congenita. *Int. J. Dermatol.* **24,** 179–180.

Feinstein et al. (1988), Schonfeld (1980), and Sivasundram et al. (1985) are three reports and reviews of pachyonychia congenita with distinct classification schemes. Everyone agrees on type I, but it is a free-for-all from there.

Gorlin, R.J., and Chaudhry, A.P. (1958). Oral lesions accompanying pachyonychia congenita. *Oral Surg. Oral Med. Oral Pathol.* **11,** 541–544.

Authors describe the mucosal changes associated with the disorder as hyperkeratotic, in contrast to the dyskeratosis of true leukoplakia.

Jackson, A.D.M., and Lawler, S.D. (1951). Pachyonychia congenita: a report of six cases in one family. *Ann. Eugen.* **16,** 142–146.

A report of a family with natal teeth, blistering of the soles, multiple skin cysts, follicular hyperkeratoses, and pachyonychia congenita. This family did not have leukoplakia.

McLean, W.H.I., Rugg, E.L., Lunny, D.P., Morley, S.M., Lane, E.B., Swensson, O., Dopping-Hepenstal, P.J.C., Griffiths, W.A. D., Eady, R.A.J., Higgins, C., Navsaria, H.A., Leigh, I.M., Strachan, T., Kunkeler, L., and Munro, C.S. (1995). Keratin 16 and keratin 17 mutations cause pachyonychia congenita. *Nat. Genet.* **9,** 273–278.

Presents mutation data and correlates clinical differences between the forms of pachyonychia congenita with specific mutations. K16 and K17 are acidic keratins that are expressed to different degrees in different tissues. K16 alterations might affect oral mucosa more (where it is expressed in greater amounts), whereas K17 alterations might be more likely to lead to epidermal cyst formation, as its expression predominates in the infundibulum of sweat glands.

Samman, P.D., and Fenton, D.A. (1986) *The nails in disease* 4th Ed. W. Heinemann Medical Books: Year Book Medical Publishers, London.

Excellent textbook. A new edition (1995, Oxford: Butterworth-Heinemann) has just come out.

Soderquist, N.A., and Reed, W.B. (1968). Pachyonychia congenita with epidermal cysts and other congenital dyskeratoses. *Arch. Dermatol.* **97,** 31–33.

In this report there was reevaluation of three of the members of the Jackson-Lawler family.

Tidman, J.N.J., Wells, R.S., and MacDonald, D.M. (1987). Pachyonychia congenita with cutaneous amyloidosis and hyperpigmentation—a distinct variant. *J. Am. Acad. Dermatol.* **16,** 935–940.

Better title: Autosomal dominant onychodystrophy with macular amyloidosis. Two pedigrees with onset of nail changes during infancy–early childhood, improving with age. Mild palmoplantar hyperkeratosis, gradual macular hyperpigmentation in axillae, neck, waist, backs of knees, thighs, buttocks, and belly. Amyloid deposition seen. No other features of pachyonychia congenita. Typifies the nonspecific use of the term *pachyonychia congenita.*

Vineyard, W.R., and Scott, R.A. (1961). Steatocystoma multiplex with pachyonychia congenita. *Arch. Dermatol.* **84,** 824–827.

Eight affected individuals in four generations with male-to-male transmission are described.

Sweat Glands

HIDRADENITIS SUPPURATIVA (MIM:142690)

DERMATOLOGIC FEATURES

MAJOR. Recurrent inflammation of apocrine sweat glands results in chronic sinus tract formation, abscesses, and scarring. Infection is secondary. Areas of involvement include the axillae, groin, perineum, buttocks, sacrum, periumbilical area, and periaureolar region. Rarely, involvement of the neck, back, scalp, and cheeks has been described. Onset is usually in the teens, but may be as late as the fourth decade.

MINOR. Acne conglobata may occur in a subset of affected individuals.

ASSOCIATED ABNORMALITIES

None.

HISTOPATHOLOGY

LIGHT. Chronic inflammatory changes in the apocrine glands with keratotic plugs in pilosebaceous follicles; scarring in the deep dermis and subcutaneous tissue. Sinus tracts are common.

EM. No information.

BASIC DEFECT

Unknown.

TREATMENT

Excision with skin grafting. No consistently positive response to isotretinoin. Chronic antibiotics may decrease episodes of secondary infection.

MODE OF INHERITANCE

Usually sporadic. Autosomal dominant when familial.

PRENATAL DIAGNOSIS

None.

DIFFERENTIAL DIAGNOSIS

Hidradenitis suppurativa occurs in patients with Dowling-Degos disease (MIM:179850) and was reported in one family with pachyonychia congenita (MIM:167200, 167210). Benign fa-

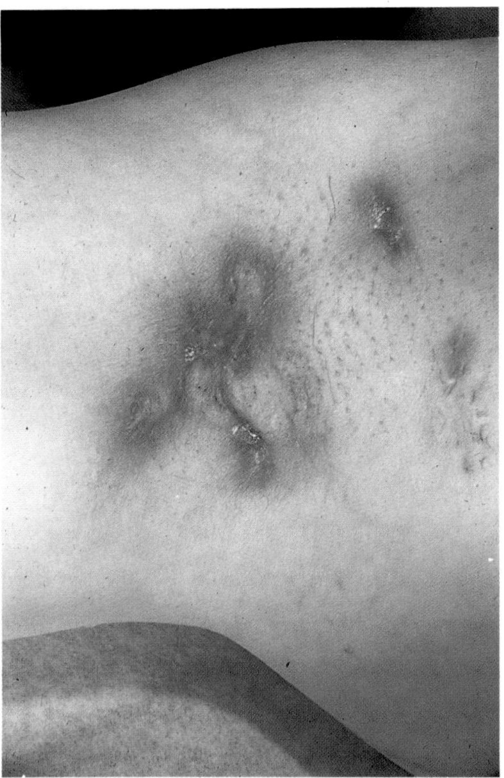

Figure 3.48. Sinus tracks and scarring in axilla. (Courtesy of Division of Dermatology, University of Washington.)

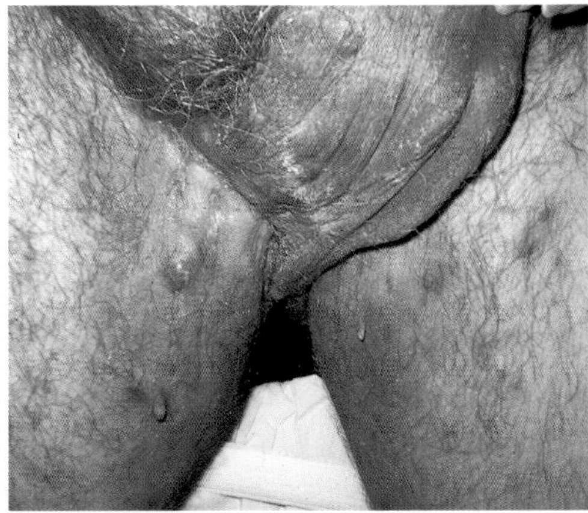

Figure 3.49. Abscesses on inner thighs and scrotum. (Courtesy of Division of Dermatology, University of Washington.)

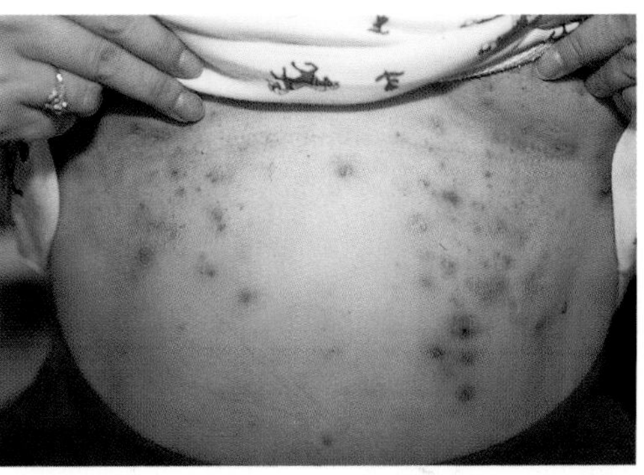

Figure 3.50. Multiple bilateral lesions under breasts and on abdomen.

milial pemphigus, Hailey-Hailey disease (MIM: 169600) is characterized by blistering in the axillae and groins; secondary infection can be confused with hidradenitis. In Fox-Fordyce disease, lesions are smaller pruritic papules rather than painful nodules and can be differentiated histologically by rupture of the intradermal portion of the apocrine gland duct.

Support Group: N.O.R.D.
P.O. Box 8923
New Fairfield, CT 06812
1-800-999-6673

SELECTED BIBLIOGRAPHY

Fitzsimmons, J.S., Fitzsimmons, E.M., and Gilbert, G. (1984). Familial hidradenitis suppurativa: evidence in favor of single gene transmission. *J. Med. Genet.* **21,** 281–285.

Fitzsimmons, J.S., and Guilbert, P.R. (1985). A family study of hidradenitis suppurativa. *J. Med. Genet.* **22,** 367–373.

Fitzsimmons, J.S., Guilbert, P.R., and Fitzsimmons, E.M. (1985). Evidence of genetic factors in hidradenitis suppurativa. *Br. J. Dermatol.* **113,** 1–8.

Eleven pedigrees with vertical transmission, one with male-to-male. Three others with probable familial occurrence. Authors suggest that delayed age of onset and reticence to admit involvement because of embarrassment may obscure the genetic nature of the disorder.

Norris, J.F.B., and Cunliffe, W.T. (1986).

Failure of treatment of familial widespread hidradenitis suppurativa with isotretinoin. *Clin. Exp. Dermatol.* **11,** 579–583.
No response to therapy in six patients from a family described by Fitzsimmons et al. (1984) coupled with worsening of the disease when the drug was stopped. The authors concisely review prior studies with the drug.

Watson, J.D. (1985). Hidradenitis suppurativa—a clinical review. *Br. J. Plast. Surg.* **38,** 567–569.
Seventy-two patients. A 54% relapse rate with excision and primary closure, 13% relapse rate with excision and skin grafting, and 19% with excision and local flap.

HYPERHIDROSIS (MIM:144110)

DERMATOLOGIC FEATURES

MAJOR. Essential hyperhidrosis is marked by excessive sweating of eccrine glands on the palms, soles, and axillae. Onset is usually in childhood, and most affected children have palmar involvement. Approximately one-half have foot involvement.

Axillary hyperhidrosis usually occurs later in adolescence. It is nonodorous because of the increased rate of flow. Essential hyperhidrosis can increase with both psychological stress and with heat.

MINOR. None.

ASSOCIATED ABNORMALITIES

None.

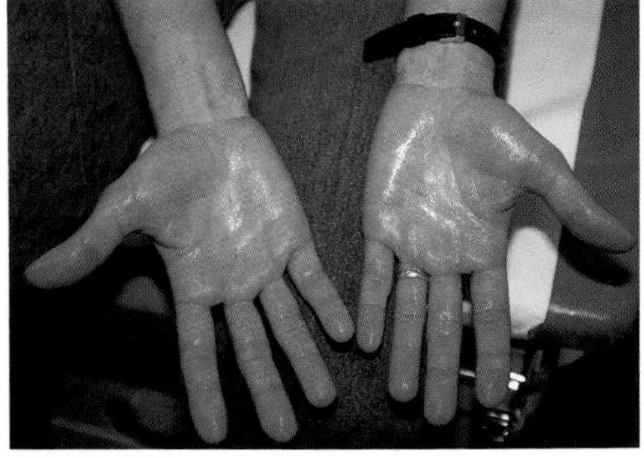

Figure 3.51. Shiny palms, slick with sweat. (Courtesy of Dr. G.F. Odland, Division of Dermatology, University of Washington.)

HISTOPATHOLOGY

LIGHT. The skin is normal.
EM. No information.

BASIC DEFECT

Unknown.

TREATMENT

Antiperspirants may help and work better in the axillae than on the palms and soles. A 6%–25% solution of aluminum chloride applied nightly under occlusion may help. Tap water iontophoresis (15—20 mAmp DC × 30 minutes 2–3 times a week) is often helpful. Sympathectomy of the T2 and T3 ganglia may be very effective but carries a risk of significant side effects, including Horner syndrome.

MODE OF INHERITANCE

Probably autosomal dominant with reduced penetrance.

PRENATAL DIAGNOSIS

None.

DIFFERENTIAL DIAGNOSIS

The diagnosis of primary hyperhidrosis is self-evident. Other conditions in which excessive sweating occur are easily distinguished by their associated features. Hyperhidrosis may occur secondary to spinal cord disease and to autonomic dysfunction. *Gustatory hyperhidrosis* refers to spontaneous sweating of the face in response to hot, spicy food. Hyperhidrosis can be seen in association with neoplasms and cardiovascular disease. Episodic hyperhidrosis in association with agenesis of the corpus callosum often occurs along with hyperthermic episodes. Familial dysautonomia (Riley-Day syndrome, MIM:223900) is often marked by excessive sweating in response to warmth.

Two sibships have been described with increased sweating after exposure to cold.

Excessive sweating at sites of specific lesions has been described in association with organoid nevi, eccrine-pilar angiomatous hamartomas, glomus tumors (MIM:138000), and blue rubber bleb nevi (MIM:112200). In one pedigree with nail-patella syndrome (MIM:161200), some affected members also had hyperhidrosis with onset in puberty. In dyskeratosis congenita (MIM:127550, 224230, 305000), there is often symmetric lividity of the palms and soles, and some patients have had palmoplantar hyperhidrosis. Böök syndrome (MIM:112300) is characterized by premature canities, premolar aplasia, and hyperhidrosis. This is a presumably autosomal dominant disease reported in one family. Hyperhidrosis can occasionally be seen in individuals with Charcot-Marie-Tooth disease (MIM:118200).

Support Group: N.O.R.D.
P.O. Box 8923
New Fairfield, CT
06812
1-800-999-6673

SELECTED BIBLIOGRAPHY

Cloward, R.B. (1957). Treatment of hyperhidrosis palmaris (sweaty hands). *Harv. Med. J.* **16,** 381–387.

Cloward R.B. (1969). Hyperhidrosis. *J. Neurosurg.* **30,** 545–551.

The author states that the condition is much more common among Hawaiian Japanese of Okinawan descent. Of his 30 patients, 25 were Japanese compared with approximately 5% in the general population. He described one affected sibling pair, one patient with an affected daughter, one family with two affected brothers, and one pedigree with five affected individuals in three generations. The follow-up paper, with a total of 82 patients, mentions an affected father and two sons. He notes that, inexplicably, foot involvement also improves after sympathectomy of T2 and T3.

Freeman, R., Waldorf, H.A., and Dover, J.S. (1992). Autonomic neurodermatology (part II): disorders of sweating and flushing. *Semin. Neurol.* **12,** 394–407.

Well written review of causes of increased and decreased sweating and flushing. One hundred sixty-four references.

James, W.D., Schoomaker, E.B., and Rodman, O.G. (1987). Emotional eccrine sweating. A heritable disorder. *Arch. Dermatol.* **123,** 925–929.

In this report, axillary sweating also started in childhood. Palms and soles showed increased sweating at birth. One affected member had involvement of the soles only. There were two obligate carriers who were symptom free.

MULTIPLE SYRINGOMAS (MIM:186600)

DERMATOLOGIC FEATURES

MAJOR. Small 1–5 mm skin-colored to yellow, occasionally shiny papules develop in childhood around puberty, or in adult life.

Two patterns of distribution are described. One is primarily periocular. The other, termed *eruptive,* involves the neck, face, anterior trunk, folds, and inner thighs. Both patterns are described in individuals within the same family, and it is unclear if they are distinctive. More circumscribed distribution (e.g., vulvar, linear) has also been described but does not appear to be specific.

MINOR. One mother–daughter pair had palmar and plantar pits as well as syringomas around the eyes.

ASSOCIATED ABNORMALITIES

The skin changes are common in Down syndrome (trisomy 21).

HISTOPATHOLOGY

LIGHT. Cystic lesions with epithelial cords abound in the upper reticular dermis. Cysts can be filled with keratinous material and may be thick or thin walled.

EM. The lumen of the cysts is lined by short microvilli. Multivesicular dense bodies are found in the cytoplasm of the inner cells.

BASIC DEFECT

Unknown.

TREATMENT

Success with carbon dioxide laser reported in one patient.

MODE OF INHERITANCE

Probably autosomal dominant. Three pedigrees with affected siblings; one father–daughter pair; two mother–daughter pairs; one grandfather, sister, and proband; one father with two daughters; and one set of identical twins. Most case reports do not describe family history.

PRENATAL DIAGNOSIS

None.

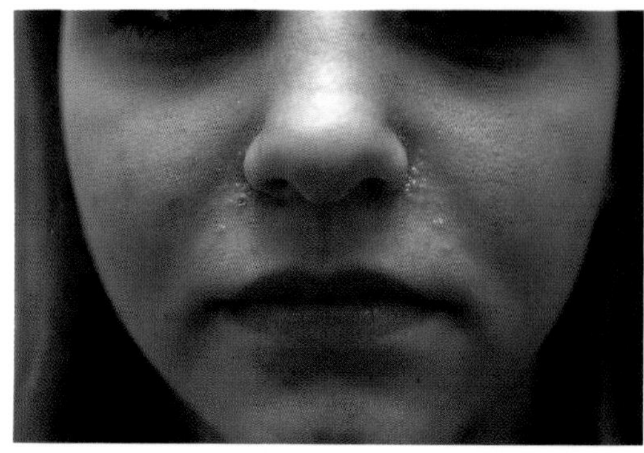

Figure 3.52. Small, flesh-colored, almost translucent papules around nares. (From Yesudian and Thambiah, 1975.)

DIFFERENTIAL DIAGNOSIS

Syringomas can mimic milia if keratinaceous material is also contained within them. Eruptive clear cell syringomas are associated with diabetes mellitus. Flat warts, angiofibromas, trichoepitheliomas, xanthelasma, and lichen planus may be confused. The initial lesions of basal cell nevus syndrome (MIM:109400) can appear similar. Biopsy will differentiate among all these possibilities.

Support Group: N.O.R.D.
P.O. Box 8923
New Fairfield, CT 06812
1-800-999-6673

SELECTED BIBLIOGRAPHY

Butterworth, T., Strean, L.P., Beerman, H., and Word, M.G. (1964). Syringoma and mongolism. *Arch. Dermatol.* **90,** 483–487.

Thirty-seven of 200 patients with Down sydrome had syringomas. Biopsy confirmed the diagnosis in 14. Females were twice as likely as males to have syringomas (26%:13%).

Carter, D.M., and Jegasothy, B.V. (1976). Alopecia areata and Down syndrome. *Arch. Dermatol.* **112,** 1397–1399.

Authors examined 214 individuals with Down syndrome, all residents at a training school, and found syringomas clinically in 58% of females and 27% of males (39% overall). Confirmed by biopsy in three. Alopecia areata was present in 9%, xerosis in 85%, atopy in 57%, and seborrheic dermatitis in 36%. There were no cases of elastosis perforans serpiginosa.

Hashimoto, K., Blum, D., Fukaya, T., and Eto, H. (1985). Familial syringoma. Case history and application of monoclonal antieccrine gland antibodies. *Arch Dermatol.* **121,** 756–760.

Father and two daughters are examined. Family history stated that the proband's father and one sister (of three siblings) had lesions also. If true, proves autosomal dominant inheritance. Authors propose lesions derived from the eccrine duct precursors.

Pruzan, D.L., Esterly, N.B., and Prose, N.S. (1989). Eruptive syringoma. *Arch. Dermatol.* **125,** 1119–1120.

Four cases, one of whom had an affected mother. Emphasizes appearance in childhood.

SEBACEOUS GLANDS

ERUPTIVE VELLUS HAIR CYSTS (MIM:None)

DERMATOLOGIC FEATURES

Major. Asymptomatic, grouped and isolated small papules that may be reddish-brown to dark brown in color develop on the upper chest, flexor and extensor surfaces of the extremities, the back, and the face. These can be present at birth, but usually develop within the first to second decades. Some lesions can be hyperkeratotic or appear more comedone-like. Mild surrounding redness has been described.

Minor. None.

A

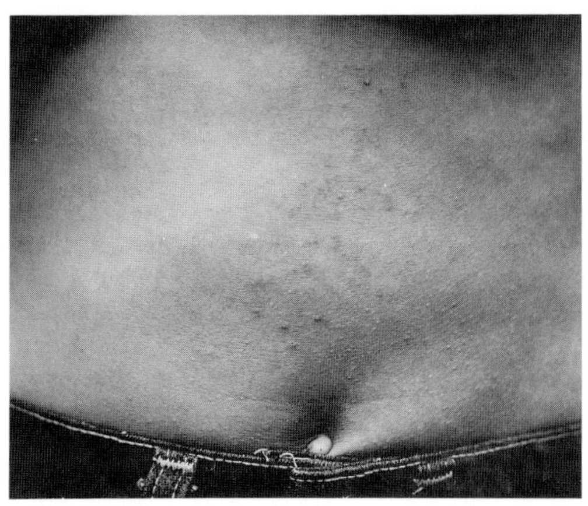

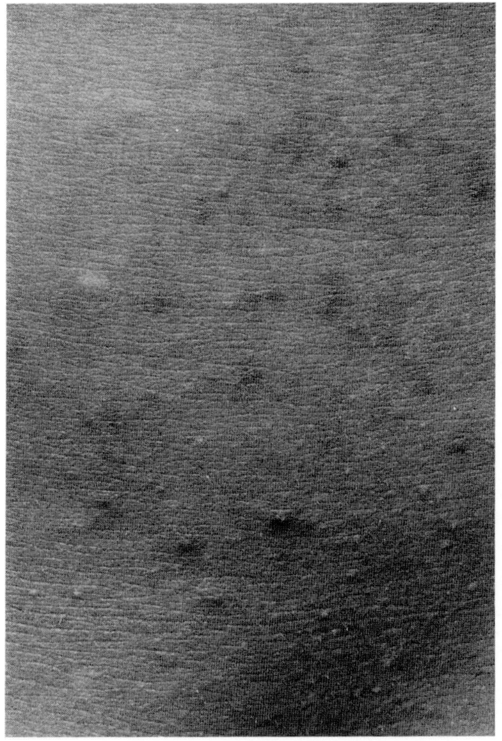

B

Figure 3.53. **(A)** Small papules. (Courtesy of Dr. M. Piepkorn, Seattle, Washington.) **(B)** Close-up shows central plug in several. (From Piepkorn et al., 1981.)

ASSOCIATED ABNORMALITIES

None.

HISTOPATHOLOGY

LIGHT. Cysts in the mid-dermis containing multiple vellus hairs embedded in laminated keratinous material. Rudimentary follicles may be contained within the wall of the cyst.
EM. No information.

BASIC DEFECT

Unknown.

TREATMENT

None Spontaneous resolution has occurred. One patient reported 50% response to Lac-Hydrin.

MODE OF INHERITANCE

Autosomal dominant.

PRENATAL DIAGNOSIS

None.

DIFFERENTIAL DIAGNOSIS

Steatocystoma multiplex (MIM:184500) may appear identical clinically; histology can usually, but not always, separate the two. Individuals with both steatocystoma multiplex and eruptive vellus hair cysts have been reported.

The papules of *keratosis pilaris* are usually flesh colored; lesions of *comedonal acne* may offer some confusion. *Milia* are usually more superficial.

Support Group: N.O.R.D.
P.O. Box 8923
New Fairfield, CT
06812
1-800-999-6673

SELECTED BIBLIOGRAPHY

Esterly, N.B., Fretzin, D.F., and Pinkus, H. (1977). Eruptive vellus hair cysts. *Arch. Dermatol.* **113,** 500–503.

A total of four patients, two with a negative family history, two with unknown family history. Lesions discovered in one child as part of a routine physical examination, suggesting that incidence may be higher, but not brought to medical attention because asymptomatic.

Mayron, R., and Grimwood, R.E. (1988). Familial occurrence of eruptive vellus hair cysts. *Pediatr. Dermatol.* **5,** 94–96.

Male-to-male transmission. Reviews treatment, including tretinoin, Lac-Hydrin, CO_2 laser, abrasion, and urea cream.

Sanchez-Yus, E., Aguilar-Martinez, A., Cristobal-Gil, M.C., Urbina-Gonzalez, F., and Guerra-Rodriguez, P. (1988). Eruptive vellus hair cyst and steatocystoma multiplex: two related conditions? *J. Cutan. Pathol.* **15,** 40–42.

Jerasutus, S., Suvanprakorn, P., and Sombatworapat, W. (1989). Eruptive vellus hair cyst and steatocystoma multiplex. *J. Am. Acad. Dermatol.* **20,** 292–293.

Two patients with multiple lesions and a positive family history, one from Spain (Sanchez-Yus et al., 1988) and one from Thailand (Jerasutus et al., 1989), showed both steatocystoma multiplex and eruptive vellus hair cysts on biopsies. Authors postulate both disorders represent a developmental defect arising from different portions of the hair follicle.

Stiefler, R.E., and Bergfeld, W.F. (1980). Eruptive vellus hair cysts—an inherited disorder. *J. Am. Acad. Dermatol.* **3,** 425–429.

Mother and four of four children affected.

FAMILIAL DYSKERATOTIC COMEDONES (MIM:120450)

Includes Nevus Comedonicus

DERMATOLOGIC FEATURES

MAJOR. Papules with central firm brown keratotic plugs, which clinically resemble open comedones, may develop on all body surfaces except the mucosa and the glans penis. Involvement of the penile shaft does occur. Inflammation and pruritis are inconstant findings. Occasionally, infection and recurrent cysts with sinuses can develop. In the sporadic form, involvement is more usually unilateral and does not cross the midline. The lesions have been described at birth but more commonly develop in childhood and rarely have not appeared until adult life.

MINOR. Although review articles often state that nevus comedonicus can be seen in association with ichthyosis, there has actually been only one report of a patient with localized ichthyosis developing in adulthood who developed a nevus comedonicus in uninvolved skin.

There is a single case report of a 69-year-old male with a unilateral lesion containing both dyskeratotic comedones and basal cell nevi. Another individual developed tricholemmal cysts in his extensive nevus comedonicus.

ASSOCIATED ABNORMALITIES

One patient with a unilateral nevus comedonicus with onset at age 9 years had an ipsilateral congenital cataract. Other case reports of scoliosis and vertebral anomalies with nevus comedonicus are rare. One patient with a Sturge-Weber/Klippel-Trenaunay-Weber phenotype and a nevus comedonicus has also been described.

HISTOPATHOLOGY

LIGHT. Follicle-like epidermal invaginations are filled with lamellated keratinous material with focal areas of acantholysis and dyskeratosis in the base of the lesions. There is no sebaceous material in the lesions. In some instances, the changes of epidermolytic hyperkeratosis have been described.

EM. In a familial case, a lesion from a hair-bearing surface showed decreased desmosomal attachments within the stratum malpighii, tonofilament aggregations surrounding the nuclei, and dyskeratotic cells with dense perinuclear keratohyalin and tonofilament aggregation, typical of Darier-White disease. A palmar lesion from a sporadic case showed dilated abnormal sweat ducts plugged with parakeratotic filiform material.

BASIC DEFECT

Unknown.

TREATMENT

Wide excision is the only effective therapy and may not be feasible. Limited excision may result in recurrence.

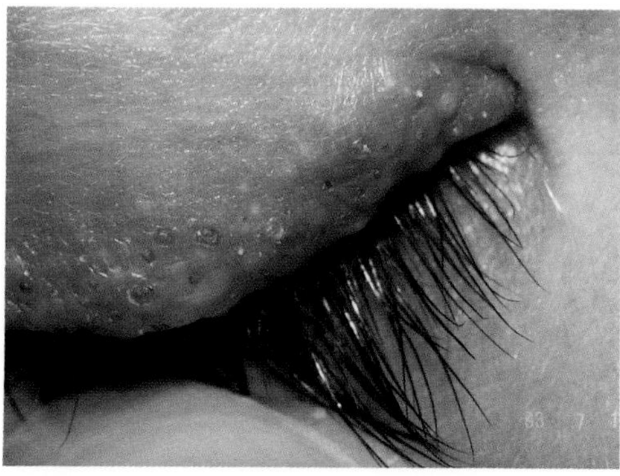

Figure 3.54. Lesions along the eyelid with multiple open and closed comedones.

A

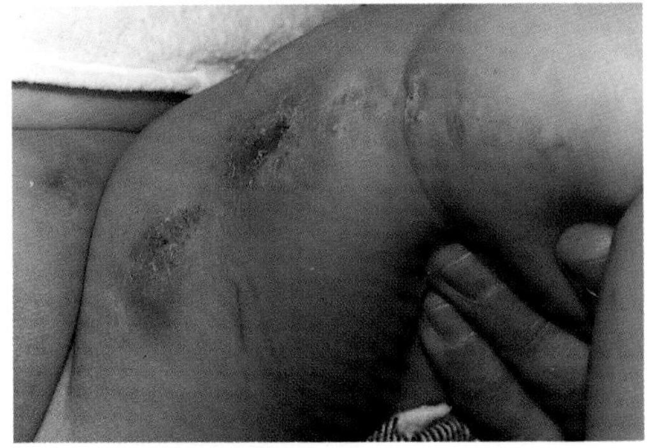

B

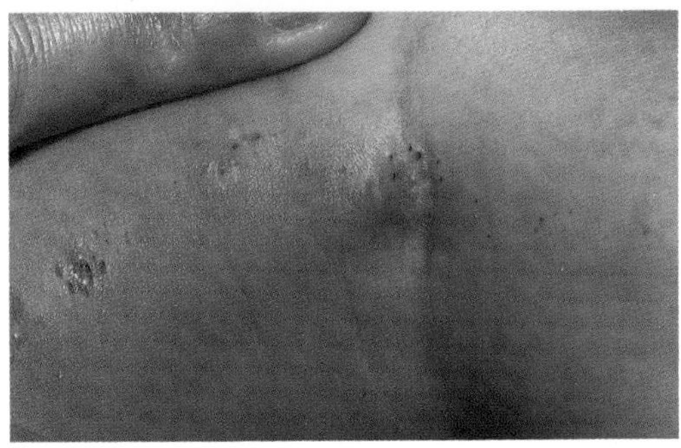

Figure 3.55. **(A)** Involvement of labia majora and thigh, with cyst formation and drainage. **(B)** Areas of comedones and scarring in same patient.

MODE OF INHERITANCE

Autosomal dominant with male-to-male transmission or sporadic. Sporadic cases predominate in the literature, appear to be more likely characterized by lesions that have cribriform scarring, and are more often unilateral and localized, suggestive of nevi resulting from postzygotic mutations. In several families, the probands were unaware of their positive family history Perhaps more of the sporadic cases are familial than is appreciated.

PRENATAL DIAGNOSIS

None.

DIFFERENTIAL DIAGNOSIS

Lesions in Darier-White disease (MIM:124200) do not have an extractable central plug. Nail changes and mucous membrane involvement do not occur in familial dyskeratotic comedones.

Differentiating between familial dyskeratotic comedones and sporadic nevus comedonicus may be difficult. Although the lesions in the latter are usually more limited in distribution, this is not invariable.

Support Group: N.O.R.D.
P.O. Box 8923
New Fairfield, CT
06812
1-800-999-6673

SELECTED BIBLIOGRAPHY

Bedi, T.R., and Bhutani, L.K. (1974). Familial comedones (a case report). *Indian J. Dermatol.* **20,** 6–7.

A four generation family with one instance of male-to-male transmission.

Carneiro, S.J.C., Dickson, J.E., and Knox, J.M. (1972). Familial dyskeratotic comedones. *Arch Dermatol.* **105,** 249–251.

A mother and three of her seven children had lesions characterized by keratin plugs and dyskeratosis. The authors suggest the term *familial dyskeratotic comedones.*

Cantú, J.M., Gómez-Bustamente, M.O., González-Mendoza, A., Sánchez-Corona, J. (1978) Familial comedones. Evidence for autosomal dominant inheritance. *Arch. Dermatol.* **114,** 1807–1809.

Sixteen affected family members. Male to male transmission. Onset was early as 10 years, findings worsened with age. Males were more severely affected than females.

Hall, J.R., Holder, W., Knox, J.M., Knox, J.M., and Verani, R. (1987). Familial dyskeratotic comedones. A report of three cases and review of the literature. *J. Am. Acad. Dermatol.* **17,** 808–814.

A father and his adult son and daughter with diffuse comedones are described. Onset in the father was during his thirties but during the first decade in his children. There was no response to retinoid therapy. The authors compare and contrast this disorder with Darier-White disease and with nevus comedonicus.

Leppard, B.J. (1982). Familial dyskeratotic comedones. *Clin. Exp. Dermatol.* **7,**329–332.

The male proband denied a family history; when other family members were visited by the author, no less than one-half of three generations were found to be similarly affected. None had sought medical advice because the condition was minimally bothersome. The gene had to have been inherited from the proband's father, but no one living could confirm that he had been affected. Leppard believed that the cases of Rodin et al. (1967) and Cantu et al. (1978) represented different entities because of more diffuse involvement and absence of dyskeratosis histologically. However, no micrographs are published by Rodin et al.

Lookingbill, D.P., Ladda, R.L., and Cohen, C. (1983). Generalized epidermolytic hyperkeratosis in the child of a parent with nevus comedonicus. *Arch. Dermatol.* **112,** 223–226.

The father of this girl with classic bullous congenital ichthyosiform erythroderma had two discrete patches of dyskeratotic comedones. He had not brought these to his physicians' attention when questioned about skin disease in the family, and they were only discovered on total skin examination of both parents. The authors suggest that careful examination of parents is warranted and that self-reporting is unreliable. The presumption is that this possibly represents somatic mosaicism in the father for BCIE.

Rodin, H.H., Blankenship, M.K., and Bernstein, C. (1967). Diffuse familial comedones. *Arch. Dermatol.* **95,** 145–146.

A woman with diffuse involvement was reported at a meeting. Although consistently referred to in the literature as an example of familial occurrence, the presenters only stated that the patient reported that her mother and grandmother's family were affected and that her father might also have been, as he had diffuse comedones of the face. No family members were examined to confirm her history.

ORAL-FACIAL-DIGITAL SYNDROME TYPE I (MIM:311200)

(OFD-I; Papillon-Leage-Psaume Syndrome;
Oro-Facial-Digital Syndrome; Oro-Facio-Digital Syndrome; Orofaciodigital Syndrome)

DERMATOLOGIC FEATURES

MAJOR. Multiple milia—fine, small, pearly papules—develop on the face, scalp, pinna, and back of the hands. These may resolve, leaving pitted scarring. Milia are often not mentioned in case descriptions, and it is not clear what proportion of patients actually have them. The skin is variably described as dry or granular in appearance. Coarse, thin, sparse hair is common. The hairs are brittle and break easily. The nails appear to be normal. Oral mucosae are marked by the presence of multiple frenulae that divide the gum ridges. Whitish nodules on the tongue are typical. Bifid tongue, lobulated tongue, and tongue-tie are also described.

MINOR. None.

ASSOCIATED ABNORMALITIES

Cleft lip and cleft palate and pseudocleft of the palate and lip are frequently seen. There may be absence of the lateral incisors and/or supernumerary canine teeth.

The hands are marked by polydactyly that is usually unilateral. Syndactyly, both cutaneous and bony, and brachydactyly have also been described. The toes are less commonly involved. The facies are marked by frontal bossing in approximately one-third of patients, and dystopia canthorum has also been noted. Mental retardation is described in approximately one-half of affected individuals. Ten percent or more have structural brain changes, including cortical atrophy, porencephaly, hydrocephaly, and agenesis of the corpus callosum. It is stated

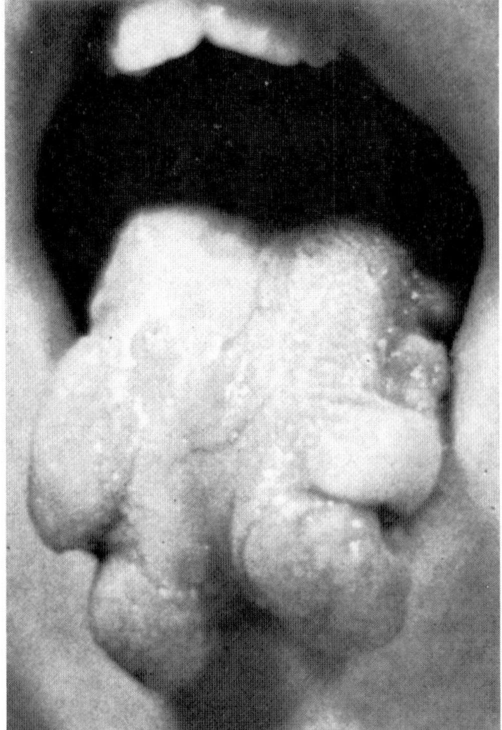

Figure 3.56. Lobulated tongue. (From Gorlin and Psaume, 1962.)

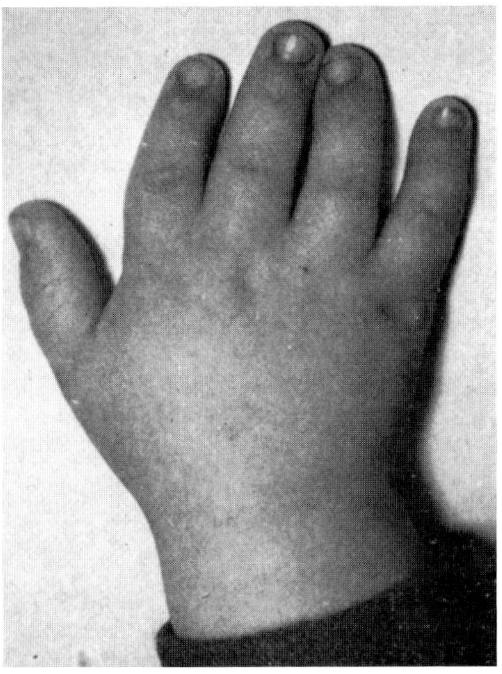

Figure 3.57. Short fingers with clinodactyly and syndactyly. (From Gorlin and Psaume, 1962.)

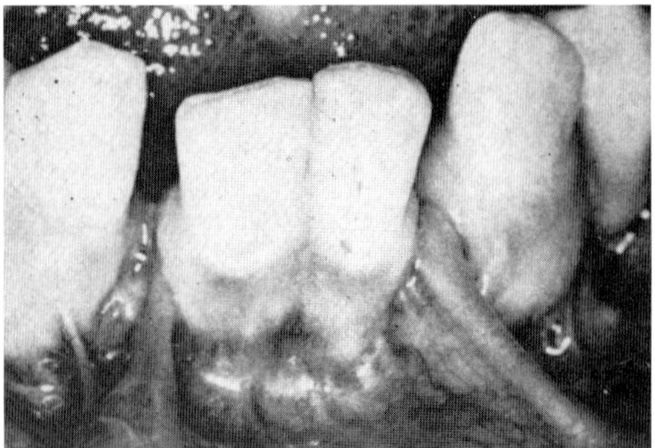

Figure 3.58. Accessory frenulae. (From Gorlin and Psaume, 1962.)

that the mental retardation tends to be mild, but supporting evidence for this contention is not in the literature. Polycystic kidney disease, usually of adult onset, may develop in as many as one-half of affected individuals. There is argument about the nature of the cysts, whether they are similar or dissimilar to those of adult onset polycystic kidney disease.

HISTOPATHOLOGY

LIGHT. The milia are epidermal cysts filled with keratinaceous material, lined with very thin walls. There is a decrease in the number of sebaceous glands. Variation in hair shaft diameter and decreased number of follicles is also described. The nodules on the tongue are connective tissue hamartomas with salivary gland tissue, fat, and muscle.
EM. No information.

BASIC DEFECT

Unknown.

TREATMENT

None for skin findings. Appropriate orthopedic management with oral surgical intervention for structural problems.

A

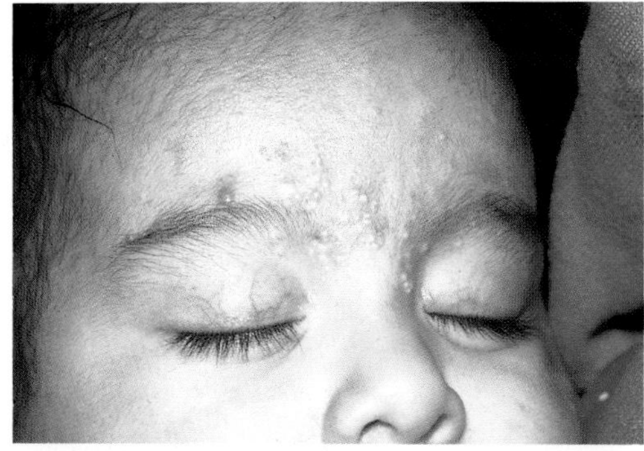

B

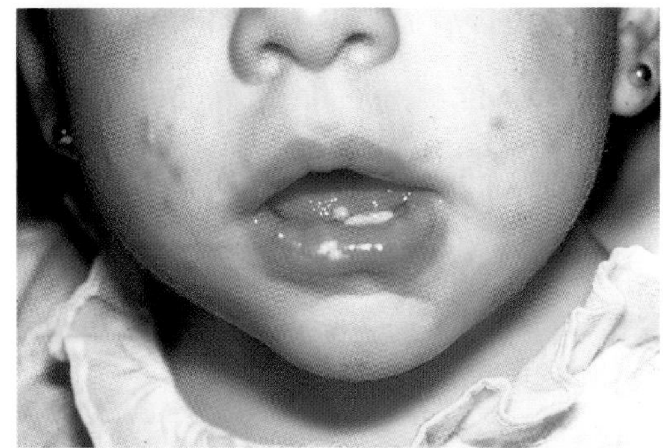

C

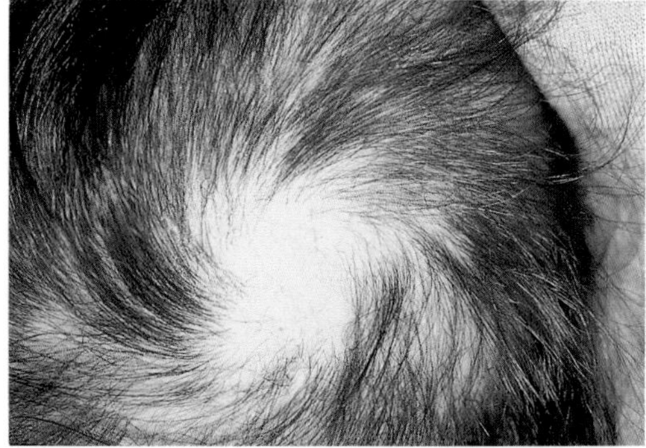

Figure 3.59. **(A)** Multiple milia. **(B)** Milia; abnormal lesion on tongue. **(C)** Scarring alopecia. (Courtesy of Dr. M. Levy, Houston, Texas.)

MODE OF INHERITANCE

X-linked dominant. There are rare reports of male survivors.

PRENATAL DIAGNOSIS

None.

DIFFERENTIAL DIAGNOSIS

OFD-II (Mohr syndrome, MIM:252100) is characterized by absence of milia, bilateral duplication of the hallux (which is extremely rare in OFD-I), short stature, abnormal central incisors, fewer oral frenulae, and usually normal intelligence. Brain malformations have been described in some patients with OFD-II. There is some overlap of OFD-I with OFD-III (Sugarman syndrome, MIM:258850), which is characterized by see-saw winking and is an autosomal recessive disorder. OFD-IV (Mohr-Majewski syndrome, MIM:258860) is the term applied to an autosomal recessive condition of short-limbed dwarfism with polydactyly and tibial dysplasia. These patients share the oral lesions in common with OFD-I. Many other isolated case reports have been labeled as OFD-V, -VI, -VII, and so forth. They share in common with OFD-I oral frenulae or oral lesions and hand malformations. They all appear to be unique disorders. The autosomal dominant popliteal pterygium syndrome (MIM: 119500) and the autosomal recessive Bartsocas-Papas lethal popliteal syndrome (MIM:263650) share multiple oral frenulae in common with OFD-I. All other features are distinct.

Support Group: N.O.R.D.
P.O. Box 8923
New Fairfield, CT
06812
1-800-999-6673

SELECTED BIBLIOGRAPHY

Curry, N.S., Milutinovic, J., Grossnickle, M., and Munden, M. (1992). Renal cystic disease associated with orofaciodigital syndrome. *Urol. Radiol.* **13,** 153–157.

Intrigued by reports of 15 patients with OFD and polycystic kidney disease in the literature, the authors screened three families. Four of six females with OFD-I had renal cysts. The two patients without cysts were 18 months and 13 years old. One affected 30-year-old female had mild hypertension. No other patients were symptomatic. They review the case reports to date.

Gorlin, R.J., and Psaume, J. (1962). Orodigitofacial dysostosis—a new syndrome. A study of 22 cases. *J. Pediatr.* **61,** 520–530.

Reviews the literature. Tabular presentation of findings. The authors describe the skin changes as seborrheic. They state that 1% of individuals with cleft palate will have OFD.

Meinecke, P., and Hayek, H. (1990). Orofacio-digital syndrome type IV (Mohr-Majewski syndrome) with severe expression expanding the known spectrum of anomalies. *J. Med. Genet.* **27,** 200–202.

Case description with photos and radiographs.

Rimoin, D.L., and Edgerton, M.T. (1967). Genetic and clinical heterogeneity in the oral-facial-digital syndromes. *J. Pediatr.* **71,** 94–102.

The authors describe a brother and sister with OFD. They delineate two distinct disorders, OFD-I and OFD-II, with a tabular explanation of the similarities and differences, including mode of inheritance, between them.

Ruess, A.L., Pruzansky, S., and Lis, E.F. (1965). Intellectual development and the OFD syndrome: a review. *Cleft Palate J.* **2,** 350–356.

Nicely sets out the inadequacy of descriptions of intelligence in case reports. They review their own experience. Four of 12 patients were clearly mentally retarded. IQs ranged from single digits to 64. Four patients appeared to have normal intellect, and four did not have formal testing, but were functioning normally. The authors caution against sweeping prognostication for affected newborns.

Salinas, C.F., Pai, G.S., Vera, C.L., Milutinovic, J., Hagerty, R., Cooper, J.D., and Cagha, D.R. (1991). Variability of expression of the orofaciodigital syndrome type I in black females: six cases. *Am. J. Med. Genet.* **38,** 574–582.

The authors point out several differences in the occurrence of specific malformations in OFD between whites and blacks. These may reflect genetic susceptibility. For example, cleft palate is reported in 25% of blacks with OFD-I but in 80% of whites. Similarly, cleft lip occurred in no blacks and in 45% of white patients. As the number of affected individuals is small, these findings need to be interpreted with caution.

Smith, R.A., and Gardner-Medwin, D. (1993). Orofaciodigital syndrome type III in two sibs. *J. Med. Genet.* **30,** 870–872.

Describes cases, contrasting with previous reports, of OFD-VI and Joubert syndrome.

Solomon, L.M., Fretzin, D., and Pruzansky, S. (1970). Pilosebaceous dysplasia in the oral-facial-digital syndrome. *Arch. Dermatol.* **102,** 598–602.

Describes in dermatologic terms skin changes in eight patients.

STEATOCYSTOMA MULTIPLEX (MIM:184500, 184510)

DERMATOLOGIC FEATURES

MAJOR. Oval, firm dermal nodules appear anywhere on the skin surface. There is a preference for the face, upper trunk, and arms. In the majority, lesions begin appearing during puberty, but onset may be later. There is usually no punctum found in the nodule. Lesions range in size from a few millimeters to several centimeters and in color from flesh to yellowish. They may appear superficial or deep.

MINOR. In a minority of patients, recurrent abscesses and inflammation are a problem. An 18-month-old child presented with nodulocystic acne. She had a positive family history for both steatocystoma multiplex and acne.

Lesions occurring within the breast can mimic cystic or malignant disease.

Malignant degeneration was reported only once, and it is not clear if the patient had epidermal inclusion cysts rather than steatocystoma multiplex.

ASSOCIATED ABNORMALITIES

Hypobetalipoproteinemia and cerebellar ataxia were described in several members of a kindred

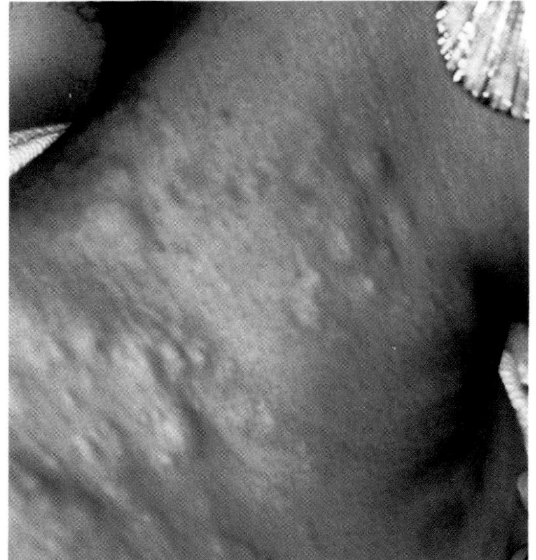

A

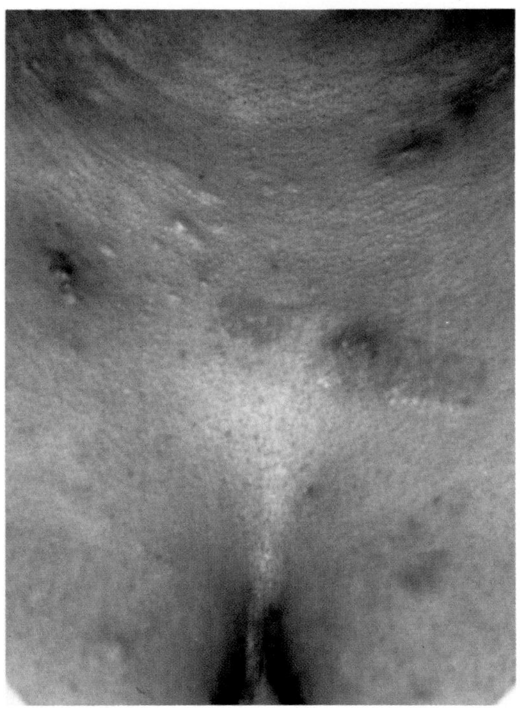

B

Figure 3.60. (A) Flesh-colored lesions on neck. **(B)** Numerous lesions on chest with abscess formation. (From Magrid, 1989.)

with steatocystoma multiplex. Not all members with skin involvement had neurologic and lipid abnormalities and vice versa, so the genetic relationship of features is unclear. Association with natal teeth was described in two families. The nails in these families were normal, suggesting that members did not have a variant of pachyonychia congenita. Preauricular sinuses were described in another pedigree with steatocystoma multiplex.

HISTOPATHOLOGY

Light. Cysts are lined by thin stratified squamous epithelium without evidence of inflammation and filled with a cheesy, oily material. Flattened sebaceous glands are often seen within or near the cyst walls. Occasionally hairs can be found in the lumen.

EM. The cyst walls are composed of keratinizing cells, with decreased keratohyalin.

BASIC DEFECT

In two families with steatocystoma multiplex, mutations in K17 have been identified. In one of these families, some individuals had nail dystrophy suggestive of pachyonychia congenita. Whether alterations in K17 underlie all instances of steatocystoma multiplex remains an open question.

TREATMENT

Treatment with isotretinoin has given inconsistent results. Surgical excision is effective, but its utility may be limited if lesions are extensive.

MODE OF INHERITANCE

Autosomal dominant.

PRENATAL DIAGNOSIS

None.

DIFFERENTIAL DIAGNOSIS

Approximately 5% of patients with pachyonychia congenita (MIM:167200, 167210) have steatocystoma multiplex. Other dermal and subcutaneous nodules such as lipomas, epidermal inclusion cysts, and neurofibromas can be confused clinically. Eruptive vellus hair cysts (MIM:None) are clinically identical and may also be inherited as an autosomal dominant trait. On histopathology, typically there are no sebaceous gland elements within the cyst wall in eruptive vellus hair cysts, and steatocystoma multiplex cysts usually do not contain hairs. However, there appears to be overlap, and it is not clear to me that one can always distinguish between eruptive vellus hair cysts and steatocystoma multiplex.

Support Group: N.O.R.D.
P.O. Box 8923
New Fairfield, CT
06812
1-800-999-6673

SELECTED BIBLIOGRAPHY

Noojin, R.O., and Reynolds, J.P. (1948). Familial steatocystoma multiplex. Twelve cases in three generations. *Arch. Dermatol. Syphilol.* **57,** 1013–1018.

Reviews literature regarding familial cases.

Plewig, G., Wolff, H.H., and Braun-Falco, O. (1982). Steatocystoma multiplex: anatomic reevaluation, electron microscopy, and autoradiography. *Arch. Dermatol. Res.* **272,** 363–380.

An extraordinary paper with three-dimensional reconstruction of cysts. Demonstrates connecting cords between the cyst and the epidermis. They claim their 6-year-old is the youngest patient, apparently unaware of Sachs' claims of congenital onset. They also found entrapped vellus hairs.

Sachs, W. (1938). Steatocystoma multiplex congenitale. Ten cases in three generations. *Arch. Dermatol. Syphilol.* **38,** 877–880.

Lesions present since birth in all 10 affected individuals; small superficial papules that on histopathology showed remnants of hairs. Perhaps eruptive vellus hair cysts and not steatocystoma multiplex?

ECTODERMAL DYSPLASIA SYNDROMES

The ectodermal dysplasias are a group of inherited disorders that share in common developmental defects of two or more of the following: hair; teeth; nails; sweat glands; other ectodermal structures. An exhaustive review and classification system can be found in Freire-Maia, N., and Pinheiro, M. (1984). *Ectodermal Dysplasias: A Clinical and Genetic Study.* Alan R. Liss, New York.

I have limited the scope of this section to those conditions that are more common and are of greater interest to me. Single case reports are not dealt with. If your patient does not appear to fit within one of the entities here, I refer you to the above text. I have not included or adhered to the numerical classification scheme of Freire-Maia and Pinheiro, as I do not personally find it useful in practice, although it can aid in rapid categorization of new syndromes.

Many conditions that involve malformations of the ectodermal structures are not classically defined as ectodermal dysplasias, because these features are neither cardinal nor major. It is helpful, therefore, to look in Appendix B for other syndromes that might have the same ectodermal manifestations as your patient, but may be described in other sections in this text.

AEC SYNDROME (MIM:106260)

(Ankyloblepharon-Ectodermal Dysplasia-Clefting; Hay-Wells)

DERMATOLOGIC FEATURES

MAJOR. At birth, 90% of affected infants present with red, cracking, peeling skin, giving the appearance of collodion membrane, and with erosions suggestive of denuded bullae. The membrane sheds within 1–2 weeks, and the underlying skin is dry and thin in appearance.

The scalp is almost always involved and often develops erosions, crusting, secondary infection, and granulation tissue. About two-thirds of patients have persistent scalp erosions, and in four-fifths recurrent scalp infections occur. Scalp hair is usually coarse and wiry, often light in color. Patchy alopecia is common. Absence or sparseness of body hair is typical.

Ankyloblepharon filiforme adenatum—cutaneous strands between the eyelids—are a herald feature, but are noted in only 70% of patients. These may lyse spontaneously and be overlooked. Conjunctivitis and blepharitis may occur. Lacrimal duct atresia or obstruction is described in about two-thirds of patients.

Nails may be hyperconvex and thickened,

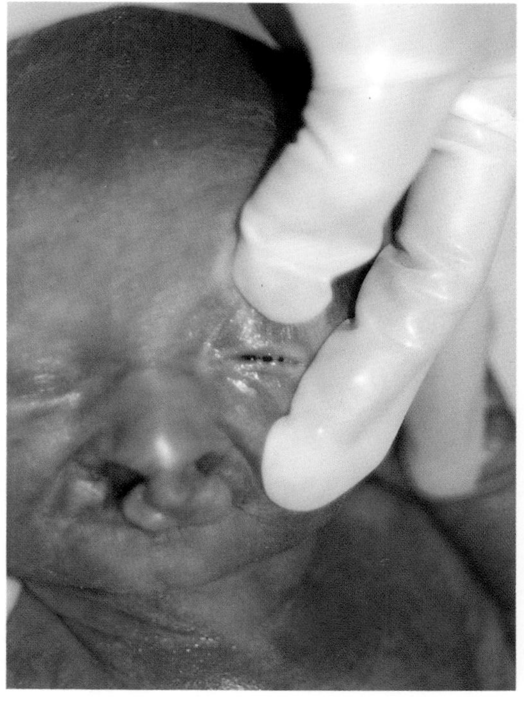

Figure 3.61. Newborn with bilateral cleft lip/palate, ankyloblepharon, and eroded areas on upper chest.

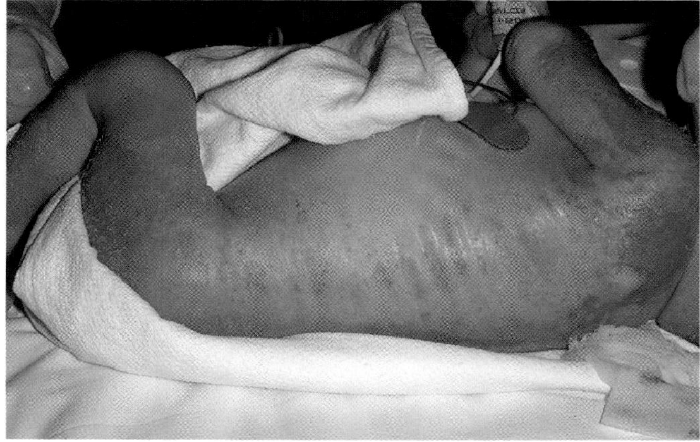

Figure 3.62. Cracking collodion membrane and erosions. (From Vanderhooft et al., 1993.)

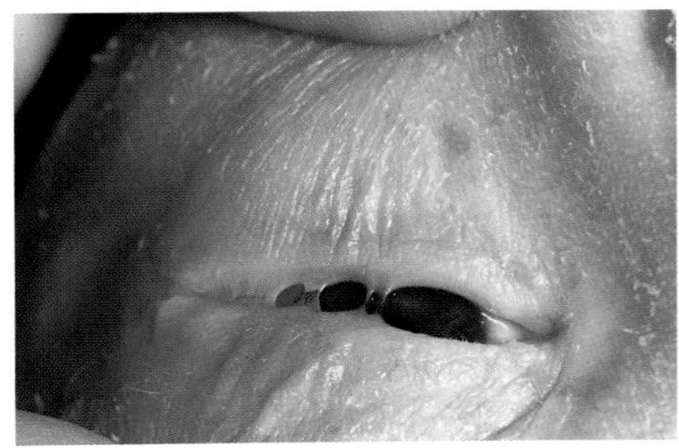

Figure 3.63. Ankyloblepharon filiforme adnatum prior to surgical lysis.

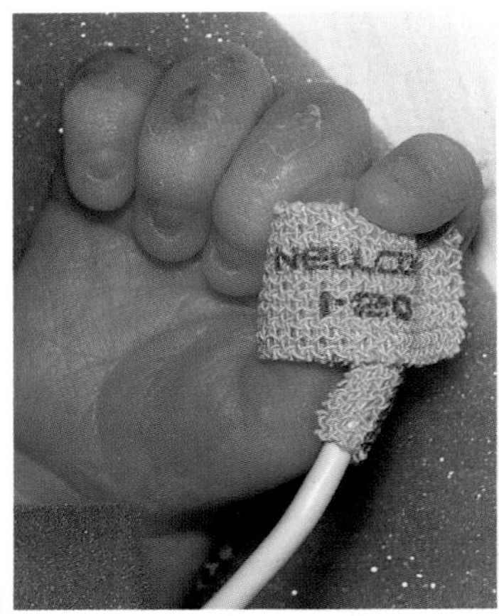

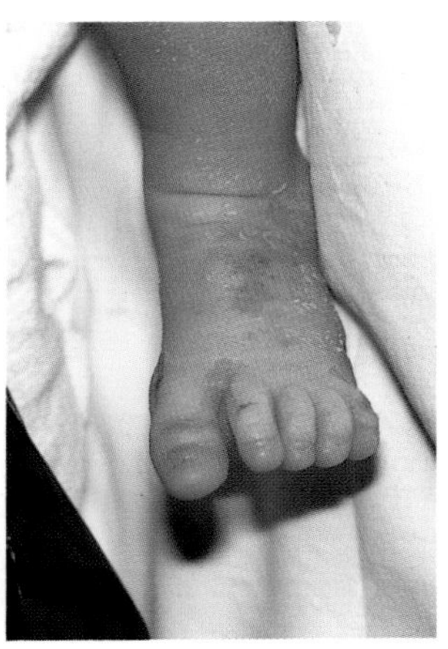

Figure 3.64. Hand **(A)** and foot **(B)** with short deep-set nails, peeling membrane, and erosions.

absent, or partially dystrophic and/or normal in the same individual.

Sweating is usually normal, although subjective heat intolerance has been described.

MINOR. Supernumerary nipples and ectopic breast tissue are occasional findings, as is mild cutaneous syndactyly of toes 2 and 3. Cleft palate with or without cleft lip occurs in 80% of affected individuals. Hypospadias has been described in several males. There may be hypodontia with missing or poorly modeled teeth. Malformed auricles with reduction of the superior pinna is noted in a few. Tortuous external ear canals are also typical, and most patients have recurrent otitis media and secondary conductive hearing loss.

HISTOPATHOLOGY

LIGHT. Decrease in number of sweat glands in some.

EM. On scanning electron microscopy there is a defective cuticular structure of the hairs, a decrease in keratins in the basal and superbasal layers of the epidermis, and disorganized keratin filaments in the stratum corneum.

BASIC DEFECT

Unknown.

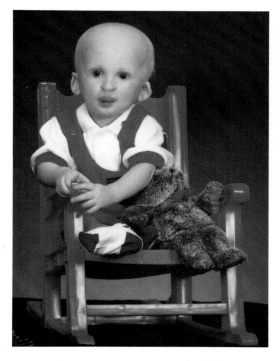

Figure 3.65. Same patient as in Fig. 3.61, now at age 1 year, after cleft repair. (From Vanderhooft et al., 1993.)

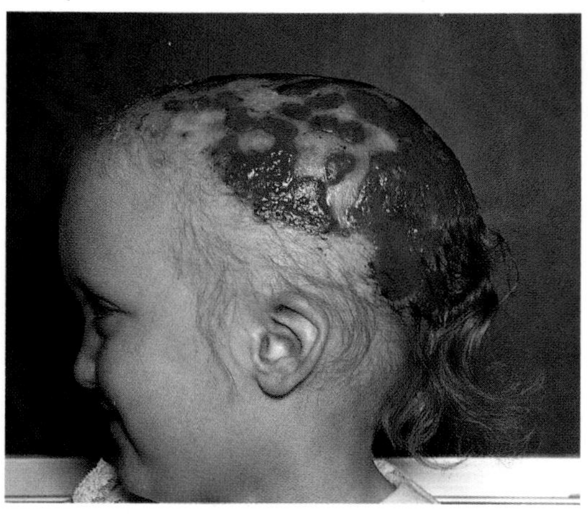

Figure 3.66. Severe scalp erosions in older patient. Flat profile with maxillary hypoplasia. (From Vanderhooft et al., 1993.)

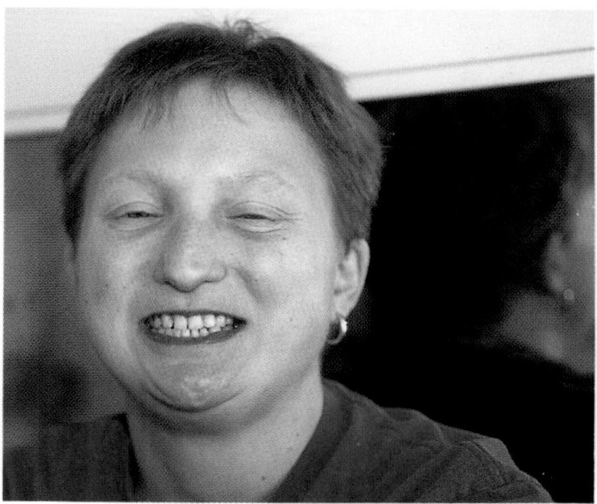

Figure 3.67. More mildly affected adult wearing dentures. Repaired cleft palate, no cleft lip. Periorbital wrinkling, sparse eyebrows, and absent eyelashes.

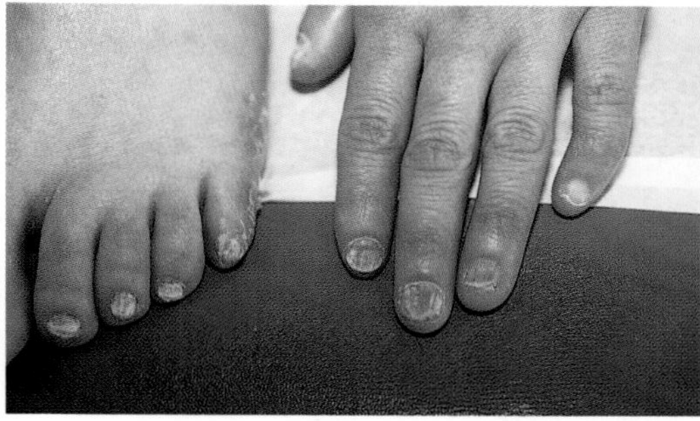

Figure 3.68. Same patient as in Fig. 3.67. Hand shows primary nail dystrophy; toenails have secondary onychomycosis. Clinodactyly of the fifth finger.

TREATMENT

The ankyloblepharon may lyse spontaneously or may require surgical correction.

Light emollients should be used until the collodion membrane sheds.

Vigorous and aggressive scalp care with prompt antibiotic treatment for infection is important.

Appropriate surgical correction of cleft lip and cleft palate.

MODE OF INHERITANCE

Autosomal dominant.

PRENATAL DIAGNOSIS

May be possible by ultrasound for cleft palate with or without cleft lip; this is not highly sensitive.

DIFFERENTIAL DIAGNOSIS

In Rapp-Hodgkin syndrome (MIM:129400), no ankyloblepharon are present, and scalp erosions and infection are much rarer. Skin erosions at birth have led to the misdiagnosis of epidermolysis bullosa simplex and epidermolysis bullosa letalis (MIM:131900, 226700). Peeling skin has led to misdiagnosis of bullous congenital ichthyosiform erythroderma (MIM:113800) and lamellar ichthyosis/nonbullous congenital ichthyosiform erythroderma (MIM:242100). Ankyloblepharon can occur in isolation, in association with chromosomal aneuploidy, and are seen in Bartsocas-Papas (lethal popliteal pterygium syndrome, MIM:263650), the autosomal dominant popliteal pterygium syndrome (MIM:119500), and CHANDS (MIM:214350).

Support Group: N.F.E.D.
219 E. Main, Box 114
Mascoutah, IL 62258-0114
1-618-566-2020.

SELECTED BIBLIOGRAPHY

Fosko, S.W., Stenn, K.S., and Bolognia, J.L. (1992). Ectodermal dysplasias associated with clefting: significance of scalp dermatitis. *J. Am. Acad. Dermatol.* **27,** 249–256.

Reviews the differential of ectodermal dysplasia with cleft palate and cleft lip. Emphasizes the scalp involvement in AEC.

Hay, R.J., and Wells, R.S. (1976). The syndrome of ankyloblepharon, ectodermal defects and cleft lip and palate: an autosomal dominant condition. *Br. J. Dermatol.* **94,** 277–289.

Three pedigrees, one with male-to-male transmission, demonstrating patchy loss of sweat glands.

Vanderhooft, S., Stephan, M.J., and Sybert, V.P. (1993). Severe skin erosions and scalp infections in AEC syndrome. *Pediatr. Dermatol.* **10,** 334–340.

Presentation of 8 new cases and a review of 14 others in the literature. A fine paper!

CLOUSTON SYNDROME (MIM:129500)

(Hidrotic Ectodermal Dysplasia; Jacobsen Syndrome; Waldeyer-Fischer Syndrome; Fischer-Jacobsen-Clouston Syndrome)

DERMATOLOGIC FEATURES

MAJOR. Scalp hair is patchy, wiry, brittle, and pale in color. Hair loss may be progressive, and total alopecia can occur. Body hair is also affected. There is varying severity among family members. Nails may appear milky-white in early childhood, becoming gradually more dystrophic. Nail plates are thick, short, slow growing, and separated distally from the nail bed. The nails are easily lost. Anonychia has been described. In a single individual nails may be affected to varying degrees. Sweating is normal. Palmoplantar hyperkeratosis that increases in severity with age is typical.

MINOR. Malignant degeneration of the palmoplantar keratoderma has been reported, but must be very rare. Darker pigmentation of knuckles, elbows, axillae, areolae, and bony prominences has been described. Oral leukoplakia has been noted in a minority of families. Eccrine poromatosis was reported in one patient.

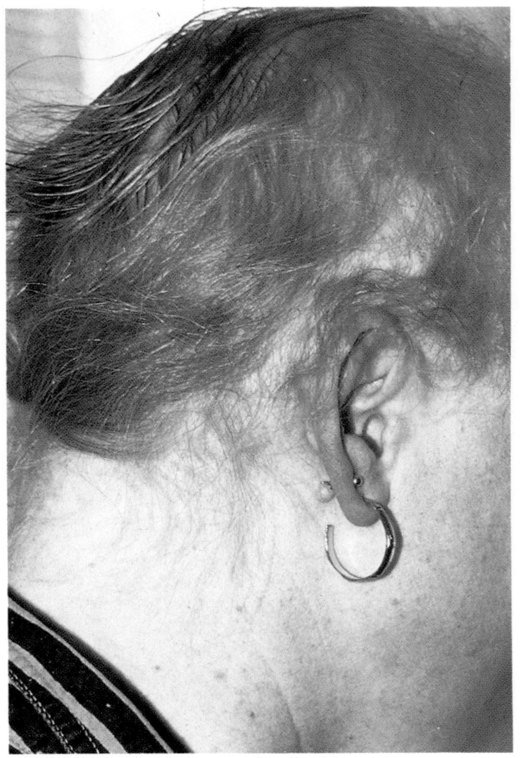
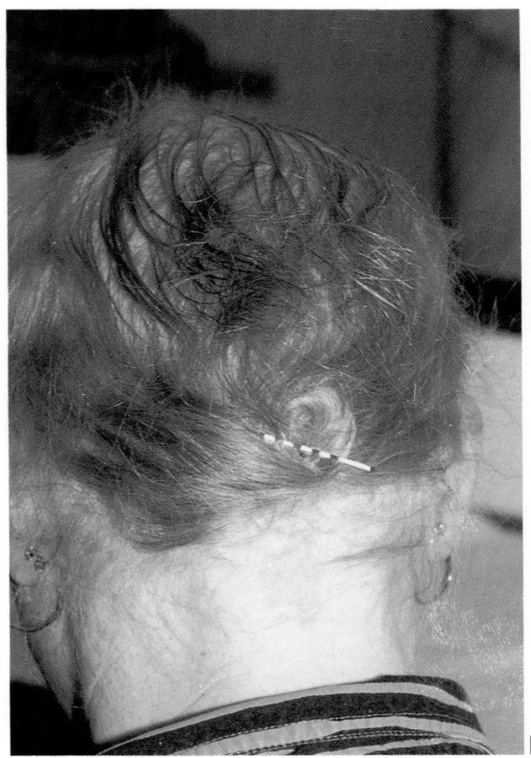

Figure 3.69. (A,B) Patchy alopecia. Hairs are coarse and blond.

ASSOCIATED ABNORMALITIES

Teeth are normal. The only dental abnormality described is caries, which may have been due to hygiene and not to a primary enamel defect.

Conjunctivitis and blepharitis, possibly secondary to absence of protection from eyelashes, is a common complaint. Other eye findings reported in the literature are probably unrelated to the underlying disease. A thickened calvarium was described by Clouston (1929) in six of six patients x-rayed. He also noted tufting of the terminal phalanges that was not present in all patients.

HISTOPATHOLOGY

LIGHT. Orthohyperkeratosis of the palms and soles with a normal granular layer. Abnormal hairs with nonspecific narrowing and fraying.

EM. No specific alterations in the skin from the palms and soles. There is an increased number of desmosomes in the stratum corneum and an abnormal irregular cuticular pattern in the hairs.

BASIC DEFECT

Unknown.

TREATMENT

Nail ablation is sometimes warranted.

MODE OF INHERITANCE

Autosomal dominant. Linkage to keratin gene clusters on chromosomes 12 and 17 has been

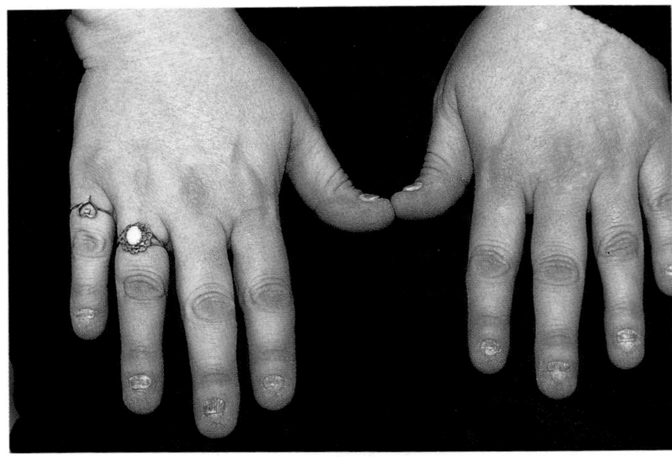

Figure 3.70. Nails are short, thickened, and striated.

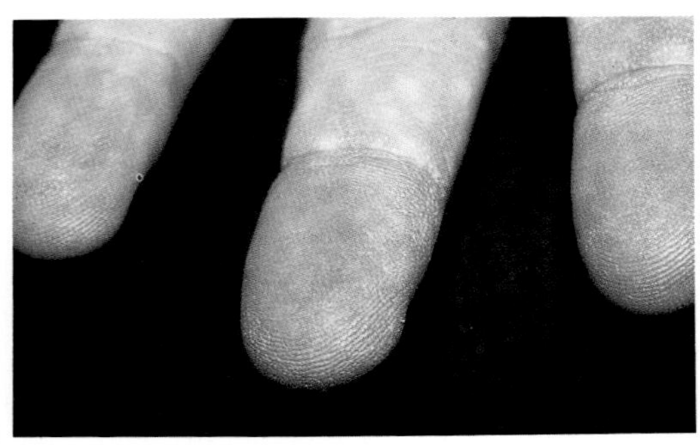

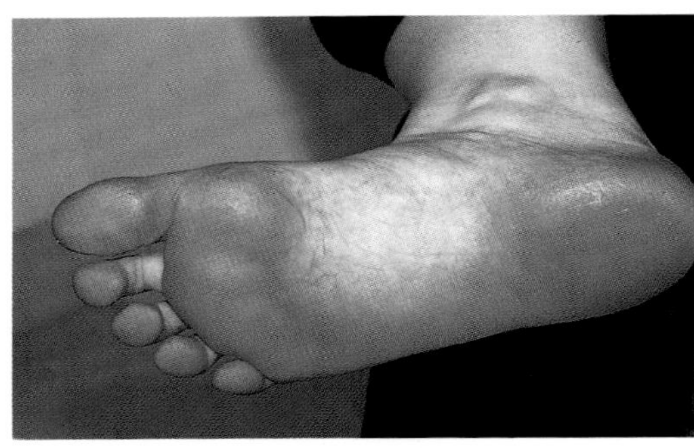

Figure 3.71. (A) Fingerpads are thickened. **(B)** Moderate plantar thickening over the weightbearing surface.

excluded, and linkage to the pericentric region of chromosome 13 has been demonstrated.

PRENATAL DIAGNOSIS

None.

DIFFERENTIAL DIAGNOSIS

Infants with Coffin-Siris syndrome (MIM: 135900) have sparse hair and hypoplasia to absence of the fifth fingernails and toenails. The coarse features and mental retardation of Coffin-Siris are not part of Clouston syndrome. Even in the absence of a positive family history, the two disorders should be easy to distinguish.

Rapp-Hodgkin syndrome (MIM:129400) shares nail and hair abnormalities, but cleft palate with or without cleft lip is not seen in Clouston syndrome.

In pachyonychia congenita (MIM:167200) the hair is usually normal in distribution.

Support Group: N.F.E.D.
219 East Main, Box 114
Mascoutah, IL 62258-0114
1-618-566-2020

SELECTED BIBLIOGRAPHY

Clouston, H.R. (1929). A hereditary ectodermal dysplasia. *Can. Med. Assoc. J.* **21,** 18–31.
A must read for its detail and its homilies.

Rajagopalan, K., and Tay, C.H. (1977). Hidrotic ectodermal dysplasia. Study of a large Chinese pedigree. *Arch. Dermatol.* **113,** 481–485.
Five generations with male-to-male transmission in a Malaysian-Chinese family.

EEC SYNDROME (MIM:129900)

(Ectrodactyly-Ectodermal Dysplasia-Cleft Lip/Palate Syndrome; Split Hand-Split Foot-Ectodermal Dysplasia-Cleft Lip/Palate Syndrome)

DERMATOLOGIC FEATURES

MAJOR. The ectodermal dysplasia is mild and consists of sparse fine scalp hair. Axillary and pubic hair may also be sparse. The nails may be dystrophic and pitted, even on the normal digits. This is in addition to absent or dystrophic nails overlying abnormal phalanges. Sweating is usually normal.

MINOR. Occasionally hyperkeratosis of the lower extremities and dry skin are reported.

ASSOCIATED ABNORMALITIES

Anodontia and/or hypodontia with premature loss of secondary teeth is described. Ectrodactyly (lobster claw deformity) occurs in 80%–100% of patients, depending on the series. Foot involvement is more constant than hand involvement. Cleft palate with or without cleft lip is described in 70%–100% of cases. Genitourinary abnormalities including hydronephrosis and structural renal or genital malformations are found in about one-third of affected individuals. Mental retardation is stated to occur in as many as 5%–10% of patients, but most cited cases are either atypical or have chromosomal aneuploidy or other possible causes for mental retardation (e.g., prematurity with a severe neonatal course, a positive family history of dull intellect). Choanal atresia has been reported in two patients. The lacrimal puncta and ducts are often malformed or atretic. Excessive tearing, photophobia, and inflammation are reported in 80% of affected individuals. Hearing loss occurs in about 15%; it is unclear if it is primary or secondary to recurrent otitis media.

HISTOPATHOLOGY

LIGHT. No information.
EM. No information.

BASIC DEFECT

Unknown.

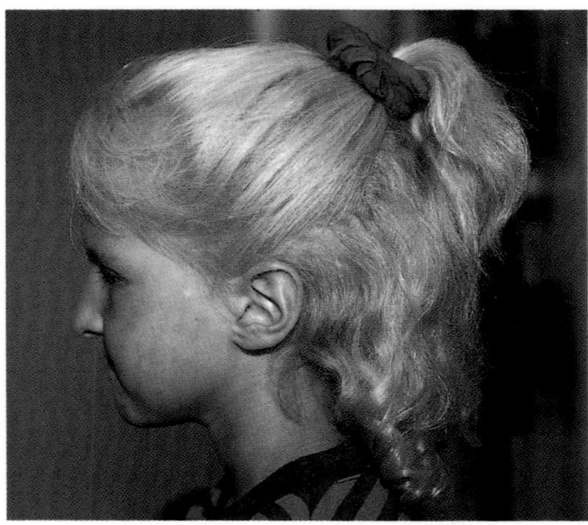

Figure 3.72. Sparse, blond, coarse hair; some are spangled; chronic blepharitis due to abnormal tearing; flat profile.

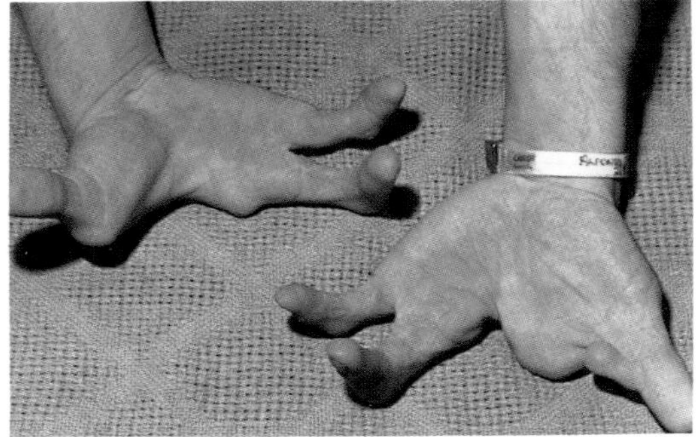

A

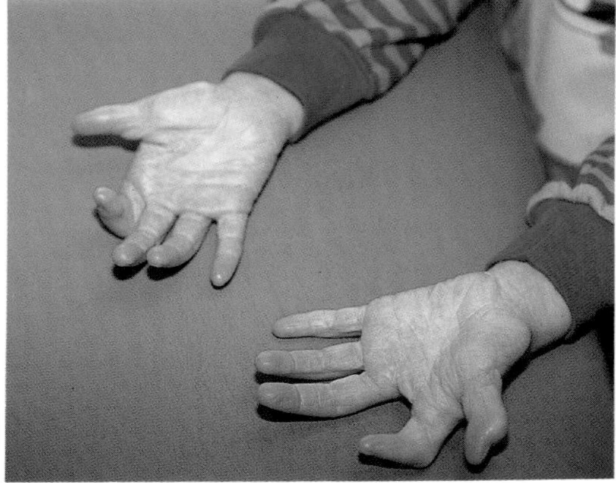

B

Figure 3.73. **(A,B)** Variability in hand malformations.

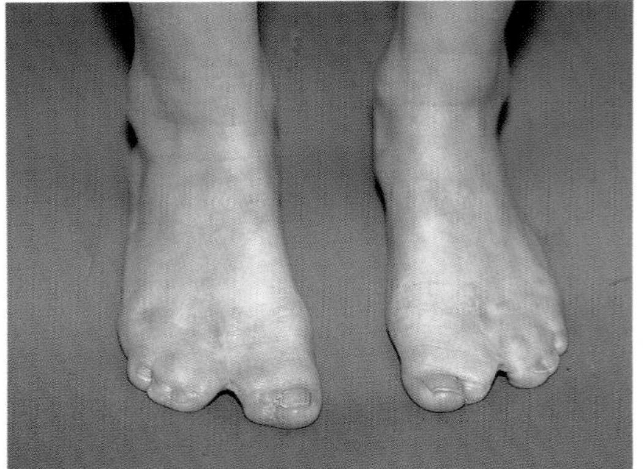

A

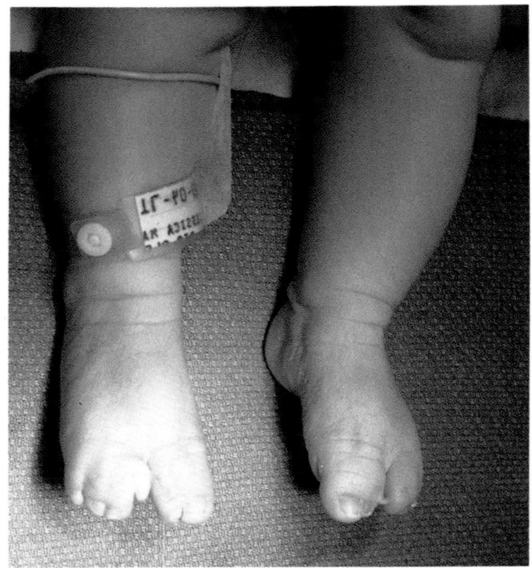

B

Figure 3.74. **(A,B)** Feet showing deep median cleft and syndactyly.

TREATMENT

None.

MODE OF INHERITANCE

Autosomal dominant with marked variability in expression and evidence for reduced penetrance. It has been suggested that EEC may be a contiguous gene syndrome with a deletion at 7q21.3–7q22.1. Locus heterogeneity demonstrated for split hand-split foot based on linkage studies.

PRENATAL DIAGNOSIS

Possibly by ultrasound for limb defects and palatal defects. It is likely to be unreliable. Potentially by linkage analysis.

DIFFERENTIAL DIAGNOSIS

All four limbs are involved in the odontotrichomelic syndrome (MIM:273400), with severe absence deformities. Aplasia cutis congenita with limb defects (Adams-Oliver syndrome, MIM:100300) can be associated with ectrodactyly. No ectodermal defects other than aplasia cutis congenita occur. Other forms of ectodermal dysplasia with cleft palate with or without cleft lip include Rapp-Hodgkin syndrome (MIM:129400), Hay-Wells (ankyloblepharon-ectodermal dysplasia-cleft lip/palate) syndrome (MIM:106260), and rarer conditions. These all need to be considered in the differential. The ECP syndrome (ectrodactyly with cleft palate, MIM:129830) lacks ectodermal abnormalities. Individuals with focal dermal hypoplasia of Goltz (MIM:305600) can have ectrodactyly and cleft palate and cleft lip. The skin features are distinctive, with atrophoderma and hypoplasia to absence of the dermis.

Support Group: N.F.E.D.
219 East Main, Box 114
Mascoutah, IL 62258-0114
1-618-566-2020

SELECTED BIBLIOGRAPHY

Qumsiyeh, M.B. (1992). EEC syndrome (ectrodactyly, ectodermal dysplasia and cleft lip/palate) is on 7p11.2–q21.3. *Clin. Genet.* **42,** 701.

There is a typo in the title—the deletion is at 7*q*11.2.–q21.3. This letter cites eight reports of deletions or translocation in this chromosomal region that are associated with EEC syndrome.

Rodini, E.S.O., and Richieri-Costa, A. (1990). EEC syndrome: report on 20 new patients, clinical and genetic considerations. *Am. J. Med. Genet.* **37,** 42–53.

Nine familial cases demonstrate extreme intrafamilial variability. Excellent discussion of differential diagnosis with descriptions of rare case reports. Unfortunately, this article is difficult to read due to the *American Journal of Medical Genetics* citation style. For example, one paragraph includes 10 words of text that are embedded in 13 lines of citations.

Trueb, R.M., Bruckner-Tuderman, L., Wyss, M., Widmer, M., Wuthrich, B., and Burg, G. (1995). Scalp dermatitis, distinctive hair abnormalities and atopic disease in the ectrodactyly-ectodermal dysplasia-clefting syndrome. *Br. J. Dermatol.* **132,** 621–625.

Isolated case, female with ectrodactyly, cleft lip and palate, and severe scalp involvement, quite atypical for EEC. In addition, she had bilateral inguinal hernias and a rectovaginal fistula, absence of sweating, and heat intolerance. Unusual in the severity of the ectodermal defects.

Wallis, C.E. (1988). Ectrodactyly (split-hand/split-foot) and ectodermal dysplasia with normal lip and palate in four generation kindred. *Clin. Genet.* **34,** 252–257.

A family with tooth abnormalities, variable sparse hair, and ectrodactyly. Authors argue for a distinct autosomal dominant disorder from EEC because of the lack of palatal clefting. It is not clear to me that this is a warranted assumption.

FOCAL FACIAL ECTODERMAL DYSPLASIA (MIM:136500, 227260)

(Brauer Syndrome; Bitemporal Aplasia Cutis Congenita; Facial Ectodermal Dysplasia)

Includes Setleis Syndrome

DERMATOLOGIC FEATURES

Major. Bilateral, but not necessarily symmetric, scarring of the temples is present at birth. Small, round, depressed areas may range in number from 1 to 10 and in size up to 1 cm. These are often described as hyperpigmented or purplish. There is absence of sweating over the defects. The lateral one-third of the eyebrows is sparse, and there are linear vertical wrinkles of the forehead. In the autosomal recessive form, lower eyelashes are usually absent with doubling of the upper lashes.

Minor. In Setleis syndrome, full lips and coarse facies are described. There are deep rugations of the skin around the lips and chin.

ASSOCIATED ABNORMALITIES

None.

HISTOPATHOLOGY

LIGHT. Absence of hair follicles and sebaceous glands with sparse sweat glands; an atrophic dermis with a thin atrophic epidermis.
EM. No information.

BASIC DEFECT

Unknown.

TREATMENT

None.

MODE OF INHERITANCE

Autosomal dominant with male-to-male transmission documented. A number of sibships with normal parents have been described as autosomal recessive. However, given the subtlety of expression that can be associated with the gene, minimal changes in a parent may have been overlooked. I have seen one family in which a mother with small bitemporal scars and a lovely visage, albeit with a full nose, had a daughter with extreme findings of classic Setleis. She reported that her father looked just like his granddaughter. Thus, my experience parallels that of DiLernia et al. (1991).

PRENATAL DIAGNOSIS

None.

DIFFERENTIAL DIAGNOSIS

This disorder is unlikely to be confused with any other and is more likely to be overlooked in an otherwise healthy child. It may be misdiagnosed as being caused by forceps or as aplasia cutis congenita (MIM:Many). Skin defects in MLS (microphthalmia with linear skin defects) or MIDAS (microphthalmia, dermal aplasia, and sclerocornea, MIM:309801) syn-

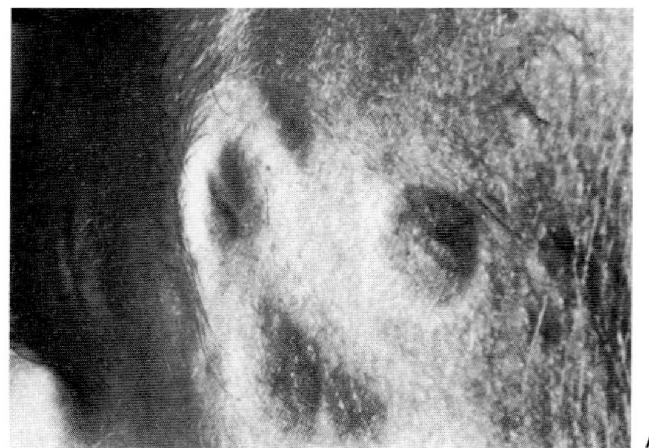
A

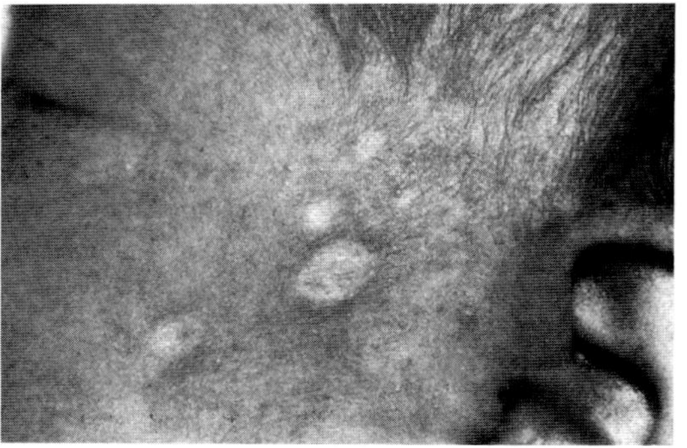
B

Figure 3.75. **(A)** Round atrophic "defects" on temple. (From Jensen, 1971.) **(B)** Lesions on cheek in different individual. (From Kowalski and Fenske, 1992.)

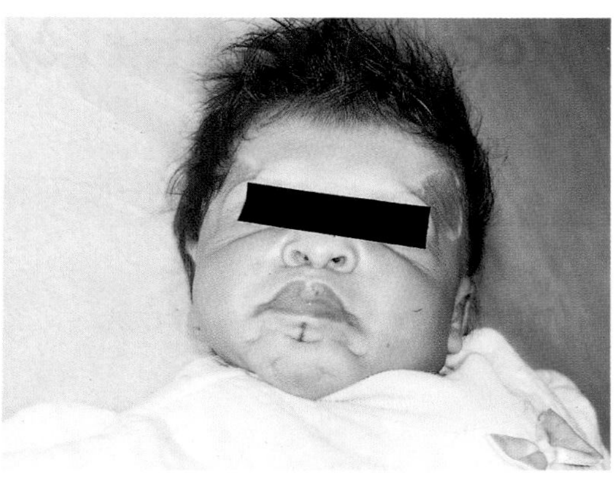

Figure 3.76. Full fleshy nose and chin with bilateral temple scars. There is a linear defect on the chin. This patient's mother had minimally apparent temporal scars. (Courtesy of Dr. M. Cunningham, Seattle, Washington.)

drome consist of areas of erosion on the face similar to lesions of aplasia cutis congenita. These go on to heal as scars. This condition is due to a chromosomal deletion and/or point mutation at Xp22.1.

Support Group: N.O.R.D.
P.O. Box 8923
New Fairfield, CT 06812
1-800-999-6673

SELECTED BIBLIOGRAPHY

DiLernia, V., Neri, I., and Patrizi, A. (1991). Focal facial dermal dysplasia: two familial cases. *J. Am. Acad. Dermatol.* **25,** 389–391.

A mother with bilateral temporal scars, absence of lower eyelashes, who had a son with full lips, bitemporal scars, absence of lower lashes, sparse eyebrows, and a facies typical of Setleis syndrome. The authors suggested that the unaffected parents reported by Setleis et al. (1963) might have had lesions that were overlooked. In the Setleis et al. report, however, the parents appear to have been well examined, although one purportedly unaffected mother had the same nasal configuration as her affected children.

Jensen, N.E. (1971). Congenital ectodermal dysplasia of the face. *Br. J. Dermatol.* **84,** 410–416.

Two pedigrees, one with autosomal dominant inheritance in five generations with male-to-male transmission, one with three of seven siblings affected. A double row of upper eyelashes was present in the latter.

Kowalski, D.C., and Fenske, N.A. (1992). The focal facial dermal dysplasias: report of a kindred and a proposed new classification. *J. Am. Acad. Dermatol.* **27,** 575–582.

Reviews the literature. Proposes three types of focal dermal dysplasia, one autosomal dominant (Brauer), one autosomal recessive, and one autosomal recessive with other facial abnormalities (Setleis). However, three affected siblings in the family they describe presented with preauricular, not temporal, lesions, suggesting a fourth entity!

Magid, M.L., Prendiville, J.S., and Esterly, N.B. (1988). Focal facial dermal dysplasia: bitemporal lesions resembling aplasia cutis congenita. *J. Am. Acad. Dermatol.* **18,** 1203–1207.

The authors argue that Setleis and Brauer syndromes are the same based on photos of a pedigree published by McGeoch et al. (*Arch. Dermatol.* **107,** 591–595, 1974), in which a patient from an autosomal dominant pedigree had the same chin clefting as one the Setleis et al. patients. However, the patient's lips were normal, as were the eyelashes.

Setleis, H., Kramer, B., Valcarcel, M., and Einhorn, A.H. (1963). Congenital ectodermal dysplasia of the face. *Pediatrics* **32,** 540–548.

Two siblings in two sibships and a fifth unrelated patient, all Puerto Rican. All patients had a striking nasal configuration.

GAPO SYNDROME (MIM:230740)

(Growth Retardation-Alopecia-Pseudoanodontia-Optic Atrophy)

DERMATOLOGIC FEATURES

MAJOR. This is a very rare disorder. The scalp hair and eyebrows are present at birth, but are lost after the first year. Eyelashes and body hair are also involved. There is a doughy appearance to the facial skin with coarse wrinkling of the forehead, cheeks, and neck.

MINOR. None.

ASSOCIATED ABNORMALITIES

Failure of both primary and secondary teeth to erupt results in a cherubic appearance to the jaws. Abnormal facies with frontal bossing, mild midfacial hypoplasia, full lips, and coarse features with a large persistent anterior fontanelle are typical.

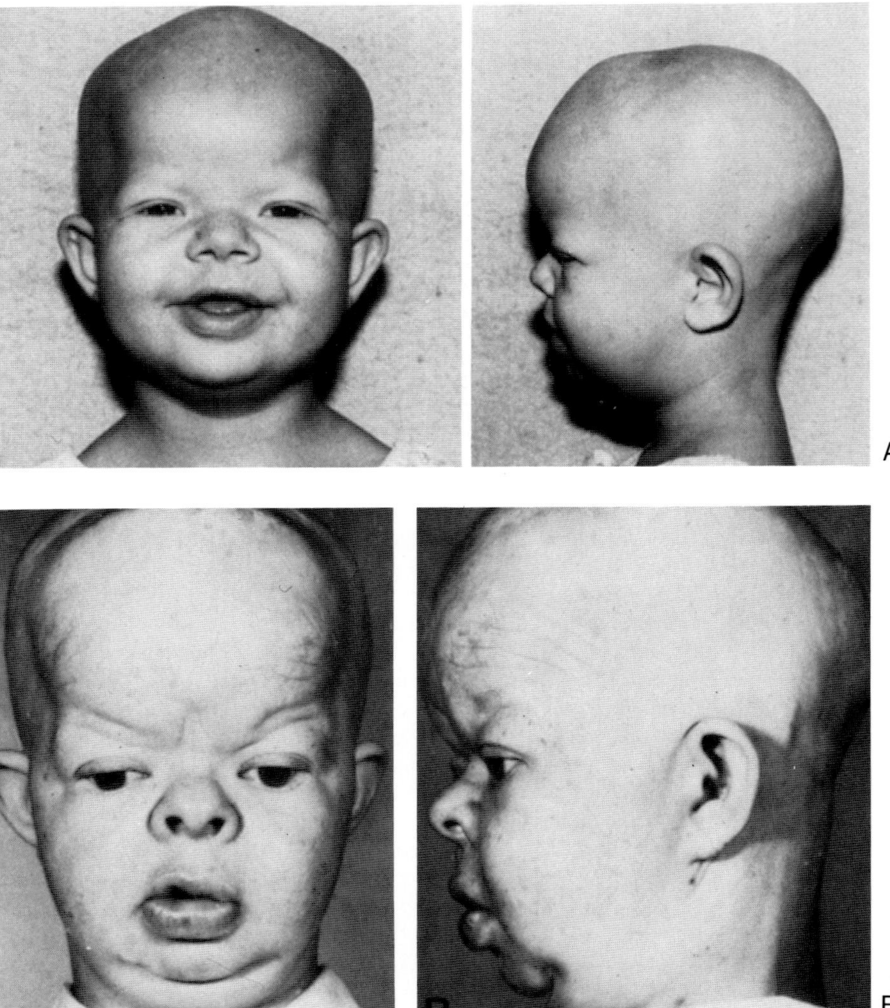

Figure 3.77. **(A)** Two-year-old with full lips and total alopecia. **(B)** Older individual showing progressive thickening of skin. (From Tipton and Gorlin, 1984.)

Proportionate short stature is a primary feature. While puberty may be normal, secondary hypogonadism with irregular menses or oligospermia has been described.

Optic atrophy occurs during childhood and in adult life and is described in half of reported patients. Keratoconus and glaucoma have been described in some. Atherosclerosis was described in two patients who died at ages 35 and 39 years. Based on these two patients it has been suggested that lifespan is decreased.

HISTOPATHOLOGY

LIGHT. The epidermis is thin with absence of ridges. There are clumps of PAS-positive hyalin material in the dermis. The hair follicles are

C
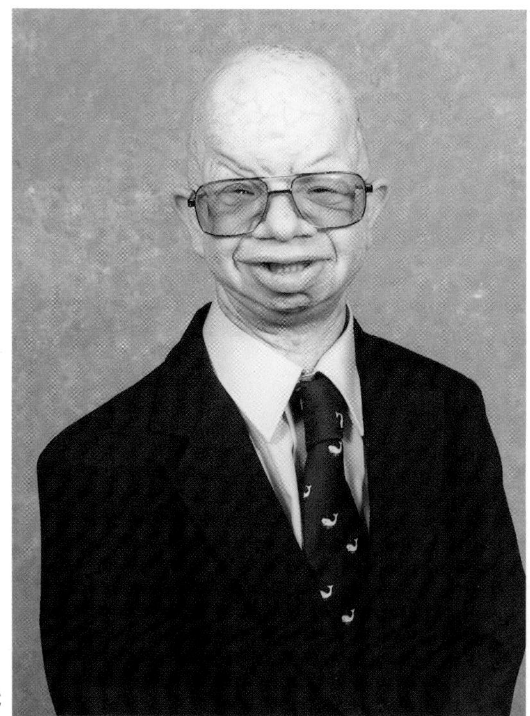

Figure 3.77C. 18 year-old, exhibiting typical features. (Courtesy of the family.)

surrounded by similar material. This is based on the study of one patient. Similar deposits were described in other organs from the same individual.

EM. No information.

BASIC DEFECT

Unknown. Believed to be a storage disorder with progressive deposition of PAS-positive hyalin material.

TREATMENT

None.

MODE OF INHERITANCE

Autosomal recessive with affected siblings and consanguinity.

PRENATAL DIAGNOSIS

None.

DIFFERENTIAL DIAGNOSIS

Failure of tooth eruption can occur in a number of syndromes, all of which are easily clinically distinguished. GAPO is so striking that misdiagnosis is unlikely. Cleidocranial dysostosis (MIM: 119600) shares a large anterior fontanelle and failure of tooth eruption, but is readily distinguished by normal hair and clavicular abnormalities.

Support Group: N.F.E.D.
219 East Main, Box 114
Mascoutah, IL 62258-0114
1-618-566-2020

SELECTED BIBLIOGRAPHY

Tipton, R.E., and Gorlin, R.J. (1984). Growth retardation, alopecia, pseudoanodontia and optic atrophy—the GAPO syndrome: report of a patient and review of the literature. *Am. J. Med. Genet.* **19,** 209–216.

A nicely written case report with follow-up photos of patient originally reported in 1947.

Wajntal, A., Koiffmann, C.P., Mendonca, B.B., Epps-Quaglia, D., Sotto, M.N., Rati, P.B.M., and Opitz, J.M. (1990). GAPO syndrome (McKusick 23074)—A connective tissue disorder: report on two affected sibs and on the pathologic findings in the older. *Am. J. Med. Genet.* **37,** 213–223.

A detailed review of two siblings, subjects of three previous reports, and a postmortem evaluation of one.

HYPOHIDROTIC ECTODERMAL DYSPLASIA (MIM:305100)

(Christ-Siemens-Touraine Syndrome; Anhidrotic Ectodermal Dysplasia)

DERMATOLOGIC FEATURES

MAJOR. At birth, affected males often have peeling skin, which may be severe enough to be mistaken for a collodion membrane. Scalp hair is sparse, fine, and blonde. It may thicken and darken at puberty. Sexual hairs may be normal, including the beard. Other body hair is usually sparse or absent.

Sweating is absent or markedly inadequate; sweat pores are absent on visual examination of fingertips. Bouts of fever because of inabil-

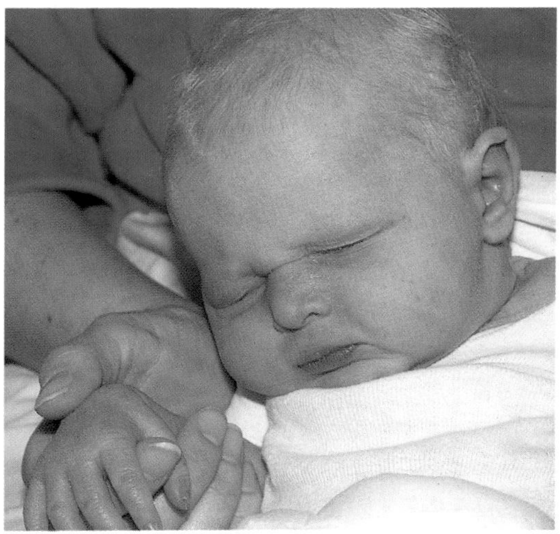

A

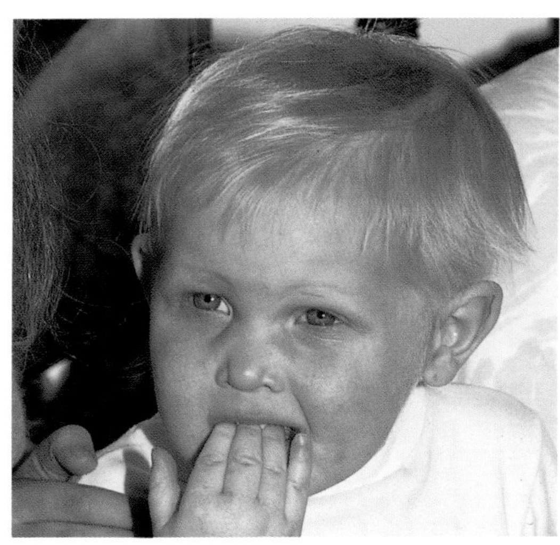

B

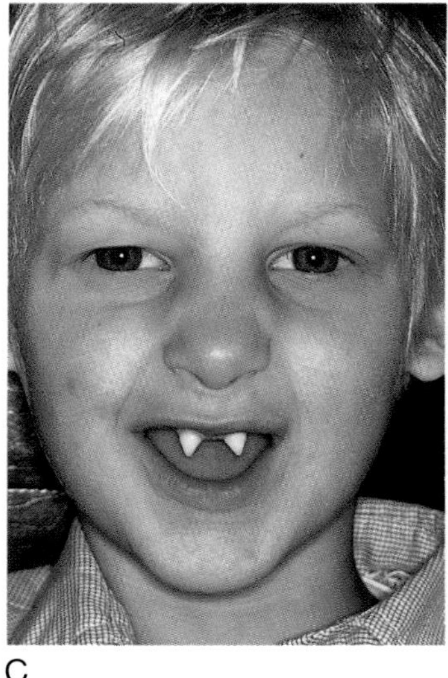

C

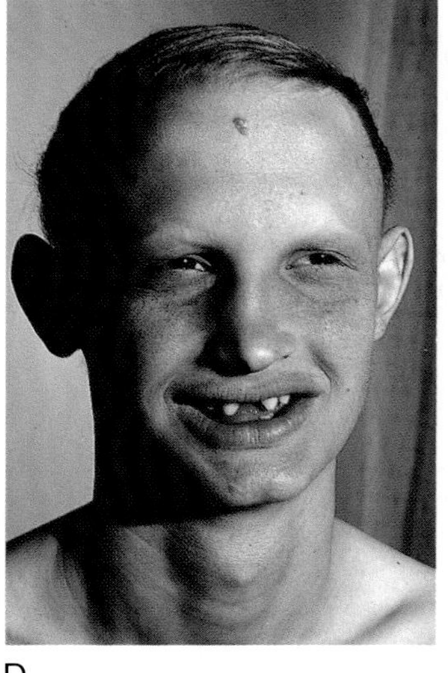

D

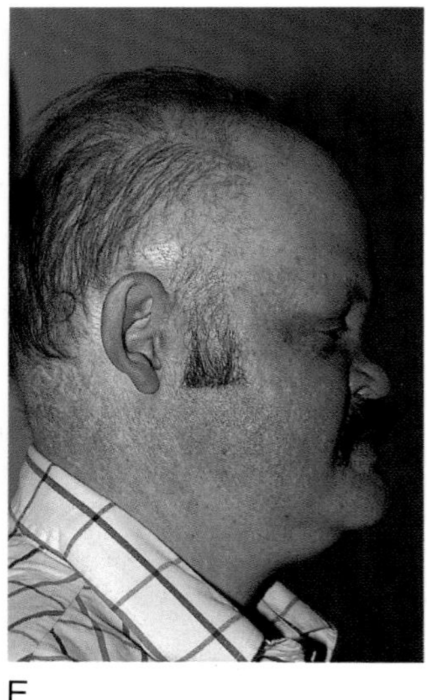

E

Figure 3.78. Newborn **(A)**, toddler, **(B)**, child **(C)**, and adult **(D)** males with hypohidrotic ectodermal dysplasia. Profile **(E)** shows saddled nose deformity and normal facial hair.

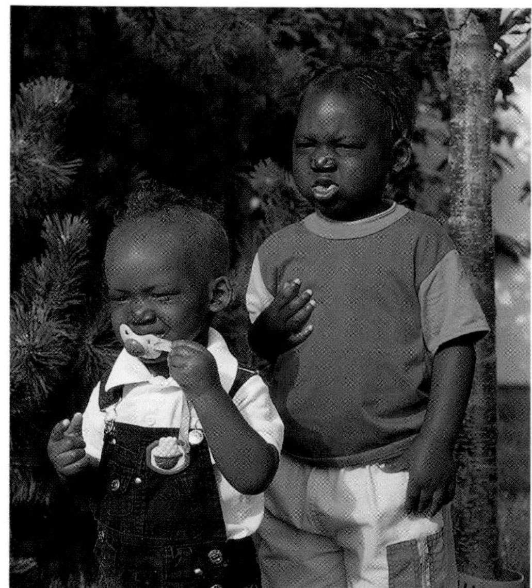

Figure 3.79. Affected brothers with periorbital wrinkling, sparse hair, unusual nasal configuration, and full lips.

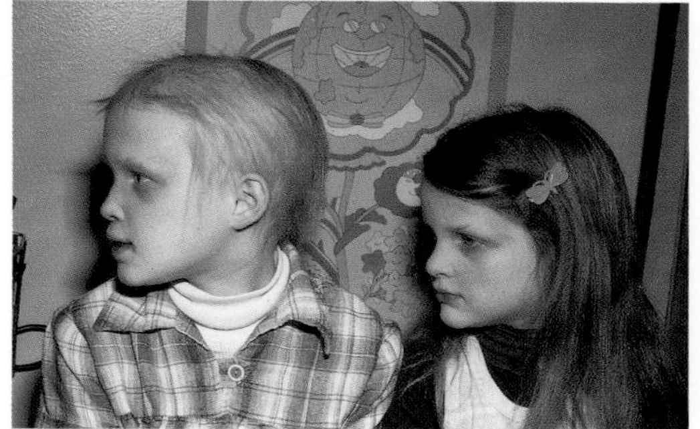

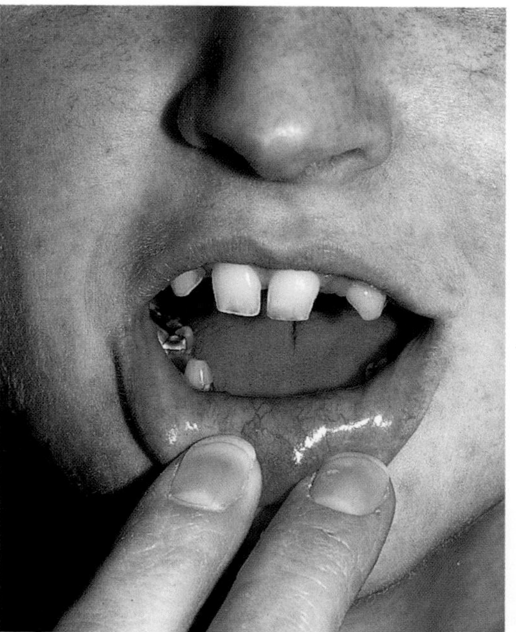

Figure 3.80. (A) Sisters expressing to different degrees. (From Sybert, 1989.) (B) Peg-shaped and missing teeth in a carrier mother.

ity to maintain effective body cooling are typical during infancy and early childhood.

The nails are essentially normal; occasional descriptions of friable and thin nails do not fall convincingly outside the range of normal.

Periorbital hyperpigmentation and fine wrinkling around the eyes is classic. Eczema is typical (70%) and may be difficult to manage. The skin may also be pale and translucent in appearance.

Minor. Absent, simple, or accessory nipples in the male (one-third); also seen in female carriers. Milia-like facial lesions that represent enlarged sebaceous glands are not uncommon.

ASSOCIATED ABNORMALITIES

The facies are typical with relative frontal bossing, a concave midface, and saddle nose. Variable hypodontia to anodontia with peg-shaped primary and secondary teeth is typical. The alveolar ridges are hypoplastic, giving rise to the typical configuration of full, everted lips.

Otolaryngologic complications include thick secretions, oezena, impacted cerumen, sinusitis, recurrent upper respiratory tract infections, decreased saliva production, hoarse voice, and an increased tendency to develop pneumonia. Gastroesophageal reflux appears to be more common than expected and may be severe, with failure to thrive occurring in upwards of 20% of affected males. Height and weight appear compromised in childhood but seem to normalize in adult life. Asthma and wheezing occur in about two-thirds of patients.

Mortality in infancy, based on literature stud-

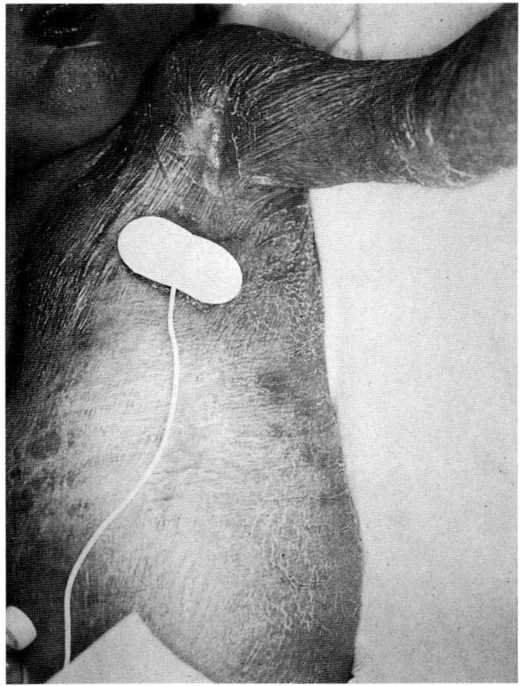

Figure 3.81. Scaling, peeling skin in a newborn, readily misdiagnosed as ichthyosis. (From National Foundation for Ectodermal Dysplasias, 1989.)

ies, may approach 30%. Whether there is an increased incidence of SIDS is unclear.

HISTOPATHOLOGY

LIGHT. There is hypoplasia to absence of sweat glands with hypoplasia to absence of pilosebaceous units.

EM. No information.

BASIC DEFECT

Unknown. One patient with a deletion at locus DXS732 has been described. The tabby mouse appears to be homologous.

TREATMENT

Environmental control for temperature stability is paramount. Aggressive and early dental restoration with early dentures and, ultimately, placement of dental implants. Ear, nose, and throat management and good ophthalmologic and dermatologic care are important.

MODE OF INHERITANCE

X-linked recessive. The gene has been mapped to Xq12–q13.1 and recently cloned. Reports of autosomal recessive inheritance of hypohidrotic ectodermal dysplasia *clinically indistinguishable* from hypohidrotic ectodermal dysplasia are mostly unconvincing. Many severely affected females from kindreds with clear-cut X-linked recessive inheritance are described in the literature. Recurrence risk counseling for parents of affected females should emphasize the likelihood of X-linked recessive inheritance.

Carrier detection requires careful physical examination with special attention to patchy distribution of body hairs and sweat pores as well as evidence for hypodontia. Carrier detection by linkage studies is possible in informative families.

PRENATAL DIAGNOSIS

Possible in some families by linkage. Fetal skin biopsy demonstrating absence of hair follicles is also diagnostic.

DIFFERENTIAL DIAGNOSIS

Passarge syndrome (MIM:224900) can be distinguished by hypertelorism, hearing loss, and hypoplastic sweat pores that are reduced in number in affected individuals rather than absent or patchy. At birth, scaling may lead to misdiagnosis of X-linked ichthyosis (MIM: 308100) or lamellar ichthyosis (MIM:242100).

Support Group: N.F.E.D.
219 East Main, Box 114
Mascoutah, IL 62258-0114
1-618-566-2020

SELECTED BIBLIOGRAPHY

Blecher, S.R., Kapalanga, J., and Lalonde, D. (1990). Induction of sweat glands by epidermal growth factor in murine X-linked anhidrotic ectodermal dysplasia. *Nature* **345,** 542–544.

Injections of epidermal growth factor for 7 days after birth resulted in development of sweat glands and dermal ridges in the tabby mouse. Treatment for 30 days resulted in sweating that persisted after treatment was stopped.

Clarke, A., Phillips, D.I.M., Brown, R., and Harper, P.S. (1987). Clinical aspects of X-linked hypohidrotic ectodermal dysplasia. *Arch. Dis. Child.* **62,** 989–996.

Authors have surveyed the population of Wales, and this is an excellent review of the less commonly appreciated clinical features of the disorder.

Executive and Scientific Advisory Boards of the National Foundation of Ectodermal Dysplasias (1989). Scaling skin in the neonate: a clue to the early diagnosis of X-linked hypohidrotic ectodermal dysplasia (Christ-Siemens-Touraine syndrome). *J. Pediatr.* **114,** 600–602.

Reviews the experience of National Foundation of Ectodermal Dysplasias families. Seventy percent of 81 males with hypohidrotic ectodermal dysplasia had marked scaling of the skin in the newborn period.

Passarge, E., Nuzum, C.T., and Schubert, W.K. (1966). Anhidrotic ectodermal dysplasia as an autosomal recessive trait in an inbred kindred. *Humangenetik* **3,** 181–185.

Cited as original suggestion that autosomal recessive and X-linked recessive hypohidrotic ectodermal dysplasia were clinically identical. All but one affected individual were deaf, and all had true hypertelorism.

Sybert, V.P. (1989). Hypohidrotic ectodermal dysplasia: argument against an autosomal recessive form clinically indistinguishable from X-linked hypohidrotic ectodermal dysplasia (Christ-Siemens-Touraine syndrome). *Pediatr. Dermatol.* **6,** 76–81.

Reviews case reports of sibships with affected females and concludes the evidence for autosomal recessive inheritance of classic hypohidrotic ectodermal dysplasia is minimal. Forty-six references.

Zonana, J., Gault, J., Davies, K.J.P., Jones, M., Browne, D., Litt, M., Brockdorff, N., Rastan, S., Clarke, A., and Thomas, N.S.T. (1993). Detection of a molecular deletion at the DXS732 locus in a patient with X-linked hypohidrotic ectodermal dysplasia (EDA), with identification of a unique junctional fragment. *Am. J. Hum. Genet.* **52,** 78–84.

An affected male and carrier mother with a deletion at this locus; they also found that the maternal aunt and grandmother carried the deletion, but not the proband's sister. The proband had typical hypohidrotic ectodermal dysplasia and was normal intellectually.

RAPP-HODGKIN SYNDROME (MIM:129400)

DERMATOLOGIC FEATURES

MAJOR. Affected individuals describe decrease in sweating with relative heat intolerance, but hyperpyrexia is usually not a problem. The hypohidrosis is marginal with or without decrease in number of sweat pores.

The hair is coarse, wiry, slow growing, and may be sparse. Hair shafts may be normal microscopically or show irregular twisting or pili trianguli et canaliculi. Progressive hair loss begins in the teens, and total alopecia may ensue. Eyelashes and eyebrows, body hair, and secondary sexual hairs may be involved. The lateral one-third of the eyebrows is typically absent.

The nails are thickened proximally and often absent distally, and they may be discolored and small or markedly hypoplastic. The nail bed may be thickened.

MINOR. The skin may appear dry.

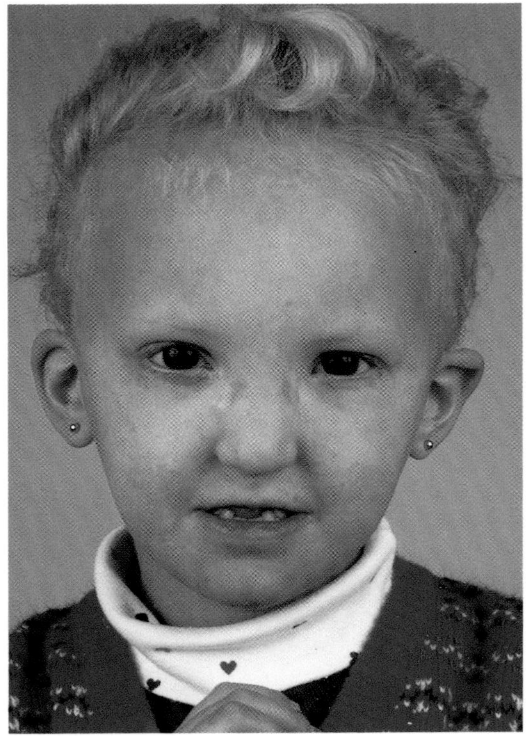

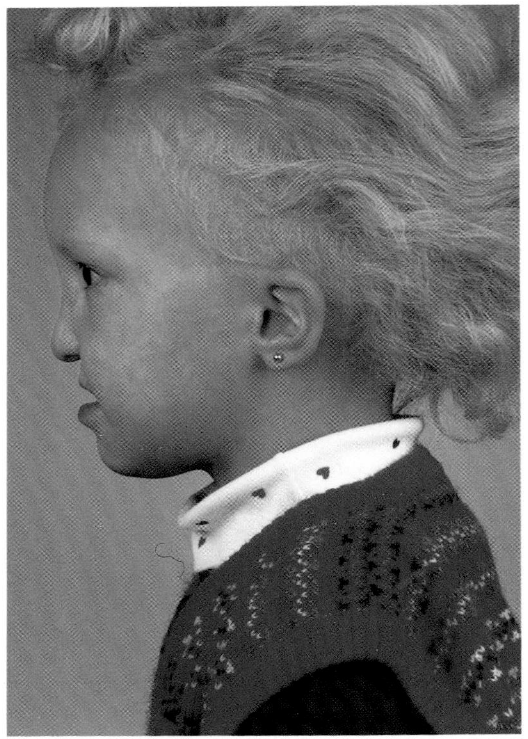

Figure 3.82. **(A)** Sparse coarse hair with abnormal eyebrows and eyelashes and blepharitis. Typical nasal configuration. **(B)** Profile shows maxillary hypoplasia. (From Schroeder and Sybert, 1987.)

ASSOCIATED ABNORMALITIES

Cleft palate with or without cleft lip is typical, and velopalatal insufficiency is common after repair. A submucous cleft may be overlooked when cleft lip is absent. Recurrent otitis media is typical.

The facies are characterized by a very short columella of the nose and maxillary hypoplasia. The upper lip is usually thin, the lower lip everted. Ears may be dysplastic. Teeth are small, may be conical, and prone to caries. Hypodontia is also reported. Aplasia of the lacrimal puncta occurs in about one-third of patients; corneal opacities and neovascularization are less common. Hypospadias has been described in 40% of reported males; hypoplasia of the labia minora and absence of the vaginal orifice have been described in one female.

HISTOPATHOLOGY

LIGHT. No information.
EM. No information.

BASIC DEFECT

Unknown.

TREATMENT

Secondary complications of cleft palate and dental restoration require the most attention.

MODE OF INHERITANCE

Autosomal dominant.

A

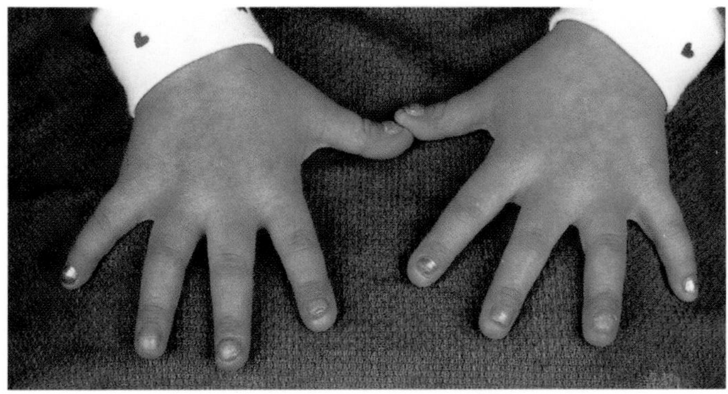

B

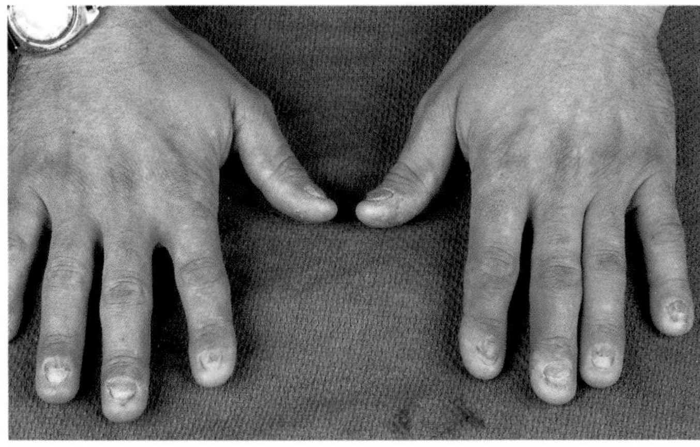

Figure 3.83. Fingernails of daughter (**A**) and father (**B**). (From Schroeder and Sybert, 1987.)

PRENATAL DIAGNOSIS

None. Potentially by ultrasound detection of cleft lip and palate, but likely to be unreliable.

DIFFERENTIAL DIAGNOSIS

There is significant overlap with the Hay-Wells syndrome (AEC, MIM:106260) and, in the absence of the ankyloblepharon filiforme adnatum typical of Hay-Wells syndrome, it may be difficult to categorize patients correctly. Scalp involvement is usually more severe in AEC. Individuals with EEC without ectrodactyly (MIM:129900) may also be confused. The hair in these patients is usually fine and sparse and not coarse. Although the facies of Rapp-Hodgkin are purportedly classic, photographic documentation is strikingly absent in a number of case reports.

Support Group: N.F.E.D.
219 East Main, Box 114
Mascoutah, IL 62258-0114
1-618-566-2020

SELECTED BIBLIOGRAPHY

Salinas, C.F., and Montes-G., G.M. (1988). Rapp-Hodgkin syndrome: observations on ten cases and characteristic hair changes (pili canaliculi). *Birth Defects* **24(2),** 149–168.

Two pedigrees, one with male-to-male transmission. Hair shaft abnormalities striking in irregularity, unlike true pili torti or true pili canaliculi et trianguli. The authors suggest that hair analysis will differentiate Rapp-Hodgkin syndrome from other ectodermal dysplasias, but to my knowledge similar hair analysis has not been done for AEC or EEC.

Schroeder, H.W., Jr., and Sybert, V.P. (1987). Rapp-Hodgkin ectodermal dysplasia. *J. Pediatr.* **110,** 72–75.

A father and daughter described, with a review of the literature.

Walpole, I.R., and Goldblatt, J. (1991). Rapp-Hodgkin hypohidrotic ectodermal dysplasia syndrome. *Clin. Genet.* **39,** 114–120.

A three generation family, with review of the previous literature.

TOOTH AND NAIL SYNDROME (MIM:189500)

(Witkop Syndrome; Hypodontia with Nail Dysgenesis)

DERMATOLOGICAL FEATURES

Major. Thin, small, friable nails with koilonychia are present at birth. The toenails are more severely involved than the fingernails. Nail changes may improve with age to the point where in adult life they may appear normal.

Minor. Thin, fine hair has been described in a few individuals.

ASSOCIATED ABNORMALITIES

The primary teeth are usually normal, although they may be somewhat small. Secondary teeth fail to erupt. There may be partial or total absence of the permanent teeth. Mandibular incisors, second molars, and maxillary canines are most often missing. The disorder is often not diagnosed until a child is evaluated at age 6 or 7 years because the primary teeth have not been lost.

The facies are generally normal. The gum ridges are well formed, and there usually is adequate mandibular and maxillary development, in contrast to the facies of hypohidrotic ectodermal dysplasia, where the absence of teeth is accompanied by bony hypoplasia.

Sweating is normal in this condition, and there is no significant heat intolerance.

HISTOPATHOLOGY

Light. No information.

EM. No information.

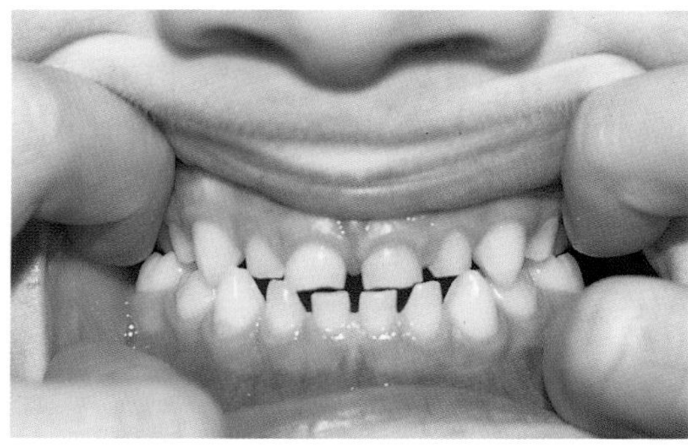

Figure 3.84. Retained primary teeth at age 12 years.

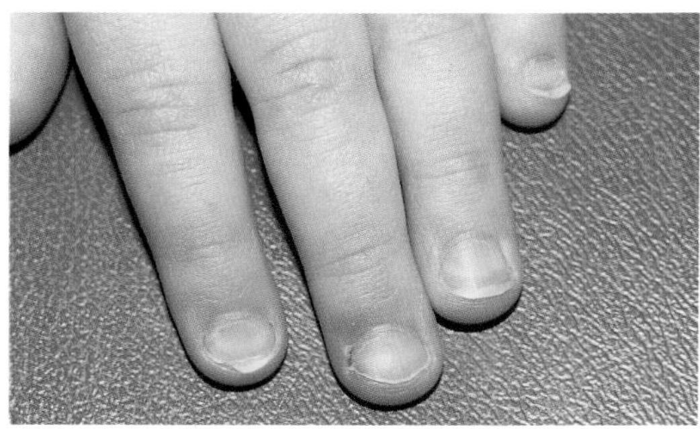

Figure 3.85. Mild koilonychia; fourth fingernail is more normal in shape and shows very high lunula.

BASIC DEFECT

Unknown.

TREATMENT

Dental restoration.

MODE OF INHERITANCE

Autosomal dominant.

PRENATAL DIAGNOSIS

None.

DIFFERENTIAL DIAGNOSIS

The diagnosis of tooth and nail syndrome is easy to miss. The nail changes can be subtle and unappreciated by family or physician. The involvement of permanent dentition and sparing of deciduous teeth, coupled with normal facies and sweating, easily exclude the diagnosis of hypohidrotic ectodermal dysplasia (Christ-Siemens-Touraine syndrome, MIM:305100). The few patients I have seen with tooth and nail syndrome were referred for evaluation for possible hypohidrotic ectodermal dysplasia.

Support Group: N.F.E.D
219 East Main, Box 114
Mascoutah, IL 62258-0114
1-618-566-2020

SELECTED BIBLIOGRAPHY

Hudson, C.D., and Witkop, C.J., Jr. (1975). Autosomal dominant hypodontia with nail dysgenesis. Report of 29 cases in six families. *Oral Pathol.* **39,** 409–423.

This is a report of six families with vertical and male-to-male transmission. It demonstrates the range of severity within and between families. In one family, one member showed mildly diminished sweating. The other affected family members sweated normally. Hypohidrosis is not a significant feature of this condition.

CHAPTER 4

DISORDERS OF PIGMENTATION

Disorders of pigmentation result from abnormal migration, distribution, or function of melanocytes. The pigmentary disturbances may be generalized, as in the oculocutaneous albinisms, or localized, as in the multiple lentigines (LEOPARD syndrome). In some disorders there can be both local and general involvement. For example, not only do individuals with neurofibromatosis have café-au-lait spots, they also exhibit generalized hypermelanosis.

For the disorders of pigmentation, as is being proved true for most inherited conditions, genetic heterogeneity exists both between disease entities and within diseases. Historically, differentiation among the oculocutaneous albinisms was based on clinical features. With the advent of molecular techniques, the underlying basis for clinical heterogeneity is becoming clear. Some clinical distinctions will continue to prove useful; others may fade into oblivion.

HYPERPIGMENTATION

DOWLING-DEGOS DISEASE (MIM:179850)

(Reticular Pigmented Anomaly of the Flexures)

Includes Kitamura Disease and Haber Syndrome

DERMATOLOGIC FEATURES

Major. Onset and gradual progression of asymptomatic macular hyperpigmentation in a reticular lacey pattern occurs in adult life. The areas of predilection include the axillae, groin, scrotum, perineal, and perianal areas. Occasionally the pigment change can be palpable.

Minor. Perioral pitted scars and comedone-like lesions on the upper eyelids are described in about one-third of patients. Hidradenitis suppurativa was mentioned in two case reports. Abscesses in the groin and axillae were described in five. One patient developed squamous cell carcinoma within the area of hidradenitis. One patient had multiple keratoacanthomas.

ASSOCIATED ABNORMALITIES

Several cases reportedly with mental retardation; most patients are intellectually normal.

HISTOPATHOLOGY

Light. Acanthosis with an increase in pigment present in thin, branching, elongated epidermal pegs.

EM. An increase in the number of normal-appearing melanosomes. These are widely dispersed in the epidermal keratinocytes.

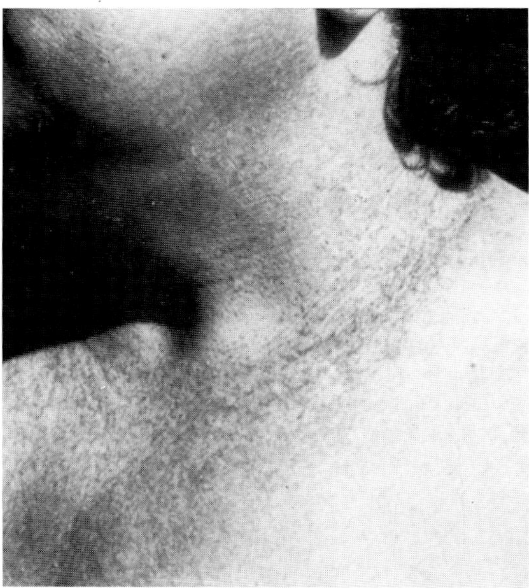

Figure 4.1. Reticular hyperpigmentation on the neck and upper chest. (From Crovato et al., 1983a.)

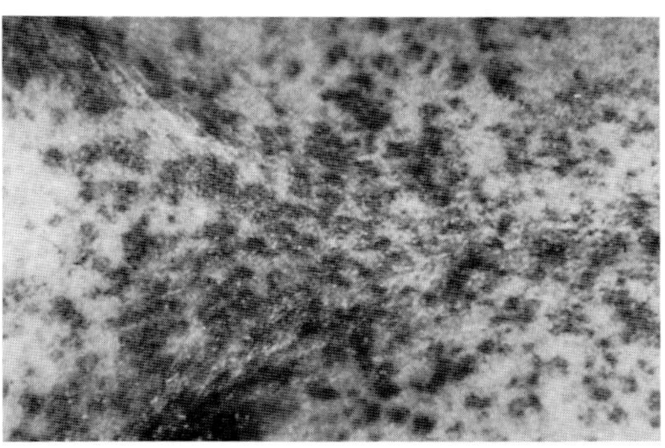

Figure 4.2. Close-up of macular hyperpigmentation. (From Crovato et al., 1983b.)

BASIC DEFECT

Unknown.

TREATMENT

None.

MODE OF INHERITANCE

?Autosomal dominant. Pedigrees with multiple generations but no male-to-male transmission.

PRENATAL DIAGNOSIS

None.

DIFFERENTIAL DIAGNOSIS

In acanthosis nigricans (MIM:100600), which might be confused very early in the disease process, the pigment is usually more diffuse and papular rather than macular and lacy. Linear and whorled nevoid hypermelanosis generally occurs earlier and is more widespread.

The axillary freckles of neurofibromatosis (MIM:162200) are individual lesions, usually lighter in color without a reticular pattern, and the lentigines of the LEOPARD syndrome (MIM:151100) are also distinct and discrete.

Eponymous confusion with Degos disease (malignant atrophic papulosis) is to be avoided. In malignant atrophic papulosis, asymptomatic pea-sized pink lesions that develop atrophic white centers and surrounding pink telangiectatic borders appear on any skin surface. Biopsy material shows atrophy with hyperkeratosis and mucin in the dermis with endothelial proliferation within deep dermal vessels. Internal organs may or may not be involved.

In reticulate acropigmentation of Kitamura, the pigment change is found primarily on the hands and feet, and there is mild atrophy of the skin. There is an increased number of melanocytes on biopsy. Some argue that the diseases are the same, as families with features of both Dowling-Degos and reticulate acropigmentation have been described.

Haber disease has similar skin changes with an acne rosacea-like facial erythema. Arguments have been raised that the disease is the same as Dowling-Degos, part of the spectrum of a single disorder.

Support Group: N.O.R.D.
P.O. Box 8923
New Fairfield, CT
06812
1-800-999-6673

SELECTED BIBLIOGRAPHY

Crovato, F., Nazzari, G., and Rebora, A. (1983). Dowling-Degos disease (reticulate pigmented anomaly of the flexures) is an autosomal dominant condition. *Br. J. Dermatol.* **108,** 473–476.

Eleven affected family members in four generations. Only two patients were examined. No male-to-male transmission occurred.

Rebora, A., and Crovato, F. (1984). The spectrum of Dowling-Degos disease. *Br. J. Dermatol.* **110,** 627–630.

Authors believe the histologic picture of epidermal budding with proliferation of follicular cells is a marker for a group of autosomal dominant disorders that show some overlap but have distinct features. They propose to use Dowling-Degos as an appellation for the entire group rather than a single subset. I do not find this particularly helpful; perhaps coining a new term rather than redefining an old one would be more useful.

Wilson Jones, E., and Grice, K. (1978). Reticulate pigmented anomaly of the flexures. *Arch. Dermatol.* **114,** 1150–1157.

Extensive report of 10 cases with review of the literature. Wilson Jones is unhyphenated. In citations he is referenced as both Wilson-Jones, E., and Jones, E.W.

DYSKERATOSIS CONGENITA (MIM:127550, 224230, 305000)

(Zinsser-Cole-Engman)

Includes Scoggins Type

DERMATOLOGIC FEATURES

MAJOR. Reticulate greyish-brown hyperpigmentation of the neck, upper chest, arms, and axillae begins in midchildhood. There is often a telangiectatic component. The pigment can progress to involve all of the folds and the lower extremities.

Nail dystrophy starts as longitudinal ridging and splitting and progresses to pterygia formation and nail loss. The skin changes may precede nail alterations or vice versa.

Oral leukoplakia is typical. Other mucosa, including conjunctival, urethral, and genital, may be affected. Involvement of the lacrimal puncta can lead to chronic blepharitis and excessive tearing.

Malignant skin and mucosal tumors develop between the ages of 20 and 50 years. These are primarily squamous cell carcinomas.

MINOR. Premature graying, hyperhidrosis, palmoplantar hyperkeratosis, and occasional patches of atrophic skin without hyperpigmentation have all been described. Sparse scalp hair and easy blistering of the hands and feet occur in response to trauma; periodontitis and tooth loss have also been noted.

ASSOCIATED ABNORMALITIES

Marrow failure begins in the teen years with anemia or thrombocytopenia and progresses to pancytopenia in about one-half of reported patients.

Infection is a major cause of death, as are hemorrhage and malignancy, and death before age 40 years is typical.

Dysphagia without obvious cause is a frequent complaint.

Although mental retardation is stated to occur in approximately 10% of cases, the actual likelihood appears to be much lower. Cases cited as showing mental retardation include patients with IQs of 79, 85, 93, or low-normal intelli-

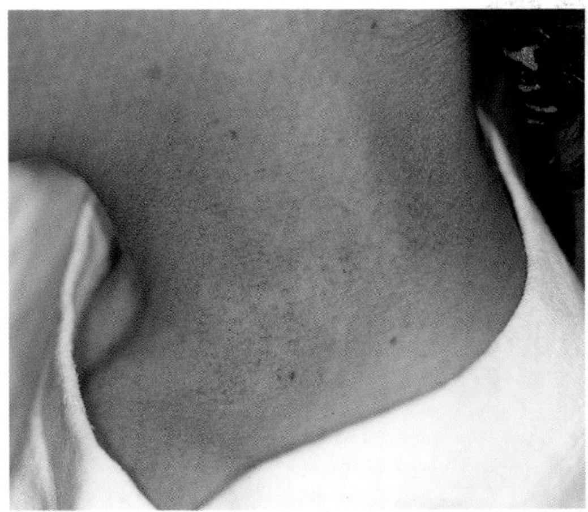

Figure 4.3. Hyperpigmented macules with telangiectases on the neck. (Courtesy of Dr. S. Vanderhooft, Salt Lake City, UT.)

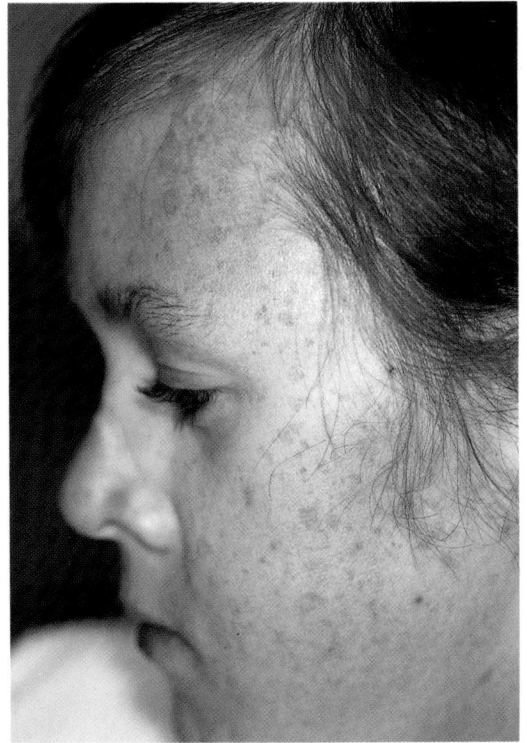

Figure 4.4. Reticulate hyperpigmentation on the face. (Courtesy of Dr. S. Vanderhooft, Salt Lake City, UT.)

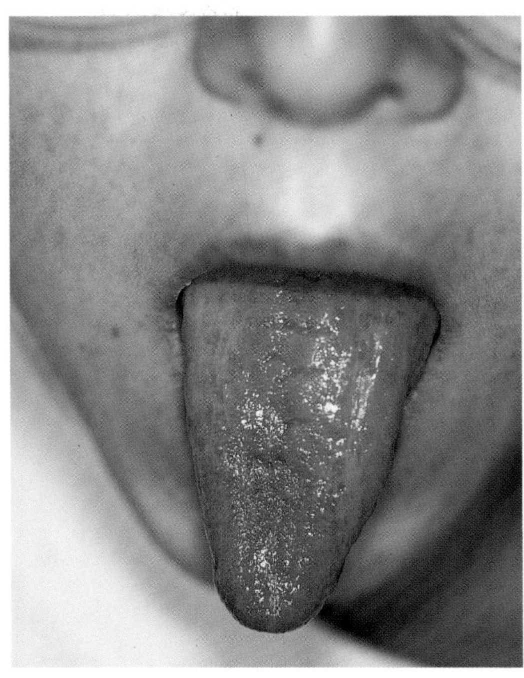

Figure 4.5. Leukoplakia, most noticeable at the sides of the tongue. (Courtesy of Dr. S. Vanderhooft, Salt Lake City, UT.)

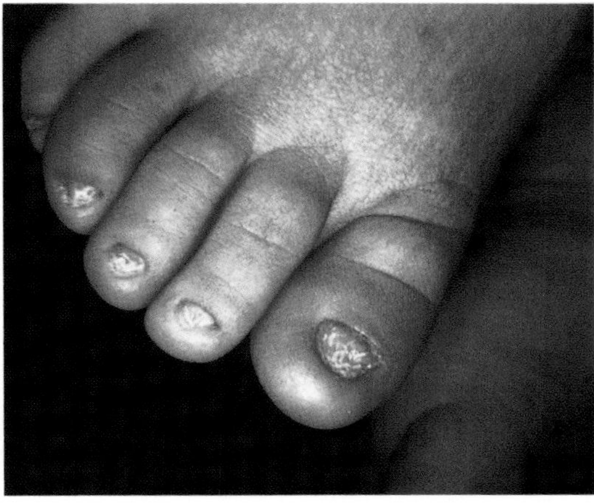

Figure 4.6. Nail changes with pterygia formation and alterations in nail plate. (Courtesy of Dr. J. Halloran, Division of Dermatology, University of Washington.)

gence. Statements such as "slightly dull," "leads the life of a normal child," "intelligence less than normal," "average," "three years of high school, trouble with math, garage mechanic" are the only descriptors given in case reports of other patients labeled as mentally retarded. There is only one pedigree with well-documented mental retardation and a few sporadic cases with other atypical features that include mental retardation.

Growth retardation is an inconstant feature. Increased chromosome fragility is reported in some cases. As there is phenotypic overlap with Fanconi anemia, it is difficult to know whether these case reports represent correct diagnoses of dyskeratosis congenita or missed diagnoses of Fanconi.

HISTOPATHOLOGY

LIGHT. Epidermal atrophy with macrophages loaded with pigment in the upper dermis.
EM. No information.

BASIC DEFECT

Unknown.

TREATMENT

Etretinate may control the leukoplakia.

Bone marrow transplantation for marrow failure has been successful but does not alter the course of other features of the disease.

MODE OF INHERITANCE

X-linked recessive. Linkage to Xq28 has been reported.

In autosomal dominant dyskeratosis congenita (Scoggins type), the onset is usually later in life. This mode of inheritance is based on one published abstract.

Autosomal recessive inheritance is claimed based on reports of females with dyskeratosis congenita. Many of the females have very atypical features and/or later onset than in the classic X-linked recessive form. It appears that the diagnosis of dyskeratosis congenita has been made in many of these patients for lack of a better diagnostic niche.

PRENATAL DIAGNOSIS

None.

DIFFERENTIAL DIAGNOSIS

In Fanconi anemia (MIM:227650, 227660) hyperpigmentation is typically more diffuse, but in many respects the disorders are similar. Nail changes and oral involvement are not typical of Fanconi anemia, and radial ray defects are not reported in dyskeratosis congenita, nor are structural renal defects. Overlap has been reported, and correct diagnosis may not be possible in some situations. Chromosomal breakage is more typical of Fanconi anemia.

Epidermolysis bullosa with mottled hyperpigmentation (MIM:131960) and Kindler syndrome (MIM:173650) share poikiloderma and acral blistering with dyskeratosis congenita, but patients do not have marrow failure. Patients with these syndromes typically do not have leukoplakia or such striking nail dystrophy.

Congenital erythropoietic porphyria (MIM: 263700) can present with blisters and pigment change. Photosensitivity is not part of dyskeratosis congenita.

Nail changes of dyskeratosis congenita are similar to those of lichen planus, and oral leukoplakia can also occur in lichen planus. Reticulate hyperpigmentation distinguishes the two conditions.

The progeric syndromes Rothmund-Thomson (MIM:268400), Werner (MIM:277700), and Bloom (MIM:210900) are marked by more telangiectatic and poikilodermatous changes and lack the nail and oral mucosal involvement associated with dyskeratosis congenita.

Chronic graft versus host disease can give

identical dermatologic changes, including the nails.

Support Group: N.O.R.D.
P.O. Box 8923
New Fairfield, CT
06812
1-800-999-6673

SELECTED BIBLIOGRAPHY

Davidson, H.R., and Connor, J.M. (1988). Dyskeratosis congenita. *J. Med. Genet.* **25,** 843–846.

Review of 104 cases in the literature with a table of presenting features. Excellent overview. They noted that the feature of intracranial calcifications was present in only two brothers, who were reported three times.

Drachtman, R.A., and Alter, B.P. (1992). Dyskeratosis congenita: clinical and genetic heterogeneity. Report of a new case and review of the literature. *Am. J. Pediatr. Hematol. Oncol.* **14,** 297–304.

Rather arbitrary categorization of literature reports into X-linked, autosomal dominant, and autosomal recessive categories, but useful in sorting out different clinical presentations and life expectancy. Typical of nondermatologic reports, the term *hyperpigmentation* is used without further descriptors for a variety of pigment changes. Their female patient had atypical skin color changes. One hundred thirteen references.

Nazzaro, P., Argentieri, R., Bassetti, F., Leonetti, F., Topi, G., and Valenzano, L. (1972). Dyskératose congénitale de Zinsser-Cole-Engmann. *Bull. Soc. Fr. Dermatol. Syphiligr.* **79,** 242–244.

This is a pedigree with questionable dominant inheritance. The statement is made that there is a varying degree of disease in five family members, including two females, but there are no further details given. In the 45- and 47-year-old brothers described, there is mild leukoplakia of the tongue only, anodontia, and absence of marrow involvement. These features suggest that this is a different disease than classic dyskeratosis congenita, despite similarities in skin and nail changes.

Phillips, R.J., Judge, M., Webb, D., and Harper, J.I. (1992). Dyskeratosis congenita: delay in diagnosis and successful treatment of pancytopenia by bone marrow transplantation. *Br. J. Dermatol.* **127,** 278–280.

Reviews the outcome of seven cases with marrow transplantation to date. Four of the seven died. Authors argue that improved outcome is possible with avoidance of pretransplant irradiation.

Tchou, P.-K., and Kohn, T. (1982). Dyskeratosis congenita: an autosomal dominant disorder. *J. Am. Acad. Dermatol.* **6,** 1034–1039.

A multiply consanguineous pedigree with two generations, five affected females, and one affected male related through unaffected transmitting males. The patients have atypical disease with no marrow failure in females and total marrow failure in only one male. Minimal nail changes are present (no nail changes in one anemic male). The pedigree is unconvincing genetically and clinically.

FANCONI ANEMIA (MIM:227650, 227660)

(Fanconi Pancytopenia)

Recognition of Fanconi anemia is usually based on typical hematologic findings or radial ray defects. However, I had one patient come to diagnosis through dermatologic consultation. The presence of classic skin changes may help to direct evaluation of patients who present with some of the other features of Fanconi anemia.

DERMATOLOGIC FEATURES

MAJOR. Diffuse or patchy brown hyperpigmentation, café-au-lait spots, and unusual freckling have been described in about 65% of patients.

MINOR. Patchy hypopigmentation along with

hyperpigmentation is occasionally mentioned. Sweet syndrome (neutrophilic dermatosis) has been reported in several children with Fanconi anemia. The lesions present as tender, red nodules that may ulcerate.

ASSOCIATED ABNORMALITIES

Hematopoietic: Failure of the bone marrow may begin with thrombocytopenia only or present as florid aplastic anemia. The median age of onset is in midchildhood.

Malignancies are common. Leukemia and hepatocellular carcinoma are the major types of cancer. Squamous cell carcinoma has been reported more often than expected for the general population.

Orthopedic: Radial ray defects ranging from triphalangeal thumbs to absence of the radial ray of the arm occur in approximately one-half of individuals with Fanconi anemia. Intrauterine growth retardation is common, and short stature is described in two-thirds to four-fifth of individuals. Often the presenting complaint is failure to thrive. Although growth hormone deficiency has been found in some, response to growth hormone treatment has been poor. Sterile, multifocal osteomyelitis may occur.

Others: Structural renal malformations including agenesis of the kidney, ectopic kidney, horseshoe kidneys, and duplication of the collecting system are found in one-third to one-half of patients.

Microcephaly is seen in 30%–50% of the patients in reported series. Mental retardation occurs in about 25% and is usually associated with small head size.

Ophthalmologic abnormalities include strabismus (in 20%) and microphthalmia (15%–30%).

Conductive deafness due to ossicle malformation occurs in about 15% of patients, and complementation studies. Abnormal pinnae are described in a similar proportion.

Hypogenitalism in males with small phallus and testes, and failure to go through puberty in both males and females, with irregular menses

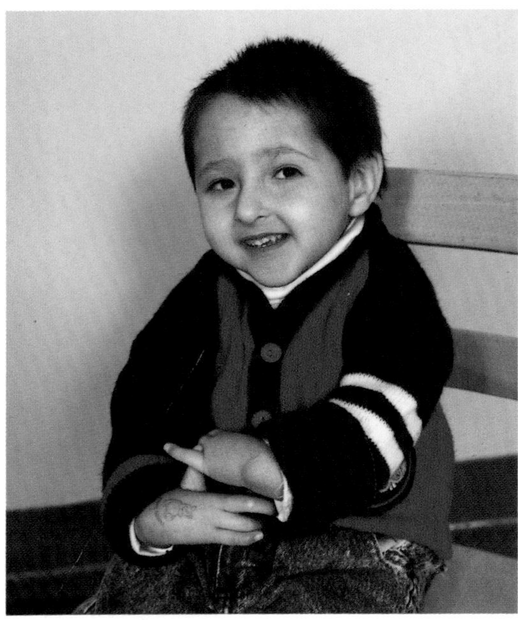

Figure 4.7. Five-year-old with radial clubhands, bilateral absence of the radii and thumbs, and microcephaly. (Courtesy of Dr. R.A. Pagon, Seattle, Washington.)

in females, is probably on the basis of primary gonadal failure rather than hypogonadotrophic. There have been a small number of pregnancies to women with Fanconi anemia; most of these patients had atypical Fanconi syndrome.

The diagnostic feature of Fanconi anemia is an increase in the number of chromatid breaks, rearrangements, and formation of quadriradials in the chromosomes of cultured lymphocytes and skin fibroblasts when exposed to diepoxybutane (DEB) or similar DNA cross-linking agents.

HISTOPATHOLOGY

LIGHT. In one patient a hyperpigmented macule showed increased amounts of melanin and "derangement of keratinocytes." In others, there have been no distinguishing histologic features.

EM. No information.

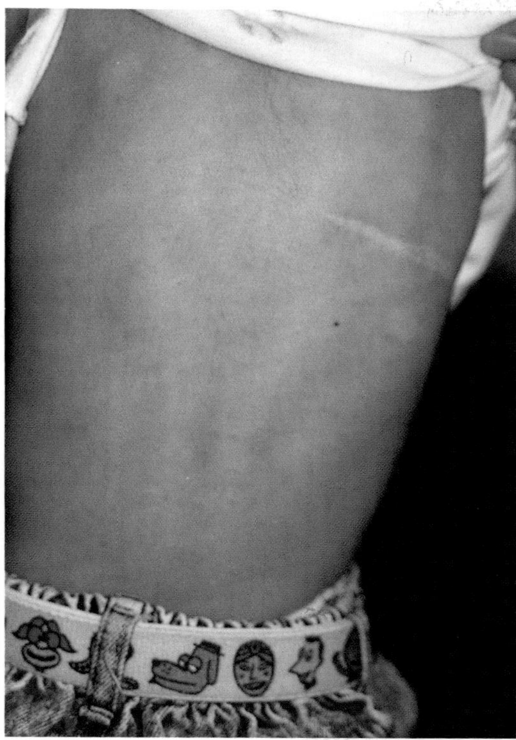

Figure 4.8. Generalized hyperpigmentation; several hypopigmented areas, one on left scapula, one below scar. (Courtesy of Dr. R.A. Pagon, Seattle, Washington.)

BASIC DEFECT

Unknown. The gene for complementation group C has been isolated *(FACC)*. Its product and function remain unknown.

TREATMENT

Androgen therapy combined with prednisone is the major treatment for marrow failure. Bone marrow transplantation has been performed with variable success.

MODE OF INHERITANCE

Autosomal recessive. The gene *FACC* maps to 20q. Genetic heterogeneity exists, based on complementation studies. Homozygosity for the same mutant alleles and compound heterozygosity for different mutant alleles have been demonstrated in patients with mutations at the *FACC* locus.

PRENATAL DIAGNOSIS

Chromosome breakage studies of chorionic villus cells or cultured amniocytes are accurate. As mutations are identified, molecular diagnosis will become possible.

DIFFERENTIAL DIAGNOSIS

In the thrombocytopenia-absent radius syndrome (MIM:274000), normal thumbs with absence of the radii are the rule, and marrow abnormalities appear limited to thrombocytopenia. Holt-Oram syndrome (MIM:142900) has similar limb changes associated with congenital heart disease, with none of the other features of Fanconi anemia. Patients with Aase syndrome (MIM:205600), which may be the same as Blackfan-Diamond syndrome (MIM:205900), have triphalangeal thumbs and red blood cell anemia. IVIC (MIM:147750) is an autosomal dominant disorder characterized by radial ray hypoplasia, deafness, external ophthalmoplegia, and thrombocytopenia. In individuals with aplastic anemia and growth failure, Fanconi syndrome must be excluded by DEB studies. The absence of associated malformations is not adequate to exclude the diagnosis.

Numerous chromosomal aneuploidy and deletion-duplication syndromes have similar findings. The diagnosis of the VATER association (MIM:192350) in a newborn should always carry with it the recognition that Fanconi syndrome may be the underlying diagnosis, and appropriate cytogenetic testing with DEB studies may be warranted if microcephaly is present or growth failure, or anemia develop.

There are numerous multiple malformation syndromes associated with growth failure and patchy hyperpigmentation that bear some resemblance to Fanconi anemia, including Bloom syndrome (MIM:210900) and Rothmund-

Thomson syndrome (MIM:268400). None of these has the hemapoietic findings of Fanconi syndrome

Support Group: International Fanconi Anemia Registry
c/o Dr. Arleen Auerbach
1230 York Avenue
New York, NY 10021
1-212-327-7533

Fanconi Anemia Research Fund, Inc.
1902 Jefferson Street, Suite 2
Eugene, OR 97405-2402
1-503-687-4658

SELECTED BIBLIOGRAPHY

Auerbach, A.D., Min, Z., Ghosh, R., Pergament, E., Verlinsky, Y., Nicolas, H., and Boue, J. (1986). Clastogen-induced chromosomal breakage as a marker for first-trimester prenatal diagnosis of Fanconi anemia. *Hum. Genet.* **73,** 86–88.

The diagnosis of Fanconi anemia was made in two pregnancies at risk and excluded in eight pregnancies at risk by DEB studies of cultured chorionic villus cells. Previous work in amniocytes gave similar results.

Auerbach, A.D., Rogatko, A., and Schroeder-Kurth, T.M. (1989). International Fanconi Anemia Registry. relation of clinical symptoms to diepoxybutane sensitivity. *Blood* **73,** 391–396.

The authors evaluated DEB-positive and DEB-negative patients for discriminating clinical features. Presence of four or more of the following correlated with positive DEB status in all but one patient: growth retardation, birthmarks, urinary tract abnormalities, microphthalmia, learning disabilities, thrombocytopenia, radial ray defects, and other skeletal abnormalities. The authors offer a "simplified" scoring system that seems complicated to me. The bottom line is that overuse of DEB testing is probably better than underutilization.

Baron, F., Sybert, V.P., Andrews, R.G. (1989) Cutaneous and extracut aneous neutrophilic infiltrates (Sweet syndrome) in three patients with Fanconi anemia. *J. Pediatr.* **115,** 726–729.

Response to prednisone was rapid and uniform. None of the patients had malignancy at the time of onset of Sweet syndrome.

Berkovitz, G.D., Zinkham, W.H., and Migeon, C.J. (1984). Gonadal function in two siblings with Fanconi's anemia. *Horm. Res.* **19,** 137–141.

Elevated gonadotrophins and low testosterone levels were found in the male sibling; elevated gonadotrophins were found in the female. Estrogen levels were not measured. The authors concluded that primary gonad failure is the cause for the hypogenitalism in Fanconi anemia.

Deal, J.E., Barratt, T.M., and Dillon, M.J. (1990). Fanconi syndrome, ichthyosis, dysmorphism, jaundice and diarrhea—a new syndrome. *Pediatr. Nephrol.* **4,** 308–313.

Beware. This syndrome, the subject of this and other reports, consists of renal Fanconi syndrome, which is generalized aminoaciduria. Fanconi anemia is not associated with ichthyosis.

Gibson, R.A., Hajianpour, A., Murer-Orlando, M., Buchwald, M., and Mathew, C.J. (1993). A nonsense mutation exon-skipping in the Fanconi anemia group C gene. *Hum. Mol. Genet.* **2,** 797–799.

The affected individual was homozygous for a nonsense mutation in exon 6 of the coding sequence.

Milner, R.D.G., Khallouf, K.A., Gibson, R., Hajianpour, A., and Mathew, C.G. (1993). A new autosomal recessive anomaly mimicking Fanconi's anaemia phenotype. *Arch. Dis. Child.* **68,** 101–103.

Three siblings with growth retardation, beaked nose, microcephaly, radial ray defects, and guttate hypopigmentation had negative DEB studies, and linkage to 20q was excluded.

Whitney, M.A., Saito, H., Jakobs, P.M., Gibson, R.A., Moses, R.E., and Grompe, M. (1993). A common mutation in the FACC gene causes Fanconi anemia in Ashkenazi Jews. *Nat. Genet.* **4,** 202–205.

Two Ashkenazic Jewish patients were homozygous for a single splice mutation in exon 4. Twenty-one additional families were studied; three had affected individuals with homozygosity. All individuals with the exon 4 splice mutation allele were Ashkenazi Jews.

HEMOCHROMATOSIS (MIM:235200)

DERMATOLOGIC FEATURES

Major. Between 66% and 100% of patients with hemochromatosis have increased skin color. This is usually described as metallic gray, but may be bronze or brown. The increased pigment is usually generalized and may be more evident in sun-exposed areas. The genitalia, skinfolds, and areolae may be involved. Mucosal hyperpigmentation and perilimbic conjunctival pigmentation occur in about 20% of patients. The skin color improves with treatment.

Thinning of pubic and body hair occurs in almost 75% of affected individuals and alopecia is complete in approximately 12%.

Dry scaling skin occurs in about 50% of patients. Severity ranges from mild xerosis to frank ichthyosis vulgaris. The dry skin also improves with treatment. Skin atrophy, most marked on the shins, is appreciated clinically in about 40%.

The nails are also affected. Half of patients are described as having koilonychia. Linear striations and leukonychia occur in approximately 10% each.

Minor. Palmar erythema is described in 15% of affected individuals.

ASSOCIATED ABNORMALITIES

Patients often present with liver and cardiac failure as a consequence of unrecognized and untreated disease. Males usually present in their forties and fifties, females in their fifties and sixties, after menopause. The ratio of affected males to females is 5:1. Liver disease is characterized by hepatomegaly, abnormal liver function tests, fibrosis and cirrhosis, and ultimately hepatocellular carcinoma. Approximately 30% of affected individuals have had hepatic malignancies.

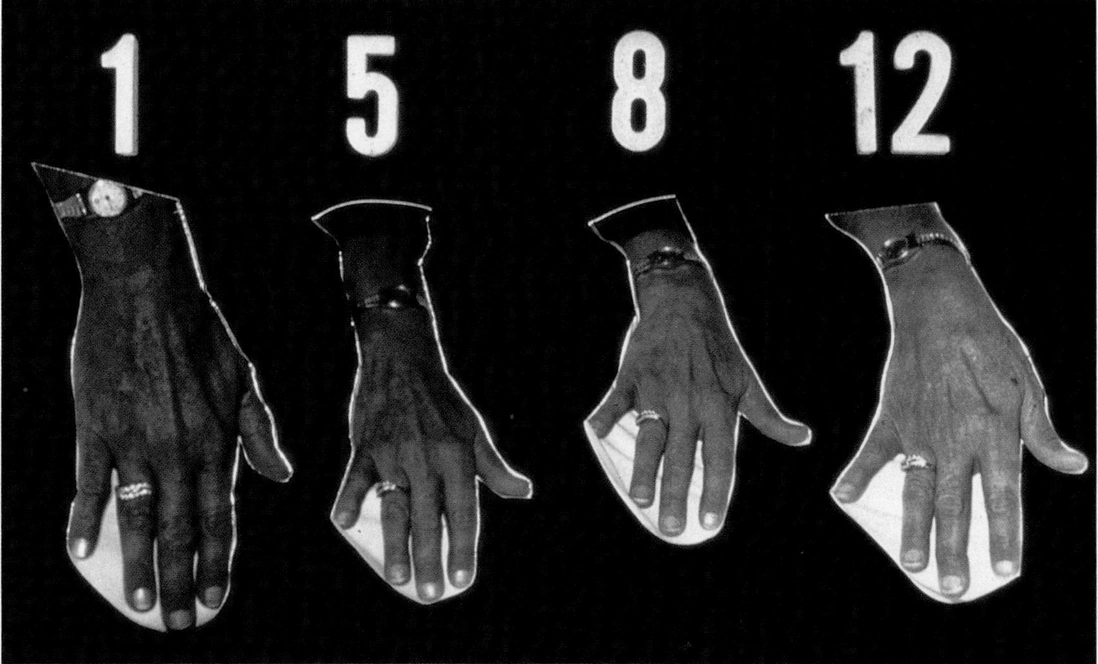

Figure 4.9. Normalization of color changes in the skin of a patient with secondary hemochromatosis, following dialysis treatment. (From Held et al., 1993.)

Hypogonadism is a common complaint in untreated males. Twenty to 40% of affected individuals complain of loss of libido; 70%–80% of weakness and lethargy.

Approximately 70% of patients develop arthropathy primarily involving small joints of the hands. Joint involvement is symmetric and painful, and the joints are swollen. In later stage disease large joints become involved. Over 75% of untreated affected individuals develop diabetes mellitus.

Once liver damage presents, the course of the disease is irreversible, although it may be slowed by treatment. Even with appropriate treatment, the arthritis and the hypogonadism do not improve, although diabetes mellitus and congestive heart failure do.

HISTOPATHOLOGY

LIGHT. There is an increase in melanin and hemosiderin. The generalized increase in pigmentation is thought to be due to melanin and not to hemosiderin. When the skin tone appears bronze, there is an increase in the melanin in the epidermis. If the skin appears gray, there seems to be an increase in iron in the eccrine sweat glands. There is a decrease in the thickness of the epidermis, and dermal atrophy may be present.

EM. No information.

BASIC DEFECT

Unknown. There is an increase in iron uptake across the gut and a decrease in secretion.

TREATMENT

The treatment of choice is phlebotomy. When treatment is initiated, the frequency of blood-letting is one to two times per week. Three to four phlebotomies per year is the usual maintenance regimen.

Liver transplantation has been performed.

MODE OF INHERITANCE

Autosomal recessive. The gene carrier frequency in the Caucasian population is estimated at 1 in 10 to 1 in 20, with 1 in 400 affected homozygotes. The gene is closely linked to the HLA locus on chromosome 6, with linkage disequilibrium. Twenty-five percent of heterozygotes will have abnormal liver function tests.

PRENATAL DIAGNOSIS

None.

DIFFERENTIAL DIAGNOSIS

The only difficulty in making the diagnosis of hemochromatosis is to suspect it in the first place. Patients often go undiagnosed for long periods of time because of the multiplicity of complaints. The skin changes can be mimicked by argyria. The diagnosis of hemochromatosis can be made by finding a serum transferrin saturation level (serum iron divided by total iron binding capacity) of greater than 55% coupled with an elevated fasting ferritin level.

Disease states that require multiple transfusions, such as thalassemia major, can result in iatrogenic hemochromatosis.

Support Group: Hemochromatosis Foundation, Inc.
P.O. Box 8569
Albany NY 12208
1-518-489-0972

Iron Overload Diseases Association, Inc.
433 Westwind Drive
North Palm Beach, FL 33408
1-407-840-8512

SELECTED BIBLIOGRAPHY

Alper, J.S., Geller, L.N., Barash, C.I., Billings, P.R., Laden, V., and Natowicz, M.R. (1994). Genetic discrimination and screening for hemochromatosis. *J. Public Health Policy* **15,** 345–358.

These authors detail instances of denied coverage for hemochromatosis and raise concern that institution of general screening tests may result in loss of insurability to currently healthy individuals. I am uncertain that this argument is legitimate, as their vignettes concern individuals undergoing treatment for symptomatic disease. Insurance companies appear ready to deny coverage any time it is needed, and I am not sure this behavior should proscribe our screening for a condition that is eminently treatable and potentially lethal if ignored until an affected individual is symptomatic.

Chevrant-Breton, J., Simon, M., Bourel, M., and Ferrand, B. (1977). Cutaneous manifestations of idiopathic hemochromatosis. *Arch. Dermatol.* **113,** 161–165.

This article reviews the skin manifestations in 100 patients. Histologic findings are interesting in that increased amounts of melanin, with or without iron, did not correlate with the degree of skin pigmentation, and the amount of melanin did not correlate with the amount of iron or vice versa.

Knisely, A.S. (1992). Neonatal hemochromatosis. *Adv. Pediatr.* **39,** 383–403.

This possibly autosomal recessive, usually lethal cause of neonatal liver failure appears to be genetically distinct from hemochromatosis. This is an exhaustive review with 108 references.

Olynyk, J.K. (1994). Genetic haemochromatosis—preventable rust. *Aust. N.Z. J. Med.* **24,** 711–715.

A succinct and clear review of the clinical features, diagnostic evaluation, and management of hemochromatosis.

Phatak, P.D., Guzman, G., Woll, J.E., Robeson, A., and Phelps, C.E. (1994). Cost-effectiveness of screening for hereditary hemochromatosis. *Arch. Intern. Med.* **154,** 769–776.

They recommend screening males over 30 years of age by serum transferrin saturation. Based on the likelihood of false positives, false negatives, the cost of a liver biopsy, the likelihood of compliance with therapy, and so forth, the authors try to vary their cost/benefit analysis using different assumptions for each of these parameters.

INCONTINENTIA PIGMENTI (MIM:308300, 308310)

(Bloch-Sulzberger; Bloch-Siemens)

DERMATOLOGIC FEATURES

MAJOR. Incontinentia pigmenti classically presents at birth or in the newborn period with blisters. These blisters are small, grouped on an erythematous base, and scattered over the body surface in a swirly, patchy pattern along the lines of Blaschko. The scalp may be involved. The blisters resolve and the second phase of raised, warty, hyperkeratotic lesions on a red base begins. Their distribution is similar to the first stage, but is not necessarily identical. These lesions also go on to disappear. The third phase is characterized by macular hyperpigmentation in whorls and streaks, also along the lines of Blaschko, and it also may be in areas unaffected by previous stages. This tan, brown, or slate gray pigmentation usually fades and in adult life is replaced by hypopigmented, slightly atrophic skin in which hair follicles and sweat glands may be absent. The face is usually spared.

All four phases may occur simultaneously or overlap, and patients may present first with any stage, the earlier changes presumably having occurred in utero. While the blisters usually occur in the immediate perinatal and postnatal period and resolve by 6 months or sooner, I have seen them persist in some patients beyond 18 months. They can be exacerbated or precipitated by heat and sun exposure. I have had two patients who first presented with initial onset of classic hyperpigmented and erythematous lesions at 15 months of age with no antecedent lesions. The pigment changes may resolve within the first few years or persist into adulthood.

MINOR. Congenital scarring alopecia (similar

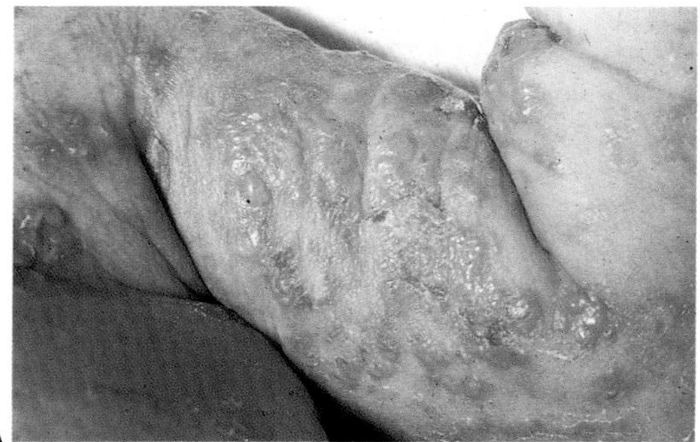

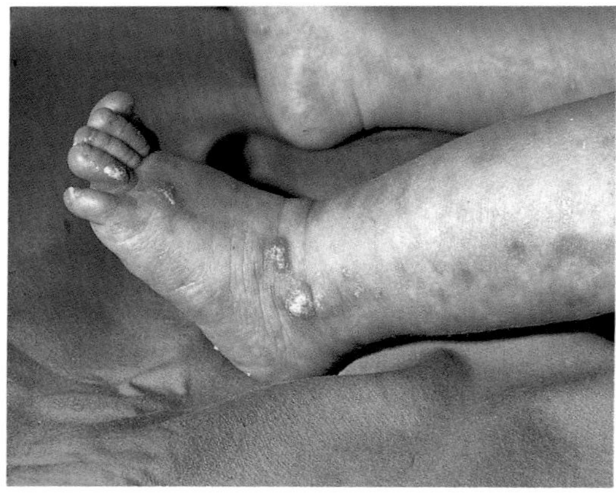

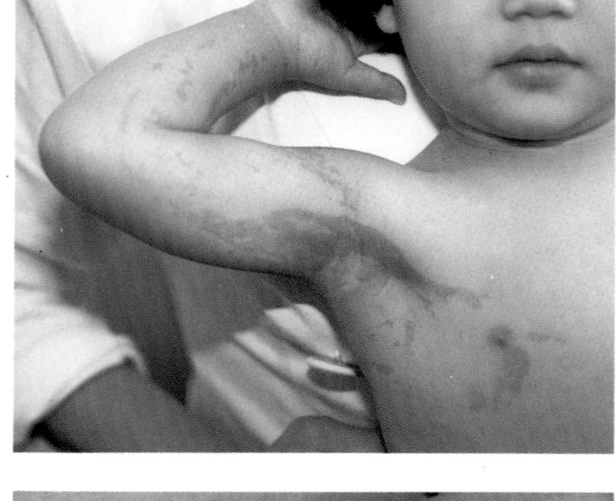

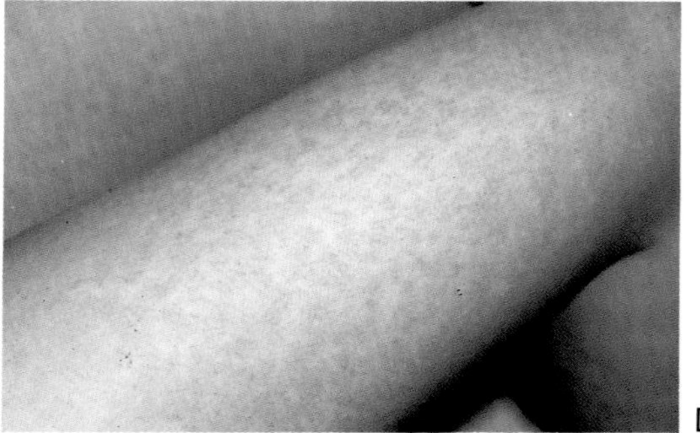

Figure 4.10. **(A)** Vesicles of stage 1. (From Sybert and Holbrook, 1987.) **(B)** Verrucous lesions of stage 2. **(C)** Hyperpigmented streaks, stage 3. **(D)** Hypopigmented areas, stage 4. (B–D, from Francis and Sybert, 1995.)

to pseudopelade or aplasia cutis congenita); nail dystrophy.

ASSOCIATED ABNORMALITIES

Dental abnormalities include oligodontia, hypodontia, peg-shaped teeth, and microdontia of primary or secondary teeth. Delayed eruption of teeth is also common. Dental abnormalities may be the only obvious finding in adult life.

Blood eosinophilia or leukocytosis may occur and resolves with age.

The reported ocular abnormalities are many. The single most important, and likely only specific, finding is retinal vascular proliferation. If untreatable or left untreated it can result in retinal detachment and loss of vision. There appear to be abnormal arteriovenous anastomoses with aneurysms. Vascular insufficiency in the retina may also occur. These changes are found within the first few months of life and have not developed de novo in any of our patients with normal retinal examinations at 1 year.

Mental retardation, seizures, and spastic diplegia, hemiplegia, or quadriplegia can be devastating consequences of the disorder. Almost 20% of reported patients have some type of neurologic deficit. This may reflect biased reporting of more significantly handicapped children.

There are occasional reports of a variety of structural malformations, including skull deformities, short stature, cleft lip with or without cleft palate, and clubfoot, which may be incidental findings and not part of the syndrome. The same is true for reported defects in neutrophil chemotaxis and lymphocyte dysfunction.

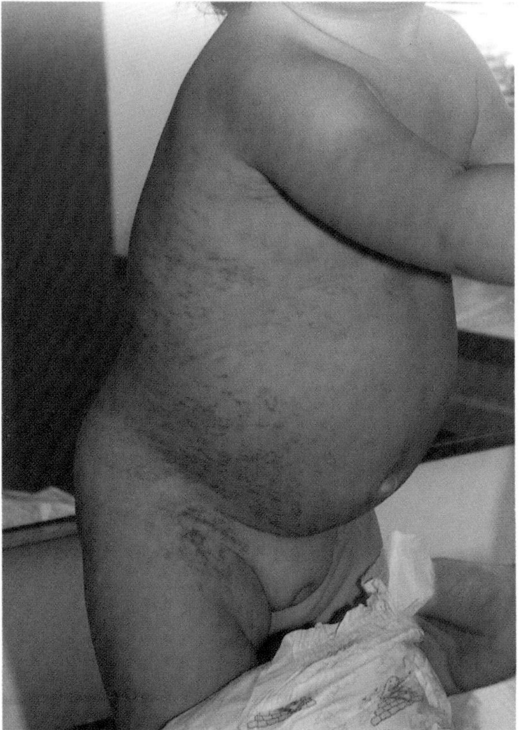

Figure 4.11. Dappling of hyperpigmentation on trunk and in groin along the lines of Blaschko.

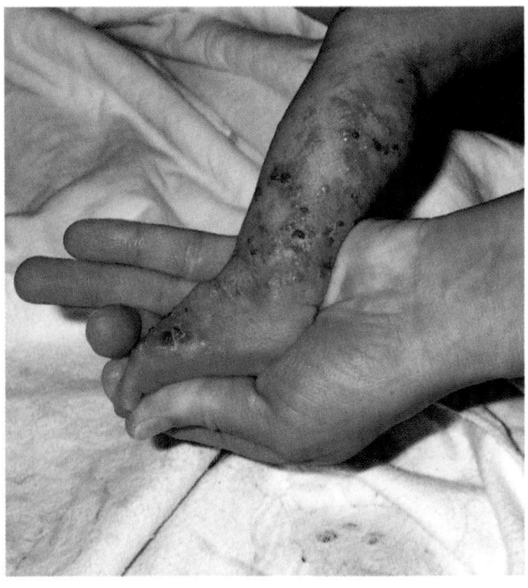

Figure 4.12. Marked crusting and blistering, easily mistaken for severe bullous impetigo.

HISTOPATHOLOGY

Light. The histopathology depends on the stage of the disorder. In the inflammatory, blistering phase, there are intercellular edema and intraepidermal vesicles. Eosinophils are prominent in the vesicles throughout the epidermis and dermis. There are clusters of dyskeratotic keratinocytes. Hyperkeratosis, papillomatosis, and mild dyskeratosis are seen in the verrucous lesions.

The pigmentary phase shows degeneration of the basal cells and melanin-loaded macrophages in the dermis, hence the term *incontinence* of pigment.

EM. Macrophages (melanophages) in the dermis, containing melanosome complexes and dyskeratotic material, are found in stages I to III.

BASIC DEFECT

Unknown. Incontinentia pigmenti is a fascinating disorder without a unifying hypothesis. There may be tissue-specific selection against the mutant gene as demonstrated in vitro in fibroblasts and lymphocytes, which selectively express the normal X chromosome.

TREATMENT

No treatment is required for the skin lesions. The blisters usually heal rapidly, without sequelae. The verrucous phase is also short lived. Dental restoration may be necessary. Ophthalmologic examination including indirect ophthalmoloscopy by a physician familiar with incontinentia pigmenti should be performed at the time of diagnosis and every 3 to 6 months thereafter for the first few years of life. Laser ablation of abnormal vessels may be indicated.

Although incontinentia pigmenti can be a serious disorder, parents can be reassured that the majority of affected girls do well, without compromise to their health and function in adulthood.

MODE OF INHERITANCE

X-linked dominant, lethal in males. When the disease occurs in a male, it is thought to have arisen as a postzygotic mutation or as the result of a "half-chromatid" mutation so that some of the cells have a normal gene on the X, allowing survival. There is one report of an affected brother and sister born to a carrier mother. The description of the male is unconvincing. Carrier women usually, but not invariably, express the disorder clinically. Pedigrees are characterized by an increased incidence of miscarriages (of presumably affected males), a distorted sex ratio of 2:1 female-to-male offspring of carriers, and female-to-female transmission. The patchy distribution of the skin lesions is thought to result from tissue mosaicism secondary to random X-inactivation, the normal and abnormal genes being active in uninvolved and involved skin, respectively. The gene has been mapped to Xq28.

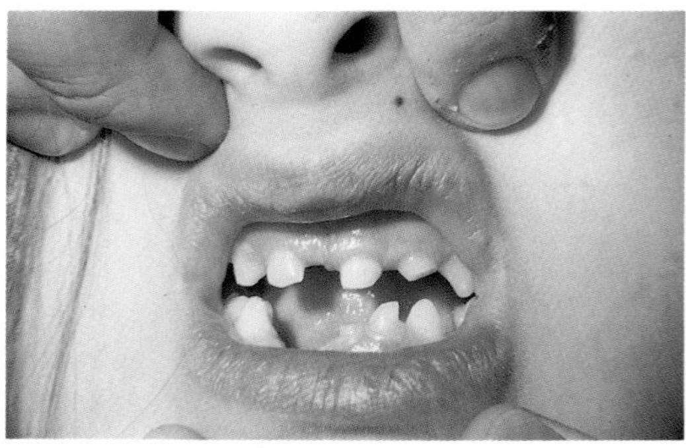

Figure 4.13. Abnormal teeth. (From Francis and Sybert, 1995.)

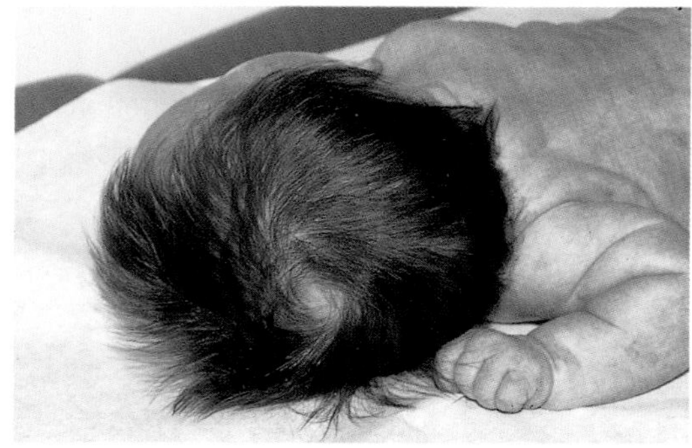

Figure 4.14. Area of congenital alopecia. (From Francis and Sybert, 1995.)

PRENATAL DIAGNOSIS

Unreliable. The inconsistent distribution of skin lesions precludes accurate diagnosis by skin biopsy.

DIFFERENTIAL DIAGNOSIS

In focal dermal hypoplasia of Goltz (MIM: 305600), while the associated malformations are similar, the skin lesions are distinct.

Similar-appearing blisters in the newborn period can result from infection (herpes, varicella, *Staphylococcus,* or *Streptococcus*) or epidermolysis bullosa, especially the Dowling-Meara or herpetiformis type (MIM:131760).

The verrucous lesions bear some resemblance to linear epidermal nevi; biopsy will differentiate between them if history of previous blistering does not.

Hypomelanosis of Ito, or incontinentia pigmenti achromians (MIM: 146150), should not be confused with incontinentia pigmenti. Although the distribution of the hypopigmentation of hypomelanosis of Ito is similar to the hyperpigmentation of incontinentia pigmenti, there are no preceding bullous or verrucous lesions.

Incontinentia pigmenti 1 (MIM:308300) is the term that has been used to describe a group of children with X-autosome translocations involving a breakpoint at Xp11. Almost all these case reports involve chromosomal mosaicism and a phenotype typical of hypomelanosis of Ito, not incontinentia pigmenti. The blisters of bullous congenital ichthyosiform erythroderma (MIM:113800, 146800) are usually larger, there is generalized rather than patchy erythema, and the hyperkeratosis is quite distinctive from the verrucous lesions of incontinentia pigmenti.

Congenital bullous mastocytosis may show blisters, but is easily distinguished clinically and histologically by the classic appearance of the mast cell tumors.

The Naegeli syndrome (MIM:161000) has similar pigment changes, which develop in the second or third year of life, but is distinguished by palmoplantar hyperkeratosis and yellow teeth. I have never seen a patient with this disorder.

Support Group: National Incontinentia Pigmenti Foundation
41 East 57th Street, 5th Floor
New York, NY 10022
1-212-207-4636

SELECTED BIBLIOGRAPHY

Carney, R.G., Jr. (1976). Incontinentia pigmenti: a world statistical analysis. *Arch. Dermatol.* **112,** 535–542.
An excellent review article of the clinical reports of incontinentia pigmenti. The clinical spectrum of the disease has not been significantly broadened since its publication.

Francois, J. (1984). Incontinentia pigmenti (Bloch-Sulzberger syndrome) and retinal changes. *Br. J. Ophthalmol.* **68,** 19–25.
Reviews the eye findings and gives a general overview.

Sybert, V.P. (1994). Incontinentia pigmenti nomenclature. *Am. J. Hum. Genet.* **55,** 209–211.
I argue for the death of the terms and concept of IP1 and IP2.

Watzke, R.C., Stevens, T.S., and Carney, R.G., Jr. (1976). Retinal vascular changes of incontinentia pigmenti. *Arch. Ophthalmol.* **94,** 743–746.
Discusses retinal changes in detail.

Wieacker, P., Zimmer, J., and Ropers, H.-H. (1985). X-inactivation patterns in two syndromes with probable X-linked dominant, male lethal inheritance. *Clin. Genet.* **28,** 238–242.
Reports the apparent selection either in vitro or in vivo against cells in which the X-chromosome bearing the incontinentia pigmenti gene is active.

LEOPARD SYNDROME (MIM:151100)

(Cardiomyopathic Lentiginosis; Moynahan Syndrome; Cardiocutaneous Syndrome; Lentiginosis Profusa)

Includes Centrofacial Lentiginosis

DERMATOLOGIC FEATURES

MAJOR. The *L* of the LEOPARD syndrome is for lentigines. These dark brown small macules develop over the face, neck, upper chest, back, and upper arms, where they are profuse. They are less densely present elsewhere. Palms, soles, and genitalia may also be involved. The lentigines may be present at birth, but usually develop over the first few months to years of life and increase with time. There is no recognized relationship with sun exposure.

MINOR. Larger (one to several centimeters in diameter) dark spots (referred to as *cafe-noir spots* by Gorlin et al., 1969) may develop on the trunk. These are usually few in number.

ASSOCIATED ABNORMALITIES

E is for echocardiographic abnormalities that are nonspecific and can include axis deviation, shortened PR intervals, bundle branch block, complete heart block, and so forth. Sudden death, presumably due to arrhythmia, has been reported in affected individuals. *O* is for ocular hypertelorism, the primary eye finding. Ptosis, epicanthal folds, and irregular iris pigmentation have also been described. *P* is for pulmonic stenosis, which is seen in some, but far from all, patients. Aortic stenosis and mitral stenoses have also been reported, as has hypertrophic cardiomyopathy. *A* is for abnormal genitalia, which are appreciated most readily in males with hypospadias, cryptorchidism, and pubertal delay. Delay of menarche in females has been described. *R* is for retardation of growth. Although there are statements in the literature that adult height is generally less than the 25th percentile, it appears that stature below the 3rd percentile occurs almost exclusively in males with genital abnormalities. This may reflect the absence of testosterone effect rather than a primary growth failure or skeletal dysplasia. Most affected females are normal in height, as are affected males who do not have testicular abnormalities. Winging of the scapulae, pectus deformities, and small joint hypermobility are common findings. *D* is for deafness, which is sensorineural and congenital. It is present in 15%–20% of patients.

Mental retardation is reported in numerous instances. Some suggest the *R* of LEOPARD should refer to psychomotor rather than somatic retardation.

In most families the acronym is not fully realized in all affected individuals.

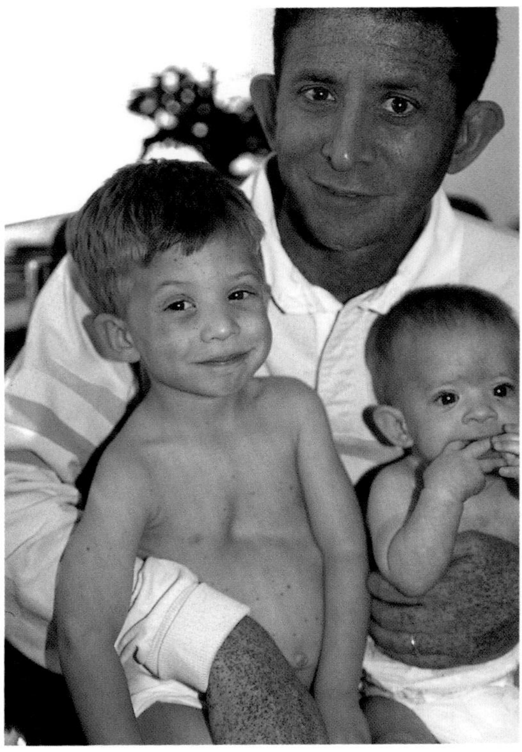

Figure 4.15. Multiple lentigenes in father; milder involvement in son. No other clinical features of LEOPARD syndrome.

HISTOPATHOLOGY

Light. Increased number of melanocytes with increase in melanin and elongation of the rete ridges.

EM. Giant melanosomes can be demonstrated but are neither a specific nor a constant feature. Most melanosomes are normal.

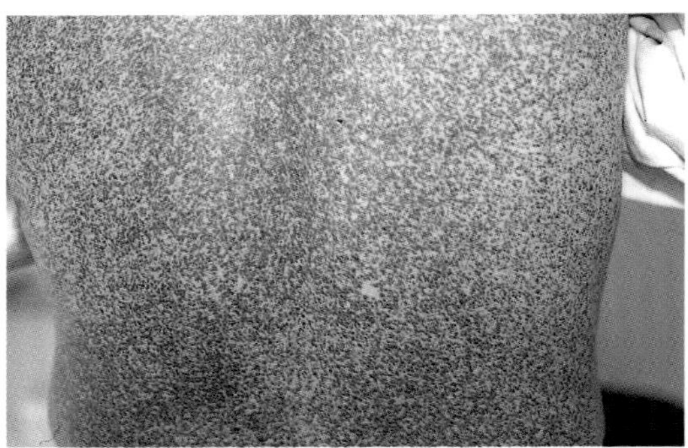

Figure 4.16. Wall-to-wall lentigenes in father.

BASIC DEFECT

Unknown.

TREATMENT

Case reports of successful obliteration of lentigines with dermabrasion and cryotherapy dot the literature.

A cardiac evaluation including electrocardiogram, screening hearing tests, and appropriate urologic and endocrinologic management of patients with genital abnormalities should all be part of routine care.

MODE OF INHERITANCE

Autosomal dominant.

PRENATAL DIAGNOSIS

None.

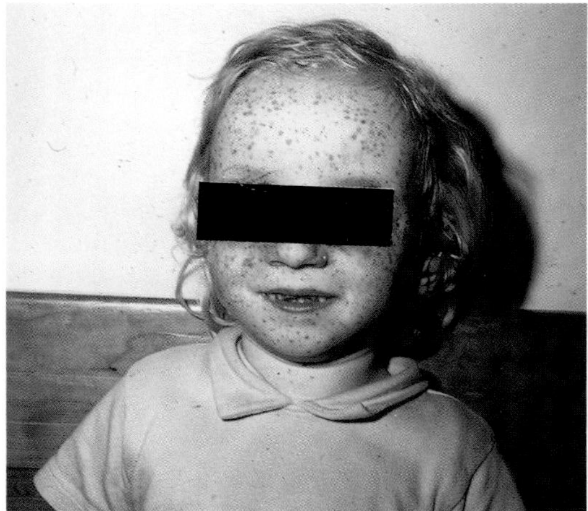
A

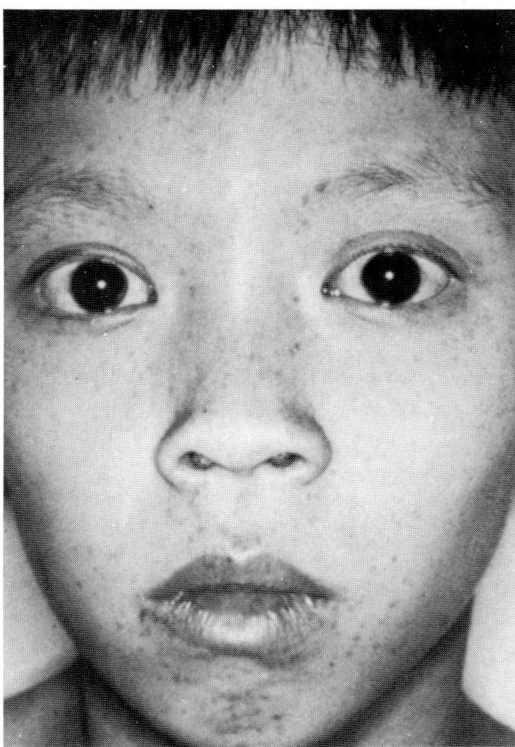
B

Figure 4.17. (A,B) Hypertelorism and lentigenes in patients with LEOPARD syndrome. (A, courtesy of Dr. J.G. Hall, Vancouver, British Columbia; B, from Ting and Ng, 1983.)

DIFFERENTIAL DIAGNOSIS

The list of syndromes associated with multiple brown pigmented macules is legion. Although there have been several reports of families with multiple lentigines without any other somatic abnormalities, full evaluation (e.g., electrocardiogram, facial measurements) for the associated features of LEOPARD syndrome was not performed in most. Thus, I am unsure if isolated autosomal dominant multiple lentigines exist, or whether such individuals represent limited expression of the gene for LEOPARD syndrome and are at risk for offspring with the full-blown condition.

Centrofacial lentiginosis (CFL) refers to a pattern of lentigines over the nose and cheeks that develops in early childhood and may fade in adult life. Two pedigrees of American families of African descent with centrofacial lentiginosis have been published. In these, pigmented lesions were also seen on the buttocks, hands, and feet. Most cases of CFL are sporadic and have been associated with neurologic and psychomotor abnormalities. This association may reflect the population screened for the skin changes (e.g., vocational training schools and psychiatric facilities).

The NAME/Carney/LAMB syndrome(s) (MIM:160980) share multiple lentigines in common with LEOPARD syndrome. Cardiac involvement in Carney complex is marked by atrial myxomas, and other cutaneous lesions include blue nevi, freckles, and myxomas.

Noonan syndrome (MIM:163950) shares some facial features, genital abnormalities, growth abnormalities, intellectual problems, and cardiac lesions with LEOPARD syndrome. The dermatologic feature associated with Noonan syndrome is ulerythema ophryogenes. The cutaneous features of the LEOPARD syndrome are not seen in patients with Noonan syndrome.

Watson syndrome (MIM:193520), which is allelic with neurofibromatosis, is characterized by café-au-lait spots, not lentigines. The typical heart lesion is pulmonic stenosis. Patients share short stature and some facial features in common with the LEOPARD syndrome.

Partial unilateral lentiginosis is a sporadic condition. There are no associated abnormalities. The distribution of lesions is usually on the upper part of the body. There are no reports of affected persons having reproduced to address whether segmental distribution of lesions might represent somatic mutation for neurofibromatosis or LEOPARD syndrome. Some case reports in the literature of this condition were mistakenly labeled as having LEOPARD syndrome.

Nevus phakomatosis pigmentovascularis refers to a group of conditions that appear to be sporadic and are characterized by pigmented and vascular birthmarks, including patches of lentigines, mongolian spots, nevus spilus, port wine stains, blue nevi, and large café-au-lait spots. Reported primarily among the Japanese (who are already more likely to have extensive mongolian spots), the associated noncutaneous abnormalities range from none to profound neurologic handicap. Individuals with LEOPARD syndrome have widespread lentigines in contrast to the focal distribution of pigment in these patients.

In the Peutz-Jeghers syndrome (MIM: 175200), lentigines are primarily on the mouth, on the mucosa, around the anus, and occasionally on the fingers, toes, palms, and soles. Widespread lentiginosis is not seen. Polyposis coli is not a feature of LEOPARD syndrome.

Freckles and junctional nevi can appear clinically similar to lentigines. Freckles are generally limited to sun-exposed areas. Junctional nevi are usually flat and darkly pigmented and not as numerous as lentigines. They may show some epidermal change. Junctional nevi can be easily differentiated histologically.

Support Group: N.O.R.D.
P.O. Box 8923
New Fairfield, CT
06812
1-800-999-6673

SELECTED BIBLIOGRAPHY

Colomb, D., and Morel, J.-P. (1984). Le syndrome des lentigines multiples. A propos de deux observations. Étude critique du syndrome LEOPARD. *Ann. Dermatol. Venereol.* **111,** 371–381.

Reviews 38 case reports along with two of the authors' own patients. One hundred percent had lentigines; 80%, electrocardiographic abnormalities and/or murmurs; 35%, mental retardation; 27%, deafness; 50%, ocular hypertelorism; 42%, short stature; 29%, genital abnormalities (present only in the males); 60%, a variety of skeletal abnormalities.

Gorlin, R.J., Anderson, R.C., and Blaw, M. (1969). Multiple lentigines syndrome. Complex comprising multiple lentigines, electrocardiographic conduction abnormalities, ocular hypertelorism, pulmonary stenosis, abnormalities of genitalia, retardation of growth, sensorineural deafness, and autosomal dominant hereditary pattern. *Am. J. Dis. Child.* **117,** 652–662.

Identical twins, each with two affected children. Both mothers had no lentigines, normal hearing, normal stature, with hypertelorism and cardiac abnormalities.

O'Neill, J.F., and James, W.D. (1989). Inherited patterned lentiginosis in blacks. *Arch. Dermatol.* **125,** 1231–1235.

Ten patients. Two reported a positive family history with multiple generations and male-to-male transmission. Histopathologic specimen was consistent with freckles rather than lentigines.

Touraine, A. (1941). Une nouvelle neuroectodermose congenitale. La lentiginose centrofaciale et ses dysplasies associees. *Ann. Dermatol. Syphiligr. (Paris)* **8,** 453–473.

Details of numerous cases. Mother-to-child(ren) transmission in four families; affected siblings in four; affected first cousins in one. No instances of male-to-male transmission.

Voron, D.A., Hatfield, H.H., and Kalkhoff, R.K. (1976). Multiple lentigines syndrome. Case report and review of the literature. *Am. J. Med.* **60,** 447–456.

The authors review 79 cases in the literature plus one of their own. Table of numbers of patients with each feature needs to be interpreted with caution, as not all case reports of individuals with lentigines represent LEOPARD syndrome, and not all case reports are complete. They suggest a minimum diagnostic criteria of (1) lentigines plus two other features or (2) in patients without lentigines, three features plus a relative who fulfills the first criterion.

LINEAR AND WHORLED NEVOID HYPERMELANOSIS (MIM:None)

DERMATOLOGIC FEATURES

Major. Brown macular pigmentation in streaks and whorls is distributed along the lines of Blaschko. It first appears in infancy and gradually spreads to involve major portions of the body. It is relatively symmetric and asymptomatic. The extent of involvement usually stabilizes by age 2 years. In some individuals it lightens over time and may disappear by adult life; in others it remains unchanged.
Minor. None.

ASSOCIATED ABNORMALITIES

There have been a few case reports of individuals described as having linear and whorled nevoid hypermelanosis who have had congenital anomalies. Chromosome studies to look for mosaicism were not performed in them.

HISTOPATHOLOGY

Light. There is an increase in pigment in the epidermis with some increase in the number of melanocytes. No giant melanosomes are found. There is mild elongation of the rete ridges.
EM. The melanosomes appear normal, as do the melanocytes. In darker areas of skin there appear to be increased numbers of normal-appearing melanosomes.

BASIC DEFECT

Unknown.

TREATMENT

None described. Bleaching agents might be effective in offering temporary relief, but there is no published information regarding this.

MODE OF INHERITANCE

Unknown. There is one mother–daughter pair reported.

PRENATAL DIAGNOSIS

None.

DIFFERENTIAL DIAGNOSIS

The skin changes of linear and whorled nevoid hyperpigmentation are clinically indistinguishable from those of incontinentia pigmenti (MIM:308300). In affected females it may be

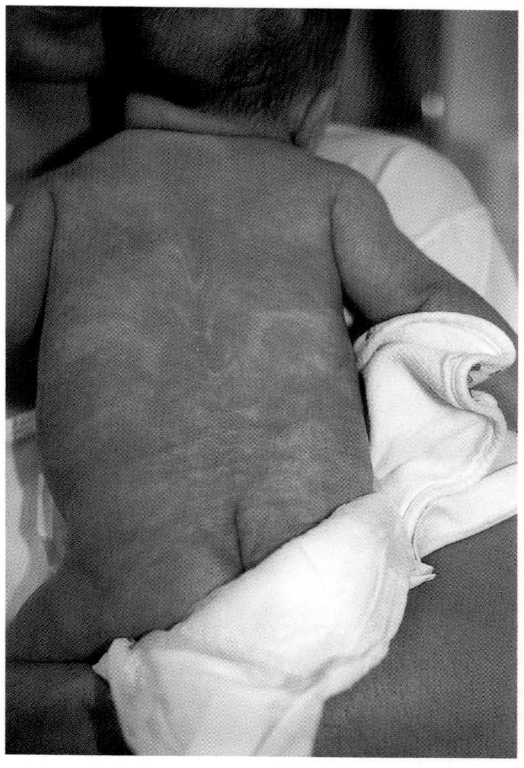

Figure 4.18. Hyperpigmentation distributed along the lines of Blaschko.

very difficult to exclude incontinentia pigmenti, as there are rare reports of incontinentia pigmenti first presenting with stage III (pigmentary) changes without preceding blistering or verrucous (stage I and stage II) lesions. Histologically, the hyperpigmented areas of incontinentia pigmenti usually show melanin incontinence and dermal melanophages, features not seen in nevoid hypermelanosis.

Chromosomal mosaicism can result in variegation of pigment, either increased or, more commonly, decreased, distributed along the lines of Blaschko (hypomelanosis of Ito). In an otherwise normal child with linear and whorled nevoid hypermelanosis, karyotyping may not be indicated, but this should be determined on a case by case basis.

Epidermal nevi may begin as macular lesions, but almost always become palpable relatively quickly. A biopsy will differentiate between these two conditions.

Lichen striatus is an acquired disorder characterized by flat-topped papules distributed along the lines of Blaschko. It can be hyperpigmented, although it is more usually pale or yellowish. The pigment change in linear and whorled nevoid hypermelanosis is macular. Lichen striatus is a palpable condition.

Progressive cribiform and zosteriform hyper-

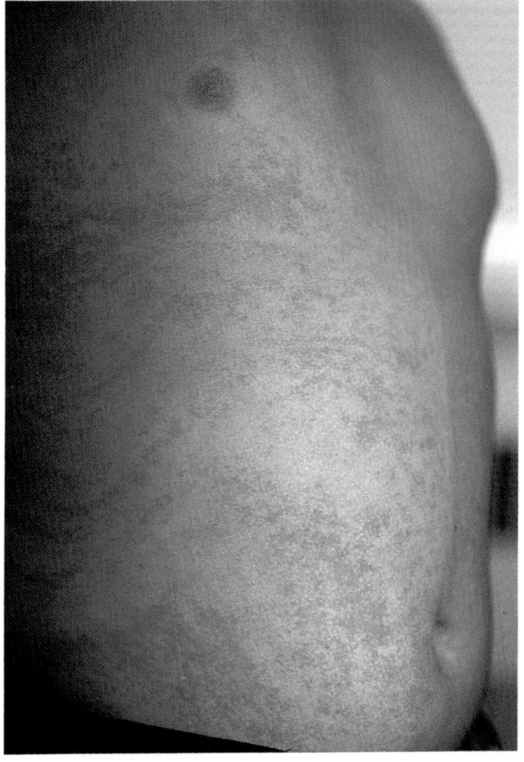

Figure 4.19. Fascinating patient with contrasting sides: one with light on dark, one with dark on light. Skin changes were noted during infancy. Patient is otherwise healthy.

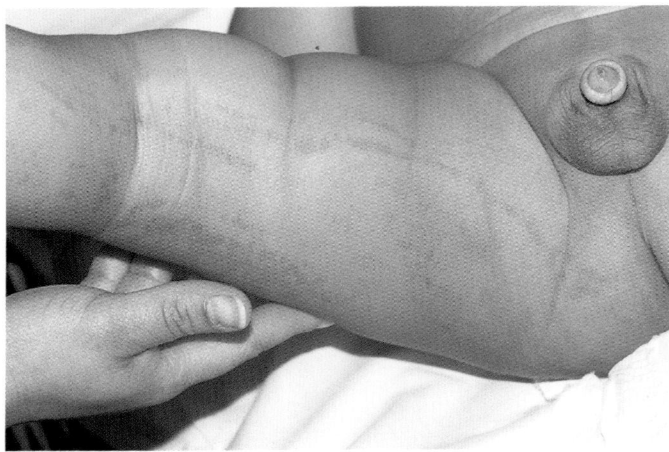

Figure 4.20. Linear hyperpigmented streaks on the leg along the lines of Blaschko in patient of African and European descent.

pigmentation has a later onset (usually around puberty) and usually is localized. Its cause is also unknown.

Support Group: N.O.R.D.
P.O. Box 8923
New Fairfield, CT
06812
1-800-999-6673

SELECTED BIBLIOGRAPHY

Akiyama, M., Aranami, A., Sasaki, Y., Ebihara, T., and Sugiura, M. (1994). Familial linear and whorled nevoid hypermelanosis. *J. Am. Acad. Dermatol.* **30,** 831–833.

A 33-year-old mother and her 3-year-old daughter. Both had onset of pigment change a few weeks after birth. They had no other problems. Biopsy did not show incontinence of pigment.

Iijima, S., Naito, Y., Naito, S., and Uyeno, K. (1987). Reticulate hyperpigmentation distributed in a zosteriform fashion: a new clinical type of hyperpigmentation. *Br. J. Dermatol.* **117,** 503–510.

Describes two patients. There is a table with a differential diagnosis that is useful.

Kalter, D.C., Griffiths, W.A., and Atherton, D.J. (1988). Linear and whorled nevoid hypermelanosis. *J. Am. Acad. Dermatol.* **19,** 1037–1044.

Presents two cases with progressive swirly hyperpigmentation that stabilized at 1 to 2 years of age. Electron microscopy and histology were thought to be nondiagnostic. Chromosome studies of skin and blood in both patients were normal. One patient had mild eosinophilia. Includes a succinct review of the literature to date.

Kanwar, A.J., Dhar, S., Ghosh, S., and Kaur, S. (1993). Letter: linear and whorled nevoid hypermelanosis. *Int. J. Dermatol.* **32,** 385–386.

Unilateral involvement in a male was described.

Wend, G. W., and Bauckus, H. H. (1919). A hitherto undescribed generalized pigmentation of the skin appearing in infancy in a brother and sister. *J. Cutan. Dis.* **37,** 685–701.

Onset occurred in early childhood with gradual disappearance in late childhood and development of guttate hypomelanosis. Affected children had variegation of color in both hair and skin.

McCUNE-ALBRIGHT SYNDROME (MIM:174800)

(Polyostotic Fibrous Dysplasia with Café-Au-Lait Spots)

DERMATOLOGIC FEATURES

MAJOR. Large, dark café-au-lait-spots, usually, but not invariably, with irregular margins, tend to be unilateral or segmental without crossing the midline. The lesions may be congenital or develop in infancy. Bone changes are usually but not consistently on the same side as the skin changes.

Skin changes are not invariably present, as only two of the triad of signs (skin, bone, endocrine) are required for diagnosis. Approximately one-third of patients diagnosed to have McCune-Albright syndrome have skin changes.

MINOR. Multiple benign soft tissue myxomas have been described in 12 patients with polyostotic fibrous dysplasia, six of whom had other features of McCune-Albright syndrome. The myxomas are usually near the most severely affected bones.

Linear epidermal nevi have been reported several times in patients with McCune-Albright.

Alopecia secondary to full-thickness fibrous hyperplasia of the scalp with ectopic bone formation was described in one patient. It was stable in early childhood but enlarged in middle age. This patient also had a lymphangioma, absence of the eyelashes on the right, paucity of pubic and axillary hair on the right, and a large café-au-lait spot on the right scapula that disappeared in adulthood. None of these changes has been reported in other patients.

ASSOCIATED ABNORMALITIES

There are distorting lucent areas (polyostotic fibrous dysplasia) in the long bones that are often unilateral and/or monomelic. In descending order of frequency, the femur, ilium, tibia, pubis, humerus, radius, scapula, and clavicle are involved, Deformity, bowing, pain, and fractures are the common presenting features. Sclerosis of the base of the skull is a common finding as well. Some claim that the bone changes stabilize in adult life with a cessation of fractures; others state that they continue to occur.

Precocious puberty occurs almost invariably only in females and appears to be under autonomous ovarian control; it is rare in males with McCune-Albright syndrome. Pituitary functions are normal, as are levels of releasing factors and suppression of pituitary function with luteinizing hormone-releasing hormone antagonists does not alter the clinical state. Approximately one-third of female patients will have precocious puberty, often associated with the presence of recurrent ovarian cysts. Fertility appears normal, and stature does not appear to be shortened, as might be expected.

Other endocrinopathies including hyperthyroidism, acromegaly, hyperprolactinemia, Cushing syndrome, endocrine adenomas, and hypophosphatemia occur. The hyperthyroidism is also under local control, and successful treatment usually requires ablation of the thyroid.

Breast carcinoma has been reported in two female patients, one aged 11 and one aged 35.

One patient with coarctation of the aorta and one with multiple arteriovenous malformations, both with polyostotic fibrous dysplasia and café-au-lait spots, are detailed in the literature. The patient with coarctation also had a malformed left kidney.

Neonatal jaundice resolving during infancy was noted in a few case reports. There were no details given regarding possible causes for jaundice.

Malignant degeneration of the bone lesions has been reported in a minority of patients with polyostotic fibrous dysplasia, at least four of whom had the cutaneous changes of McCune-Albright. The estimated risk for malignant change ranges from less than 5% to less than 1%. Of 29 cases of malignancy, 12 received prior radiation treatment to the bony lesions, suggesting that radiotherapy of benign lesions should be avoided.

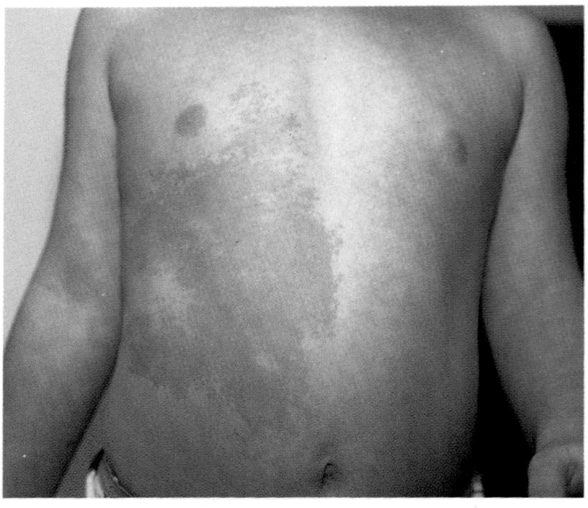

Figure 4.21. Large, irregular café-au-lait patch, respecting the midline.

HISTOPATHOLOGY

LIGHT. Polyostotic fibrous displasia: Spicules of bone and islands of cartilage interspersed in the matrix of collagenous tissue characterize the bony lesions.

The café-au-lait spots are indistinguishable histologically from typical café-au-lait spots or those associated with neurofibromatosis.

EM. A decreased number of giant pigment granules has been described but this is not a consistent finding.

BASIC DEFECT

Different mutations in exon 8 of the G_S-alpha gene have been demonstrated in patients with McCune-Albright syndrome. These alterations result in a functional increase in activity of the G_S-alpha protein and increased cyclic AMP activity. This protein is also altered in acquired endocrine tumors.

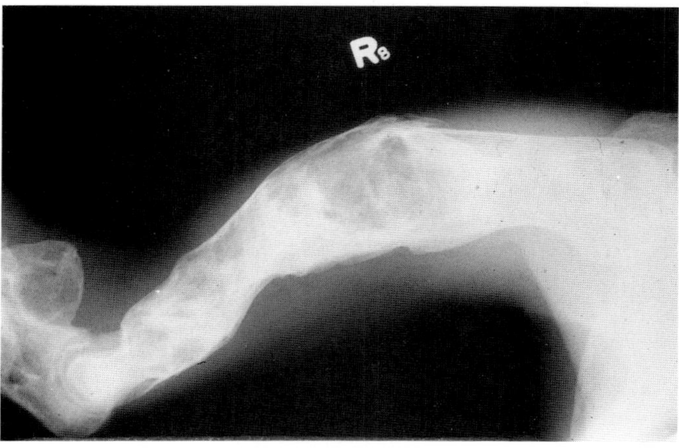

Figure 4.22. Severe bony changes of polyostotic fibrous dysplasia. (Courtesy of Dr. J.G. Hall, Vancouver, British Columbia.)

TREATMENT

Bone changes: Bony alterations may require surgical amputation, rodding, grafting, and so forth. Radiotherapy should be avoided. Intravenous pamidronate has had preliminary success in controlling bone pain and reducing fractures.

Sexual precocity: It is unclear if any treatment is useful. Testolactone, which blocks estrogen synthesis, has been successful in suppressing pubertal changes, but its use is still investigational. It is important to reassure families regarding ultimate stature and fertility. Psychological support for the premature maturation may be helpful.

Hyperthyroidism: Ablative therapy is necessary.

Acromegaly: Growth hormone over production has been successfully suppressed with treatment with Octreotide, a somatostatin analog.

MODE OF INHERITANCE

Sporadic. McCune-Albright appears to result from a postzygotic mutation of an autosomal dominant gene. Support for this comes from molecular studies that demonstrated different amounts of mutant G_S-alpha protein from different tissues in the same individual. There are two reports of classic McCune-Albright in one of two monozygotic twins and minor manifestations in the second. These are not convincing to me. The minor manifestations in the second twin could be considered normal variation. No instance of familial transmission of McCune-Albright syndrome has been documented.

PRENATAL DIAGNOSIS

None.

DIFFERENTIAL DIAGNOSIS

In the newborn or young infant, the presence of an isolated giant café-au-lait spot may be the harbinger of segmental neurofibromatosis, neurofibromatosis, or McCune-Albright syndrome or have no medical significance. Mutational analysis of the G_S-alpha gene might help to diagnose McCune-Albright syndrome, but it is not currently clinically available. Although smooth (neurofibromatosis) versus serrated (McCune-Albright) borders of the spots are supposedly distinctive, either configuration of café-au-lait spots can be found in either of the two disorders.

The bone changes of McCune-Albright syndrome are distinct from the pseudoarthroses of neurofibromatosis. Axillary freckling is absent, and neurofibromas do not occur in McCune-Albright. It may be difficult to differentiate between the two conditions in the young infant or child with a single giant café-au-lait spot. The presence of giant melanosomes is not pathognomonic for either, although they are more common in café-au-lait spots from normal individuals and those with neurofibromatosis than those with McCune-Albright.

Polyostotic fibrous dysplasia limited to the craniofacies with autosomal dominant inheritance has been described. Of 13 affected family members, none had other features of McCune-Albright syndrome.

There is a single report of a male with three melanotic patches, diffuse (panostotic) fibrous dysplasia and recurrent fractures, hypophosphatemia, and hyperphosphatasemia.

Support Group: MAGIC Foundation for Children's Growth
1327 North Harlem Avenue
Oak Park, IL 60302
1-800-362-4423

SELECTED BIBLIOGRAPHY

Benedict, P.H., Szabo, G., Fitzpatrick, T.B., and Sinesi, S.J. (1968). Melanotic macules in Albright's syndrome and in neurofibromatosis. *JAMA* **205,** 72–80.

Giant melanosomes were found in café-au-lait spots from 18 neurofibromatosis patients and only one of 10 patients wiht McCune-Albright syndrome. There is a wonderful triptych of photos depicting the classic features of McCune-Albright cafe-au-lait spots, with the coast of Maine margins and unilateral distribution, all three from patients with neurofibromatosis.

Happle, R. (1986). The McCune-Albright syndrome: A lethal gene surviving by mosaicism. *Clin. Genet.* **29,** 321–324.

The observation of the distribution of the café-au-lait spots along the lines of Blaschko in one patient led Happle to review previous reports in which he noticed similar features. He postulated somatic mosaicism as a cause for variable findings in McCune-Albright. This is a nice example of clinical acumen leading to predictive hypothesis.

Harris, W.H., Dudley, H.R., Jr., and Barry, R.J. (1962). The natural history of fibrous dysplasia. An orthopedic, pathological, and roentgenographic study. *J. Bone Joint Surg. Am.* **44A,** 207–233.

Extensive follow-up of polyostotic and monoostotic fibrous dysplasia. Two cases of malignancy in McCune-Albright syndrome, both with prior radiation. Details the spectrum of the disorder.

Hibbs, R.E. and Rush, H.P. (1952). Albright's syndrome. *Ann. Intern. Med.* **37,** 587–593.

Case report of an affected mother with the full triad. Her healthy 13-year-old daughter had a single bony lesion of the upper left radius that showed fibrous dysplasia on tissue from a biopsy performed at age 12.

Lee, P.A., Van Dop, C., and Migeon, C.J. (1986). McCune-Albright syndrome. Long-term follow-up. *JAMA* **256,** 2980–2984.

This is a follow-up study of 15 patients (6 were 18 years of age older), 13 of whom were female. Fractures occurred only during childhood, but four of six adults developed deafness secondary to temporal bone involvement. Two adult females had normal offspring.

Liens, D., Delmas, P.D., and Meunier, P.J. (1994). Long-term effects of intravenous pamidronate in fibrous dysplasia of bone. *Lancet* **343,** 953–954.

Three day infusions every 6 months. Nine patients treated, with good results in most; follow-up time was 18–48 months. Toxicity and difficulty of administration may limit use.

McCune, D. J., and Bruch, H. (1937). Osteodystrophia fibrosa. *Am. J. Dis. Child.* **54,** 806–848.

Albright, F., Butler, A.M., Hamptom, A.O., and Smith, P. (1937). Syndrome characterized by osteitis fibrosa disseminata, areas of pigmentation and endocrine dysfunction, with precocious puberty in females. *N. Engl. J. Med.* **216,** 727–746.

McCune reported his patient at a meeting; Albright mentioned his in the ensuing discussion and returned to Boston subsequently to publish five cases, beating McCune and Bruch to the publication punch.

Rustin, M.H.A., Bunker, C.B., Gilkes, J.J.H.,

Robinson, T.W.E., and Dowd, P.M. (1989). Polyostotic fibrous dysplasia associated with extensive linear epidermal naevi. *Clin. Exp. Dermatol.* **14,** 371–375.

A 35-year-old male with polyostotic fibrous dysplasia and extensive linear nevus on the right humerus, left arm, and left hand. Treatment with etretinate improved the skin lesions.

Weinstein, L.S., Shenker, A., Gejman, P.V., Merino, M.J., Friedman, E., and Spiegel, A.M. (1991). Activating mutations of the stimulatory G protein in the McCune-Albright syndrome. *N. Engl. J. Med.* **325,** 1688–1695.

Four of six patients with McCune-Albright studies (plus four others not reported in detail) were found to have mutations in Arg^{201}, substituting cystine or histidine. The proportion of mutant and normal proteins varied among tissues. Tissue from all three germ layers contained the mutation. The accompanying, very clearly written and helpful editorial (Levine, M. A. *N. Engl. J. Med.* **325,** 1738–1740, 1991) points out that mutations in the same gene that result in downregulation of expression of the G_S-alpha protein have been implicated in Albright hereditary osteodystrophy. This is the same Albright and the same gene, but different mutations and phenotypes.

NAEGELI SYNDROME (MIM:161000)

(Naegeli-Franceschetti-Jadassohn)

DERMATOLOGIC FEATURES

Major. Brown-gray reticulate hyperpigmentation begins in early childhood (3 months to 5 years) and progresses. It stabilizes and starts to regress during puberty. The abdomen, neck, trunk, flexures, and perioral and periocular skin are involved in decreasing frequency. A decreased ability to sweat with heat intolerance is a constant feature and varies in severity.

Palmoplantar hyperkeratosis begins in late childhood and is characterized by diffuse distribution of punctate lesions. Absence of dermatoglyphics is typically noted.

Minor. Nail abnormalities include brittle nails and malalignment of the great toenails, subungual hyperkeratosis, and onycholysis. Transient blistering of the soles during the newborn period has been described in a few individuals.

ASSOCIATED ABNORMALITIES

The teeth are yellow with enamel defects, carious, and prone to early loss.

HISTOPATHOLOGY

Light. Eccrine glands may be normal, reduced in number, or absent. There may be an increase in chromatophores or melanophages in the dermis. The changes are not diagnostic.

EM. No information.

BASIC DEFECT

Unknown.

TREATMENT

Emollients may ameliorate the palmoplantar keratoderma. Environmental control to avoid hyperthermia is important.

MODE OF INHERITANCE

Autosomal dominant. Male-to-male transmission has been documented.

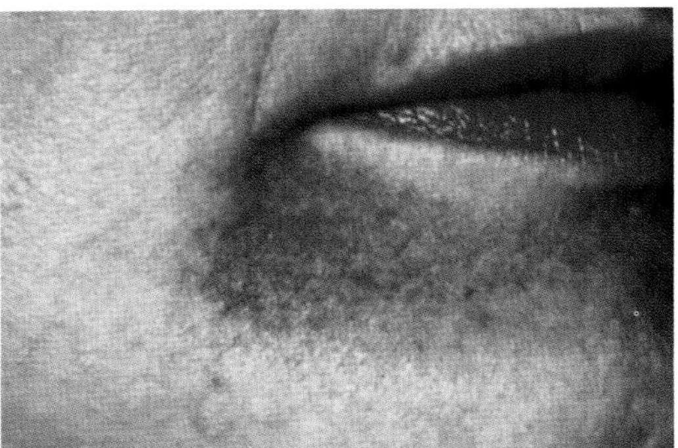

Figure 4.23. Hyperpigmentation under lips. (From Itin et al., 1993.)

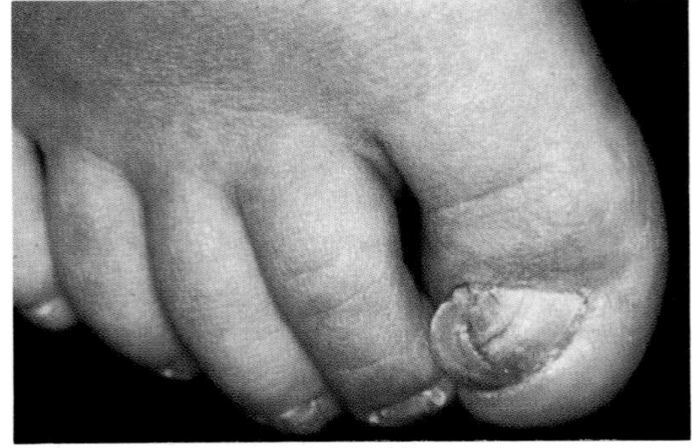

Figure 4.25. Malalignment of great toenail; hyperpigmentation of the skin. (From Itin et al., 1993.)

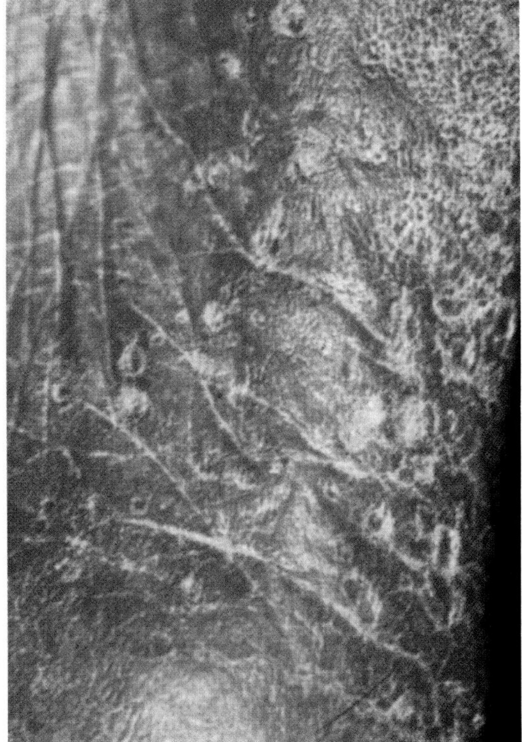

Figure 4.24. Punctate keratoderma. (From Itin et al., 1993.)

PRENATAL DIAGNOSIS

None.

DIFFERENTIAL DIAGNOSIS

In incontinentia pigmenti (MIM:308300), the hyperpigmented lesions are preceded by bullous, erythematous, and verrucous stages, palmoplantar hyperkeratosis is absent, and inheritance is X-linked.

Absence of dermatoglyphics can be isolated (MIM:136000, 125540), accompany junctional epidermolysis bullosa progressiva (MIM: 226500), or be seen with other conditions in which palmoplantar hyperkeratoses occur (MIM:Many).

Congenital malalignment of the great toenails may be inherited as an isolated autosomal dominant disorder (MIM:None).

In dermatopathia pigmentosa reticularis (MIM:None), the pigment changes do not fade, and there is scarring alopecia of the scalp, eyebrows, and axillary hair. The teeth are normal. Otherwise the disorders are quite similar. Dermatopathia pigmentosa reticularis has been reported in siblings.

Kindler-Weary syndrome (MIM:137650) and epidermolysis bullosa with mottled hyperpigmentation (MIM:131960) are similar but are marked by atrophy of the skin and poikiloderma and absence of heat intolerance.

Dyskeratosis congenita (MIM:305000) also

presents with diffuse streaky hyperpigmentation and may have similar nail changes. Leukoplakia, palmar hyperhidrosis, and anemia are distinguishing features of dyskeratosis congenita, as is X-linked inheritance.

Support Group: N.F.E.D.
219 East Main, Box 114
Mascoutah, IL 62258-0114
1-618-566-2020

SELECTED BIBLIOGRAPHY

Franceschetti, A., and Jadassohn, W. (1954). A propos de l' "incontinentia pigmenti" délimitation de deux syndromes différents figurant sous le même terme. *Dermatologica* **8,** 1–28.

Reexamination of Naegeli's patient and descendants. Recognized distinction between incontinentia pigmenti and Naegeli syndrome. Good color plate of skin changes.

Heimer, W.L. II, Brauner, G., and James, W.D. (1992). Dermatopathia pigmentosa reticularis: a report of a family demonstrating autosomal dominant inheritance. *J. Am. Acad. Dermatol.* **26,** 298–301.

There was no opportunity for male-to-male transmission in a five generation pedigree. Affected individuals in all the generations that reproduced were female.

Itin, P.H., Lautenschlager, S., Meyer, R., Mevorah, B., and Rufli, T. (1993). Natural history of the Naegeli-Franceschetti-Jadassohn syndrome and further delineation of its clinical manifestations. *J. Am. Acad. Dermatol.* **28,** 942–950.

Follow-up of Naegeli's original family. The authors examined 10 of 14 affected members of a 62 person, six generation pedigree. The age range was 6 to 78 years. They classify the disorder as a true ectodermal dysplasia.

NAME/CARNEY/LAMB COMPLEX (MIM:160980)

(Myxoma, Spotty Pigmentation, Endocrine Overactivity)

DERMATOLOGIC FEATURES

MAJOR. The acronyms NAME and LAMB stand for, respectively, *N*evi, *A*trial myxoma, *M*yxoid neurofibromata, *E*phelides; and *L*entigines, *A*trial myxoma, *M*yxoid tumors, *B*lue nevi.

In early childhood, diffuse, discrete to confluent, pale brown to black macules develop everywhere, including the lips and mucosa. Small bluish domed papules with a smooth surface also develop over time.

Myxoid cutaneous tumors of many histologic types present as subcutaneous nodules or swelling. They can involve any skin surface, including the mucosa. These may develop during childhood and throughout adult life.

MINOR. Red hair and pale complexion have been reported in a number of patients.

Pigmentation of the conjunctiva has also been described.

ASSOCIATED ABNORMALITIES

Atrial myxomas develop during childhood and cause progressive atrial hypertrophy. Affected individuals may complain of chest pain, dyspnea on exertion, and weakness. Myxomas of the ventricular wall and other intracardiac sites have occurred. Lesions may be single or multiple and recurrence after excision can occur. Central nervous system infarct and death due to tumor emboli are major complications of the cardiac tumors.

Some authors would expand the *E* to represent endocrine disturbances. The development of Cushing syndrome due to adrenocortical pigmented nodular hyperplasia, acromegaly due to pituitary adenoma, and tumors of the Sertoli cells of the testes have been reported. Ductal fibroadenomas of the breasts are also a feature of the condition. Patients with breast lesions may present with complaint of discharge from the nipple, or the lesions may be asymptomatic.

In the Carney complex, pigmented lesions on the conjunctiva and in the caruncle (the mucosal pad in the nasal corner of the eye) and myxomas of the eyelid are additional features.

HISTOPATHOLOGY

LIGHT. The pigmented macules are ephelides (freckles), with a normal number of melanocytes and normal rete ridges. There is increased melanin in the basal layer. In darker lesions there may be melanin in the suprabasal layers as well. Other reports have found histologic evidence supportive of lentigines; others report histologic features of both freckles and lentigines.

The blue lesions are cellular blue nevi.

The dermal nodules are composed of stellate and spindle-shaped cells in a mucoid basophilic matrix, primarily composed of proteoglycans. The number of mast cells is increased.

EM. In the dermal nodules there are scattered Schwann cells and mast cells, aggregates of fine granular material, and islands of degenerating collagen.

BASIC DEFECT

Unknown.

TREATMENT

Excision of cutaneous myxomas if desired. Evaluation for and excision of cardiac tumors when necessary.

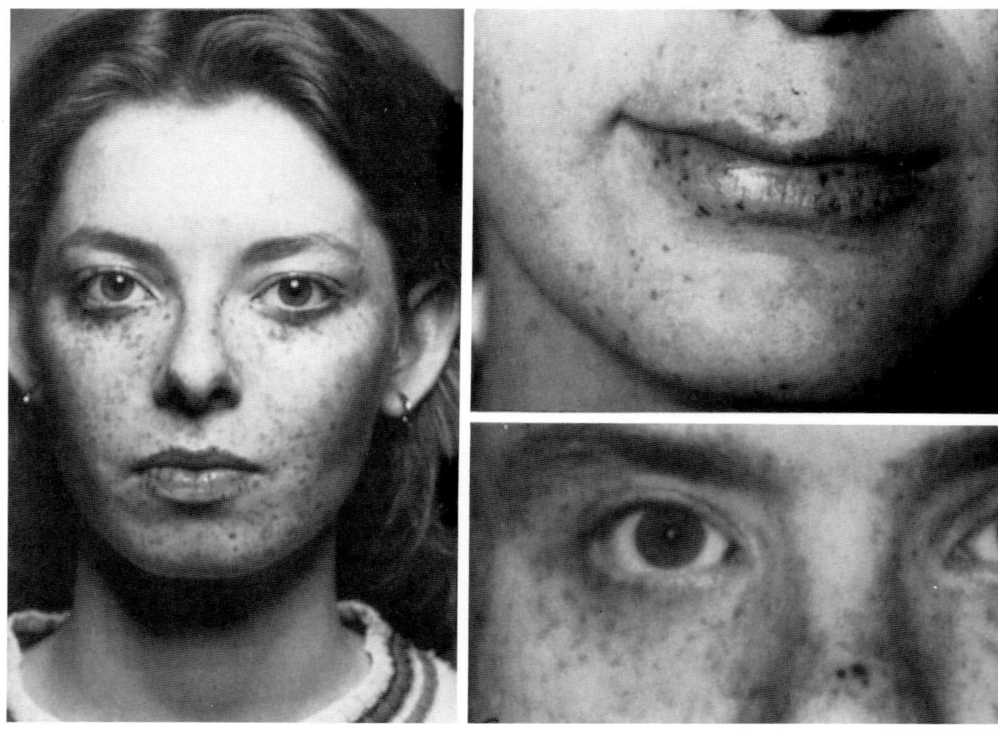

Figure 4.26. **(A)** Lentigines on face; myxoma on right lower lid. **(B)** Multiple pigmented spots in a different patient. **(C)** Pigmented lesion in the corner of the right eye. (From Carney et al., 1985.)

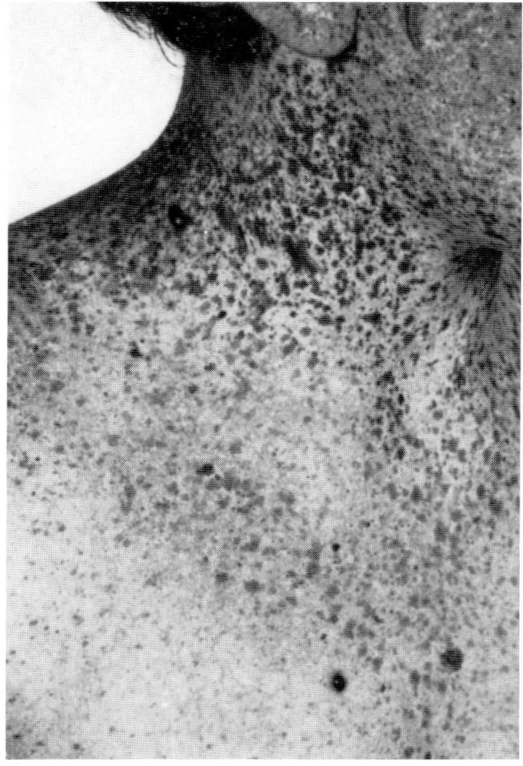

Figure 4.27. Multiple lentigines, domed blue nevi on neck and chest. (From Atherton et al., 1980.)

MODE OF INHERITANCE

Autosomal dominant. Tentatively mapped to 2p16.

PRENATAL DIAGNOSIS

None.

DIFFERENTIAL DIAGNOSIS

LEOPARD syndrome (MIM:151100) and Peutz-Jeghers syndrome (MIM:175200) need to be excluded. While sharing in common the multiple pigmented macules, other associated features can readily distinguish them. Disorders of photosensitivity such as xeroderma pigmentosa (MIM:278700), in which abnormal freckling occurs, can easily be distinguished by association with sun exposure. The melanotic lesions of NAME syndrome do not appear to be particularly associated with sun exposure. Atrophy, xerosis, and telangiectasias will also help to distinguish the disorders of photosensitivity from NAME syndrome.

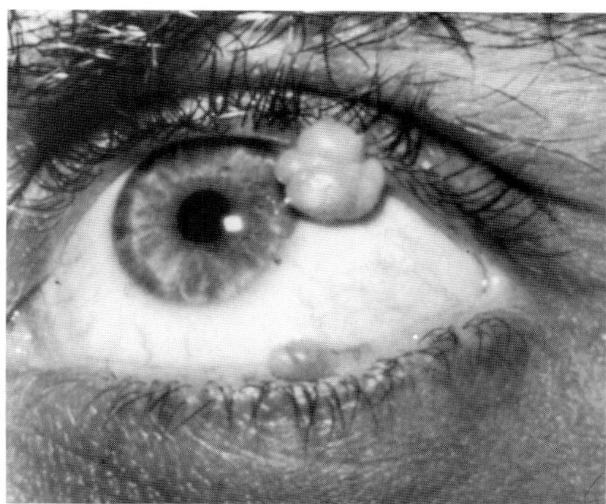

Figure 4.28. Focal mucinosis of the eyelid. (From Koopman and Happle, 1991.)

Neurofibromatosis (MIM:162200) is easily differentiated clinically by the presence of café-au-lait spots and freckling limited to axillae, groins, and inframammary regions.

Atrial myxomas can be sporadic; skin changes should be looked for in any patient with a cardiac myxoma. Centrofacial lentiginosis can be isolated and seen in association with neurologic abnormalities outside of NAME syndrome. Patients with centrofacial lentiginosis should be evaluated for other features of the Carney complex.

Support Group: N.O.R.D.
P.O. Box 8923
New Fairfield, CT
06812
1-800-999-6673

SELECTED BIBLIOGRAPHY

Atherton, D.J., Pitcher, D.W., Wells, R.S., and MacDonald, D.M. (1980). A syndrome of various cutaneous pigmented lesions, myxoid neurofibromata, and atrial myxoma: The NAME syndrome. *Br. J. Dermatol.* **103,** 421–429.

Single patient with a negative family history. The histology was consistent with freckles.

Carney, J.A., Gordon, H., Carpenter, P.C., Shenoy, B.V., and Go, V.L.W. (1985). The complex of myxomas, spotty pigmentation, and endocrine overactivity. *Medicine* **64,** 270–283.

Vidaillet, H.J., Jr., Seward, J.B., Fyke, E., III, and Tajik, A.J. (1984). NAME syndrome (nevi, atrial myxoma, myxoid neurofibromata, ephelides): a new and unrecognized subset of patients with cardiac myxoma. *Minn. Med.* **67,** 695–696.

Carney et al. (1985) reviewed patients with Cushing syndrome from the Mayo Clinic, noticed the co-occurrence of atrial myxomas, then reviewed patients with atrial myxomas, and recognized that a subset had pigmentary changes and cutaneous tumors. Concurrently Vidaillet and colleagues (1984) reviewed atrial myxomas and recognized the same associations. There have been multiple publications by both groups and others at the Mayo Clinic using the same database. Caution should be exercised in generating statistics regarding natural history and expression of this condition, recognizing that the same patient pool has been published in various permutations with occasional addition of new case reports.

Goksel, S., and Kural, T. (1989). Lentiginosis and right atrial myxoma. *Eur. Heart J.* **10,** 769–771.

A 21-year-old female with unilateral speckled hyperpigmentation of the trunk and right arm, with a few lesions on her nose, had a right atrial myxoma. Her father was also reported to have lentigines but was not examined.

Koopmann, R.J., and Happle, R. (1990). Autosomal dominant transmission of the NAME syndrome (nevi, atrial myxoma, mucinosis of the skin, and endocrine overactivity). *Hum. Genet.* **86,** 300–304.

An affected father with an affected son and daughter. The authors propose changing the meaning of the acronym NAME to include endocrine abnormalities.

Rhodes, A.R., Silverman, R.A., Harrist, T.J., and Perez-Atayde, A.R. (1984). Mucocutaneous lentigines, cardiomucocutaneous myxomas, and multiple blue nevi: the LAMB syndrome. *J. Am. Acad. Dermatol.* **10,** 72–82.

Case report. Histology and electron microscopy of tumors and pigmented lesion. The authors preferred the acronym LAMB because they felt the dermal tumors represented myxomas, not neurofibromas, and histopathology of the pigmented lesions showed lentigines.

NEUROFIBROMATOSIS (MIM:162200)

(Von Recklinghausen Disease; NF1)

Includes Watson Syndrome; NF-Noonan; Familial Multiple Café-au-lait Spots

Among the most common of autosomal dominant disorders, neurofibromatosis has been the subject of numerous books, monographs, and articles. I have attempted to include here only what I consider to be important basic facts, and there are far better sources for in-depth information.

DERMATOLOGIC FEATURES

Major. Café-au-lait spots are flat, round or oval, light tan to darker brown patches. These are the hallmark of the disorder. They may be present at birth or appear in infancy. They increase in number during childhood and adolescence. Some authors argue that all of the spots are present within the first few years of life. My experience has been otherwise. Six café-au-lait spots greater than 1.5 cm in diameter in an individual are highly suggestive of the diagnosis of neurofibromatosis. Five or six café-au-lait spots greater than 0.5 cm in young children also almost invariably indicate neurofibromatosis. The number of spots does not correlate with the severity of the disease. They

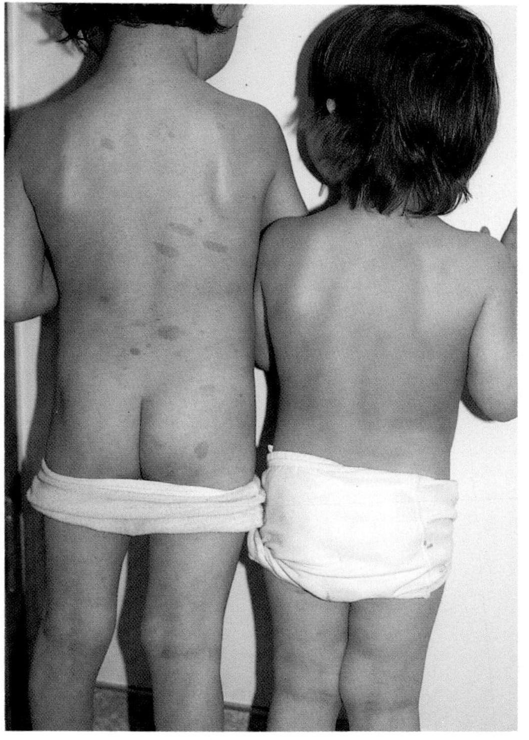

Figure 4.29. Multiple café-au-lait spots (unaffected brother insisted on participating).

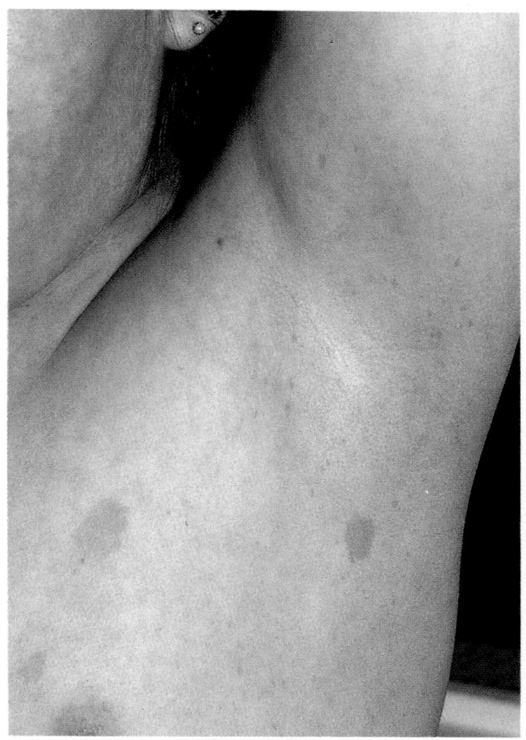

Figure 4.30. Crowe's sign—axillary freckling. Café-au-lait spots also visible.

grow in proportion to the body, and they may disappear in the elderly. The palms, soles, and genitalia are usually not involved. Freckling, comprised of small café-au-lait macules in nonsun-exposed areas, such as the axilla, the inguinal area, the inframammary region, and under the chin onto the anterior neck, is typical of the disorder. Crowe's sign (axillary freckling) usually develops in middle to late childhood. Approximately 80% of adult patients will have freckling in the folds.

Peripheral neurofibromas protrude from the skin surface. They may be flesh colored or pink, smooth or more nipple-like, with soft epidermal rugations. Sometimes one can appreciate "buttonholing"—the ability to push the nodule back into the plane of the skin. Peripheral neurofibromas usually begin developing in middle to late childhood or may not appear until puberty.

Small peripheral plexiform neurofibromas are soft, pinkish-red-purple papules that rise little above the skin surface. The finger falls into them; they are soft and squishy and do not buttonhole. The epidermis appears thinned. I believe that these are the lesions that are described by others when they use the term *pseudoatrophic macules*.

MINOR. Generalized melanosis with a darker tinge to the skin is a feature often overlooked.

Large disfiguring plexiform neurofibromas can occur anywhere and often involve the face. While these present significant medical handicap and are extremely difficult to manage, they occur only in a minority of patients.

Giant café-au-lait spots can be seen. They often overlie areas that go on to develop plexiform neurofibromas.

Multiple juvenile xanthogranulomas, yellowish-pink firm papules and nodules, develop in a minority of patients and may presage the development of leukemia. Hypopigmented

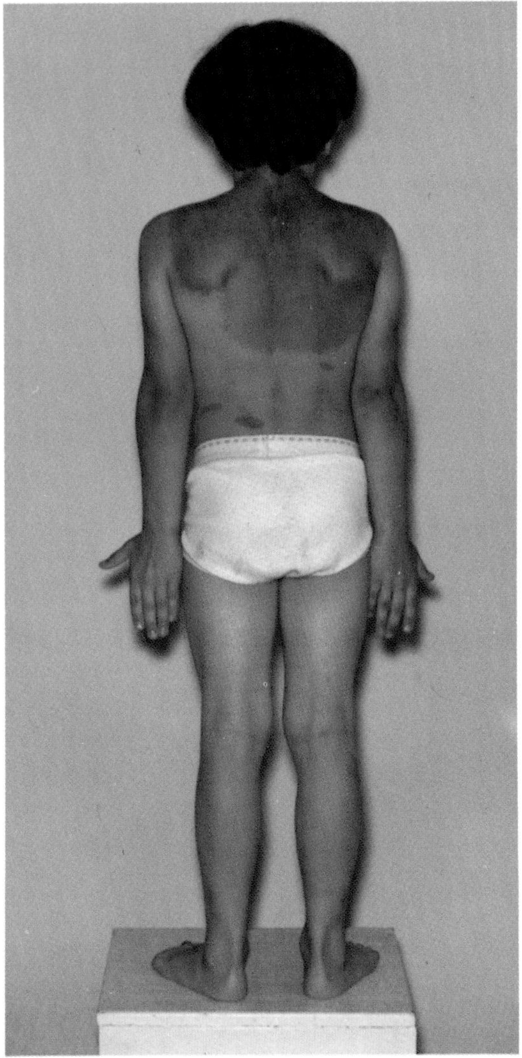

Figure 4.31. Giant café-au-lait spot over back and shoulders, along with more typical macules.

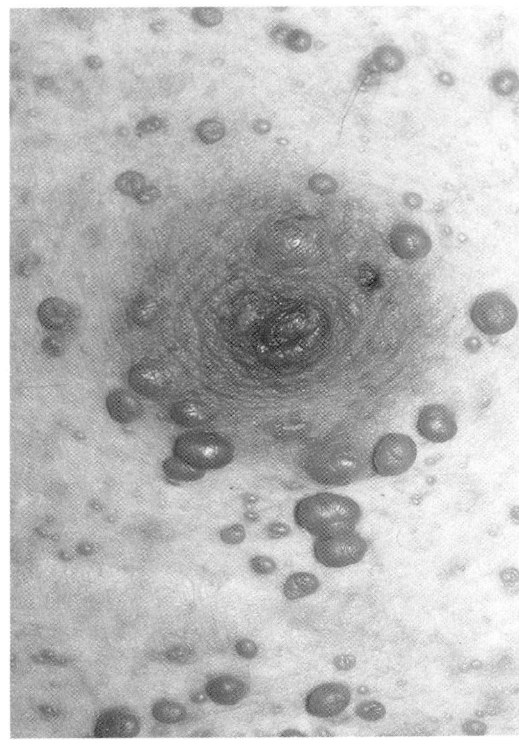

Figure 4.32. Multiple peripheral neurofibromas around areola and over chest wall.

patches, similar to those of tuberous sclerosis, and guttate hypomelanosis have also been described.

ASSOCIATED ABNORMALITIES

Central nervous system: Mental retardation occurs in approximately 5%–10% of patients. Brain tumors, both benign and malignant, have been reported. There is a decrement in IQ score compared with unaffected siblings and an increased occurrence of learning problems.

Eye: Lisch nodules are iris hamartomas that can be appreciated best with slit-lamp examination. They may be few or many in number. They are seen in fewer than 10% of patients younger than 6 years of age but are found in 50% of affected individuals by age 20 years and in more than 90% by midadult life.

Optic gliomas may be present in up to 15% of affected individuals; however, they become symptomatic in less than 5%.

Ear: Acoustic neuromas are a feature of neurofibromatosis type 2 (NF2) and do not appear to be a major feature of neurofibromatosis type 1 (NF1).

Cardiovascular: Hypertension on an idiopathic or renovascular basis can occur. Pulmonary fibrosis has been reported in a minority of patients.

Orthopedic: Scoliosis is seen in upwards of

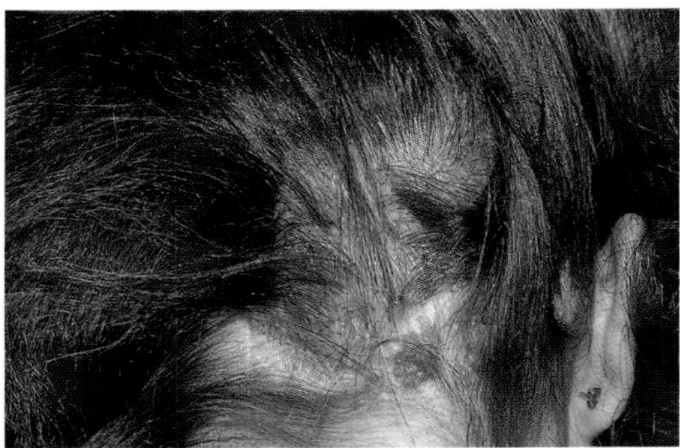

Figure 4.33. Plexiform neurofibroma of scalp.

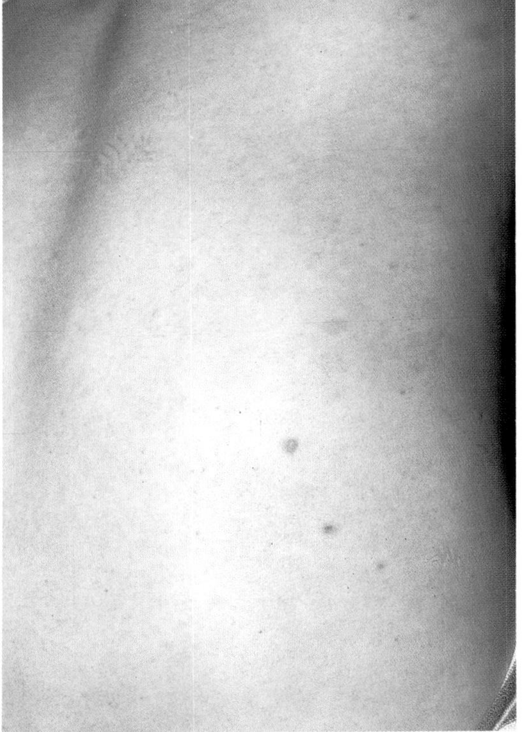

Figure 4.34. "Pseudoatrophic macules"—slightly bluish-purple spots. Café-au-lait spots are also obvious.

60% of patients, but severe scoliosis occurs in less than 10%.

Pseudoarthroses, bowing of the long bones, most often the tibia, occur in 3% or less of patients and are usually present at birth or within the first 6 months of life.

Other orthopedic features that are considered diagnostic of the disorder include sphenoid dysplasia, which is often unilateral, and scalloping of the dorsal surface of the vertebral bodies. Sprengel's deformity has also been noted more frequently in this group of patients.

Endocrine: Precocious puberty occurs in less than 5% of patients and is almost always associated with the presence of a pituitary adenoma or optic glioma. Delay of puberty also happens. The basis of this is unknown. Pheochromocytoma has been reported in less than 1% of patients.

Malignancy: Leukemia, malignant schwannoma, and neurofibrosarcoma are all increased in occurrence in individuals with neurofibromatosis. There may be an increased risk for other malignancies, but that is less clear.

There are a host of complications that can occur in any and all organ systems secondary to the growth of neurofibromas.

HISTOPATHOLOGY

LIGHT. Not specific to the disorder. The neurofibromas and café-au-lait spots of NF1 show changes similar to similar lesions from individuals without NF1.

EM. The café-au-lait spots of neurofibromatosis do not have distinctive features. Giant melanosomes or melanin-related macroglobules are not specific to these lesions.

BASIC DEFECT

The gene is approximately 300 kilobases long with many exons. It codes for "neurofibromin," a protein that appears to act as a negative feedback control for the *ras* protooncogene.

TREATMENT

Specific to the complication. Removal of peripheral neurofibromas for cosmetic reasons is practiced by some. No controlled studies of outcome (e.g., regrowth, unacceptable scarring, paresthesia) have been performed.

MODE OF INHERITANCE

Autosomal dominant with marked allelic heterogeneity. The gene maps to 17q11.2. Approximately 50% of the patients represent new mutations. There are rare instances of presumed gonadal mosaicism with recurrent transmission of NF1 by an unaffected parent.

PRENATAL DIAGNOSIS

Available by linkage analysis and in some instances mutational analysis.

DIFFERENTIAL DIAGNOSIS

Multiple café-au-lait spots have been described in a host of syndromes, for example, Bloom syndrome (MIM:210900) and Bannayan-Riley-Ruvalcaba syndrome (MIM:153480). In reality, these disorders do not present difficulty in diagnosis and should never be confused with neurofibromatosis. It is the person with numerous café-au-lait spots and no other clinical findings who presents the dilemma, "is this neurofibromatosis?"

Familial multiple café-au-lait spots is an autosomal dominant condition far less common than neurofibromatosis. Affected individuals have multiple typical café-au-lait macules, usually do not have axillary or inguinal freckling, and lack the other neural crest involvement of NF1. In the absence of a positive family history for multiple café-au-lait spots, individuals with multiple café-au-lait spots should be followed as if they had NF1 until proven otherwise, i.e., no other features of neurofibromatosis by adulthood.

Segmental neurofibromatosis, presumably due to postzygotic mutations in the NF1 gene, has been reported in many individuals. Affected individuals have disease limited to a quadrant or sector, defined by the lines of Blaschko.

Schimke immuno-osseous dysplasia (MIM: 242900) is characterized by nephrotic syndrome or focal segmental glomerulosclerosis, coupled with spondyloepiphyseal dysplasia, failure to thrive, and lymphopenia. Pigmented lesions have been noted in all cases, variably described as café-au-lait spots, lentigines, or moles. In the patient I have seen, the spots were typical of the inguinal freckling of NF1, scattered over the abdomen. Onset of these spots was after several years of age.

Neurofibromatosis—Noonan syndrome refers to patients with neurofibromatosis and a Noonan-like physiognomy (ptosis, downslanting palpebral fissures, broad neck, widespaced nipples and mild short stature), and has been described numerous times. The condition may be allelic to NF1, with affected individuals possessing large deletions of the NF1 gene, or may be the result of a contiguous gene syndrome. I had one patient with neurofibromatosis— Noonan syndrome whose mother had Noonan syndrome and father had NF1, so the explanations may be even be more complicated. Watson syndrome (MIM:193520) also appears to be allelic to neurofibromatosis. Patients again have short stature, pulmonic stenosis, and dull intelligence, in addition to the routine features of NF1.

NF2 (MIM:101000) is marked by fewer cutaneous changes and bilateral acoustic neurinomas. Crowe's sign is absent, and Lisch nodules are rare.

The freckles of neurofibromatosis can resemble the lentigines of the autosomal dominant disorders, multiple lentigines/LEOPARD syndrome (MIM:151000) and individuals with multiple lentigines/LEOPARD may have larger spots similar to café-au-lait spots, although the former are often darker *(café noir)*. The widespread distribution of lentigines and the associated abnormalities of the LEOPARD syndrome can distinguish these conditions from neurofibromatosis.

In McCune-Albright syndrome (MIM: 139320), the giant café-au-lait spots may be mistaken for the spots of NF1 that presage the development of plexiform neurofibromas. The absence of other features of NF1 and the presence of polyostotic fibrous dysplasia point to the diagnosis of McCune-Albright syndrome.

In the young child with an isolated giant café-au-lait spot there is currently, in my opinion, no way to distinguish among NF1, segmental neurofibromatosis, McCune-Albright syndrome, or an isolated birthmark. The patient should be monitored with all possibilities in mind. By age 5, NF1 will usually become apparent. By puberty, the bony changes of McCune-Albright are likely to develop. With the advent of molecular and biochemical markers, accurate and early diagnosis of these conditions will become possible.

Small plexiform neuromas can be misconstrued as nevi, either pigmented or vascular, and I have seen several patients in whom the diagnosis of neurofibromatosis has been missed because the clinician was not aware of the significance of these lesions. This was despite the presence of multiple café-au-lait spots.

Support Group: National Neurofibromatosis Foundation, Inc. (NNFF)
95 Pine Street, 16th Floor
New York, New York 10005
1-800-323-7938

SELECTED BIBLIOGRAPHY

Arnsmeier, S.L., Riccardi, V.M., and Paller, A.S. (1994). Familial multiple café-au-lait spots. *Arch. Dermatol.* **130,** 1425–1426.

Adds three families to a handful in the literature. In one pedigree, affected individuals had Lisch nodules and Crowe's sign in addition to café-au-lait spots, but no other manifestations of classic NF1. While the distinction between NF1 and familial multiple café-au-lait spots may be difficult to draw, I would have classified this one family as NF1. Mutational analysis will ultimately resolve these issues.

Benjamin, C.M., Colley, A., Donnai, D., Kingston, H., Harris, R., and Kerzin-Storrar, L. (1993). Neurofibromatosis type 1 (NF1): Knowledge, experience, and reproductive decisions of affected patients and families. *J. Med. Genet.* **30,** 567–574.

This is an interesting study of subjective assessment of disease severity by patients. Their assessment of the severity of the disease did not correlate at all with the medical assessment of severity. There was a relative lack of understanding of the genetics of the disorder (understanding was better if patients had received genetic counseling, but was still poor). While severity did not correlate with the decision to reproduce, the desire for prenatal diagnosis was great, despite lack of intent to terminate affected pregnancies on the part of most individuals.

Ehrich, J.H.H., Burchert, W., Schirg, E., Krull, F., Offner, G., Hoyer, P.F., and Brodehl, J. (1995). Steroid resistant nephrotic syndrome associated with spondyloepiphyseal dysplasia, transient ischemic attacks and lymphopenia. *Clin. Nephrol.* **43,** 89–95.

Reviews previously reported cases plus two new ones. Interestingly, the pigment changes, which are striking, are mentioned only in passing.

Gutmann, D.H., and Collins, F.S. (1993). Neurofibromatosis type 1: beyond positional cloning. *Arch. Neurol.* **50,** 1185–1193.

Gutmann, D.H., and Collins, F.S. (1993). The NF type 1 gene and its protein product, neurofibromin. *Neuron* **10,** 335–343.

Review molecular data and discuss possible function of neurofibromin.

Korf, B.R. (1992). Diagnostic outcome in children with multiple café-au-lait spots. *Pediatrics* **90,** 924–927.

Of 41 children with six or more café-au-lait spots presenting to neurofibromatosis clinic, age range 1 month to 14 years, 24 went on to develop other signs of neurofibromatosis, including axillary freckling, Lisch nodules, or peripheral neurofibromas. Six appeared to have segmental disease; three were recognized to have other syndromes.

Lubs, M.-L.E., Bauer, M. S., Formas, M.E., and Djokic, B. (1991). Lisch nodules in neurofibromatosis type 1. *N. Engl. J. Med.* **324,** 1264–1266.

Seventy-three percent of 167 patients had Lisch nodules. Less than 5% of children under 3 had them. All adults over 21 years had Lisch nodules. Subsequent studies have found a somewhat lower prevalence.

Morier, P., Merot, Y., Paccaud, D., Beck, D., and Frenk, E. (1990). Juvenile chronic granulocytic leukemia, juvenile xanthogranulomas, and neurofibromatosis. *J. Am. Acad. Dermatol.* **22,** 962–965.

A case report and review. The authors found 23 cases in the literature. The association may be independent in that some individuals with NF1 will have juvenile xanthogranulomas without leukemia, some individuals with leukemia without NF1 will have juvenile xanthogranulomas, and some patients with neurofibromatosis will have leukemia without juvenile xanthogranulomas.

Westerhof, W., and Konrad, K. (1982). Blue-red macules and pseudoatrophic macules. Additional cutaneous signs of neurofibromatosis. *Arch. Dermatol.* **118,** 577–580.

Red-blue macules overlay subcutaneous neurofibromas and show thick-walled blood vessels in the papillary dermis. Pseudoatrophic lesions show decreased collagen and aberrant neuroid tissue.

Crowe, F.W., and Schull, W.J., Neel, J.V. (1956) A clinical, pathological, and genetic study of multiple neurofibromatosis. Springfield, IL. Charles C. Thomas

Whitehouse, D. (1966). Diagnostic value of the café-au-lait spot in children. *Arch. Dis. Child.* **41,** 316–319.

Obringer, A.C., Meadows, A.T., and Zackai, E.H. (1989). The diagnosis of neurofibromatosis 1 in the child under the age of 6 years. *Am. J. Dis. Child.* **143,** 717–719.

Both Obringer et al. and Whitehouse (1966) deal with the diagnosis in children. Whitehouse chose a smaller diameter café-au-lait spot than Crowe et al. (1956) because he felt that one was unlikely to confuse smaller spots with freckles or solar damage in children. Crowe et al. (1956) were concerned about this in adults, which is why they chose a diameter of 1.5 cm or greater for the café-au-lait spot. Two of 365 children had five or more café-au-lait spots greater than 0.5 cm in diameter. One had a family history of neurofibromatosis. The child with four café-au-lait spots had a positive family history for café-au-lait spots. Whitehouse evaluated both white and black children but did not give the absolute numbers of each population. Obringer et al. looked at 160 children. With a family history, 80% fulfilled NIH criteria. In the absence of a family history only 30% did. This supports the clinical impression that most young children with NF1 will have limited clinical features.

NEVUS PHAKOMATOSIS PIGMENTOVASCULARIS (MIM:None)

(Adamson-Best; Takano-Krüger-Doi; Kobori-Toda)

Includes Types I, II, III, and IV

DERMATOLOGIC FEATURES

Major. Type I: Multiple flame nevi that are lightly colored port wine stains or salmon patches in conjunction with nevus pigmentosus et verrucosus—a pigmented irregular epidermal nevus

Type II: The nevus flammeus is seen in association with aberrant Mongolian spots.

Type III: Nevus flammeus in association with nevus spilus, which is a flat brown patch, café-au-lait colored, with stippling of darker pigment or freckles or lentigo-like lesions within it.

Type IIIb: Changes similar to Klippel-Trenaunay-Weber.

Type IV: Nevus flammeus, aberrant Mongolian spots, nevus spilus with or without nevus anemicus, a pale area of abnormal vasoconstriction that does not flare with rubbing.

All four of the conditions subsumed in the heading "nevus phakomatosis pigmentovascularis" share in common flame nevi. They are distinguished by the other skin changes that they have. No individuals have had a positive family history. There appear to be no consistent findings outside of the skin, and the case reports are very few in number.

The condition is most commonly described among the Japanese, which may reflect the baseline increased likelihood of having aberrant Mongolian spots in that population.

Minor. One patient had multiple granular cell tumors in addition to a nevus flammeus and

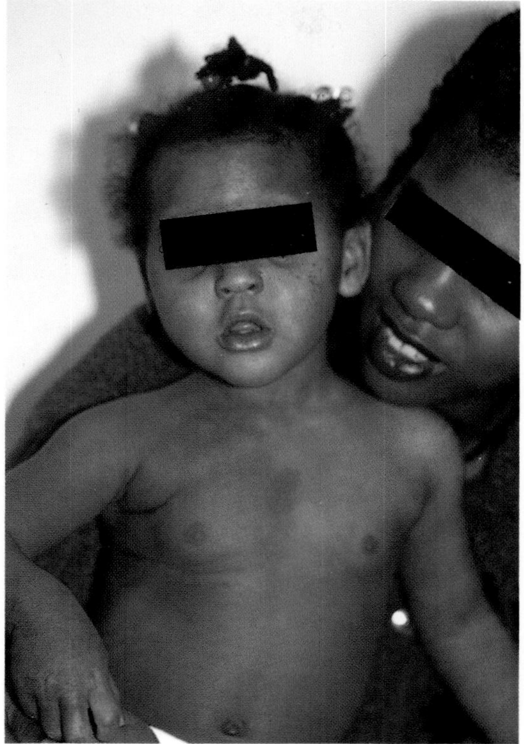

Figure 4.35. Café-au-lait over abdomen, nevus of Ota bilaterally, port wine stain over right breast, extensive Mongolian spots, and nevus spilus on left cheek.

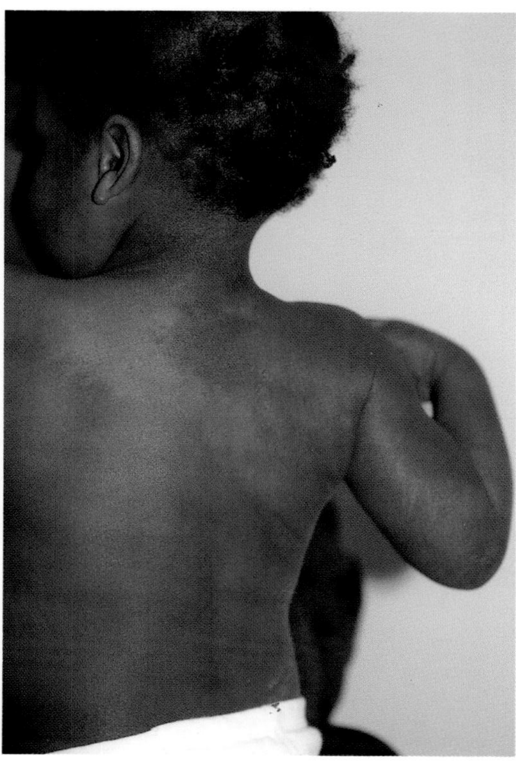

Figure 4.36. Widespread Mongolian spots on back and down arm, port wine stain over right scapula, and large café-au-lait spot on left back.

nevus spilus, another patient had café-au-lait spots, another patient had café-au-lait spots and nevus spilus and nevus flammeus.

ASSOCIATED ABNORMALITIES

Iris mammillations were reported in one patient with type II.

HISTOPATHOLOGY

Light. The blue spots show few fusiform melanocytes and melanin granules in the middle and lower dermis, all typical of a normal Mongolian spot. The brown macules show increased pigment in the basal layer, typical of a nevus spilus. The nevus flammeus of this condition shows irregular endothelial cell nuclei, thickened fibrous lamina of the nucleus, slight flattening of the endothelial cells, and peripheral nervous elements in perivascular regions.

EM. No information.

BASIC DEFECT

Unknown.

TREATMENT

None.

MODE OF INHERITANCE

Unknown. There is one Japanese pedigree in which a mother with a flame nevus on the palm and a nevus spilus and a father with a nevus spilus had two children, one of whom had Mongolian spots, the other who had a nevus spilus, nevus flammeus, and Mongolian spot. The probands' lesions were fairly widespread. A maternal aunt had a brown macule on the right leg. It is hard to know what to make of this.

PRENATAL DIAGNOSIS

None.

DIFFERENTIAL DIAGNOSIS

Familial flame nevi (MIM:163000) can be inherited as an autosomal dominant condition without any of the other pigmented changes associated with nevus phakomatosis pigmentovascularis. I think it is reasonable to invoke the diagnosis of nevus phakomatosis pigmentovascularis when one is confronted with a child who has a variety of pigmented and vascular lesions, without systemic findings, for which there is no other explanation. I think this diagnosis is very much of the "we see this" variety. We can describe it without understanding it.

Support Group: N.O.R.D.
P.O. Box 8923
New Fairfield, CT
06812
1-800-999-6673

SELECTED BIBLIOGRAPHY

Gilliam, A.C., Ragge, N.K., Perez, M.I., and Bolognia, J.L. (1993). Phakomatosis pigmentovascularis type IIb with iris mammillations. *Arch. Dermatol.* **129,** 340–342.

The authors point out that the iris lesions differ from Lisch nodules. They are smaller, stellate, darker, more numerous, and regular in distribution. They show photographs contrasting both lesions. Their patient also had a nevus of Ota, a lesion associated with iris mammillations.

Hasagawa, T., and Yasuhara, M. (1985). Phakomatosis pigmentovascularis type IVa. *Arch. Dermatol.* **121,** 651–655.

They divide these conditions into types A and B. In A, changes are limited to the skin. In B, children have systemic features such as mental retardation or seizures.

PEUTZ-JEGHERS SYNDROME (MIM:175200)

(Peutz-Touraine-Jeghers; Hamartomatous Intestinal Polyposis)

DERMATOLOGIC FEATURES

MAJOR. Flat brown to black small macules develop on the fingers, palms, soles, lips, buccal mucosa, tongue, and perioral, periorbital, and perinasal skin. Lesions are multiple and may become confluent. They appear in early childhood. Although lesions on the skin are said to fade with puberty and disappear in adult life, most case descriptions do not mention this feature. It appears to occur only in a minority of patients. The mucosal lesions persist in all patients. Lips are involved in almost all affected individuals; not all patients have the skin changes. Fingertips are involved in approximately two-thirds. The size of the macules tends to be smaller on skin surfaces and larger on mucosa. The oral lesions may appear dark brown to purple. The pigment changes can also involve the eyelids and palpebral conjunctiva.

MINOR. In two case reports, oral telangiectases, in addition to pigmented lesions, were described. These do not appear to be common features.

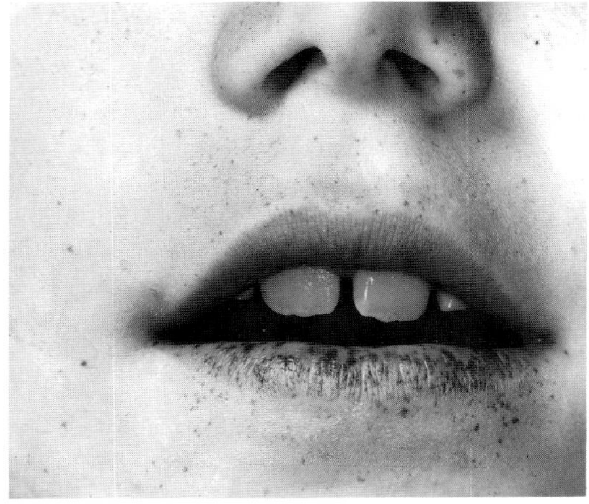

A

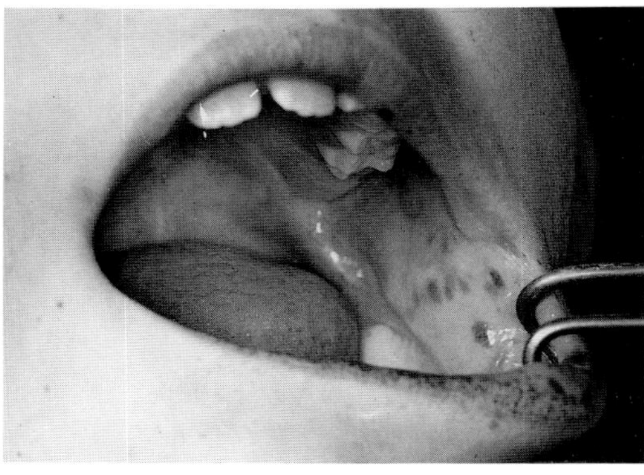

B

Figure 4.37. Lentigines on philtrum, nose, and mouth **(A)** and on buccal mucosa **(B).** (Courtesy of Dr. J.G. Hall, Vancouver, British Columbia.)

ASSOCIATED ABNORMALITIES

Gastrointestinal: Hamartomatous polyps in the jejunum, ileum, colon, rectum, stomach, and duodenum develop throughout life. These result in colicky abdominal pain, intussusception, rectal bleeding, and rectal prolapse (even in infancy and early childhood). Case descriptions are impressive in the degree to which nonmalignant bowel complications can cause morbidity. Intestinal bleeding can lead to anemia.

Risks for cancer: Adenocarcinomas of the breast, cervix, pancreas, and uterus and ovaries can occur at relatively young ages. Ovarian sex cord tumors and Sertoli cell testicular tumors can develop. Testicular tumors can develop in prepubertal males. Cancer of the gall bladder has also occurred.

In the gastrointestinal tract, cancers are thought to arise on the hamartomatous substrate of the polyps. Estimated frequency of gastrointestinal malignancy ranges from 2% to 13%, and the overall risk of cancer approaches 50%. Arguments about misdiagnosis of malignant change for cellular atypia vie with well-documented case reports of death from metastases. Statements in the literature that malignancy is rare in Peutz-Jeghers are followed by risk estimates of approximately 10%, which hardly qualifies as rare, in my opinion. In a series of 66 patients followed over a period of time, 16 developed malignancies, and, of these, 15 died.

Precocious puberty and gynecomastia have been reported in children associated with Sertoli tumors or ovarian sex cord tumors, and the occurrence of precocious puberty should always invoke a search for gonadal malignancy in these patients.

HISTOPATHOLOGY

LIGHT. There is an increase in pigment in the basal keratinocytes, with elongation of the rete ridges. These changes are typical of lentigines.
EM. Findings are uncertain. One reference (unavailable to me) was quoted as showing an increased number of melanocytes with melanosomes filling the dendrites.

BASIC DEFECT

Unknown.

TREATMENT

There are no reports of effective treatment for the pigment changes. Whether laser treatment will be useful is an open question. Recommendations for management of bowel involvement are divergent and include semiannual endoscopy and colonoscopy with removal of polyps, semiannual small bowel follow-through, and yearly Pap smears, and mammograms in females. Affected individuals should be taught self-examination of breasts or testicles.

MODE OF INHERITANCE

Autosomal dominant. Tentative assignment of the gene to chromosome 1.

PRENATAL DIAGNOSIS

None.

DIFFERENTIAL DIAGNOSIS

Late acquired melanotic macules without gastrointestinal polyposis have been described in a few elderly patients, occurring in association with malignancy. None of these individuals has had a positive family history. Unfortunately, these cases have been labeled as atypical Peutz-Jeghers syndrome or forme fruste Peutz-Jeghers syndrome, which can create confusion.

In the Moynahan or LEOPARD syndrome (MIM:151100), lentigines develop from head to toe, clustering over the upper trunk and neck. Associated features are hypertrophic cardiomyopathy, developmental delays, and hypogenitalism.

In partial unilateral lentiginosis, the distribution of skin lesions is localized to one side of the body.

The NAME/Carney/LAMB complex (MIM: 160980) shares cutaneous brown macules in common with Peutz-Jeghers syndrome. Histologically, the lesions in this disorder may look like freckles or lentigos. The associated abnormalities, including atrial myxomas, blue nevi, and other myxoid tumors, are not found in Peutz-Jeghers syndrome.

Normal freckling can occasionally involve the lips and periorbital area, but is not seen on the mucosa.

In darkly pigmented races, pigmented bands or spots can be occasionally seen on the mucosa, but not in association with cutaneous lentigines. Patterned lentiginoses is a condition described in blacks. Patients with this condition have lesions primarily on the buttocks, and there is no mucosal involvement.

Bannayan-Riley-Ruvalcaba syndrome (macrocephaly, multiple lipomas, and hemangiomas; MIM:153480) is an autosomal dominant disorder in which affected individuals have macrosomia at birth, mental retardation (50%), and hamartomas in the small and large intestine (50%). They also appear to have a lipid storage myopathy. Affected individuals develop brown macules on the penis, but not elsewhere.

The presence of facial lentigines is almost universal in early childhood in Peutz-Jeghers syndrome and should quickly eliminate other familial polyposis coli syndromes from further consideration.

Support Group: Intestinal Multiple Polyposis and Colorectal Cancer (IMPACC)
P.O. Box 11
Conyngham, PA 18219
1-717-788-3712

SELECTED BIBLIOGRAPHY

Dormandy, T.L. (1957). Gastrointestinal polyposis with mucocutaneous pigmentation (Peutz-Jeghers syndrome). *N. Engl. J. Med.* **56,** 1093–1103, 1141–1146, 1186–1190.

Massive review. Several case descriptions are especially telling: A 22-year-old with bowel complaints came into hospital and had exploratory surgery during which polyposis was found. "Only then were pigment changes specifically looked for, and these now appeared fairly obvious." In another instance, "though awareness of the syndrome was not lacking, her mucosal pigmentation passed unnoticed." The last paragraph on page 1189 is a classic example of social Darwinism. The case descriptions in this very long review are wonderful.

Foley, R.T., McGarrity, T.J., and Abt, A.B. (1988). Peutz-Jeghers syndrome: a clinicopathologic survey of the "Harrisburg Family" with a 49-year follow-up. *Gastroenterology* **95,** 1535–1540.

Two of Jeghers' original patients from a single pedigree. The presumed progenitor died at age

69 with cancer of the pancreas, but had no pigment changes and no polyps. Though the authors state that he was not affected, of his seven children one had Peutz-Jeghers syndrome and two others died of bowel intussusception in their teens. The same family was also reviewed by others in *Surg. Gynecol. Obstet.* **115,** 1–11, 1962.

Jeghers, H., McKusick, V.A., and Katz, K.H. (1949). Generalized intestinal polyposis with melanin spots of the oral mucosa, lips and digits. A syndrome of diagnostic significance. *N. Engl. J. Med.* **241,** 993–1005, 1031–1036.

A detailed review with many photographs. This article set Peutz-Jeghers out as a distinct inherited entity.

Ohshiro, T., Maruyama, Y., Nakajima, H., and Mima, M. (1980). Treatment of pigmentation of the lips and mucosa in Peutz-Jeghers syndrome using ruby and argon lasers. *Br. J. Plast. Surg.* **33,** 346–349.

Three children who were teased (they were called "cannibals" and "sesame seed lips" by playmates) desired treatment of lip lesions. Initial results were promising.

Shepherd, N.A., Bussey, H.J.R., and Jass, J.R. (1987). Epithelial misplacement in Peutz-Jeghers polyps. A diagnostic pitfall. *Am. J. Surg. Pathol.* **11,** 743–749.

Evaluating polyps from the St. Mark's Hospital registry, the authors try to explain the controversy regarding the risk for malignant degeneration in Peutz-Jeghers polyps by a confusion of a benign histologic feature characteristic of the disorder with malignant adenomatous invasion. Unfortunately, this explanation is not convincing, as 3 of the 25 patients died of gastrointestinal malignancy.

Spigelman, A.D., Murday, V., and Phillips, R.K.S. (1989). Cancer and the Peutz-Jeghers syndrome. *Gut* **30,** 1588–1590.

Data regarding 72 patients with Peutz-Jeghers syndrome, part of a large polyposis registry in London, were reviewed. The authors calculated that the risk of death from carcinoma by age 57 in these patients was 48%. This was similar to a study published in *N. Engl. J. Med.* **316,** 1511–1514, 1987, in which the occurrence of cancer approached 50%.

Utsunomya, J., Gocho, H., Miyanaga, T., Hamaguchi, E., Kashimure, A., Aoki, N., and Komatsu, I. (1975). Peutz-Jeghers syndrome: its natural course and management. *Johns Hopkins Med. J.* **136,** 71–82.

Two hundred twenty-two patients. Average age of diagnosis was in the third decade. Presenting complaints were gastrointestinal in 75%, cutaneous in the rest. Almost 50% of patients suffered intussusception. Twelve percent had cancer, and 7% died with it.

UNIVERSAL MELANOSIS (MIM:145250, 155800)

(Familial Progressive Hyperpigmentation; Melanosis Universalis Hereditaria; Melanosis Diffusa Congenita)

DERMATOLOGIC FEATURES

MAJOR. Different patterns of progressive hyperpigmentation have been described in a handful of families. The coloration may be congenital or appear soon after birth; sometimes its appearance is delayed until childhood. It may progress centrally from acral locations. It may be diffuse and confluent or diffuse and patchy, and it is always asymptomatic. In some affected individuals it is reticulate, in others more uniform.

In some case descriptions, patchy or guttate hypopigmentation is also described.

I am not convinced that all the "unique" descriptors (e.g., familial progressive hyperpigmentation, dyspigmentation universalis) represent different disorders. They share in common an increase in melanin in the epidermis, and the pattern of involvement of skin seems fairly variable even within a family.

MINOR. There may be discrete brown macules on the palms and soles. In two case reports, nails were described as thin with irregular surfaces.

ASSOCIATED ABNORMALITIES

None.

HISTOPATHOLOGY

Light. Conflicting reports.
EM. In one report, an increase in the number of mature melanosomes was noted..

BASIC DEFECT

Unknown.

TREATMENT

None.

MODE OF INHERITANCE

Autosomal dominant or autosomal recessive. There are reports of both affected sibships with normal parents and families with vertical and male-to-male transmission. The latter predominate in the literature.

PRENATAL DIAGNOSIS

None.

DIFFERENTIAL DIAGNOSIS

Diffuse hyperpigmentation is a feature of NF1 (MIM:162200), which is often unappreciated. Café-au-lait spots, axillary freckling, and neurofibromas are not found in familial melanosis. The pigmentation of Addison's disease and the adrenoleukodystrophies (MIM:202370, 300100) is progressive, bronze in tone, and often more exaggerated in the skinfolds and along the palmar creases. Hemochromatosis (MIM:235200) can cause a slate grayish-brown coloration to the skin. Measurement of serum transferrin saturation will give the correct diagnosis.

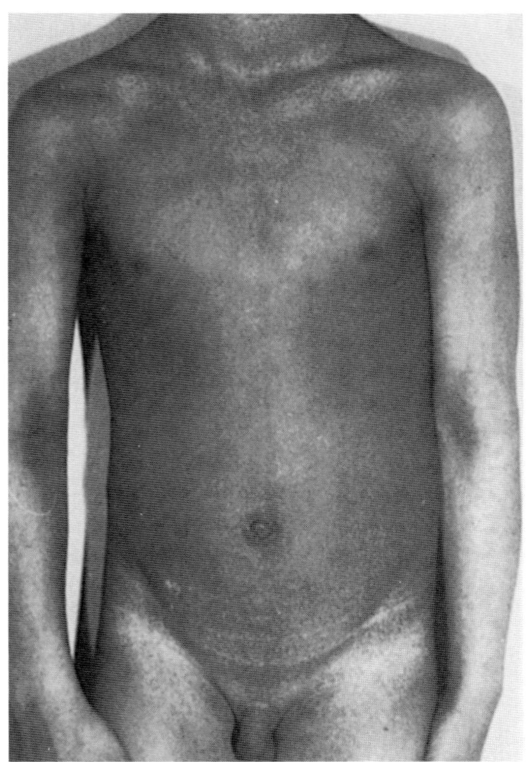

Figure 4.38. Diffuse darkening, most homogeneous on trunk. (From Kint et al., 1987.)

Melasma is usually limited to the face and seen in association with pregnancy and oral contraceptive exposure. Linear and whorled nevoid hypermelanosis can be distinguished by its distribution along the lines of Blaschko. Reticulated hyperpigmentation is a hallmark of Dowling-Degos disease (MIM:179850). Pigment change usually develops in late childhood or early adult life and tends to involve the flexures. There may be some overlap cases described in the literature as universal melanosis. Acanthosis nigricans (MIM:100600) may begin as macular or patchy hyperpigmentation but soon develops the velvety thickened texture that is its hallmark. It tends to involve the flexures and perioral areas.

The swirly hyperpigmentation of incontinentia pigmenti (MIM:308310) is generally, but not always, preceded by bullous and verrucous stages. Biopsy material will show melanin incontinence.

Erythema dyschromicum perstans is usually of later onset, and the color is bluish-gray rather than brown.

Support Group: N.O.R.D.
P.O. Box 8923
New Fairfield, CT
06812
1-800-999-6673

SELECTED BIBLIOGRAPHY

Chernosky, M.E., Anderson, D.E., Chang, J.P., Shaw, M.W., and Romsdahl, M.M. (1971). Familial progressive hyperpigmentation. *Arch. Dermatol.* **103,** 581–598.

Black family with progressive hyperpigmentation of the skin, conjunctivae, and cornea. There were some skip areas of the skin. The pigment also rubbed off on towels and on white clothing.

Debao, L., and Ting, L. (1991). Familial progressive hyperpigmentation: a family study in China. *Br. J. Dermatol.* **125,** 607.

A six generation family with male-to-male transmission was described.

Goodman, R.M., and Belcher, R.W. (1969). Periorbital hyperpigmentation. An overlooked genetic disorder of pigmentation. *Arch. Dermatol.* **100,** 169–174.

Yellowish-brown periorbital pigmentation with onset in childhood and progression with age. No associated abnormalities. Male-to-male transmission described. In one family, both parents were affected. Seven of the eight offspring were also affected, but not more severely than their parents. Biopsy showed increased amounts of melanin. The authors think that the condition is much more common than the literature would suggest and believe that it often goes unremarked upon or unnoticed by physicians.

Kint, A., Osman, C., Geerts, M.L., and Breuillard, F. (1987). Melanose diffuse congenitale. *Ann. Dermatol. Venereol.* **114,** 11–16.

Two unrelated children with progressive brown pigmentation. Biopsy material showed increase in melanosomes, both mature and immature, and melanin incontinence.

Ruiz-Maldonado, R., Tamayo, L., and Fernandez-Diez, J. (1978). Universal acquired melanosis. The carbon baby. *Arch. Dermatol.* **114,** 775–778.

One of three siblings was normal at birth and then developed progressive dark hyperpigmentation of the skin, conjunctivae, and nails. Biopsy material showed increased amounts of pigment and increased numbers of melanosomes, but no other abnormalities. The authors describe that the child's clothing turned color after it was worn, suggesting that pigment was being excreted in the sweat, as it is in alkaptonuria.

HYPOPIGMENTATION

ALBINISMS

The albinisms are inherited disorders marked by congenitally absent or reduced pigment production, in the presence of normal number, structure, and distribution of melanocytes. The albinisms have been distinguished classically by their characteristic tint of skin, hair, and irides and by their positive or negative production of pigment in hairbulbs incubated with DOPA or tyrosine. Currently, delineation of molecular defects is beginning to provide the basis for differentiation of these conditions and an explanation for overlapping phenotypes.

SELECTED BIBLIOGRAPHY

King, R.A., Hearing, V.J., Creel, D.J., and Oetting, W.S. (1995). Albinism. In *The Metabolic and Molecular Bases of Inherited Disease*. Scriver, C.R., Beaudet, A.L., Sly, W.S., and Valle, E.D. (eds.). McGraw-Hill, New York, 7th ed., pp. 4353–4392.

This is a comprehensive review chapter with both clinical information and a review of the basic biology of pigment production. There are 528 citations. The authors state that the diagnosis of albinism requires the presence of certain features in the optic system, including nystagmus, reduced iris pigment, reduced retinal pigment with foveal hypoplasia and misrouting of optic fibers at the chiasm, in addition to reduced pigment of skin and hair.

ALBINISM WITH DEAFNESS (MIM:300700)

DERMATOLOGIC FEATURES

MAJOR. The skin is marked by piebald-like changes with splotchy dotted, achromic patches interspersed with hyperpigmented areas. The buttocks tend to be very darkly pigmented compared with other areas. The hair is white, even that which grows from patches of dark scalp skin. In one individual the hair was described as straw colored. Eyebrows and eyelashes can also be involved. The pigmented areas of skin are yellow-brown to brown-black.
MINOR. None.

ASSOCIATED ABNORMALITIES

Vision is normal. Heterochromic irides can occur, but there is no iris transillumination. There is a profound congenital sensorineural deafness. Carriers vary in their degree of hearing impairment.

HISTOPATHOLOGY

LIGHT. There are no major microscopic changes seen in either the light or the dark skin. The DOPA reaction is very positive in dark skin and poor in light skin. In one patient, melanocytes appeared to be normal in both light and dark skin.
EM. No information.

BASIC DEFECT

Unknown.

TREATMENT

Early recognition of hearing impairment, sun protection.

MODE OF INHERITANCE

X-linked recessive, maps to Xq26.3–q27.1.

PRENATAL DIAGNOSIS

None.

DIFFERENTIAL DIAGNOSIS

Piebaldism (MIM:172800) can be associated with deafness. The autosomal dominant mode of inheritance of piebaldism may help to distinguish the two conditions, but in an isolated male the diagnosis may remain uncertain. Similarly, Waardenburg syndrome might be considered (MIM:193500, 193510) in the differential. Dystopia canthorum is not a feature of albinism with deafness. Skin biopsy to demonstrate distribution of melanocytes should be diagnostic. Achromic areas in piebaldism and Waardenburg are deficient in melanocytes.

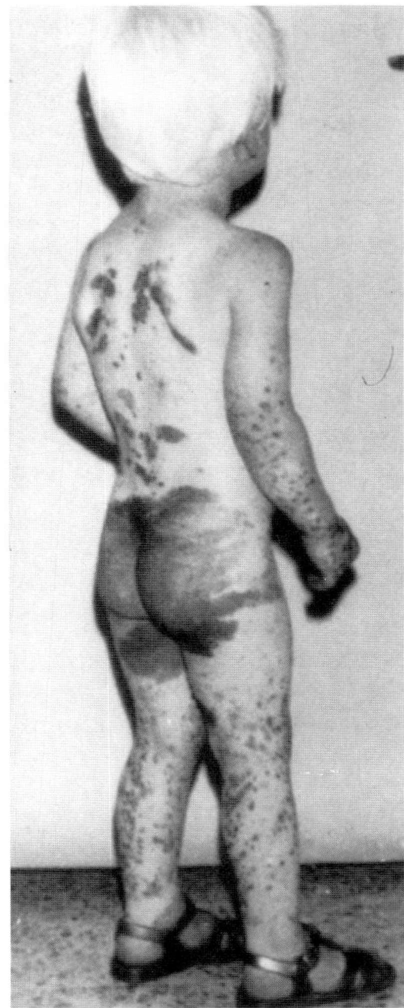

Figure 4.39. Typical changes of white hair; hypopigmented and hyperpigmented skin. (From Shiloh, 1990.)

Support Group: National Organization for Albinism and Hypopigmentation (N.O.A.H.)
1530 Locust Street,
Box 29
Philadelphia, PA 19102
1-215-545-2322

National Information Center on Deafness
Gallaudet University
800 Florida Avenue NE
Washington, DC 20002
1-202-651-5051

Hereditary Hearing Impairment Resource Registry
Boys Town National Research Hospital
555 North 30th
Omaha, NE 68131
1-402-498-6375

SELECTED BIBLIOGRAPHY

Shiloh, Y., Litvak, G., Ziv, Y., Lehner, T., Sandkayl, L., Hildesheimer, M., Buchris, V., Cremers, F.P.M., Szabo, P., White, B.N., Holden, J.J.A., and Ott, J. (1990). Genetic mapping of X-linked albinism-deafness syndrome (ADFN) to Xq26.3–q27.1. *Am. J. Hum. Genet.* **47,** 20–27.

Large Israeli pedigree. All obligate carriers (identified by pedigree analysis) had bilateral sensorineural hearing loss ranging from moderate to severe. Among the females at risk to be carriers, six had normal hearing, four had retrocochlear hearing loss of varying degrees.

Ziprkowski, L., and Adam, A. (1964). Recessive total albinism and congenital deaf-mutism. *Arch. Dermatol.* **89,** 151–155.

An apparently recessive pedigree. Cousin offspring of siblings, one married to a first cousin, and the other married to a second cousin, all related through the same progenitor. Of seven siblings with deafness, four were albino. The findings in this family could be due to two separate nonallelic mutations rather than to the effects of a single gene. Albinism was described as total, but one affected individual had pigmented patches on legs.

Ziprkowski, L., Krakowski, A., Adam, A., Costeff, H., and Sade, J. (1962). Partial albinism and deaf mutism due to a recessive sex-linked gene. *Arch. Dermatol.* **86,** 530–539.

This is a huge Israeli Sephardic Moroccan family. No features were found in obligate heterozygotes. This is the same family reported by Margolis in *Acta Genet.* **12,** 12–19, 1962, but therein it was described as originating from Egypt.

HERMANSKY-PUDLAK SYNDROME (MIM:203300)

(Albinism with Hemorrhagic Diathesis and Pigmented Reticuloendothelial Cells)

DERMATOLOGIC FEATURES

MAJOR. There is a generalized decrease in pigment involving the hair and skin. This can range from the complete absence of color typical of classic oculocutaneous albinism to a relative decrease in skin tone and hair color compared with family members or with ethnic group. Skin and hair pigmentation can increase and normalize over time. Patients can freckle.

Easy bruising with persistent ecchymoses is common.

MINOR. None.

ASSOCIATED ABNORMALITIES

Platelet dysfunction results in easy bruisability and prolonged bleeding. Menorrhagia in females is a frequent complaint, as is postpartum hemorrhage. Excessive bleeding after dental extractions is typical.

Interstitial pulmonary fibrosis has its onset in adult life. It is most common among Puerto Rican families, occurring in upwards of 80%–90% of adult patients. It was not seen in a large extended Swiss pedigree with Hermansky-Pudlak. It may be an allele-specific finding. Although cardiac involvement in Hermansky-Pudlak is referred to in reviews and in texts, it appears to be entirely secondary to end-stage pulmonary disease.

The eyes are involved with absence of retinal pigment and poor macular development. Transillumination of the irises and nystagmus similar to that in oculocutaneous albinism is seen. Photophobia is a common complaint.

Inflammatory bowel disease may also cluster within families. It has its onset in the second and third decades. Patients present with diarrhea, abdominal pain, and fever. The bowel shows ulceration with non-necrotizing granulomas.

Renal failure is not reported, despite ceroid-like deposition in the kidneys. One patient developed lupus nephritis.

HISTOPATHOLOGY

LIGHT. Pigment-laden macrophages can be demonstrated in the skin, as well as in bone marrow aspirates. These cells are filled with ceroid-like material, as are other cells of the reticuloendothelial system and the kidney.

EM. Platelets show a deficiency of dense granules. Melanocytes in the skin have immature melanosomes; some patients have decreased number of melanosomes, and others have increased number of melanosomes in melanocytes and keratinocytes. In the Swiss patients, giant melanosomes were seen. Macrophages contain ceroid-like pigment in membrane-bound structures that vary in size from 350 to 740 nm.

BASIC DEFECT

Unknown. In vitro activity of platelets is variable, with failure to aggregate in response to appropriate stimuli.

TREATMENT

Avoidance of medications that affect platelet function, including aspirin and prostaglandin blockers. Avoidance of sun exposure to prevent secondary skin damage. For patients who develop bowel disease, surgical resection is the only treatment. Steroids are of no benefit. There is no effective treatment for the pulmonary fibrosis. Local control of bleeding with platelet transfusion if bleeding is severe. Treatment with vitamin E has resulted in improvement in hemostasis in anecdotal reports.

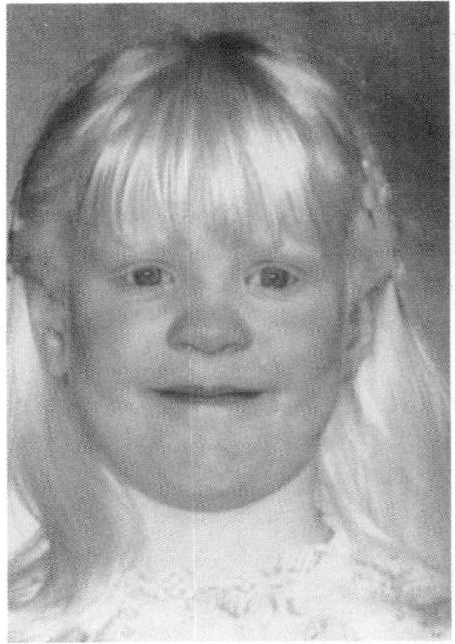
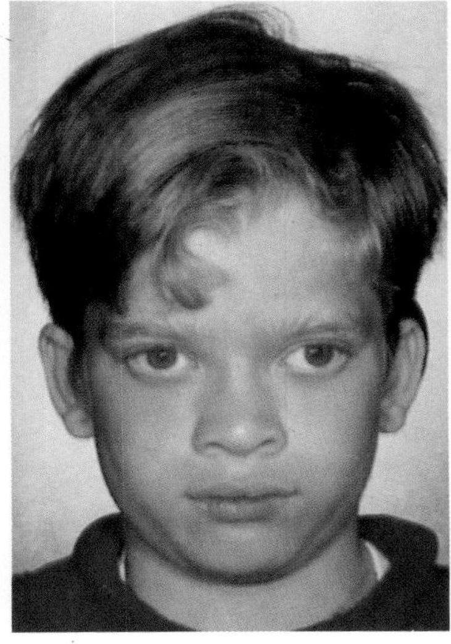
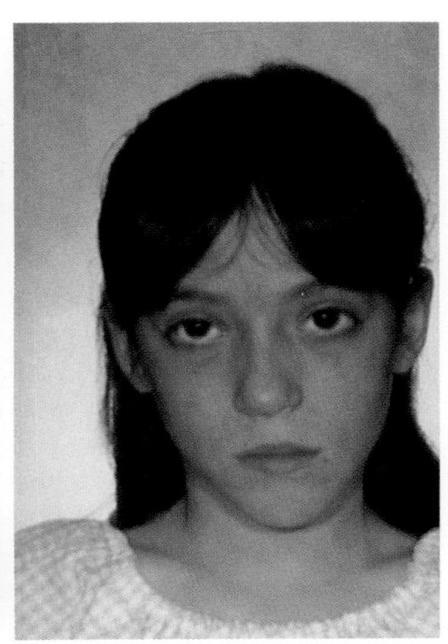

Figure 4.40. Marked variation and degree of pigment dilution in patients of Dutch-German, Madras Indian, and Puerto Rican ancestry. The last patient is unusually dark for Hermansky-Pudlak disease, even given her ethnic background. (From Witkop, 1985.)

MODE OF INHERITANCE

Autosomal recessive. Reported most commonly among Dutch and Puerto Rican populations, but also occurs in other groups. No carrier detection available. The gene tentatively maps to 10q.

PRENATAL DIAGNOSIS

None.

DIFFERENTIAL DIAGNOSIS

Oculocutaneous albinism type I and oculocutaneous albinism type II (MIM:203100, 203200, 203290) are not associated with bleeding problems. Patients with normal pigment and Hermansky-Pudlak syndrome can be misdiagnosed as having a variety of other bleeding diatheses. Because the decrease in skin and hair color may not be readily appreciated in some patients, misdiagnosis of ocular albinism (MIM:203310, 300500, 300600) is possible in patients with Hermansky-Pudlak syndrome because of eye findings.

Chediak-Higashi syndrome and Griscelli syndrome (MIM:214500, 214450) share in common decrease in pigmentation and abnormal platelets. There is no evidence for disturbed immune function in patients with Hermansky-Pudlak syndrome, and leukocytes are normal. Patients with Chediak-Higashi syndrome do not have pigment-laden macrophages.

Isolated platelet storage pool deficiency is a heterogeneous category of bleeding disorders, and affected individuals usually have normal pigment.

Support Group: Hermansky-Pudlak Syndrome Network
39 Riveria Court
Malverne, NY 11565-1602
1-800-789-9477

SELECTED BIBLIOGRAPHY

Harmon, K.R., Witkop, C.J., Jr., White, J.G., King, R.A., Peterson, M., Moore, D., Tashjian, J., Marinelli, W.A., and Bitterman, P.B. (1994). Pathogenesis of pulmonary fibrosis: platelet-derived growth factor precedes structural alterations in the Hermansky-Pudlak syndrome. *J. Lab. Clin. Med.* **123,** 617–627.

The authors screened 30 asymptomatic patients of Puerto Rican descent with Hermansky-Pudlak syndrome and nine heterozygous relatives, as well as controls, for platelet-derived growth factor–related peptides in bronchial lavage fluid and found sixfold greater values in patients. The patients were either normal physiologically or had early restrictive lung disease detected by testing only. Interestingly, over 50% of asymptomatic heterozygote relatives also had early restrictive lung changes and elevated platelet-derived growth factor–related peptides.

Hermansky, F., and Pudlak, P. (1959). Albinism associated with hemorrhagic diathesis and unusual pigmented reticular cells in the bone marrow: report of two cases with histochemical studies. *Blood* **14,** 162–169.

Both adults presented with bleeding. Both had pulmonary involvement. Both were Czechoslovakian

King, R.A., Hearing, V.J., Creel, D.J., and Oetting, W.S. (1995). Albinism. In *The Metabolic and Molecular Bases of Inherited Disease.* Scriver, C.R., Beaudet, A.L., Sly, W.S., and Valle, D. (eds.). McGraw-Hill, New York, 7th ed., pp. 4353–4392.

Comprehensive chapter on albinisms. Categorizes 10 types of oculocutaneous albinism. Hermansky-Pudlak is type VIA.

Reynolds, S.P., Davies, B.H., and Gibbs, A.R. (1994). Diffuse pulmonary fibrosis in the Hermansky-Pudlak syndrome: clinical course and postmortem findings. *Thorax* **49,** 617–618.

Case report of a woman with progressive lung involvement, onset at age 35, and death at age 51. The authors review the literature and cite 18 cases.

Summers, C.G., Knoblock, W.H., Witkop, C.J., Jr., and King, R.A. (1988). Hermansky-Pudlak syndrome. Ophthalmic findings. *Ophthalmology* **95,** 545–554.

Presents findings in 20 patients. Visual acuity ranged from 20/60 to 20/400, and authors caution that variability is the rule. Vision did not necessarily correlate with amount of skin or iris pigment. No ophthalmologic features specifically diagnostic for Hermansky-Pudlak syndrome were found.

OCULOCUTANEOUS ALBINISM TYROSINASE NEGATIVE (MIM:203100, 203280)

(Tyrosinase–Deficient Oculocutaneous Albinism; OCA1A)

Includes Temperature–Sensitive Albinism, OCA1TS; and Minimal Pigment Albinism, OCA1MP

DERMATOLOGIC FEATURES

MAJOR. The skin of individuals with oculocutaneous albinism type 1 (OCA1A) is dead or milky white, with no pigment production, failure to tan, and a complete absence of freckles and pigmented nevi, although amelanotic nevi may appear. The hair is white. If yellowing of the hair occurs, it is due to shampooing and weathering, not to pigment production.

MINOR. Malignant melanoma is a rare occurrence in individuals with OCA1A. It has been reported in less than 30 patients. It was amelanotic in three-fourths of the case reports. Squamous cell carcinomas and basal cell carcinomas are increased in frequency, ostensibly due to lack of protection against sun damage.

ASSOCIATED ABNORMALITIES

Visual disturbances in OCA1A include poor vision (often correctable to 20/50 to 20/200, but in some instances as poor as 20/400), nystagmus, poor stereovision, and photophobia. The irides are usually light gray or blue, but may have brown areas. They transilluminate readily, giving the pink appearance to the eyes. There is reduced retinal pigment and foveal

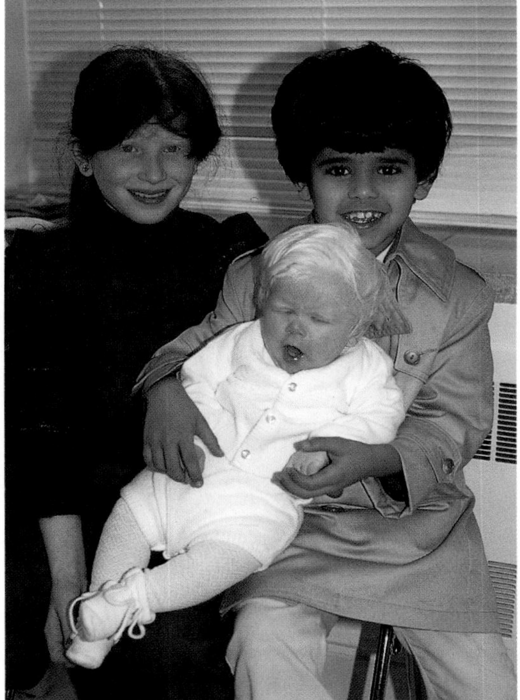

Figure 4.41. Affected infant with white hair and skin; affected sister with dyed hair and marked red reflex, normal brother.

hypoplasia. There is a paucity of uncrossed optic fibers, disorganization of the dorsal lateral geniculate nuclei, and disorganization of the connection from these to the visual cortex. All of these defects in neuronal pathway development affect vision. There is variability in the degree of ocular impairment, even between affected siblings.

Although pigmented melanocytes also populate the inner ear, and animal models with albinism show increased susceptibility to noise-induced hearing loss, affected humans show only a temporary threshold shift in hearing after exposure to noise. Despite the lack of clinical hearing problems, brain stem auditory evoked responses are often abnormal.

HISTOPATHOLOGY

LIGHT. In hair bulbs, only stage I and stage II premelanosomes are seen.

EM. The melanosome structure appears normal for developmental stages I and II.

BASIC DEFECT

Mutations in the tyrosinase gene result in an absent or defective enzyme, thus truncating melanin production. OCA1A is associated with a complete lack of enzyme activity, OCA1B with greatly reduced tyrosinase activity. In OCA1TS, the tyrosinase enzyme activity is defective at 37°C but appears to be functional at temperatures of 35°C or less.

TREATMENT

Early recognition of visual impairment and referral for appropriate visual testing and aids is most important. Sunscreen protection and protective clothing play a role.

MODE OF INHERITANCE

Autosomal recessive. There are many compound heterozygotes among affected individuals, and many mutations have been identified. OCA1A, OCA1B, OCA1MP, and OCA1TS are all allelic, and the gene is located at 11q14–21.

PRENATAL DIAGNOSIS

Previously performed successfully by fetal skin biopsy using electron microscopy evaluation of the DOPA reaction test in fetal skin. Only stage I and stage II melanosomes are found, in comparison with stages III and IV in normal fetuses of similar gestational age (19–20 weeks). Now diagnosis should be possible by molecular analysis if the mutation has been identified in the family.

DIFFERENTIAL DIAGNOSIS

In minimal pigment oculocutaneous albinism (MIM:203280), the findings in affected individuals are identical to those of classic OCA1A at birth. At puberty, however, pigmented nevi may appear, and the hair may yellow and the irises darken. Hair bulb tyrosinase activity is absent. OCA1MP may result from compound heterozygosity for allelic alterations in tyrosinase activity.

The development of pigment in the hair and skin of individuals with yellow mutant oculocutaneous albinism (MIM:203180) usually occurs within the first decade of life. Individuals with this variant of oculocutaneous albinism are clinically indistinguishable at birth from those with classic OCA1A.

White skin and white hair are also typical of OCA1TS; however, at puberty, darker hairs develop on areas of the body where the skin is cooler, such as the distal limbs. The hairs on the arms and the legs darken, whereas those of the scalp and axillae remain white. A patient with this form of oculocutaneous albinism also developed pigmented nevi in adolescence. Poor visual acuity, nystagmus, and iris transillumination are part of OCA1TS, as they are part of OCA1A.

There is a host of case reports of albinism in association with a variety of abnormalities including mental retardation, skeletal dysplasias, dysmorphic features, and deafness, to name a few. Most are individual case reports or occurrences among siblings who are offspring of consanguineous matings, suggesting that other autosomal recessive disorders might be responsible for additional features.

Support Group: National Organization for Albinism and Hypopigmentation (NOAH)
1530 Locust Street
Box 29
Philadelphia, PA 19102
1-215-545-2322

SELECTED BIBLIOGRAPHY

Creel, D.J., Summers, C.G., and King, R.A. (1990). Visual anomalies associated with albinism. *Ophthalmic Paediatr. Genet.* **11,** 193–200.

A discussion of the development of visual pathways and the perturbations caused by defects in the tyrosinase gene.

King, R.A., Townsend, D., Oetting, W., Summers, C.G., Olds, D.P., White, J.G., and Spritz, R. A. (1991). Temperature-sensitive tyrosinase associated with peripheral pigmentation in oculocutaneous albinism. *J. Clin. Invest.* **87,** 1046–1053.

At temperatures of 35°–37°C, there is loss of hair bulb tyrosinase activity. This defect is similar to that seen in Siamese cats and Himalayan mice.

King, R.A., Wertschafter, J.D., Olds, D.P., and Brumbaugh, J. (1986). Minimal pigment: a new type of oculocutaneous albinism. *Clin. Genet.* **29,** 42–50.

This is a report of sisters who were followed over many years. One developed pigment in her late teens, the other earlier in childhood. Their mother showed decreased tyrosinase activity in hair bulbs; the father's hair bulbs were normal. Two other families are referred to briefly.

Spritz, R.A. (1993). Molecular genetics of oculocutaneous albinism. *Semin. Dermatol.* **12,** 167–172.

A review of molecular data, clearly written.

OCULOCUTANEOUS ALBINISM TYSOSINASE POSITIVE (MIM: 203200)

(OCA2; Xanthism; Partial Albinism) Includes Rufous Albinism; Brown Albinism

DERMATOLOGIC FEATURES

MAJOR. There is little or no pigment in the skin and hair at birth. Pigment gradually accumulates during childhood and adolescence. The degree to which pigment develops in the hair and skin appears to correlate with the genetic background; affected individuals of

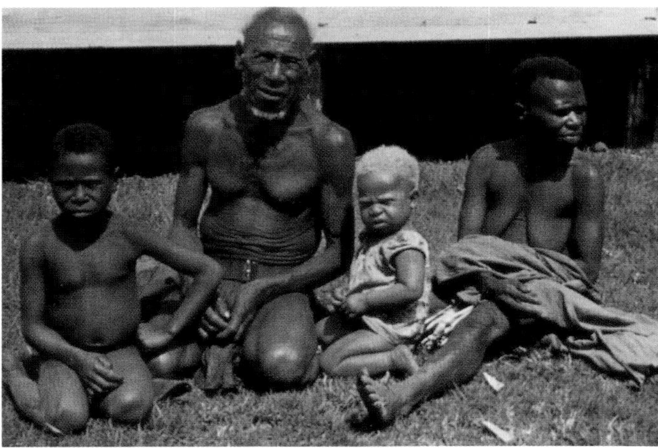

Figure 4.42. Striking hypopigmentation of affected child compared with family members. (From Walsh, 1971.)

fair-skinned populations (e.g., Scandinavian) pigment less and later than those from darker ethnic groups (e.g., Mediterraneans, Africans). The hair may be dead white, to light yellow, to golden blonde or red, and it gradually darkens with age as pheomelanin accumulates. The skin is milky-white at birth and does not appreciably change with age in tone, nor does tanning occur, although freckles and pigmented nevi may develop.

In rufous albinism (reported in Africa and New Guinea) affected individuals have reddish hair and skin. The skin has almost a copper color to it.

Minor. None.

ASSOCIATED ABNORMALITIES

The irides are blue-gray to light brown. Vision may be quite poor in early childhood, but generally improves throughout adolescence. Both acuity and nystagmus can normalize. The irises are brown to hazel in rufous albinism, and nystagmus is reported in only some individuals.

HISTOPATHOLOGY

Light. Hair bulbs will pigment when incubated with tyrosine.

EM. The melanocytes and melanosomes are normal, and stage IV melanized melanosomes will be formed on incubation with DOPA or tyrosine.

BASIC DEFECT

Approximately one-third of patients have mutations in the tyrosinase gene, suggesting that the clinical distinctions between OCA1B (yellow mutant) and OCA2 may not be reliable. Other nonallelic mutations have been identified in a gene called P. The function of the P gene product is not known, but is believed to be a melanosomal membrane transport protein that may be involved in the transport of tyrosine.

TREATMENT

Sun protection and appropriate visual aids.

MODE OF INHERITANCE

Autosomal recessive. The P gene maps to 15q11–q13. Deletions in this region are responsible for the Prader-Willi and Angelman syndromes, which are marked by hypopigmentation. However, the P locus does not appear to undergo imprinting. Thus its role in the dilution of color in these two conditions remains unexplained.

PRENATAL DIAGNOSIS

Possible by molecular techniques when the specific mutation is identified.

DIFFERENTIAL DIAGNOSIS

Caucasians with brown albinism (MIM: 203290) have golden brown hair coupled with white skin lacking pigment. Brown albinos from African populations have light brown skin that can tan, freckles, brown hair, and blue or brown eyes. Approximately 50% of individuals with brown albinism will have nystagmus, and the reduction in visual acuity is moderate (20/60 to 20/150). The gene for OCA brown remains unidentified.

There are rare reports of autosomal dominant albinism (MIM:126070), some of which may represent pseudodominance for autosomal recessive albinism. Others, presumably autosomal dominant forms, do not have associated visual disturbances. In general in these reports the skin is light in color and tans, and the hair color is light.

Support Group: National Organization for Albinism and Hypopigmentation (NOAH)
1530 Locust Street
Box 29
Philadelphia, PA 19102
1-215-545-2322

SELECTED BIBLIOGRAPHY

King, R.A., Hearing, V.J., Creel, D.J., and Oetting, W.S. (1995). Albinism. In *The Metabolic and Molecular Basis of Inherited Disease.* Scriver, C.R., Beaudet, A.L., Sly, W.S., and Valle, E.D. (eds.) McGraw-Hill, New York, 7th ed., pp. 4353–4392.

This is a comprehensive review chapter with both clinical information and a review of the basic biology of pigment production. There are 528 citations. The authors state that the diagnosis of albinism requires the presence of certain features in the optic system, including nystagmus, reduced iris pigment, reduced retinal pigment with foveal hypoplasia, and misrouting of optic fibers at the chiasm.

Walsh, R.J. (1971). A distinctive pigment of the skin in New Guinea indigenes. *Ann. Hum. Genet.* **34,** 379–388.

Although parental transmission of rufous albinism was seen, the author believes that this reflects pseudodominance of an autosomal recessive condition because of inbreeding within the pedigree.

YELLOW MUTANT ALBINISM (MIM:203180)

(OCA1B; Amish Albinism)

DERMATOLOGIC FEATURES

Major. Individuals with this form of albinism are clinically identical to those with OCA1A at birth. The hair is white, the skin creamy white. The hair may become flaxen within a few months of life or later in childhood. It may eventually darken to a light brown. In some families, the hair appears to redden. Tanning has been reported in older individuals. Pigmented nevi may also develop.

Minor. None.

ASSOCIATED ABNORMALITIES

Vision is initially poor, with nystagmus and iris transillumination. Visual acuity is similar

A
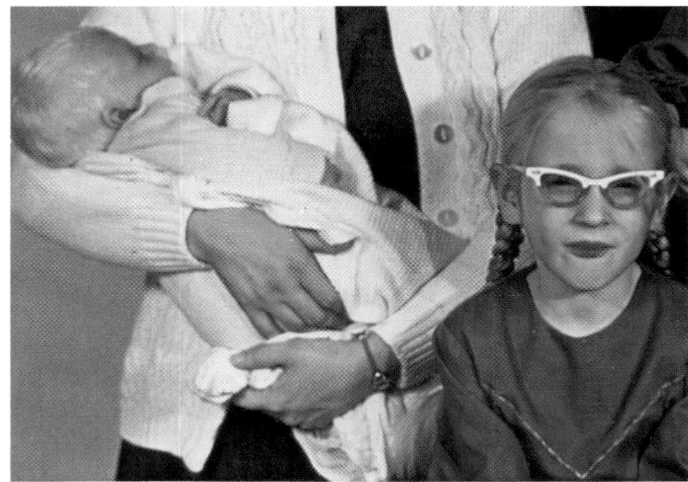

B
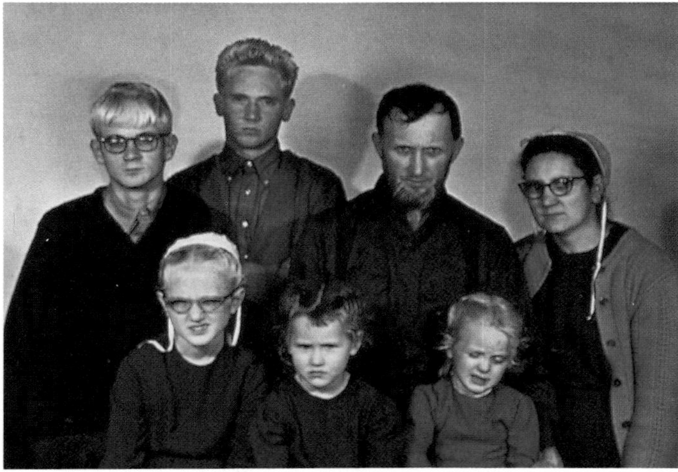

Figure 4.43. **(A)** Two affected children with white hair in infant, cornsilk color in older girl. **(B)** Parents and child in the middle front are unaffected; other four siblings affected. (From Nance et al., 1970.)

to that in OCA1A. The irises may darken with age.

HISTOPATHOLOGY

Light. There is a negative DOPA reaction in hair bulbs. There may be slight yellowing on incubation in the presence of DOPA and cystine or tyrosine and cystine.
EM. The melanocytes and hair bulbs show stages I, II, and III premelanosomes. There are no stage IV premelanosomes.

BASIC DEFECT

Mutations in the tyrosinase gene that result in greatly reduced tyrosinase function.

TREATMENT

Visual aids and sun avoidance and protection.

MODE OF INHERITANCE

Autosomal recessive. OCA1B is allelic to OCA1A, OCA1TS, and OCA1MP on 11q14.21. As the name implies, first identified among the Amish.

PRENATAL DIAGNOSIS

Presumably possible by molecular techniques or fetal skin biopsy.

DIFFERENTIAL DIAGNOSIS

Differentiation from other forms of oculocutaneous albinism may not be possible at birth in isolated cases.

Support Group: National Organization for Albinism and Hypopigmentation (N.O.A.H.)
1530 Locust Street
Box 29
Philadelphia, PA 19102
1-215-545-2322

SELECTED BIBLIOGRAPHY

Hu, F., Hanifin, J.M., Prescott, G.H., and Tongue, A.C. (1980). Yellow mutant albinism: cytochemical, ultrastructural and genetic characterization suggesting multiple allelism. *Am. J. Hum. Genet.* **32,** 387–395.
A sibship of Scottish/Irish/English descent. The authors propose that the phenotype results from heterozygosity for a yellow mutant allele and the OCA1A allele, as a maternal first cousin, once removed, had classic OCA1A albinism. One of the affected sisters also had mild platelet abnormalities.

CROSS SYNDROME (MIM: 257800)

(Oculocerebral Syndrome with Hypopigmentation; Kramer Syndrome; Cross-McKusick-Breen Syndrome)

DERMATOLOGIC FEATURES

Major. There have been a handful of case reports of children with pigmentary abnormalities, ocular abnormalities, and neurologic abnormalities. These cases share in common marked generalized hypopigmentation of the skin and hair. The hair is variably described as white, yellowish, or silvery blonde. Note has been made in several case reports of involvement of eyebrows and eyelashes with scattered, darkly pigmented hairs distributed among hairs without color.

In the originally described patients, darkly pigmented nevi were noted over the back, buttocks, and thighs. Nevi have also been described in a few other case reports.

Minor. Thin hair was described in one case report.

ASSOCIATED ABNORMALITIES

All affected individuals have had severe mental retardation with spastic diplegia or quadriplegia, seizures, and athetosis.

Ocular abnormalities have ranged from microphthalmia to cataracts to blonde fundi, abnormal electroretinograms, and nystagmus. Photophobia and iris transillumination have also been noted. Severe growth retardation and failure to thrive, presumably on a neurologic basis, is described in all patients.

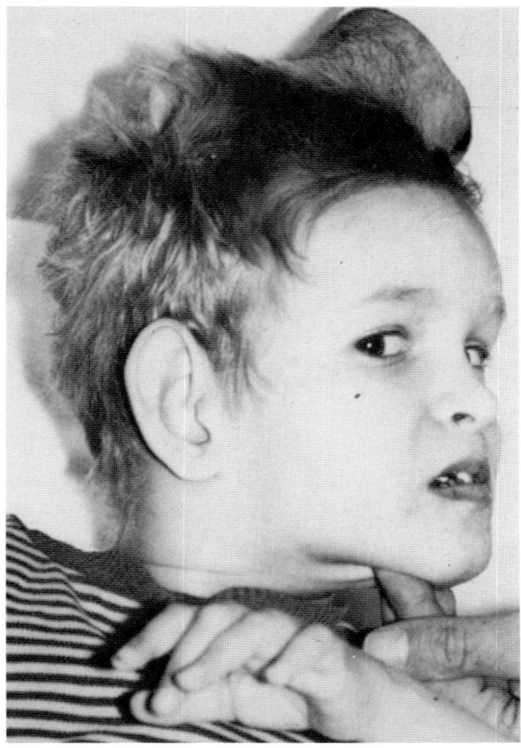

Figure 4.44. Mixture of silver and pigmented hairs on scalp. (From Fryns et al., 1988.)

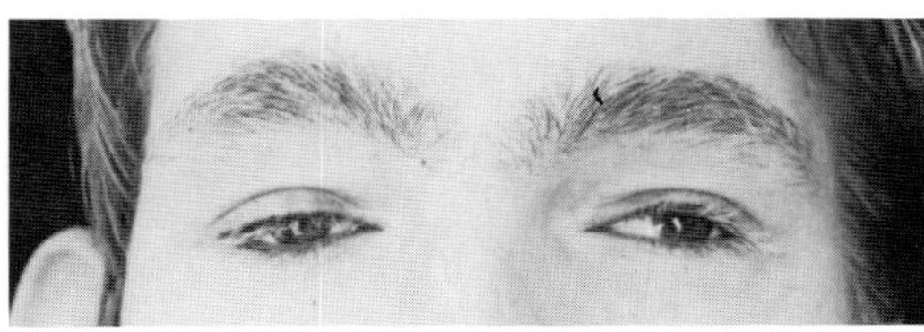

Figure 4.45. Patchy distribution of silver hairs in eyebrows and eyelashes. (From Fryns et al., 1988.)

Although osteoporosis has been noted in a few patients, it appears most likely to be secondary to nonweightbearing and chronic wasting rather than a primary feature. Gum hypertrophy was described in a few case reports and may be secondary to anticonvulsant therapy in at least some.

One patient had a posterior fossa cyst, and another had a Dandy-walker malformation. One patient was reported to have deafness and severe neutropenia.

HISTOPATHOLOGY

Light. Patchy distribution of melanocytes.
EM. A decreased number of melanocytes with few clustered melanosomes has been noted in some patients. Premelanosomes in hair bulbs appear to be normal. One patient was reported as tyrosine positive, one as tyrosine negative.

BASIC DEFECT

Unknown.

TREATMENT

None.

MODE OF INHERITANCE

Presumably autosomal recessive based on recurrences in siblings and consanguinity.

PRENATAL DIAGNOSIS

None.

DIFFERENTIAL DIAGNOSIS

It is not clear, in my opinion, that this syndrome actually represents a single entity. In the seven reports of nine affected children, variability seems to be the rule. There has been discussion in the literature suggesting that a subset of these patients (in particular, two described by Preus et al. [1983]) can be separated out (MIM: 257790.) I remain unconvinced that these children fall into either a unitary group or distinct subtypes. What distinguishes these patients from classic OCA1A is their severe neurologic compromise and their ocular abnormalities. Children with Chediak-Higashi syndrome (MIM:214500) do not have structural ocular abnormalities and do not have the neurologic alterations evident in the Cross syndrome, although the abnormalities of the hair are similar. Children with Cross syndrome do not have the immunologic abnormalities associated with Chediak-Higashi.

Support Group: N.O.R.D.
P.O. Box 8923
New Fairfield, CT
06812
1-800-999-6673

SELECTED BIBLIOGRAPHY

Cross, H.E., McKusick, V.A., and Breen, W. (1967). A new oculocerebral syndrome with hypopigmentation. *J. Pediatr.* **70,** 398–406.

Consanguineous Amish family had three children with microphthalmia, athetosis, lack of color in the hair and skin, but with darkly pigmented nevi over the lower part of the body in one of three affected siblings. There were occasional darkly pigmented strands of hair.

Fryns, J.P., Derey Maeker, A.M., Heremans, G., Marien, J., van Hauwaert, J., Turner, G., Hockey, A., and van den Berghe, H. (1988). Oculocerebral syndrome with hypopigmentation (Cross syndrome). *Clin. Genet.* **34,** 81–84.

Two of 10 offspring born to second degree cousins showed severe mental retardation and spasticity, coupled with cutaneous findings of silver blonde hair with light and dark hairs in the eyebrows and eyelashes. The affected children had nystagmus with normal fundi. The skin was pale. Skin biopsy tissue showed patchy distribution of melanocytes. The melanocytes, when present, were "stuffed with melanosomes." Interestingly, another brother had the hair and eyebrow changes but had no other problems.

Preus, M., Fraser, F.C., Wigglesworth, F.W. (1983). An oculocerebral hypopigmentation syndrome. *J. Genet. Hum.* **31,** 323–328.

Two sisters with neutropenia and anemia, nystagmus, and decreased pigment–blond hair, pale skin, blue eyes with albinoid fundi and cataracts. Growth and psychomotor retardation with progressive neurologic degeneration. Parents were consanguineous.

HYPOMELANOSIS OF ITO (MIM:146150)

(Incontinentia Pigmenti Achromians)

DERMATOLOGIC FEATURES

MAJOR. Hypopigmentation or depigmentation is distributed in swirls and patches along the lines of Blaschko. Involvement is usually generalized but may be patchy and is often asymmetric. The skin is otherwise entirely normal.

Color changes may be present at birth, but more usually become obvious in late infancy to early childhood. In one of my patients, who was carefully examined on several occasions, the pigment changes were not discernible until midchildhood.

In some instances, it may not be possible to distinguish which are the normal areas, the lighter or the darker.

MINOR. Other dermatologic abnormalities have been mentioned in case reports, but these are nonspecific and may reflect the underlying specific chromosome alteration or be unassociated.

ASSOCIATED ABNORMALITIES

A host of associated abnormalities have been described in more than 50% of all reports of hypomelanosis of Ito, as might be expected for a disorder that is highly heterogeneous in cause. Chromosomal mosaicism has been found in 50% of appropriately tested affected children.

Mental retardation, with or without seizures, and structural brain alterations are common (40%–60%). The risk for mental retardation in individuals with hypomelanosis of Ito and normal karyotypes appears to be as great as for those who are chromosomally abnormal.

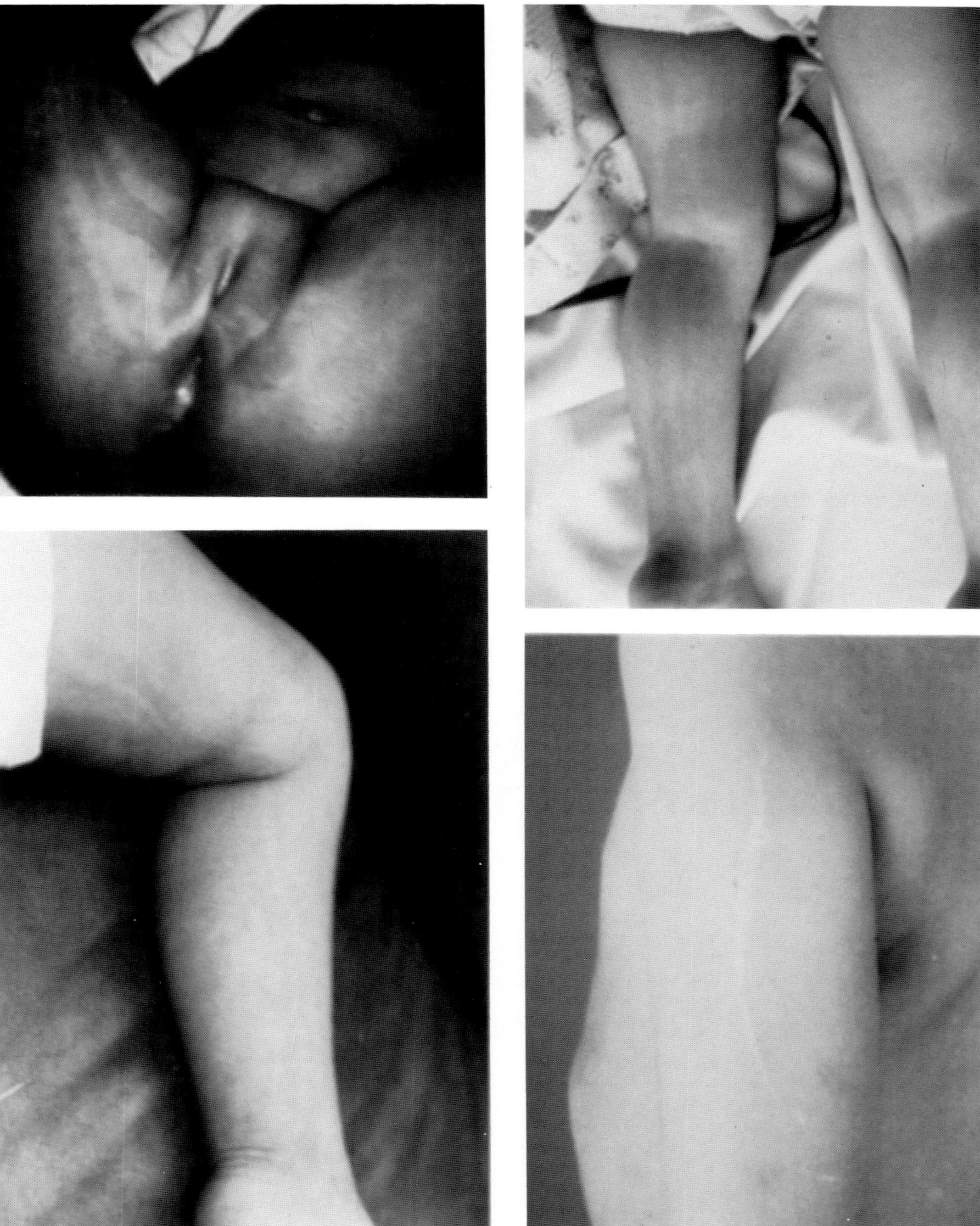

Figure 4.46. Four individuals with hypomelanosis of Ito. The top two are mosaic for chromosomal aneuploidy. The bottom two have normal karyotypes. (From Sybert et al., 1990.)

However, this may reflect bias of ascertainment in that the typical skin changes in an otherwise normal child may not be brought to medical attention. Nonetheless, faced with a young infant with these cutaneous changes and normal chromosomes, predictions for intellectual development must remain guarded.

Any organ system can be affected. Prognosis is not dependent on the diagnosis of hypomelanosis of Ito but rather upon either the specific karyotype alteration or the severity of the specific malformations.

HISTOPATHOLOGY

LIGHT. Inconstant findings include a decrease in the number of melanocytes, normal number of melanocytes but decreased melanin granules, and decrease in melanosomes. The DOPA reaction results are also inconsistent, but usually normal.

EM. Inconstant findings of a decrease in the number of melanosomes within melanocytes and a decrease in the number of fully melanized granules in the keratinocytes are described.

BASIC DEFECT

The phenotype of hypomelanosis of Ito appears to be nonspecific for chromosomal mosaicism and has been reported in a host of distinct karyotype alterations, including chimerism, triploidy, X-chromosome abnormalities, autosomal deletions and duplications (7, 12, 13, 14, 15, 18), and mosaic trisomies (8, 13, 14, 18, 22). Not all patients will have karyotype alterations.

TREATMENT

None specific.

MODE OF INHERITANCE

Chromosomal/unknown. No convincing familial transmission has been reported. Where familial recurrence appears to have occurred, the correct diagnosis has been incontinentia pigmenti, not hypomelanosis of Ito.

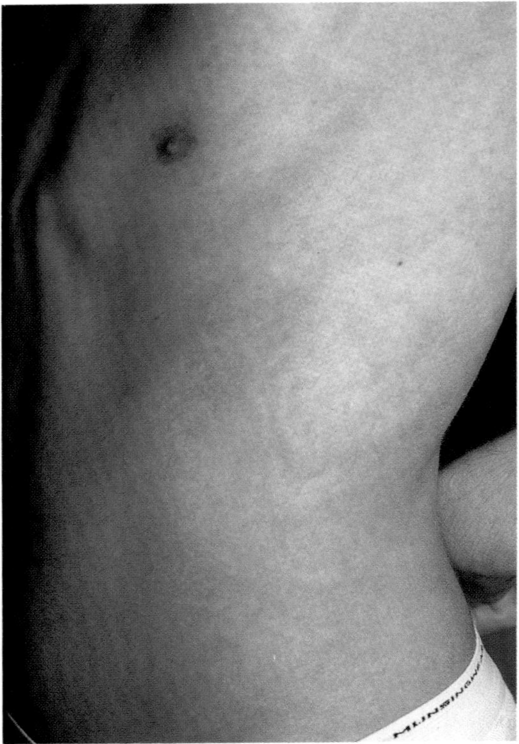

Figure 4.47. Hypopigmentation along the lines of Blaschko in a patient mosaic for Trisomy 8.

PRENATAL DIAGNOSIS

Only for cases due to familial translocations in which karyotyping of chorionic villus cell samples or amniotic cells is possible.

DIFFERENTIAL DIAGNOSIS

It is sometimes difficult to distinguish which skin color is normal, the darker or the lighter; thus linear and whorled nevoid hypermelanosis, in which swirly hyperpigmentation occurs, must be considered in the differential. In linear and whorled nevoid hypermelanosis, males and females are affected with equal frequency, and there are no other abnormalities, in contrast to hypomelanosis of Ito. In both conditions the color change may become more widespread and pronounced with time. Skin biopsies in nevoid hypermelanosis have demonstrated increased numbers of melanocytes or increase in the basal layer pigmentation, but these features are probably not useful to distinguish the two conditions.

Although guttate hypomelanosis has been described in tuberous sclerosis (MIM:191100), the swirly pattern of hypopigmentation along Blaschko lines typical of hypomelanosis of Ito has not been.

In the Waardenburg syndrome (MIM: 193500) and in piebaldism (MIM:172800), there is the dead white appearance of true depigmentation, which is rare in hypomelanosis of Ito. The changes of piebaldism are usually distributed in symmetric patches, not along the lines of Blaschko, and often on flexor surfaces. It is also usually congenital. Islands of normally pigmented skin within the depigmented areas are typical of piebaldism and are not seen in hypomelanosis of Ito.

Nevus depigmentosus has a distribution similar to hypomelanosis of Ito. While it is usually present at birth, this is not invariable. Ito's (Ito, 1952) patient was described by him as having a nevus depigmentosus although her lesions were acquired. Some patients with nevus depigmentosus have had structural and neurological abnormalities. It is probably reasonable to karyotype such patients.

In the final adult stages of incontinentia pigmenti, (MIM: 308300), hypopigmented areas similar to hypomelanosis of Ito may occur. In incontinentia pigmenti these areas are devoid of hairs and sweat glands, in contrast to the normal appendages of hypopigmented skin in hypomelanosis of Ito. Hypomelanosis of Ito is not preceded by either the bullous or verrucous changes of incontinentia pigmenti.

Support Group: N.O.R.D.
P.O. Box 8923
New Fairfield, CT
06812
1-800-999-6673

SELECTED BIBLIOGRAPHY

Donnai, D., Read, A.P., McKeown, C., and Andrews, T. (1988). Hypomelanosis of Ito: a manifestation of mosaicism or chimerism. *J. Med. Genet.* **25,** 809–818.

Ohashi, H., Tsukahara, M., Murano, I., Naritomi, K., Nishioka, K., Susumu, M., and Kajii, T. (1992). Pigmentary dysplasia and chromosomal mosaicism, report of nine cases. *Am. J. Med. Genet.* **43,** 716–721.

Ritter, C.L., Stele, M.W., Wenger, S.L., and Cohen, B.A. (1990). Chromosomal mosaicism in hypomelanosis of Ito. *Am. J. Med Genet.* **35,** 14–17.

Sybert, V.P., Pagon, R.A., Donlan, M., and Bradley, C.N. (1990). Pigmentary abnormalities and mosaicism for chromosomal aberration: association with clinical features similar to hypomelanosis of Ito. *J. Pediatr.* **116,** 581–586.

Donna, et al. (1988), Ohashi et al. (1992), Ritter et al. (1990), and Sybert et al. (1990) report one or more patients and review the literature, all with the same emphasis: hypomelanosis of Ito is a descriptive term, not a diagnostic one, and cytogenetic studies of lymphocytes, and fibroblasts where lymphocyte cultures are karyotypically normal, are mandatory.

Ito, M. (1952). Studies on melanin. XI. Incontinentia pigmenti achromians: a singular case of a nevus depigmentosus systematicus bilateralis. *Tohoku. J. Exp. Med.* (suppl) **55,** 57–59.

Description of 22 year old female, with depigmentation along lines of Blaschko. Ito also noted slight atrophy. Histopathology evaluation showed absence of melanin granules. Loss of pigment began in childhood and continued to expand gradually.

Sybert, V.P. (1990). Hypomelanosis of Ito. Editorial. *Pediatr. Dermatol.* **7,** 74–76.

In this editorial, I reviewed the published literature of familial cases and argue against a Mendelian mode of inheritance for hypomelanosis of Ito. Although it is possible that some cases may represent new dominant mutations, the recurrence risk for hypomelanosis of Ito is essentially nil, outside of families with balanced translocations as the cause for chromosomal mosaicism.

Sybert, V.P. (1994) Hypomelanosis of Ito: a description, not a diagnosis. *J. Invest. Dermatol.* **103,** 141S–143S

Of 115 individuals in the medical literature in

whom karyotyping was performed, abnormalities were detected in 60. Most were mosaic, either for chromosomally normal and abnormal cell lines, or for two or more different chromosomally abnormal cell lines. Tables contain all previous reports.

Vormittag, W., Ensinger, C., and Raff, M. (1992). Cytogenetic and dermatoglyphic findings in a familial case of hypomelanosis of Ito (IPA). *Clin. Genet.* **41,** 309–314.

A mother with seizures, leg length asymmetry, scoliosis, radial head dysplasia, and unilateral ocular abnormalities had skin findings of hypomelanosis of Ito that on biopsy showed decreased to absent pigment in the light areas, normal to increased pigment in the dark areas. Her 4-year-old daughter had similar skin changes and "depigmentation" of the irises. The mother was mosaic diploid/triploid/tetraploid in skin only. The daughter was karyotypically normal in lymphocytes; skin fibroblast culture was not done. The relationship of the hypopigmentation to the karyotype abnormality thus remains unclear.

PIEBALDISM (MIM:172800)

(White Spot Disease)

DERMATOLOGIC FEATURES

MAJOR. Dead white, often strikingly symmetric, patches of skin are the classic feature of piebaldism. The midforehead, chest, abdomen, and extremities are typical sites for involvement. The central back is usually spared, as are the hands and feet. The shoulder girdle and hips are also usually, but not invariably, spared. A triangular- or diamond-shaped white forelock is present in approximately 90% of affected individuals and may extend to involve the medial third of the eyebrows. The chin is also often involved. Intrafamilial variability in the degree of involvement is great. Within depigmented areas there may be islands of hyperpigmentation, and the margins of lesions are also often hyperpigmented and surrounded by little droplets or rosettes of color.

Surprisingly, islands of repigmentation have developed in some affected individuals after sun exposure.

In one family, gain and loss of areas of involvement of the skin over time was reported.

MINOR. None.

ASSOCIATED ABNORMALITIES

Hirschsprung disease has been reported in some families, as has deafness. Occasionally heterochromia iridis is described. Whether these are features truly associated with piebaldism or whether these case reports represent misdiagnosis of Waardenburg syndrome is uncertain.

HISTOPATHOLOGY

LIGHT. Absence of melanocytes in involved skin.

EM. Melanocytes from normal skin have had some abnormalities, including abnormal melanosomes, and irregular cytoplasmic vesicles. These changes are not diagnostic. Langerhans cells are increased in number in both normal and lesional skin. Melanocytes in involved skin appeared "empty" (one patient).

BASIC DEFECT

Mutations in the *KIT* protooncogene affect melanocyte proliferation and/or migration during embryogenesis. The gene codes for the tyrosine kinase cell surface receptor for mast and stem cell growth factor. The homologous locus in the mouse is dominant white spotting.

TREATMENT

Essentially none. One report of minigrafting of autologous normal skin in one patient, and one

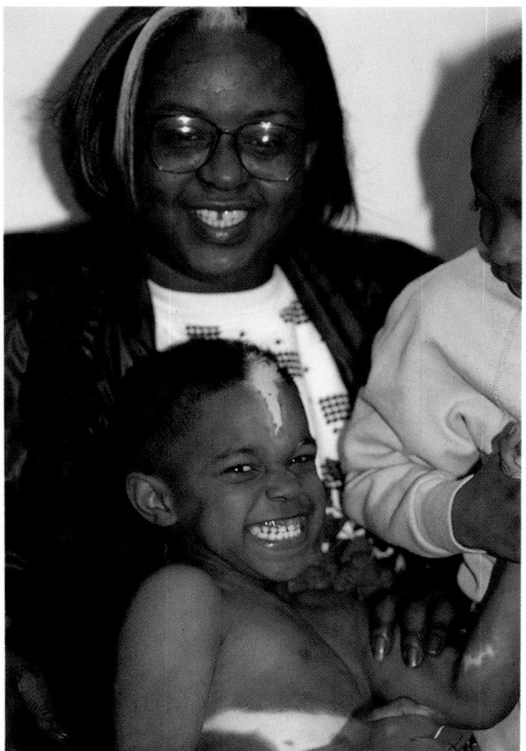

Figure 4.48. Grandmother and grandson—white forelock only in grandmother, depigmented skin patches in grandson.

report of psoralen plus ultraviolet light of the A wavelength (PUVA) with minimal results in another patient.

MODE OF INHERITANCE

Autosomal dominant with allelic heterogeneity. The gene maps to 4q11–q12, and there has been no locus heterogeneity to date.

PRENATAL DIAGNOSIS

Not attempted. Presumably possible using molecular techniques.

DIFFERENTIAL DIAGNOSIS

Vitiligo (MIM:193200) is usually an acquired disorder. Rarely, patients with vitiligo can present with congenital patches of pigment loss. In piebaldism, pigment loss is usually not progressive, and the margins of the lesions have increased numbers of melanocytes. Although rare, repigmentation in piebaldism similar to that seen in vitiligo can occur, so there may be instances in which confusion between the two disorders may arise.

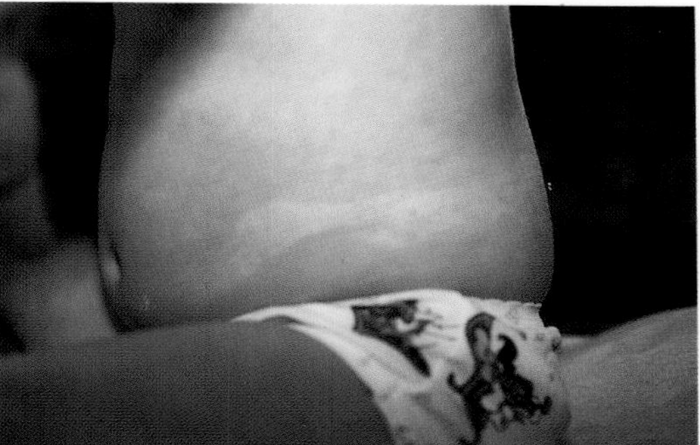

Figure 4.49. Nevus depigmentosus is less strikingly white because of baseline fairness of skin.

Without a family history, piebaldism may be indistinguishable clinically from Waardenburg type II (MIM:193510).

The color loss is absolute in piebaldism, in contrast to the hypopigmentation of hypomelanosis of Ito (MIM:146150). Melanocytes are present in the hypopigmented areas of hypomelanosis of Ito. The distribution of affected areas is swirly, along the lines of Blaschko, in hypomelanosis of Ito, and usually patchy in piebaldism.

A nevus depigmentosus may be a small localized lesion or generalized. It also occurs along the lines of Blaschko. In some instances it may not be possible to distinguish between piebaldism and nevus depigmentosus in an isolated case, although the depigmented patches in piebaldism tend to be more geometric blotches rather than swirling.

Isolated white forelock is inherited as an isolated autosomal dominant trait. It can be an isolated finding in some individuals in families with piebaldism. It may or may not be a genetically distinct entity. A white forelock has also been reported in a sibship with a combination of other malformations (MIM:277740), including transverse terminal limb defects, congenital heart defects, and ocular hypertelorism.

Support Group: N.O.R.D.
P.O. Box 8923
New Fairfield, CT
06812
1-800-999-6673

SELECTED BIBLIOGRAPHY

Dippel, E., Haas, N., Grabbe, J., Schadendorf, D., Hamann, K., and Czarnetzki, B.M. (1995). Expression of the *c-kit* receptor in hypomelanosis: a comparative study between piebaldism, naevus depigmentosus and vitiligo. *Br. J. Dermatol.* **132,** 182–189.

Epidermis from lesional skin of five patients with vitiligo failed to stain with *c-kit* protein and showed no immunoreactivity to TA99, a melanosome-specific antibody; lesional tissue from two patients with piebaldism had weak staining with TA99 and no *c-kit* staining; in one patient with nevus depigmentosus, *c-kit* staining was positive, TA99 faint. Thus the authors conclude that in diagnostically difficult situations, these techniques may help. Beware the small numbers!

Falabella, R. (1978). Repigmentation of leukoderma by minigrafts of normally pigmented autologous skin. *J. Dermatol. Surg. Oncol.* **4,** 916–919.

Color photos before and after grafting with 1–2 mm pinch minigrafts in a patient with piebaldism. The results are impressive, but the appearance is still far from normal. Perhaps that is why I have found no other publications of attempts to replicate this treatment.

Fleischman, R.A., Saltman, D.L., Stastny, V., and Zneimer, S. (1991). Deletion of the *c-kit* protooncogene in the human developmental defect piebald trait. *Proc. Natl. Acad. Sci. U.S.A.* **88,** 10885–10889.

Of seven patients studied, one was deleted for *c-kit*. Striking photos of affected child and affected mouse, both with similar leukodermic patches. The authors suggest mutations in other genes, such as the ligand for *c-kit,* which is abnormal in the steel mouse, could be causal in some patients with piebaldism.

Froggatt, P. (1959). An outline, with bibliography, of human piebaldism and white forelock. *Ir. J. Med. Sci.* **398,** 86–94.

A wonderful review of piebaldism through history. One Italian family with piebaldism reported in 1877 and revisited in 1924 had the surname Bianconcini, which means whitelock. Froggatt infers that isolated white forelock is not a distinct entity, but represents variable expression of piebaldism.

Hulten, M.A., Honeyman, M.M., Mayne, A.J., and Tarlow, M.J. (1987). Homozygosity in piebald trait. *J. Med. Genet.* **24,** 568–571.

Child of first cousin parents with piebaldism had severe developmental delay, was thought to be deaf, had absence of pigmentation of the hair and the skin, blue irises, brachycephaly, synophrys, and a broad nasal root. The authors theorized that the patient was homozygous for piebaldism. Unfortunately, the family was not adequately evaluated to rule out hearing problems. This patient, alluded to in a subsequent paper, died of unclear cause, precluding molecular proof of the homozygosity hypothesis.

Jimbow, K., Fitzpatrick, T.B., Szabo, G., and Hori, Y. (1975). Congenital circumscribed hypomelanosis: a characterization based on electron microscopic study of tuberous sclerosis, nevus depigmentosus, and piebaldism. *J. Invest. Dermatol.* **64,** 50–62.

Contrasting features of tuberous sclerosis, nevus depigmentosus, and piebaldism, these authors found that the normally pigmented skin in piebaldism contains melanocytes that produce both normal and abnormal melanosomes. No melanocytes were seen in the unpigmented areas.

Spritz, R.A. (1994). Molecular basis of human piebaldism. *J. Invest. Dermatol.* **103,** 137S–140S.

Succinct review.

Spritz, R.A., Holmes, S.A., Ramesar, R., Greenberg, J., Curtis, D., and Beighton, P. (1992). Mutations of the *KIT* (mast/stem cell growth factor receptor) proto-oncogene account for a continuous range of phenotypes in human piebaldism. *Am. J. Hum. Genet.* **51,** 1058–1065.

Presents two different mutations with different clinical severity and reviews previously published mutations. The authors try to correlate genotype with phenotype, contrasting loss of function alleles with mutations that have a dominant negative effect. Errata in *Am. J. Hum. Genet.* **52,** 654, 1993, deal with methods.

Winship, I., Young, K., Martell, R., Ramesar,

R., Curtis, D., and Beighton, P. (1991). Piebaldism: an autonomous autosomal dominant entity. *Clin. Genet.* **39,** 330–337.
Photo documentation of variability of involvement among affected relatives. Although affected males and females were examined in the flesh and described in the text, apparently only the females allowed themselves to be photographed.

PREMATURE CANITIES (MIM:139100)

(Early Graying of Hair)

DERMATOLOGIC FEATURES

MAJOR. Although in general premature graying is defined as 50% gray hairs before age 50, the term *premature canities* is usually reserved for significant graying or whitening of the hair before age 20 in whites and before age 30 in blacks. Despite its apparent common occurrence (personal observation in shopping malls), reports of documented pedigrees are rare in the literature. The family studied by Hare (1929) is the only one cited in most publications that discuss inheritance. In pursuit of families with premature canities for study, I asked individuals with early graying about their family histories. All had, at most, one or two affected relatives. Often it was a second degree, not first degree, relative. Perhaps the condition is not as commonly familial as believed, or perhaps it is not a simple autosomal dominant trait

MINOR. None.

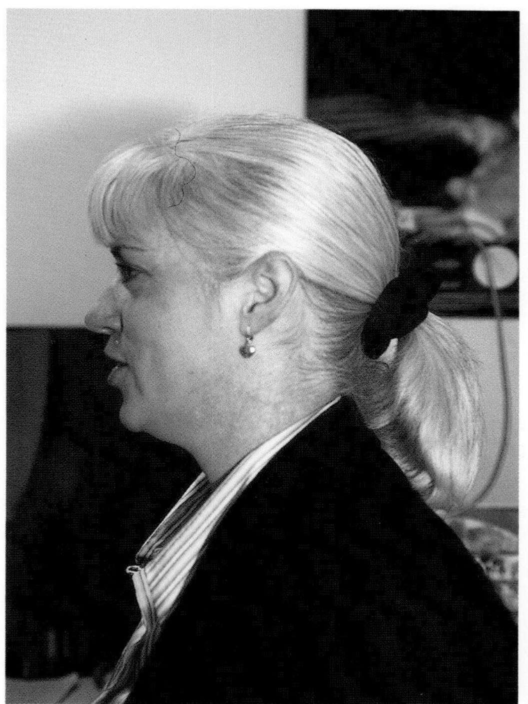

A

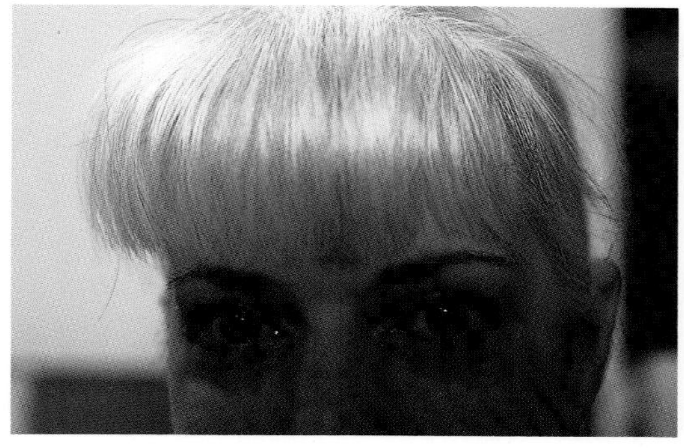

B

Figure 4.50. (A,B) Early loss of color of scalp hair; color preserved in eyebrows and eyelashes.

ASSOCIATED ABNORMALITIES

Individuals with premature canities may have one or more of the disorders associated with vitiligo, including thyroid disease and pernicious anemia.

The suggestion has been made that early graying has been associated with early mortality from premature cardiovascular disease. This has not been substantiated in well-designed studies. One study suggested a relationship of early graying with osteopenia, but all patients were ascertained from a Metabolic Bone Clinic, and this relationship is also not proven.

HISTOPATHOLOGY

Light. No information.
EM. No information.

BASIC DEFECT

Unknown.

TREATMENT

Dyeing of the hair.

PRENATAL DIAGNOSIS

None.

DIFFERENTIAL DIAGNOSIS

In vitiligo (MIM:193200) loss of color of the hair can occur. Often it is patchy. In premature canities, loss of color does not occur elsewhere on the body. There can be patchy loss of hair color in systemic lupus erythematosus (MIM:152700). The correct diagnosis should be readily apparent. In alopecia areata, pigmented hairs are more susceptible to loss, and white hairs are usually spared. It is this phenomenon that is believed to account for "the hair turned white over night." In premature canities, the graying of the hair is gradual, whereas in alopecia areata the loss of the normal pigmented hairs occurs fairly rapidly over a period of weeks. Premature graying of the hair has been reported in association with absence of the bicuspids and hyperhidrosis (Böök syndrome, MIM:112300).

Support Group: N.O.R.D.
P.O. Box 8923
New Fairfield, CT 06812
1-800-999-6673

SELECTED BIBLIOGRAPHY

Hare, H.J.H. (1929). Premature whitening of hair. *J. Hered.* **20,** 31–32.

This is a five generation pedigree with evidence of male-to-male transmission. Of interest is the author's statement that two of the affected individuals, upon noticing their early graying, underwent treatment to prevent loss of color: "by taking exceptional care of the hair, the development of the abnormal condition was checked, and she now has a fine head of black hair. No dyes were used . . ." It makes one wonder what that special care might have been. One also ought to note the happy juxtaposition of the author's surname and subject.

Keogh, E.V., and Walsh, R.J. (1965). Rate of greying of human hair. *Nature* **207,** 877–878.

By age 25, 25% of individuals have some gray hairs; 1 in 1,000 females and 1 in 500 males are completely gray. By age 35, 60%–61% of males and 66% of females have some gray hair; 2.2% of males and 1.6% of females are entirely gray. By age 45, 88% have some gray hair; 12.6% of males and 10% of females are completely gray. By age 55, 94%–96% of Caucasian human beings will have some gray hair, and almost 30% of both sexes will be completely gray.

VITILIGO (MIM:193200)

DERMATOLOGIC FEATURES

Major. Leukoderma, or white patches of skin, are the defining feature of vitiligo. Different distribution patterns of pigment loss have been appreciated and specifically named, i.e., localized, generalized, segmental, or acrofacial vitiligo, but do not offer prognostic

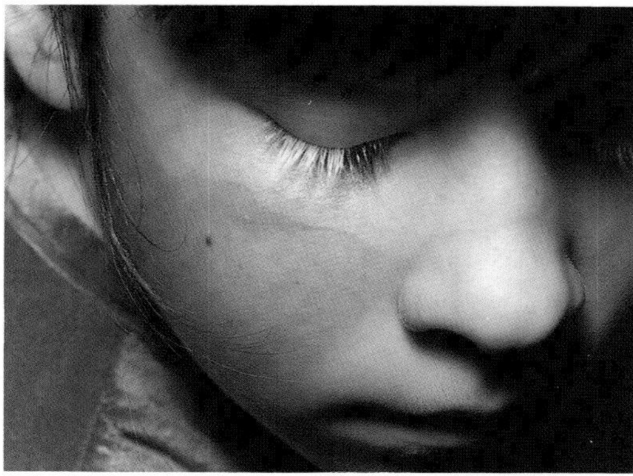

Figure 4.51. Involvement around eye; eyelashes also affected.

or causal distinctions. Initially, patches may be hypopigmented rather than completely depigmented. The margins of involved areas are usually sharply defined and may be hyperpigmented. The pigment may be retained around hair follicles, and repigmentation often occurs at these sites as well, giving a "freckled" or stippled appearance to the patches. The term *trichome,* in reference to vitiligo, describes the hyperpigmented brown margins, the lighter newer areas of involvement, and the dead white areas of older involvement, which can be seen in a lesion.

The face and the periorbital, perinasal, perioral, and periaureolar areas are sites of predilection, as are the naval and the genitalia. Bony prominences such as the elbows and wrists are also often involved. In individuals affected with vitiligo areas of trauma may develop pigment loss (Koebnerization). The term *poliosis* refers to the loss of color in eyebrows, eyelashes, and patches of hair on the scalp. Halo nevi, loss of pigment around congenital or acquired nevocytic moles, is a common occurrence.

Onset of vitiligo occurs before age 20 in approximately 50% of affected individuals. There are rare reports of newborns presenting with vitiligo. Females are more commonly affected than males. Segmental vitiligo is more common in children than in adults.

Minor. Premature graying of the hair can occur in affected individuals and may be a finding in otherwise asymptomatic relatives.

The patches of vitiligo may be warmer and sweat more than surrounding skin. The physiologic basis for this is not known.

ASSOCIATED ABNORMALITIES

Other autoimmune disorders are believed to be associated with vitiligo, including alopecia areata, thyroid disease, diabetes mellitus, pernicious anemia, and Addison disease. These associated disorders are unusual in children with vitiligo.

Thyroid disease is most common in older women presenting with pigment loss. When patients with vitiligo are studied for thyroid abnormalities, approximately 50% have subclinical evidence of disease. Frank thyroid disease occurs in about 25%.

Retinal changes, including atrophy of the retinal pigment epithelium, can occur and is usually asymptomatic. Uveitis has been reported.

Vitiligo can develop in the setting of melamona. Thus, adult patients should be examined carefully for this tumor. This is not a recognized risk factor in children.

HISTOPATHOLOGY

Light. At the margins, melanocytes often appear large. Within the body of the lesion, there is absence of melanocytes.

EM. In patches from long-standing disease, no melanocytes are found. In early disease, junctional melanocytes with cellular abnormalities have been noted.

BASIC DEFECT

Unknown. The disorder is thought to be mediated on an autoimmune basis.

TREATMENT

Treatment is aimed at repigmentation if areas of involvement are small or depigmentation if

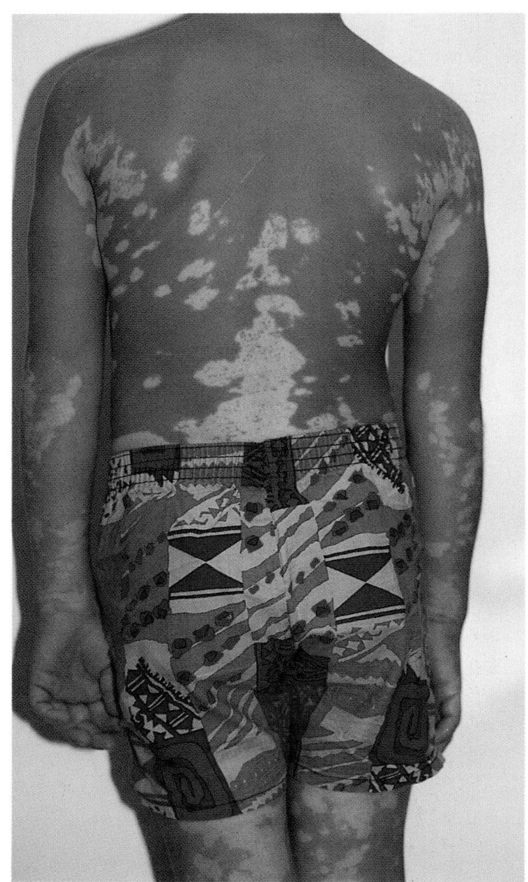

A

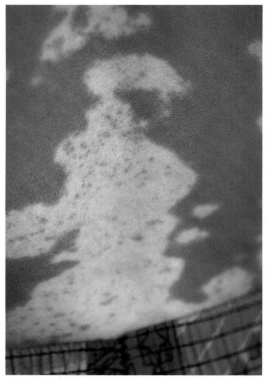

B

Figure 4.52. (A) Extensive disease. Contrast between affected and unaffected regions aggravated by tanning. **(B)** Spotty repigmentation from hair follicles.

a greater proportion of the body is affected. It is the contrast between normal and abnormal pigment that is unacceptable, not the absence of pigment itself. Vitiligo can spontaneously resolve, and in some instances no treatment is appropriate. Psoralen with ultraviolet light has been used with success in appropriate patients. Pinch grafting with melanocytes has been done. Results, in my opinion, are variable. Use of bleaches, such as the monobenzones, is usually reserved for those patients who have greater than 70% body surface area involved.

MODE OF INHERITANCE

Unknown. Approximately 30% of patients with vitiligo will have a positive family history, and about 20% will have an affected first degree relative. Accurate recurrence risk figures are not available.

PRENATAL DIAGNOSIS

None.

DIFFERENTIAL DIAGNOSIS

The white patches, or ash leaf spots, of tuberous sclerosis (MIM:191100) are hypopigmented, not depigmented, and do not fluoresce as brightly on Woods light examination. Typically, in tuberous sclerosis, ash leaf spots appear within the first few years. Lesions have smooth borders without surrounding hyperpigmentation and do not show the typical distribution of vitiligo. The distinction between tuberous sclerosis and vitiligo is usually straightforward.

In piebaldism (MIM:164920), Waardenburg syndrome (MIM:193500), and nevus depigmentosus, amelanotic patches are evident at birth. Congenital presentation with vitiligo is rare, but can occur, especially in the setting of a positive family history. In the absence of history, the clinical picture of piebaldism and vitiligo may be indistinguishable.

Scars may be amelanotic, and vitiligo can occur secondary to exposure to certain chemicals, including thiols, phenols, quinones, mercaptoamines, and catechols. History should quickly rule out exogenous causes. Vogt-Koyanagi-Harada syndrome is an acquired disorder of hyperacusis, poliosis, iritis, and vitiligo. It is also thought to be autoimmune in cause. I have never seen this in children. Any adult presenting with vitiligo should be appropriately examined for the associated features of Vogt-Koyanagi-Harada syndrome.

Premature graying of the hair (MIM:139100) may be an entity distinct from vitiligo. It can be seen both in individuals with vitiligo and in their relatives without cutaneous pigment loss.

Support Group: National Vitiligo
Foundation, Inc.
P.O. Box 6337
Tyler, TX 75711-6337
1-903-534-2925

SELECTED BIBLIOGRAPHY

Grimes, P.E., Kelly, A.P., Cline, D.J., Nordlund, J.J., Jareatt, M.T., Rogers, M., Treadwell, P.A., Burgdorf, W.H., and Kenney, J.A., Jr. (1986). Management of vitiligo in children. *Pediatr. Dermatol.* **3,** 498–510.

Nine pediatric dermatologists outlined their approach to the diagnosis and management of vitiligo in children. This is a very helpful compilation of opinions.

Majumder, P.P., Nordlund, J.J., and Nath, S.K. (1993). Pattern of familial aggregation of vitiligo. *Arch. Dermatol.* **129,** 995–998.

Sixty-five percent of 300 questionnaires sent to randomly selected members of the National Vitiligo Association were returned. None of the probands belonged to the same family. Limited analysis of 160 Caucasian families was performed. Thirty-one percent had a positive family history, and 20% had affected first degree relatives. The relative risk to siblings was approximately 11, to offspring 19–37. The usual caveat needs to be applied, that the findings are based on hearsay and not on direct examination.

Nordlund, J. J., Halder, R. M., and Grimes, P. (1993). Management of vitiligo. *Dermatol. Clin.* **11,** 27–33.

Concise review of approach, diagnostic evaluation, and treatment.

Tosti, A., Bardazzi, F., Tosti, G., and Monti, L. (1987). Audiologic abnormalities—cases of vitiligo. *J. Am. Acad. Dermatol.* **17,** 220–223.

This is a very intriguing study. Of 200 patients with vitiligo, the authors selected 50 individuals less than 40 years of age who had no known exposure to environmental agents known to affect hearing. None of the individuals complained of hearing problems. They compared this group with 40 controls. Sixteen percent of patients with vitiligo had hypoacusis compared with none of the controls. Six of eight patients with hearing loss also had fluorescein angiography performed. Four had loss of retinal pigment epithelium. This was similar to the proportion of patients with retinal abnormalities and vitiligo without hearing loss.

WAARDENBURG SYNDROME TYPES 1, 2, AND 3 (MIM:193500, 193510, 148820)

(Klein-Waardenburg Syndrome)

Includes Shah-Waardenburg Syndrome

DERMATOLOGIC FEATURES

The clinical characterization of the Waardenburg syndromes is rapidly being superseded by the delineation of molecular heterogeneity, both among and within the clinical categories. Traditionally, type 1 Waardenburg syndrome and type 2 share in common all features except dystopia canthorum. Type 3 refers to a heterogeneous group of individuals with a type 1 phenotype and skeletal abnormalities (Klein-Waardenburg). Shah-Waardenburg (type 4) syndrome refers to an autosomal recessive condition consisting of the pigment changes of Waardenburg syndrome, plus or minus deafness, no dystopia canthorum and long segment Hirschsprung disease or microcolon.

Major. While patchy areas of amelanosis are a cardinal sign of all types of Waardenburg syndrome, they are actually reported in only about 15% of patients. Within the unpigmented areas, brown macules are often found.

A white forelock may be present at birth or develop later. It is seen in about 30% of affected individuals with both types 1 and 2. When congenital, it is often lost with shedding of the newborn hairs and replaced by normally pigmented hairs. Patches of white hair may occur in other areas of the scalp as well.

Early graying (premature canities) in the late teens and early twenties is a feature in 10% of affected individuals with either type 1 or type 2. The graying can involve all body hair. Premature whitening of the hair without other aspects of Waardenburg syndrome has been reported (MIM:193800).

Minor. Synophrys is described in two-thirds of patients with type 1 and about one fourth with type 2.

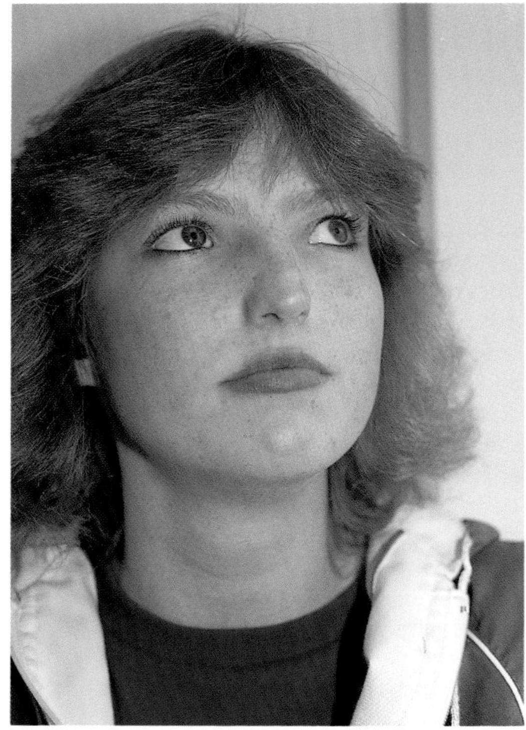

Figure 4.53. Heterochromia iridis, dystopia canthorum, and typical thin-pinched nose.

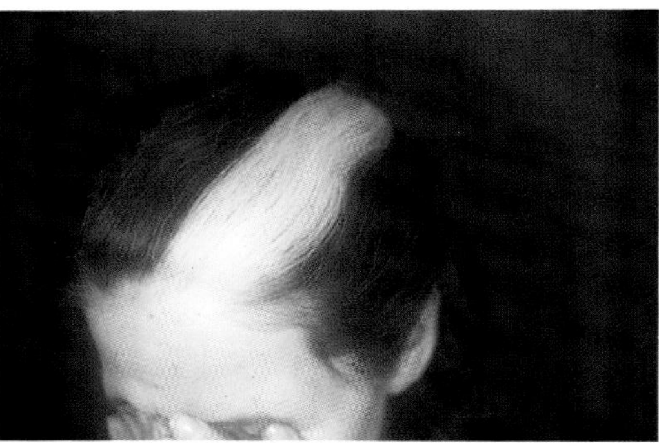

Figure 4.54. White forelock. (Courtesy of Division of Dermatology, University of Washington.)

ASSOCIATED ABNORMALITIES

The heterochromia iridis observed in Waardenburg syndrome is believed to result from abnormal migration of neural crest cells during embryogenesis. It is found in 30%–40% of affected persons with either type 1 or type 2. Different parts of the same iris may be multicolored, or the two irises may be different in color. Heterochromia iridis may not be evident at birth, as iris pigmentation is not complete until around age 2 years. Hypoplasia of the iris stroma is not uncommon, and the eyes are often blue when heterochromia iridis is not present. The fundi may also be hypopigmented.

Waardenburg syndrome has been subdivided primarily into two types. In the first, dystopia canthorum (displacement of the inner canthi without true hypertelorism, giving rise to short palpebral fissures) is a major feature. The tear ducts of the lower lid are medially displaced. Also seen are pinched, hypoplastic alae nasi, with the columella of the nose prominently visible. In type 2, the facies are either entirely normal, or, while features such as synophrys may be present, dystopia canthorum is always absent.

Deafness is a feature of type 1, type 2, and type 3 Waardenburg syndrome and has been reported in some individuals with piebaldism. It is believed to result from failure of normal migration of neural crest cells into the organ of Corti and the cochlea. Severity of the hearing loss can range from mild to profound. Deafness may be more frequent among type 2 patients, occurring in about 50% of type 2 and only 25% of type 1 patients. It is also a variable finding within families. Waardenburg syndrome accounts for 1%–2% of all individuals with deafness.

Hirschprung disease, aganglionosis of the colon, is reported in about 10% of persons with Waardenburg syndrome and has been reported in both type 1 and type 2. Again, failure of normal migration of neural crest cells, in this instance to the gut, is believed to be the cause.

Cleft lip with or without cleft palate has been reported in 1% of patients with the Waardenburg syndrome.

Myelomeningocele may occur more often than expected by chance alone, but absolute risk is small.

The eponym *Klein-Waardenburg* (MIM: 148820) has sometimes mistakenly been used interchangeably with the term *Waardenburg syndrome*. In 1947, Klein reported a girl with the features of Waardenburg syndrome and arthrogryposis of the upper extremities with absence of muscle, axillary pterygia, and camptodactyly of the fingers. She had hypoplasia of the first and second ribs and fusions of the carpal bones. Subsequently, several other similarly affected patients were described. As limb defects are extremely rare in Waardenburg syndrome, it has been suggested that Klein-Waardenburg syndrome is a separate genetic disorder; it is sometimes referred to as Klein-Waardenburg type 3. Klein (1983) more recently reported a family in which the father had classic Klein-Waardenburg type 3 and his son had Waardenburg type 1 with skeletal changes limited to a Sprengel's deformity, supporting the converse hypothesis that types 1 and 3 represent variable expression of the same allele rather than genetic heterogeneity. Association of Klein-Waardenburg with chromosomal deletions in the *PAX3* region suggests that it might be a contiguous gene syndrome, i.e., Waardenburg + plus.

HISTOPATHOLOGY

LIGHT. In the unpigmented areas of the skin there is absence of melanocytes.

EM. In the normally pigmented skin of affected individuals, both normal melanocytes and melanocytes with abnormal unmelanized melanosomes and short dendrites are found. No melanocytes are present in the unpigmented skin.

BASIC DEFECT

The basic defects in Waardenburg syndromes are believed to reside in the control of migration and differentiation of neural crest cells, including melanocytes, ganglion cells of the colon, and hair cells in the organ of Corti in the ear.

TREATMENT

Protection from exposure to ultraviolet light and avoidance of sunburning is important. Surgical correction of the aganglionic segment of bowel may be necessary. Establishing the diagnosis of Waardenburg syndrome should lead to early detection of hearing loss and appropriate intervention.

MODE OF INHERITANCE

Autosomal dominant with reduced penetrance. Preus et al. (1983) estimated penetrance of type 1 at 85%, using clinical findings of dystopia canthorum, hearing loss, white forelock, and premature graying of the hair with or without circumscribed depigmentation of the skin. Penetrance was 83% if dystopia canthorum alone was used. Thus the other features did not add significantly to the ability to detect gene carriers. As evidenced by clinical distinction into type 1 and type 2 and linkage and molecular data, genetic heterogeneity exists. Not all families with Waardenburg type 1 show linkage to *PAX3*, provisional location of which is at 2q25–37. No family with pure Waardenburg type 2 has shown linkage to *PAX3*, but in many families demonstrating linkage to *PAX3* not all affected members have had dystopia canthorum. Linkage to the microphthalmia gene (*MITF*) on 3p12 has been shown based on two families, and mutations in *MITF* have been identified in some type 2 families. From a counseling vantage, the distinction between types 1 and 2 is an unimportant issue, as the natural history of type 1 and type 2 are the same. For purposes of prenatal diagnosis, this distinction is vital. One family with type 3 had a mutation in *PAX3* also.

PRENATAL DIAGNOSIS

Possible by chorionic villi sampling and mutation analysis or linkage if molecular defect in a family is identified. Fetal skin biopsy is likely to be unreliable as distribution of melanocytes is patchy.

DIFFERENTIAL DIAGNOSIS

Piebaldism (MIM:172800): I am not convinced that one can always clearly distinguish clinically between Waardenburg type 2 and piebaldism. Both are autosomal dominant conditions. Many reports of piebaldism mention deafness in affected individuals. Some describe heterochromia iridis, and some mention Hirschsprung disease. These cases may represent misdiagnosis of true Waardenburg syndrome, allelic variation, or the same mutation with variable expression. Assignment of isolated piebaldism to the *c-KIT* protooncogene on 4q24 suggests that there is a distinct mutation responsible for pigment change alone. However, I am not comfortable assuring a patient with piebaldism that his or her offspring are not at risk for hearing loss or for Hirschsprung disease unless there is a clear-cut family history of only pigment abnormalities in several generations.

Nevus depigmentosus: The distribution of unpigmented areas in nevus depigmentosus may be quite localized; when generalized it tends to occur along the lines of Blaschko. In piebaldism and the Waardenburg syndromes, the pigmentary abnormalities are much more patchy.

Vitiligo (MIM:193200): This is not usually congenital but acquired. In early stages, a skin biopsy of a depigmented area demonstrating presence of melanocytes and an inflammatory infiltrate can distinguish between vitiligo and the Waardenburg syndrome, in which there is an absence of melanocytes. In late vitiligo, the histopathology is indistinguishable. Vitiligo represents true depigmentation, i.e., loss of pigment production that was previously normal.

Isolated white forelock: Isolated white forelock is inherited as an isolated autosomal dominant trait. It can be an isolated finding in some individuals from families with piebaldism. It may or may not be a genetically distinct entity. A white forelock has also been reported in a sibship with a combination of other malformations (MIM:277740), including terminal transverse limb defects, congenital heart disease, and ocular hypertelorism.

Shah-Waardenburg syndrome (Waardenburg type 4, MIM:277580): There are reports of siblings, born to healthy parents, affected with white forelock, eyebrows, and eyelashes, isochromia iridis, and microcolon. Hearing loss has been noted in some affected individuals. In some of the families with consanguinity, both parents or both branches of the family had heterochromia iridis or pigment change. Homozygosity for mutations in the endothelin-3 gene (*EDN3*) or the endothelin-receptor B gene (*EDNRB*), which map to 20q13.2-q13.3 and 13q22 respectively, has been found. Heterozygous carriers of *EDN3* may show premature graying of the hair.

Miscellaneous: Patchy pigmentary abnormalities that result from abnormal migration of neural crest cells are described in innumerable case reports of unique, possibly private, syndromes. Individuals with such skin findings should be carefully evaluated for hearing deficits. Intensive search for chromosomal mosaicism in both blood and skin is warranted (see hypomelanosis of Ito) in those patients with multiple congenital anomalies.

Support Group: National Organization for Albinism and Hypopigmentation (N.O.A.H.)
1530 Locust Street
Box 29
Philadelphia PA 19102
1-215-545-2322

National Information Center on Deafness
Gallaudet University
800 Florida Avenue NE
Washington, DC 20002
1-202-651-5051

Hereditary Hearing Impairment Resource Registry
Boys Town National Research Hospital
555 North 30th
Omaha, NE 68131
1-402-498-6375

SELECTED BIBLIOGRAPHY

Arias, S. (1971). Genetic heterogeneity in the Waardenburg syndrome. *Birth Defects* **7,** 87–101.

Distinguishes between Waardenburg syndrome type 1 and Waardenburg syndrome type 2. Mentions occurrence of "black" forelock as a possible feature of Waardenburg syndrome. Arias also describes a different type 3 Waardenburg syndrome (not Klein-Waardenburg) characterized by unilateral ptosis, heterochromia iridis, and deafness in one family. It is not convincing to me that this is truly a distinct disorder.

Baldwin, C.T., Hoth, C.F., Macine, R.A., and Milunsky, A. (1995). Mutations in *PAX3* that cause Waardenburg syndrome type I: ten new mutations and review of the literature. *Am. J. Med. Genet.* **58,** 115–122.

The authors describe mutations in *PAX3* and review previous data. Two families, reported by others and reviewed here, with mutations in *PAX3* resulted in a phenotype of Klein-Waardenburg (Waardenburg type III).

Brown, K.S., Bergsma, D.R., and Barrow, M.V. (1971). Animal models of pigment and hearing abnormalities in man. *Birth Defects* **7,** 102–109.

A detailed discussion of the "blue-eyed, white cat," which may be a model for Waardenburg syndrome.

Farrer, L.A., Grundfast, K.M., Amos, J., Arnos, K.S., Fisher, J.H. Jr., Beighton, P., Diehl, S.R., Fex, J., Foy, C., Friedman, J.B., Greenberg, J., Holt, C., Marazita, M., Milunsky, A., Morell, R., Nance, W., Newton, V., Ramesar, R., San Augustin, T.B., Skare, J., Stevens, C.A., Wagner, R.G. Jr., Wilcox, E.R., Winship, I., and Read, A.P. (1992). Waardenburg syndrome (WS) type I is caused by defects at multiple loci, one of which is near *ALPP* on chromosome 2: first report of the WS consortium. *Am. J. Hum. Genet.* **50,** 902–913.

A formula for determining normal or abnormal placement of the inner canthi (W score) has been determined by the Waardenburg Consortium to try to assign families (patients) definitively to Waardenburg type I or Waardenburg type II. Linkage to 2q demonstrated in 45% of families. Diagnostic criteria used for Waardenburg type I are listed.

Foy, C., Newton, V., Wellesley, D., Harris, R., and Read, A.P. (1990). Assignment of the locus for Waardenburg syndrome type I to human chromosome 2q37 and possible homology to the splotch mouse. *Am. J. Hum. Genet.* **46,** 1017–1023.

Possible linkage to the placental alkaline phosphatase locus with a lod score of 4.76 and recombination fraction of 0.023 in five families is demonstrated.

Hageman, M.J., and Delleman, J.W. (1977). Heterogeneity in Waardenburg syndrome. *Am. J. Hum. Genet.* **29,** 468–485.

A Herculean literature review of 1,285 patients, from which they culled 276 with type 1, 159 with type 2, in addition to 34 of their own, with emphasis on the occurrence of deafness. They state risk for deafness is 25% in type 1, 50% in type 2. Two hundred eighteen references.

Klein, D. (1947) Albinisme partiel (leucisme) accompagné de surdimutité, d'ostéomyodysplasie, de raideurs articulaires congénitales multiples et d'autres malformations congénitales. *Arch. Klaus. Stift. Vererb. Forsch.* **22,** 336–342.

Klein, D. (1950) Albinisme partiel (leucisme) avec surdi-mutité, blepharophimosis et dysplasie myo-ostéo-articulare. *Helv. Paediatr. Acta.* **5,** 38–58.

Initial and subsequently detailed reports of a very abnormal appearing child with piebaldism-like pigment, pterygia of axillae, arthrogryposis, blepharophimosis, skeletal abnormalities, deafness and abnormal facies. Were she to be seen now, karyotyping for a contiguous gene deletion involving the *PAX-3* locus would be indicated!

Klein, D. (1983). Historical background and evidence for autosomal dominant inheritance of the Klein-Waardenburg syndrome (type III). *Am. J. Med. Genet.* **14,** 231–239.

The subtext of this reevaluation of Klein-Waardenburg type III deals with the history of appropriate or inappropriate attribution of the "first" description of Waardenburg syndrome. It is an interesting example of the problems posed by eponyms, especially when egos are involved.

Ortonne, J.-P. (1988). Piebaldism, Waardenburg's syndrome and related disorders: "Neural crest depigmentation syndromes"? *Dermatol. Clin.* **6,** 205–215.

Reviews mechanisms for lack of pigment production in the animal models for Waardenburg syndrome and discusses the differential diagnosis of Waardenburg syndrome.

Pasteris, N.G., Trask, B.J., Sheldon, S., and Gorski, J.L. (1993). Discordant phenotype of two overlapping deletions involving the *PAX3* gene on chromosome 2q35. *Hum. Mol. Genet.* **2,** 953–959.

A patient with Waardenburg syndrome, microcephaly, mental retardation, and skeletal abnormalities had a deletion of chromosome 2 at q35–q36, suggesting that Klein-Waardenburg may be a contiguous gene syndrome. The authors discuss overlap of the phenotypes of Waardenburg syndromes 1, 2, and 3, all of which have been associated with molecular changes in *PAX3* in some individuals.

Preus, M., Linstrom, C., Polomeno, R.C., and Milot, J. (1983). Waardenburg syndrome—penetrance of major signs. *Am. J. Med. Genet.* **15,** 383–388.

Using data from the literature from 18 families with 150 affected individuals, a penetrance of 85% was calculated. This type of study must always be interpreted with caution, as it depends on the accuracy of the examination and reporting of diagnostic features by the original authors of the tabulated reports.

Shah, K.N., Dalal, S.J., Desai, M.P., Sheth, P.N., Joshi, N.C., and Ambani, L.M. (1981). White forelock, pigmentary disorder of irides, and long segment Hirschsprung disease: possible variant of Waardenburg syndrome. *J. Pediatr.* **99,** 432–435.

Evidence from five families for autosomal recessive inheritance of this constellation of features. Several pedigrees are suggestive of piebaldism in parents with affected children demonstrating homozygosity for the piebald gene.

Tassabehji, M., Newton, V.E., Liu, X.-Z., Brady, A., Donnai, D., Krajewska-Walasek, M., Murday, V., Norman, A., Obersztyn, E., Reardon, W., Rice, J.C., Trembath, R., Wieacker, P., Whiteford, M., Winter, R., Read, A.P. (1995). The mutational spectrum in Waardenburg syndrome. *Hum. Molec. Genet.* **4,** 2131–2137.

The authors screened 134 families with Waardenburg syndrome or possible neurocristopathies. Twenty of 25 families with type 1 Waardenburg were found to have mutations in *PAX3,* as was one of three families with type 3. Seven families had mutations in *MITF;* five of these families appeared to have type 2 Waardenburg. In 18 families with type 2, no mutations in either gene were found. Discussion of genetic and clinical heterogeneity is helpful.

Waardenburg, P.J. (1951). A new syndrome combining developmental anomalies of the eyelids, eyebrows and nose root with pigmentary defects of the iris and head hair and with congenital deafness. *Am. J. Hum. Genet.* **3,** 195–253.

Detailed and exhaustive review of the literature up to that time and presentation of clinical features and genetics of the disorder based on both the literature and the author's experience.

CHAPTER 5

DISORDERS OF THE DERMIS

COLLAGEN

AINHUM (MIM:103400)

DERMATOLOGIC FEATURES

Major. There is confusion in the literature because the term *ainhum,* which is from a Brazilian-African dialect and means "to saw" or "file," is used for acquired deep grooves of the digits, constricting amniotic bands, and transverse terminal defects of the digits with deep residual grooves.

Ainhum proper refers to a deep groove that occurs primarily on the fifth toes, most commonly in adult Africans from both West Africa and South Africa. Putative causes include a congenital vascular malformation with secondary circulatory compromise, trauma, and infection.

The term *pseudo-ainhum* has been coined to apply to all other instances of constricting bands. The deep groove usually occurs over the first interphalangeal joint, most commonly of the fifth toe. All toes can be involved.

Minor. None.

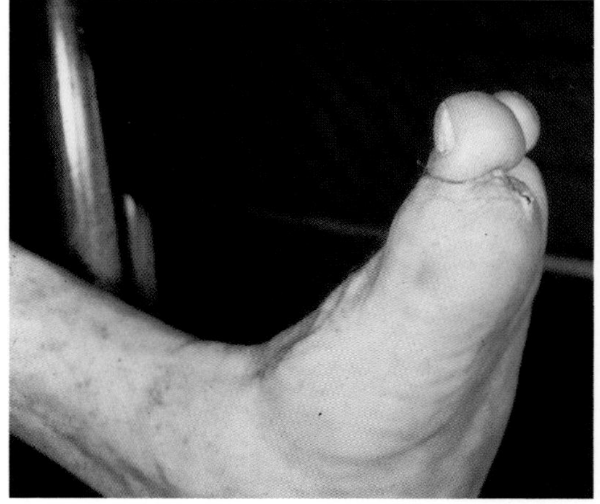

Figure 5.1. Ainhum of great toe with distal swelling. (Courtesy of Division of Dermatology, University of Washington.)

ASSOCIATED ABNORMALITIES

None.

HISTOPATHOLOGY

Light. Features are unclear for the genetic forms. There is hyperparakeratosis with acanthosis and mild inflammation in the dermis along with fibrosis in the acquired form of the disorder. In late stages, fatty degeneration with loss of connective tissue is seen.

EM. No information.

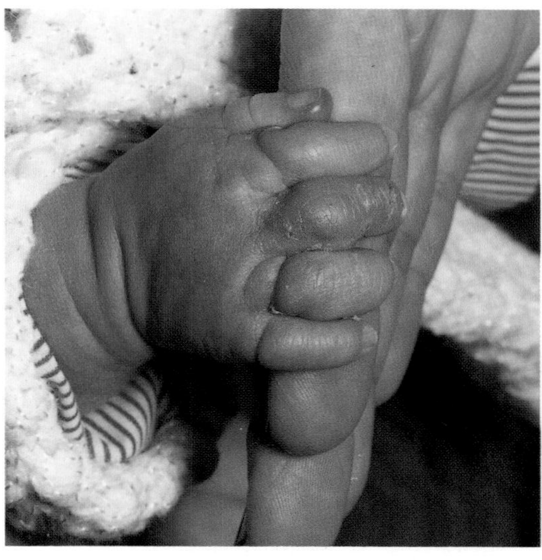

Figure 5.2. Pseudoainhum due to amniotic bands.

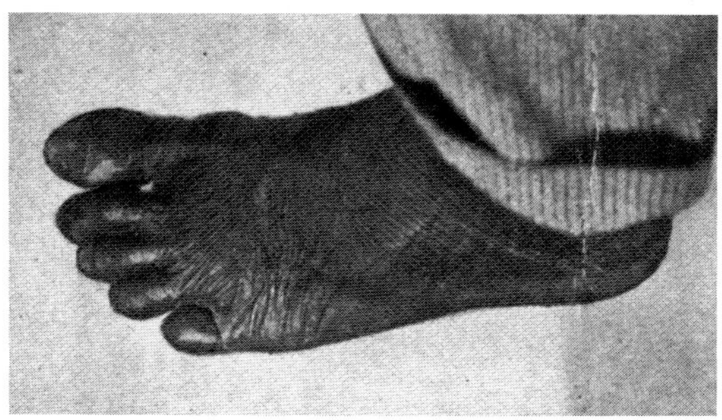

Figure 5.3. Constriction band around small toe in 46-year-old male. His son was also affected. (From Weinstein, 1913.)

BASIC DEFECT

Unknown.

TREATMENT

One report of classic acquired ainhum was successfully treated with intralesional steroids. Surgical amputation or autoamputation is curative, without proximal recurrence.

MODE OF INHERITANCE

Uncertain. There are very few details about family history given in the literature.

PRENATAL DIAGNOSIS

None.

DIFFERENTIAL DIAGNOSIS

In the mutilating keratodermas (MIM:Many), constriction bands of the digits can occur. These are usually the result of markedly thickened epidermis, although in Vohwinkel syndrome (MIM:124500), they appear to develop independently of the hyperkeratosis. Acquired infections such as syphilis, leprosy, and yaws can also result in constriction bands and amputation. Trauma and scleroderma can also be implicated.

Constriction bands have been described in patients with sensory and autonomic neuropathy (MIM:223900), presumably secondary to repeated trauma.

Support Group: N.O.R.D.
P.O. Box 8923
New Fairfield, CT
06812
1-800-999-6673

SELECTED BIBLIOGRAPHY

Da Silva Lima, J.F. (1880). On ainhum. *Arch. Dermatol. (N.Y.).* **6,** 367–376.

A delightful discourse on the etymology, pronunciation, and spelling: *agnoumin* in French, *añum* in Spanish, and *aynyoon* in English. The author makes no mention of familial occurrence, but stated that the disorder has predilection for Brazilian negroes of West African origin.

Dent, D.M., Fataar, S., and Rose, A.G. (1981). Ainhum and angiodysplasia. *Lancet.* **ii,** 396–397.

Four adult patients with classic disease; two of these had affected aunts. All showed absence of the plantar branch of the posterior tibial artery. The authors posit that remaining circulation from the dorsalis pedis put these individuals at increased risk for vascular compromise, but they could not determine if the abnormality was congenital or acquired, causal or only coincidentally associated.

Raque, C.J., Stein, K.M., Lane, J.M., and Ruse, E.C., Jr. (1972). Pseudoainhum constricting bands of the extremities. *Arch. Dermatol.* **105,** 434–438.

Nice table outlining causes of constricting bands.

Tunstall, M. (1974). An investigation into the prevalence and geographical distribution of ainhum in the Tsolo district of the Transkei. *S. Afr. Med. J.* **48,** 2409–2411.

In the Transkei, where prevalence of ainhum is high (1%–2%), one-third of 127 patients had affected first degree relatives. Interpretation of the data is complicated by discrepancies between terms used to describe genetic relationships and social relationships. For example, the word *brother* can refer to a biologic brother, a brother-in-law, or a cousin. The author offered multifactorial inheritance as the best fit.

Weinstein, H. (1913). A description of ainhum as seen on the Canal Zone, with report of interesting cases occurring in one family. *South. Med. J.* **6,** 651–656.

The pedigree presented had two affected brothers, each of whom had an affected son.

AMNIOTIC BANDS (MIM:217100)

(Streeter's Bands; Congenital Constriction Bands Syndrome; Early Amnion Rupture Sequence)

DERMATOLOGIC FEATURES

Major. Tight constriction bands or indentations in the soft tissue, often accompanied by distal amputation, are seen in the limbs. There may be syndactyly, bony fusion, or bone loss. Marked swelling distal to the constriction bands can occur. Occasionally fibrous bands or adhesions are found within the constrictions. The hands and feet are more commonly involved than the body and face. Involvement may be asymmetric. When body wall defects accompany these findings, the condition is referred to as *limb–body-wall* defects. The affected limb is usually ipsilateral to the abdominal-thoracic involvement.

A

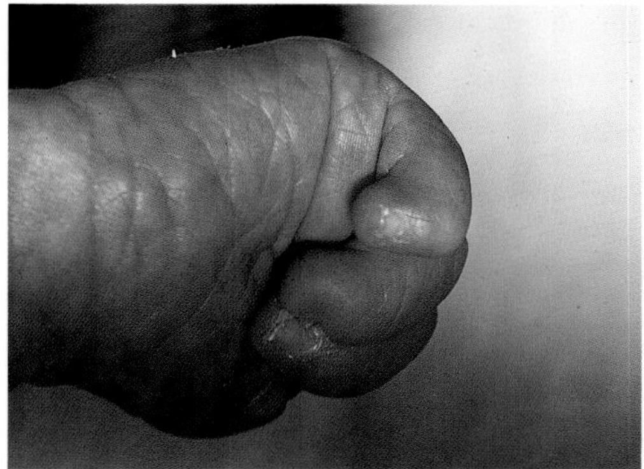

B

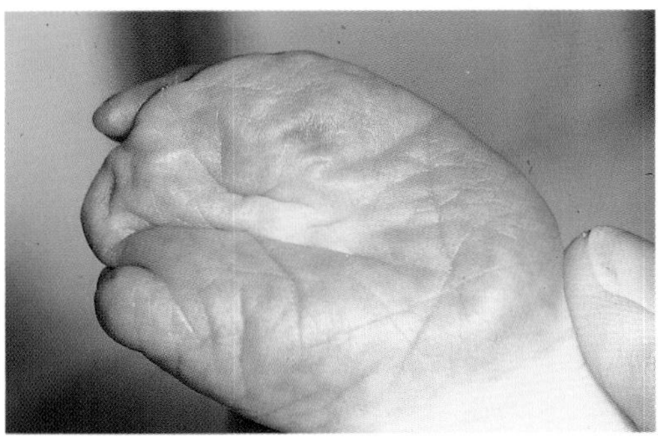

Figure 5.4. **(A)** Hand with fusion; partial loss of distal phalanx and nail on fourth finger. **(B)** More marked deformation.

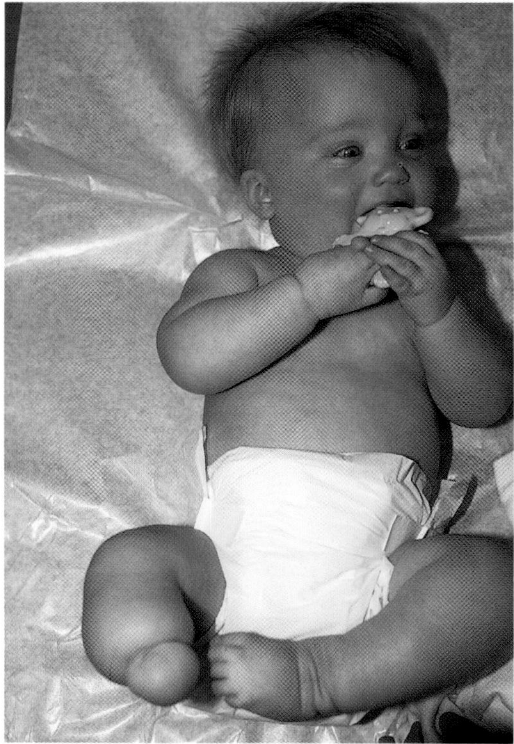

Figure 5.5. Left leg with circumferential band and distal ball of tissue.

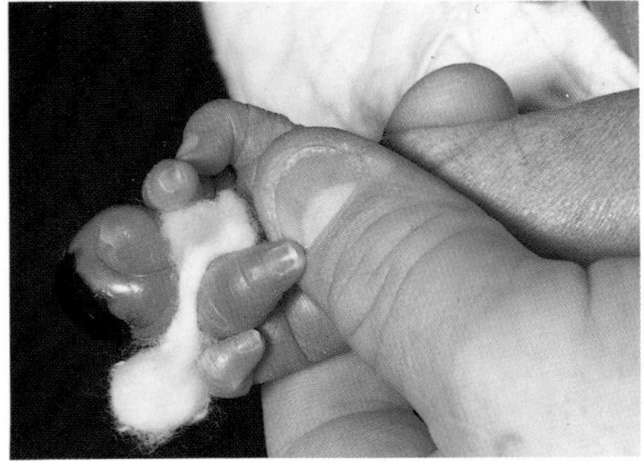
A

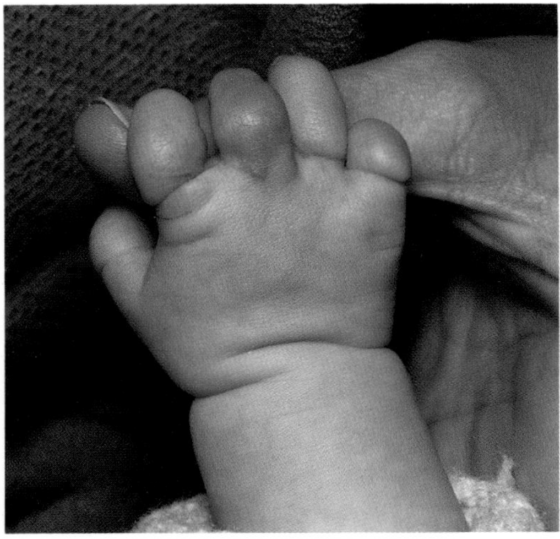
B

Figure 5.6. **(A)** Swollen third finger with necrosis. **(B)** After lysis of band. Circumferential depression and scar.

Deep grooves above the ankle are almost invariably present.

These defects are rare, occurring in 1 in 5,000 to 1 in 10,000 liveborns, and have generated more than their fair share of attention in the literature.

MINOR. A variety of skin and scalp defects have also been described.

ASSOCIATED ABNORMALITIES

Approximately one-third of the cases have clubfoot deformities.

Bizarre facial clefting in a nonanatomic (that is, not along the planes of closure) distribution has been reported. Occasionally residual tissue strands can be seen within these clefts.

Structural eye abnormalities and encephaloceles can also be associated.

HISTOPATHOLOGY

LIGHT. Various descriptions include amorphous tissue, normal skin, fibrous tissue, degenerating amnion, and fibrous amnion.

EM. No information.

BASIC DEFECT

Unknown. Experimental rupture of the amnion in mice and rats produces a similar phenotype. There are many hypotheses regarding causation, but none has been proven.

TREATMENT

Surgical correction when possible.

MODE OF INHERITANCE

Sporadic. There are a handful of familial recurrences, almost all of which describe only involvement of the distal digits.

PRENATAL DIAGNOSIS

Amniotic bands extending from the amnion can be detected by ultrasound. If there is no attachment of the fetus to the band and normal fetal movement, as well as absence of visible fetal malformations, the risk of abnormal outcome of pregnancy is extremely low.

DIFFERENTIAL DIAGNOSIS

Ainhum (MIM:103400) is an acquired, not a congenital, condition, usually involving the little toes in which constriction bands develop. Some cases of aplasia cutis congenita of the body wall with limb defects (MIM: 107600) may be indistinguishable from amniotic band syndrome. It may not be possible to offer specific recurrence risks. In Adams-Oliver syndrome (MIM:100300)—terminal transverse limb defects with aplasia cutis congenita of the scalp—there can be constriction bands and distal swelling of the involved extremities. One should examine the scalp very carefully in all putative cases of amniotic band syndrome. Familial transverse terminal limb defects without aplasia cutis congenita have also been reported.

The Michelin tire baby syndrome (MIM: 156610) is characterized by symmetric, circumferential deep grooves on the extremities and puffiness of the intervening soft tissue. These gradually resolve, and there are no associated limb defects or amputations.

Support Group: N.O.R.D.
P.O. Box 8923
New Fairfield, CT 06812
1-800-999-6673

SELECTED BIBLIOGRAPHY

Baker, C.J., and Rudolph, A.J. (1971). Congenital ring constrictions and intrauterine amputation. *Am. J. Dis. Child.* **121,** 393–400.

Clearly written exegis of Streeter's (1930) proposal of endogenous causes versus Torpin's work (1965) imputing the syndrome to the mechanical effects of amniotic bands.

Burton, D.J., and Filly, R.A. (1991). Sonographic diagnosis of the amniotic band syndrome. *A.J.R.–Am. J. Roentgenol.* **156,** 555–558.

Reviews ultrasound findings. Points out that amniotic sheets are not predictive of fetal abnormality and that the diagnosis of amniotic band syndrome requires ultrasound evidence of fetal deformity.

Etches, P.C., Stewart, A.R., and Ives, E.J. (1982). Familial congenital amputations. *J. Pediatr.* **101,** 448–449.

Describes familial occurrence of unilateral loss of digits 2 and 3 with constriction bands. Mother, son, maternal great-aunt on the grandmaternal side, and a paternal cousin on the grandpaternal side were all affected. There is no mention of examination of the scalp to rule out Adams-Oliver syndrome.

Streeter, G.L., (1930). Focal deficiencies in fetal tissues and their relation to intrauterine amputation. *Contrib. Embryol. Carneg. Inst.* **22,** 1–44.

Streeter states, "In conclusion, it may be stated that no evidence has been found that intrauterine amputation is due to amniotic bands or adhesions or other mechanical constriction. Amniotic bands do exist and are sometimes associated with malformations, but where this occurs, the two participate in the same disturbance and the latter are not mechanically produced by the former."

Torpin, R. (1965). Amniochorionic mesoblastic fibrous strings and amniotic bands. *Am. J. Obstet. Gynecol.* **91,** 65–79.

Torpin was studying placentas, filling placental sacs with water. He discovered one in which the amnion had ruptured. He postulated the effects on the fetus. He drove to the home of an infant whose placenta he had examined and discovered that the baby had, indeed, the predicted limb defects. He went on to repeat this experiment with a second placenta and subsequently followed up 11 infants. Seven had placental defects with limb defects, constricting bands, and clubfeet. Four had intact membranes and no constricting bands or clubfeet.

Van Allen, M.I., Siegel-Bartelt, J., Dixon, J., Zuker, R.M., Clarke, H.M., and Toi, A. (1992). Constriction bands and limb reduction defects in two newborns with fetal ultrasound evidence for vascular disruption. *Am. J. Med. Genet.* **44,** 598–604.

One infant with a dead co-twin, a second with hepatic vein emboli, both with limb defects and constriction bands. One had a cleft palate and cleft lip in addition. There was no evidence of amniotic bands. The authors argue for vascular compromise as a possible cause of the amniotic band sequence in some. Irrespective of causal hypothesis, recurrence risk appears to be very low.

Winter, R.M., and Donnai, D. (1989). A possible human homologue for the mouse mutant disorganisation. *J. Med. Genet.* **26,** 417–420.

Suggests that some cases of amniotic band syndrome might represent genetic alterations in a gene homologous to the disorganisation (*Ds*) locus in the mouse. This is a semidominant gene that causes multiple malformations similar to those reported in some infants with amniotic band syndrome.

BUSCHKE-OLLENDORFF SYNDROME (MIM:166700)

(Dermatofibrosis Lenticularis Disseminata; Dermatoosteopoikilosis)

DERMATOLOGIC FEATURES

Major. Asymptomatic small yellow papules develop during early childhood and can appear anywhere on the skin. Sites of predilection are the thighs, buttocks, and abdomen. Congenital lesions have been reported. Lesions can coalesce to form linear raised plaques. Lesions can be asymmetric or grouped and symmetric.
Minor. Scaling, dryness of the skin, and keratosis pilaris similar to ichthyosis vulgaris has been mentioned in several case reports.

ASSOCIATED ABNORMALITIES

Osteopoikilosis: This refers to asymptomatic radiographic densities seen within the carpal, tarsal, and phalangeal bones. They may also develop in the long bones and in the pelvis.

HISTOPATHOLOGY

Light. Thickened interlacing elastin fibers are seen within the dermis. These appear to "entrap" collagen bundles in lesional skin.
EM. There is an increase in elastin with variable changes in collagen and in the microfibrillar component of elastin. The broad elastic fibers are found near fibroblast-like cells that are marked by a dilated rough endoplasmic reticulum.

BASIC DEFECT

Unknown.

TREATMENT

None.

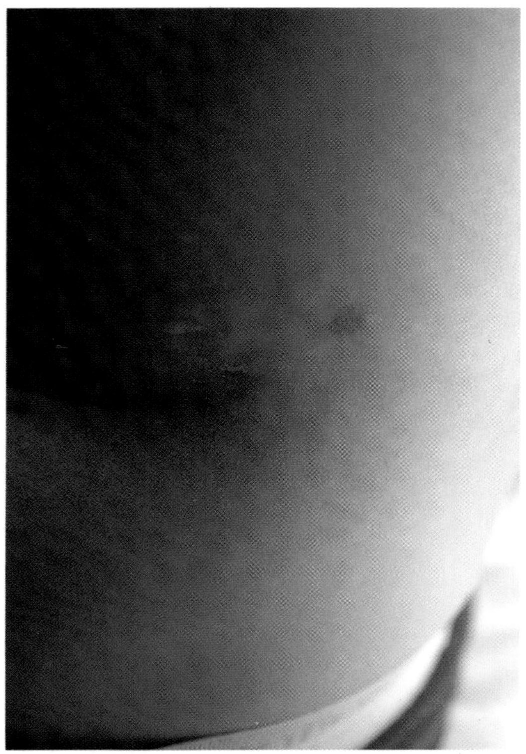

A

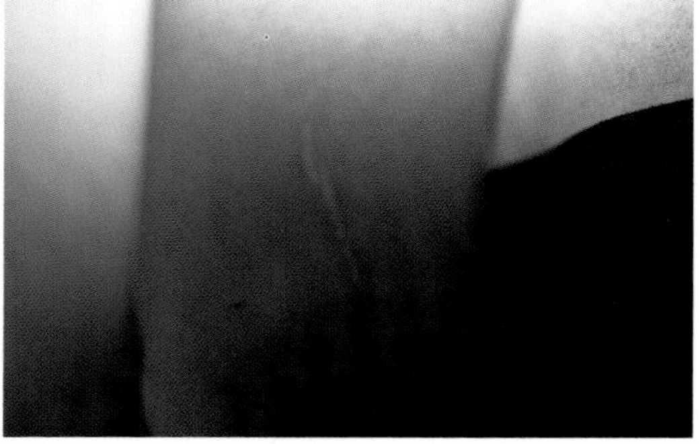

B

Figure 5.7. **(A)** Subtle flesh-colored thickening of the skin. The biopsy site is still inflamed. **(B)** Thickening in area of trauma. (Courtesy of Drs. L. Hudgins and R. Pagon, Seattle, Washington.)

MODE OF INHERITANCE

Autosomal dominant. Affected individuals within a family may show skin changes or bone changes or both.

PRENATAL DIAGNOSIS

None.

DIFFERENTIAL DIAGNOSIS

The connective tissue nevi or shagreen patches of tuberous sclerosis (MIM:191100) may be clinically similar. These show an increase in collagen and a decrease in elastin on histopathology. Other connective tissue nevi can also appear clinically similar. Hypertrophic varicella scars may also give a similar clinical appearance. These should be distinguishable by histopathology.

Support Group: N.O.R.D.
P.O. Box 8923
New Fairfield, CT
06812
1-800-999-6673

SELECTED BIBLIOGRAPHY

DeCroix, J., Frankhart, M., Pollet, J.-Cl., and Bourlond, A. (1988). Syndrome de Buschke-Ollendorff. Six observations dans une famille. *Ann. Dermatol. Venereol.* **115,** 455–458.
Variability of expression nicely demonstrated.

Giro, M.G., Duvic, M., Smith, L.T., Kennedy, R., Rapini, R., Arnett, F.C., and Davidson, J.M. (1992). Buschke-Ollendorff syndrome associated with elevated elastin production by affected skin fibroblasts in culture. *J. Invest. Dermatol.* **99,** 129–137.
Authors found a two- to eightfold increase in tropoelastin production.

Verbov, J, and Graham, R. (1986). Buschke-Ollendorff syndrome—disseminated dermatofibrosis with osteopoikilosis. *Clin. Exp. Dermatol.* **11,** 17–26.
A review article with 32 references.

DERMATOSPARAXIS (MIM:None)

(Ehlers-Danlos Syndrome Type VIIC)

DERMATOLOGIC FEATURES

Major. The skin is soft, doughy, and avulses with minimal trauma. Inguinal tears at birth have been described. The skin may sag and appear puffy around the eyes. These sites heal normally, with normal scars.
Minor. Easy bruising.

ASSOCIATED ABNORMALITIES

Premature rupture of the membranes with premature birth occurred in the three infants reported with this syndrome. Micrognathia, joint laxity and umbilical hernias are also features.

HISTOPATHOLOGY

Light. No specific changes.
EM. There are ribbon-like collagen fibrils with a "hieroglyphic-like" appearance to the fibrils on cross section.

BASIC DEFECT

There is a defect in the activity of type I procollagen N-proteinase.

TREATMENT

None.

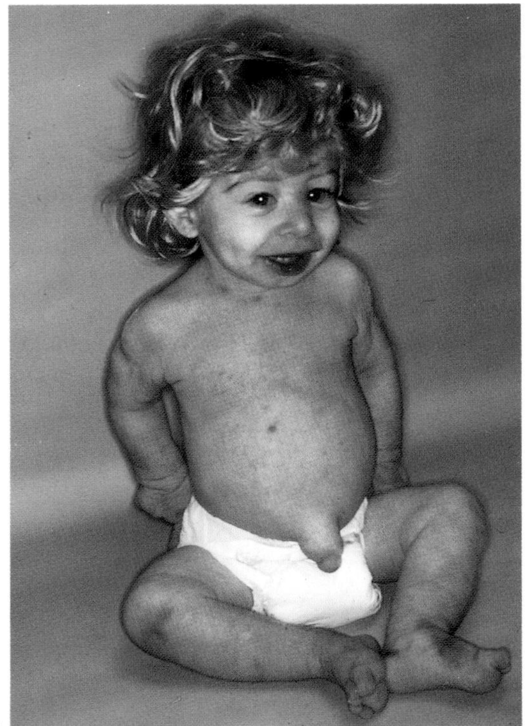

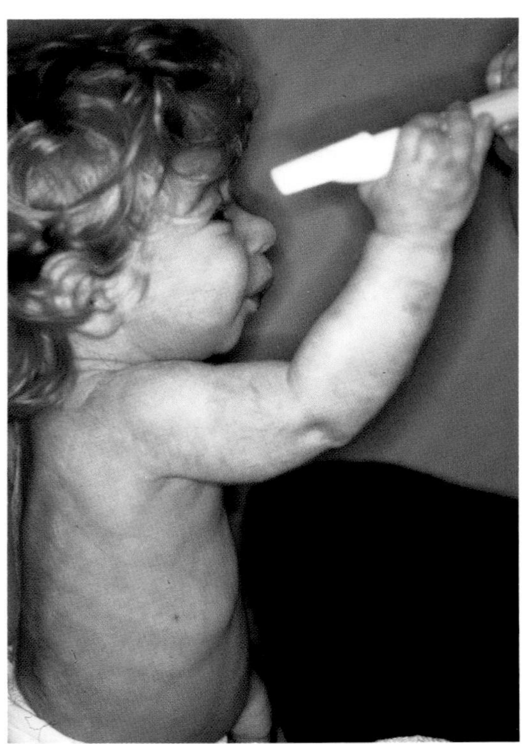

Figure 5.8. **(A)** Blue sclera, umbilical hernia, bruises on ankles and knees, and wrinkly skin (From Petty et al., 1993.) **(B)** Micrognathia and facial hirsutism (Courtesy of Dr. E. M. Petty, Ann Arbor, Michigan, and Dr. P. H. Byers, Seattle, Washington, and the family.)

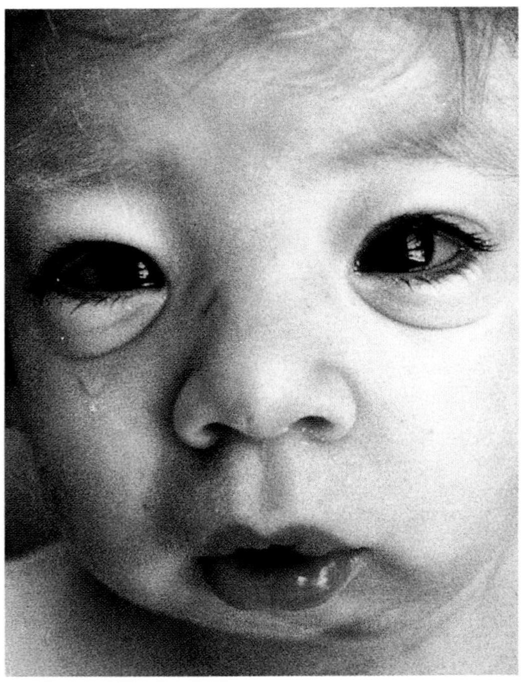

Figure 5.9. Strikingly similar facial appearance in a different child. (Courtesy of Dr. W. Wertelecki, Mobile, Alabama, and the family.)

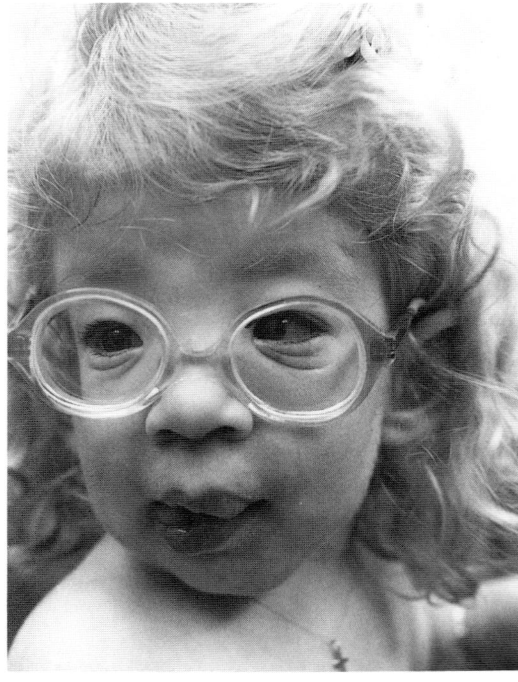

Figure 5.10. Same child as in Fig. 5.9. showing progressive changes. (Courtesy of Dr. W. Wertelecki, Mobile, Alabama, and the family.)

MODE OF INHERITANCE

Autosomal recessive.

PRENATAL DIAGNOSIS

Yet to be attempted.

DIFFERENTIAL DIAGNOSIS

The clinical features are striking, and biochemical studies are diagnostic. Cutis laxa (MIM: Many) might be confused with this early on.

Support Group: Ehlers-Danlos National Foundation
P.O. Box 1212
Southgate, MI 48195
1-800-990-3363

SELECTED BIBLIOGRAPHY

Wertelecki, W., Smith, L.T., and Byers, P. (1992). Initial observations of human dermatosparaxis: Ehlers-Danlos syndrome type VIIC. *J. Pediatr.* **121,** 558–564.

Smith, L.T., Wertelecki, W., Milstone, L.M., Petty, E.M., Seashore, M.R., Braverman, I.M., Jenkins, T.G., and Byers, P.H. (1992). Human dermatosparaxis: a form of Ehlers-Danlos syndrome that results from failure to remove the amino-terminal propeptide of type I procollagen. *Am. J. Hum. Genet.* **51,** 235–244.

Clinical description of a single patient (Wertelecki et al., 1992) followed by biochemical and ultrastructural evaluation of both her and a second patient (Smith, et al., 1992).

EHLERS-DANLOS TYPES I, II, AND III (MIM:130000, 130010, 130020)

(Ehlers-Danlos Syndrome [EDS] Gravis; EDS Mitis; Benign Familial Hypermobility)

DERMATOLOGIC FEATURES

MAJOR. EDS-I and -II share similar skin findings. The difference is in degree, with type II more mild than type I. EDS-III is marked by minimal skin changes and noticeable joint involvement.

The skin is thin, soft, doughy, or velvety to the touch. It stretches readily and snaps back. Easy bruising is typical. The skin is fragile, splitting on mild trauma with gaping wounds that heal slowly and leave cigarette paper atrophic scars. Violaceous hyperpigmentation of scars, possibly due, in part, to hemosiderin deposition, is common. Scarring of the forehead due to repeated falls in the toddler years is typical.

MINOR. Molluscoid pseudotumors are fleshy, raised papules that occur over areas of repeated trauma.

Spheroids are small, hard, freely moveable

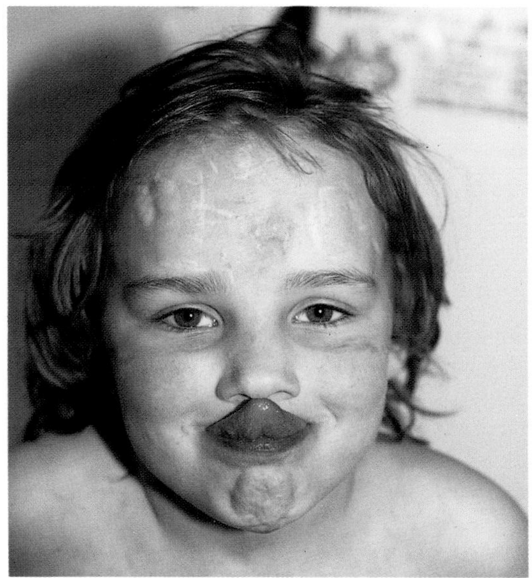

Figure 5.11. Scarring on forehead; hyperextensible tongue.

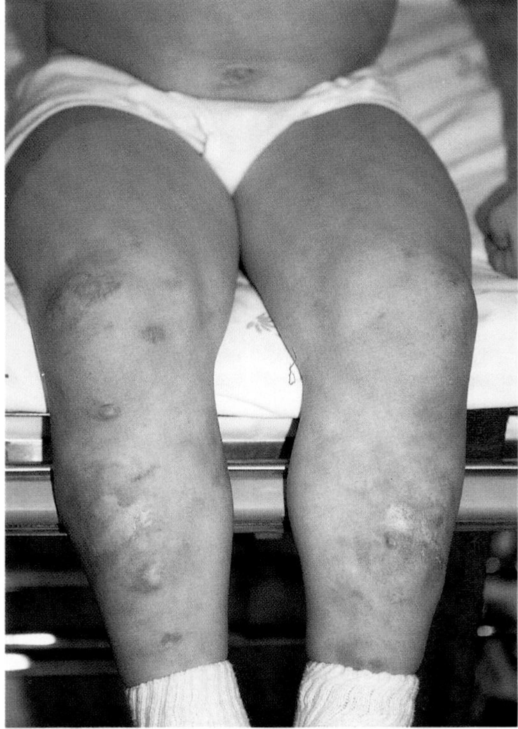

Figure 5.12. Multiple scars on shins with hemosiderin staining.

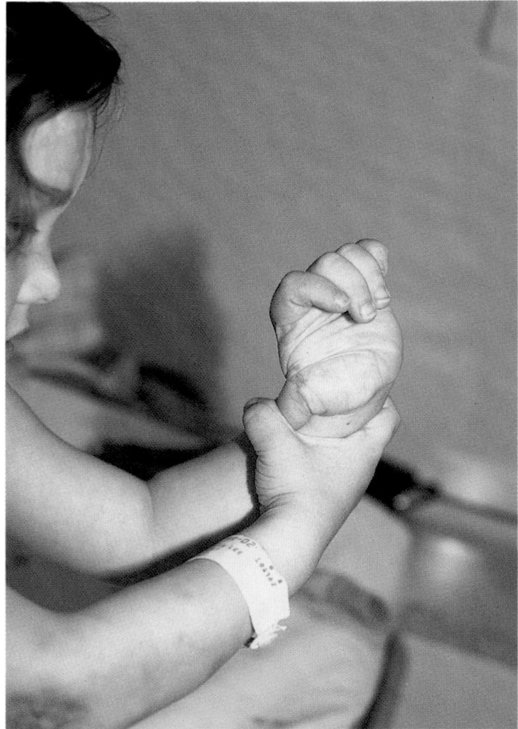

Figure 5.13. Joint hypermobility, scars on elbow, loose skin on palm.

rice grain-like nodules in the subcutaneous tissue usually found over the bony prominences of the arms and legs.

Knuckle pads have been described, as have painful piezogenic papules on the heels.

ASSOCIATED ABNORMALITIES

Joint laxity with recurrent dislocation is common to all of these three forms of EDS. It is the major feature of EDS-III and is least marked in EDS-II. Ligamentous laxity may result in delay of motor milestones, as stabilization of feet, ankles, and knees is difficult. Osteoarthritis is a late complication and may occur in as many as 80% of patients over the age of 40 years.

Premature rupture of the membranes with premature birth occurs commonly in EDS-I and EDS-II, and uterine prolapse or rupture can occur in pregnant women with EDS-I. Misdiagnosis of child abuse because of gaping wounds and bruising of the skin has occurred with both EDS-I and EDS-II. Floppy mitral valve may be more common in EDS-I and EDS-II than in the general population.

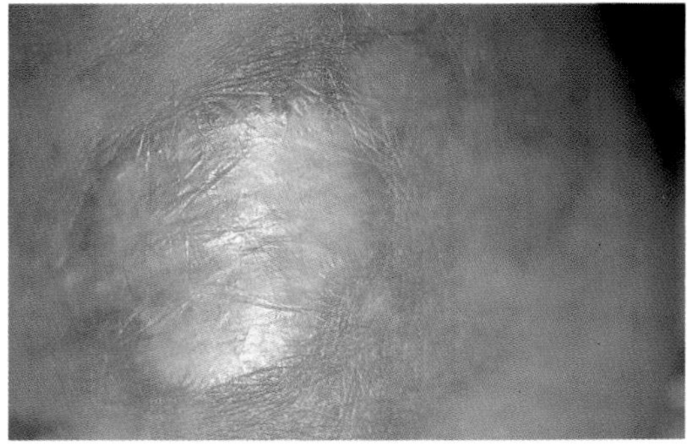

Figure 5.14. Atrophic thinned epidermis at site of healing, along with hemosiderin staining.

HISTOPATHOLOGY

LIGHT. No diagnostic changes.
EM. Large irregular collagen fibrils are seen in all three types.

BASIC DEFECT

Tight linkage to and mutations in the alpha-1 chain of type 5 collagen (*COL5A1*) have been identified in some families with EDS types I and II. Type 5 collagen is distributed in all tissues, including the uterus, placenta and chorion.

TREATMENT

Orthopedic management of joint laxity with physical therapy, bracing, and orthotics. Surgical correction of joint laxity is usually fraught with recurrence. Protection of the skin with appropriate padding and meticulous suturing of wounds with delayed removal of sutures may decrease scarring.

MODE OF INHERITANCE

Autosomal dominant. Locus heterogeneity is likely. The gene *COL5A1* maps to 9q34.3 and linkage to this locus has been excluded in some EDS type II families.

PRENATAL DIAGNOSIS

None.

DIFFERENTIAL DIAGNOSIS

In cutis laxa (MIM:Many) the skin is lax, not hyperelastic, and hangs in folds rather than snapping back easily. Easy bruising may lead to the misdiagnosis of a bleeding diathesis in some patients with EDS; recognition of the other skin changes will make the diagnosis clear. Children with Lowe syndrome (oculocerebrorenal syndrome, (MIM:309000) have extremely soft skin and ligamentous laxity, similar to EDS-III. Their failure to thrive, cataracts and glaucoma, renal tubular dysfunction, and mental retardation readily differentiate them.

Support Group: Ehlers-Danlos National Foundation
P.O. Box 1212
Southgate, MI 48195
1-800-990-3363

SELECTED BIBLIOGRAPHY

Holbrook, K.A., and Byers, P.H. (1982). Structural abnormalities in the dermal collagen and elastic matrix from the skin of patients with inherited connective tissue disorders. *J. Invest. Dermatol.* **79,** 7s–16s.
Beautiful electron micrographs.

Steinmann, B., Royce, P.M., and Superti-Furga, A. (1993). The Ehlers-Danlos syndrome. In *Connective Tissue and Its Heritable Disorders*. Royce, P.M., and Steinmann, B. (eds.). Wiley-Liss, New York, pp. 351–407.
This exhaustive and very clear discourse on the Ehlers-Danlos syndromes offers historical perspective, 491 references, and is the best review I have read to date.

EHLERS-DANLOS TYPE IV (MIM:130050, 225350, 225360)

(Acrogeria de Gottron; Arterial EDS; Sack-Barabas EDS; Ecchymotic EDS)

DERMATOLOGIC FEATURES

MAJOR. Thinning, translucence, and a prematurely aged appearance of the skin with a prominent vascular pattern is classic. The skin is not hyperelastic, and joint hypermobility is generally absent except in the fingers. Bruising is typical, and repeated ecchymoses result in

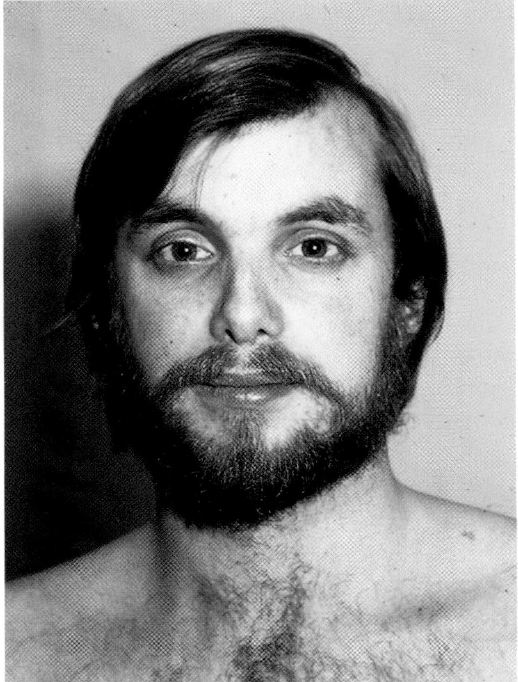

Figure 5.15. Fine features. Deep-set eyes with periorbital redness; pinched, sculpted appearance to nose.

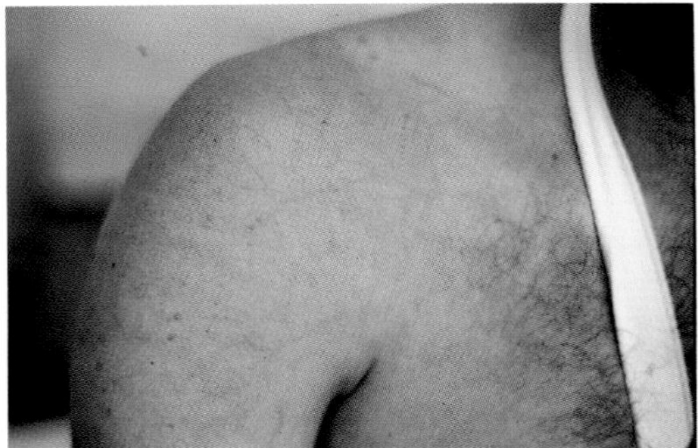

Figure 5.16. Venous pattern readily seen through thin skin.

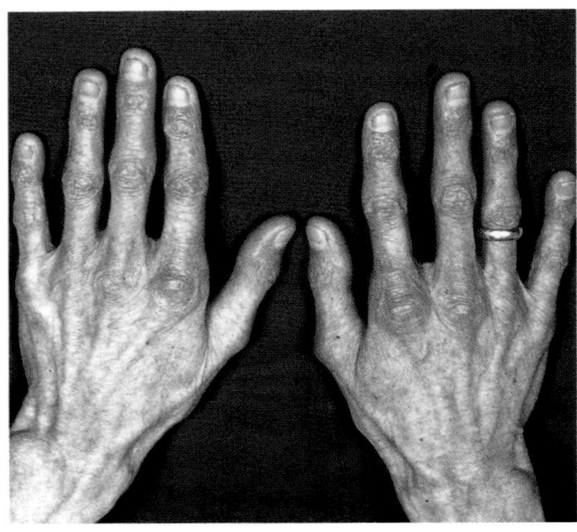

Figure 5.17. Acrogeric hand changes. (Courtesy of Dr. P. H. Byers, Seattle, Washington.)

chronically hyperpigmented areas. Healing is normal.

Minor. There is an "acrogeric" appearance of the hands and feet, with thin wrinkled skin.

Elastosis perforans serpiginosa has been described. This is marked by grouped hyperkeratotic papules that are in an annular or circular pattern. The lesions bleed when unroofed and may extrude material spontaneously.

ASSOCIATED ABNORMALITIES

The major features of EDS-IV are rupture of bowel (both large and small intestine) or major arteries and uterine rupture during pregnancy. Although biased by ascertainment, the mean age of death is between 35 and 40 years of age.

The facies are typically marked by a thin, pinched nose, thin lips, prominent eyes, and a general lack of subcutaneous tissue.

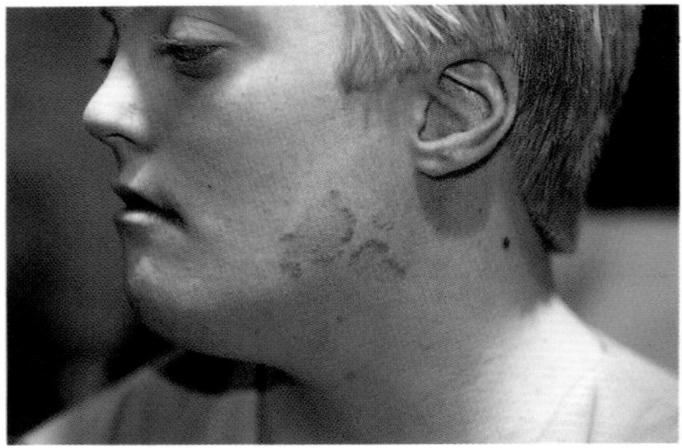

Figure 5.18. Elastosis perforans serpiginosa in a patient with trisomy 21.

HISTOPATHOLOGY

Light. There is thinning of the dermis.
EM. Small collagen fibers, variable collagen fibrils. Storage of type III collagen within fibroblasts in some.

BASIC DEFECT

Defects in type III collagen (*COL3A1*) including decreased secretion and structurally abnormal molecules.

TREATMENT

Recognition of catastrophic rupture with immediate surgical intervention when possible.

MODE OF INHERITANCE

Autosomal dominant with marked allelic heterogeneity. Gene mapped to 2q31. The basis for an autosomal recessive mode of inheritance is lacking. Somatic mosaicism has been documented in at least one instance of an "unaffected parent."

PRENATAL DIAGNOSIS

Available by biochemical analysis of type III collagen, direct mutational analysis, and/or linkage in chorionic villus samples.

DIFFERENTIAL DIAGNOSIS

Because of easy bruising, the misdiagnosis of a bleeding disorder is not uncommon. Individuals with familial arterial aneurysms (MIM: 120180.0004) due to a defect in *COL3A1* do not have any abnormal skin findings.

Support Group: Ehlers-Danlos National Foundation
P.O. Box 1212
Southgate, MI 48195
1-800-990-3363

SELECTED BIBLIOGRAPHY

Byers, P.H., Holbrook, K.A., McGillivray, B., MacLeod, P.M., and Lowry, R.B. (1979). Clinical and ultrastructural heterogeneity of type IV Ehlers-Danlos syndrome. *Hum. Genet.* **47,** 141–150.

Outdated biochemically, this paper still gives good clinical and ultrastructural information with excellent photographs.

Steinmann, B., Royce, P.M., and Superti-Furga, A. (1993). The Ehlers-Danlos syndrome. In *Connective Tissue and Its Heritable Disorders*. Royce, P.M., and Steinmann, B. (eds.). Wiley-Liss, New York, pp. 351–407.

This exhaustive and very clear discourse on the Ehlers-Danlos syndrome offers historical perspective, 491 references, and is the best review I have read to date.

EHLERS-DANLOS TYPE VI (MIM:225400)

(Lysyl Hydroxylase Deficiency; Ocular-Scoliotic Form)

DERMATOLOGIC FEATURES

Major. This is a very rare condition. There is bruising with mild to moderate thinning of the skin and widening of scars. The skin is mildly hyperextensible. Molluscoid pseudotumors have been described.
Minor. None.

ASSOCIATED ABNORMALITIES

Muscle hypotonia is a presenting feature at birth and persists. Moderate to severe joint laxity with kyphoscoliosis, which also can be present at birth, is typical, as are recurrent joint dislocations. Scoliosis can be severe enough to lead to cardiopulmonary insufficiency.

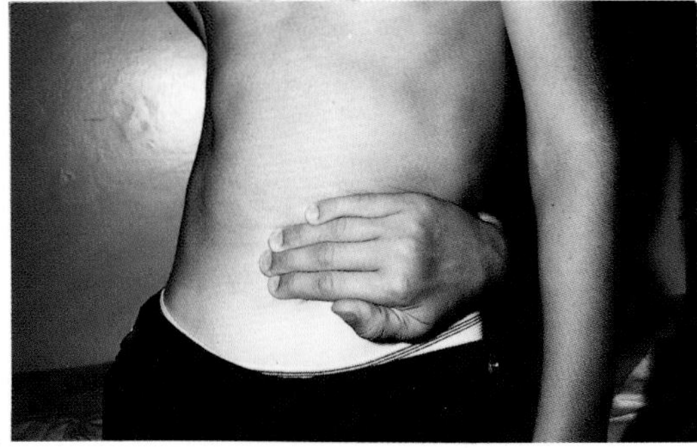

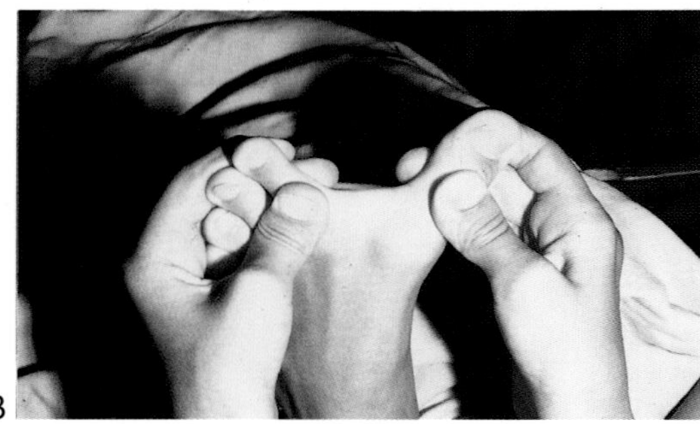

Figure 5.19. (A, B) Marked hyperextensibility of joints and skin. (Courtesy of Dr. S. Pinnell, Durham, North Carolina.)

Myopia is common and often severe. Glaucoma and retinal detachment have been described. Ocular rupture after trauma is also a feature.

Arterial rupture (intracranial, vertebral, femoral, and aortic) has been a major cause of death.

Inguinal hernias and bladder diverticuli are also reported.

HISTOPATHOLOGY

LIGHT. Not specific.
EM. EM findings are variable, with both small and large collagen fibrils described.

BASIC DEFECT

Deficiency of lysyl hydroxylase in type VIA. The term type VIB refers to patients with clinical features of EDS-VI and no demonstrable abnormalities in lysyl hydroxylase.

TREATMENT

Unclear if vitamin C has any effect.

MODE OF INHERITANCE

Autosomal recessive.

PRENATAL DIAGNOSIS

Lysyl hydroxylase activity in amniotic fluid cells can be measured.

DIFFERENTIAL DIAGNOSIS

The congenital hypotonias (MIM:Many) may be excluded by the joint laxity and easy bruising of EDS-VI. The presence of hypotonia should help to rule out EDS-I and EDS-II (MIM: 130000, 130010).

Support Group: Ehlers-Danlos National Foundation
P.O. Box 1212
Southgate, MI 48195
1-800-990-3363

SELECTED BIBLIOGRAPHY

Steinmann, B., Royce, P.M., and Superti-Furga, A. (1993). The Ehlers-Danlos syndrome. In *Connective Tissue and Its Heritable Disorders*. Royce, P.M., and Steinmann, B. (eds.). Wiley-Liss, New York, pp. 351–407.

This exhaustive and very clear discourse on the Ehlers-Danlos syndrome offers historical perspective, 491 references, and is the best review I have read to date.

Wenstrup, R.J., Murad, S., and Pinnell, S.R. (1989). Ehlers-Danlos syndrome type VI: clinical manifestation of collagen lysyl hydroxylase deficiency. *J. Pediatr.* **115:** 405–409.

Review of 10 patients with this disorder. Points out that ocular fragility occurs in a minority of patients.

EHLERS-DANLOS TYPE VIII (MIM:130080)

(Periodontal Ehlers-Danlos Syndrome)

DERMATOLOGIC FEATURES

MAJOR. Skin changes are similar to EDS-II, with velvety hyperextensible skin and moderate fragility and spreading of scars. Excessive wrinkling of the palms and soles, with marked hyperpigmentation and atrophy of skin on the shins.

MINOR. None.

ASSOCIATED ABNORMALITIES

Periodontitis with onset in early teens is the hallmark of this disorder, with alveolar bone

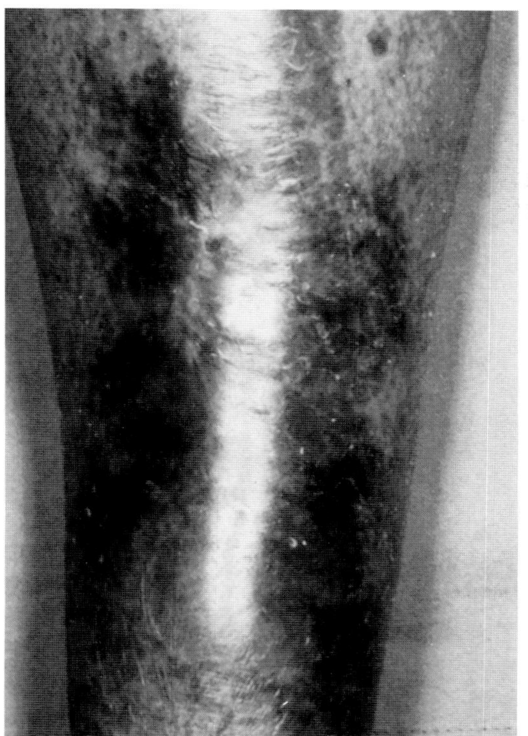

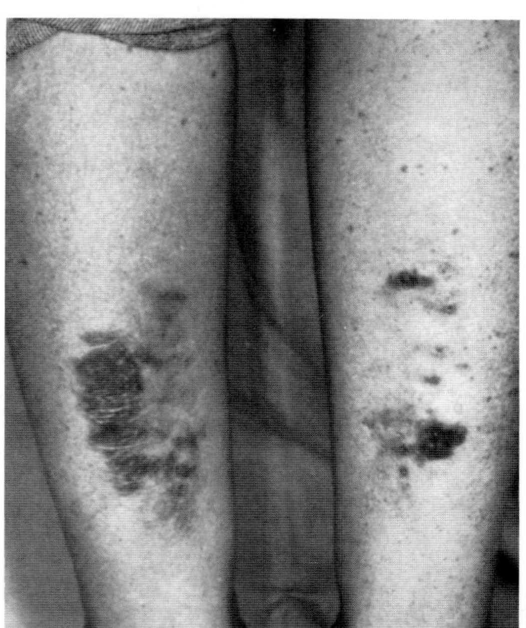

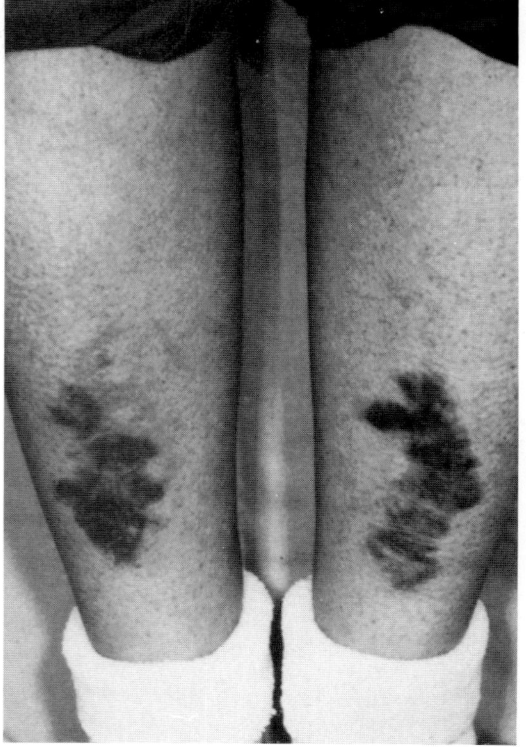

Figure 5.20. Shiny atrophic skin over the shins in a 70-year-old woman **(A)** and her 18-year-old **(B)** and 19-year-old **(C)** granddaughters. Changes are similar to those seen in pretibial epidermolysis bullosa dystrophica. (From Nelson and King, 1981.)

regression, resorption, and tooth loss occurring in the twenties. Mild joint laxity is present.

HISTOPATHOLOGY

Light. No information.
EM. Mixed population of collagen fibrils with large and small diameters.

BASIC DEFECT

Unknown.

TREATMENT

None.

MODE OF INHERITANCE

Autosomal dominant.

PRENATAL DIAGNOSIS

None.

DIFFERENTIAL DIAGNOSIS

Juvenile periodontitis (MIM:170650) is not associated with skin changes. EDS-I and EDS-II (MIM:130000, 130010) do not have gum disease.

In Papillon-Lefèvre syndrome (MIM: 245000), periodontitis is associated with palmoplantar hyperkeratosis.

Support Group: Ehlers-Danlos National Foundation
P.O. Box 1212
Southgate, MI 48195
1-800-990-3363

SELECTED BIBLIOGRAPHY

Nelson, D.L., and King, R.A. (1981). Ehlers-Danlos syndrome type VIII. *J. Am. Acad. Dermatol.* **5,** 297–303.
Three generation family is presented.
Steinmann, B., Royce, P.M., and Superti-Furga, A. (1993). The Ehlers-Danlos syndrome. In *Connective Tissue and Its Heritable Disorders*. Royce, P.M., and Steinmann, B. (eds.). Wiley-Liss, New York, pages 351–407.
This exhaustive and very clear discourse on the Ehlers-Danlos syndrome offers historical perspective, 491 references, and is the best review I have read to date.

REACTIVE PERFORATING COLLAGENOSIS (MIM:216700)

DERMATOLOGIC FEATURES

Major. Individual pinhead-sized keratotic papules appear and grow slowly to 5–10 mm in size over a 4–5 week period. They develop a central umbilication with a thick hard plug. The plug is gradually lost, the papules flatten, and ultimately disappear. The entire cycle takes 8–10 weeks.

Lesions tend to occur over the backs of the hands, the arms, legs, upper thighs, and trunk. They may koebnerize, developing in areas of trauma. Lesions may develop along stretch marks and in insect bites. In one affected individual, lesions developed on the lips and in the mouth. The papules usually begin appearing in childhood, although in one affected individual the process started at 1 month of age.
Minor. None.

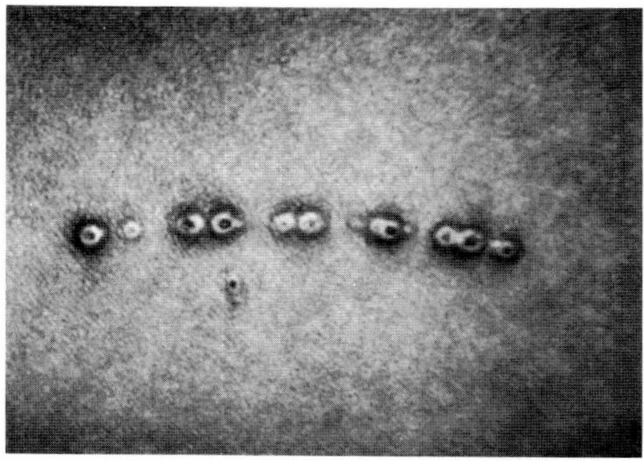

Figure 5.21. Umbilicated lesions in linear array. (From Mehregan, 1970.)

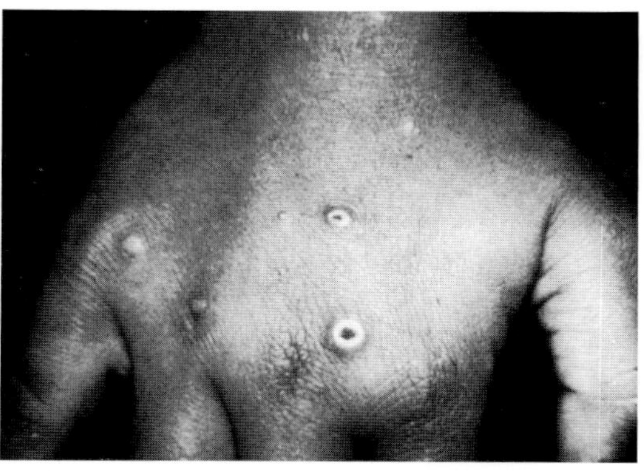

Figure 5.22. Multiple lesions at different stages of development. (From Mehregan, 1970.)

ASSOCIATED ABNORMALITIES

None.

HISTOPATHOLOGY

LIGHT. Findings change depending on the stage of the lesion. Early lesions are marked by a dilated papilla filled with necrobiotic connective tissue. Umbilicated lesions show a central cup-shaped epidermal dell with thickened columns of parakeratotic keratin and inflammatory cells. Extrusion of collagen bundles may occur.

EM. Absence of the basal lamina beneath the plug. The collagen fibers appear normal.

BASIC DEFECT

Unknown.

TREATMENT

Topical retinoid therapy was reported to be successful in one case.

MODE OF INHERITANCE

?Autosomal recessive. Most reports are of affected sibships; there is one uncle–niece (paternal) pair. There is another report of a two generation, highly inbred kindred, consistent with autosomal recessive inheritance and pseudodominance.

PRENATAL DIAGNOSIS

None.

DIFFERENTIAL DIAGNOSIS

Reactive perforating collagenosis can be acquired, most commonly seen in association with diabetes mellitus complicated by renal failure and need for dialysis. Other perforating diseases such as Kyrle disease (MIM:149500) and elastosis perforans serpiginosa (MIM: 130100) may initially be confused. Percutaneous perforation rarely occurs in association with granuloma annulare. Biopsy will differentiate among these possibilities.

Support Group: N.O.R.D.
P.O. Box 8923
New Fairfield, CT
06812
1-800-999-6673

SELECTED BIBLIOGRAPHY

Kanan, M.W. (1974). Familial reactive perforating collagenosis and intolerance to cold. *Br. J. Dermatol.* **91,** 405–414.

Two pedigrees, one with a nice example of pseudodominance. Underscores the role of trauma in producing lesions.

Nair, B.K.H., Sarojini, P.A., Basheer, A.M., and Nair, C.H.K. (1974). Reactive perforating collagenosis. *Br. J. Dermatol.* **91,** 399–403.

A father and his three affected children were described in this Indian pedigree. This paper is repeatedly cited as supporting autosomal dominant inheritance, but the pedigree is clearly consistent with autosomal recessive inheritance with pseudodominance. The mother of these three children was the unaffected sister of an affected individual, and the father was her affected first cousin.

Trattner, A., Ingber, A., and Sandbank, M. (1991). Mucosal involvement in reactive perforating collagenosis. *J. Am. Acad. Dermatol.* **25,** 1079–1080.

Two affected brothers; one had lesions in the oral cavity and on the lips, and the other did not.

ELASTIN

COSTELLO SYNDROME (MIM:218040)

Includes Facio-Cutaneous-Skeletal Syndrome

DERMATOLOGIC FEATURES

Major. Loose, redundant skin of the neck, backs of the hands, and tops of the feet is noticeable at birth. The palm and sole skin is thickened with deep creases, but is not hyperkeratotic. Over time, acanthosis nigricans develops in a typical distribution around the neck and in the folds. Papillomas around the nose and mouth make their appearance in early to middle childhood. These papillomas arise at other sites as well.

Typically the hair is curly and sparse.

Nails are brittle, with koilonychia.

Minor. Acrochordons, or skin tags, on the neck are described in a number of patients.

ASSOCIATED ABNORMALITIES

Mental retardation has been a feature in all reported cases and ranges from moderate to severe. Head circumference is usually normal. Infants have normal birth weight and birth length, but this is followed by postnatal growth failure with short stature. Poor feeding may complicate infancy.

Generalized joint hypermobility is common, as are congenital clubfeet. Despite generalized joint laxity, tight achilles tendons are also seen.

The facial features are coarse, with thick full lips, depressed nasal bridge, thick pinnae, and a short neck. The voice is described as hoarse.

It is unclear if cardiac involvement is a feature of the disorder. Several patients, each with different cardiac lesions, including thickened mitral valve, cardiac arrhythmias, and hypertrophic cardiomyopathy, have been reported.

HISTOPATHOLOGY

Light. The papillomas have changes typical of warts with acanthosis and papillomatosis.

EM. Evaluation of a biopsy from one patient showed elastic fibers with irregular borders and a porous central zone. The elastic fibers were

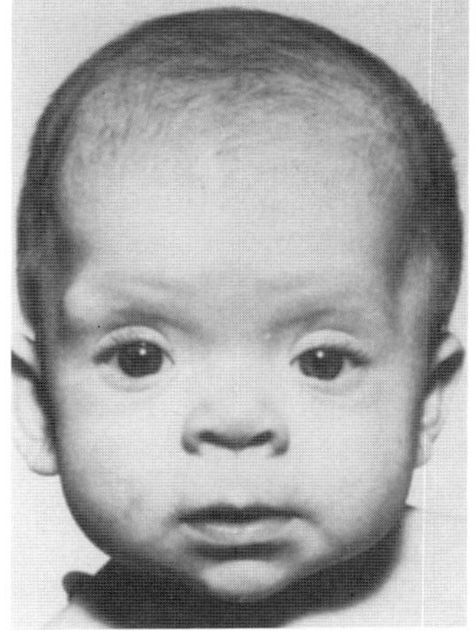

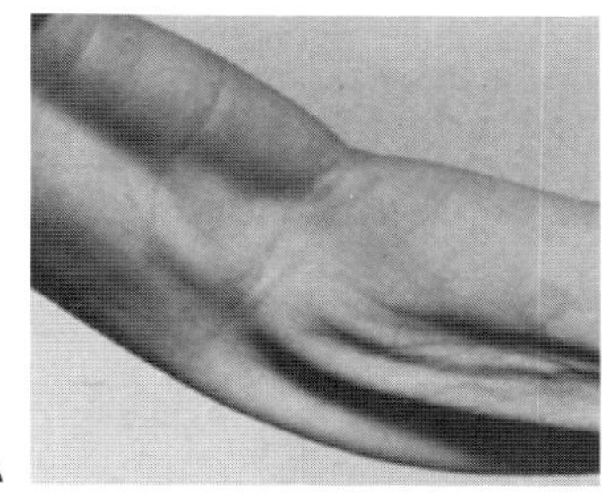

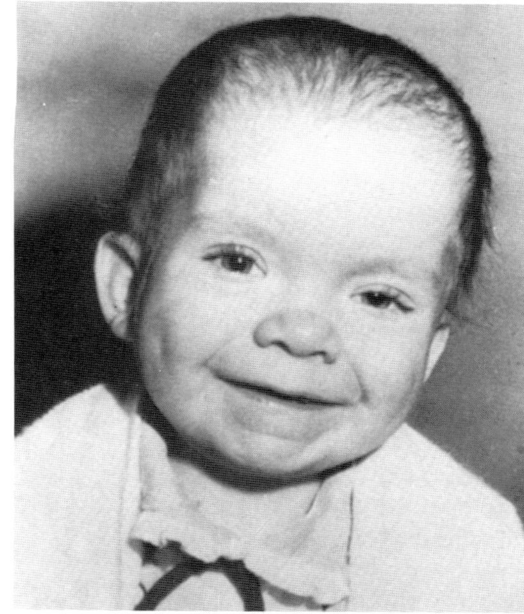

Figure 5.23. Facial appearance of patient at 8 months **(A),** 2½ years **(B),** and 10 years **(C).** Redundant skin on arm **(A).** (From Davies and Hughes, 1994.)

C

described as appearing immature. In a second patient there appeared to be a decrease in collagen with normal elastin.

BASIC DEFECT

Unknown.

TREATMENT

None.

MODE OF INHERITANCE

Autosomal recessive. Most cases are sporadic. There have been two sibling pairs and single affected offspring from two consanguineous, highly inbred Druze families.

PRENATAL DIAGNOSIS

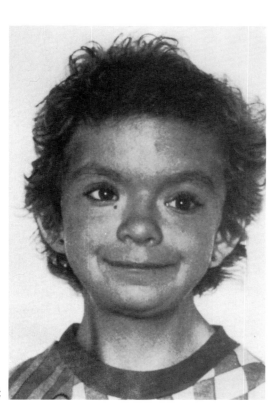

None.

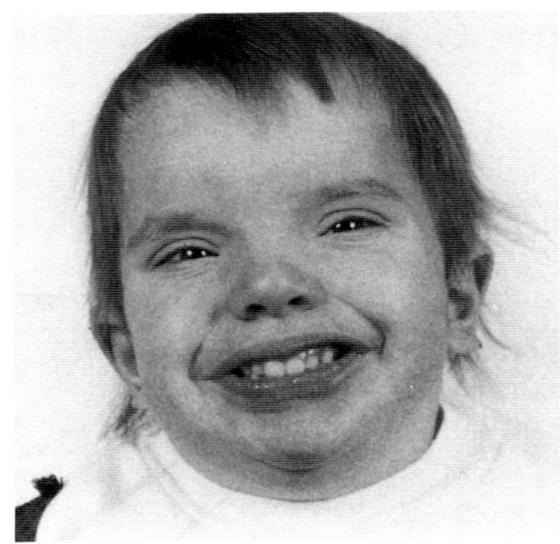

Figure 5.24. Second patient. Full lips, sparse hair, and wide-spaced eyes. (From Costa et al., 1994.)

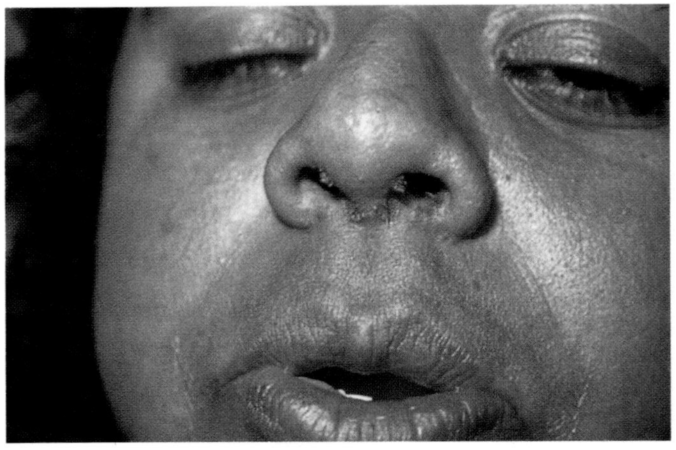

Figure 5.25. Papillomas around nose and on cheeks. (From Costa et al., 1994.)

DIFFERENTIAL DIAGNOSIS

Lipoid proteinosis (MIM:247100) shares facial papules and plaques and a hoarse voice in common with Costello syndrome. Individuals with lipoid proteinosis do not have redundant skin or the facies and hair changes of Costello syndrome.

The cutis laxa syndromes (MIM:123700, 219100, 304150) might present some confusion, as children with Costello syndrome have loose redundant skin. Individuals with cutis laxa do not have thickened palms and soles and do not develop facial papules.

Leprechaunism (Donohue syndrome, MIM: 246200) shares in common loose skin and acanthosis nigricans with the Costello syndrome, but lacks the facial papules and facial features.

Some patients with Noonan syndrome (MIM: 163950) will show a similar hair pattern and redundant nuchal skin. The facial changes are quite distinctive.

Support Group: N.O.R.D.
P.O. Box 8923
New Fairfield, CT
06812
1-800-999-6673

SELECTED BIBLIOGRAPHY

Costello, J.M. (1977). A new syndrome: mental subnormality and nasal papillomata. *Aust. Paediatr. J.* **13,** 114–118.

Describes two unrelated children who were also discussed in his original abstract in 1971. They are fully described in this publication.

Davies, S.J., and Hughes, H.E. (1994). Costello syndrome: natural history and differential diagnosis of cutis laxa. *J. Med. Genet.* **31,** 486–489.

Nice review of a patient with Costello syndrome who was originally described as having congenital cutis laxa with retardation of growth and development. The authors point out that another patient who carried that diagnosis also subsequently was recognized to have Costello syndrome. The discussion outlines the ease of confusion of Costello syndrome with Noonan/cardio-facial-cutaneous syndrome, leprechaunism, and cutis laxa.

Lurie, I.W. (1994). Genetics of the Costello syndrome. *Am. J. Med. Genet.* **52,** 358–359.

The author argues against autosomal recessive inheritance, reviewing 28 cases in 26 families. He invokes new dominant mutation as causal in most and gonadal mosaicism responsible for the recurrences in families.

CUTIS LAXA (MIM:123700, 219100, 219150, 219200, 235360, 304150)

(Generalized Elastolysis)

Includes Occipital Horn Syndrome; Ehlers-Danlos Type IX; Wrinkly Skin; SCARF

DERMATOLOGIC FEATURES

MAJOR. *Cutis laxa* is a term applied to a heterogeneous group of conditions that share the clinical finding of loose, lax skin. The skin is droopy, not hyperelastic, and often gives a prematurely aged "hound-dog" appearance to the face. Skin fragility and healing are normal in the autosomal dominant and autosomal recessive forms. In X-linked cutis laxa (occipital horn disease), the skin may be more velvety and bruise more easily than normal. Scars may be atrophic. Skin flaccidity may be present at birth, more common in the X-linked recessive and autosomal recessive forms, or may develop during childhood, adolescence, or adult life (more typical of autosomal dominant disease).

MINOR. In addition to the laxity of facial skin, the nasal tip is often flattened with a short columella. It appears on profile as if there is a deficiency in the terminal cartilage of the distal septum so that the slope of the nose flattens precipitously as it comes off the bony prominence.

ASSOCIATED ABNORMALITIES

Other organ systems may be affected. In general, the autosomal dominant form of cutis laxa involves only the skin, although inguinal and abdominal hernias have been described.

Early emphysema is a frequent feature of the autosomal recessive forms of cutis laxa. Late bronchiectasis developing in midlife has been described in the autosomal dominant form.

Bladder diverticuli are common in the X-linked form (occipital horn disease, also known as Ehlers-Danlos type IX). Gastrointestinal diverticuli may also occur.

Diaphragmatic, inguinal, and abdominal hernias are common features of the autosomal

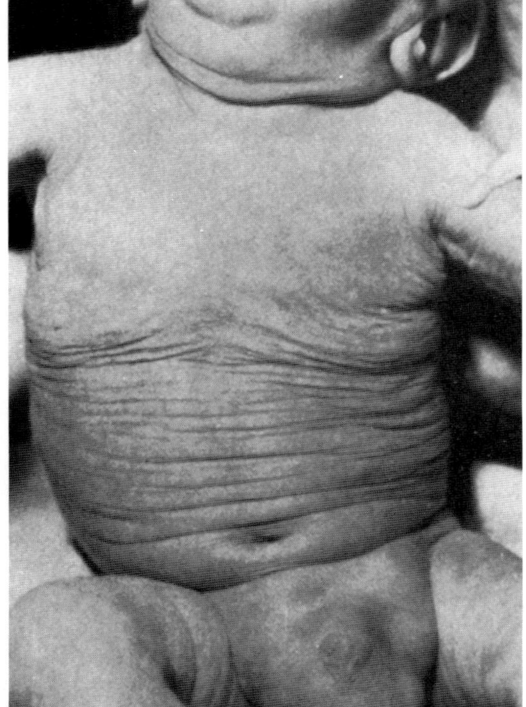

A

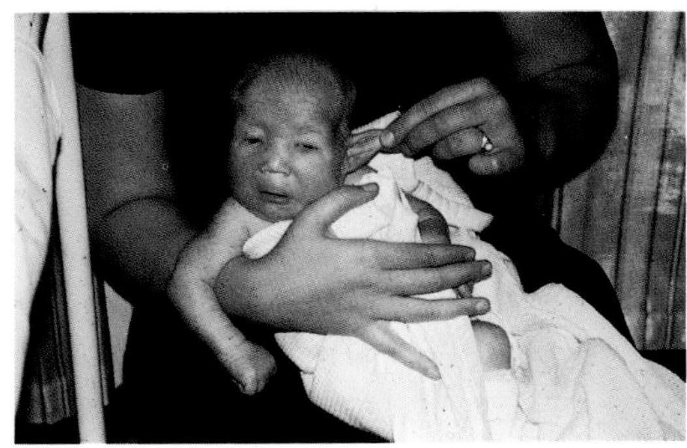

B

Figure 5.26. (A) Wrinkled, lax skin in newborn with bilateral inguinal hernias. (From Phillips, 1978.) **(B)** Droopy face, stretchy pinnae in infant.

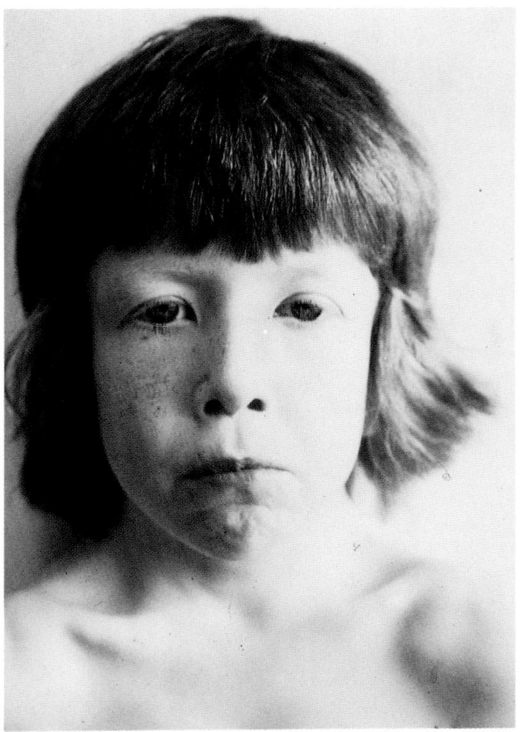

Figure 5.27. Ptosis. Slightly sagging jowls in a male with occipital horn disease (X-linked cutis laxa).

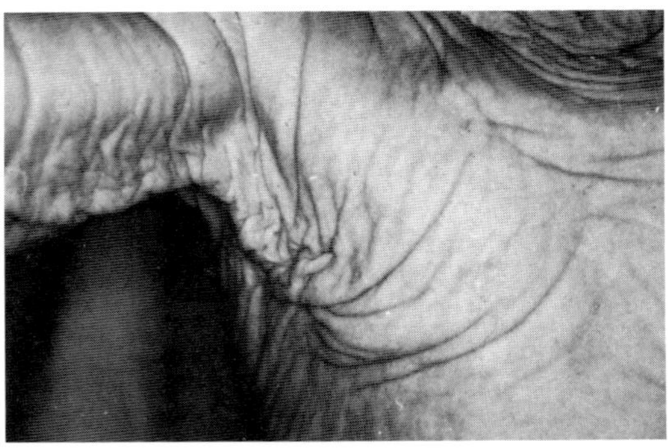

Figure 5.28. Marked sagging, flaccid skin in 2-year-old. (From Ledoux-Corbusiere, 1983.)

recessive forms. Inguinal hernias are also reported in the X-linked form. Chronic diarrhea is a common complaint in X-linked cutis laxa.

Generalized joint laxity can be seen in all types of cutis laxa. Bony changes include occipital horns (X-linked form), delayed closure of the fontanelles, and congenital dislocation of the hips. A delayed bone age is more typical of unusual syndromes associated with cutis laxa and is reported more commonly in those children who have mental retardation as well. The term *occipital horn syndrome* refers specifically to X-linked cutis laxa in which bony prominences extend down from the occiput bilaterally. They represent ectopic bone formation in

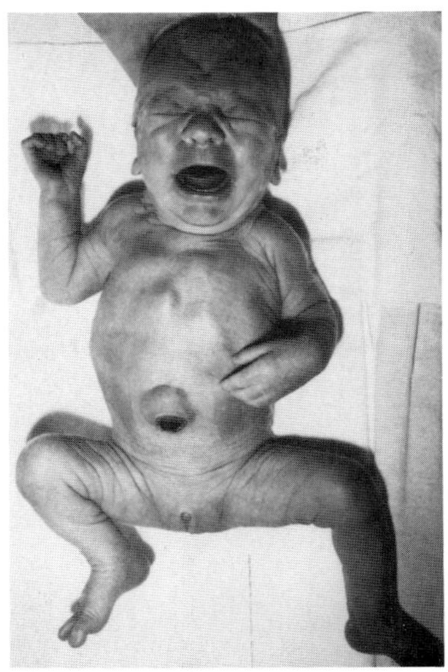

the aponeuroses of the sternocleidomastoid and trapezius muscles. X-linked cutis laxa is also marked by a more generalized skeletal dysplasia with broad clavicles and shortening of the long bones, abnormal elbows, coxa valga, genu valgum, flattening of the vertebral bodies, and generalized osteopenia.

Developmental delay has been described in a few families with autosomal recessive cutis laxa, but is not consistently present in all affected siblings. In X-linked cutis laxa, mild intellectual deficits are common, but not invariable.

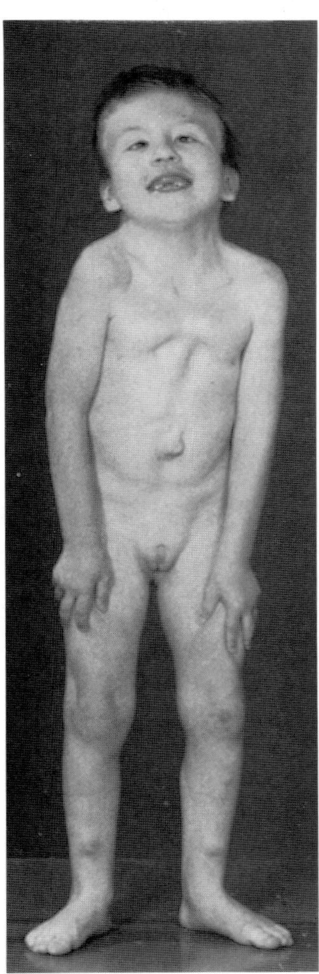

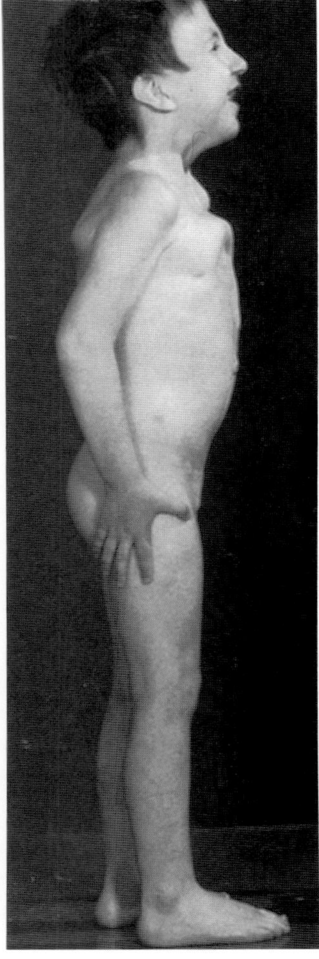

Figure 5.29. Patient with SCARF at birth **(A)** and age 5½ years **(B)**. (From Koppe et al., 1989.)

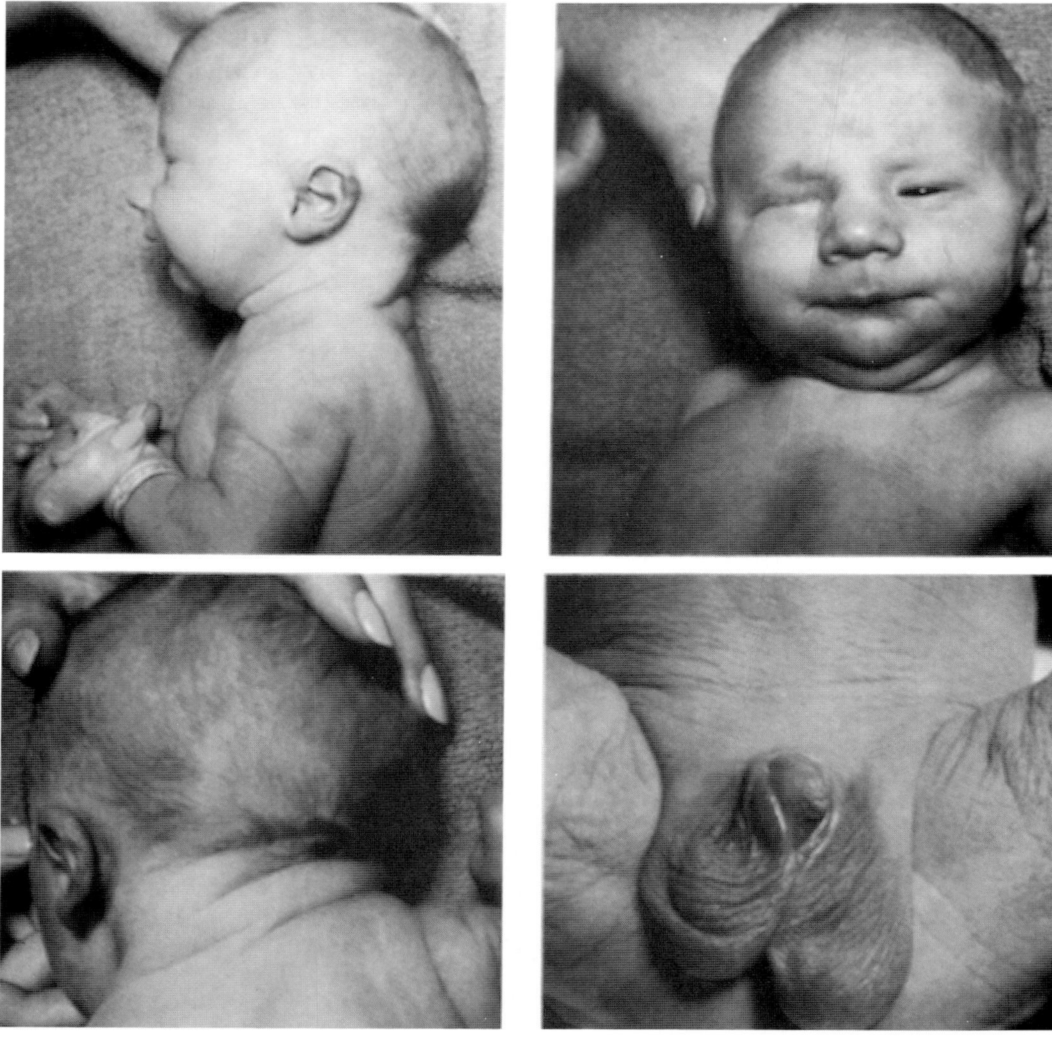

Figure 5.30. Wrinkled redundant skin; facial and genital abnormalities in SCARF. (From Koppe et al., 1989.)

HISTOPATHOLOGY

LIGHT. A decrease in to absence of elastic fibers in the dermis. Remaining elastic fibers are fragmented and clumped.

EM. In the X-linked form there are large densely packed collagen fibrils with normal-appearing elastic fibers. In other forms of cutis laxa there is a decrease in elastin with abnormality of the dense amorphous component and an apparently normal microfibrillar component. There is some variation in collagen fibril diameter and occasional collagen flowers.

BASIC DEFECT

In the X-linked form of cutis laxa, mutations in the *MNK* gene cause defective uptake of copper and secondary deficiency of copper-dependent enzymes, such as lysyl oxidase. This results in abnormal cross-link formation in collagen. Serum copper and ceruloplasmin levels are low in males with the X-linked form of cutis laxa.

The basic defects in the autosomal forms are unknown.

TREATMENT

None specific. Plastic surgery has been recommended for cosmesis. Patients should be followed for genitourinary involvement and lung involvement. Whether copper histidine supplementation will be useful in occipital horn syndrome remains to be demonstrated.

MODE OF INHERITANCE

Autosomal dominant: usually involves the skin only.

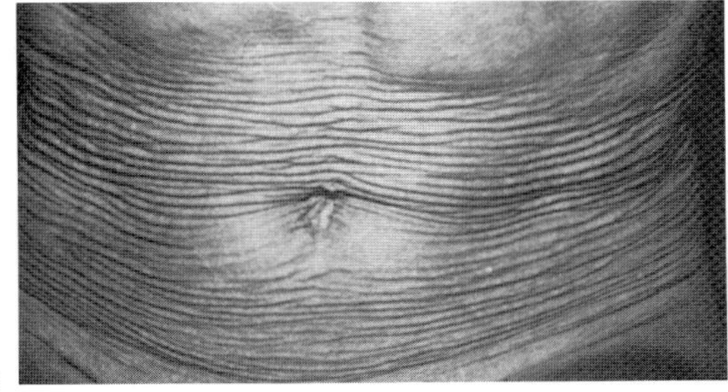

Figure 5.31. Abdomen **(A)** and hands **(B–E)** of patients with wrinkly skin syndrome. B and C are the hands of a 9 year old; D and E are those of a $5^{1}/_{2}$ year old. (A, from Hurvitz et al., 1990; B, from Gazit et al., 1973.)

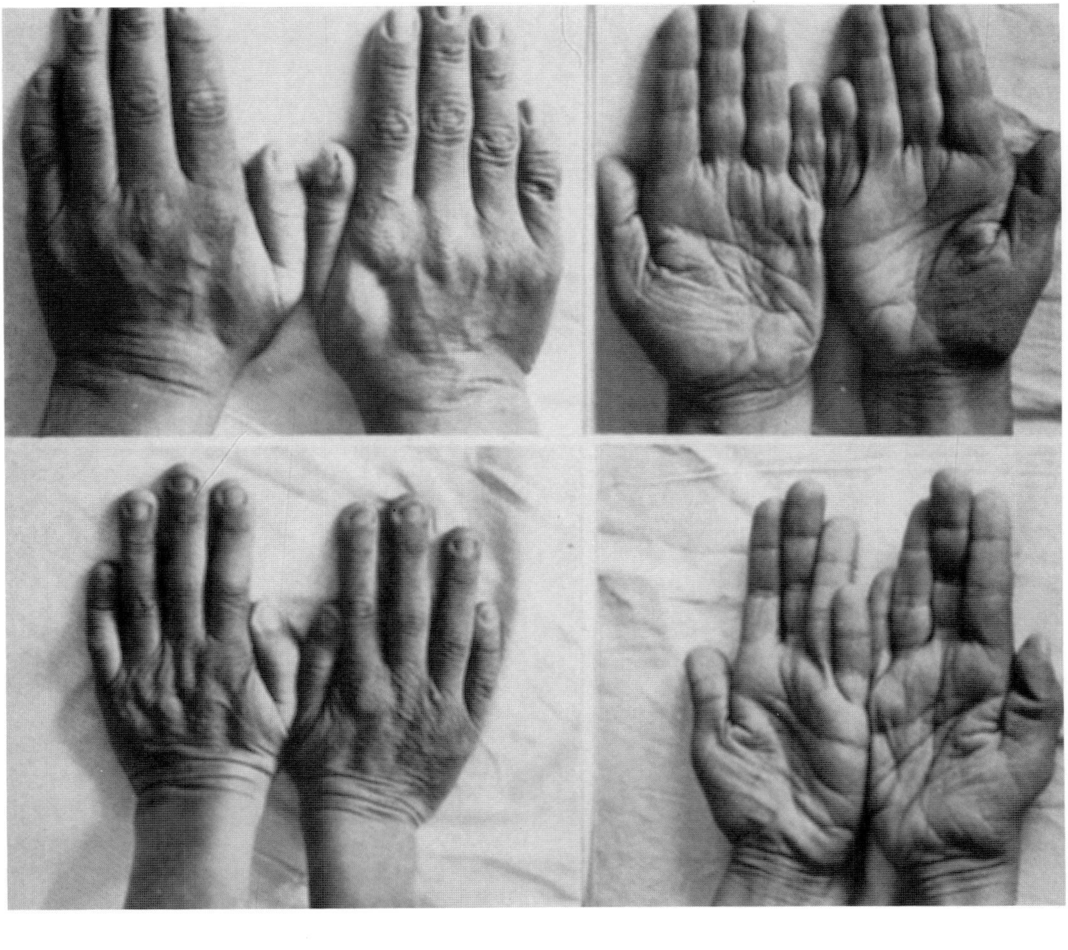

A

B

C

D

E

Autosomal recessive: usually is associated with emphysema and is the most severe.

X-linked recessive: presents with both skin and systemic changes. The gene is mapped to Xq13.3.

PRENATAL DIAGNOSIS

For the X-linked form, direct mutational analysis is now possible.

DIFFERENTIAL DIAGNOSIS

Loose, thin skin can be seen in Lenz-Majewski dwarfism (MIM:151050), redundant fixed folds of skin in the Beare-Stevenson syndrome (MIM:None), and redundant loose skin in the Costello syndrome (MIM:218040). Two male cousins with craniostenosis and ambiguous genitalia, mental retardation, and unusual facial features also had loose skin, which resolved over time (SCARF syndrome, MIM:None). Cutis laxa can be seen in de Barsy syndrome (MIM:219150), which is marked by cloudy corneas, mental retardation, and athetoid movements in addition to the skin changes. Maternal ingestion of penicillamine has resulted in cutis laxa in the newborn. The Michelin tire baby (MIM:156610) has redundant-appearing skin with deep folds; the skin is not lax but full and firm.

In the autosomal recessive wrinkly skin syndrome (MIM:278250), the skin of the hands, feet, and abdomen is covered with fine wrinkles, there are increased palmar and plantar lines, hypotonia, congenital dislocation of the hip, and winged scapulae, along with laxity of the skin. While mental retardation and microcephaly have also been described, they are not consistently found among affected siblings. In a single biopsy specimen each from two patients elastic fibers were described as normal on light microscopy, and in one of two biopsy specimens from a third patient the elastic fibers were described as short and decreased in number.

Infants with neonatal Marfan syndrome (MIM:154700) have, in addition to lax skin, marked arachnodactyly, severe cardiac valve insufficiency and aortic dilation, joint contractures, and crumpled ears.

Acquired generalized elastolysis is a rare disease of adult life. Common to some cases of acquired cutis laxa are exposure to penicillin and development of a preceding erythematous rash. Pulmonary and cardiovascular involvement can also occur, along with gastrointestinal and genitourinary complications. Elastolysis can also follow a variety of inflammatory skin problems, including erythema multiforme and chronic urticaria.

Support Group:

Ehlers-Danlos National Foundation
P.O. Box 1212
Southgate, MI 48195
1-800-990-3363

Corporation for Menke's Disease
5720 Buckfield Court
Fort Wayne, IN 46804
1-219-436-0137

SELECTED BIBLIOGRAPHY

deBarsy, A.M., Moens, E., and Dierckx, L. (1968). Dwarfism, oligophrenia and degeneration of the elastic tissue in skin and cornea. A new syndrome? *Helv. Paediatr. Acta* **23,** 305–313.

Single case report in a female. Histopathology showed decreased elastic fibers.

Fitzsimmons, J.S., Fitzsimmons, E.M., Guiberts, P.R., Zaldua, V., and Dodd, K.L. (1985). Variable clinical presentation of cutis laxa. *Clin. Genet.* **28,** 284–295.

Report of four patients with cutis laxa. The descriptions typify the difficulty in sorting out the heterogeneity of this syndrome; others might classify these patients differently based on the clinical precis provided.

Gazit, E., Goodman, R.M., Bat-Miriam Katznelson, M., and Rotem, Y. (1973). The wrinkly skin syndrome: a new heritable disorder of connective tissue. *Clin. Genet.* **4,** 186–192.

Differentiates the wrinkly skin syndrome from

cutis laxa on a somewhat shaky basis—lack of facial involvement, lack of typical nasal configuration (patients are 9 years, 5 1/2 years, and 3 months old, respectively), and normal light microscopy of elastic fibers in one biopsy specimen from one patient.

Herman, T.E., McAlister, W.H., Boniface, A., and Whyte, M.P. (1992). Occipital horn syndrome. Additional radiographic findings in two new cases. *Pediatr. Radiol.* **22,** 363–365.

Describes two cases, brief review of the literature. Good radiographs.

Hurvitz, S.A., Baumgarten, A., and Goodman, R.M. (1990). The wrinkly skin syndrome: a report of a case and review of the literature. *Clin. Genet.* **38,** 307–313.

Excellent table. Suffers from lack of histologic confirmation of normal elastin to exclude the diagnosis of cutis laxa.

Koppe, R., Kaplan, P., Hunter, A., and MacMurray, B. (1989). Ambiguous genitalia associated with skeletal abnormalities, cutis laxa, craniostenosis, psychomotor retardation and facial abnormalities (SCARF syndrome). *Am. J. Med. Genet.* **34,** 305–312.

It is a stretch to get from AGSACLCSPRFA to SCARF, but these authors manage it.

Kreuz, F.R., and Wittwer, B.H. (1993). Del(2q)—cause of the wrinkly skin syndrome? *Clin. Genet.* **43,** 132–138.

Mother and two sons with clinical features of del(2q) and wrinkly skin. No other patients with 2q deletions have been described with these skin changes.

Ledoux-Corbusiere, M. (1983). Cutis laxa, congenital form with pulmonary emphysema: an ultrastructural study. *J. Cutan. Pathol.* **10,** 340–349.

Beautiful electron micrographs and clinical photos in this case report.

Hamer, D.H. (1993). "Kinky hair" disease sheds light on copper metabolism. *Nat. Genet.* **3,** 3.

Levinson, B., Gitschier, J., Vulpe, C., Whitney, S., Yang, S., and Packman, S. (1993). Are X-linked cutis laxa and Menkes disease allelic? *Nat. Genet.* **3,** 6.

Vulpe, C., Levinson, B., Whitney, S., Packman, S., and Gitschier, J. (1993). Isolation of a candidate gene for Menkes disease and evidence that it encodes a copper-transporting ATPase. *Nat. Genet.* **3,** 7–13.

Chelly, J., Tumer, Z., Tonnesen, T., Petterson, A., Ishikawa-Brush, Y., Tommerup, N., Horn, N., and Monaco, A.P. (1993). Isolation of a candidate gene for Menkes disease that encodes a potential heavy metal binding protein. *Nat. Genet.* **3,** 14–19.

Mercer, J.F.B., Livingston, J., Hall, B., Paynter, J.A., Begy, C., Chandrasekharappa, S., Lockhart, P., Grimes, A., Bhave, M., Siemieniak, D., and Glover T.W. (1993). Isolation of a partial candidate gene for Menkes disease by positional cloning. *Nat. Genet.* **3,** 20–25.

Chelly et al. (1993), Hamer (1993), Levinson et al. (1993), Vulpe et al. (1993), and Mercer et al. (1993) are back to back reports from three laboratories of isolation and identification of a candidate gene with an accompanying editorial and letter suggesting the allelic nature of Menkes and X-linked cutis laxa.

Sakati, N.O., Nyhan, W.L., Shear, C.S., Kattan, H., Akhtar, M., Bay, C., Jones, K.L., and Schackner [sic], L. (1983). Syndrome of cutis laxa, ligamentous laxity and delayed development. *Pediatrics* **72,** 850–856.

Six case reports with good discourse on the clinical overlap of genetically distinct forms of cutis laxa. The authors suggested X-linked dominant inheritance because there had been to date no reports of affected males. In a follow-up letter, Karrar (*Pediatrics* **74,** 903, 1984) substantiated autosomal recessive inheritance in one family, and, in subsequent papers, affected males have been described.

Sephel, G.C., Byers, P.H., Holbrook, K.A., and Davidson, J.M. (1989). Heterogeneity of elastin expression in cutis laxa fibroblast strains. *J. Invest. Dermatol.* **93,** 147–153.

No consistent correlation of biochemical findings and clinical presentation in six cases of presumed autosomal recessive cutis laxa, five of whom had both skin and systemic findings.

PSEUDOXANTHOMA ELASTICUM (MIM:177850, 177860, 264800, 264810)

(Gronblad-Strandberg)

Includes Elastosis Perforans Serpiginosa

DERMATOLOGIC FEATURES

MAJOR. Small, yellow confluent papules coalesce to form plaques at the nape, in the axillae, and the antecubital and popliteal fossae. Periumbilical and inguinal areas may also be involved. The skin changes mimic those of solar elastosis. The skin may develop a cobblestoned or plucked chicken skin appearance. The skin changes are usually not recognized until puberty or later, although they may develop unnoticed earlier. The skin can become loose and inelastic. The nasolabial and perioral folds can become exaggerated.

Similar changes can occur in the mucosa. These consist of yellowish cobblestoning of all mucosal surfaces. The gastrointestinal mucosa can also be involved.

MINOR. Elastosis perforans serpiginosa occurs in about 4% of patients with pseudoxanthoma elasticum (PXE). Elastosis perforans serpiginosa consists of annular grouped papules that bleed when unroofed and extrude a calcified material.

Calcinosis cutis has also been described. Pruritis is an occasional complaint.

ASSOCIATED ABNORMALITIES

Angioid streaks in the retina are red-gray to yellow thin lines resembling vessels, but do not originate in the optic disc. They occur in over 90% of patients. More than 50% of patients with angioid streaks will have PXE. A peau d'orange fundus with mottling is found in almost all patients. These changes are usually present by age 30 years and are rare before age 10 years.

Drusen are described in approximately 50% of patients. Visual loss due to subretinal hemorrhage occurs in about 30% of patients.

Gastrointestinal manifestations include ulcers and hemorrhage. Eight percent of patients will have suffered a gastrointestinal hemorrhage by age 30 years.

Cardiovascular abnormalities include arteriosclerosis, angina, hypertension, and claudication. Their frequency varies markedly among studies.

Cerebrovascular complications are rare. Approximately 1% of patients in the literature have had strokes. There have been a number of reports describing neuropsychiatric symptoms, but an increase in psychiatric disease has not been demonstrated in unselected series.

HISTOPATHOLOGY

LIGHT. Calcified and irregular fragmented elastic fibers in the lower papillary and reticular dermis along with calcium deposition is typical. These features are common to the vessels and the dermis. Calcification in the vessels involves both the elastic media and the intima, and involvement is usually patchy.

EM. Fine, granular calcification of elastic fibers. Electron dense septae criss-cross the center of the fibers. Collagen florettes were described in one study.

BASIC DEFECT

Unknown.

TREATMENT

None. Restriction of dietary calcium has been proposed because two studies have suggested a

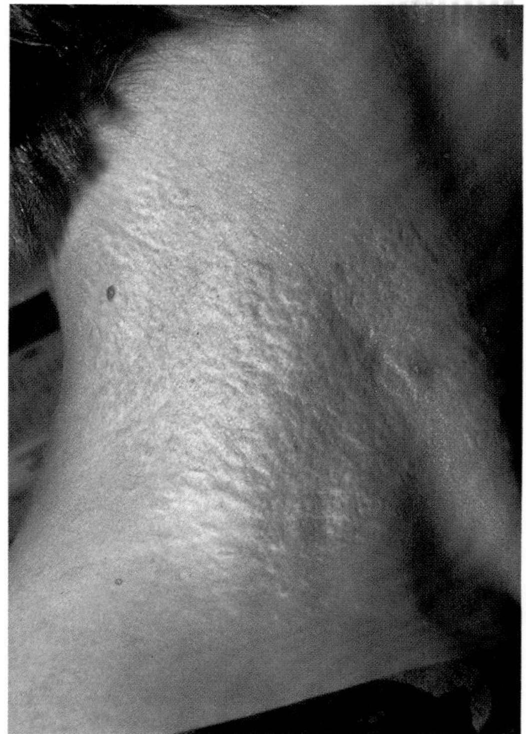
A

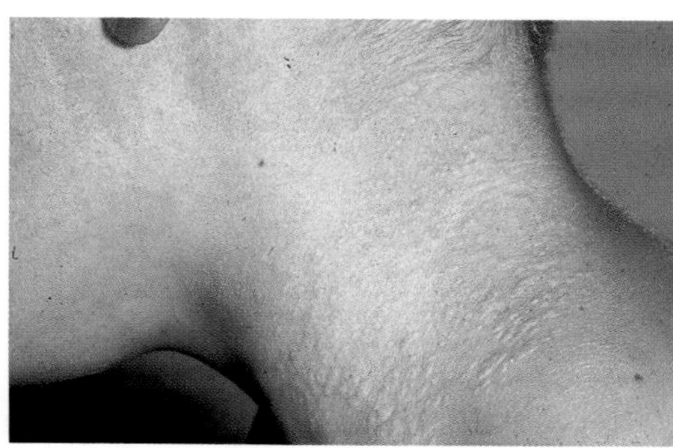
B

Figure 5.32. Severe **(A)**, moderate **(B)**, and subtle **(C)** changes. (Courtesy of Division of Dermatology, University of Washington.)

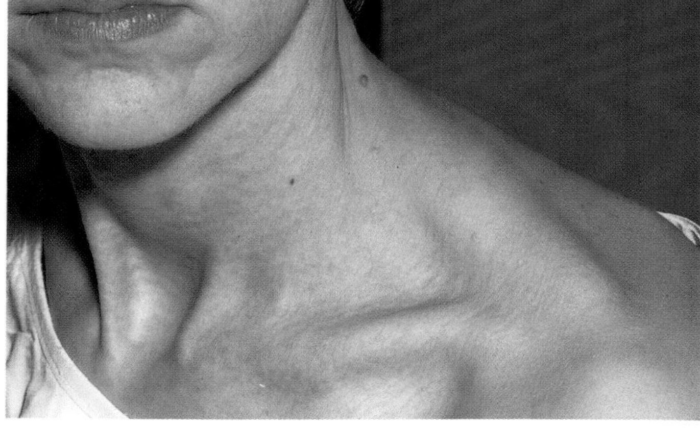
C

correlation of severity with a history of high calcium intake in childhood and adolescence. There is, however, no correlation of severity with calcium intake in adult life. No long-term studies of calcium restriction have been published. Cosmetic surgery for skin changes has been successful. Laser therapy for ocular involvement may be of benefit in some instances.

MODE OF INHERITANCE

Heterogeneous. Autosomal dominant and autosomal recessive. The delineation by Pope (1975) into four distinct groups (two autosomal recessive, two autosomal dominant) has not been substantiated by others. There are numerous pedigrees with recurrence among siblings born to unaffected parents, as well as pedigrees

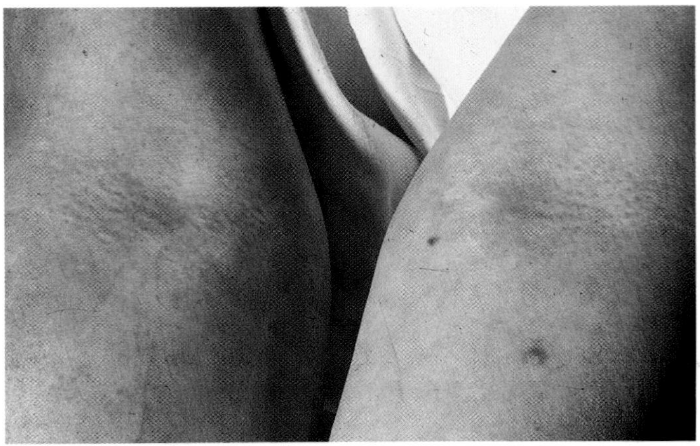

Figure 5.33. Subtle thickening of skin of the antecubital fossa. (Courtesy of Division of Dermatology, University of Washington.)

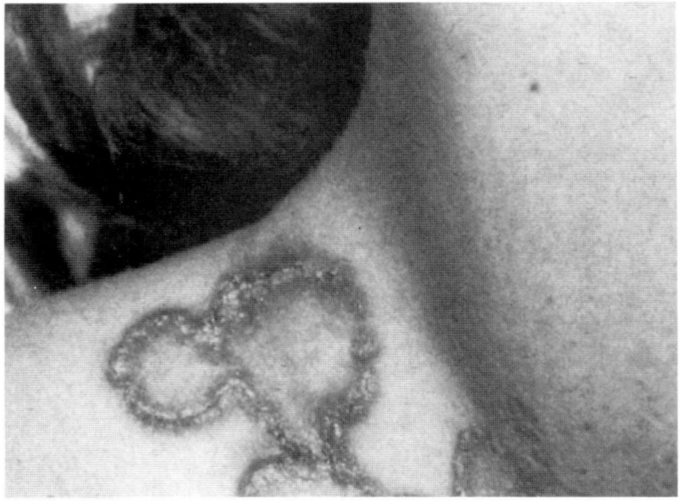

Figure 5.34. Elastosis serpignosa perforans. (From van Joost et al., 1988.)

that show vertical transmission. There appears to be a distinct subset of PXE within a population in South Africa for which a founder effect has been postulated.

PRENATAL DIAGNOSIS

None.

DIFFERENTIAL DIAGNOSIS

Angioid streaks can be isolated or seen in association with other systemic diseases. They are rarely reported in senile or solar elastosis, which would be the only dermatologic condition in which concern for PXE might be raised. Solar elastosis is indistinguishable from PXE, but changes occurring in nonsun-exposed areas would suggest the latter diagnosis. Elastosis perforans serpiginosa (MIM:130100) can be seen in Marfan syndrome (MIM:154700) and has also been described in Ehlers-Danlos syndrome type IV (MIM:130050). A few families have been described with possible autosomal dominant or recessive inheritance of elastosis perforans serpiginosa alone. Other clinical features should easily eliminate these other conditions.

L-tryptophan–induced eosinophilia-myalgia syndrome and D-penicillamine therapy can be associated with similar skin changes.

Support Group: National Association for Pseudoxanthoma Elasticum (NAPE)
1420 Ogden Street
Denver, CO 80218-1910
1-303-832-5055

SELECTED BIBLIOGRAPHY

Aessopos, A., Savvides, P., Stamatelos, G., Rombos, I., Tassiopoulos, T., Karagiorga, M., Kaklamanis, P., and Fessas, P. (1992). Pseudoxanthoma elasticum-like skin lesions and angioid streaks in beta-thalassemia. *Am. J. Hematol.* **41,** 159–164.

Twenty-six of 100 individuals with β-thalassemia had angioid streaks or PXE changes or both. Presence of features correlated with increasing age. The causal relationship between these findings remains unexplained.

Hauser, I., and Anton-Lamprecht, I. (1991). Early preclinical diagnosis of dominant pseudoxanthoma elasticum by specific ultrastructural changes of dermal elastic and collagen tissue in a family at risk. *Hum. Genet.* **87,** 693–700.

Despite the authors' claims, reliability of preclinical diagnosis by ultrastructure evaluation remains, in my opinion, quite uncertain. Others have not been as successful as these authors.

Neldner, K.H. (1988). Pseudoxanthoma elasticum. *Clin. Dermatol.* **6,** 1–159.

The entire volume is devoted to pseudoxanthoma elasticum. This is a study of 100 individuals specifically referred for the disease. There are many color photos of varying quality. The author claims that 90% of the patients had a family history consistent with autosomal recessive disease, but he included in this number all isolated cases. Of 88 families, nine parent pairs were consanguineous, seven sibships had more than one affected member, and three had affected cousins. There were three parent–offspring pairs and nine other with possible parental involvement. It is impossible from the description given to actually generate appropriate proportions for dominant and recessive inheritance. Neldner argues against Pope's (1975) classification. He suggests that the severity of the skin findings correlates with the severity of involvement of other organs. Recommendations for care are given.

Pope, F.M. (1975) Historical evidence for the genetic heterogeneity of pseudoxanthoma elasticum. *Br. J. Dermatol.,* **92,** 493–509.

One of a series of articles by Pope. He believes that differences in skin findings and severity of eye findings can distinguish 4 subtypes of pseudoxanthoma elasticum.

Viljoen, D.L., Beatty, S., and Beighton, P. (1987). The obstetric and gynaecological implications of pseudoxanthoma elasticum. *Br. J. Obstet. Gynaecol.* **94,** 884–888.

An increased risk of first trimester loss, but otherwise no significant adverse outcomes noted in 54 pregnancies. The limitation of the study is that all patients were from a South African population, a subset of which the authors believe have a distinct form of PXE. The information regarding the origin of this population is not presented in the paper cited but in another paper by the authors. All probands had presumably autosomal recessive PXE.

VASCULAR

ATAXIA TELANGIECTASIA (MIM:208900)

(Louis-Bar Syndrome)

DERMATOLOGIC FEATURES

Major. Telangiectases of the face and bulbar conjunctiva first appear at about age 3 years and increase in number throughout life. The conjunctiva are usually the first to be involved. The telangiectases are symmetric and involve the canthal areas overlying the sclerae. The cutaneous telangiectases are often in a butterfly distribution across the face, on the eyelids, and on the ears, developing first in sun-exposed regions. The neck, hands, feet, and popliteal and antecubital fossae may become involved over time.

Minor. Premature graying of the hair is described in more than 50% of the reported patients. Mottled hyperpigmentation and hypopigmentation and poikiloderma are common.

Café-au-lait spots have been described in some patients, but are probably not a significant or specific feature.

Seborrheic dermatitis, atopic dermatitis, and xerosis are more common among patients with ataxia telangiectasia than in the general population. Smith and Conerly (1985) suggest that these features may be more frequent in chronic central nervous system disorders in general and may not be specific for ataxia telangiectasia.

ASSOCIATED ABNORMALITIES

Cerebellar ataxia is often the first presenting sign of ataxia telangiectasia, with onset at about 1 year of age and progression thereafter. Loss of developmental milestones usually does not occur, but intellectual progress may plateau before adolescence. Some studies suggest a gradual decline in intellectual function. Most adolescents and adults are wheelchair bound. Choreoathetoid movements are the rule, and the diagnosis of cerebral palsy is often mistakenly applied until the classic skin lesions manifest and are recognized. Dysarthria is common. The ataxia is believed to be caused by white matter degeneration. The brain shows loss of Purkinje cells, granular cells, and basket cells in the cerebellum, along with degeneration of the dentate and olivary nuclei. The spinal cord may show loss of anterior horn cells and posterior and lateral column degeneration.

Nystagmus, strabismus, and abnormal eye movements are found in the majority of patients.

Immunodeficiency is the rule in ataxia telangiectasia, the basis of which is unknown. There are defects in IgA, IgE and cellular immunity. Lymphopenia is common. Recurrent infections, especially upper respiratory, are common, reported in 50%–80% of patients.

Generalized lymphadenopathy is typical. Lymphoreticular malignancy (leukemia, lymphoma) occurs in 10% of patients; 90% of these develop before age 20 years. Liver, ovarian, and brain tumors have also occurred. Patients with ataxia telangiectasia have increased susceptibility to γ-radiation, evidenced clinically by a high incidence of cancer after irradiation and in vitro by a variety of defects in DNA repair and increased cell death after radiation. Spontaneous chromosome breakage in cultured cells with resultant translocations, rings, markers, and rearrangement is more frequent in ataxia telangiectasia cells than in normal cells. These spontaneous rearrangements often involve chromosomes 7 and 14. A variety of malignancies in ataxia telangiectasia patients are also often associated with translocations involving chromosomes 7 and 14. It has been

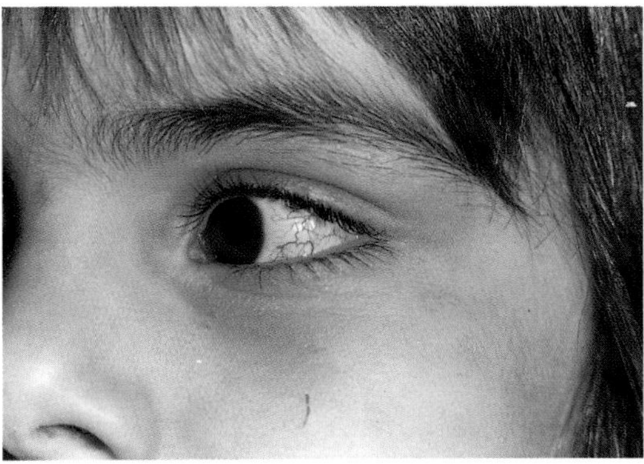

Figure 5.35. Telangiectases on bulbar conjunctiva in 6 year old.

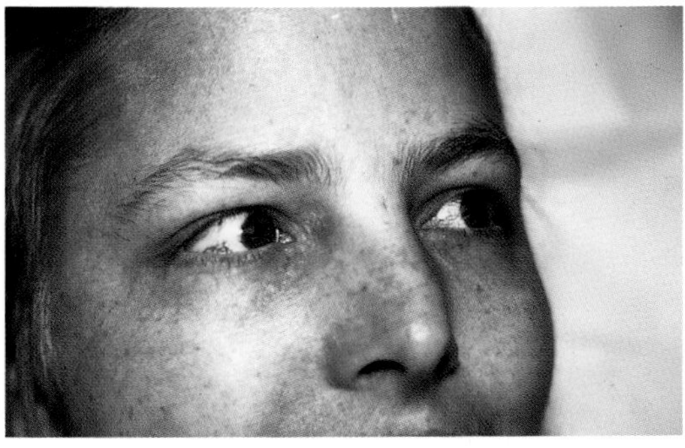

Figure 5.36. Cutaneous and conjunctival telangiectases. (Courtesy of Dr. H. Ochs, Seattle, Washington.)

suggested that heterozygotes for ataxia telangiectasia (estimated at 2.8% [0.6%–7.7%] of the population) may be at increased risk to develop cancer, especially of the breast.

Serum α-fetoprotein is elevated. It has been proposed that there is a general defect in mesodermal–endodermal interactions in ataxia telangiectasia, manifested by an immature liver that produces α-fetoprotein throughout life, persistence of carcinoembryonic antigen, and an immature thymus.

Insulin resistance and glucose intolerance are reported in over 50% of patients.

Mortality in the first two decades is the rule, caused by malignancy, infection, or progressive neurologic deterioration. A handful of patients have survived into their forties and fifties.

HISTOPATHOLOGY

Light. There are numerous, greatly dilated vessels in the upper dermis that arise from the subpapillary venous plexus.
EM. No information.

BASIC DEFECT

Unknown. Linkage to 11q22–23 has been established for all ataxia telangiectasia complementation groups, and mutations in a candidate gene, *ATM,* have been identified.

TREATMENT

None specific. Avoidance of exposure to irradiation is important. Administration of levamisole to improve immune function has been tried with minimal and anecdotal success.

Thymosin F-5, which stimulates T-cell production, did not alter the course of the disease in three patients with ataxia telangiectasia.

Good pulmonary toilet may be helpful in patients with chronic obstructive pulmonary disease.

MODE OF INHERITANCE

Autosomal recessive. Carrier detection by increased susceptibility of cultured cells to x-rays and bleomycin, a radiomimetic chemical, may not be accurate, as there is overlap with the low normal range.

PRENATAL DIAGNOSIS

Prenatal diagnosis has been performed for ataxia telangiectasia based on elevated levels of a "clastogenic factor" in amniotic fluid and increased chromosome breakage and a translocation involving chromosome 14 in amniotic cell culture. γ-radiation of both chorionic villus tissue and derived chorionic villus cell cultures from a fetus at risk demonstrated normal levels compared with an ataxia telangiectasia control.

Normal findings were confirmed by amniocyte and subsequent lymphocyte studies. Concern has been raised about the potential for false-positive results in heterozygous fetuses. With identification of the gene, both linkage and direct DNA studies should be possible.

DIFFERENTIAL DIAGNOSIS

Bloom syndrome (MIM:210900), Rothmund-Thomson syndrome (MIM:268400), essential or hereditary telangiectasia (MIM:187260), Cockayne syndrome (MIM:216400, 216410, 216411), Fanconi anemia (MIM:227650, 227660), systemic lupus erythematosus (MIM: 152700), and hereditary hemorrhagic telangiectasia (MIM:187300) all share facial telangiectasia in common with ataxia telangiectasia; none of them is associated with ataxia. The telangiectasia of hereditary hemorrhagic telangiectasia do not usually involve the bulbar conjunctiva. Hemorrhage and bleeding are not usually seen in ataxia telangiectasia, whereas they are common in hereditary hemorrhagic telangiectasia.

Other cerebellar ataxias (MIM:Many) can be difficult to differentiate from ataxia telangiectasia prior to the onset of skin manifestations. The presence of low IgA levels, high carcinoembryonic antigen and α-fetoprotein levels and other immunologic abnormalities of ataxia telangiectasia may help to distinguish it from other hereditary ataxias.

Support Group:

A-T Children's Project
21645 Cartagena Drive
Boca Raton, FL 33428
1-800-543-5728

National Ataxia Foundation (NAF)
15500 Wayzata Blvd., No. 750
Wayzata, MN 55391
1-612-473-7666

SELECTED BIBLIOGRAPHY

Bridges, B.A., and Harnden, D.G. (eds.) (1982). *Ataxia Telangiectasia: A Cellular and Molecular Link Between Cancer, Neuropathology, and Immune Deficiency.* John Wiley & Sons, New York.

Report of a workshop on ataxia telangiectasia held in 1980. Several review chapters dealing with different aspects of ataxia telangiectasia are included in addition to the presented papers.

Foroud, T., Wei, S., Ziv, Y., Sobel, E., Lange, E., Chao, A., Goradia, T., Huo, Y., Tolun, A., Chessa, L., Charmley, P., Sanal, O., Salman, N., Julier, C., Concannon, P., McConville, C., Taylor, A.M.R., Shiloh, Y., Lange, K., and Gatti, R.A. (1991). Localization of an ataxia telangiectasia locus to a 3-cM interval on chromosome 11q23: linkage analysis of 111 families by an international consortium. *Am. J. Hum. Genet.* **49,** 1263–1279.

One hundred eleven families from England, Israel, Italy, Turkey, and the United States were analyzed for linkage. Ataxia telangiectasia complementation groups A, C, and D appear to be linked to this region.

Jaspers, N.G., and Bootsma, D. (1982). Genetic heterogeneity in ataxia-telangiectasia studied by cell fusion. *Proc. Natl. Acad. Sci. U.S.A.* **79,** 2641–2644.

Suggested nonallelic heterogeneity in ataxia telangiectasia by virtue of correction of defects in vitro by co-culturing of cells from different patients. Apparently a secondary phenomenon, if newer molecular work identifying a single locus proves true.

Savitsky, K., Bar-Shira, A., Gilad, S., Rotman, G., Ziv, Y., Vanagaite, L., Tagle, D.A., Smith, S., Uziel, T., Sfez, S., Ashkenazi, M., Pecker, I., Frydman, M., Harnik, R., Patanjali, S.R., Simmons, A., Clines, G.A., Sartiel, A., Gatti, R.A., Chessa, L., Sanal, O., Lavin, M.F., Jaspers, N.G.J., Taylor, A.M.R., Arlett, C.F., Miki, T., Weissman, S.M., Lovett, M., Collins, F.S., and Shiloh, Y. (1995). A single ataxia telangiectasia gene with a product similar to PI-3 kinase. *Science* **268,** 1749–1753.

The identified gene encodes a protein similar to yeast and mammalian phosphatidylinositol-3 kinases that are involved in mutagenic signal transduction, meiotic recombination, and cell cycle control. Mutations in the *ATM* gene were found in ataxia telangiectasia complementation groups A, C, D, and E. Compound heterozygotes were identified as well as homozygotes. Authors believe that there is only one ataxia telangiectasia locus and no locus heterogeneity.

Shaham, M., Voss, R., Becker, Y., Yarkoni, S., Ornoy, A., and Kohn, G. (1982). Prenatal diagnosis of ataxia telangiectasia. *J. Pediatr.* **100,** 134–137.

Prenatal diagnosis reported and confirmed by demonstration of increased susceptibility to x-ray in amniotic membrane cells cultured post-termination.

Smith, L.L., and Conerly, S.L. (1985). Ataxia-telangiectasia or Louis-Bar syndrome. *J. Am. Acad. Dermatol.* **12,** 681–696.

Report of two sisters and review article with 70 references. The difference in severity between the siblings was striking, both were severely neurologically involved, but only one had recurrent infections.

Swift, M., Morrell, D., Cromartie, E., Chamberlin, A.R., Skolnick, M.H., and Bishop, D.T. (1986). The incidence and gene frequency of ataxia-telangiectasia in the United States. *Am. J. Hum. Genet.* **39,** 573–583.

An attempt to identify all United States cases with ataxia telangiectasia between 1970 and 1977 and 1980 and 1984 to estimate gene frequency.

Swift, M., Morrell, D., Massey, R.B., and Chase, C.L. (1991). Incidence of cancer in 161 families affected by ataxia telangiectasia. *N. Engl. J. Med.* **325,** 1831–1836.

Prospective study (mean 6.4 years) of 1,599 blood relatives and 821 spouses. Risk of cancer in female relatives was 5.1 for breast and 3.5 for all compared with controls; for male relatives, relative risk for cancer was 3.8. Female relatives with breast cancer had significantly greater exposure to ionizing radiation than female relatives without cancer. First and second degree relatives were included; great-grandparents were included in consanguineous families. Concerns regarding methodology are voiced in letters (*N. Engl. J. Med.* **326,**1357–1361, 1992).

Woods, C.G., Bundey, S.E., and Taylor, A.M.R. (1990). Unusual features in the inheritance of ataxia telangiectasia. *Hum. Genet.* **84,** 555–562.

A study in West Midlands found prevalence to be 1 in 514,000, with a birth frequency of 1 in 300,000. Evaluation of 47 families including three with "atypical" disease revealed less than the expected number of consanguineous matings and fewer than expected affected siblings. The authors posit other modes of inheritance, such as new dominant mutations, for some individuals with ataxia telangiectasia. The statistical methods are confusing to me, and I am not sure how compelling their data are.

BLUE RUBBER BLEB NEVUS SYNDROME (MIM:112200)

(Bean Syndrome)

DERMATOLOGIC FEATURES

MAJOR. The rubbery, compressible blue-purple nodules of this syndrome are unusual vascular malformations with dilated vascular spaces. These are pathognomonic in their clinical appearance. When compressed, they are wrinkled, empty sacs, and there is a palpable defect in the underlying soft tissue. They rapidly refill. They range in size from millimeters to centimeters. Although occasionally present at birth, the nodules usually appear in childhood. New lesions develop throughout life and may number in the hundreds.

MINOR. Hyperhidrosis of the overlying skin has been an inconstant finding, as has been spontaneous pain. Significant soft tissue enlargement can occur and has led to amputation in a minority of cases.

ASSOCIATED ABNORMALITIES

Visceral involvement is common. The small bowel is the usual site, but the entire gastrointestinal tract may be affected. Gastrointestinal bleeding can occur. At autopsy, one affected

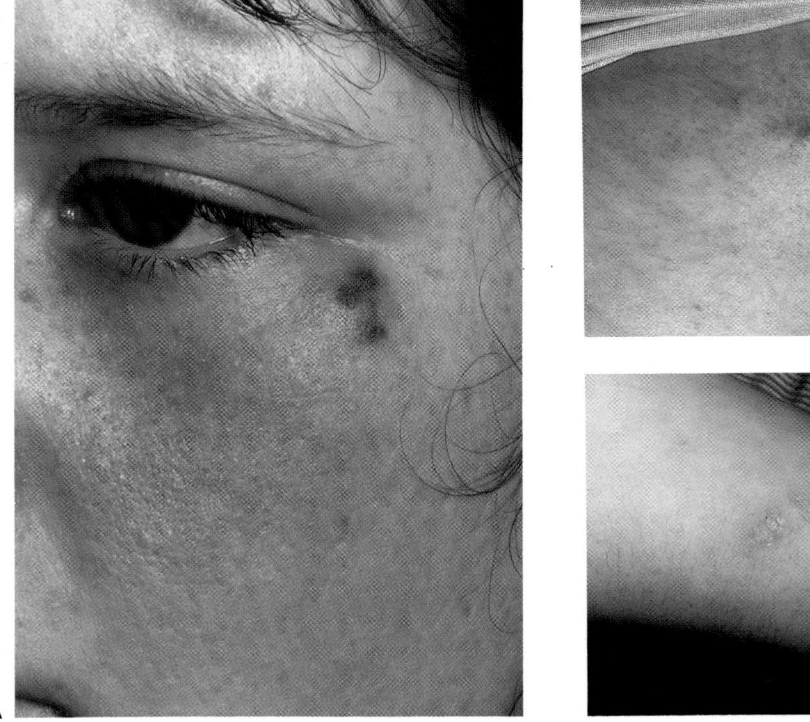

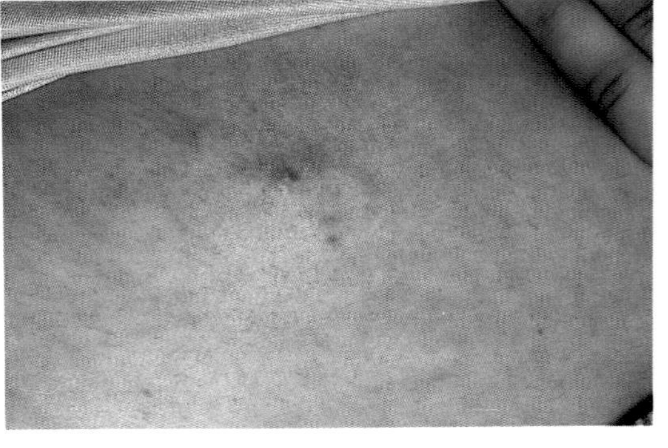

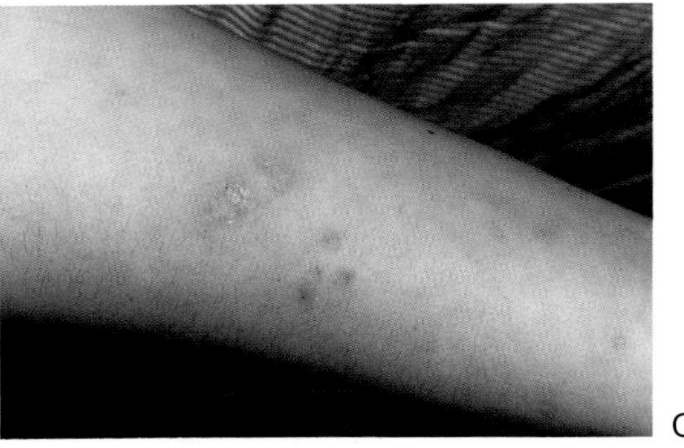

Figure 5.37. Young girl with scattered lesions on face **(A)**, trunk **(B)**, and arm **(C)**. Scaly patches on arm are unrelated.

individual had lesions in lung, pleura, peritoneum, and skeletal muscle. Another had similar vascular malformations on the cerebral surface, in the heart, and in the pericardium.

HISTOPATHOLOGY

Light. Lesions are histiologically cavernous vascular malformations marked by dilated vascular spaces lined by a thin endothelial layer and a thin rim of fibrous tissue that appears almost epithelial. They are separated by smooth muscle or connective fibrous tissue. They may be in the dermis or subcutaneous tissue. There may be increased numbers of sweat glands.

EM. Marked elongation of endothelial cells and pericytes. Cell organelles appear normal.

BASIC DEFECT

Unknown.

TREATMENT

Surgical excision of individual lesions is possible. Successful ablation with the carbon dioxide laser has been reported. Periodic stool guaiac testing to detect occult bleeding that might result in chronic anemia is reasonable. Unless patients are symptomatic, excision of lesions is not warranted.

MODE OF INHERITANCE

Autosomal dominant. Sporadic cases are more common than familial and probably represent new dominant mutations.

PRENATAL DIAGNOSIS

None.

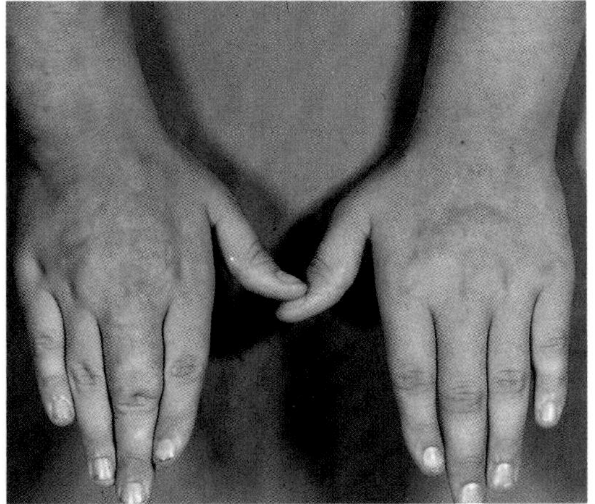

A

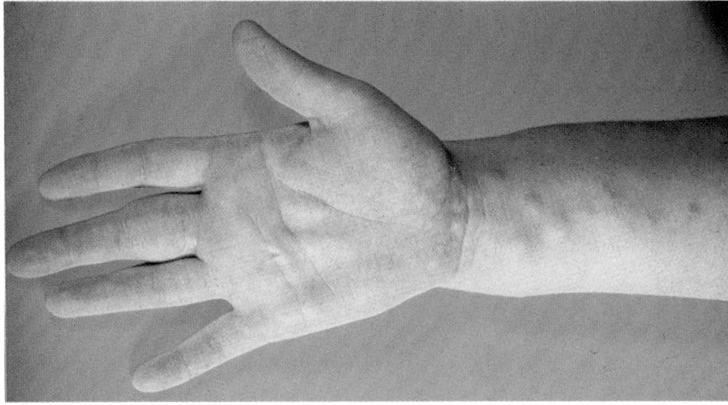

B

Figure 5.38. **(A)** Adult with enlargement of middle finger; larger vascular mass is on hand. **(B)** Color of lesions on the arm is not as strikingly blue.

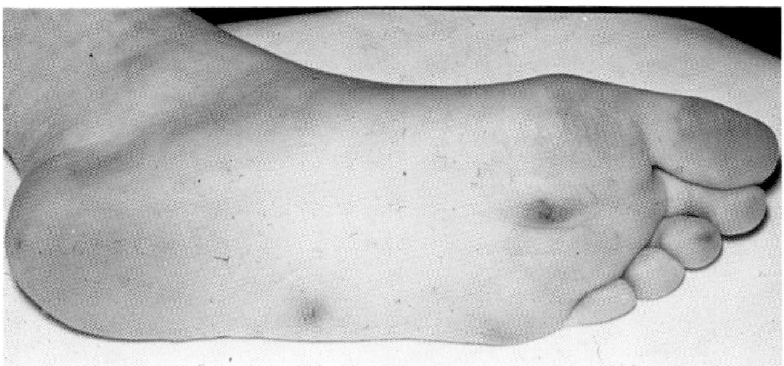

Figure 5.39. Foot lesions in a third patient. (Courtesy of Division of Dermatology, University of Washington.)

DIFFERENTIAL DIAGNOSIS

Hereditary hemorrhagic telangiectasia (Osler-Weber-Rendu, MIM:187300): The skin lesions of hereditary hemorrhagic telangiectasia are flat to slightly raised and not the compressible sacs of the blue rubber bleb nevus syndrome.

Multiple glomus tumors (MIM:138000): The glomus tumors may appear clinically similar, but are often spontaneously painful and do not compress through dermal defects as do blue rubber bleb nevi.

Maffucci syndrome (MIM:166000): The hemangiomas of Maffucci syndrome (enchondromatosis with multiple hemangiomas) may give a similar appearance to blue rubber blebs. The bony abnormalities of Maffucci are distinctive.

Klippel-Trenaunay-Weber syndrome (MIM: 149000): Can be confused with severe blue rubber bleb nevus syndrome; somatic overgrowth and the lack of visceral involvement in the former and the widespread blue cutaneous lesions of the latter distinguish the two.

Support Group: N.O.R.D.
P.O. Box 8923
New Fairfield, CT 06812
1-800-999-6673

SELECTED REFERENCES

Bean, W.B. (1958). *Vascular Spiders and Related Lesions of the Skin.* Charles C. Thomas, Springfield, IL.

A wonderful book recounting Dr. Bean's experiences and observations of blood vessel changes, both normal and pathologic.

Fine, R.M., Derbes, V.J., and Clark, C.O.H., Jr. (1961). Blue rubber bleb nevus. *Arch. Dermatol.* **84,** 802–805.

Case report of one child with blue rubber bleb nevus, with an extensive description of the histopathologic features of the disorder.

Gallione, C.J., Pasyk, K.A., Boon, L.M., Lennon, F., Johnson, D.W., Helmbold, E.A., Markel, D.S., Vikkula, M., Mulliken, J.B., Warman, M.L., Pericak-Vance, M.A., and Marchuk, D.A. (1995). A gene for familial venous malformations maps to chromosome 9p in a second large kindred. *J. Med. Genet.* **32,** 197–199.

Demonstrated linkage to 9p in a second large family with venous malformations and a clinical picture similar to but not identical with blue rubber bleb nevus syndrome. Authors speculate that familial venous malformations is an umbrella diagnosis that subsumes the blue rubber bleb nevus syndrome.

Gallo, S.H., and McClave, S.A. (1992). Blue rubber bleb nevus syndrome: gastrointestinal involvement and its endoscopic presentation. *Gastrointest. Endosc.* **38,** 72–76.

Succinct review with 33 references and color photographs of intestinal lesions.

Olsen, T.G., Milroy, S.K., Goldman, L., and Fidler, J.P. (1979). Laser surgery for blue rubber bleb nevus. *Arch. Dermatol.* **115,** 81–82.

Report of one patient treated successfully with the CO_2 laser.

Talbot, S., and Wyatt, E.H. (1970). Blue rubber bleb nevi (report of a family in which only males were affected). *Br. J. Dermatol.* **82,** 37–39.

Three generations with only affected males. One female presumed heterozygote by pedigree had no findings by history. She was not examined.

Walshe, M.M., Evans, C.D., and Warin, R.P. (1966) Blue rubber bleb nevus. *Br. Med. J.* **2,** 931–932.

A report of two pedigrees with blue rubber bleb nevus syndrome.

CUTIS MARMORATA TELANGIECTATICA CONGENITA (MIM:219250)

(Congenital Generalized Phlebectasia; Nevus Vascularis Reticularis; Congenital Livedo Reticularis)

DERMATOLOGIC FEATURES

MAJOR. Cutis marmorata telangiectatica congenita (CMTC) is classically defined by the presence at birth of a persistent reticular vascular pattern resulting in a marbled appearance of the skin. The vascular markings are dark, often with overlying loss of dermal substance, so that the drop-off from normal to involved areas is palpable. Epidermal atrophy and ulceration may also occur. The pattern of involvement mimics the normal cutis marmorata of the newborn seen with exposure to cold, but differs in its constancy and actual loss of tissue substance. Its similarity to the livedo reticularis of acquired disease gives CMTC one of its synonyms. The condition improves in the first year of life, with more than 50% of patients showing diminution of the vascular markings and resolution of cutaneous atrophy and 20% showing complete resolution.

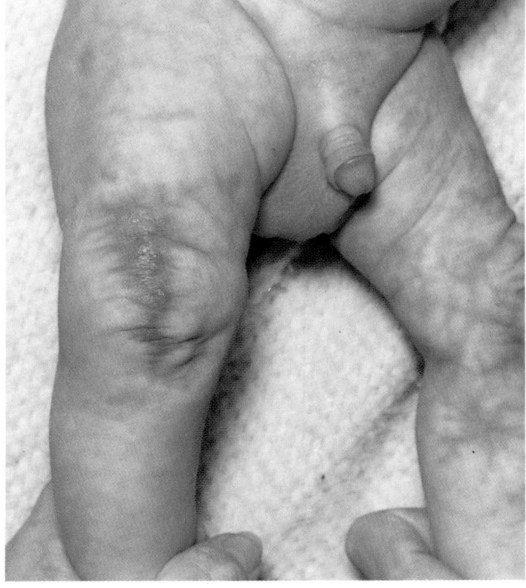

Figure 5.40. Vascular changes with overlying hyperkeratosis on the right knee. Livedo reticularis pattern on the other leg.

Males and females appear to be affected with equal frequency. Involvement is often unilateral and limited to a single extremity, but bilateral and truncal involvement is not unusual. In approximately 10% of reported cases, atrophy of the involved limb has been described; this feature may also ameliorate with time.

It is my impression, from the literature and personal experience with a handful of patients, that there is a subtype of CMTC that is clinically distinct but difficult to appreciate. Such affected children appear to have widespread telangiectatic-like lacy capillary vascular malformations more like a diffuse nevus flammeus than cutis marmorata. The configuration of the lesions is similar to the pattern of CMTC, but the lesions differ in that there is no atrophy and no significant resolution, and associated hypertrophy of the involved area can be seen. When involving the first branch of the trigeminal nerve, glaucoma has been reported. It may be that these children actually have a variation of the Klippel-Trenaunay-Weber or Sturge Weber syndromes, but clinical categorization into one or the other category is difficult.

This separation of CMTC into two types is

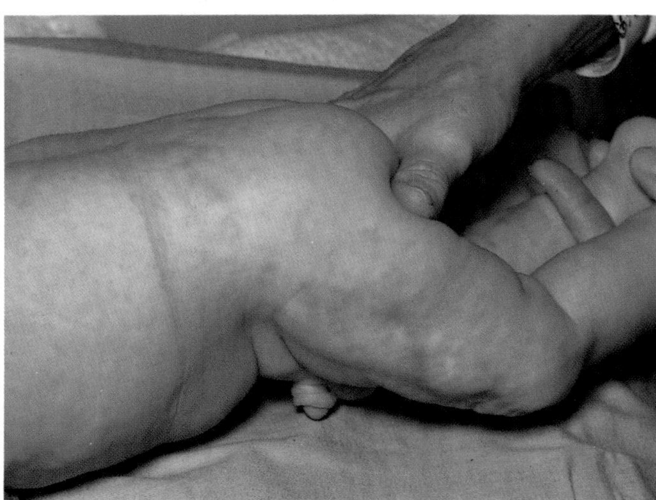

Figure 5.41. Loss of substance on thigh in same patient as in Fig. 5.40.

not generally accepted, and in most reviews of the condition they are lumped together. This results in mistakenly predicting a risk for hemihypertrophy in classic CMTC. When the finer diffuse capillary changes are present, the risk is greater for overgrowth, glaucoma, seizures, and mental retardation. When the larger, darker vascular pattern more typical of livedo reticularis is present, atrophy is more likely and the other complications are rarer.

MINOR. Hyperkeratosis and hyperpigmentation have been described in one patient with the nevus flammeus variant of CMTC.

Angiokeratomas were described in one patient whose clinical description does not fit, in my opinion, with CMTC, despite being given the diagnostic label.

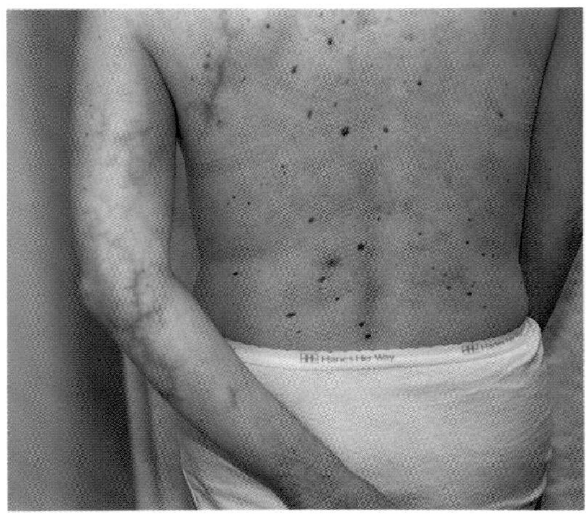

Figure 5.42. Persistence of vascular lakes and channels on arms and upper back of adult. The dysplastic nevi are an unrelated finding.

ASSOCIATED ABNORMALITIES

Hemiatrophy of the involved limb is common, seen in more than 10% of reported cases. The atrophy involves limb length and girth, is usually mild, and improves with time.

Hemihypertrophy has been noted in several case reports and subsequently referred to in reviews. However, in most, although there was overgrowth, it was of the uninvolved limb, i.e., there was atrophy of the extremity with the vascular lesion. In one patient with bilateral generalized CMTC, unilateral hypertrophy occurred. In the remaining case reports of hypertrophy where photographs were published, all had the nevus flammeus type of reticular telangiectatic vascular change, suggesting that they were variants of Klippel-Trenaunay-Weber syndrome rather than CMTC. As pointed out by Stephan et al. (1975), CMTC, Klippel-Trenaunay-Weber syndrome, and Sturge-Weber syndrome may all be part of a spectrum of malformation syndromes caused by vascular aberrations with significant overlap and artificial distinctions.

Porencephalic cysts have been reported in two patients with CMTC, one of whom also had generalized cutaneous fibromatosis. The other patient had a cerebrovascular malformation. In the absence of neurologic signs, computed tomographic scan, magnetic resonance imaging, or cranial ultrasound does not seem warranted in infants with CMTC.

Macrocephaly was reported by Stephan et al. (1975) in four patients with CMTC. One of these, however, also had multiple flame nevi, hemangiomas, and subcutaneous masses. The photos of a second child demonstrated a reticular nevus flammeus, and a third child, in addition to persistent cutis marmorata, had a widespread midline port wine stain of the face with minor involvement of the neck and thorax. Parental head circumferences were not mentioned for any of the children.

Glaucoma has been reported in several infants; in all but one there was a nevus flammeus in the distribution of the first branch of the trigeminal nerve. Both increased episcleral venous pressure and an abnormal angle structure have been imputed as causes for glaucoma. All infants with CMTC and facial lesions deserve an eye examination.

Mental retardation has been mentioned in approximately 10% of reported cases of CMTC. However, one patient also had a cleft palate, one had Turner syndrome, one had a porencephalic cyst, and two had large midline facial port wine stains, one of whom was a 33 week premature who developed hydrocephalus requiring shunt placement. Two cases were

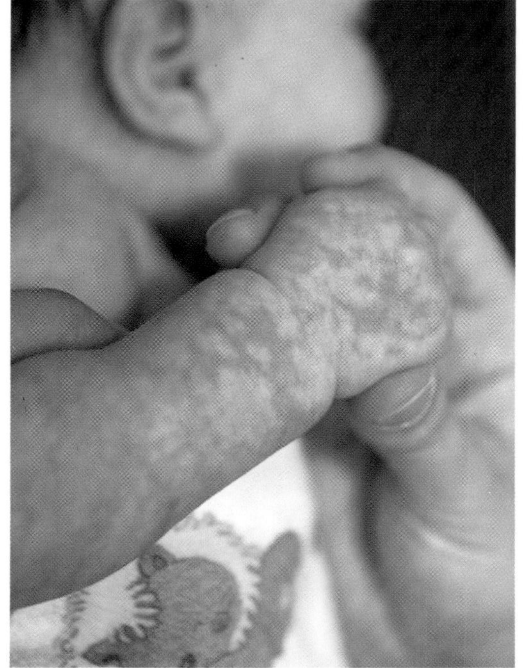

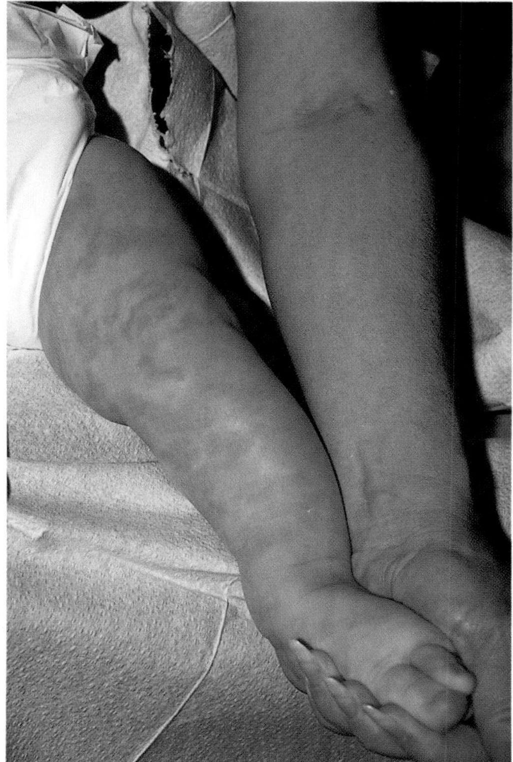

Figure 5.43. **(A)** Arm and **(B)** leg of patient showing lacy reticular vascular pattern.

brothers who developed progressive dementia in adult life and corticomeningeal angiomatosis, hyper- and hypopigmentation of the skin, abnormal patches of body hair, and telangiectatic vascular lesions distributed along the lines of Blaschko. The diagnosis of CMTC in these brothers (which was not made by the authors but applied in subsequent reviews) seems inappropriate. One infant who at 14 months was normal on Denver Developmental Screening except for a "five month delay in language" has been characterized as mentally retarded in subsequent reviews, but no follow-up data are available. The risk for mental retardation in classic CMTC is probably less than the 10% cited and appears to be greatest in those infants with facial port wine stains or with features outside the usual scope of CMTC.

HISTOPATHOLOGY

LIGHT. The findings are nonspecific. The epidermis is usually spared, but atrophy, acanthosis, and hyperkeratosis have been described. Dilated vascular spaces, both capillary and venous, lined by swollen epithelial cells, are seen in the dermis. Lymphatic channels may also be dilated, and vascular fibrosis can be seen.

EM. Vascular spaces are lined by primitive embryonic cells without an investing basement membrane or can appear to be normal. One report described an increase in the number of pericytes; in another, vacuolated Weibel-Palade granules in the endothelial cells were described.

BASIC DEFECT

Unknown. This condition is most likely causally heterogeneous. Causal hypotheses have included environmental agents and postzygotic mutations for otherwise lethal dominant mutations.

TREATMENT

Rarely, skin ulceration can become a chronic problem requiring treatment. Examination for glaucoma is appropriate in all infants with facial involvement. Orthopedic management of limb asymmetry.

MODE OF INHERITANCE

Sporadic. There has been one report of two affected sisters. Kurczynski (1982) reported an affected female whose father and paternal grandmother had had similar findings. Another report mentioned an aunt with hemiatrophy of a limb, another with an aunt with "a facial birthmark," and a third report noted a grandfather with a "facial birthmark." No further details were provided. The evidence for a genetic component is thus not compelling. It has been suggested that CMTC might be the result of a postzygotic lethal mutation. As generalized involvement is not rare, this hypothesis is not as well supported as it is for disorders that manifest only in a patchy distribution. The patchy appearance of CMTC may reflect more the structure of the vascular bed than the effect of tissue mosaicism. I am unaware of any follow-up studies of reproductive outcomes for individuals with CMTC.

PRENATAL DIAGNOSIS

None.

DIFFERENTIAL DIAGNOSIS

CMTC can be seen in association with aplasia cutis congenita (MIM:100300, 107600, 207700, 207730, 207731). All affected infants should be evaluated for scalp defects and/or limb defects.

Transient cutis marmorata is common in prematures and newborns and may be somewhat more persistent in infants with Down syndrome and other malformation syndromes. In all of these, the vascular pattern rapidly disappears with warming of the infant.

Diffuse genuine phlebectasia is confusing only in terminology. Clinically it is entirely distinct, marked by progressive enlargement of the limb with deep and superficial varicosities.

Klippel-Trenaunay-Weber syndrome (MIM: 149000) and Sturge-Weber syndrome (MIM: 185300) show considerable overlap with CMTC and may be difficult to differentiate from the telangiectatic form of CMTC. Overgrowth is far more common in Klippel-Trenaunay-Weber syndrome, as are lymphangiomas, varicosities, and subcutaneous hemangiomas. Seizures, mental retardation, and glaucoma, along with the typical port wine stain, define Sturge-Weber syndrome but may be seen in CMTC as well.

Support Group:

The Sturge-Weber Foundation
P.O. Box 418
Mt. Freedom, NJ 07970-0418
1-800-627-5482

Klippel-Trenaunay Support Group
4610 Wooddale Avenue
Edina, MN 55424
1-612-925-2596

The National Vascular Malformations Foundation
8320 Nightingale
Dearborn Heights, MI 48127-1202
1-313-274-1243

SELECTED BIBLIOGRAPHY

Gelmetti, C., Schianchi, R., and Ermacora, E. (1987). Cutis marmorata telangiectatica congenita. Quatre nouveaux cas et revue de la litterature. *Ann. Dermatol. Venereol.* **114,** 1517–1528.

This is an exhaustive but uncritical review of the literature. Many useful tables, but caution in interpreting numbers must be exercised, as many cases that are clinically dissimilar to CMTC (e.g., the third patient of Way, the brothers with meningeal angiomatosis) are included.

Kruczynski, T.W. (1982) Hereditary cutis

marmorata telangiectatic congenita. *Pediatr.* **70,** 52–53.

Four year old girl presented to hospital for dehydration associated with a viral syndrome. Skin findings were noted incidentally. By history, father and paternal grandmother affected; in both, improvement occurred by adulthood.

Piscascia, D.D., and Esterly, N.B. (1989). Cutis marmorata telangiectatica congenita: report of 22 cases. *J. Am. Acad. Dermatol.* **20,** 1098–1104.

This is a well-written review of the authors' experience and of the literature.

Powell, S.T., and Su, W.P.D. (1984). Cutis marmorata telangiectatica congenita. Report of nine cases and review of the literature. *Cutis* **34,** 305–312.

Pictures of two cases with telangiectatic nevus flammeus, atrophie blanche, and recurrent ulcerations are shown. One patient had mucosal involvement, which is extremely rare in CMTC.

Stephen, M.J., Hall, B.D., Smith, D.W., Cohen, M.M.Jr (1975). Macrocephaly in association with unusual cutaneous angiomatosis. *J. Pediatr.* **87,** 353-359.

Report of ten patients, four of whom were categorized as CMTC, three as Klippel-Trenaunay-Weber syndrome and three as Klippel-Trenaunay-Weber plus Sturge-Weber syndrome.

Way, B.H., Hermann, J., Gilbert, E.F., Johnson, S.A.M., and Opitz, J.M. (1974). Cutis marmorata telangiectatica congenita. *J. Cutan. Pathol.* **1,** 10–25.

Case reports, one with typical CMTC and atrophy, and one with unilateral telangiectatic port wine stain and hemihypertrophy, and a last with diffuse angiokeratomas and subcutaneous venous hemangiomata. All three patients were different clinically, and all are lumped together under the rubric CMTC. The paper includes a tabular review of the literature.

FABRY SYNDROME (MIM:301500)

(Angiokeratoma Corporis Diffusum; α-Galactosidase A Deficiency)

DERMATOLOGIC FEATURES

MAJOR. The vascular lesions of this disorder, which give it one of its names, appear in mid-childhood, often in the bathing trunks region. They are small macules and papules, bluish to red to dark purple-black in color. They rarely occur on the hands, feet, or face. The surface of the papules may appear slightly scaly or with a fine translucent, parchment-like wrinkling of the overlying epidermis.

The oral mucosa may also be involved; the top of the tongue is usually spared, while the underside is involved.

Vasomotor function of the skin is abnormal, with acquired hypohidrosis and heat intolerance reported in upwards of two-thirds of affected males.

MINOR. Edema, with onset prior to renal and cardiac disease, may be the first presenting sign.

ASSOCIATED ABNORMALITIES

Episodic pain and paresthesia of the extremities, primarily in the fingers and toes, and acute intermittent abdominal pain are classic features that often begin in childhood. These complaints are also common in heterozygote females.

Neurologic involvement may be primary, due to damage from storage of glycosphingolipids within the neuronal cytoplasm, or secondary, caused by premature cerebrovascular disease, possibly on the basis of vascular occlusion or thrombosis. Neurologic symptoms include vertigo, tinnitus, hearing loss, and long tract signs.

Renal involvement leads ultimately to renal failure, a major cause of death, the mean age of which is in the forties. Cardiac abnormalities, including conduction defects, infiltration of cardiac muscle, and valvular disease, are typical in early adult life. Asymptomatic corneal dystrophy (cornea verticullata) with fine opacities is common in affected males and in carrier females. There is decreased fertility in males.

HISTOPATHOLOGY

LIGHT. There is minimal hyperkeratosis with dilation of capillaries in the dermal papillae and lipid deposition in the endothelial cells and pericytes.

EM. Many cell types contain intracytoplasmic electron-dense granules, some of which are membrane bound with a regular lamellar structure.

BASIC DEFECT

Deficiency of α-galactosidase due to multiple allelic mutations. Glycosphingolipids (primarily ceramide trihexoside) accumulate in many tissues, with predilection for the vascular endothelium.

TREATMENT

1. Phenytoin or cabamazepine can be given for pain.
2. The benefit of renal transplantation is uncertain. Recurrence of involvement of a transplanted kidney was reported in one patient.
3. Angiokeratomas respond to both argon and copper vapor lasers.

MODE OF INHERITANCE

X-linked recessive. The gene has been mapped to Xq22 and has been sequenced.

PRENATAL DIAGNOSIS

Possible by enzyme assay of amniocytes or chorionic villi; linkage and mutation analyses using chorionic villi.

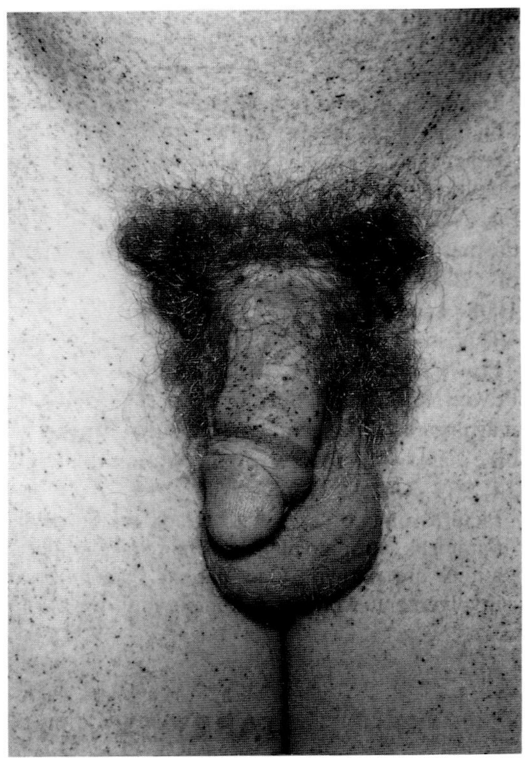

Figure 5.44. Angiokeratomas over thighs, penis, on scrotum and perineum. (From Sybert and Holbrook, 1987.)

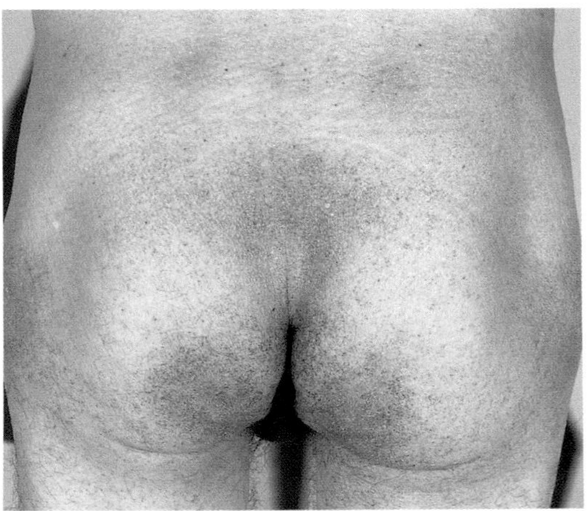

Figure 5.45. Lesions on buttocks, sacrum, and iliac crest. (Courtesy of Dr. G. F. Odland, Division of Dermatology, University of Washington.)

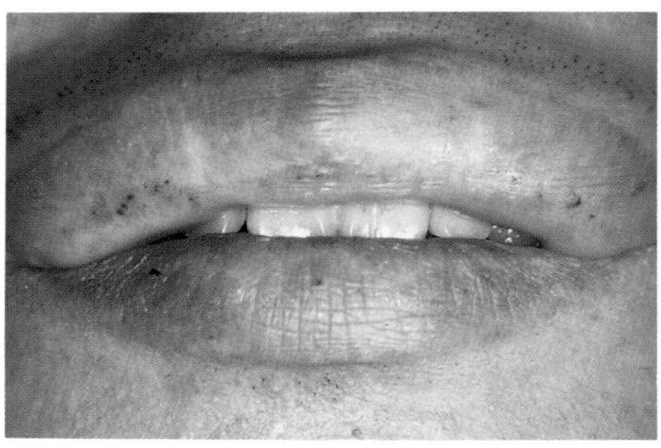

Figure 5.46. Spots on lips. (Courtesy of Dr. G. F. Odland, Division of Dermatology, University of Washington.)

DIFFERENTIAL DIAGNOSIS

Angiokeratomas may be isolated or multiple, without a recognized genetic or syndromic component. They are also seen in association with other lysosomal storage diseases, including fucosidosis (MIM:230000), G_{M1} gangliosidosis (MIM:230500), adult type neuraminidase deficiency (MIM:256540), and late infantile galactosialidosis (MIM:256540.0001). In angiokeratoma of Mibelli, lesions are acral in distribution and have more of a hyperkeratotic appearance, and affected individuals have no systemic symptoms. Angiokeratomas of the scrotum or labia (Fordyce disease) and cherry or senile angiomas appear later in life, tend to be fewer in number, and are rarely keratotic. Angiokeratoma circumscripta is usually marked by grouped lesions in single or contiguous areas. Only in angiokeratoma corporis diffusum (Fabry) are electron-dense granules found.

Among other vascular lesions, verrucous hemangiomas are usually larger, isolated, and show vascular dilatation and proliferation deep into the subcutaneous tissue. The lesions of angioma serpiginosum (MIM:106050) are typically flatter, without epidermal changes, as are the telangiectases of Osler-Weber-Rendu (MIM:187300). In Osler-Weber-Rendu the vascular lesions typically involve the top of the tongue, whereas in Fabry it is the underside that is affected.

Acute episodes of inexplicable pain can be part of familial Mediterranean fever (MIM: 249150) and acute intermittent porphyria (MIM: 176000). These conditions are not marked by angiokeratomas. Attacks of pain, numbness, and tingling of the extremities in individuals with Fabry syndrome may be misdiagnosed as multiple sclerosis, especially in heterozygous females.

The hypohidrosis of Fabry syndrome is acquired, which readily differentiates it from the hypohidrotic ectodermal dysplasias (MIM: Many).

Support Group: N.O.R.D.
P.O. Box 8923
New Fairfield, CT
06812
1-800-999-6673

SELECTED BIBLIOGRAPHY

Calzavara-Pinton, P.G., Colombi, M., Carlino, A., Zane, C., Gardella, R., Clemente, M., Facchetti, F., Moro, L., Zoppi, N., Caimi, L., Barlati, S., and De Panfilis, G. (1995). Angiokeratoma corporis diffusum and arteriovenous fistulas with dominant transmission in the absence of metabolic disorders. *Arch. Dermatol.* **131,** 57–62.

Large family with cutaneous angiokeratomas. Some affected individuals had asymmetry with hyperhidrosis of a leg, with evidence of arteriovenous fistulas. No abnormalities in lysosomal enzymes were found.

Eng, C.M., Resnick-Silverman, L.A., Niehaus, D.J., Astrin, K.H., and Desnick, R.J. (1993). Nature and frequency of mutations in the α-galactosidase A gene that causes Fabry disease. *Am. J. Hum. Genet.* **53,** 1186–1197.

Private mutations were in the majority. A hot spot at codon 227 was identified, and genotype: phenotype correlations, with some mutations conferring milder disease, were noted.

Kousseff, B.G., Beratis, N.G., Strauss, L., Brill, P.W., Rosenfield, R.E., Kaplan, B., and Hirschhorn, K. (1976). Fucosidosis type 2. *Pediatrics* **57,** 205–213.

Authors believe that the presence of angiokeratomas distinguishes a specific subtype of fucosidosis.

Levade, T., Giordano, F., Maret, A., Marguery, M.-C., Bazex, J., and Salvayre, R. (1991). Different phenotypic expression of Fabry disease in female monozygote twins. *J. Inherit. Metab. Dis.* **14,** 105–106.

Marguery, M.-C., Giordano, F., Parant, M., Samalens, G., Levade, T., Salvayre, R., Maret, A., Calvas, P., Bourrouillou, G., Cantala, P., and Bazex, J. (1993). Fabry's disease: heterozygous form of different expression in two monozygous twin sisters. *Dermatology* **187,** 9–15.

Levade et al. (1991) and Marguery et al. (1993) report on the same twins. The later report does not cite the prior. Markedly discordant expression of Fabry syndrome, presumably secondary to random X inactivation.

Marriott, P.J., Dowling, D.M., and Ryan, T. (1975). Angioma serpiginosum—familial incidence. *Br. J. Dermatol.* **93,** 701–705.

Two families, one with two affected generations (no male-to-male transmission), the other with two of four sisters affected, had onset in early childhood with progression of asymptomatic punctate red-purple macules in a serpiginous distribution.

Touraine, J.L., Malik, M.C., Traeger, J., Perrot, H., and Maire, I. (1979). Attempt at enzyme replacement by fetal liver transplantation in Fabry's disease (Letter). *Lancet* **i,** 1094–1095.

Touraine, J.L., Malik, M.C., Maire, I., Veyron, P., Zabot, M.T., Rolland, M.O., and Mathieu, M. (1982). Fetal liver transplantation in congenital enzyme deficiencies in man. *Exp. Hematol.* **10 (suppl. 10),** 46–47.

Touraine et al. (1979, 1982) report on three patients with Fabry syndrome who received fetal liver transplants; all improved. The follow-up time was 28–77 months. Sweating was restored, pain disappeared, and renal involvement stabilized. To date I am aware of no follow-up to these studies.

Wise, D., Wallace, H.J., and Jellinek, E.H. (1962). Angiokeratoma corporis diffusum. A clinical study of eight affected families. *Q. J. Med.* **31,** 177–207.

A beautifully detailed clinical and historical review with evaluation of eight families and four sporadic cases.

HEREDITARY GLOMUS TUMORS (MIM:138000)

(Barre-Masson Syndrome)

DERMATOLOGIC FEATURES

MAJOR. Multiple small bluish to purple to red subcutaneous or cutaneous nodules, single or grouped, occur primarily on the distal extremities, but may develop on any cutaneous surface. They can be compressed easily, often with tenderness. Although their presence has been recorded at birth or in early childhood, they usually appear in later childhood and adolescence and continue to develop throughout adult life. In contrast, the average age of occurrence for an isolated glomus tumor is in the early thirties. Tumors can range in number from less than 10 to several hundred. They can vary in size from that of a pea to several centimeters.

Spontaneous pain is a hallmark of isolated glomus tumors. Its occurrence in inherited glomus tumors is not invariable. It has been suggested that in the familial form tumors are rarely painful. However, this contention is not supported by numerous case reports or by my clinical experience. While spontaneous pain is not consistent, pain to pressure is fairly typical.

MINOR. None.

ASSOCIATED ABNORMALITIES

Shortness of the fourth and fifth metacarpals has been occasionally reported. As this is a

A

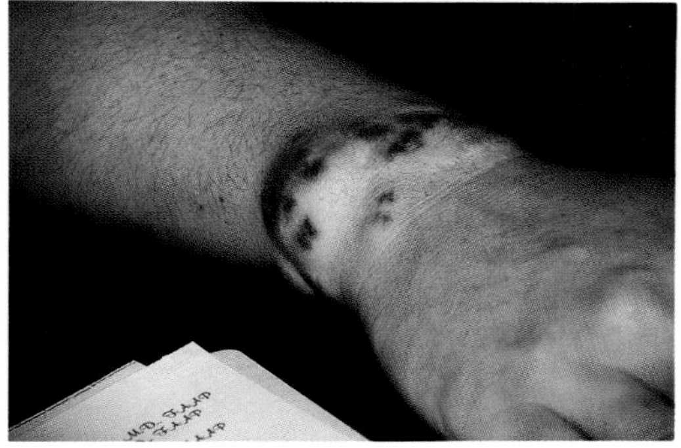

B

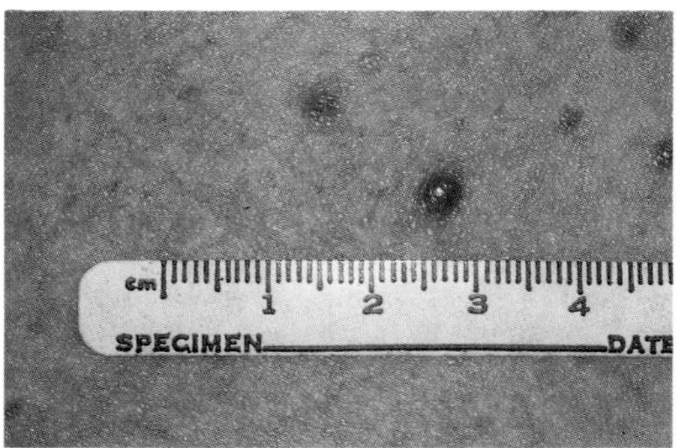

Figure 5.47. **(A)** Grouped dark purple lesions on wrists. **(B)** Individual red papules in another patient.

common finding in the general population, this finding may not reflect a true association with the disorder.

HISTOPATHOLOGY

LIGHT. Numerous endothelial lined vascular spaces arrayed in unencapsulated but well-circumscribed tumors at the dermoepidermal junction, surrounded by one to several rows of glomus cells, is the typical picture. Histologically these lesions can resemble cavernous hemangiomas. Isolated nonfamilial lesions are usually, but not always, encapsulated and have narrower vascular spaces and more glomus cells.

EM. Glomus cells from both solitary and multiple tumors show the same electron microscopic characteristics. The glomus cells have irregular rounded outlines, are closely aligned in rows, and are surrounded by bundles of collagen and finer filaments. Within the glomus cells there are numerous microfilaments and abundant mitochondria. The cells have the appearance of modified smooth muscle cells.

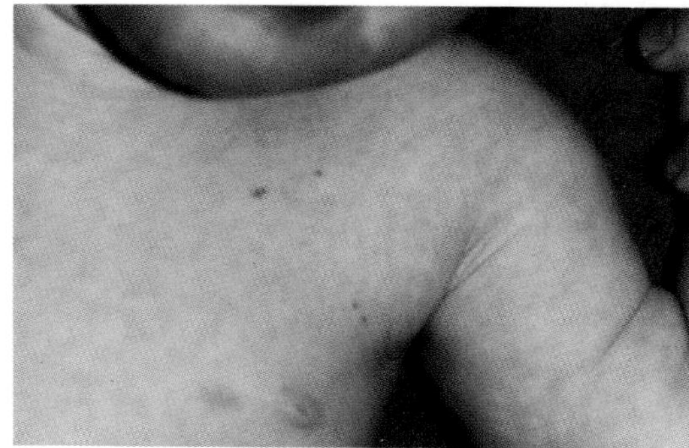

Figure 5.48. Son of patient in Fig. 5.47. He has very early lesions on the upper chest.

BASIC DEFECT

Unknown. The tumors arise from the *glomus body,* a term used in dermatology to refer to the arteriovenous anastamoses situated in the reticular dermis. These are most numerous in the extremities and are believed to be important in thermal regulation. The glomus cells in the glomus body are believed to arise from smooth muscle precursors; thus, the glomus tumor is a hamartoma of smooth muscle origin.

TREATMENT

Surgical excision can be effective; incomplete removal results in recurrence.

Successful ablation of and relief of pain from superficial lesions with use of the argon and carbon dioxide lasers have been reported. Use of the pulsed dye laser has not been reported but is likely to be effective only for very superficial lesions.

MODE OF INHERITANCE

Autosomal dominant. There are some documented obligate gene carriers who have not expressed the disorder. Confusion has been generated regarding the inheritance of this entity, because there are two distinct inherited conditions that enjoy the term *glomus tumors.* The dermatologic condition is clearly autosomal dominant with male-to-male transmission. The glomus tumor that arises from the glomus bodies in the jugular, middle ear, tympanic branches of cranial nerves IX and X and in the carotid is a neurosurgical disorder of neural crest origin that, when familial (MIM:168000), demonstrates an unusual inheritance pattern in which affected females do not transmit the disorder but are at risk for affected grandchildren who have inherited the gene through a carrier father. This mode of inheritance is mistakenly attributed to the dermatologic condition, to which it does not apply.

PRENATAL DIAGNOSIS

None.

DIFFERENTIAL DIAGNOSIS

In the blue rubber bleb nevus syndrome (MIM:112200), the vascular lesions are not usually spontaneously painful or particularly painful on palpation. Blue rubber bleb nevi are usually firmer and more protuberant than glomus tumors. Although both types of lesions compress easily, there is no dermal defect in multiple glomus tumors as there is in the blue rubber bleb nevus syndrome. Blue rubber blebs can involve the viscera and other internal organs; multiple glomus tumors usually do not. The two disorders can be distinguished histologically by the absence of glomus cells in blue rubber bleb nevi.

Single glomus tumors are sporadic, usually subungual, and very painful. There have been several reports of isolated congenital infiltrating glomus tumors that clinically resemble venous varicosities.

The telangiectases of hereditary hemorrhagic telangiectasia (Osler-Weber-Rendu, MIM: 187300) are clinically distinguishable from the lesions of multiple glomus tumors.

Cutaneous hemangiomas can be confused with glomus tumors and, when part of benign familial hemangiomatosis, may have to be differentiated histologically.

The blue lesions of cutaneous melanoma and blue nevi are easily distinguished clinically.

Support Group:

N.O.R.D.
P.O. Box 8923
New Fairfield, CT 06812
1-800-999-6673

National Vascular Malformations Foundation
8320 Nightingale
Dearborn Heights, MI 48127-1202
1-313-274-1243

SELECTED BIBLIOGRAPHY

Conant, M.A., and Wiesenfeld, S.L. (1971). Multiple glomus tumors of the skin. *Arch Dermatol.* **103,** 481–485.

Description of a three-generation family with good color photographs.

Pepper, M.C., Laubenheimer, R., and Cripps, D.J. (1977). Multiple glomus tumors. *J. Cutan. Pathol.* **4,** 244–257.

The father in this family was misdiagnosed to have blue rubber bleb nevus syndrome and was subsequently recognized to have multiple glomus tumors after the correct diagnosis was made in his son. There is a very readable exposition of the embryology and pathology of these lesions and good histopathology figures.

Sluiter, J.T.F., and Postma, C. (1959). Multiple glomus tumours of the skin. *Acta Dermatol Venereol.* **39,** 98–107.

The authors propose the term *glomangioma* rather than *glomus tumor*. I think this would be an excellent cure for the glomus tumor (dermatology)/glomus tumor (neurology) confusion. Conversely, we could reserve glomus tumor for the former and use the term *paraganglioma* for the latter.

van der Mey, A.G.L., Maaswinkel-Mooy, P.D., Cornelisse, C.J., Schmidt, P.H., and van

de Kamp, J.J.P. (1989). Genomic imprinting in hereditary glomus tumors: evidence for new genetic theory. *Lancet* **i,** 1291–1294.
Exhaustive review of pedigrees with inherited paragangliomas. This paper cites few instances of female-to-offspring inheritance of the disease and posits that imprinting plays a role in inheritance. This paper deals with inherited paragangliomata and not the multiple glomus tumors of cutaneous origin.

HEREDITARY HEMORRHAGIC TELANGIECTASIA (MIM: 187300)

(Osler-Weber-Rendu; Rendu-Osler-Weber; OWR1; OWR2)

Includes Hereditary Benign Telangiectasia; Angioma Serpiginosum

DERMATOLOGIC FEATURES

MAJOR. Red to purple telangiectases begin as pinpoint macules and progress to papules and nodules. The nail beds, palms, lips, tongue, ears, face, and chest are most commonly involved, but any skin surface may be affected. Cutaneous lesions usually begin appearing in the second and third decades, but presentation with systemic signs in infancy has occurred.

Mucosal involvement is primary, and epistaxis is often the only complaint, occurring in four-fifths of individuals. Nosebleeds predate skin findings in most patients. Nosebleeds may start in infancy but more commonly begin in childhood or adolescence. These episodes can result in fatal hemorrhage. Telangiectases can be seen on the nasal mucosa, palate, tongue, and buccal mucosa. True spider angiomas with pulsation are rare. Mat angiomas mimicking vascular malformations have been reported.

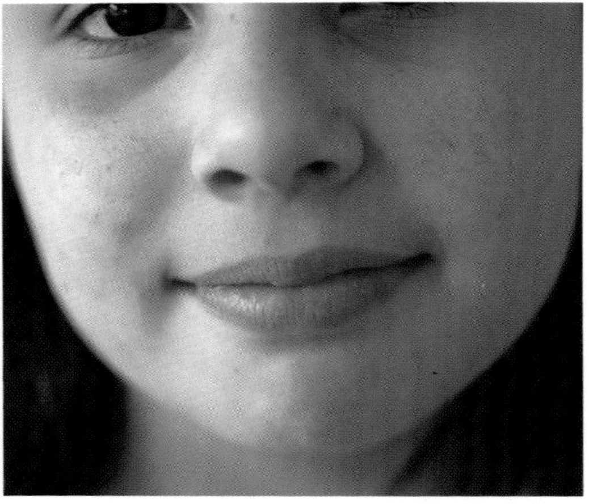

Figure 5.49. Multiple fine telangiectases on cheeks.

MINOR. Conjunctival involvement can occur, and conjunctival bleeds have been documented.

ASSOCIATED ABNORMALITIES

By age 30 years, 10%–15% of patients with hereditary hemorrhagic telangiectasia have internal involvement. From 40% to 50% of patients over the age of 60 years will have complications due to vascular involvement of organs other than the skin.

Central nervous system: From 15% to 20% of patients with pulmonary arteriovenous malformations present with stroke secondary to embolic abscesses. Strokes caused by bleeding of arteriovenous malformations in the brain are also reported. Vascular lesions may be present in the spinal cord. Of 12 patients with multiple central nervous system arteriovenous malformations investigated by one group, five had Osler-Weber-Rendu Syndrome.

Lungs: Arteriovenous malformations in the lungs can cause shunting, leading to hypoxia, high output failure, and death. Pulmonary insufficiency in childhood has been well documented. It has been suggested that patients with hereditary hemorrhagic telangiectasia and pulmonary arteriovenous malformations have a higher risk for secondary central nervous system complication than those with pulmonary arteriovenous malformations alone. A greater

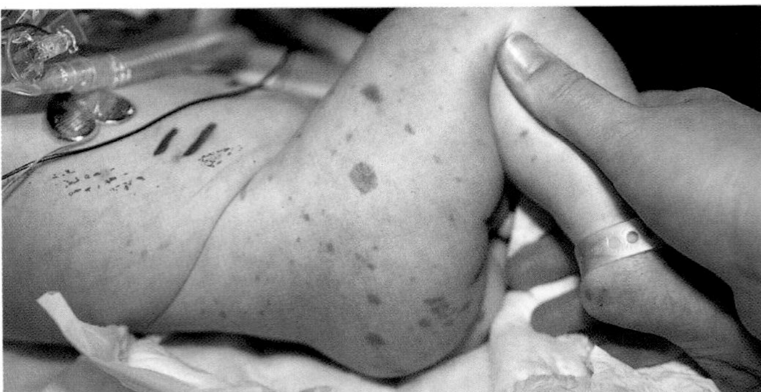

Figure 5.50. Too numerous to count mat telangiectases on trunk and extremities.

risk for pulmonary involvement may distinguish families with OWR1. There are as yet insufficient data to be able to predict a specific risk for this complication in a given individual.

Gastrointestinal: Liver involvement with telangiectases with fibrosis resulting in portal hypertension and esophageal varices and hepato-porto-systemic encephalopathy has been described. Gastrointestinal hemorrhage secondary to mucosal lesions in the gut occurs in about 20% of affected individuals.

Hematologic: Iron deficiency anemia secondary to recurrent hemorrhage, both gastrointestinal and nasal, is common. Bleeding appears to be worse in premenstrual or postmenopausal (natural or surgical) women and decreases during pregnancy.

Other: Involvement of practically every organ, including bone, has been described at least once in hereditary hemorrhagic telangiectasia. The frequency of specific complications reflects the specialty of the reporting physician. Neurologists report a higher proportion of patients with central nervous system disease; pulmonologists tout the frequency of lung involvement. I have seen children present with each of the major complications—central nervous system bleed, pulmonary insufficiency, gastrointestinal hemorrhage—prior to recognition of the diagnosis of hereditary hemorrhagic telangiectasia.

HISTOPATHOLOGY

LIGHT. Thin-walled, dilated vessels in the papillary and subpapillary dermis, lined by flat-

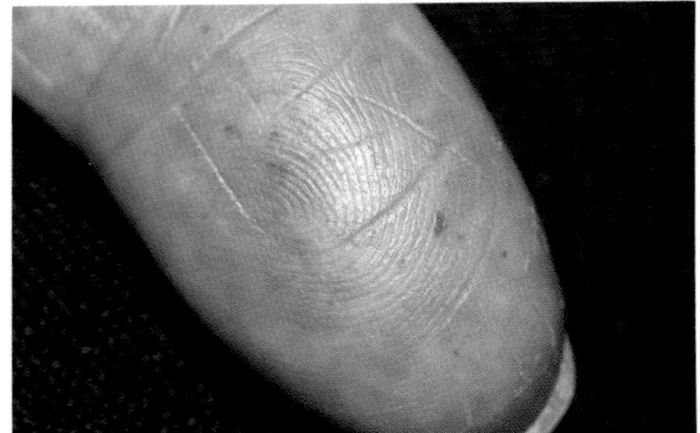

A

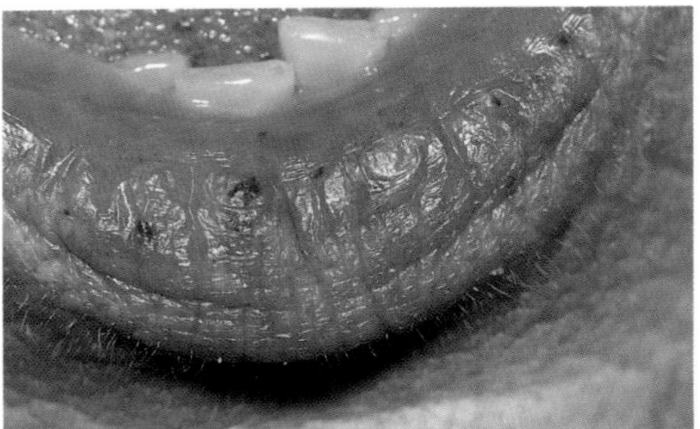

B

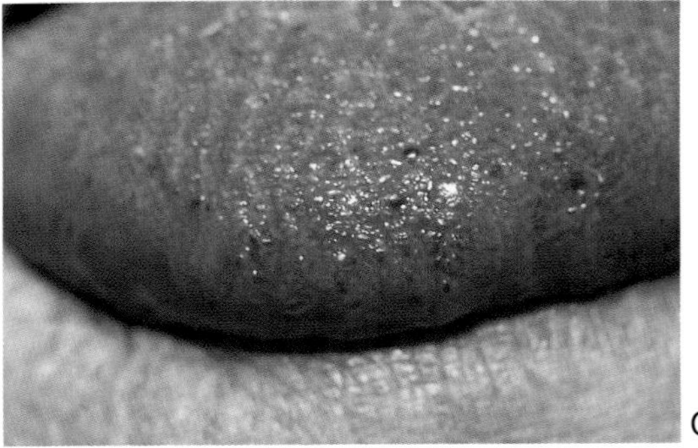

C

Figure 5.51. Telangiectases on fingertips **(A)**, lip **(B)**, and tongue **(C)**.

tened epithelial cells without pericytes, characterize the telangiectases that develop from postcapillary venules. The arteriovenous malformations show dilated tortuous vessels involving both arteries and veins without a capillary bed. This results in shunting. It has been suggested that the arteriovenous malformations in hereditary hemorrhagic telangiectasia represent the end stage of development of telangiectases. In the liver, arteriovenous malformations are embedded in dense fibrous tissue, which can entrap normal liver.

EM. The cells lining the dilated capillaries appear normal, and the vessels are surrounded by several layers of smooth muscle cells.

BASIC DEFECT

Unknown. Alterations in the transforming growth factor-β (TGF-β) ligand–receptor complex may be responsible in OWR1; mutations in activin receptor–like kinase 1 (*ALK1*) may underlie OWR2.

TREATMENT

Use of laser therapy for vascular ablation has had good results. The carbon dioxide, argon, pulsed dye, Nd-Yag, and KTP lasers have all been used. Laser therapy coupled with septodermoplasty with buccal mucosa has been suggested as the most successful for treatment of recurrent severe epistaxis. Repeated treatment is often necessary. Use of high-dose estrogen has questionable efficacy and significant side effects. In one patient, discontinuity of the endothelial surface in small venules was found. These gaps were filled by thrombi. These sites or gaps were reduced in number with estrogen therapy. This, coupled with the natural history of improvement during pregnancy and worsening in the absence of normal ovarian hormones, suggests that the use of birth control pills or low-dose estrogen and progesterone regimens may be helpful.

Antibiotic prophylaxis against subacute bacterial endocarditis similar to the regimen for cardiac valvular disease is appropriate.

Surgical excision of large or symptomatic arteriovenous malformations may be necessary. We have had one child with hereditary hemorrhagic telangiectasia come to lung transplant because of pulmonary involvement. Magnetic resonance imaging to look for brain lesions and magnetic resonance imaging or ultrasound to evaluate liver involvement may be useful for prospective management but is not warranted as a general screening tool. Screening by oximetry and chest radiographs for pulmonary arteriovenous malformations has been suggested. Management needs to be individually tailored.

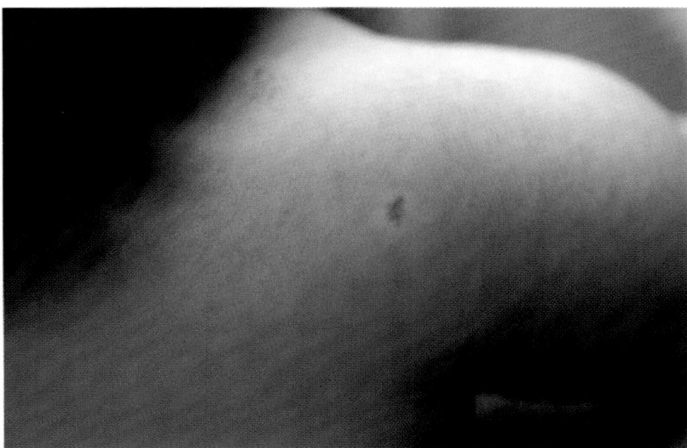

Figure 5.52. Halo of vasoconstriction around mat telangiectases.

MODE OF INHERITANCE

Autosomal dominant with variable expression. Penetrance approaches 100% in adult life. There is no evidence for increased severity in subsequent generations, different severity of expression between the genders, or parental imprinting. There is locus heterogeneity, with the gene mapping to 9q33–q34 in some families (*OWR1* or *HHT1*). Mutations in a TGF-β binding protein, endoglin, have been identified in some of these kindreds. A second locus has been identified in the pericentric region of chromosome 12. A candidate gene, *ALK1*, has been proposed. Genetic linkage to von Willebrand disease (a disorder that has been reported in five pedigrees with hereditary hemorrhagic telangiectasia) has been excluded.

Homozygosity has been reported once. A female presented at birth with an angioma of the thyroid; she developed innumerable telangiectases over her body and died at age 2 1/2 months of anemia. All of her organs had vascular changes.

PRENATAL DIAGNOSIS

Now possible by direct DNA techniques in families with identified mutations.

DIFFERENTIAL DIAGNOSIS

Hereditary benign telangiectasia (MIM: 187260): Changes in this disorder are limited to the skin, and there is far less mucosal involvement. There is no internal involvement. One cannot really differentiate between the two conditions from skin evaluation alone. Spider angiomas are more common in hereditary benign telangiectasia and rarer in hereditary hemorrhagic telangiectasia. The onset of skin lesions in hereditary benign telangiectasia may be at a younger age, but this is not always true. The skin lesions increase in severity in pregnancy in hereditary benign telangiectasia, whereas they improve in hereditary hemorrhagic telangiectasia.

Ataxia telangiectasia (MIM:208900): There is earlier onset of telangiectases in this condition than in hereditary hemorrhagic telangiectasia. The presence of ataxia also usually occurs earlier than the skin manifestations of hereditary hemorrhagic telangiectasia. Bulbar conjunctival involvement is far more common in ataxia telangiectasia.

Generalized essential telangiectasia: This condition usually involves the lower extremities, is of adult onset, far more common in females, and characterized by sheets of linear telangiectases. Bleeding is rare.

Unilateral nevoid telangiectasia: The skin changes are usually in a limited region, most often the upper face, neck, chest, and arms. Although the condition may be congenital, it is usually acquired. Again, it is not associated with significant bleeding.

Congenital vascular malformations: Although large mat vascular malformations have been reported in hereditary hemorrhagic telangiectasia, they do not occur in isolation, and the other skin changes of hereditary hemorrhagic telangiectasia will ultimately distinguish the isolated vascular malformation from the systemic disorder.

Although *spider angiomas* are usually solitary, they can be multiple. They usually have marked central pulsations that are often absent in the telangiectases of hereditary hemorrhagic telangiectasia.

CREST: The cutaneous telangiectases of CREST are clinically similar, but the associated clinical features of cutis calcinosis, Raynaud Syndrome, and scleroderma are not part of hereditary hemorrhagic telangiectasia.

Fabry syndrome (Angiokeratoma corporis diffusum) (MIM:301500): The lesions of this X-linked disorder of α-galactosidase deficiency are usually flat-topped and often hyperkeratotic. They do not usually bleed spontaneously, and they are usually darker than the vascular papules of hereditary hemorrhagic telangiectasia. The genitals, thighs, and abdomen are sites of preference for the angiokeratomas in contrast to the distribution of the telangiectasias of hereditary hemorrhagic telangiectasia. The underside of the tongue is usually involved in Fabry syndrome, the top surface in hereditary hemorrhagic telangiectasia. The underside of the tongue is usually involved in Fabry, the top surface in hereditary hemorrhagic telangiectasia.

Angioma serpiginosum (MIM:106050): In angioma serpiginosum, pinpoint purple papules develop progressively, usually on the lower extremities. These appear to be telangiectases on biopsy. Most cases are sporadic; there have been a few pedigrees reported with no clear-cut pattern of inheritance.

Support Group: HHT Foundation International, Inc.
P.O. Box 8087
New Haven, CT 06530
1-800-448-6389

SELECTED BIBLIOGRAPHY

Braverman, I.M., Keh, A., and Jacobson, B.S. (1990). Ultrastructure and three-dimensional organization of the telangiectasias of hereditary hemorrhagic telangiectasia. *J. Invest. Dermatol.* **95,** 422–427.

Intriguing three-dimensional computer modeling of cutaneous telangiectases in hereditary hemorrhagic telangiectasia as they develop. Authors propose that the lesions start as dilatations in the postcapillary venules, which enlarge and anastomose with dilated arterioles via capillaries. The capillaries drop out as lesions enlarge, leaving the arteriovenous connection. A perivascular lymphocytic infiltrate is typical.

Frain-Bell, W. (1957). Angioma serpiginosum. *Br. J. Dermatol.* **69,** 251–268.

Eleven cases, 10 female. There were no familial occurrences, and none were noted in accompanying review of literature.

Marriott, P.J., Munro, D.D., and Ryan, T. (1975). Angioma serpiginosum—familial incidence. *Br. J. Dermatol.* **93,** 701–705.

Two pedigrees, one with two siblings, one with two generations. There was no male-to-male transmission.

McAllister, K.A., Grogg, K.M., Johnson, D.W., Gallione, C.J., Baldwin, M.A., Jackson, C.E., Helmbold, E.A., Markel, D.S., McKinnon, W.C., Murrell, J., McCormick, M.K., Pericak-Vance, M.A., Heutink, P., Oostra, B.A., Haitjema, T., Westerman, C.J.J., Porteous, M.E., Guttmacher, A.E., Letarte, M. and Marchuk, D.A. (1994). Endoglin, a TGF-β binding protein of endothelial cells, is the gene for hereditary haemorrhagic telangiectasia type 1. *Nat. Genet.* **8,** 345–351.

Authors demonstrate three distinct mutations in the gene for endoglin, a member of the TGF-β receptor complex. Suggest mutations for other genes in this complex responsible for other subsets of hereditary hemorrhagic telangiectasia and have paper in preparation of a family with hereditary hemorrhagic telangiectasia demonstrating linkage to 3p22, where TGF-β II receptor is located.

Menefee, M.G., Flessa, H.G., Glueck, H.I., and Hogg, S.P. (1975). Hereditary hemorrhagic telangiectasia (Osler-Weber-Rendu disease), an electron microscopic study of the vascular lesions before and after therapy with hormones. *Arch. Otolaryngol.* **101,** 246–251.

Lesions from two of eight individuals with Osler-Weber-Rendu Syndrome who were treated with Enovid (norethynodrel and mestranol) were biopsied before and after treatment. With therapy, there was no evidence for endothelial cell damage, and the gaps between cells were no longer present.

Peery, W.H. (1987). Clinical spectrum of hereditary hemorrhagic telangiectasia (Osler-Weber-Rendu disease). *Am. J. Med.* **82,** 989–997.

This is a very nice review with 89 references.

Plauchu, H., de Chadarevian, J.P., Bideau, A., and Robert, J.-M. (1989). Age-related clinical profile of hereditary hemorrhagic telangiectasia in an epidemiologically recruited population. *Am. J. Med. Genet.* **32,** 291–297.

A study of 324 of 1,270 patients identified from 520 families. The criteria for diagnosis required any two of the following: epistaxis, telangiectases other than nasal, positive family history, or visceral involvement. Even this population-based study has limitations; only clinically evident complications were tabulated, and minimally affected individuals may not have satisfied clinical criteria and thus have been excluded. The study underscores the variability in expression in this disorder among individuals and over time.

Porteous, M.E.M., Burn, J., and Proctor, S.J. (1992). Hereditary hemorrhagic telangiectasia: a clinical analysis. *J. Med. Genet.* **29,** 527–530.

Ascertained patients in northern region of Britain. Evaluated 98. Frustrating to read because many details left out, e.g., 97% were symptomatic by age 35 years, but how many features they showed is not given. Authors were unable to examine most patients' entire body surfaces, and statements regarding distribution of skin lesions are based on a "limited number."

Richtsmeier, W., Weaver, G., Streck, W., Jacobson, H., Dewell, R., and Olson, J. (1984). Estrogen and progesterone receptors in hereditary hemorrhagic telangiectasia. *Otolaryngol. Head Neck Surg.* **92,** 564–570.

Four individuals, two each from two families with hereditary hemorrhagic telangiectasia (in one of which EDS-III was also segregating), were biopsied. Tissues from two females in one family were found to have estrogen and progesterone receptors in increased numbers similar to those in breast carcinoma. The tissues from the two males in the other family showed only a modest increase in progesterone receptors, which was still significantly greater than that of controls. Whether these differences reflected gender or genetic heterogeneity remains uncertain. The authors recommend treatment with progesterone.

Siegel, M.B., Keane, W.M., Atkins, J.P., Jr., and Rosen, M.R. (1991). Control of epistaxis in patients with hereditary hemorrhagic telangiectasia. *Otolaryngol. Head Neck Surg.* **105,** 675–679.

A clearly written review of the therapeutic options for control of nasal bleeding. No single treatment is optimum. The authors suggest that use of laser coupled with septodermoplasty with buccal mucosal grafts gives the longest (24.4 months) relief.

Willinsky, R.A., Lasjaunias, P., Terbrugge, K., and Burrows, R. (1990). Multiple cerebral arteriovenous malformations (AVMs). Review of our experience from 203 patients with cerebrovascular lesions. *Neuroradiology* **32,** 207–210.

Five of 203 individuals with cerebral arteriovenous malformations had Osler-Weber-Rendu syndrome. The authors state that in no patient with Osler-Weber-Rendu syndrome did new arteriovenous malformations develop and that all lesions were congenital, in contrast to the vascular lesions of the skin. They do not substantiate this claim with long-term prospective data.

KLIPPEL-TRENAUNAY-WEBER SYNDROME (MIM:149000)

(Naevus Vasculosus Osteohypertrophicus; Angioosteohypertrophy Syndrome; Congenital Angiodysplasia)

Includes Cobb Syndrome; Familial Flame Nevi

The literature abounds with arguments about the nomenclature for this group of vascular malformations. The term *Klippel-Trenaunay syndrome* is generally used for those individuals without significant arteriovenous malformations or lymphangiomas. Weber's name is added when those features are present. There has been too much time and far too much energy, as far as I am concerned, spent on lumping and splitting condition(s) that we do not understand at any biologic level. The presence of a major arteriovenous malformation makes a difference in prognosis; beyond this, eponymous distinctions seem moot.

DERMATOLOGIC FEATURES

Major. This condition of vascular malformations is characterized by the presence of macular vascular patches (nevus flammeus). These port wine stains may be small or extensive. In addition to the nevus flammeus changes, there may be a marked venous pattern and frank varicosities. Involvement is usually, but not always, unilateral and generally involves the extremities. The body wall may also be involved.

There may be absence, hypoplasia, or ob-

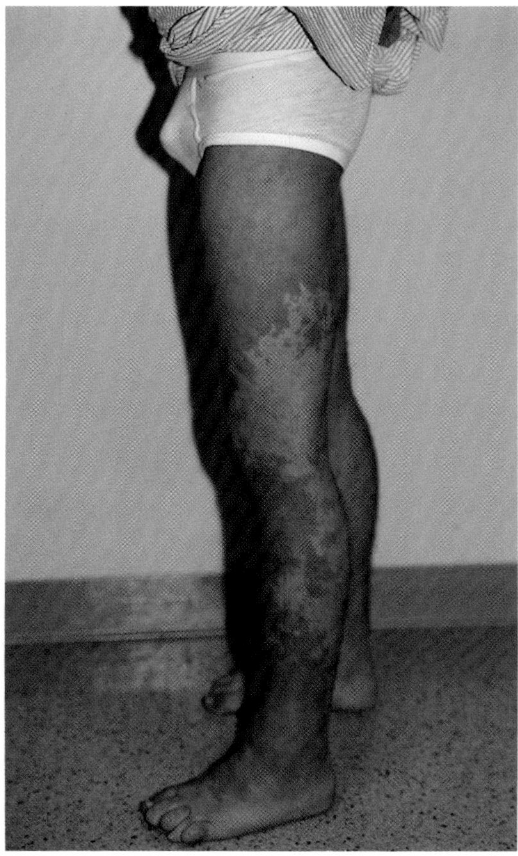

Figure 5.53. Involvement of leg with port wine stain; overgrowth of ankle and some toes. (Courtesy of Dr. J. Francis, Seattle, Washington.)

struction of the deep venous system resulting in, over time, significant lymphedema.

Angiokeratoma circumscripta can develop on the surface of the skin. This condition is marked by small, raised, red to purple papules, many of which appear to be vesicular with a hemorrhagic component. The term *frog spawn* has been used because they resemble clutches of frog eggs.

Arteriovenous malformations can occasionally be seen. These are manifest by pulsating warm areas. A palpable thrill may be found.

Lymphangiomas are common and may be small or large.

MINOR. Secondary changes of edema, phlebitis, thrombosis, and cellulitis typically develop as patients get older. Stasis dermatitis and ulcers can also occur. There may be hyperhidrosis of involved areas.

ASSOCIATED ABNORMALITIES

There is often soft tissue hypertrophy, and there may be bony hypertrophy as well. Bony abnormalities such as macrodactyly and syndactyly have been described infrequently. Overgrowth of a leg may lead to development of compensatory scoliosis. There may be erosion of bone underlying a vascular malformation. There are a host of other orthopedic complications, in addition to overgrowth, that have been described.

Pulmonary hypertension and high output failure have been described, as has subacute bacterial endocarditis, presumably due to vascular shunts. Paresthesias of involved limbs have also occurred in some patients. The major problems associated with the disorder are due to the mechanical difficulty induced by asymmetry of the limbs and the changes of chronic lymphedema and stasis.

There have been many isolated individual case reports with angiomatous involvement of other organs, including the retina, intestine, spleen, liver, brain, and kidney. These are the exception rather than the rule.

HISTOPATHOLOGY

LIGHT. Depends on the nature of the vascular lesion.

EM. Changes of nevus flammeus in the port wine stains.

BASIC DEFECT

Unknown. In some individuals there appears to be an absence of deep venous channels; in others there may be obstruction to deep venous drainage. The condition appears to be the result of a primary defect in development of the vascular and lymphatic channels.

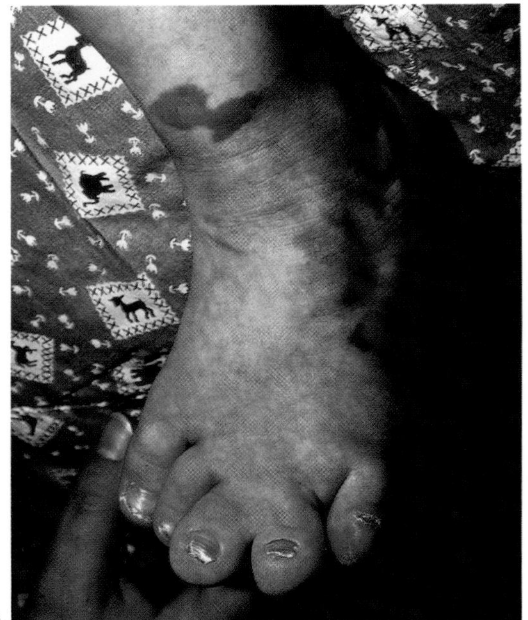

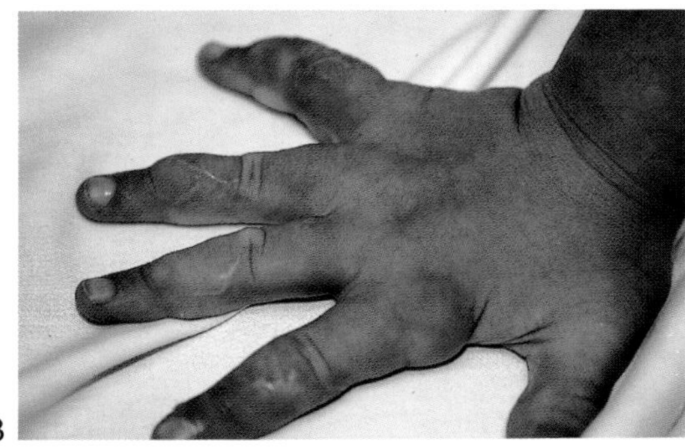

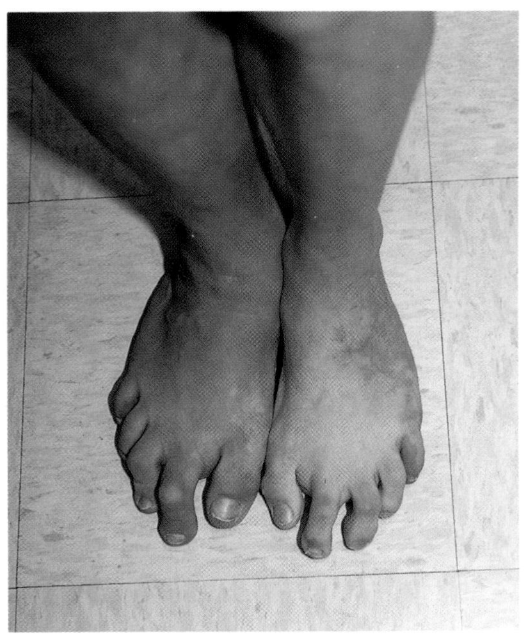

Figure 5.54. **(A)** Marked malformation of toes with complex vascular malformation. **(B)** Overgrowth of parts of fingers with overlying port wine stain. Surgical scars at sites of attempted excision. **(C)** Vascular malformation greater on right; bony malformations bilaterally.

TREATMENT

Use of magnetic resonance imaging has been advocated to document the extent and type of vascular malformation. It may or may not be warranted based on the clinical examination and symptoms.

If warranted, pulsed dye laser for port wine stains—recognizing that lesions on the lower extremity respond less well to treatment and that the cosmetic aspect of the superficial vascular lesion may be minimal in the context of overgrowth, edema, and varicosities.

Support hosiery and, when necessary, use of Jobst intermittent pressure pumps, along with careful orthopedic management. Treatment of bony overgrowth by epiphysiodesis is sometimes warranted.

MODE OF INHERITANCE

The condition appears not to be genetic. There is one report of an affected brother and sister.

PRENATAL DIAGNOSIS

There was a fortuitous prenatal diagnosis by ultrasound of a fetus presenting with hydrops and limb asymmetry.

DIFFERENTIAL DIAGNOSIS

Syndromes that share asymmetric overgrowth include Proteus syndrome (MIM:176920), which is differentiated by discrete soft tissue masses that are usually not vascular but rather lipomas or epidermal nevi.

Isolated hemihypertrophy (MIM:235000) without vascular involvement is usually nongenetic, although there are a few familial cases reported.

The Beckwith-Wiedemann syndrome (MIM: 130650), while marked by hemihypertrophy, has no associated vascular changes of the skin. Individuals with Klippel-Trenaunay-Weber do not have omphaloceles, macroglossia, or hypoglycemia.

In the Maffucci syndrome (MIM:166000), characterized by enchondromas and hemangiomas, the bony lesions are distinctive.

Cutis marmorata telangiectatica congenita (MIM:219250) is marked by a livedo pattern of vascular changes and usually atrophy, not hypertrophy, of the involved limb. I think that there is some overlap of Klippel-Trenaunay-Weber syndrome with the fine, lacy variant of cutis marmorata telangiectatica congenita (*vide infra*).

It may not be possible to determine in early childhood if a child with an extensive port wine stain/nevus flammeus of an extremity will have problems with hemihypertrophy or varicosities. There are rare infants who are born with multiple vascular malformations involving the skin and internal organs and who uniformly die. Some of these cases have been published under the heading of Klippel-Trenaunay-Weber syndrome, and others have been published as having diffuse hemangiomatosis. The cutaneous lesions are usually very uniformly dark. There is always internal involvement, and hypertrophy is usually evident at birth. Often there are other structural malformations as well.

The Cobb syndrome (MIM:106670), or cutaneomeningeal angiomatosis, is marked by cutaneous vascular malformations overlying spinal and dural hemangiomatosis. Klippel-Trenaunay-Weber syndrome usually does not involve the trunk, and Cobb syndrome does not involve the limb. In one report of a male with paraplegia secondary to vertebral and epidermal vascular malformations, the cutaneous lesion involved an arm and shoulder and extended across the midline of the upper back at C4 through T2.

In autosomal dominant familial flame nevi (MIM:163000), the vascular lesions are usually small and inconsequential. They are usually on the glabella, eyelids, shoulders, and trunk. There are no other associated abnormalities. The lesions are typical nevus flammeus or storkbite vascular malformations and differ from sporadic lesions only in their multiplicity.

Support Group: Klippel-Trenaunay-Weber Syndrome Support Group
4610 Wooddale Avenue
Edina, MN 55424
1-612-925-2596

SELECTED BIBLIOGRAPHY

Lindenauer, S. M. (1965). The Klippel-Trenaunay syndrome: varicosity, hypertrophy and hemangioma with no arteriovenous fistula. *Ann. Surg.* **162,** 303–313.

There is a great table. The author reports experience with 18 patients. He prefers to separate Klippel-Trenaunay-Weber from Klippel-Trenaunay syndrome and argues forcibly against surgical intervention. Eleven of 18 patients had bony hypertrophy, two had atrophy, and five had no bony changes. Fourteen of 18 had soft tissue hypertrophy, 2 of 18 had soft tissue atrophy, and 2 had no soft tissue findings. Seventeen of the 18 patients had a leg involved; one an arm. Three of the 18 had no cutaneous vascular changes. Ligation of abnormal veins with vein stripping was attempted in 12 patients, 11 of whom were worse after surgery. In the twelfth, there was no benefit from surgery.

McGrory, B.J., Amadio, P.C., Dobyns, J.H., Stickler, G.B., and Unni, K.K. (1991). Anomalies of the fingers and toes associated with Klippel-Trenaunay syndrome. *J. Bone Joint Surg. (Am.)* **73A,** 1537–1546.

Twenty-nine of 108 patients with Klippel-Trenaunay syndrome had digital abnormalities. Most had macrodactyly. Ten had syndactyly. Five of the patients had metatarsus primus varus. One-third of the malformations involved a limb without cutaneous vascular lesions.

Pasyk, K.A., Argenta, L.C., and Erickson, R.P. (1984). Familial vascular malformations.

Report of 25 members of one family. *Clin. Genet.* **26,** 221–227.

A family in which individuals had multiple vascular lesions. The authors refer to these as cavernous hemangiomas, but histopathology and behavior were typical of vascular malformations, not hemangiomas. Lesions were at different sites in different individuals, some with one, some with several. Some had mucosal involvement. The disorder was presumably autosomal dominant. Some affected individuals presented at birth, and some developed their lesions later. In none did the vascular lesions regress.

Selmanowitz, V.J. (1968). Nevus flammeus of the forehead. *J. Pediatr.* **73,** 755–757.

Shuper, A., Merlob, P., Garty, B., and Varsario, I. (1984). Familial multiple naevi flammei. *J. Med. Genet.* **21,** 112–113.

Two generation family with flame nevi on the glabella (Shuper et al. 1984) and a similar three generation family (Selmanowitz, 1968). There has been one instance of male-to-male transmission, but the transmitting father did not express. Another instance of male-to-male transmission in the literature was not documented by examination. I have seen a family with multiple flame nevi at the glabella and other sites who were oblivious to how interesting they were. The family was not bothered by the birthmarks, why should I be? They had come to clinic for unrelated reasons, and an astute resident picked up on the unusual skin findings. Perhaps this is a more common condition than appreciated.

Weber, F.P. (1907). Angioma-formation in connection with hypertrophy of limbs and hemihypertrophy. *Br. J. Dermatol.* **19,** 231–235.

Weber, F.P. (1918). Haemangiectatic hypertrophy of limbs—congenital phlebarteriectasis and so-called congenital varicose veins. *Br. J. Child. Dis.* **15,** 13–17.

In perpetuity, F. Parkes Weber will be held accountable for citing Thomas Smith's case of a woman with an arteriovenous malformation and tortuous vascularity of the hand, which has resulted in the separation of Klippel-Trenaunay syndrome from Klippel-Trenaunay-Weber syndrome. In this review, he describes the gamut of vascular malformations, reviewing multiple cases presented by others, many with typical Klippel-Trenaunay syndrome. The single case with the arteriovenous malformation did not have a superficial nevus flammeus. None of the patients Weber described were his own. He noted that arteriovenous malformations are not a typical feature of "genuine diffuse phlebarteriectasis," and I see no reason for perpetuating the distinct eponyms of Klippel-Trenaunay-Weber versus Klippel-Trenaunay syndrome.

You, C.K., Rees, J., Gillis, D.A., and Steves, J. (1983). Klippel-Trenaunay syndrome: a review. *Can. J. Surg.* **26,** 399–403.

Nice description of the historical delineation of Klippel-Trenaunay syndrome versus Klippel-Trenaunay-Weber syndrome. The authors present a classification scheme attributed to Bourde, but give no citation. The classification seems very functional to me: I = mild, II = varicosities, III = negligible arteriovenous malformation, IV = important but surgically excisable arteriovenous malformation, V = inoperable arteriovenous malformation. The patients in the last category tended to require amputation. This classification is based on prognosis rather than on causality.

MAFFUCCI SYNDROME (MIM:166000)

(Dyschondroplasia [Ollier Disease] and Hemangiomatosis; Enchondromatosis and Hemangiomatosis; Osteochondromatosis)

DERMATOLOGIC FEATURES

MAJOR. Soft tissue cavernous vascular malformations develop and progress during infancy and childhood. Rarely, lesions may be present at birth. There may be significant deformity and loss of function due to these vascular lesions without concomitant bony involvement. Varicosities may be present. The vascular lesions usually stabilize by adult life. They are usually deep in the dermis and subcutaneous tissue and bluish in color, although more "strawberry-like"

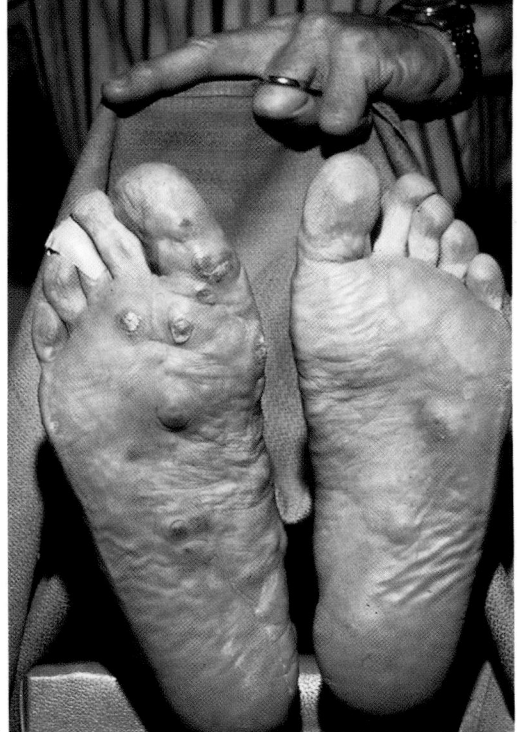

A

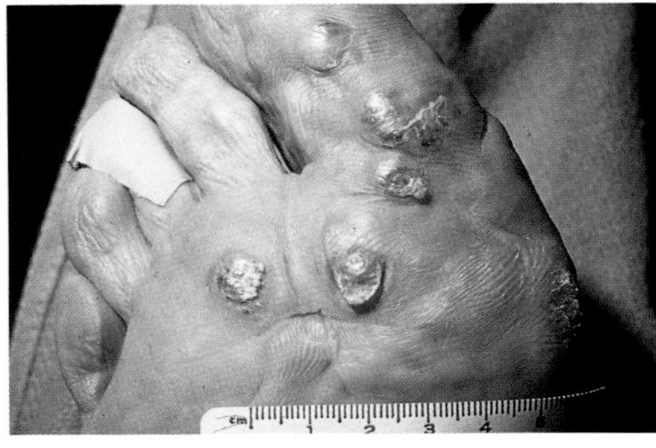

B

Figure 5.55. **(A)** Vascular malformation on feet. **(B)** Close-up shows hyperkeratosis overlying some. (Courtesy of Division of Dermatology, University of Washington.)

superficial capillary lesions have been described, as well as lesions resembling blue rubber bleb nevi. Phleboliths are common within the vascular lesions. The overlying skin may be hyperkeratotic or hyperhidrotic.

The viscera may also be involved, as may oral mucosa. Intracerebral hemangiomas have also been reported.

Approximately 15% of patients with enchondromatosis have clinically obvious hemangiomatosis.

Unilateral involvement is seen in about 50% of all cases, and, when involvement is bilateral, it is usually more marked on one side than the other. The distribution of vascular lesions is independent of the location of the enchondromas.

MINOR. Although lymphangiomas in Maffucci syndrome are alluded to in the discussions in many papers, they are rare in actual clinical descriptions.

Patchy vitiligo was described in two patients; one was the subject of two separate reports. This individual also had increased hair growth over the varicosities, which has not been reported in other patients.

ASSOCIATED ABNORMALITIES

During childhood, multiple areas of cystic change in the bones (enchondromas) develop and may increase in number and size until adulthood, when they usually stabilize. Any bone can be involved; metacarpals, phalanges, and metatarsals are preferred sites. Fractures, which may heal poorly and recur, are common, as are bony deformity and asymmetric short stature. The progressive deformity of the long bones can be quite marked.

Malignant degeneration of enchondromas has been reported in about 25% of patients with Ollier disease by age 40 years. Of these tumors, approximately 50% are chondrosarcomas. Some authors assert that the risk for malignant degeneration in Maffucci syndrome approaches 100%. Malignant change is usually marked clinically by rapid growth and pain, in contrast to the slow painless growth of enchondromas.

Tumors of the ovary—juvenile granulosa cell and Sertoli-Leydig cell—have been reported at least 10 times in association either with Maffucci syndrome or with Ollier disease. The youngest patient with a germ-line tumor was 1 year old. Juvenile granulosa cell tumors of the testis have not been reported in males with Maffucci syndrome.

Other reported malignant tumors have included pancreatic adenocarcinoma, hepatic adenocarcinoma, glioma, hemangiosarcoma, lymphangiosarcoma, and fibrosarcoma. Second malignancies are not rare. The occurrence of malignancy does not appear to correlate with unilateral versus bilateral bony involvement.

Three patients developed aneurysms, two carotid, one mesenteric.

HISTOPATHOLOGY

LIGHT. The vascular tumors are cavernous hemangiomas, usually located in the middle to lower dermis and in the subcutaneous fat. Thrombi and phleboliths are common.

The enchondromas are islands of cartilagenous tissue within the bony matrix of the metaphyses.

EM. No information.

BASIC DEFECT

Unknown.

TREATMENT

Surgical excision of troublesome vascular overgrowth, including amputation, may be required. Limb lengthening was described in two patients. In one, the course of surgeries took over 7 years, with the patient spending a total of 5 years in casts. She was still left with a significant residual limb length discrepancy.

Careful monitoring for the development of both internal malignancies and sarcomatous degeneration of enchondromas is prudent. Any rapidly enlarging or painful lesion should be evaluated. Magnetic resonance imaging is useful in differentiating benign from malignant bony lesions.

MODE OF INHERITANCE

All cases have been sporadic. Most patients have not reproduced. Among those few who have, there have been no recurrences. The possibility of mosaicism for a semilethal or lethal gene is supported by several reports of unilateral involvement of bony changes, hemangiomas, and ovarian malignancies.

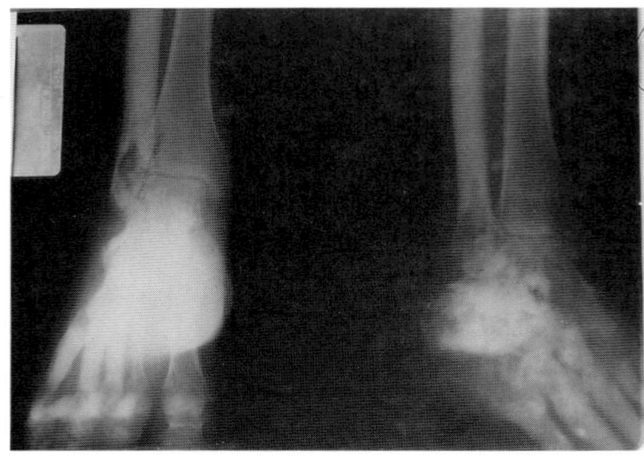

Figure 5.56. Enchondromas.

PRENATAL DIAGNOSIS

None.

DIFFERENTIAL DIAGNOSIS

In Klippel-Trenaunay-Weber syndrome (MIM: 149000), enchondromas do not occur, although bony asymmetry may. Port wine stains, common in Klippel-Trenaunay-Weber syndrome, are not part of Maffucci syndrome. The vascular changes of Klippel-Trenaunay-Weber syndrome are usually present at birth, although they too may progress with time.

Isolated enchondromas and widespread enchondromatosis (Ollier disease) can occur without hemangiomatosis. The distinction between Maffucci syndrome and Ollier disease is unclear. In one case report of a child diagnosed at age 5 years with Ollier disease, a hemangioma subsequently developed at age 10, resulting in a change of diagnosis. In another case report, at autopsy a 68-year-old male with a diagnosis of Ollier disease and osteosarcoma was found to have hemangiomas in the subcutaneous tissue of the chest wall and on the stomach, suggesting that the difference between a diagnosis of Ollier disease and a diagnosis of Maffucci syndrome is the presence of readily visible cutaneous vascular lesions. The two disorders may represent a contiguous gene syndrome or a continuum of developmental and regulatory defects rather than two distinct disorders.

Although the majority of case reports of Ollier disease with malignancy state that cancer is a far more common occurrence in Maffucci syndrome, the number of patients with Ollier disease alone and malignancy is impressive. Similar malignancies occur in both diseases, and the relative incidence of malignant change really cannot be determined by case reports.

Although vascular lesions similar to those of blue rubber bleb nevus syndrome (MIM: 112200) have been described in a small number of patients with Maffucci syndrome, the presence of enchondromas should allow for correct diagnosis.

Support Group: Ollier's Disease Self-Help Group
P.O. Box 52616
Shaw Air Force Base
Sumter, SC 29152-1521
1-803-775-1757

SELECTED BIBLIOGRAPHY

Carleton, A., Elkington, J.St.C., Greenfield, J.G., and Robb-Smith, A.H.T. (1942). Maffucci's syndrome (dyschondroplasia with hemangeiomata). *Q. J. Med.* **11,** 203–228.

This article contains a spectacular array of historical illustrations and photographs. The opening sentence, "The study of rare disorders has a scientific justification in addition to that of giving aesthetic pleasure to the clinical collector" must give one pause! A wonderful discursive paper. The authors dismiss the report of affected brothers (Steudel. *Beitr. Z. Klin. Chir.* **8,** 503–521.) as poorly documented.

Halal, F., and Azouz, E.M. (1991). Generalized enchondromatosis in a boy with only platyspondyly in father. *Am. J. Med. Genet.* **38,** 588–592.

This article contains a useful table with the differential diagnosis of enchondromas.

Kessler, H.B., Recht, M.P., and Dalinka, M.K. (1983). Vascular anomalies in association with osteodystrophies—a spectum. *Skeletal Radiol.* **10,** 95–101.

A clear exposition of the differential diagnosis of syndromes with both bony and vascular malformations.

Lewis, R.J., and Ketcham, A.S. (1973). Maffucci's syndrome: functional and neoplastic significance. Case report and review of the literature. *J. Bone Joint Surg. Am.* **55A,** 1465–1479.

This article reviews the literature; there are useful tables and an assessment of severity. There are 88 references. Their case was a 22-year-old female with grotesque deformity who succumbed to a second chondrosarcoma of the leg 6 years after a forequarter amputation for her first bony malignancy.

Schwartz, H.S., Zimmerman, N.B., Simon, M.A., Wroble, R.R., Millar, E.A., and Bonfiglio, M. (1987). The malignant potential of enchondromatosis. *J. Bone Joint Surg. Am.* **69A,** 269–274.

Seven of 44 patients with enchondromatosis had Maffucci syndrome. These were ascertained by investigating medical records of patients diagnosed with enchondromas as children. Of these seven, four developed seven malignant bone tumors subsequent to diagnosis. Three of these four also had nonskeletal malignancies, a pancreatic adenocarcinoma, biliary adenocarcinoma, and a frontal lobe astrocytoma. Malignancies developed in the third, fourth, and fifth decades. Death occurred from the nonskeletal malignancies.

Tanaka, Y., Sasaki, Y., Nishihira, H., Izawa, T., and Nishi, T. (1992). Ovarian juvenile granulosa cell tumor associated with Maffucci's syndrome. *Am. J. Clin. Pathol.* **97,** 523–527.

Case report and review of the literature. This is a very readable paper with a useful table summarizing previous case reports.

STURGE-WEBER SYNDROME (MIM:185300)

(Encephalotrigeminal Angiomatosis; Oculomeningeal Nevus Flammeus)

Includes Familial Cavernous Angiomas; Diffuse Cortical Meningeal Angiomatosis of Divry and van Bogaert; Wyburn-Mason Syndrome

DERMATOLOGIC FEATURES

MAJOR. Port wine stains—flat red patches involving at least the first branch (ophthalmic), with or without involvement of branches II and III, of the trigeminal nerve—present at birth. This lesion may be overlooked in the plethoric newborn. Involvement is usually unilateral, but can be bilateral, and there may be skip areas; for example, involvement of the upper cheek with sparing of the lateral forehead and involvement of the midforehead. When the skin of the distribution area of the first branch of the trigeminal nerve is spared, the risk for the other two features of the Sturge-Weber triad is very low. Clinically, this translates to sparing of the palpebral fissure and above. There may be more extensive involvement with a port wine stain on other areas of the body and some overlap with Klippel-Trenaunay-Weber syndrome. Males and females appear to be affected with equal frequency.

MINOR. None.

ASSOCIATED ABNORMALITIES

Ocular: If the first and/or second branches of the trigeminal nerve are involved, the choroid of the eye may be as well, and there is an increased risk for glaucoma, buphthalmos, and retinal detachment.

Central nervous system: Leptomeningeal and dural involvement with angiomatous malformation occurs primarily in those patients with involvement of the first branch of the trigeminal nerve. The risk estimates for central nervous system involvement range from 8% to 50% if the port wine stain occurs in the distribution of the first branch of the trigeminal nerve. Similar central nervous system vascular changes have been documented in some patients who have no cutaneous port wine stain. Calcification ("railroad tracking") occurs within the cortex proper, beneath the abnormal vessels, and may also occur within the vessels themselves. This calcification may be detected as early as 3 weeks of age and usually develops by age 2 to 3. The underlying brain may be atrophic. Seizures usually begin prior to age 2, and mental retardation is typical. Seizures can occasionally be delayed until later in childhood. Central nervous system involvement may be progressive, with worsening of seizures and deterioration of intellect. Earlier onset of seizures has worse prognosis for intellectual outcome, and seizures within the first month of life carry very poor prognosis for cognition and an increased likelihood of intractable seizures and hemiplegia. The central nervous system findings are usually ipsilateral to the skin changes, occasionally contralateral, and may be bilateral. Hemianopsia, hemiplegia, and hemiatrophy can all occur, usually contralateral to skin involvement. Magnetic resonance imaging is a better test for determining abnormal vessels; computed tomographic scan is better for detecting calcification.

HISTOPATHOLOGY

LIGHT. Vascular malformations are typical port wine stains showing thin-walled dilated small vessels. In older lesions, vessel walls may be thick and fibrotic.

EM. The endothelial cells are normal. There is multiplication of basal lamina investing the endothelial cells and several layers of muscle cells around them. Fine collagen fibers surround the vessel walls.

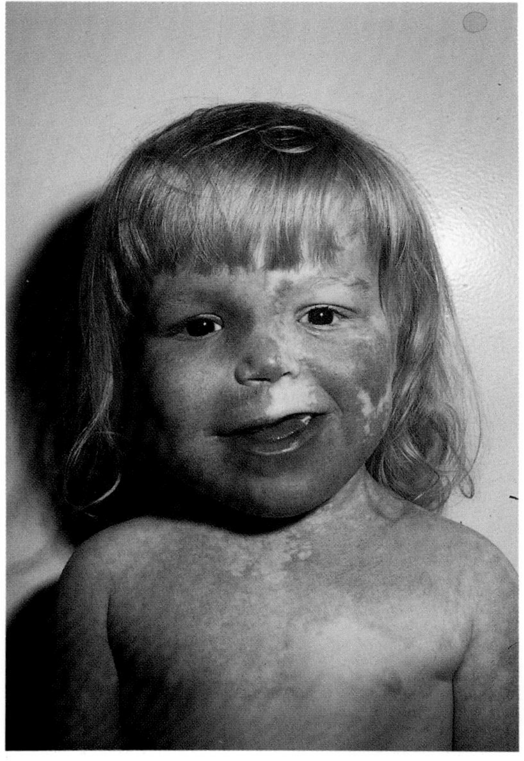

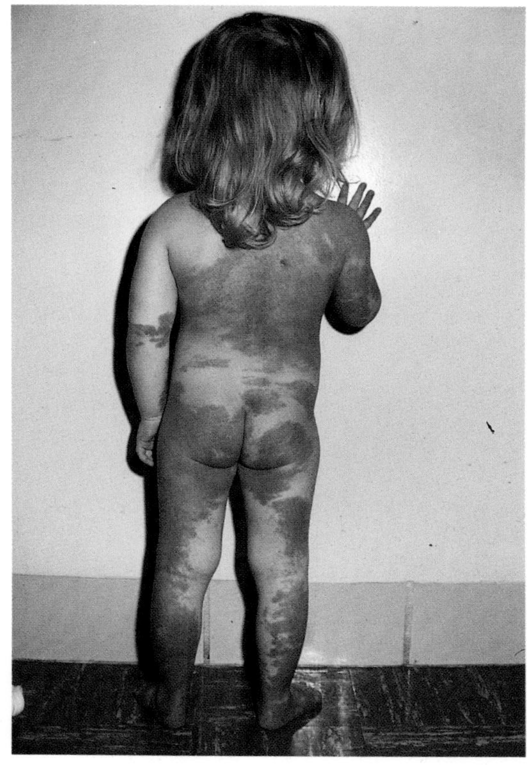

Figure 5.57. **(A)** Widespread bilateral involvement with soft tissue overgrowth. **(B)** Port wine stains on body on same patient showing overlap with Klippel-Trenaunay-Weber syndrome.

BASIC DEFECT

Unknown.

TREATMENT

Unilateral hemispherectomy is indicated for uncontrolled seizures. Use of the pulsed dye laser for cosmetic relief is indicated for some patients.

MODE OF INHERITANCE

Not genetic. There are rare instances of a parent with a port wine stain having an infant with Sturge-Weber syndrome. This is probably coincidental. There is one report of an infant with Sturge-Weber syndrome who had a maternal aunt with a port wine stain of her face. No further information was given.

PRENATAL DIAGNOSIS

None.

DIFFERENTIAL DIAGNOSIS

The isolated nevus flammeus of the glabella and/or eyelids should give no confusion with Sturge-Weber syndrome. Prominent and extensive flame nevi of the glabella, nasal tip, philtrum, and even to the chin are frequently associated with syndromes that affect the limbs, including skeletal dysplasias such as achondroplasia (MIM:100800), limb reduction disorders such as hypoglossia/hypodactylia (MIM:

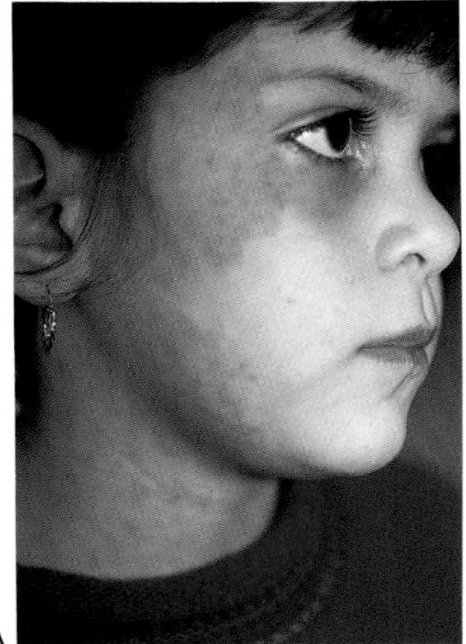

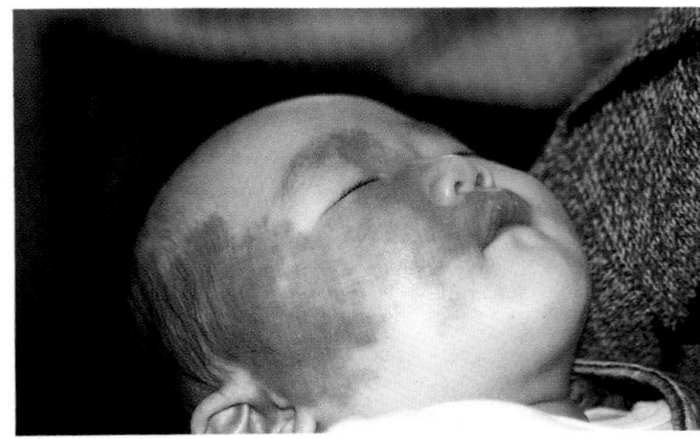

Figure 5.58. **(A)** Although first and second branches of trigeminal nerve are involved, patient is normal neurologically. (Courtesy of Dr. J. Francis, Seattle, Washington.) **(B)** Involvement in distribution of second and part of the third branches of the trigeminal nerve, with sparing of the eyelid.

103300), and movement disorders such as the arthrogryposes (MIM:Many).

The major problem in making the diagnosis of Sturge-Weber syndrome is to recognize those patients who have only a port wine stain versus those who are at risk for central nervous system and ophthalmologic involvement. The Wyburn-Mason syndrome (MIM:193300) is marked by congenital vascular malformations including arteriovenous malformations. There is a unilateral increase in number of vessels and tortuosity in the vessels of the retina. There may be associated arteriovenous malformations of the thalamus and midbrain. Some affected individuals have also had a cutaneous port wine stain. In the Cobb syndrome (MIM:106070), or hereditary neurocutaneous angioma, there are vascular lesions of the skin overlying and in association with dural or spinal cord vascular lesions. The vascular malformations include arteriovenous malformations, hemangiomas, and angiomas.

In von Hippel-Lindau disease (MIM:193300) there are rare reports of individuals with facial port wine stains. Von Hippel-Lindau is characterized by retinal angiomas, cerebellar hemangioblastomas, and renal lesions.

Familial flame nevi (MIM:163000) is characterized by typical stork bites or salmon patches over the glabella, eyelids, and elsewhere on the body. There is no association with central nervous system abnormalities, and the condition is entirely benign. It is autosomal dominant.

Diffuse cortical meningeal angiomatosis of Divry and Van Bogaert (MIM:206570) refers to two pedigrees of siblings with vascular malformations of the leptomeninges. Some affected individuals had marbling of the skin, similar to that seen in cutis marmorata telangiectatica congenita. Patients had no port wine stains and no intracranial calcifications.

In familial cavernous angiomas (MIM: 116860), affected individuals have vascular lesions in the central nervous system that may be multiple, and onset of seizures may be delayed by many years. There are reports of cutaneous vascular lesions in some affected individuals. These have been described as hemangiomas or angiomas, not as port wine stains.

Support Group: The Sturge-Weber Foundation (SWF)
P.O. Box 418
Mt. Freedom, NJ 07970-0418
1-800-627-5482

SELECTED BIBLIOGRAPHY

Bebin, E.M., and Gomez, M.R. (1988). Prognosis in Sturge-Weber disease: comparison of unihemispheric and bihemispheric involvement. *J. Child Neurol.* **3,** 181–184.

One hundred two Mayo Clinic charts reviewed. Eighty-eight patients with unilateral involvement, 14 with bilateral. Seizures occurred in 75% of the unilateral patients, 95% of those with bilateral involvement. Almost 50% of the unilateral patients had normal intelligence; less than 10% of those with bilateral disease did. No patient without seizures had mental retardation.

Cobb, S. (1915). Haemangioma of the spinal cord associated with skin naevi of the same metamere. *Ann. Surg.* **62,** 641–649.

Patchy port wine stains were present bilaterally on the back and abdomen in an 8-year-old who presented with sudden onset of paralysis and a hemangioma (angioma) involving the pia. Lesions can occur at any level in the central nervous system.

Enjolras, O., Riche, M.C., and Merland, J.J. (1985). Facial port wine stains and Sturge-Weber syndrome. *Pediatrics* **76,** 48–51.

Tallman, B., Tan, O.T., Morelli, J.G., Piepenbrink, J., Stafford, T.J., Trainor, S., and Westin, W.L. (1991). Location of port wine stains and the likelihood of ophthalmic and/or central nervous system complications. *Pediatrics* **87,** 323–327.

Stevenson, R.F., Thomson, H.G., and Morin, J.D. (1974). Unrecognized ocular problems associated with port wine stain of the face in children. *Can. Med. Assoc. J.* **111,** 953–954.

Enjolras et al. described 50 children. Twenty-six had V_1 and V_2 involvement. Of these, 45% had visual problems with glaucoma or suspected glaucoma. Of 42 with V_2 or V_3 port wine stains, none had glaucoma. Tallman et al. (1991) discuss 310 patients. Those who had involvement of V_3 alone had no ocular problems. If V_1 or V_2 was involved, the risk was 8%. Tallman et al. defined V_1 as upper lid, V_2 as lower lid. They state that Enjolras et al. defined V_1 as both. This is true based on the diagram in the Enjolras et al. article, but not as described in the text. Stevenson et al. (1974) reported 106 patients with facial port wine stains, of whom 12 had Sturge-Weber complex. Four of 106 had glaucoma alone; 4 of 106 had glaucoma and Sturge-Weber complex. If V_2 only was involved, there was no risk for eye findings. The differences in the findings among these three studies may relate to differences in defining the distribution pattern of the branches of the trigeminal nerve.

Louis-Bar, D. (1946–1947). IV. Sur l'heredité de la maladie de Sturge-Weber-Krabbe. *Confinia Neurol.* **7,** 238–244.

Reviews the literature and states that there is no compelling evidence for single-gene inheritance.

Roach, E.S., Riela, A.R., and Chugani, H.T. (1994). Sturge-Weber syndrome: recommendations for surgery. *J. Child Neurol.* **9,** 190–192.

Surgery may be appropriate for patients with medically unresponsive seizures, in hopes of preserving normal tissue. Corpus callectomy recommended for intractable seizures in patients who cannot be surgically approached.

MIXED

APLASIA CUTIS CONGENITA (MIM:107600, 207700, 107730, 100300, 181250, 181270)

Includes Adams-Oliver Syndrome, Scalp-Ear-Nipple Syndrome

DERMATOLOGIC FEATURES

MAJOR. The term *aplasia cutis congenita* encompasses a heterogeneous group of conditions that share in common focal absence of the skin. The defect may be limited to the epidermis, involve the full thickness of the skin, or include bony defects as well. Cutaneous defects heal rapidly, leaving a residual scar. The bony defects also ultimately close.

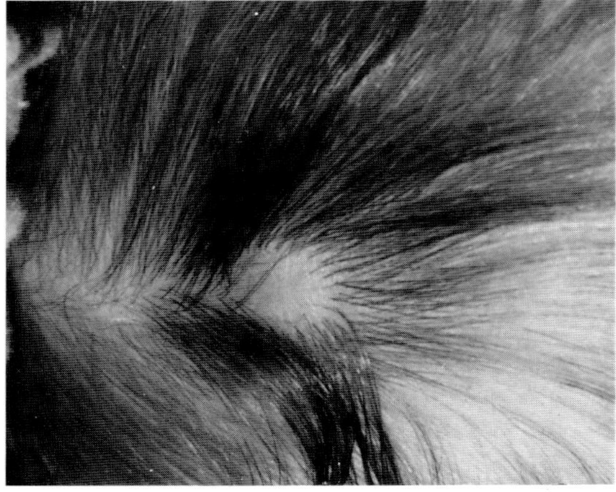

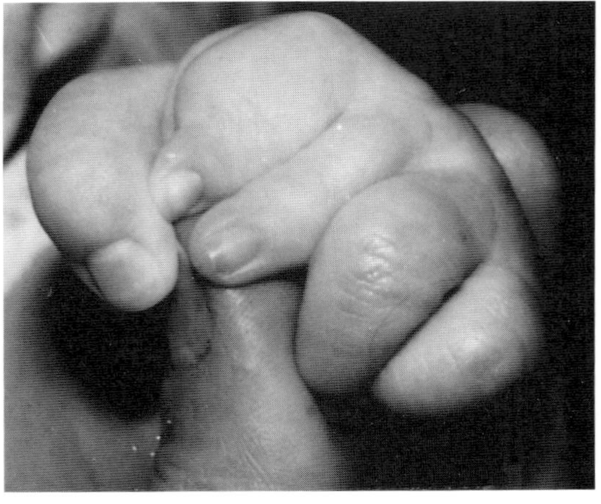

A B

Figure 5.59. **(A)** Infant with healed scalp defect. **(B)** Hand deformities with tapered index finger and short middle finger. (From Sybert, 1985.)

The most common site of involvement is the vertex of the scalp. Lesions can range from dime sized to involving the entire scalp. They may be single or multiple. Aplasia cutis congenita of the body wall is also reported.

At birth, the involved area is often a shiny, red, glistening defect that is mistakenly attributed to injury, placement of a fetal scalp monitor, or forceps mark.

The following classification of aplasia cutis congenita is formulated to allow for accurate diagnosis and genetic counseling. There is probably heterogeneity within each category as well.

Type I: Defect limited to the scalp and skull without associated abnormalities.
Type II: Aplasia cutis congenita limited to the scalp with limb defects.
Type III: Skin defects of the body wall with or without scalp involvement, with or without limb defects.
Type IV: Epidermolysis bullosa with aplasia cutis congenita (includes junctional epidermolysis bullosa and dystrophic epidermolysis bullosa).
Type V: Syndromic/teratogenic/nonspecific associations.

MINOR. Cutis marmorata is frequently reported in affected infants. It is seen more often in association with larger scalp defects and defects of the body wall. It usually resolves.

ASSOCIATED ABNORMALITIES

Type I: None.

Type II: Limb defects in association with aplasia cutis congenita of the scalp appear to comprise a group of genetically distinct conditions, each characterized by a specific limb defect that breeds true within a pedigree. Reported limb defects include reduction defects (Adams-Oliver syndrome, MIM:100300), polydactyly, (MIM:101250), zygodactyly syndactyly, ectrodactyly, and brachydactyly. Limb involvement is often asymmetric, and gene carriers may show aplasia cutis congenita or limb defects, both, or none.

Whether these conditions represent tight linkage of a gene for aplasia cutis congenita and one for limb defects (in which multiple allelic mutations in the latter result in the different limb defects), allelic mutations in a single gene, or nonallelic single-gene mutations is not known.

Type III: A variety of limb defects have been reported in a subset of children with aplasia cutis congenita of the body wall.

Type IV: Aplasia cutis congenita present at birth has been reported in both junctional and dystrophic forms of epidermolysis bullosa (MIM:Many). It has been suggested that two infants reported by Carmi et al. (1982) (MIM:207730) with aplasia cutis congenita and pyloric atresia represent a genetically distinct disorder. I believe they are instances of epidermolysis bullosa letalis with aplasia cutis congenita and pyloric atresia (MIM:226730), a well-recognized association.

Type V: Infants with chromosomal aberrations may have aplasia cutis congenita. It is reported most often in trisomy 13 and 4p− syndrome.

Aplasia cutis congenita can be a feature of focal dermal hypoplasia of Goltz (MIM: 305600) and Johanson-Blizzard syndrome (MIM:243800) and has been reported in many other malformation syndromes as an occasional or rare feature. The scalp-ear-nipple syndrome (MIM:181270) is an autosomal dominant disorder marked by aplasia cutis congenita of the vertex, abnormal teeth, malformed pinnae, and hypoplasia of the nipples and sometimes breasts.

Exposure to maternal methimazole use is associated with aplasia cutis congenita, as are intrauterine herpes simplex and varicella infections.

HISTOPATHOLOGY

LIGHT. Complete absence of any to all layers of the skin in new lesions. After healing, sites show a flattened epidermis, absence of adnexal structures, new capillaries, and fibroblasts in a loose connective tissue stroma consistent with a scar.

EM. No information.

BASIC DEFECT

Type I: Unknown.

Type II: Unknown.

Type III: The presence of a fetus papyraceous in a significant proportion of cases with type III aplasia cutis congenita prompted Mannino et al. (1977) to postulate a vascular or thrombotic cause for this category. They theorized that the dead twin released clots or clotting factors that entered the circulation of the survivor and resulted in vascular occlusion, cell death, and

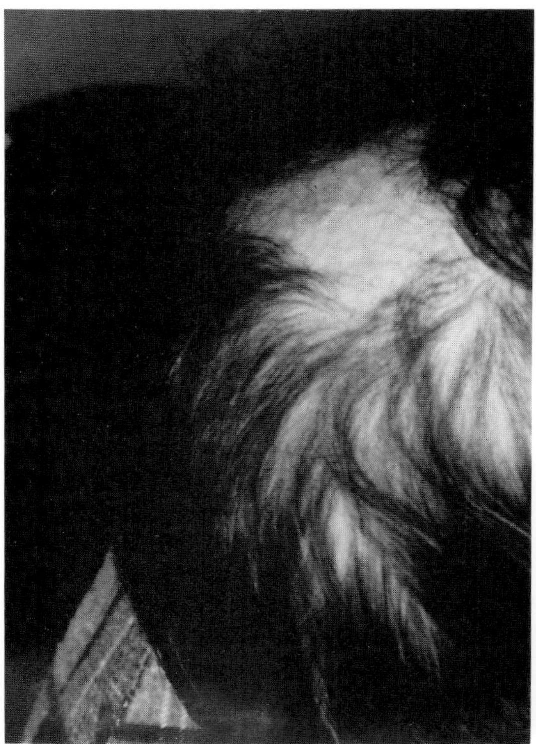
A

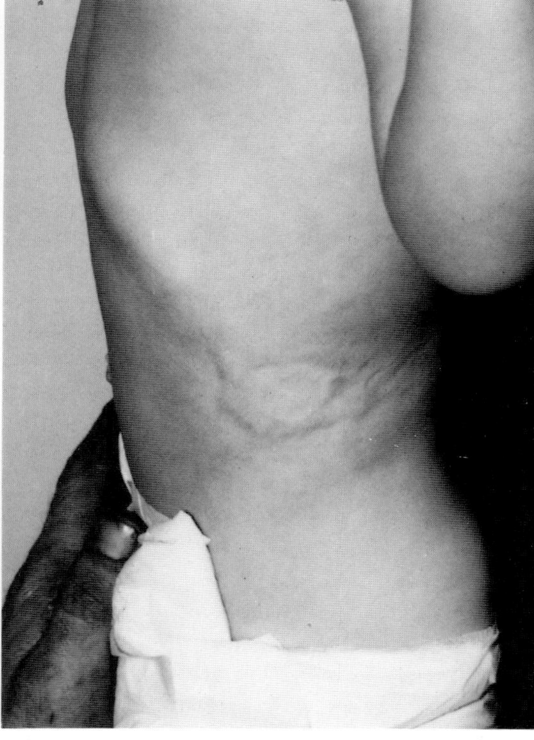
B

Figure 5.60. Scalp **(A)** and body wall **(B)** defects. (From Sybert, 1985.)

tissue necrosis. Amniotic bands have been reported in some cases of type III aplasia cutis congenita. It probably represents a causally heterogeneous group.

Type IV: Experimental evidence from the chick embryo showed that if the epidermis is separated from the dermis early in embryogenesis it does not differentiate to form feather buds, suggesting that dermoepidermal contact is necessary for the induction of epidermal appendages. It is possible that blistering of fetal skin in the third to fourth month of gestation could result in failure of appendageal formation, causing the defects seen in aplasia cutis congenita associated with epidermolysis bullosa, rather than attributing the scarring to loss of skin on the basis of blistering and erosion alone.

Type V: Unknown.

TREATMENT

Treatment is usually not required. The defects heal rapidly, leaving hairless scars. The skull defects usually fill in, although very large lesions may not completely ossify. If the scalp defect is very large and the superior sagittal sinus is exposed, there is risk for thrombosis, and these defects should be closed with a pedicle or flap graft. Split thickness grafts invariably fail. Hemorrhage from large lesions can occur; careful monitoring and conservative management are appropriate.

MODE OF INHERITANCE

Type I: Many cases appear to be sporadic. When the family history is positive, almost all

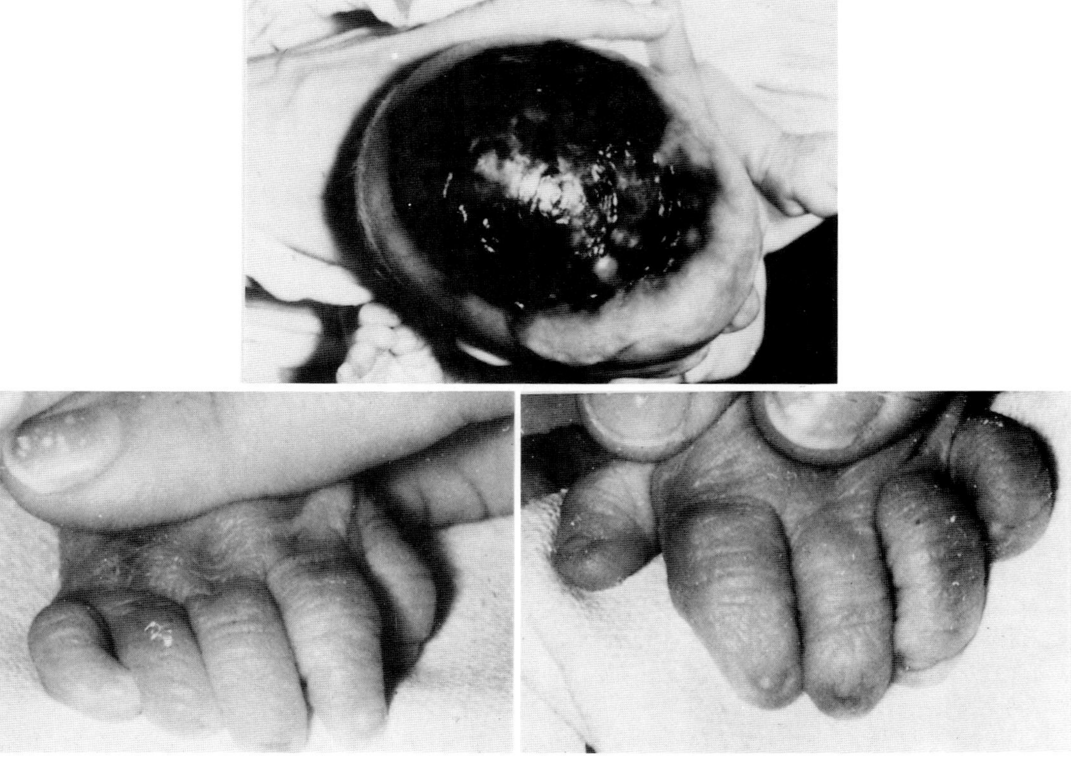

Figure 5.61. (A) Huge scalp defect covered by necrosing skin graft. **(B,C)** Short distal phalanges with small nails. (From Sybert, 1985.)

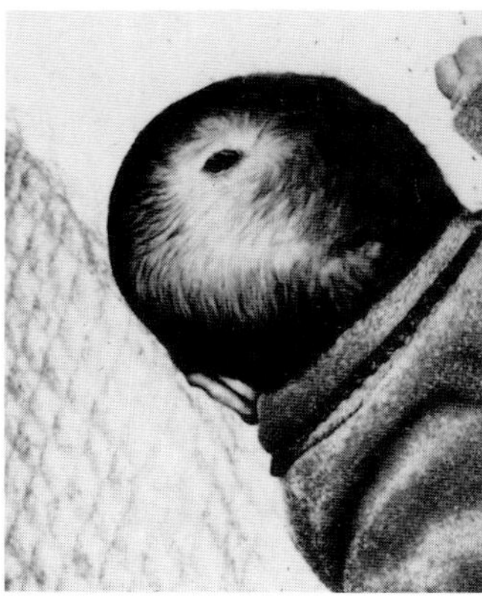

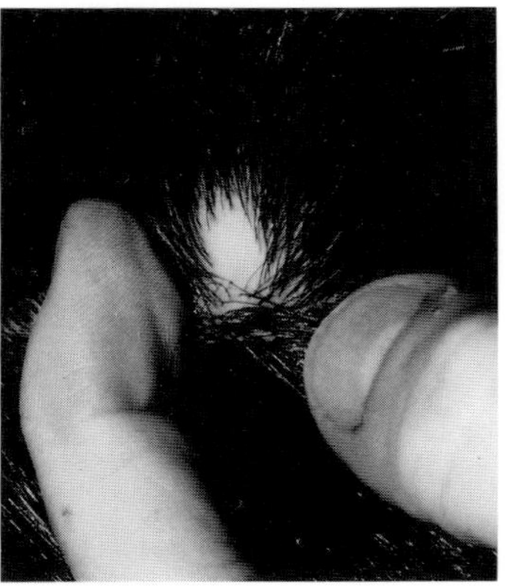

Figure 5.62. (A) Ulcer present at birth in infant. **(B)** Healed site in mother. She was unaware of defect. (From Sybert, 1985.)

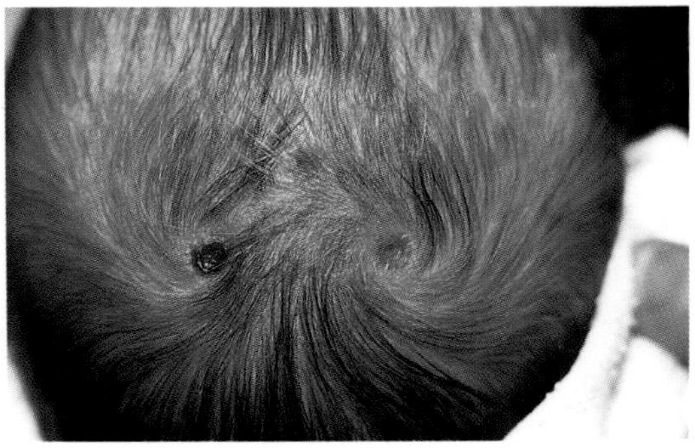

Figure 5.63. Three scalp defects in infant with trisomy 13. (From Sybert, 1985.)

pedigrees are consistent with autosomal dominant inheritance with reduced penetrance and variable expressivity. Reports consistent with autosomal recessive inheritance are not convincing, as in most instances parents were not examined. Healed scalp defects are easily overlooked, and in several families I have seen parents were unaware of their own lesions of aplasia cutis congenita. Analysis of our pedigrees suggested penetrance of approximately 60%, but this probably is an underestimate due to inaccurate reporting and my inability to examine personally all obligate heterozygotes. All first degree relatives of sporadic cases should be carefully examined for aplasia cutis congenita. If no one other than the proband is found to be affected, counseling for the possibility of a new dominant mutation should be given.

Type II: Most demonstrate autosomal dominant inheritance with reduced penetrance and variable expressivity. The pedigrees supporting autosomal recessive inheritance are not compelling.

Type III: There is no recurrence risk if associated with fetus papyraceous. The placenta and membranes should be carefully examined in all newborns with aplasia cutis congenita of the body wall.

Pedigrees consistent with both autosomal dominant and autosomal recessive inheritance for type III aplasia cutis congenita in the absence of a fetus papyraceous have been reported.

Type IV: Inheritance is specific for the type of epidermolysis bullosa with which the aplasia cutis congenita is associated. Although I do not believe that pyloric atresia and aplasia cutis congenita is an entity distinct from junctional epidermolysis bullosa letalis with pyloric atresia, others disagree. Inheritance for both conditions appears to be autosomal recessive; thus genetic counseling issues are not affected by this disagreement.

Type V: Depends on cause.

PRENATAL DIAGNOSIS

Available for epidermolysis bullosa by fetoscopy and fetal skin biopsy and mutation analysis or linkage and for chromosome abnormalities by chorionic villous sampling and amniocentesis. Directed level 2 ultrasound examination and α-fetoprotein levels were normal during a pregnancy at risk that subsequently resulted in a male infant with a large scalp defect. These techniques thus cannot be used reliably for prenatal diagnosis of aplasia cutis congenita.

DIFFERENTIAL DIAGNOSIS

Nevus sebaceous of the scalp, congenital nevocytic nevi of the scalp, and hemangiomas can give a similar clinical picture of a hairless, discolored area. These can usually be distinguished by examination; biopsy and histopathology will be diagnostic in difficult cases. Neuroectodermal rests or ectopic neural tissue can appear as purple or red hairless areas at the vertex, often surrounded by a ring of dark, long hairs. Surrounding rings of hair can also accompany aplasia cutis congenita and nevi. If doubt exists, appropriate studies (computed tomography or magnetic resonance imaging) should be performed to determine any connection through the dura.

Support Group: Specific for cause:
D.E.B.R.A. (EB)
40 Rector Street, 8th Floor
New York, NY 10006
1-212-693-6610

S.O.F.T. (Trisomy 13, 4p−)
2982 South Union Street
Rochester, NY 14624-1926
1-800-716-7638

N.O.R.D.
P.O. Box 8923
New Fairfield, CT 06812
1-800-999-6673

SELECTED BIBLIOGRAPHY

Adams, F.H., and Oliver, C.P. (1945). Hereditary deformities in man due to arrested development. *J. Hered.* **36,** 2–7.

Report of a large pedigree with several generations and male-to-male transmission of aplasia cutis congenita and terminal transverse defects of the limbs. Variable expression well described.

Carmi, R., Sofer, S., Karplus, M., Ben–Yakar, Y., Mahler, D., Zirkin, H, Bar–Ziv, J. (1982). Aplasia cutis congenita in two sibs discordant for pyloric atresia. *Amer. J. Med. Genet.* **11,** 319–328.

Products of consanguineous parents; one with pyloric atresia, one without. Skin sloughed readily.

Edwards, M.J., McDonald, D., Moore, P., and Rae, J. (1994). Scalp-ear-nipple syndrome: additional manifestations. *Am. J. Med. Genet.* **50,** 247–250.

Reviews 13 published cases and 11 of their own in a large kindred. Some decrease in apocrine sweating.

Frieden, I.J. (1986). Aplasia cutis congenita. A clinical review and proposal for classification. *J. Am. Acad. Dermatol.* **14,** 646–660.

Excellent review of aplasia cutis congenita with emphasis on both genetic and nongenetic forms. Her classification scheme differs from mine.

Mannino, F.I., Jones, K.L., and Benirschke, K. (1977). Congenital skin defects and fetus papyraceous. *J. Pediatr.* **91,** 559–564.

Reviews the findings of fetus papyraceous in a significant proportion of infants with aplasia cutis congenita of the body wall. Proposes a vascular occlusion mechanism for causation.

Sybert, V.P. (1985). Aplasia cutis congenita: a report of twelve new families and review of the literature. *Pediatr. Dermatol.* **3,** 1–14.

Discusses 14 families with aplasia cutis congenita and sets out classification scheme that I have revised here. Focuses on genetic aspects.

FOCAL DERMAL HYPOPLASIA (MIM:305600)

(Goltz Syndrome)

Includes MIDAS Syndrome

DERMATOLOGIC FEATURES

Major. The dermatologic features are the basis for making the diagnosis of focal dermal hypoplasia. Other associated malformations may or may not be present and are not necessary to make the diagnosis. The skin findings include the following.

Linear, streaky, punctate cribiform atrophy often occurs with telangiectases and hyperpigmentation. These linear areas of multiple, almost pinpoint, "pore-like" depressions in the skin are typical of the disorder. In my experience, they are more common and distinctive than the classic subcutaneous tissue herniation.

Patchy thinning to absence of the dermis results in herniation of the subcutaneous fat up into the epidermis, causing small, yellow, pouching areas that are soft and easily depressed;

Fleshy or vascular papillomas that develop with age are seen most frequently on mucosal, perioral, perigenital, and intertriginous surfaces.

Nail hypoplasia, dystrophy, or aplasia is a common finding.

Minor. Patchy alopecia, brittle hair, sparse hair; hyperkeratotic papules on palms and soles; hyperhidrosis; and aplasia cutis congenita have been described occasionally.

ASSOCIATED ABNORMALITIES

Other organ systems commonly involved are the ocular, dental, and skeletal.

A host of eye abnormalities has been described, the most common of which are strabismus, nystagmus, colobomas, microphthalmia, and photophobia. The diagnosis of focal dermal hypoplasia should prompt a complete ophthalmologic evaluation.

Dental abnormalities include oligodontia, dysplastic teeth, and enamel defects. I do not routinely obtain dental radiographs of an infant with focal dermal hypoplasia, but advise parents that a screening examination by a knowledgeable dentist at about age 2–3 years is reasonable. If primary teeth are very late to erupt, earlier evaluation may be appropriate.

Skeletal defects are legion. Parallel vertical banding (striated osteopathy) is seen in radiographs of the long bones. The clinical significance of these lines is unknown. Cutaneous or bony syndactyly is relatively common. Hypoplasia and aplasia of the digits can occur. Short stature, body and facial asymmetry, and a variety of other skeletal defects are reported in a minority of patients.

Cardiac malformations, abdominal wall defects, omphalocele, sensorineural hearing loss, renal malformations, and other defects have occurred in a minority of individuals. These may be true manifestations of the syndrome, coincidental findings, or features of disorders other than focal dermal hypoplasia sharing the same cutaneous findings that cannot be clinically differentiated. There are no physical features that would exclude the diagnosis of focal dermal hypoplasia in the presence of typical skin findings.

Mental retardation with or without microcephaly has been reported in about 15% of patients.

HISTOPATHOLOGY

Light. There is diminution to absence of the collagenous connective tissue of the dermis, with adipose cells extending up to the epidermis, separated by only a thin band of connective tissue. When collagen bundles are present, the fibers appear thinned or fragmented.

EM. Collagen fibers are small, but normally striated.

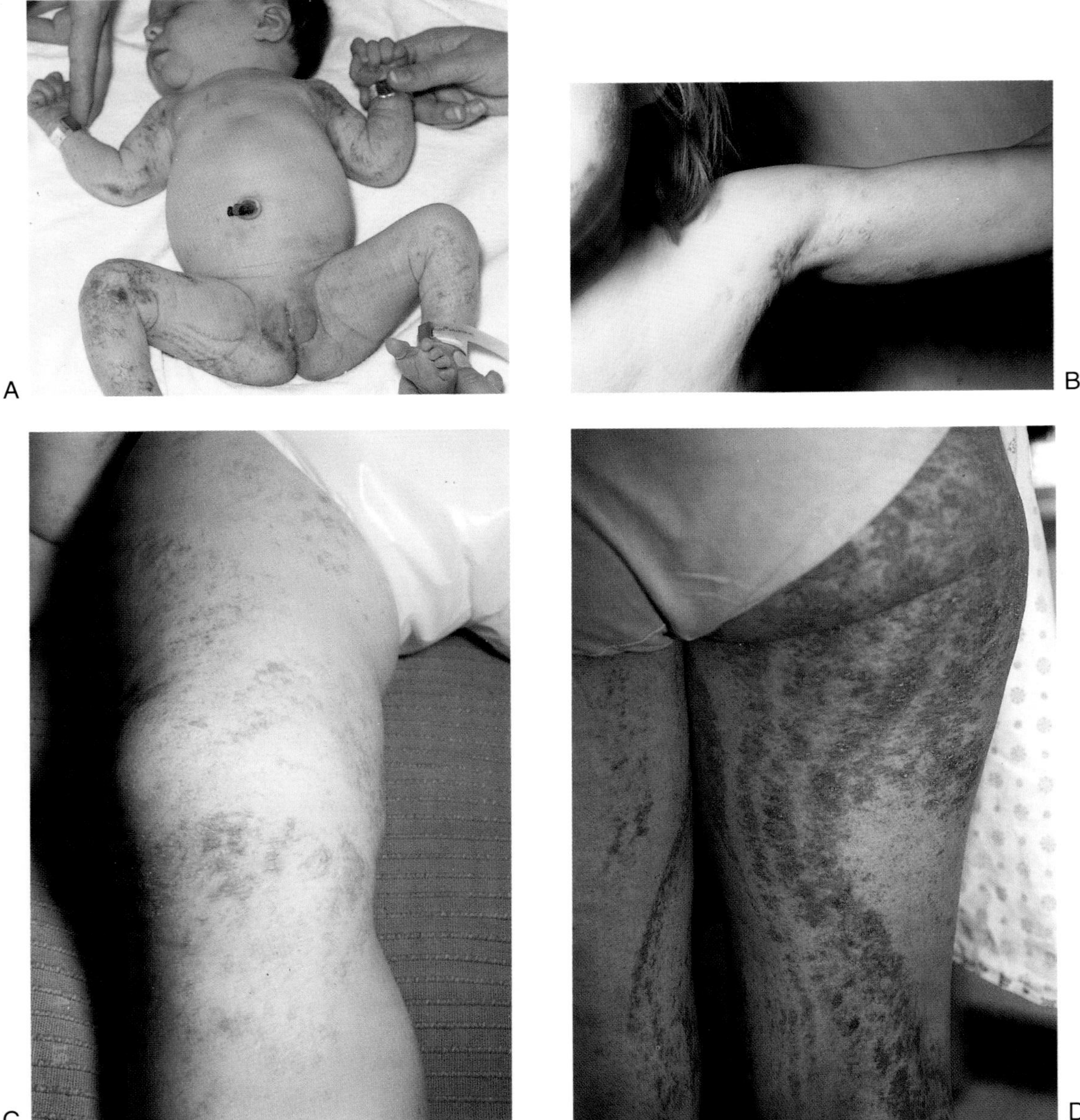

Figure 5.64. (A) Newborn with streaks and patches. **(B,C)** Same child at age 2 years, now with marked atrophy and outpouching of subcutaneous tissue. **(D)** Same patient at 19 years, with marked erythema and atrophy.

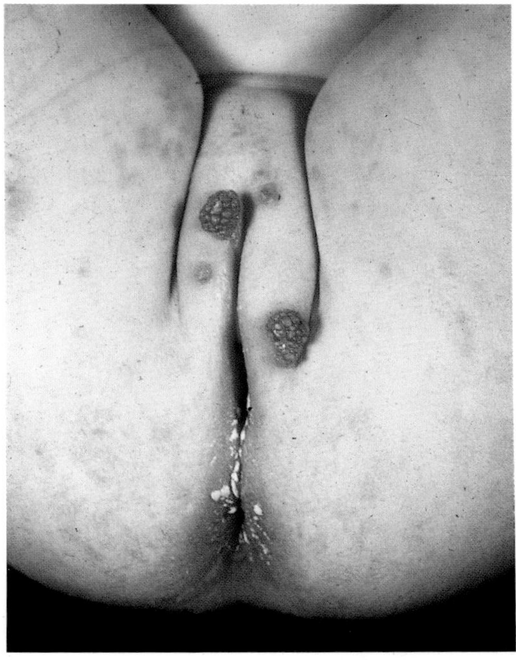

Figure 5.65. Papillomas on labia majora.

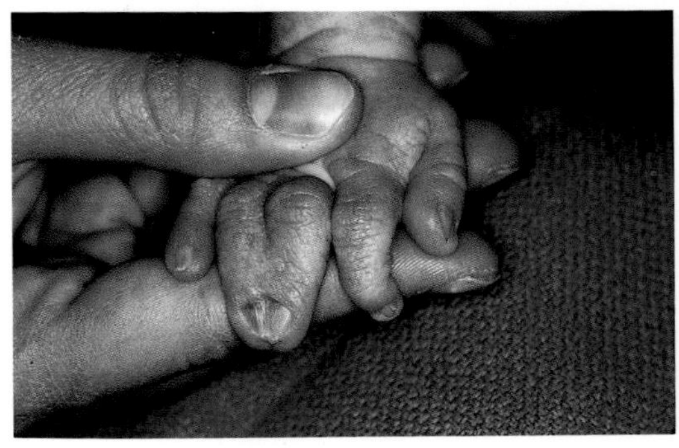

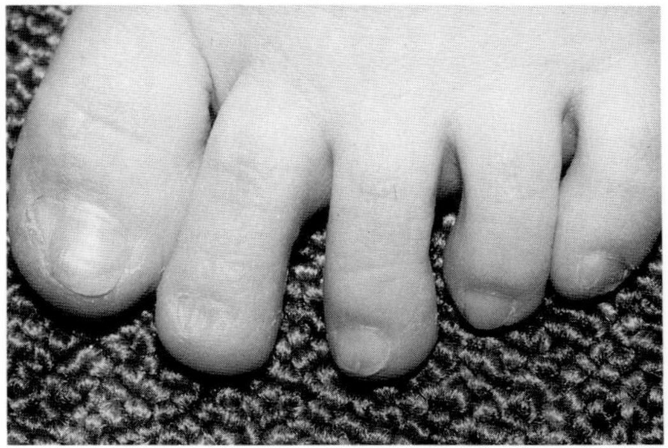

Figure 5.66. **(A)** Cutaneous and bony fusion with nail dystrophy. **(B)** Mild nail changes in another patient.

BASIC DEFECT

Unknown. Structures of both mesodermal and ectodermal origin are involved in the disorder. The variability in expression of focal dermal hypoplasia and the patchy distribution of skin findings is thought to be due to random X-inactivation (lyonization). There are animal models that may be homologous: bare patches and striated in the mouse and streaked hairlessness in cattle.

TREATMENT

There are no specific therapies for focal dermal hypoplasia. Excision of symptomatic papillomas may be desirable. Treatment for associated malformations (ocular, dental, and skeletal anomalies) may be required. Laser ablation of telangiectases may provide some cosmetic relief.

MODE OF INHERITANCE

X-linked dominant. Of more than 200 reported cases, only a few have been males. Most cases are sporadic, but inheritance through female relatives has been documented.

PRENATAL DIAGNOSIS

Not available. Although skin changes may be present in utero, their patchy distribution precludes accurate diagnosis by fetal skin biopsy.

DIFFERENTIAL DIAGNOSIS

There is some similarity of some skin lesions to the atrophic lesions of incontinentia pigmenti

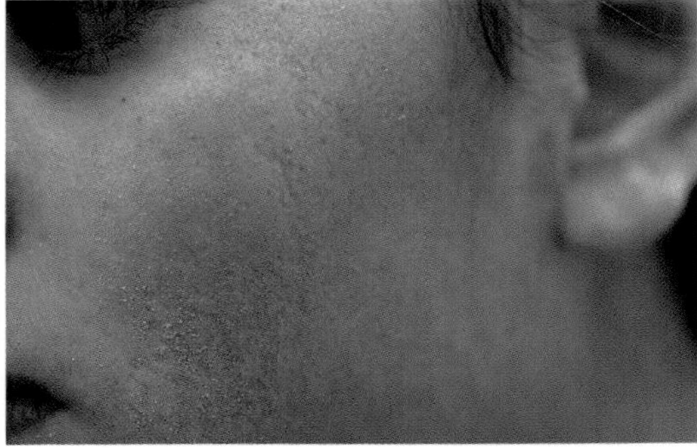

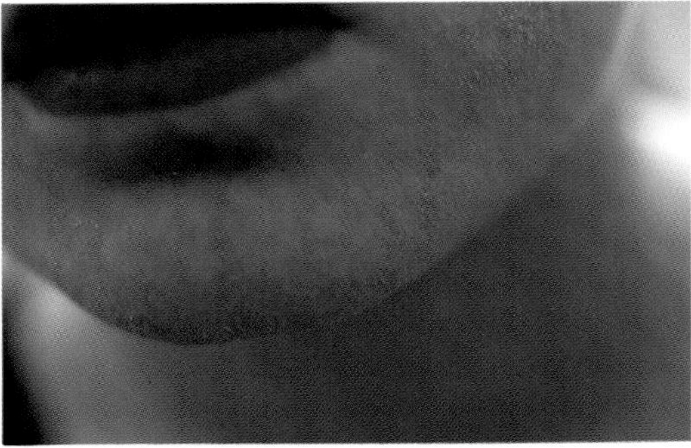

Figure 5.67. Icepick scarring and erythema.

(MIM:308300, 308310) and overlap of systemic features; focal dermal hypoplasia does not have the pigmentary change of incontinentia pigmenti. Although there is some overlap with the features of Rothmund-Thomson syndrome (poikiloderma congenitale, MIM:268400), there is no sun sensitivity in focal dermal hypoplasia. The atrophic lesions are clinically dissimilar to those of aplasia cutis congenita (MIM:107600, 207700, 207730). The follicular atrophoderma of chondrodysplasia punctata (MIM:302960), the X-linked dominant form, is similar to the cribiform lesions of focal dermal hypoplasia. The stippling of epiphyses in the former can distinguish between the two disorders. *M*icrophthalmia, *D*ermal *A*plasia, and *S*clerocornea comprise the MIDAS syndrome, or MLS (microphthalmia and linear skin defects, MIM:309801), a possibly X-linked dominant disorder tentatively mapped to X22.1–22.3. The skin lesions are more typical of aplasia cutis congenita with atrophic scars of the face and neck. There is no herniation of subcutaneous fat and none of the other skin manifestations of focal dermal hypoplasia of Goltz.

Support Group:

N.F.E.D.
219 East Main, Box 114
Mascoutah, IL 62258-0114
1-618-566-2020

N.O.R.D.
P.O. Box 8923
New Fairfield, CT 06812
1-800-999-6673

SELECTED BIBLIOGRAPHY

Goltz, R.W., Henderson, R.R., Hitch, J.M., and Ott, J.E. (1970). Focal dermal hypoplasia syndrome. A review of the literature and report of two cases. *Arch. Dermatol.* **101,** 1–11.

Review article with tables of frequency of abnormal features.

Goltz, R.W., Peterson, W.C., Jr., Gorlin, R.J., and Ravits, H.G. (1962). Focal dermal hypoplasia. *Arch. Dermatol.* **86,** 707–717.

Review of three patients with linear hypoplasia of the dermis. Refers to two previously reported cases, one in 1934 (reported as atrophoderma linearis maculosa et papillomatosis congenitalis) and one in 1941 (reported as a mesodermal and ectodermal defect syndrome of an anhidrotic type). Discusses differential of Rothmund-Thomson syndrome and nevus lipomatosus cutaneous superficialis of Hoffmann and Zuehelle.

Hall, E.H., and Terezhalmy, G.T. (1983). Focal dermal hypoplasia syndrome. Case report and literature review. *J. Am. Acad. Dermatol.* **9,** 443–451.

Case report of an affected male and review of the literature. Tables of associated malformations and skin findings are helpful.

Temple, I.K., Hurst, J.A., Hing, S., Butler, L., and Baraitser, M. (1990). De novo deletion of Xp22.2-pter in a female with linear skin lesions of the face and neck, microphthalmia, and anterior chamber eye anomalies. *J. Med. Genet.* **27,** 56–58.

Al-Gazali, L.I., Mueller, R.F., Caine, A., Antonlou, A., McCartney, A., Fitchett, M., and Dennis, N.R. (1990). Two 46,XX,t(X;Y) females with linear skin defects and congenital microphthalmia: a new syndrome at Xp22.3. *J. Med. Genet.* **27,** 59–63.

This article and that of Temple et al. (1990) report infants with the MIDAS syndrome. Skin lesions start as erosions and heal to scars and/or hyperpigmentation.

TUBEROUS SCLEROSIS (MIM:191100, 191092)

(Bourneville Disease)

DERMATOLOGIC FEATURES

MAJOR. Ash leaf shaped, hypopigmented macules occur in almost 90% of patients diagnosed with tuberous sclerosis. They may be present at birth or develop or increase in number during the first 2 years of life. I have had patients in whom lesions were documented to occur after 1 year of age, in direct contradiction to statements in the literature that the hypopigmented macules are present within the first few months of life. The lesions are not the dead white of vitiligo and fluoresce moderately with ultraviolet light (Wood's lamp). There is no change in the texture of the skin. The hypopigmented patches are usually on the trunk,

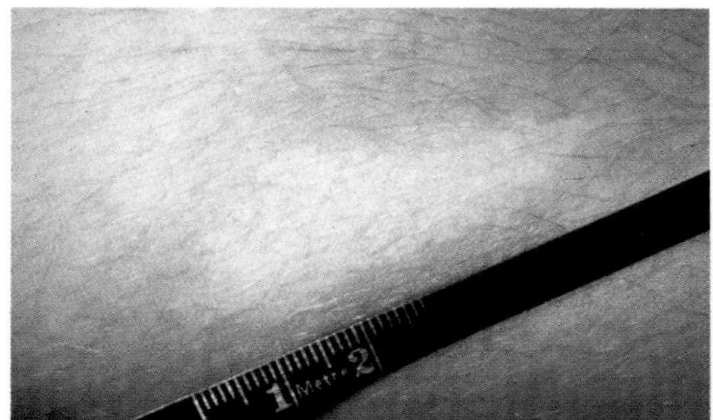

A

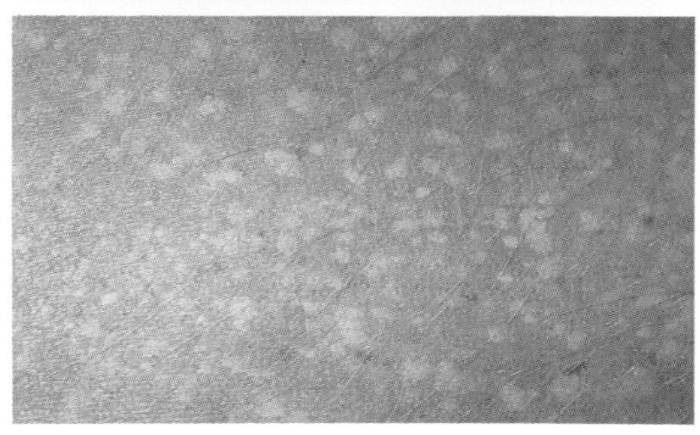

B

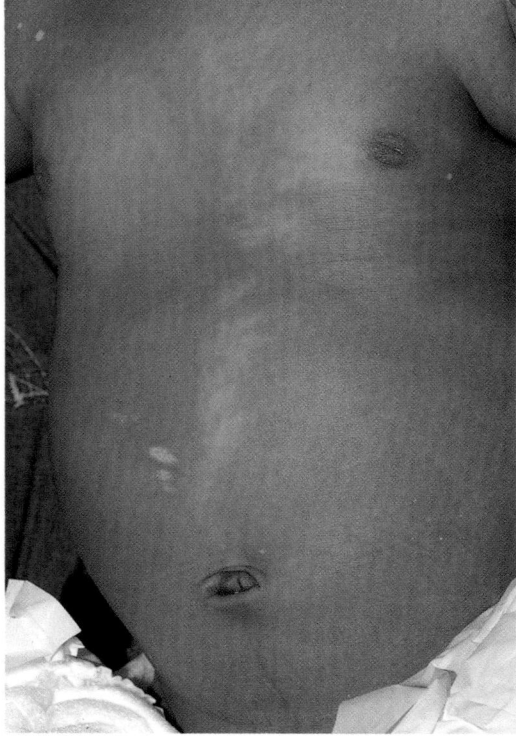

C

Figure 5.68. **(A)** Ash-leaf macule. **(B)** Confetti hypopigmentation. **(C)** Widespread distribution of hypopigmentation mimicking hypomelanosis of Ito.

buttocks, and extremities and are rare on the face. When on the scalp, the hair may be white.

Raindrop or guttate hypopigmented macules distributed in a confetti-like configuration have also been reported in some individuals with tuberous sclerosis.

Angiofibromas (adenoma sebaceum) are small discrete papules that can become confluent and fungating. They may be flesh colored if the fibrous component prevails or red if the vascular elements are more prominent. They tend to cluster on the face, cheeks, and nose and around the mouth. They are described in 50% of patients, but, as they develop in midchildhood or later, the actual occurrence may be higher. Gomez considers them pathognomonic for tuberous sclerosis; however, we have had two families who have had multiple facial angiofibromas without any other signs of tuberous sclerosis.

Shagreen patches or collagenomas are raised, firm, flesh colored to pink, yellow, or whitish plaques. Typical locations for these are the forehead and the sacrum, but they can appear anywhere. The skin appears thickened and coarse. Shagreen patches are described in approximately 20% of individuals with tuberous sclerosis, but, as they are easily overlooked, the prevalence may be higher. The onset of shagreen patches tends to be around the time of puberty.

Periungual fibromas (Könen tumor) are found in about 20% of affected individuals. These also develop later in childhood, puberty, and adult life. These fleshy growths occur around or under the nailplate. They may be reddish or flesh colored. The toenails are usually more involved than the fingernails. The growths may distort the nail. The periungual fibromas have normal epidermal skin lines, which helps to differentiate them from warts. They are also considered pathognomonic features of tuberous sclerosis.

Minor. Large fibromata can occur on the forehead. These are raised, rubbery, smooth, flesh-colored masses. *Molluscum fibrosum pendulum* is the term used for typical acrochordons or skin tags, which occur in typical locations,

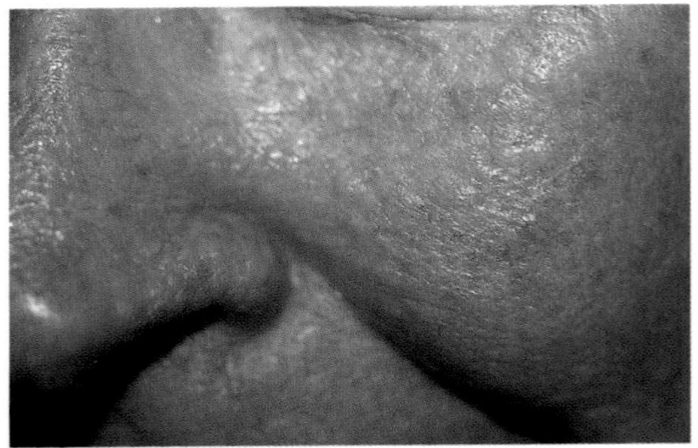
A

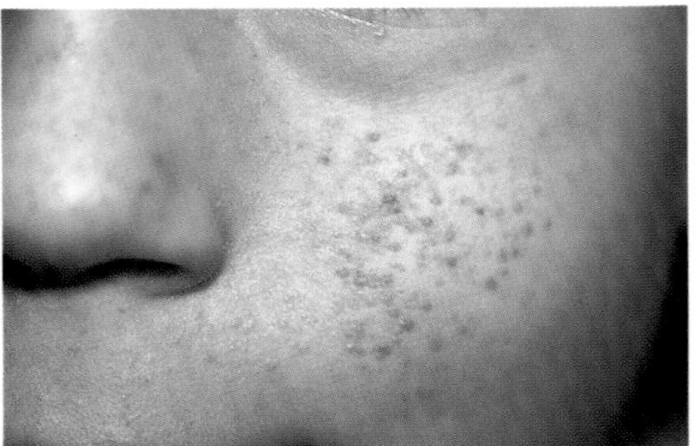
B

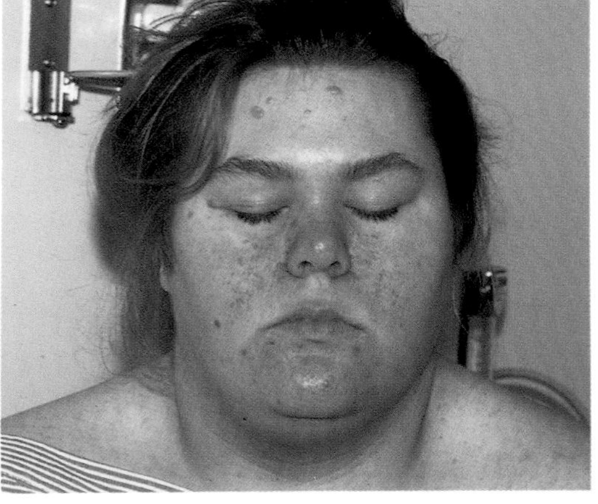
C

Figure 5.69. **(A)** Flesh-colored angiofibromas in an older individual. **(B)** Reddish angiofibromas. **(C)** Widespread distribution mimicking acne. Larger fibromas on forehead.

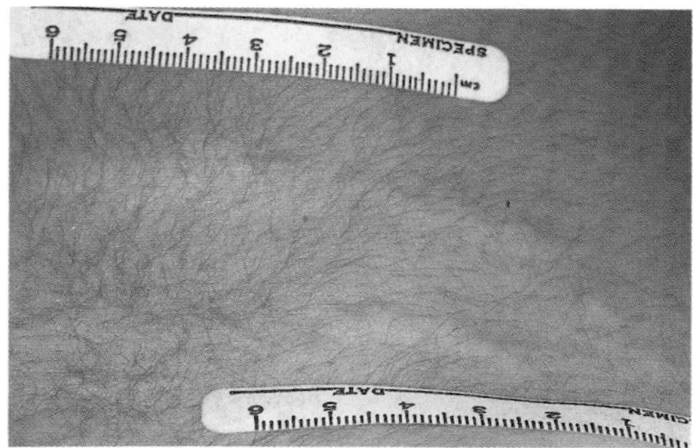

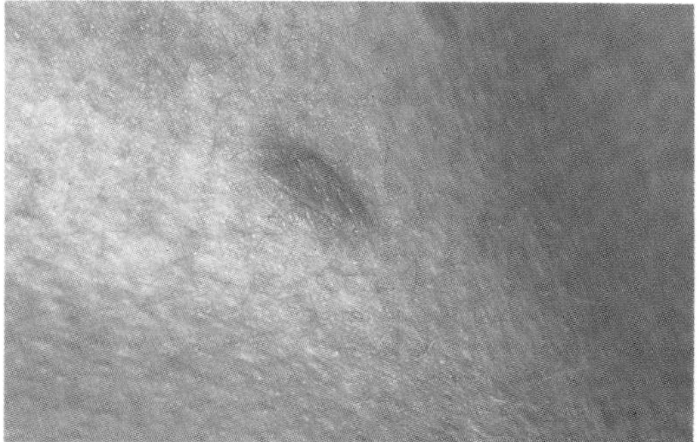

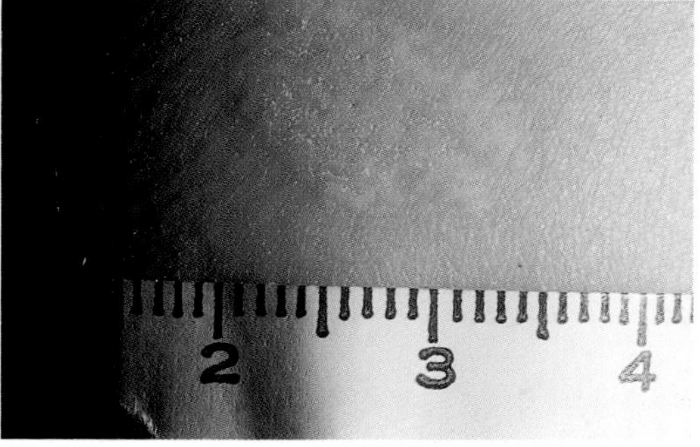

Figure 5.70. Shagreen patches.

the neck and axillae, in some patients with tuberous sclerosis. Small papules occurring on the trunk and neck, simulating gooseflesh, have been described in some patients. Fibromata of the gums can also occur.

ASSOCIATED ABNORMALITIES

Hamartomas, cortical and subcortical white matter tubers that are composed of abnormal giant astrocytes, are found in 90% of affected individuals. They are pathognomonic for tuberous sclerosis. Subependymal glial nodules that calcify are typical. Magnetic resonance imaging may be the best diagnostic test when looking for central nervous system involvement. Intracranial aneurysms have been reported in a handful of patients, as has the development of astrocytomas in childhood and the teen years.

Seizures develop in 84% of patients brought to diagnosis. The actual incidence may be less, as individuals with mild skin disease may be overlooked. The seizures usually begin in infancy, and the classic pattern is one of hypsarrhythmia or infantile spasms, but partial complex seizures and other patterns can also be seen. Estimates of mental retardation range from 30% to 65%, and the severity ranges from mild to severe. It has been suggested that autistic behavior may be a common feature, even in the absence of seizures or retardation. Of patients with mental retardation, all have seizures. Of patients with normal intelligence, about 65% have seizures.

Rhabdomyomas are congenital cardiac lesions that may be detectable by prenatal ultrasound and can be symptomatic in utero. They can arise anywhere in the myocardium. They may obstruct outflow and result in arrhythmias and syncope. They can also cause congestive heart failure because of inadequate myocardial function. They appear to resolve spontaneously over time. Wolf-Parkinson-White syndrome with and without rhabdomyomas has also been reported. Pulmonary involvement is uncommon in tuberous sclerosis. Cysts in the lungs and lymphangiomyomatosis have been described in 1% of patients. The onset of these problems is usually in adult life. Renal involvement includes angiomyolipomas that are multiple, bilateral, and usually asymptomatic. They can cause pain and bleeding. Cysts occur in approximately 20% of patients and can be severe and result in renal insufficiency. Renal failure can ensue, and renal disease may be the leading cause of death. Cysts of the kidney may be more common in tuberous sclerosis type 2, which is closely linked to the locus for adult onset polycystic kidney disease, but they also occur in tuberous sclerosis type 1. The risk for renal clear cell carcinoma, bilateral disease and onset in the twenties, may approach 4%. Renal transplantation has been performed successfully.

Eye involvement includes hamartomas of the retina, or classic mulberry lesions, which are similar to the lesions in the brain. These lesions may be flat or raised and may be multiple. They can calcify over time. Hypopigmented patches can also be seen. Visual loss is rare. Orthopedic involvement is marked by areas of sclerosis in the skull and vertebrae. Bony cysts in the hands and periosteal new bone formation along the metatarsals have been described.

Defects in enamel appear as small pits scattered over the teeth. They are not frequent in children, but almost invariably present in adults.

Angiomyolipomas can develop in the adrenal glands and are often asymptomatic. Thyroid papillary adenomas have also been described. A few patients have precocious puberty. Any organ may develop cysts or vascular proliferation.

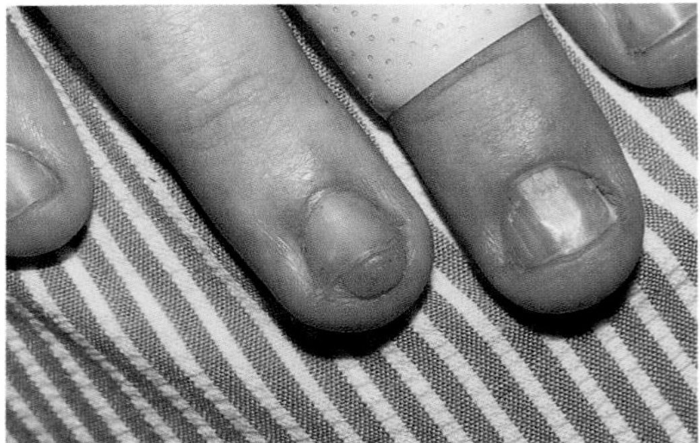

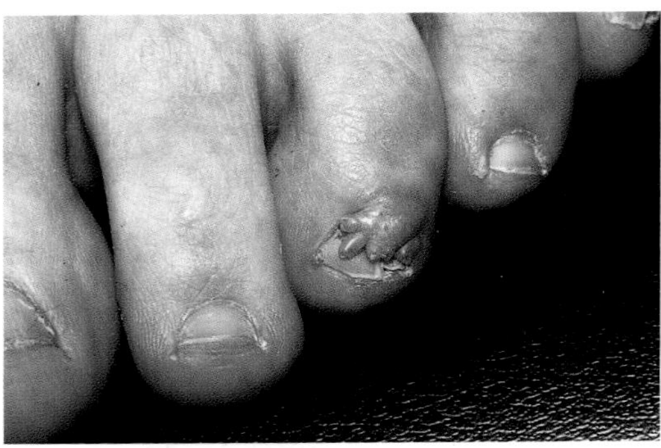

Figure 5.71. Periungual fibromas.

HISTOPATHOLOGY

LIGHT. The white spots appear normal on light microscopy. There may be decreased DOPA staining. The angiofibromas and periungual fibromas show dermal fibrosis and vasodilation with absence of elastic tissue. The fibroblasts may be large and stellate. The fibrous plaques show similar fibrotic changes without alterations of the vascular elements. The shagreen patch and connective tissue nevi show an increase in collagen and elastin.

EM. The hypopigmented macules show "effete" melanosomes with a decrease in number and size and melanization. It is not at all clear that this finding is limited to the white spots of tuberous sclerosis, as comparison to hypopigmented spots in normal controls has not been done. The angiofibromas show dermal vessels lined by a single layer of endothelial cells with poorly formed luminal microvilli. The shagreen patches show thickened and irregular collagen bundles in the lower dermis.

BASIC DEFECT

Unknown. The protein product of *TSC2* is tuberin. It has homology to a GTPase-activating protein, GAP3. Tuberin may act as a tumor suppressor.

TREATMENT

For angiofibromas, shave excision, dermabrasion, and CO_2 laser all give a modicum of short-term (months to years) cosmetic improvement. Fibromas can be excised but recurrence is likely. Treatment of seizures and other neurologic complications is problematic. Careful monitoring of renal involvement is important, and screening of young infants for rhabdomyomas is appropriate.

MODE OF INHERITANCE

Autosomal dominant. The condition shows locus heterogeneity. Tuberous sclerosis complex 1 (*TSC1*) appears to be linked to 9q34.3. *TSC2* is linked to 16p13.3, close to the adult onset polycystic kidney disease locus. There may be other families in whom other genes may be causal. There have been a few recurrences to siblings born of unaffected parents, the mechanism of which may be either gonadal mosaicism or decreased penetrance.

PRENATAL DIAGNOSIS

Possible by linkage in informative families and by ultrasound looking for cardiac rhabdomyomas between 22 and 24 weeks.

DIFFERENTIAL DIAGNOSIS

Isolated ash leaf spots occur in 5% of the general population. The white patches of pityriasis alba can also be confused. In tuberous sclerosis the hypomelanotic macules usually spare the face. In pityriasis alba the face is typically involved, and fine scaling may be apparent. In hypomelanosis of Ito (MIM: 146150) there is hypopigmentation distributed along the lines of Blaschko and not in ash leaf spots. In piebaldism (MIM:164920), Waardenburg syndrome (MIM:193500), and vitiligo (MIM:193200), loss of color results in depigmentation, not hypopigmentation. A nevus anemicus is an area of pallor due to increased vasomotor tone. These patches do not pinken with stroking, whereas an ash leaf spot will.

Angiofibromas can be misdiagnosed as acne vulgaris and acne rosacea. The pustules of the latter two conditions are distinct from the vascular papules of angiofibromas. Multiple trichoepitheliomas (MIM:190345) may look similar. Biopsy will differentiate between the two. Connective tissue nevi are part of the Buschke-Ollendorff syndrome (MIM:166700) and are seen in association with osteopoikilosis. Connective tissue nevi also occur in otherwise normal individuals. The periungual fibromas can be misdiagnosed as infantile digital fibromatosis, fibrokeratosis, and warts. In a relative at risk without any other signs of tuberous sclerosis, a biopsy may be necessary to differentiate a periungual fibroma from these other lesions. Isolated periungual fibromas can occur outside the setting of tuberous sclerosis.

Band heterotopias is a neuronal migration defect in which periventricular heterotopias occur. They do not calcify. Affected patients have seizures. This also can occur in families. The genetics of this condition are unclear.

Support Group: National Tuberous Sclerosis Association, Inc. (NTSA)
8000 Corporate Drive, Suite 120
Landover, MD 20785
1-800-225-6872

SELECTED BIBLIOGRAPHY

Ahlsen, G., Gillberg, I.C., Lindblom, R., and Gillberg, C. (1994). Tuberous sclerosis in western Sweden. A population study of cases with early childhood onset. *Arch. Neurol.* **51,** 76–81.

In this population survey, the authors demonstrate autism to be a feature common in children with tuberous sclerosis (a more detailed discussion is found in *Dev. Med. Child Neurol.* **36,** 50–56, 1994). They suggest that from 4% to 12% of children with autism have tuberous sclerosis. They argue that epilepsy and autism should always trigger an evaluation for tuberous sclerosis.

Bender, B.L., and Yunis, E.J. (1982). The pathology of tuberous sclerosis. *Pathol. Annu.* **17,** 339–382.

Describes clinical features and histopathology of tuberous sclerosis. Very complete and detailed.

Gomez, M.R. (ed.) (1988). *Tuberous Sclerosis*. Raven Press, New York, 2nd ed.

This detailed and useful second edition deals extensively with all the manifestations of tuberous sclerosis and is a must-read for anyone interested in the disorder. The clinical review is based on 300 patients in the author's Mayo Clinic population. He credits Von Recklinghausen with the first case description. The introduction by McDonald Cutchley is a good read about good riddance to the terms *epiloia* and *phakomatosis*. Chapter Two outlines criteria for definitive and presumptive diagnosis.

Johnson, W.G., and Gomez, M.R. (eds.) *Ann. N.Y. Acad. Sci.* **615,** 1–397, 1991.

The entire volume is devoted to tuberous sclerosis. There is a short entry by Osborn, Friar, and Wells (pp. 125–127) that suggests a recurrence risk of 2% if both parents are normal. This was based on three instances of recurrences to normal individuals.

Northrup, H., Wheless, J.W., Bertin, T.K., and Lewis, R.A. (1993). Variability of expression in tuberous sclerosis. *J. Med. Genet.* **30,** 41–43.

Three families illustrated extraordinary intrafamilial variation and the difficulty of determining carrier status of parents.

Petrikovsky, B.M., Vintzileos, A.M., Cassidy, S.B., and Egan, F.F.X. (1990). Tuberous sclerosis in pregnancy. *Am. J. Perinatol.* **7,** 133–135.

Two cases of their own with four from the literature of pregnancies to patients with tuberous sclerosis. Pregnancy is clearly underreported in these patients, and biased recognition of those pregnancies with complications is inevitable. Nonetheless, the authors suggest that renal status is a major predictor of high risk in pregnancy to these patients and recommend that women with tuberous sclerosis be evaluated for renal involvement prior to undertaking pregnancy.

Shepherd, C.W., Gomez, M.R., Lie, J.T., and Crowson, C.S. (1991). Causes of death in patients with tuberous sclerosis. *Mayo Clin. Proc.* **66,** 792–796.

Three hundred fifty-five patients. Forty-nine died, 40 of causes attributable to tuberous sclerosis. Two deaths were due to cardiac involvement (rhabdomyomas in a 3-day-old, rupture of a thoracic aneurysm in a 3-year-old), 11 of renal involvement (all older than 10 years of age). Ten patients developed astrocytomas. Lymphangiomatosis of the lung resulted in the death of four individuals over the age of 40 years. Thirteen individuals with severe mental retardation died in status epilepticus with bronchopneumonia.

Stapleton, F.B., Johnson, D., Kaplan, G.W., and Griswold, W. (1980). The cystic renal lesion in tuberous sclerosis. *J. Pediatr.* **97,** 574–579.

Three infants with polycystic kidneys; two were diagnosed as adult onset polycystic kidney disease manifesting in infancy, one was diagnosed with infantile polycystic kidney disease prior to onset or recognition of other stigmata of tuberous sclerosis.

Van Baal, J.G., Smits, N.J., Keeman, J.N., Lindhout, D., and Verhoef, S. (1994). The evolution of renal angiomyoplipomas in patients with tuberous sclerosis. *J. Urol.* **152,** 35–38.

A 5-year follow-up of 20 patients with renal angiomyolipomas. Seven had experienced renal hemorrhage requiring hospital admission. One died. In four patients, the lesions increased in size. An increased risk for bleeding was associated with size of tumor greater than 3.5 cm. The authors recommend periodic screening for and embolization of large lesions. The 20 patients were culled from 30 tuberous sclerosis patients originally screened.

OTHER DISORDERS OF THE DERMIS

ALBRIGHT HEREDITARY OSTEODYSTROPHY (MIM:103580, 203330, 300800)

(Pseudohypoparathyroidism; Pseudopseudohypoparathyroidism)

Includes Osteoma Cutis (Familial Ectopic Ossification, MIM:166350)

DERMATOLOGIC FEATURES

MAJOR. The skin lesions of osteoma cutis usually develop in infancy and early childhood. Skin-colored to bluish, hard papules to nodules commonly develop in areas of trauma, such as immunization sites and pressure points. The lesions may coalesce to form plaques; this is a feature seen almost exclusively in Albright hereditary osteodystrophy. There is often overlying erythema.

MINOR. Ulceration of skin lesions can occur.

ASSOCIATED ABNORMALITIES

The terminology for the disorders that have been labeled as *Albright hereditary osteodystrophy* (AHO) is at best confusing. With the recent delineation of molecular defects, some clinical and biochemical correlations can be made. In most patients, pseudohypoparathyroidism Ia (PHP-Ia) results from a defect in the α-subunit of the G_s protein (guanine nucleotide-binding protein). G_s activity is approximately 50% of normal in affected individuals. All patients with this defect have Albright hereditary osteodystrophy with the skeletal changes of short stature, short fourth and fifth metacarpals and metatarsals, short distal phalanges, and a round face. They may have a decreased sense of smell. Mental deficiency is common in this group, as is obesity. Resistance to thyroid-stimulating hormone and glucagon, along with gonadal dysfunction, is common. Hypogonadism and hypothyroidism have been the presenting features in some infants. In families with PHP-Ia some affected individuals may have the changes of AHO alone, without hormone resistance. It is for these individuals that the term pseudopseudohypoparathyroidism (PPHP) is reserved.

In pseudohypoparathyroidism Ib (PHP-Ib), affected individuals have normal G_s activity. They do not have mental retardation. They have no resistance to pituitary hormones other than parathormone hormone, and only 15% have AHO.

In different series, between 50% and 100% of individuals with AHO who were examined showed basal ganglia calcification.

Metabolic problems of hypocalcemia and hyperphosphatemia are common. In both PHP-Ia and -Ib there is a decreased urinary secretion of cyclic AMP in response to parathormone infusion.

Pseudohypoparathyroidism type II is not a familial condition and is marked by resistance to parathormone alone. Urinary cyclic AMP production is normal.

HISTOPATHOLOGY

LIGHT. Osteoblast-like cells are present in an osteoid matrix. There is positive staining for calcium, which is organized in a lamellar bone-like pattern.

EM. Cells appear to be osteocytes. There is globular or needle-like deposition consistent with calcium phosphate and hydroxyapatite deposition.

BASIC DEFECT

Mutations in the *GNAS1* gene in some. There is end-organ resistance to parathormone, which results in the skeletal changes.

TREATMENT

Vitamin D treatment with or without calcium supplementation may be effective. Affected individuals need to be monitored carefully for hypothyroidism.

MODE OF INHERITANCE

PHP-Ia, uncertain. The gene *GNAS1* is mapped to 20q13.11. In some pedigrees the condition is clearly autosomal dominant based on molecular studies. Some variants appear to be autosomal recessive, and there is suggestion of X-linked or sex-limited expression. Imprinting has been proposed and then refuted. Although this chromosomal region is imprinted in the mouse, there is no evidence for this in humans. Most cases of type Ib are sporadic. When familial, the mode of inheritance has not yet been defined. Type II appears to be sporadic.

PRENATAL DIAGNOSIS

Presumably possible for PHP-Ia by molecular techniques.

DIFFERENTIAL DIAGNOSIS

Isolated osteoma cutis is rare. Infants have been described with congenital plaques of osteoma cutis.

Osteoma cutis can occur secondarily in tumors, scars, and after inflammatory disorders such as dermatomyositis and scleroderma. It has also been described within nevi, calluses, and hemangiomas. Calcinosis cutis, deposition of calcium without true bone formation in the skin, can also be seen secondary to trauma, in scars, and in association with collagen vascular disease. A biopsy may be necessary to distinguish between calcinosis cutis and osteoma cutis. In myositis ossificans progressiva (MIM: 135100), ectopic bone forms in the muscle, not in the subcutis. COPS (calcinosis cutis, osteoma cutis, poikiloderma, and skeletal abnormalities; MIM:None) is marked by cutaneous atrophy and telangiectasias of the facial skin, in addition to the calcium deposition and ectopic bone formation.

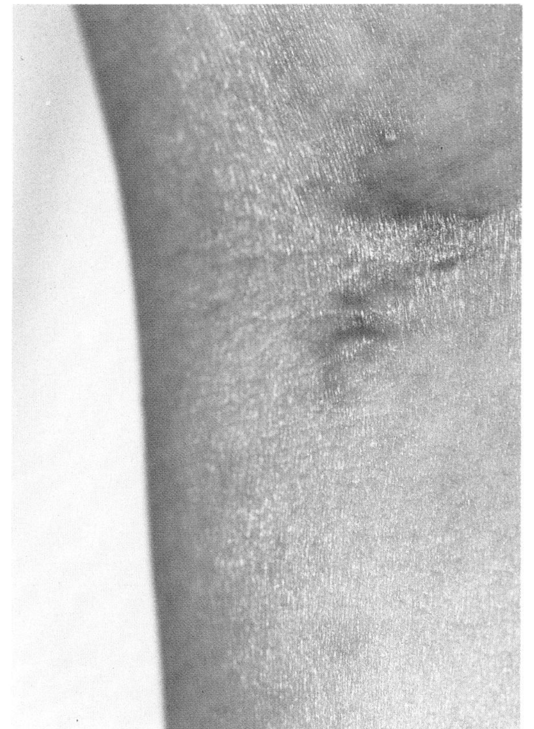

A

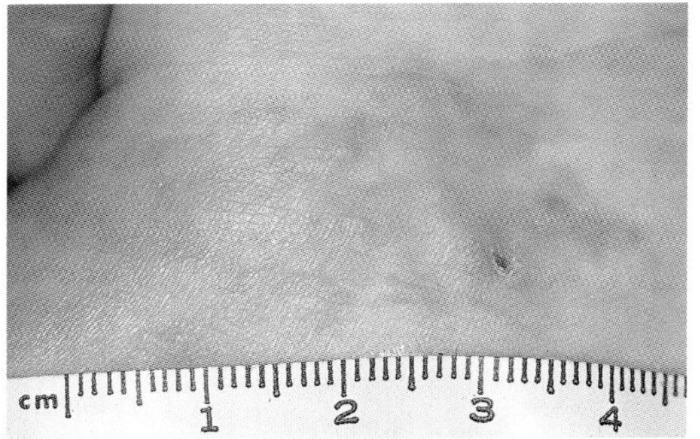

B

Figure 5.72. Osteoma cutis: **(A)** Fairly nondescript slightly red plaque. **(B)** Somewhat hyperpigmented plaque over ankle. Biopsy site at 5 o'clock. (B, courtesy of Division of Dermatology, University of Washington.)

Although McKusick lists osteoma cutis as a separate autosomal dominant entry (MIM: 166350), there are no compelling pedigrees that have excluded the possibility of AHO. Tumoral calcinosis (MIM:114120, 211900) is an autosomal recessive disorder characterized by large deep deposits of calcium that develop over the hips, buttocks, and joints. These often extrude whitish material. The lesions of AHO tend to be smaller. Biopsy will differentiate between the two conditions if the distinction is not obvious clinically.

Patients with Turner syndrome have short stature and short fourth metacarpals in common with AHO, but they don't develop osteoma cutis.

Support Group: N.O.R.D.
P.O. Box 8923
New Fairfield, CT
06812
1-800-999-6673

SELECTED BIBLIOGRAPHY

Campbell, R., Gosden, C.M., and Bonthron, D.T. (1994). Parental origin of transcription from the human GNAS1 gene. *J. Med. Genet.* **31,** 607–614.

In 13 informative fetuses, no parental-specific expression of *GNAS1* was seen. In other words, both the paternal and maternal alleles appear to be active, suggesting that imprinting does not occur at that locus consistently during gestation.

Izraeli, S., Metzger, A., Horev, G., Karmi, D., Merlob, P., Farfel, Z. (1992). Albright hereditary osteodystrophy with hypothyroidism, normal calcemia, and normal G_s protein activity: a family presenting with congenital osteoma cutis. *Am. J. Med. Genet.* **43,** 764–767.

The diagnosis in this family was made after evaluation of a newborn with multiple small, flat, hard subcutaneous plaques. More lesions appeared within the first few years. Although the skeletal changes of AHO were present, affected individuals had normal calcium, phosphorous, and alpha G_s activity.

Phelan, M.C., Rogers, R.C., Clarkson, K.B., Bowyer, F.P., Levine, M.A., Estabrooks, L.L., Severson, M.C., and Dobyns, W.B. (1995). Albright hereditary osteodystrophy and del(2)(q37.3) in four unrelated individuals. *Am. J. Med. Genet.* **58,** 1–7.

Four unrelated probands with obesity, dull normal intelligence or mental retardation, skeletal features of AHO, and no calcinosis cutis had deletions at 2q37. Authors posit a second locus for AHO.

Spiegel, A.M., and Weinstein, L.S. (1995). Pseudohypoparathyroidism. In *The Metabolic and Molecular Bases of Inherited Disease.* Scriver, C.R., Beaudet, A.L., Sly, W.S., and Valle, E.D. (eds.). McGraw-Hill, New York, 7th ed., pp. 3073–3089.

This is a great review, clear and comprehensive. The vignettes in the genetics section are most enlightening. In the premolecular era, the diagnosis was made in a father and his daughters based on full expression in the girls and short fourth metacarpals in him. After α-G_s testing, the mother was found to be affected. The father had an old fracture in his metacarpal, resulting in his bony changes. This raises a cautionary note for those who depend on pedigree analysis of reports in the literature to support the concepts of anticipation and imprinting.

CUTIS VERTICIS GYRATA (MIM:219300, 304200)

(Bulldog Scalp)

Includes Pachydermoperiostosis; Hypertrophic Osteoarthropathy, Primary (MIM:167100); Beare-Stevenson Syndrome (MIM:123790)

DERMATOLOGIC FEATURES

MAJOR. Fixed, thickened, corrugated folds of the skin of the scalp may be present at birth or develop in childhood or early adult life. The folds of skin are fixed and do not flatten with traction. The involved areas are usually normal in color. The appearance is similar to the sur-

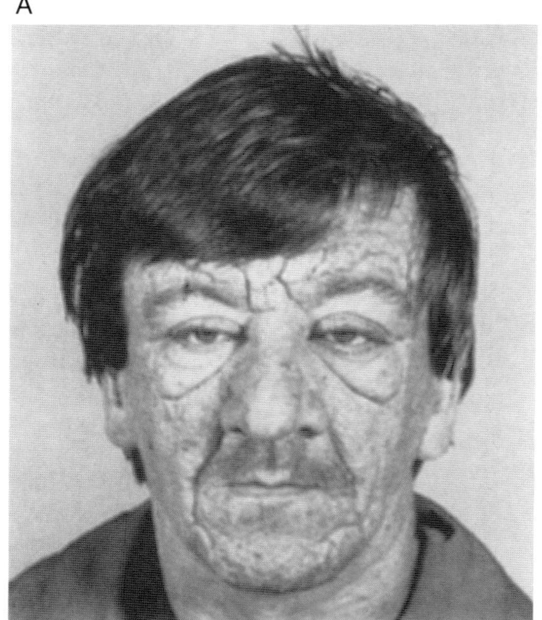

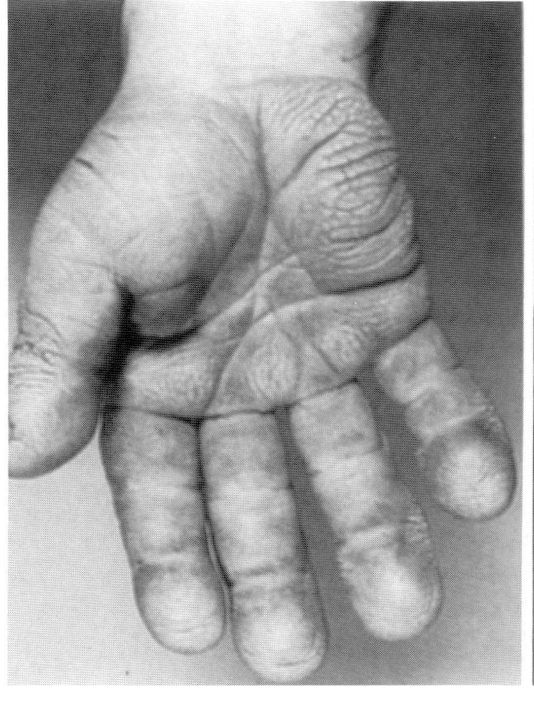

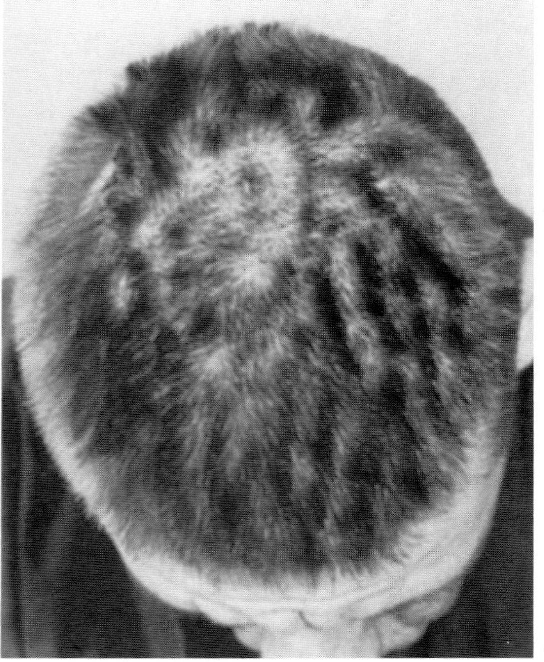

Figure 5.73. **(A)** Coarse facial skin. **(B)** Distal hypertrophy of fingers and palmar thickening. **(C)** Rugated scalp of a different individual. (From Oikarinen et al., 1994.)

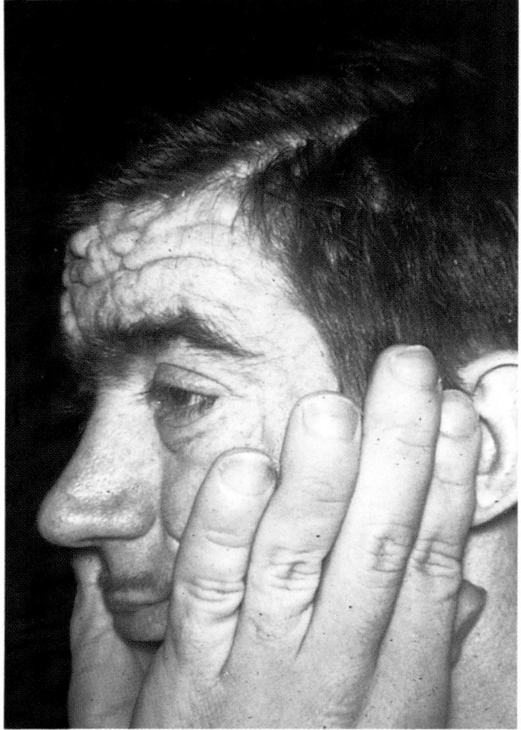

Figure 5.74. Thickened furrows on scalp; broad spatulate fingers. (Courtesy of Dr. J. Halloran, Division of Dermatology, University of Washington.)

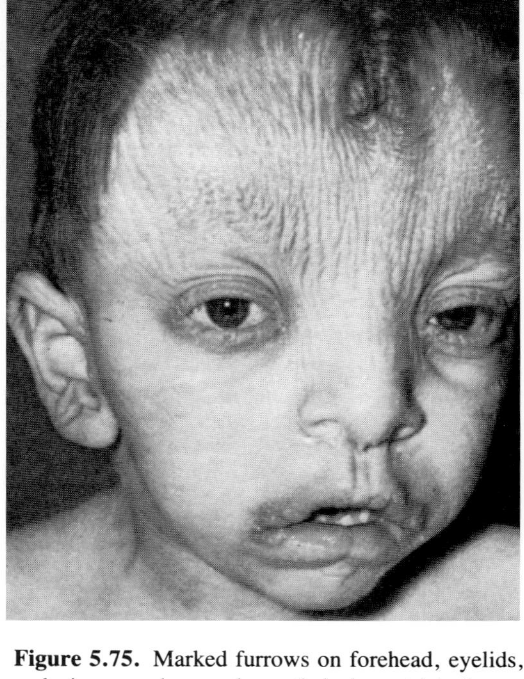

Figure 5.75. Marked furrows on forehead, eyelids, and pinnae and around mouth in hypertrichotic patient with Beare-Stevenson syndrome. (From Beare et al., 1969.)

face of the brain with gyri and sulci, hence the adjective *cerebriform*. Lesions tend to increase in size and thickness over years.

While the most common site is on the scalp, the forehead, neck, and scrotum may also be involved.

MINOR. None.

ASSOCIATED ABNORMALITIES

Primary cutis verticis gyrata can be seen in isolation, in association with mental retardation, and in the autosomal dominant disorder of pachydermoperiostosis (MIM:167100). It can be the result of ongoing dermatologic diseases such as eczema and psoriasis or a feature of systemic disease, such as acromegaly.

Mental retardation is reported in approximately 25% of the cases of cutis verticis gyrata in the literature. The presence of cutis verticis gyrata at birth does not correlate with the risk of mental retardation; in cases with mental retardation the cutis verticis gyrata is often acquired rather than congenital. Palo and colleagues (1970) found cutis verticis gyrata in 2% of 590 patients in a mental institution. In 11 of these, pneumoencephalogram revealed structural brain or calvarial abnormalities.

I have seen two patients with Turner syndrome (Mary Spraker and colleagues have seen one other) who were born with localized cutis verticis gyrata. One lesion was excised and showed normal skin. I believe the lesion resulted from in utero "pinching" of edematous skin, which resulted in fixation of redundant tissue.

There have been reports of infants with extensive cutis verticis gyrata of the face and limbs, acanthosis nigricans, and multiple malformations, including craniofacial dysostosis similar to Crouzon syndrome (Beare-Stevenson syndrome, MIM:123790). As acanthosis nigricans is a feature of Crouzon syndrome, these infants may represent a contiguous gene syndrome. All cases have been sporadic.

Pachydermoperiostosis (Touraine-Solente-Gole syndrome, MIM:167100) is characterized by progressive cutis verticis gyrata and progressive periostosis of the long bones and clubbing of the nails (Hippocratic nails). In pachydermoperiostosis, the skin changes can involve the entire face as well as the scalp and the distal extremities. In addition to the fixed rugations of cutis verticis gyrata, generalized thickening and coarsening of the skin with deep furrows are seen. The skin is described as greasy or seborrhea-like. The clubbed appearance of the distal fingers is due to soft tissue enlargement. Decreased sweating of the hands and feet has been reported.

HISTOPATHOLOGY

LIGHT. Orkin and colleagues (1974) found intradermal nests of nevus cells and neuroid elements in the deeper dermis of three patients they studied and suggested that cerebriform nevi are a common cause for the clinical appearance of isolated cutis verticis gyrata. Polan and Butterworth (1953) found no consistent histopathologic feature in cutis verticis gyrata, and in some instances no abnormalities at all were seen. The one feature they thought might be significant was an increase in the number of hair follicles. Hambrick and Carter (1966) reported hyperplasia of the epidermal appendages, proliferation of fibrocytes, and increased collagen and ground substance in two patients with pachydermoperiostosis.

EM. Not specific.

BASIC DEFECT

Unknown.

TREATMENT

Excision of the involved areas is the only effective treatment. Orkin et al. (1974) suggested obligatory removal of cerebriform intradermal nevi because of a possible risk for melanoma; the basis for this concern was not stated.

MODE OF INHERITANCE

Familial occurrence of isolated cutis verticis gyrata is rare.

Pachydermoperiostosis has familial occurrence. The genetics are unclear. Expression is extremely variable. Rimoin (1965) claimed autosomal dominant inheritance based on the presence of the full syndrome in a proband and radiologic evidence of periostosis in numerous first, second, and third degree relatives. None other than the proband had skin changes. Others have reported the occurrence of pachydermoperiostosis in siblings only, in offspring of consanguineous matings, and with vertical and male-to-male transmission.

Cutis verticis gyrata in association with mental retardation is usually sporadic, with rare recurrences in relatives.

PRENATAL DIAGNOSIS

None.

DIFFERENTIAL DIAGNOSIS

Cylindromas (MIM:123850) can mimic cutis verticis gyrata. The collagenomas of tuberous sclerosis (MIM:191100) may have a cerebriform appearance. The digit changes of secondary (pulmonary) hypertrophic osteoarthropathy are clinically identical to pachydermoperiostosis. The presence of lung tumors and absence of family history differentiate the former from the latter. Isolated clubbing (MIM: 119800) can also be familial.

Support Group: N.O.R.D.
P.O. Box 8923

New Fairfield, CT
06812
1-800-999-6673

SELECTED BIBLIOGRAPHY

Hall, B.D., Cadle, R.G., Golabi, M., Morris, C.A., and Cohen, M.M. Jr. (1992). Beare-Stevenson cutis gyrata syndrome. *Am. J. Med. Genet.* **44,** 82–89.

Review of the literature and authors' experience. Summary states that palms and soles are thickened; original report by Beare and Stevenson describes them as clear. I am not convinced by published photos or reports that the acanthosis nigricans is really present. No histopathology presented. Some photos look like skin changes of CHILD syndrome on the trunk.

Hambrick, G.W., Jr., and Carter, D.M. (1966). Pachydermoperiostosis. Touraine-Solente-Gole syndrome. *Arch. Dermatol.* **94,** 594–608.

Report of two cases and review of literature.

Oikarinen, A., Palatsi, R., Kylmaniemi, M., Keski-Oja, J., Risteli, J., and Kallioinen, M. (1994). Pachydermoperiostosis: analysis of the connective tissue abnormality in one family. *J. Am. Acad. Dermatol.* **31,** 947–953.

Authors biopsied affected father and two sons with pachydermoperiostosis. Light microscopy showed increased epidermal folding, thickened collagen bundles, and fragmented elastin fibers, along with an increase in glycosaminoglycans. Ultrastructural features included disorganization and degeneration of collagen and elastin fibers. Tenascin expression appeared to be increased in lesional and perilesional skin.

Orkin, M., Frichot, B.C., and Zelickson, A.S. (1974). Cerebriform intradermal nevus. A cause of cutis verticis gyrata. *Arch. Dermatol.* **110,** 575–582.

Discusses the subset of cutis verticis gyrata associated with dermal neuroid nevi.

Palo, J., Iivanainen, M., Blomqvist, K., and Pesonen, S. (1970). Aetiological aspects of the cutis verticis gyrata and mental retardation syndrome. *J. Ment. Defic. Res.* **14,** 33–43.

Detailed report of a survey of 590 institutionalized patients, 13 of whom were found to have cutis verticis gyrata.

Polan, S., and Butterworth, T. (1953). Cutis verticis gyrata. A review with report of seven new cases. *Am. J. Ment. Defic.* **57,** 613–629.

A detailed review of the literature with report of some cases of their own.

Rimoin, D.L. (1965). Pachydermoperiostosis (idiopathic clubbing and periostosis). Genetic and physiologic considerations. *N. Engl. J. Med.* **272,** 923–931.

Very clear review of pachydermoperiostosis. Rimoin presents pedigree data from the literature. Suggests that hereditary clubbing may represent limited expression of the gene for pachydermoperiostosis.

FAMILIAL DYSAUTONOMIA (MIM:223900)

(Riley-Day Syndrome; HSAN-III)

DERMATOLOGIC FEATURES

MAJOR. This condition is rare and seen almost always, but not exclusively, in Ashkenazi Jews. Familial dysautonomia usually presents in early infancy, but, in the absence of previously affected siblings, the correct diagnosis often is not made until several years of age.

Blotching and mottling of the skin may be the first cutaneous sign, usually seen after 1 month of age. It may not develop until a year or so of age. Patches of red skin can appear anywhere and do so often during emotional excitement.

There is increased sweating and drooling, often to inappropriate stimuli.

Self-mutilation presumably because of lack of sensation results in many of the classic skin changes in this disorder. Biting of the tongue can result in problems of speech. There may be inadvertant loss of teeth because of inappropriate biting. Burns and ulcerations of the

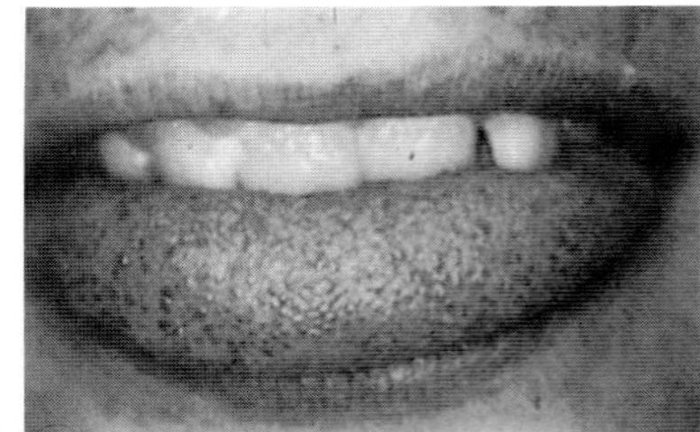

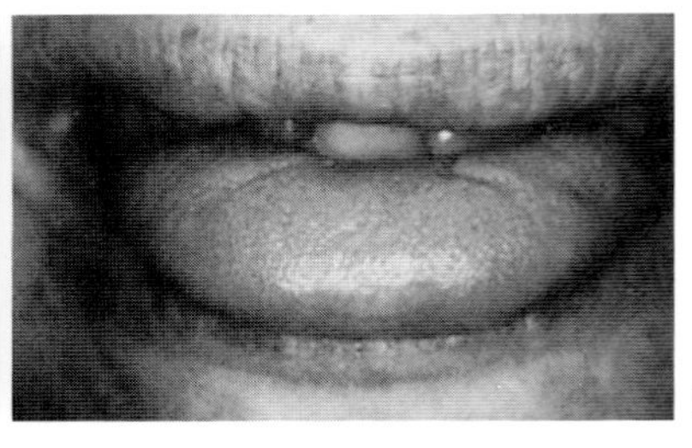

Figure 5.76. **(A)** Normal fungiform papillae are the "red" dots at the margin of the tongue. **(B)** These are absent in an individual with Riley-Day syndrome. (From Axelrod et al., 1974.)

hands and feet secondary to unrecognized injury are common.

Absence of fungiform papillae on the tongue are almost pathognomonic for the disorder. There is often a decrease in taste sensation.

There is lack of a flare response to injection of histamine (1:10,000).

MINOR. A seborrheic dermatitis-like rash involving the scalp and eyebrows has been described in some patients.

ASSOCIATED ABNORMALITIES

Approximately 25% of patients present breech at birth. Intrauterine growth retardation, hypotonia, poor respiratory efforts, and difficult feeding are typical.

Unexplained fevers and failure to thrive are seen early on, along with continued feeding problems. Pneumonias secondary to aspiration are common (greater than 65% of patients). Repeated vomiting occurs in approximately 40% of patients, and vomiting crises, possibly due to abnormal esophageal motility, occur in more than 65% of patients. Eye involvement is characterized by a decrease to absence of lacrimation and corneal hypesthesia. Secondary corneal ulcerations occur. The absence of overflow tearing may not be appreciated until infants are several months of age, as little or no overflow tearing is normal up to about 3 months of age. Neurologic features include absence of deep tendon reflexes, abnormal temperature control, delay in milestones in approximately 65% of patients, seizures in 40%, and gait ataxia. Fine motor function is usually normal. In patients with normal intelligence, there appears to be a decrement from that expected based on sibling IQs. There is a great deal of variability in intellectual development. Cardiovascular manifestations include instability of blood pressure with labile hypertension and hypotension. Orthopedic problems include the development of Charcot joints, autoamputation, osteomyelitis, and scoliosis. Short stature occurs in 80% of affected individuals.

The face is often described as having a startled appearance.

Death in infancy and childhood is not uncommon (18%). Among long-term survivors, mortality approaches 50% by age 30 years.

Some patients have delay of puberty. These tend to be those who are most poorly nourished. Enuresis may also be an ongoing problem.

HISTOPATHOLOGY

LIGHT. No pathologic changes.
EM. No information.

BASIC DEFECT

Unknown.

TREATMENT

Careful attention to feeding, placement of gastrostomy tubes, use of Thorazine for emetic crises. Attention to the possibility of and prompt treatment for pneumonia is important. Careful ophthalmologic toilet is necessary to prevent corneal damage. Protection from injury is the primary mechanism to prevent skin breakdown and ulceration.

MODE OF INHERITANCE

Autosomal recessive. The disorder is linked to 9q31–q33.

PRENATAL DIAGNOSIS

Available by linkage studies where applicable.

DIFFERENTIAL DIAGNOSIS

In congenital indifference to pain (MIM: 147430, 243000), there is muting of the pain sensation and no dysautonomia. The disorder may be congenital or present in early childhood. Patients with these conditions can develop ulcerations secondary to unappreciated injury. The histamine test, methacholine testing of pupillary constriction, and examination of the tongue for the presence of fungiform papillae will discriminate this condition from Riley-Day syndrome.

Hereditary sensory radicular neuropathy (MIM:162400) is an autosomal dominant disorder that appears usually between the ages of 10 and 30 years. This is a progressive condition, primarily involving the limbs distal to the knees and the elbows, in which there is progressive loss of sensation. Again, ulcers may occur because of injury.

Anhidrotic congenital sensory neuropathy (HSAN-IV, FD-II, MIM:256800) is characterized by absence of sweating with presence of normal sweat glands, recurrent fevers, trophic ulcers, and absence of tearing. In contrast, Riley-Day syndrome is characterized by erratic, episodic, copious sweating.

Self-mutilation is a feature of Lesch-Nyhan syndrome (MIM:308000), an X-linked disorder easily differentiated clinically by lack of dysautonomia and readily diagnosed biochemically.

Sweating abnormalities, failure to thrive, and fever of unknown origin may raise the possibility of an ectodermal dysplasia (MIM:Many). Drooling, episodic red patches of skin, and absence of fungiform papillae are discriminating markers of Riley-Day syndrome.

In cystic fibrosis (MIM:219700), patients may have feeding problems and pneumonias in infancy similar to those occurring in Riley-Day syndrome. The skin changes of Riley-Day syndrome are absent in cystic fibrosis, and the histamine test is normal.

Support Group: Dysautonomia Foundation, Inc.
20 East 46th Street, Room 302
New York, NY 10017
1-212-949-6644

SELECTED BIBLIOGRAPHY

Axelrod, F.B., Nachtigal, R., and Dancis, J. (1974). Familial dysautonomia: pathogenesis and management. *Adv. Pediatr.* **21,** 75–96.

Comprehensive review of their experience with 80 patients. Twelve percent of patients were asymptomatic at birth. Guidelines for management, including use of anesthetics, are given.

Blumenfeld, A., Slaugenhaupt, S.A., Axelrod, F.B., Lucente, D.E., Maayan, C., Liebert, C.B., Ozelius, L.J., Trofatter, J.A., Haines, J.L., Breakfield, X.O., and Gusella, J.F. (1993). Localization of the gene for familial dysautonomia on chromosome 9 and definition of DNA markers for genetic diagnosis. *Nat. Genet.* **4,** 160–163.

Twenty-six families gave a LOD score of 21.1. The authors demonstrated linkage disequilibrium. In families with one previously affected child, prenatal diagnosis is possible.

Day, R., and Klingman, W.O. (1939). The effect of sleep on skin temperature reactions in a case of acrocyanosis. *J. Clin. Invest.* **18,** 271–276.

Case report of a 6 1/2-year-old with intermittently cold, blue hands and feet. Both a positive family history and all the other signs of dysauto-

nomia were mentioned, but their significance was mostly unappreciated.
Riley, C.M., and Moore, R.H. (1966). Familial dysautonomia differentiated from related disorders. *Pediatrics* **37,** 435–446.
Outlines major and minor criteria for the diagnosis. Uses two instructive case reports to underscore the difficulty of diagnosis. Groups abnormalities by function and points out the essential features in each category.

FRANÇOIS SYNDROME (MIM:221800)

(Dermochondrocorneal Dystrophy)

Includes Blau/Jabs Syndrome

DERMATOLOGIC FEATURES

Major. There are remarkably few cases of this condition reported. Small, hard, cutaneous papules and nodules develop over the backs of the hands, clustering around joints. They also develop on the nose and ears. The nodules are whitish-gray and waxy and range in size from a few millimeters to several centimeters in diameter. Skin lesions first develop in early childhood.

Minor. Mucosal hypertrophy of the gums and the palate may occur.

ASSOCIATED ABNORMALITIES

Osteochondrodystrophy of the hands develops within the first few years of life, followed by foot involvement later in childhood. There is limited range of motion in the hands and feet due to subluxation of joints, and cystic changes in the bones occur.

Bilateral central superficial corneal opacities, white or brown in color, develop by the end of the first decade. Conjunctival pterygia also occur.

Intelligence appears to be normal.

HISTOPATHOLOGY

Light. Early: spongiocytes and lymphocytes in the dermis and no accumulation of lipid. Late changes show compact fibrosis in the dermis, hyperkeratosis, and moderate acanthosis in the epidermis.

EM. Spongiocytes are large, fibroblastoid-like cells. The collagen fiber structure appears to be normal.

BASIC DEFECT

Unknown.

TREATMENT

None.

MODE OF INHERITANCE

Autosomal recessive.

PRENATAL DIAGNOSIS

None.

DIFFERENTIAL DIAGNOSIS

Juvenile hyaline fibromatosis (MIM:228600) has onset much earlier and more severely. It is not characterized by eye findings. Histopathology shows accumulation in the dermis of glycosaminoglycans, which is not a feature of François syndrome.

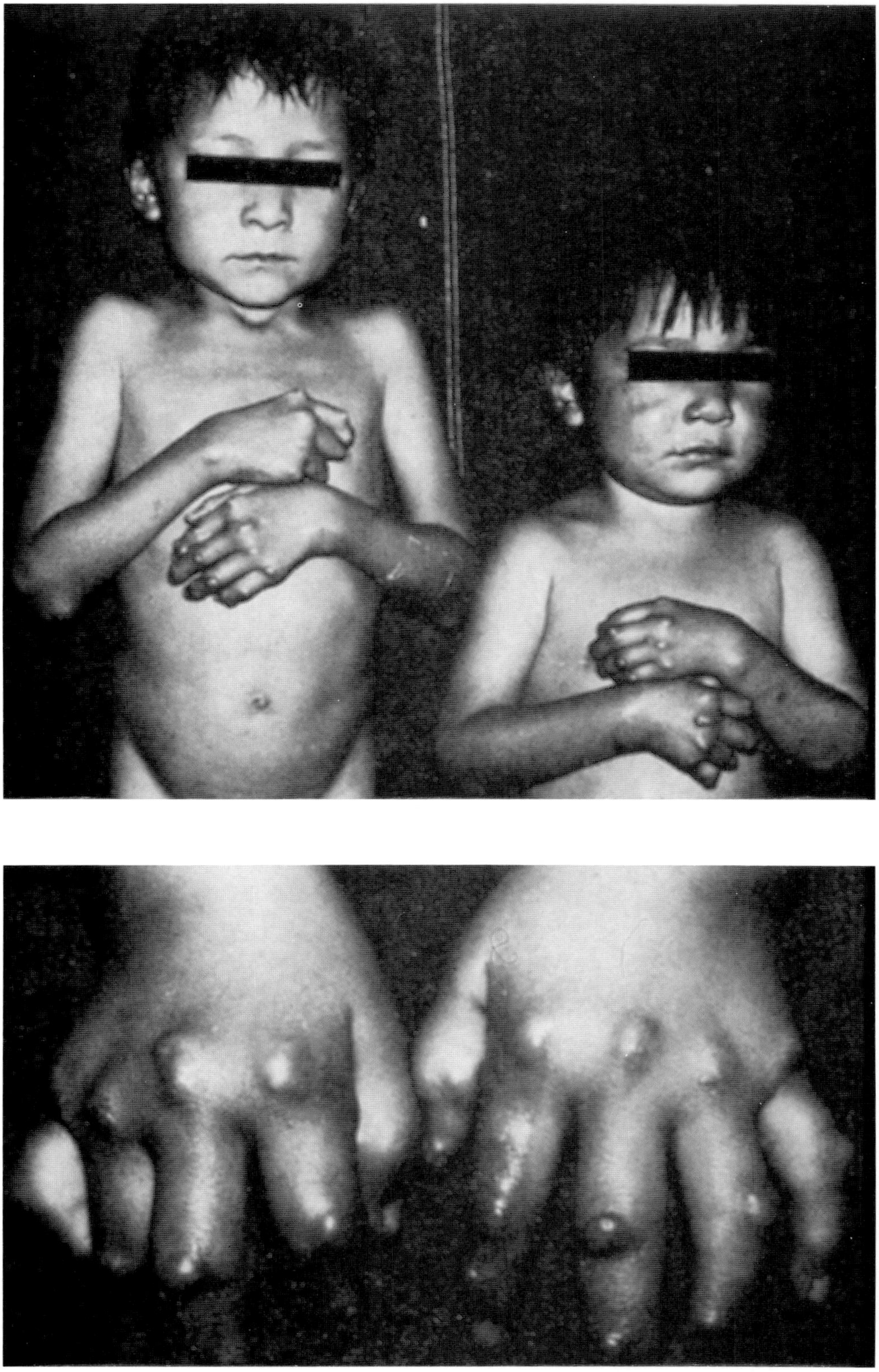

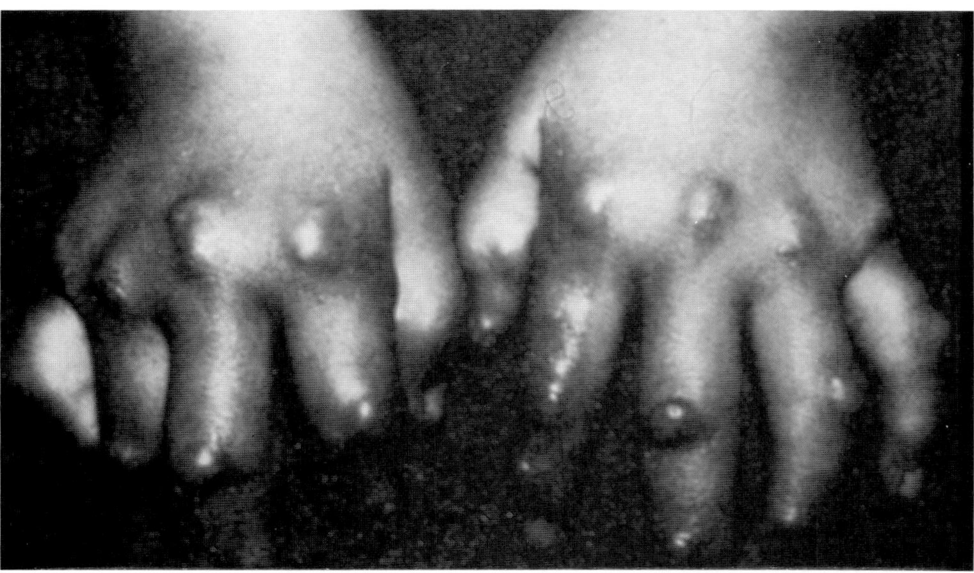

Figure 5.77. Nodules on pinnae and hands in two affected brothers. (From Ruiz-Maldonado et al., 1977.)

The familial histiocytic dermoarthritis (MIM: 142730) described by Zayid and Farraj (1973) is very similar. This condition was reported in one family with autosomal dominant (male-to-male) transmission. The skin lesions are similar. The eye findings include glaucoma, uveitis, and posterior cataracts. Arthritis may also develop. The skin nodules have a similar distribution and may be brown, violaceous, or pale. Skin biopsy tissue shows an inflammatory infiltrate and histiocytes in newer lesions, fibrosis and mild infiltrate in older lesions.

Blau syndrome or Jabs syndrome (MIM: 186580) is an autosomal dominant disorder of uveitis, polyarteritis, and multiple synovial cysts that has been described in three families. Most affected individuals do not have all features. In some affected persons there is a recurrent erythematous papular rash with onset in early childhood. Skin biopsy tissue shows noncaseating granulomas. Although joint swelling can occur in both François and Blau syndromes, they are otherwise readily distinguishable.

The multiple xanthomas of the hyperlipidemias and xanthogranulomas may appear similar to the papules of François syndrome. Biopsy will quickly distinguish these conditions, as will recognition of associated findings.

François' name has also been eponymically applied to Hallermann-Streiff syndrome (MIM:234100), which bears no clinical resemblance to dermochondrocorneal dystrophy.

Support Group: N.O.R.D.
P.O. Box 8923
New Fairfield, CT 06812
1-800-999-6673

SELECTED BIBLIOGRAPHY

Bierly, J.R., George, S.P., and Volpicelli, M. (1992). Dermochondral corneal dystrophy (of François). *Br. J. Ophthalmol.* **76,** 760–761.

Follow-up of brothers in the 1977 report of Ruiz-Maldonado et al.

Pastores, G.M., Michels, V.V., Stickler, G.B., Su, W.P.D., Nelson, A.M., and Bovenmeyer, D.A. (1990). Autosomal dominant granulomatous arthritis, uveitis, skin rash, and synoveal cysts. *J. Pediatr.* **117,** 403–408.

This is the second family with this clinical spectrum. The disease was steroid responsive. The discussion lists several families and case reports of similar conditions. They argue that Blau syndrome is distinguished from Jabs syndrome by the presence of synovial cysts.

Ruiz-Maldonado, R., Tamayo, L., and Velazquez, E. (1977). Dystrophie dermo-chondro-cornéenne familiale (syndrome de François). *Ann. Dermatol. Venereol.* **104,** 475–478.

Two siblings with onset in infancy and laryngeal involvement.

Zayid, I., and Farraj, S. (1973). Familial histiocytic dermoarthritis. A new syndrome. *Am. J. Med.* **54,** 793–800.

A father and three children were affected. Histopathology of the skin lesions showed a dense inflammatory infiltrate composed of lymphocytes and plasma cells with some histiocytes. Older lesions had a similar histologic appearance to the nodules of François syndrome.

LIPOID PROTEINOSIS (MIM:247100)

(Urbach-Wiethe Syndrome; Hyalinosis Cutis et Mucosae)

DERMATOLOGIC FEATURES

Major. The skin findings consist of waxy, yellow, discrete, and confluent dermal papules and generalized thickening. The margins of the lips and eyelids are preferentially involved. Other sites of involvement include palms, soles, axillae, elbows, knees, fingers, toes, and scrotum. The papules may become confluent. Plaques over the elbows and knees are often verrucous or wart-like in appearance. Hyperpigmentation can occur.

Vesicular lesions that crust and scar, leaving small varioliform pock marks and larger,

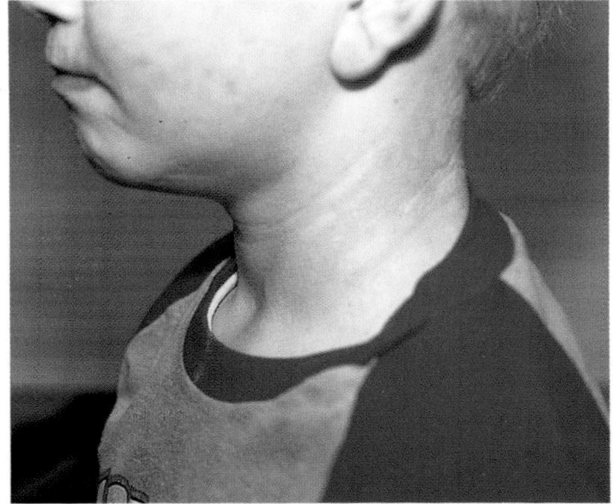

A

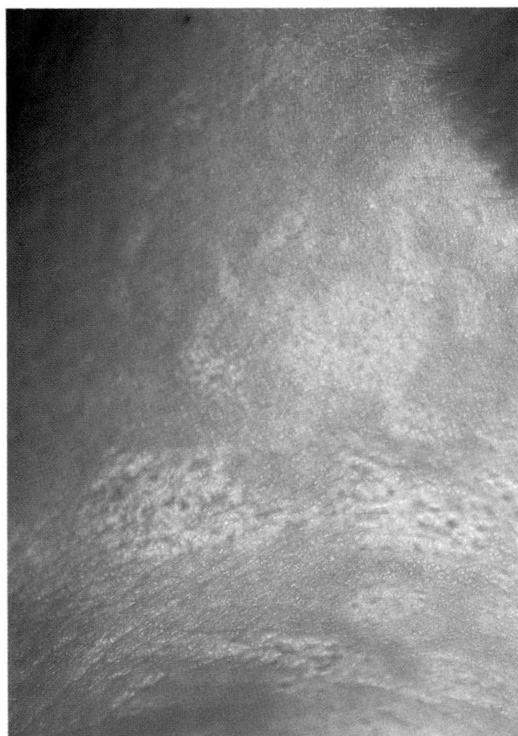

B

Figure 5.78. **(A)** Lesions on neck similar in appearance to connective tissue nevi. **(B)** Close-up of plaques.

crater-like scars are seen. Some authors state that these early lesions are often mistaken for impetigo.

Exposure to sunlight and actinic damage appear to exacerbate the skin changes.

Minor. Patchy hair loss is reported in some patients; loss of eyebrows and eyelashes has also been noted.

ASSOCIATED ABNORMALITIES

Hoarseness of the voice, caused by deposits of material in the vocal cords, develops in the first few months to years. The mucous membranes of the entire oropharynx are involved. The rectum and vagina may also be affected.

The viscera are also involved, with histopathologic evidence of depositions identical to those in the skin. These changes do not usually cause symptoms.

Asymptomatic changes in the retina of small, round, yellow-white exudates and a general granular appearance to the retina have been reported in a few patients.

Bilateral symmetric intracranial calcifications develop behind the posterior clinoid process, apparently in the hippocampal gyri. In the series of Gordon et al. (1971), 18 of 27 patients showed this finding, which was correlated with increasing age. Epilepsy has been described in a handful of patients. Intelligence is usually normal.

Hypoplasia of the lateral incisors has been reported rarely but may not be a related feature of the disease, as it is a relatively common, isolated autosomal dominant condition.

HISTOPATHOLOGY

Light. Early changes include thickening of the capillary walls with deposition of a homogeneous hyalin-like eosinophilic material. Nerves, sweat glands, and hair follicles may also show laminated deposits along the basement membrane. Late changes include hyperkeratosis of the epidermis, with the same but more pronounced hyaline deposits around the vessels throughout the dermis and the eccrine glands, which have an atrophic epithelium. The dermis is usually thickened, with bundles of pink-staining homogeneous hyaline material in the upper regions and focal deposits in the reticular dermis. In areas where there is papillomatosis of the epidermis, the hyaline bundles are often vertically arranged. The arrector pili muscles and hair follicles may also be involved. **EM.** There is marked thickening and reduplication of the basal laminae of blood vessels, appendages, smooth muscle cells, peri neuria, and Schwann cells; there are deposits of amorphous "fibrogranular" material in the upper dermis and around vessels and diminution of collagen fibrils in number and size.

BASIC DEFECT

Unknown. The hyaline deposits are PAS positive and diastase resistant, suggesting that they are composed of glycoproteins and proteoglycans. The reduplicated basement membranes appear to contain laminin and type III and type IV collagen. Olsen et al. (1988) have demonstrated a 4.5-fold increase in the mRNA levels for pro-α-1 (IV) collagen in fibroblast culture from one patient with lipoid proteinosis.

Other experimental evidence, generated from single studies of single individuals, has suggested that lipoid proteinosis is a lysosomal storage disease, that it results from a generalized increase in basement membrane collagens IV and V, that it is a disease caused by overproduction of structural noncollagenous glycoproteins, and/or that it is a condition in which there is both underproduction of fibrous collagens and overproduction of basement membrane collagens.

TREATMENT

Narrowing of the larynx and trachea may cause respiratory compromise, and repeated surgical debulking or tracheostomy may be necessary.

Dermabrasion of facial skin can provide temporary cosmetic relief.

Wong and Lin (1988) have reported clinical improvement with decrease in hoarseness, improvement in esophageal function, and smoothing of the skin in a 41-year-old patient treated orally for 3 years with 40–60 mg/kg/day of dimethylsulfoxide. The basis for this success was thought to be the ability of the drug to "dissolve collagen and scavenge hydroxyl radicals." They did not biopsy their patient after treatment to determine the histologic response to therapy.

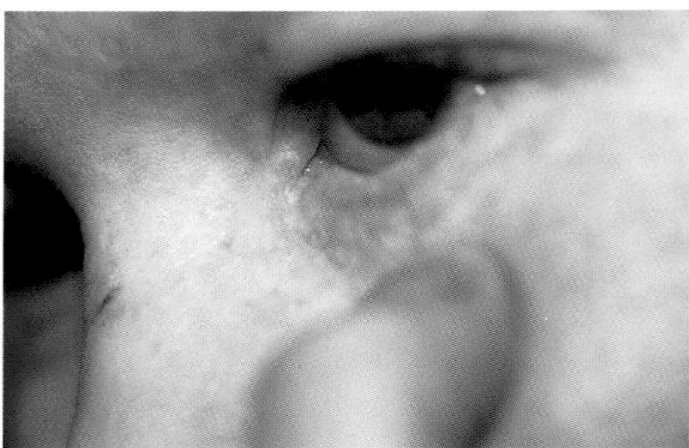

Figure 5.79. Deposition along eyelids with some loss of lower lashes. There is a yellow, waxy hue.

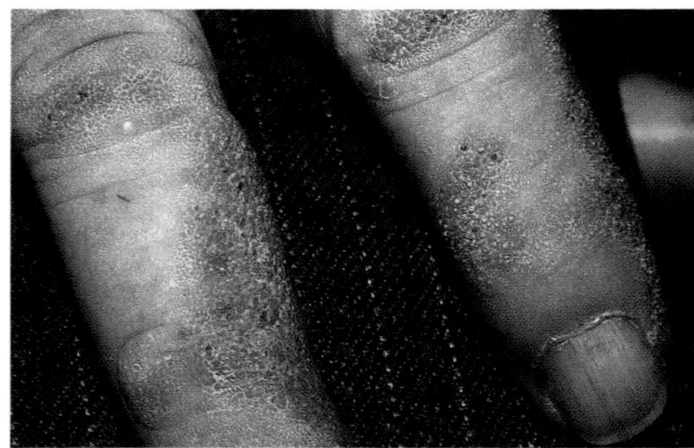

Figure 5.80. More verrucous-like plaques over fingers.

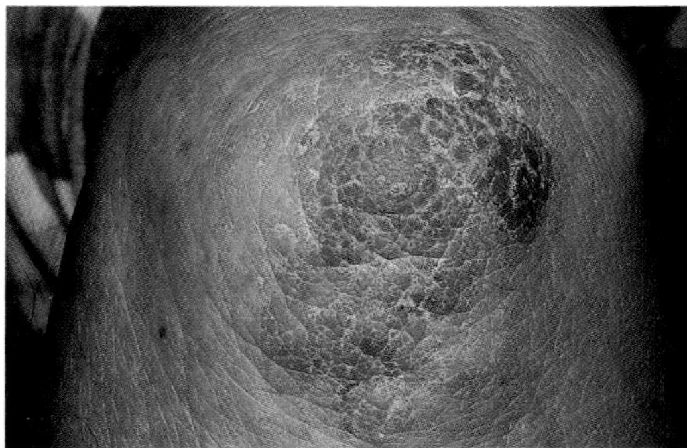

Figure 5.81. Plaque on knee somewhat similar to psoriasis.

MODE OF INHERITANCE

Autosomal recessive. There are clusters of the disease among Hottentots (inbred South Africans of European/Khoikhoi mix), Afrikaaners, and Swedes. Consanguinity is frequent among parents of patients.

PRENATAL DIAGNOSIS

None.

DIFFERENTIAL DIAGNOSIS

The early vesicular lesions of lipoid proteinosis can resemble those of erythropoietic protoporphyria (MIM:177000), as do the early histopathologic changes in which there is thickening of perivascular basement membrane in both disorders. Patients with erythropoietic protoporphyria do not have mucosal involvement and do not have hoarse voices. Excretion of porphyrins is normal in lipoid proteinosis. Some early cases of erythropoietic protoporphyria were designated as "light-sensitive lipoid proteinosis."

Some of the skin changes on the neck are reminiscent of pseudoxanthoma elasticum (MIM:177850, 177860, 264800, 264810). The presence of extensor involvement, lesions on the eyelids, hoarseness, and scarring should readily lead to the diagnosis of lipoid proteinosis, which histology will confirm.

Support Group: N.O.R.D.
P.O. Box 8923
New Fairfield, CT
06812
1-800-999-6673

SELECTED BIBLIOGRAPHY

Bauer, E.A., Santa-Cruz, D.J., and Eisen, A.Z. (1981). Lipoid proteinosis: In vivo and in vitro evidence for a lysosomal storage disease. *J. Invest. Dermatol.* **76,** 119–125.

These authors evaluated tissue and cultured fibroblasts from a 62-year-old patient. Fibroblasts in the dermis had cytoplasmic vacuolization, which also occurred in the cultured cells. These membrane-bound vacuoles contained membranous lamellar substance. They suggested that lipoid proteinosis might fall into the category of the mucolipidoses but appropriately cautioned that this was preliminary evidence from only one patient.

Gordon, H., Gordon, W., Botha, V., and Edelstein, I. (1971). Lipoid proteinosis. *Birth Defects* **VII (8),** 164–177.

Extensive clinical review of 28 cases of lipoid proteinosis among "the Colored" in Namaqualand, South Africa.

Harper, J.I., Duance, V.C., Sims, T.J., and Light, N.D. (1985). Lipoid proteinosis: an inherited disorder of collagen metabolism. *Br. J. Dermatol.* **113,** 145–151.

Study of skin from one patient with lipoid proteinosis demonstrating increased levels of types III and V collagen, with abnormal collagen cross–links.

Heyl, T. (1970). Genealogical study of lipoid proteinosis in South Africa. *Br. J. Dermatol.* **83,** 338–340.

In four white South African families, Heyl was able to trace the gene for lipoid proteinosis back to two "founders," a German brother and sister who settled in South Africa in the 17th century.

Olsen, D.R., Chu, M.-L., and Uitto, J. (1988). Expression of basement membrane zone genes coding for type IV procollagen and laminin by human skin fibroblasts in vitro: elevated α-1 (IV) collagen mRNA levels in lipoid proteinosis. *J. Invest. Dermatol.* **90,** 734–738.

Increased levels of mRNA for pro-α-1 collagen chains were found in tissue cultured from one patient. The authors posit that upregulated transcription of this gene might be a basis for the disease. mRNA for other components of the basement membrane zone were normal.

Wong, C.-K., and Lin, C.-S. (1988). Remarkable response of lipoid proteinosis to oral dimethyl sulphoxide. *Br. J. Dermatol.* **119,** 541–544.

A single case report.

MULTIPLE PTERYGIA (MIM:177980, 178110, 178200, 253290, 263650 265000, 312150)

Includes Escobar Syndrome; Popliteal Pterygium (Facio-Genito-Popliteal) Syndrome; Bartsocas/Papas Syndrome (Lethal Popliteal Pterygia); Antecubital Pterygia; Multiple Lethal Pterygia; Pena-Shokeir Type I

DERMATOLOGIC FEATURES

MAJOR. Wings of skin and subcutaneous tissue across joints characterize all of the pterygia syndromes, which are distinguished by site of involvement, mode of inheritance, and associated abnormalities. The bands are skin-covered and firm. The degree of joint fixation may increase or remain static or improve somewhat with time. Pterygia of the nails and/or hypoplastic nails have been reported in about 30% of patients.
MINOR. None.

ASSOCIATED ABNORMALITIES

See Differential Diagnosis.

HISTOPATHOLOGY

LIGHT. The wings of tissue appear to be normal skin; may contain nerves and arteries.
EM. No information.

BASIC DEFECT

Unknown. There is much debate about decrease of movement in utero resulting in formation of pterygia versus pterygia formation as the primary problem causing decreased movement.

TREATMENT

There have been several reports of surgical approaches to releasing pterygia. Results have been variable.

MODE OF INHERITANCE

Autosomal dominant; autosomal recessive; X-linked recessive.

PRENATAL DIAGNOSIS

Possible by ultrasound, but at least one false-negative result has been reported. A better marker for these conditions may be polyhydramnios rather than decreased fetal movement.

DIFFERENTIAL DIAGNOSIS

Escobar syndrome (MIM:265000) is characterized by multiple webs across joints, including

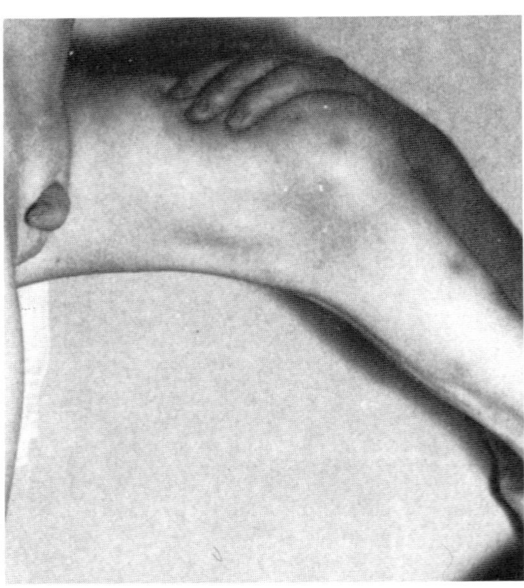

Figure 5.82. Popliteal pterygia with cryptorchidism. (From Hall et al., 1982.)

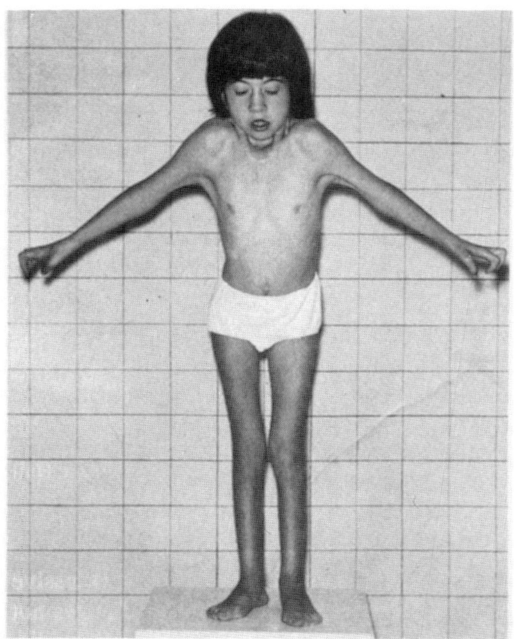

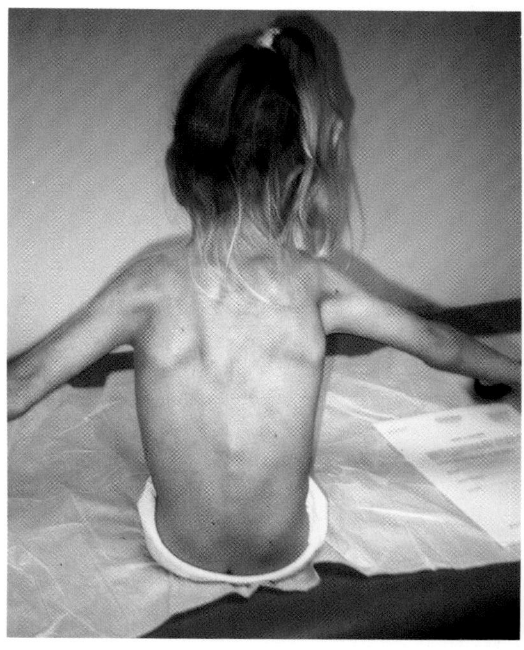

Figure 5.83. **(A)** Multiple pterygia syndrome—band across axilla. (From Hall et al., 1982.) **(B)** Abnormal winging of scapula and band across axilla. (Courtesy of Dr. L. Hudgins, Seattle, Washington.)

the neck. There are multiple joint contractures and camptodactyly. The facies are marked by ptosis and downslanting palpebral fissures. Patients have short stature, scoliosis, and vertebral abnormalities, including fusion. There may be intracrural bands and secondary cryptorchidism. Hydrops fetalis is a common feature. Many patients are described as having hearing loss. Escobar syndrome is autosomal recessive.

Pena-Shokeir syndrome type I (MIM: 208150) is similar to Escobar syndrome with the exception of absence of involvement of the neck. Patients with Pena-Shokeir type I usually do not have hydrops and do have lung hypoplasia.

Babies with multiple lethal pterygium syndrome (MIM:253290) have marked nuchal webbing and nuchal edema, intrauterine growth retardation, and facial changes. In addition, internal organs are affected. Hypoplastic lungs, heart defects, genital abnormalities, and gastrointestinal abnormalities have all been described. Some subsets of multiple lethal pterygium syndrome appear to be characterized by bony fusion. There are many case reports with unique findings, and it is uncertain whether these truly represent distinct syndromes.

Popliteal pterygium syndrome (facio-genito-popliteal, MIM:119500) is characterized most markedly by wings of tissue behind the knees. These occur in 85%–95% of all reported probands, but are actually only seen in 57% of familial cases, suggesting that the finding is not invariable. Twenty percent of patients have ankyloblepharon filiforme adnatum. Forty-five percent have lip pits, and more than 90% have cleft palate with or without cleft lip. Over 40% of patients have intraoral bands between the gums. Hypoplastic digits and syndactyly are common features. Genital abnormalities include cryptorchidism, absent or cleft scrotum, malposition of the testicles, hernias, absence of the labia majora, and apparent increase in the size of the clitoris. Crural pterygia are common. Intelligence appears to be normal in this condition. It is an autosomal dominant condition with variable expression. The differential diagnosis of this syndrome is much more broad and includes Hay-Wells syndrome (AEC syndrome, MIM:106260) which shares ankyloblepharon

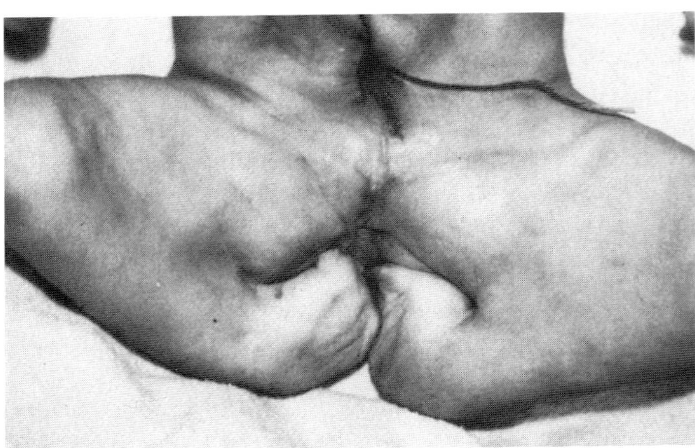

Figure 5.84. Lethal popilteal pterygia. (From Hall et al., 1982.)

filiforme adnatum in common. Individuals with popliteal pterygia syndrome do not usually have the hair abnormalities seen in AEC. Conversely, individuals with AEC do not have pterygia. Although individuals with oro-facio-digital syndrome type I (MIM:311200) share in common with popliteal pterygium multiple oral frenuli, they do not have pterygia. Van der Woude syndrome (cleft lip with or without cleft palate with lip pits, MIM:119300) is also not marked by pterygia. In an isolated case, it may not be possible to differentiate between these two conditions, as some family members with popliteal pterygia syndrome have had only lip pits or cleft palate.

Nail-patella syndrome (MIM:161200) can be marked by similar nail changes of hypoplastic nails and pterygia of the nailfold and by cleft lip with or without cleft palate. Patients with nail-patella syndrome do not have pterygia across the joints.

Bartsocas/Papas lethal popliteal pterygia syndrome (MIM:263650) is marked by death in the newborn period. Affected infants have, in addition to popliteal webs, facial clefts, oral synechiae, ankyloblepharon filiforme adnatum, and severe syndactyly of the toes and fingers, along with thumb hypoplasia. Microcephaly is typical. Hypoplastic alae nasi and labia majora are reported. Corneal aplasia is a major feature. Although usually lethal, a few affected individuals who have survived evidenced mental retardation. Babies with the autosomal recessive lethal popliteal syndrome have eye changes not seen in the dominant popliteal pterygium disorder.

The antecubital pterygia syndrome (MIM: 178200) is marked by wings of skin across the elbow joints only.

Individuals with Noonan syndrome (MIM: 163950), Turner syndrome, and Klippel-Feil syndrome (MIM:148900) can all have pterygia colli or webbed necks. Their associated features and the absence of pterygia elsewhere should readily set these disorders apart.

Support Group: AVENUES—National Support Group for Arthrogryposes
P.O. Box 5192
Sonora, CA 95370
1-209-928-3688

SELECTED BIBLIOGRAPHY

GENERAL

Hall, J.G., Reed, S.D., Rosenbaum, K.N., Gershanik, J., Chen, H., and Wilson, K.M. (1982). Limb pterygium syndromes. A review and report of eleven patients. *Am. J. Med. Genet.* **12,** 377–409.

Exhaustive review, very difficult to digest whole, but useful as a starting point. Multiple tables with details of previous case reports. Eighty-seven references.

POPLITEAL PTERYGIUM SYNDROME

Froster-Iskenius, U.G. (1990). Popliteal pterygium syndrome. *J. Med. Genet.* **27,** 320–326.

A "Syndrome of the Month" review with tabular presentation of frequency of associated malformations and the differential diagnoses.

Hunter, A. (1990). The popliteal pterygium syndrome: report of a new family and review of the literature. *Am. J. Med. Genet.* **36,** 196–208.

Extensive and clear review of the differential diagnosis with 82 references.

BARTSOCAS/PAPAS

Bartsocas, C.S., and Papas C.V. (1972). Popliteal pterygium syndrome. Evidence for a severe autosomal recessive form. *J. Med. Genet.* **9,** 222–226.

A consanguineous family with four of seven siblings affected. Severe malformations of the hands and feet, micrognathia, and mental retardation.

MULTIPLE LETHAL PTERYGIA

Hall, J.G., (1984). Editorial comment: the lethal multiple pterygium syndromes. *Am. J. Med. Genet.* **17,** 803–807.

This editorial precedes four papers (pp. 809–847) that discuss the various "forms" of multiple lethal pterygium syndrome, including Bartsocas/Papas syndrome.

ANTECUBITAL PTERYGIUM SYNDROME

Wallis, C.E., Shun-Shin, M., and Beighton, P.H. (1988). Autosomal dominant antecubital pterygium: syndromic status substantiated. *Clin. Genet.* **34,** 64–69.

An autosomal dominant pedigree. The founder had unilateral involvement (Judy Hall suggested gonadal/somatic mosaicism in a subsequent letter). Skin creases over the DIP joints were absent, although the range of motion of these joints was normal.

ESCOBAR SYNDROME

Escobar, V., Bixler, D., Gleiser, S., Weaver, D.D., and Gibbs, T. (1978). Multiple pterygia syndrome. *Am. J. Dis. Child.* **132,** 609–611.

Single report with a table reviewing case reports to that time. Authors differentiate this condition from the popliteal pterygium syndrome

SYSTEMIC HYALINOSIS (MIM:228600, 236490)

(Puretic Syndrome; Juvenile Hyaline Fibromatosis)

Includes Infantile and Juvenile Forms; Winchester Syndrome; Congenital Generalized Fibromatosis

DERMATOLOGIC FEATURES

MAJOR. The systemic hyalinoses are very rare disorders. The separation of systemic hyalinosis into infantile and juvenile subtypes may be artificial. There is overlap in the findings between the two conditions, and within sibships both "forms" have occurred, one with early onset and lethal outcome and one with a protracted and more mild course. I believe there may be a distinct entity of cutaneous hyalinosis characterized by multiple skin nodules and with a relatively benign course (see Drescher et al., 1967), but I am not convinced that juvenile and infantile hyalinosis, both of which have systemic involvement, truly differ from each other.

In the typical infantile form, thickened skin and stiff joints develop within the first weeks to months of life, and death usually ensues within the first 2 years. In the juvenile form, large subcutaneous nodules, particularly around the head and neck, develop over the course of years. Survival into adulthood is typical for the juvenile form. Although diffuse thickening of the skin is more typical of the infantile variety, it has also been reported in the juvenile form.

Both disorders share in common the development of small pearly papules on the face and abdomen.

Fleshy nodules resembling condyloma acuminata develop perianally.

Gingival hypertrophy is also reported in both.

Minor. Edema has been described in some infants. Hyperpigmentation can develop over joints. Some reports describe a fine erythematous pinpoint papular rash.

ASSOCIATED ABNORMALITIES

Failure to thrive, recurrent infections, diarrhea, and hypoproteinemia are typical of the infantile form. Intellectual development appears to be unaffected, but this is difficult to assess in babies with the infantile form, as they are unable to achieve normal motor milestones because of limitation of movement. The classic description of these babies suggests that they have significant pain, irritability, and a dislike of being handled. Hypotonia, despite joint stiffness, is fairly typical.

Joint contractures develop, and infants and children maintain a typical frog-leg position. Osteoporosis and an increased fracture rate are reported, but this may be a secondary phenomenon due to restricted movement and disuse. All of these features are severe in the infantile form and may be more mild in those with juvenile disease.

Deposition of hyalin is widespread, occurring in other organs including the intestines, heart, and adrenal glands.

In many case descriptions, a typical facial appearance with a saddle nose is described.

HISTOPATHOLOGY

Light. The papules show hyalin deposition within the papillary dermis with rarefaction of collagen bundles. No histologic changes have been noted in the skin from other areas.

EM. Fibrillogranular deposits between collagen bundles, around blood vessels, and within fibroblasts are seen. These may be composed

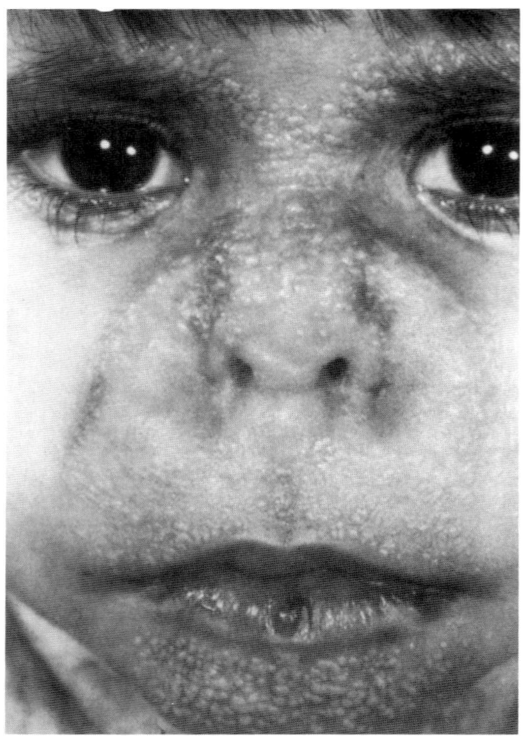

Figure 5.85. Numerous pearly papules; deeper nodules around nose. (From Glover et al., 1992.)

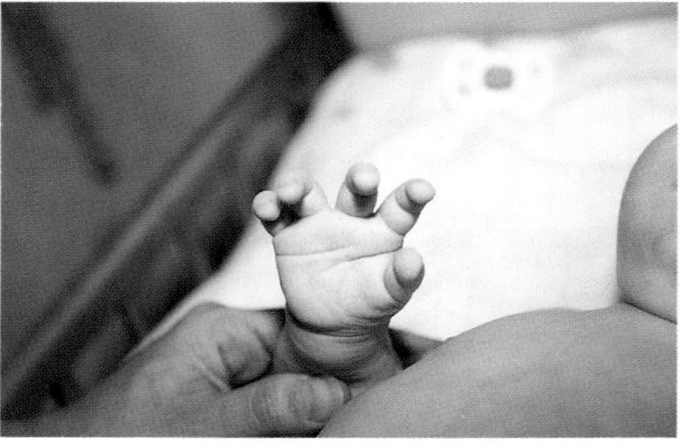

Figure 5.86. Hand held in abnormal position with fingers flexed. (Courtesy of Dr. D. Sherry, Seattle, Washington.)

→

Figure 5.87. Patient with Winchester syndrome showing joint contractures **(A)**, hirsutism over shoulder and arm **(B)**, and corneal opacity **(C)**. (From Hollister et al., 1974.)

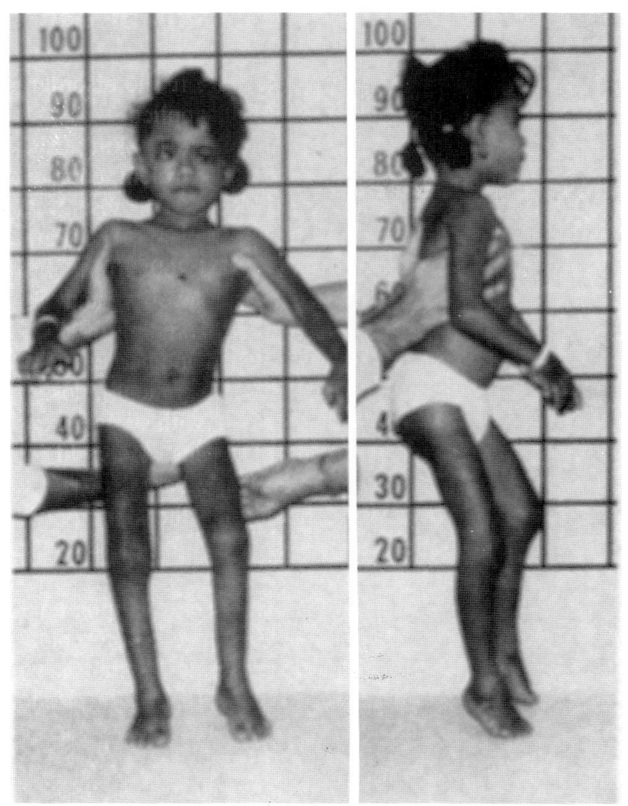

A

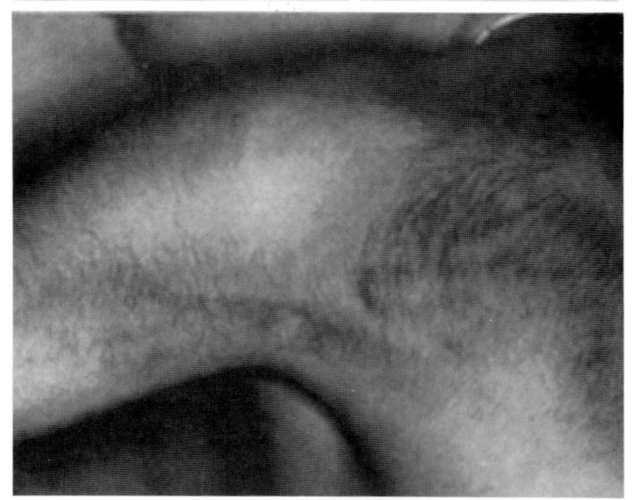

B

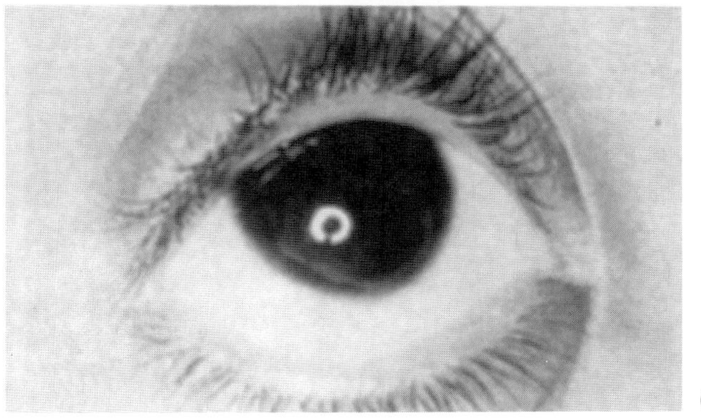

C

of glycosaminoglycans. There is variation in the size of collagen bundles. The elastin appears normal.

BASIC DEFECT

Unknown.

TREATMENT

Penicillamine was used in one patient with report of improvement in joint mobility. The patient was lost to follow-up.

MODE OF INHERITANCE

Autosomal recessive. There have been recurrences within sibships, and an increased proportion of children are the products of consanguineous matings.

PRENATAL DIAGNOSIS

None.

DIFFERENTIAL DIAGNOSIS

The Winchester syndrome (MIM:277950) shares the features of joint contractures and gingival hypertrophy. It differs in the absence of diffusely thickened skin, the presence of corneal opacities and hypertrichosis, and otherwise good health. Although dwarfing is described for children with Winchester syndrome, the changes in the bones do not seem any different from the bone changes of severe systemic hyalinosis in that they appear to be progressive and destructive due to restriction of movement. Some cases in the literature labeled as Winchester syndrome with skin findings similar to systemic hyalinosis may represent the latter condition.

If the skin changes are not recognized as distinctive, diagnoses such as protein-losing enteropathy, arthrogryposis, mixed connective tissue disease, or connective tissue disorder of unknown cause may be misapplied.

Individuals with mild stiff skin (MIM: 184900) do not have the virulent course of systemic hyalinosis. Nodules are absent, and skin involvement is less severe. The Parana variant of stiff skin (MIM:260530) is more similar. While it shares severity and joint involvement, it lacks the thickening of skin. It is marked more by tightened and hardened skin.

Infants with I-cell disease (mucolipidosis II) (MIM:252500) may present with stiff skin early on. The skin gradually softens, and mild joint contractures improve. These babies do not develop papules or nodules in the skin. A urine metabolic screen will allow for the exclusion of I-cell disease.

Infants with Farber disease (lipogranulomatosis) (MIM:228000) have a presentation identical to infantile systemic hyalinosis with severe failure to thrive with onset in infancy, joint contractures, periarticular swelling, and nodules. The bony changes are also similar. The differences are the yellowish color of the nodules in Farber disease and the absence of pearly papules. The infiltrative lesions of Farber are granulomas composed of histiocytes that store material that may also be composed of glycosaminoglycans. There is a defect in acid ceramidase activity in this disorder.

Congenital generalized multiple fibromatosis (MIM:228550) is clinically, at least in my mind, indistinguishable from infantile hyalinosis. The nodules are fibromas or myofibromas rather than hyalin deposits. There appear to be severe and mild forms, similar to the hyalinoses, with similar courses. Inheritance is also autosomal recessive.

Support Group: N.O.R.D.
P.O. Box 8923
New Fairfield, CT
06812
1-800-999-6673

SELECTED BIBLIOGRAPHY

Drescher, E., Woyke, S., Markiewicz, C., and Tegi, S. (1967). Juvenile fibromatosis in siblings (fibromatosis hyalinica multiplex juvenilis). *J. Pediatr. Surg.* **2,** 427–430.

A brother and a sister with painless, diffuse, large subcutaneous nodules showing hyalin deposition. They also had gingival hypertrophy but no other features of juvenile systemic hyalinosis. This appears to be a distinct disorder without joint involvement or skeletal changes.

Glover, M.T., Lake, B.D., and Atherton, D.J. (1991). Infantile systemic hyalinosis: newly recognized disorder of collagen? *Pediatrics* **87,** 228–234.

A description of four cases and a nice discussion of the differential diagnosis. They suggest that the infantile and the juvenile forms are the same disease. They hypothesize a defect in type VI collagen but present no biochemical or molecular evidence.

Hollister, D.W., Rimoin, D.L., Lachman, R.S., Cohen, A.H., Reed, W.B., and Westin, G.W. (1974). The Winchester syndrome: a non-lysosomal connective tissue disease. *J. Pediatr.* **84,** 701–709.

Three cases, all related to each other. Excellent photographs. Onset occurred within the first year of life. Skin thickening and hyperpigmentation developed, along with arthralgias. Affected individuals had diffuse coarseness of the skin. The corneal opacities were first noted in midchildhood. Patients also had marked hypertrichosis.

CHAPTER 6

DISORDERS OF SUBCUTANEOUS TISSUE

CEREBROTENDINOUS XANTHOMATOSIS (MIM:213700)

(CTX; Cerebral Cholesterinosis; Cholestanolosis)

DERMATOLOGIC FEATURES

MAJOR. Thick yellow or skin-colored nodules and plaques, which may become calcified, usually develop during the teen years and twenties, but can appear in childhood. A thickening of the tendons—achilles, triceps, and fingers—can develop during adolescence and is the presenting sign in more than 85% of patients. The thickenings may be smooth and even or irregular and tuberous.

Xanthelasma is a feature mentioned in many case reports.

MINOR. None.

ASSOCIATED ABNORMALITIES

Central nervous system: There is a progressive decrease in mentation. Psychiatric problems and behavioral problems may be major, and the correct diagnosis can be overlooked if the skin changes are not appreciated. There are progressive motor problems with increasing ataxia. Deep tendon reflexes are hyperreactive, and a Babinski reflex is often present. Pyramidal signs with myopathic facies are also described. Diffuse demyelinization is typical. Seizures are rare, but electroencephalographic abnormalities are common. On computed tomographic scans, cerebral atrophy, cerebellar atrophy, and loss of white matter are found.

Eye: Juvenile cataracts of the anterior and posterior lens usually appear late in the first decade or early in the second. These changes may predate the skin findings.

Cardiovascular: Accelerated development of atherosclerosis, angina, and myocardial infarction are reported in approximately 10% of patients. Respiratory involvement includes pulmonary dysfunction secondary to xanthomas, with a secondary problem of aspiration pneumonia due to neurologic degeneration.

Other: The ovaries are involved. Affected females have irregular menses and early menopause. Case reports of affected females often describe poorly developed secondary sexual characteristics. Osteopenia develops, and frequent fractures can occur. One report describes several patients who had lifelong intractable diarrhea.

Death in the disorder occurs from myocardial infarction, bulbar palsy, and/or neurologic degeneration.

HISTOPATHOLOGY

LIGHT. Increased deposits of fat, which is composed of cholestanol, foamy histiocytes, and

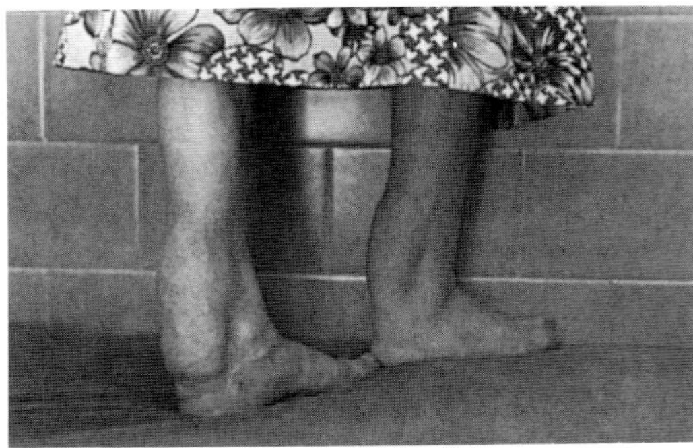

Figure 6.1. Marked thickening along Achilles tendons in patient with cerebrotendinous xanthomatosis. (From Bacchi et al., 1992.)

A

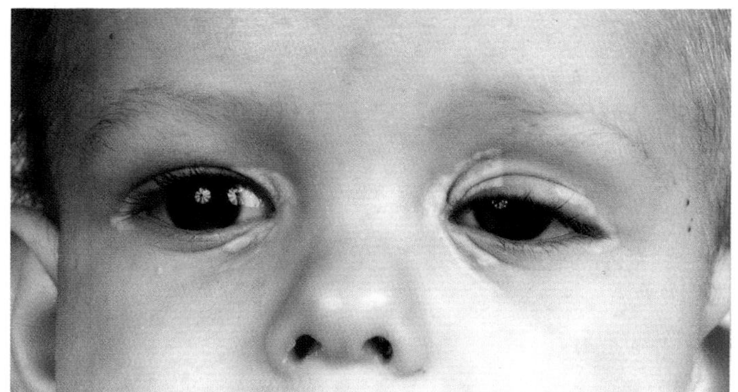

B

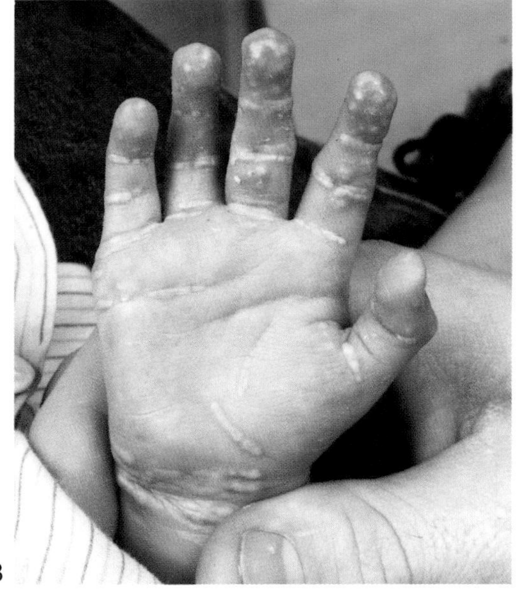

Figure 6.2. **(A)** Deposition around eyelids. **(B)** Distribution of lesions along lines of trauma and flexion (Koebner phenomenon), in addition to papules on fingertips, in a young child with hypercholesterolemia.

giant cells, are seen with extracellular crystalline deposits.

EM. No information.

BASIC DEFECT

There is a defect in sterol 27-hydroxylase, a mitochondrial enzyme that is important in bile acid metabolism. This defect leads to an increased amount of cholestanol, which is deposited in multiple tissues, including myelin.

TREATMENT

Chenodeoxycholic acid (CDCA) in doses of 750 mg per day PO decreases cholestanol production and suppresses abnormal bile acid synthesis. Remyelinization and reversal of central nervous system findings after treatment have been documented.

MODE OF INHERITANCE

Autosomal recessive. The gene (*CYP27*) has been mapped to 2q33-qter, and mutations have been identified. The carrier frequency has been estimated between 1 in 108 to 1 in 152. Carriers can be detected by provocative 2 day cholestyramine challenge, which increases endogenous bile acid synthesis resulting in excretion of bile alcohol by carriers.

PRENATAL DIAGNOSIS

Potentially by mutation analysis or linkage.

DIFFERENTIAL DIAGNOSIS

The disorder is diagnosed by elevated levels of bile alcohol in the urine. This finding is specific to cerebrotendinous xanthomatosis. Xanthomas are also a feature of the hypercholesterolemias (MIM:Many), especially familial type II hyperlipoproteinemia (MIM:144400). The central nervous system and the lungs are not involved in hypercholesterolemia.

Individuals with sitosterolemia also present

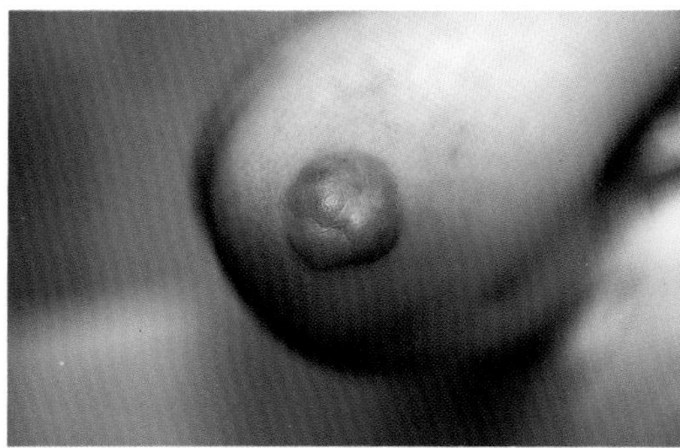

Figure 6.3. A tuberous xanthoma in a normolipemic patient.

with increased cholestanol, but have accompanying elevated levels of plant sterols. Xanthomas are also seen in cholestatic liver disease. Patients with liver disease have abnormal liver function tests and elevation of plasma cholesterol, which are not seen in cerebrotendinous xanthomatosis.

Support Group: N.O.R.D.
P.O. Box 8923
New Fairfield, CT 06812
1-800-999-6673

SELECTED BIBLIOGRAPHY

Berginer, V.M., Foster, N.M., Sadowsky, M., Townsend, J.A., III, Siegel, G.J., and Salen, G. (1988). Psychiatric disorders in patients with cerebrotendinous xanthomatosis. *Am. J. Psychiatr.* **145,** 354–357.

In reviewing cases of 35 patients, these authors found four with significant psychiatric symptoms. There was improvement with therapy with CDCA and very little response to antipsychotics.

Berginer, V.M., Salen, G., and Shefer, S. (1984). Long-term treatment of cerebrotendinous xanthomatosis with chenodeoxycholic acid. *N. Engl. J. Med.* **311,** 1649–1652.

Initial report of treatment in 17 patients. Subsequent experience supports the long-term safety and efficacy of this treatment.

Berginer, V.M., Shany, S., Alkalay, D., Berginer, J., Dekel, S., Salen, G., Tint, G.S., and Gazet, D. (1993). Osteoporosis and increased bone fractures in cerebrotendinous xanthomatosis. *Metabolism* **42,** 69–74.

Fifteen adult patients had regional bone mass measurements taken. Half the patients were being treated, half were not. Nine patients had fractures with minimal trauma. The authors postulate that this may be related to lower levels of serum 25-OH vitamin D and 24,25-$(OH)_2$ vitamin D, but the cause for the osteoporosis is actually unclear.

Cali, J.J., Hsieh, C.-L., Francke, U., and Russell, D.W. (1991). Mutations in the bile acid biosynthetic enzyme sterol 27-hydroxylase underlie cerebrotendinous xanthomatosis. *J. Biol. Chem.* **266,** 7779–7783.

Two point mutations in *CYP27,* localized to 2q33-qter, were demonstrated in two unrelated subjects. The authors suggest it is possible to devise carrier detection programs in populations in which the carrier frequency is high (e.g., Sephardic Jews of Moroccan descent) to allow for early recognition of pregnancies at risk and early institution of treatment in affected infants.

Leitersdorf, E., Reshef, A., Meiner, V., Levitzki, R., Pressman Schwartz, S., Dann, J.E., Berkman, N., Cali, J.J., Klapholz, L., and Berginer, V.M. (1993). Frameshift and splice junction mutations in the sterol 27-hydroxylase gene cause cerebrotendinous xanthomatosis in Jews of Moroccan origin. *J. Clin. Invest.* **91,** 2488–2496.

Again, two different mutations were found. Both gave rise to null alleles with no functional gene product. Clinical picture differed between siblings and among patients. One affected individual had no skin findings.

Salen, G., Shefer, S., and Berginer, V. (1991). Biochemical abnormalities in cerebrotendinous xanthomatosis. *Dev. Neurosci.* **13,** 363–370.

Clear, concise synopsis of biochemical pathway involved in cerebrotendinous xanthomatosis with a discussion of the differential diagnosis of the laboratory findings and treatment.

FAMILIAL MULTIPLE LIPOMATOSIS (MIM:151900)

(Familial Nonsymmetric Lipomatosis)

Includes Familial Angiolipomatosis; Dercum Disease

DERMATOLOGIC FEATURES

MAJOR. Multiple, nontender, small to very large, soft, subcutaneous, freely movable nodules usually appear in the teen years and increase in number throughout life. When the vascular component predominates, as in angiolipomas, the tumors are firmer and more rubbery. They tend to involve the trunk and extremities. While some reports in the literature describe severely involved individuals, the multiple growths usually remain fairly small (less than 5 cm) and often are not disfiguring.

A 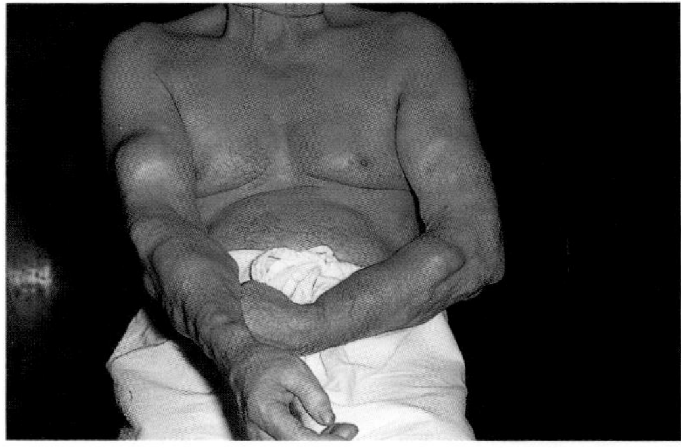

B 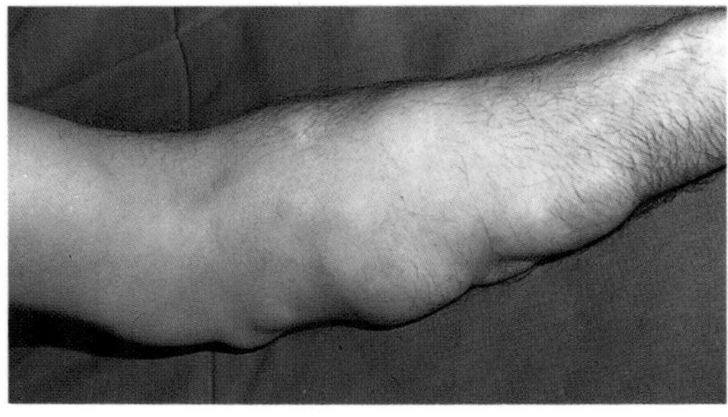

Figure 6.4. **(A)** Multiple soft tissue nodules on arms, sparing of neck and shoulders, in contrast to symmetric lipomatosis. (Courtesy of Dr. W. Baker, Division of Dermatology, University of Washington.) **(B)** Subcutaneous nodules on arm of second patient. (Courtesy of Dr. J. Halloran, Division of Dermatology, University of Washington.)

Hereditary multiple angiolipomatosis is also autosomal dominant and is clinically similar to multiple lipomatosis. The histopathologic distinction is based on the proportion of vascular elements to fatty tissue. As the diagnosis of one condition versus the other is usually based on microscopic evaluation of one or two specimens from a single proband in a family, the occurrence of both types of growths in the same individual or other family members could be easily overlooked. A systemic evaluation of multiple tumors from multiple family members has not been done for either condition. Whether multiple lipomas and multiple angiolipomas result from distinct and separate mutations or reflect variation in expression of the same mutation remains unclear.

MINOR. None.

ASSOCIATED ABNORMALITIES

In one family, concomitant elevation in cholesterol and triglyceride levels was found in affected family members. Lipid abnormalities have not been mentioned in other reports.

HISTOPATHOLOGY

LIGHT. The lipomas are encapsulated tumors composed of large fat cells. If the vascular component is 10% or less, they are termed *fibrolipomas;* if the vascular elements account for 15% or more of the specimen, the term *angiolipoma* is used. A fine capillary network interwoven in a sheath of extracellular matrix comprises the capsule of the lipomas.

EM. The cells of a lipoma are indistinguishable from normal lipocytes. The stroma is edematous and invested with many small blood vessels.

BASIC DEFECT

Unknown. These growths rarely become malignant. Numerous chromosome abnormalities in sporadic benign lipomas have been reported; these have involved chromosomes 6, 12, and 13. Abnormalities in phosphofructokinase have been demonstrated in fat cells from isolated lipomas. In the discussion section of papers reporting benign familial lipomatosis, abnormalities in cholesterol are often mentioned. All the supporting citations, however, are reports of familial cervical lipomatosis. There have been no documented, consistent, lipid abnormalities found in patients with multiple benign lipomatosis.

TREATMENT

Surgical excision is the major method of treatment. Tumors do not recur once they are removed. Liposuction has also been used, with anecdotal reports of success.

MODE OF INHERITANCE

The great majority of reports support uncomplicated autosomal dominant transmission with age of onset in late teens or later.

A complicated pedigree reported by Rabbiosi et al. (1977) was interpreted by the authors to represent autosomal recessive or polygenic inheritance, although the pattern was consistent with autosomal dominant inheritance with reduced penetrance. Dolph et al. (1980) reported a five generation family with 11 affected family members and male-to-male transmission. As one obligate heterozygote did not express the disorder, they inferred polygenic inheritance. It seems more likely that this individual was a nonexpressing carrier and that penetrance is not 100% in this disorder or that he had not yet expressed the condition because of his relatively young age.

PRENATAL DIAGNOSIS

None.

DIFFERENTIAL DIAGNOSIS

Multiple neurofibromas, leiomyomas, xanthomas, and cystic steatocystomas may be somewhat clinically similar. If the correct diagnosis cannot be established by clinical context, biopsy for histopathology will do so.

Given the common occurrence of isolated lipomas, one to three lipomas in a single older individual without a family history is not likely to be a sign of familial lipomatosis. I think familial occurrence of lipomas may be more common than appreciated. Patients often volunteer that other family members have similar growths for which no medical attention has ever been sought.

Features of Proteus syndrome (MIM:176920) include partial gigantism, usually of the hands and feet, multiple hemangiomas, epidermal nevi, and multiple lipomas, with onset in infancy and early childhood.

Individuals with the autosomal dominant Bannayan-Zonana syndrome (MIM:153480) have macrocephaly, mild mental retardation, multiple hemangiomas, lymphangiomas, and lipomas. The last often regress in later life.

In familial benign cervical or symmetric lipomatosis (MIM:151800), the unencapsulated fatty deposits occur around the neck, shoulder, and upper chest. They are histopathologically distinct from the encapsulated lipomas of familial nonsymmetric lipomatosis.

Multiple nonencapsulated angiolipomatosis (MIM:206550) has been reported in a brother and sister (Hapnes et al., 1980). The brother also had bony deformities and muscle atrophy. Histopathologically these nonencapsulated lesions differed from lipomas.

The lymphangiomatous and angiomatous malformations of Klippel-Trenaunay-Weber syndrome (MIM:149000) are easily distinguished clinically from lipomas by the visually obvious major vascular component of the former. While soft tissue and bony undergrowth and overgrowth do not always occur in Klippel-Trenaunay-Weber syndrome, when present, they distinguish Klippel-Trenauney-Weber syndrome from familial lipomatosis.

The fatty tumors in Dercum disease (adiposis dolorosa, MIM:103200) are painful and usually occur in obese, postmenopausal, middle-aged women. Familial occurrence has been reported twice. It was apparently the painful nature of the lipomas in the families of Lynch and Harlan that suggested to them that this was not familial, nonsymmetric lipomatosis but familial Dercum disease. In one family, affected males were not obese, and the lesions were not painful; the two affected females had classic adiposis dolorosa. In the other family, pain was an inconstant finding, and only one of four affected family members was obese. I am not sure these two families justify the consideration of a genetically distinct entity.

Support Group: N.O.R.D.
P.O. Box 8923
New Fairfield, CT
06812
1-800-999-6673

SELECTED BIBLIOGRAPHY

Dolph, J.L., Demuth, R.J., and Miller, S.H. (1980). Familial multiple lipomatosis. *Plast. Reconstr. Surg.* **66,** 620–622.

Report of a five generation family.

Hapnes, S.A., Bowman, H., Skeie, S.O. (1980). Familial angiolipomatosis. *Clin. Genet.* **17,** 202–208.

Bilateral involvement at wrists, knees and ankles. Onset at age 1 year in brother, age 5 years in sister, and slow progression in both. Lesions were deep, extending between muscles and joints, but non-infiltrating. No consanguinity but parental ancestors from same area in Norway.

Kumar, R., Pereira, B.J.G., Sakhuja, V., and Chugh, K.S. (1989). Autosomal dominant inheritance in familial angiolipomatosis. *Clin. Genet.* **35,** 202–204.

Multiple angiolipomas in three generations with male-to-male transmission. The proband, who inherited her disease from her father, was ascertained when she presented with adult onset polycystic kidney disease inherited from her mother.

Lynch, H.T., and Harlan, W.L. (1963). Hereditary factors in adiposis dolorosa (Dercum's disease). *Am. J. Hum. Genet.* **15,** 184–190.

Two pedigrees with affected individuals, some of whom were obese and had multiple painful lipomas, others were not obese and had painless lesions. The authors argue for an autosomal dominant entity distinct from familial lipomatosis.

Rabbiosi, G., Borroni, G., and Scuderi, N. (1977). Familial multiple lipomatosis. *Acta Dermatol. Venereol. (Stockh.)* **57,** 265–267.

Report of two pedigrees, the first of which is quite interesting. The unaffected nephew of two aunts with the disorder, the son of their unaffected brother, married an unrelated affected woman who was one of four affected sisters born to unaffected parents. Three of this couple's seven children were also affected.

Rubenstein, A., Goor, Y., Gazit, E., and Cabili, S. (1989). Nonsymmetric subcutaneous lipomatosis associated with familial combined hyperlipidemia. *Br. J. Dermatol.* **120,** 689–694.

Report of a single pedigree with 12 family members affected with multiple lipomas who had elevated levels of cholesterol and triglycerides.

FAMILIAL SYMMETRIC LIPOMATOSIS (MIM:151800)

(Familial Benign Cervical Lipomatosis; Launois-Bensaude Adenolipomatosis; Nonencapsulated Central Lipomatosis; Fetthals Disease)

DERMATOLOGIC FEATURES

MAJOR. The development of slowly enlarging, soft, subcutaneous tissue masses around the neck and the shoulders, usually occurring in the third to sixth decades of life, is described in almost all reported patients. The upper chest, breast area, abdomen and thighs may also be involved. In some patients, the masses appear distinct from the general body fat and are nodular; in others, there appears to be diffuse enlargement of subcutaneous tissue in general.

Minor. Overlying erythema and lividity with telangiectases are common findings in some surveys.

ASSOCIATED ABNORMALITIES

Hyperlipidemia, hyperuricemia, abnormal glucose tolerance, frank diabetes, and renal tubular acidosis have been reported in some affected persons.

Venous stasis and airway compromise due to mechanical compression caused by the fatty masses has occurred.

Enzi (1984) reported peripheral motor and sensory neuropathies and autonomic neuropathy in his series. The basis of these was not thought to be ethanol abuse, although many of his patients had liver disease secondary to alcohol damage. He found a "diabetic-like demyelinated neuropathy" in nerve biopsys specimens from affected individuals. All of Enzi's patients were male. In the series of Ruzicka et al. (1977), the great majority of affected individuals were alcoholic. Three patients in this group had cancer, which has also been reported in other cases of cervical lipomatosis. The malignancies are of many types.

HISTOPATHOLOGY

Light. Normal-appearing, unencapsulated fatty tissue that invades surrounding structures is typical. There appear to be increased numbers of adipocytes. Both fibrous tissue and the vascular supply may be increased.

EM. No information.

BASIC DEFECT

A defect in the adrenergic-stimulated lipolysis of fatty tissue has been demonstrated in vitro. Lipoprotein lipase activity in adipocytes from affected patients is higher than that of fat cells from normals. It has been suggested that this disorder is one of abnormal triglyceride storage.

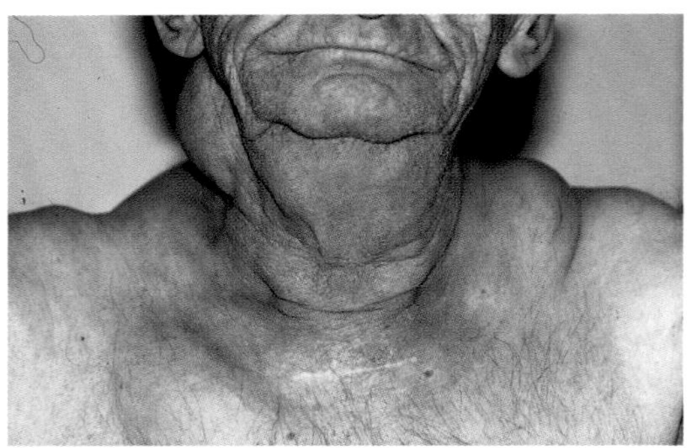

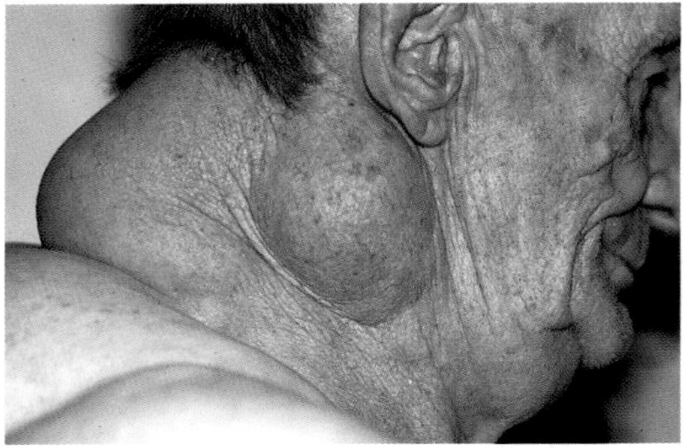

Figure 6.5. Marked cervical involvement (Courtesy of Division of Dermatology, University of Washington.)

TREATMENT

Surgical excision if the growths are life threatening. Complete extirpation is often unsuccessful because of invasion into surrounding tissues, and recurrence is common.

MODE OF INHERITANCE

Although listed as a possible autosomal dominant disorder, most cases are sporadic, and alcohol abuse is an almost invariable finding. Except for one report of an affected aunt related to the proband through an unaffected parent, the few familial cases have only involved siblings. No male-to-male transmission has occurred.

PRENATAL DIAGNOSIS

None.

DIFFERENTIAL DIAGNOSIS

The fat deposits of familial symmetric lipomatosis can appear vascular, and a superficial bluish discoloration with telangiectases has been described, giving consideration to the diagnosis of Klippel-Trenaunay-Weber syndrome (MIM:149000). The later onset of these lesions contrasts with the congenital and early childhood onset of Klippel-Trenaunay-Weber syndrome.

Support Group: N.O.R.D.
P.O. Box 8923
New Fairfield, CT
06812
1-800-999-6673

SELECTED BIBLIOGRAPHY

Enzi, G. (1984). Multiple symmetric lipomatosis: an updated clinical report. *Medicine* **63,** 56–64.

Report of 19 patients with an eight-year follow-up of nine. Striking photographs accompany the article.

Greene, M.L., Glueck, C.J., Fujimoto, W.Y., and Seegmiller, J.E. (1970). Benign symmetrical lipomatosis (Launois-Bensaude adenolipomatosis) with gout and hyperlipoproteinemia. *Am. J. Med.* **48,** 239–246.

Two sisters are presented, both of whom had gout, pes cavus, hypertriglyceridemia, and abnormal glucose tolerance. One had gouty arthritis and oligomenorrhea.

McKusick, V.A. (1962). Medical genetics 1961 (Figure 24). *J. Chronic Dis.* **15,** 417–572.

Photographs of three affected brothers are shown. Two sisters and a maternal aunt were reported to be affected. The siblings' mother was unaffected. The photographs demonstrate a collar of fat around the neck. There is a description of typical lipomas elsewhere on the body. There is not enough information given with which to evaluate the report critically.

Ruzicka, T., Vieluf, D., Landthaler, M., and Braun-Falco, O. (1987). Benign symmetric lipomatosis Launois-Bensaude. *J. Am. Acad. Dermatol.* **17,** 663–673.

Report of clinical findings in 10 patients, 5 of whom were women.

FIBRODYSPLASIA OSSIFICANS PROGRESSIVA (MIM:135100)

(Myositis Ossificans)

DERMATOLOGIC FEATURES

MAJOR. During the first decade, firm, subcutaneous nodules attached to tendons and ligaments and within skeletal muscle develop. They may be tender, red and warm, or noninflammatory. They can develop spontaneously or at sites of trauma. Lesions may also resolve spontaneously. They may first present in infancy, but occasionally may not show until adult life. Upon initial presentation they may be soft and then gradually calcify over several months. Calcification usually develops from head to foot, proximally to distally. The nodules may occur in crops. As the lesions mature, they gradually become painless.

Occasionally fever accompanies the development of new lesions.

MINOR. Diffuse thinning of the hair has been reported in about 25% of patients, including females.

ASSOCIATED ABNORMALITIES

Hallux valgus present at birth is a classic feature. Shortened metacarpals of the thumbs and

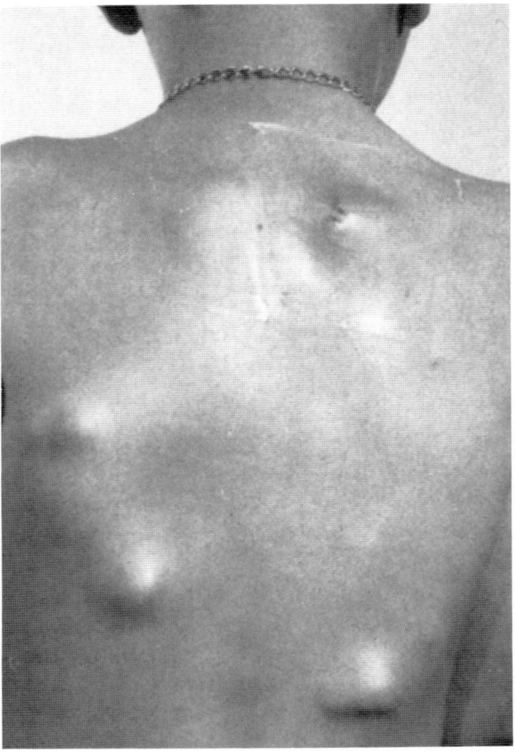

Figure 6.6. Multiple nodules on back. (From Pereyo, 1976.)

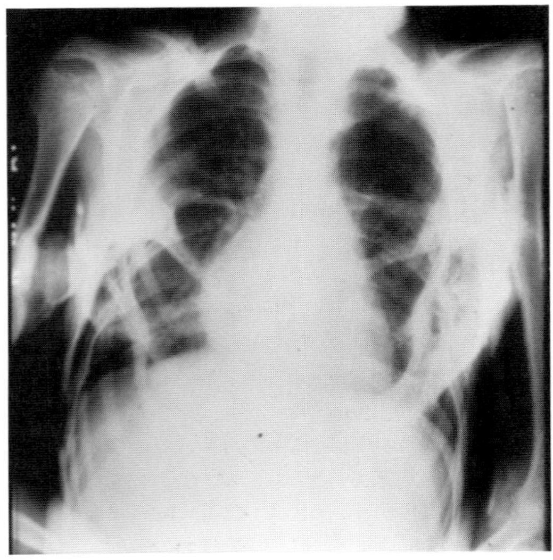

Figure 6.7. Development of osseous bridges. (Courtesy of Dr. J. G. Hall, Vancouver, British Columbia.)

metatarsals of the great toes are typical. Other fingers may also be involved. Clinodactyly of the third and fifth fingers is common. The great toes may also have shortened phalanges or a single phalanx.

The disorder is marked by progressive involvement of all soft tissues, development of bony bridges, and decreased range of motion at all joints. Sixty-five percent of affected individuals have scoliosis, which appears to be unresponsive to bracing or surgery. Osseous bridges develop between the iliac crest and the ribcage in over 50% of patients. Ossification of the paravertebral muscles and the fascia is typical. Ankylosis of the joints occurs at sites of ossification. Patients can have respiratory compromise secondary to scoliosis and restriction of ribcage excursion because of ossification. Starvation may ensue because of inability to open the mouth. Life expectancy is reduced and the mean age of death is in the forties.

A conductive hearing loss occurs in about 25% of affected individuals. Intelligence is usually normal. There is occasional mention made of early menopause in affected females. The reasons for this are not known.

HISTOPATHOLOGY

LIGHT. Early nodules show proliferation of loose myxoid connective tissue with an increase in the number of small vessles, infiltration of normal fascia, and striated muscle. Entrapped degenerating muscle fibers can be seen, along with cartilagenous foci. Late lesions show heterotopic bone formation.

EM. Normal elastic fibrils and matrix with abnormal granules within mast cells. Increased amounts of proteoglycans and glycoproteins in the dermis are seen prior to calcification.

BASIC DEFECT

Unknown.

TREATMENT

None effective. Excision of nodules leads to reoccurrence at the surgical site. It has been suggested that biopsy of soft tissue swelling may lead to increased calcification and that diagnosis by clinical means and/or radiographic evaluation is preferrable. Protection against trauma is prudent. Surgical treatment of the bony deformities also results in poor outcome in most patients.

MODE OF INHERITANCE

Autosomal dominant. Male-to-male transmission has been demonstrated, and there is older paternal age of fathers of sporadic cases. There is marked variability within the few families reported. Fitness is reduced, and there have been few adults who have reproduced. Most cases are sporadic.

PRENATAL DIAGNOSIS

None.

DIFFERENTIAL DIAGNOSIS

Early in the course of the disease, confusion with soft tissue malignancy (e.g., fibrosarcoma) often leads to biopsy. Recognition of the congenital hand and foot malformations may point to the correct diagnosis.

Support Group: International Fibrodysplasia Ossificans Progressiva Association, Inc.
P.O.B. 3578
Winter Springs, FL 32708
1-407-365-4194

SELECTED BIBLIOGRAPHY

Connor, J.M., and Evans, D.A.P. (1982). Fibrodysplasia ossificans progressiva. The clinical features and natural history of 34 patients. *J. Bone Joint Surg. (Br.)* **64B,** 76–83.

Cohen, R.B., Hahn, G.V., Tabas, J.A., Peeper, J., Levitz, C.L., Sando, A., Sando, N., Zasloff, M., and Kaplan, F.S. (1993). The natural history of heterotopic ossification in patients who have fibrodysplasia ossificans progressiva. *J. Bone Joint Surg. (Am.)* **75A,** 215–219.

Kaplan, F.S., Tabas, J.A., Gannon, F.H., Finkel, G., Hahn, G.V., and Zasloff, M.A. (1993). The histopathology of fibrodysplasia ossificans progressiva: an endochondral process. *J. Bone Joint Surg. (Am.)* **75A,** 220–230.

The first reference reports information derived from interviews of patients in Great Britain. The second resulted from a mailed questionnaire to patients in Great Britain. Therefore, there may have been some overlap, and some of the patients may have been represented twice. Both papers give broad overviews of the spectrum of the condition. The second mentions mental retardation. Only 2 of 34 patients had "low IQ." Both had severe terminal transverse defects of the limbs and baldness, along with their intellectual changes. The third reference reviews the 12 biopsies from 11 of these patients. The authors note that the biopsies were done to rule out malignancy and that the diagnosis of fibrodysplasia ossificans progressiva was not considered prior to biopsy. There are many micrographs.

Kaplan, F.S., McCluskey, W., Hahn, G., Muenke, M., and Zasloff, M.A. (1993). Genetic transmission of fibrodysplasia ossificans progressiva. Report of a family. *J. Bone Joint Surg. (Am.)* **75A,** 214–220.

An affected male, the first in his family, had two affected daughters and an affected son.

Kaplan, F.S., Tabas, J.A., and Zasloff, M.A. (1990). Fibrodysplasia ossificans progressiva: a clue from the fly? *Calcif. Tissue Int.* **47,** 117–125.

The authors suggest homology with decapentaplegic (*dpp*) in the fruitfly. The candidate genes include *BMP2A* and *BMP2B* (members of the *TGF-β* family). These are bone morphogenetic proteins that appear to induce ossification of cartilage in vivo. The senior author has published extensively on this disorder. There is also a diagram of the hands with the percentage of involvement of specific bones based on 16 patients. The *dpp* mutations in the fly are either lethal or result in limb malformations and loss of wing patterns and antennae, proboscis, and eyes.

Ludman, H., Hamilton, E.B.D., and Eade, A.W.T. (1968). Deafness in myositis ossificans progressiva. *J. Laryngol. Otol.* **82,** 57–63.

Authors review three cases of their own and six from the literature. Conductive deafness developed in four, sensorineural hearing loss in two. In one patient, surgical exploration revealed normal ossicles. There is a very sad vignette—one patient had only one hearing aid, as she could reach only one ear because of joint immobility caused by the disorder.

Rosenstirn, J. (1918). A contribution to the study of myositis ossificans progressiva. *Ann. Surg.* **68,** 485–520, 591–637.

The author reviewed 119 cases from the literature and one of his own in great detail. Family history was negative in all but two. He noted the features of the abnormal great toes and thumbs and emphasized that failure to recognize clinical features significantly biases the reported prevalence of the feature.

Shah, P.B., Zasloff, M.A., Drummond, D., and Kaplan, F.S. (1994). Spinal deformity in patients who have fibrodysplasia ossificans progressiva. *J. Bone Joint Surg. (Am.)* **76A,** 1442–1450.

Forty patients. Twenty-six had scoliosis. Five patients had operative repairs of their scoliosis, which either failed or resulted in heterotopic calcification at other sites. The authors argue that surgery is not a good choice. There are painfully detailed case reports underscoring the horrific consequences of this disorder.

LIPOGRANULOMATOSIS (MIM:228000)

(Farber Disease)

DERMATOLOGIC FEATURES

MAJOR. Flesh-colored nodules develop overlying the joints, in the larynx, on the scalp, and less frequently, on the trunk. Onset is usually within the first year of life, but it may be delayed until several years of age.

MINOR. None.

ASSOCIATED ABNORMALITIES

Mental retardation and failure to thrive, affecting both ponderal and linear growth, are typical. In middle to late infancy, painless joint swelling occurs, resulting in limited range of motion and subsequent atrophy of muscles. Systemic involvement can include hepatosplenomegaly, pulmonary infiltrates, lymphadenopathy, and both central nervous system and peripheral nervous system findings. A cherry red spot has been described in the retina. Death usually occurs by age 3 years.

HISTOPATHOLOGY

LIGHT. Lesions are deep within the dermis and show accumulation of histiocytes with foamy cytoplasm. A moderate lymphoplasmacytic infiltrate can be seen. Capillaries are dilated, with swollen endothelial cells.

EM. Foamy cells with membrane-bound inclusions of curvilinear tubular bodies. Other typical inclusions are "banana bodies" and "zebra-like bodies," and these are limited to the peripheral and central nervous systems. Fibroblasts show storage; epidermal cells do not.

BASIC DEFECT

Acid ceramidase deficiency.

TREATMENT

None.

MODE OF INHERITANCE

Autosomal recessive.

PRENATAL DIAGNOSIS

A decrease in ceramidase activity can be demonstrated in cultured amniocytes.

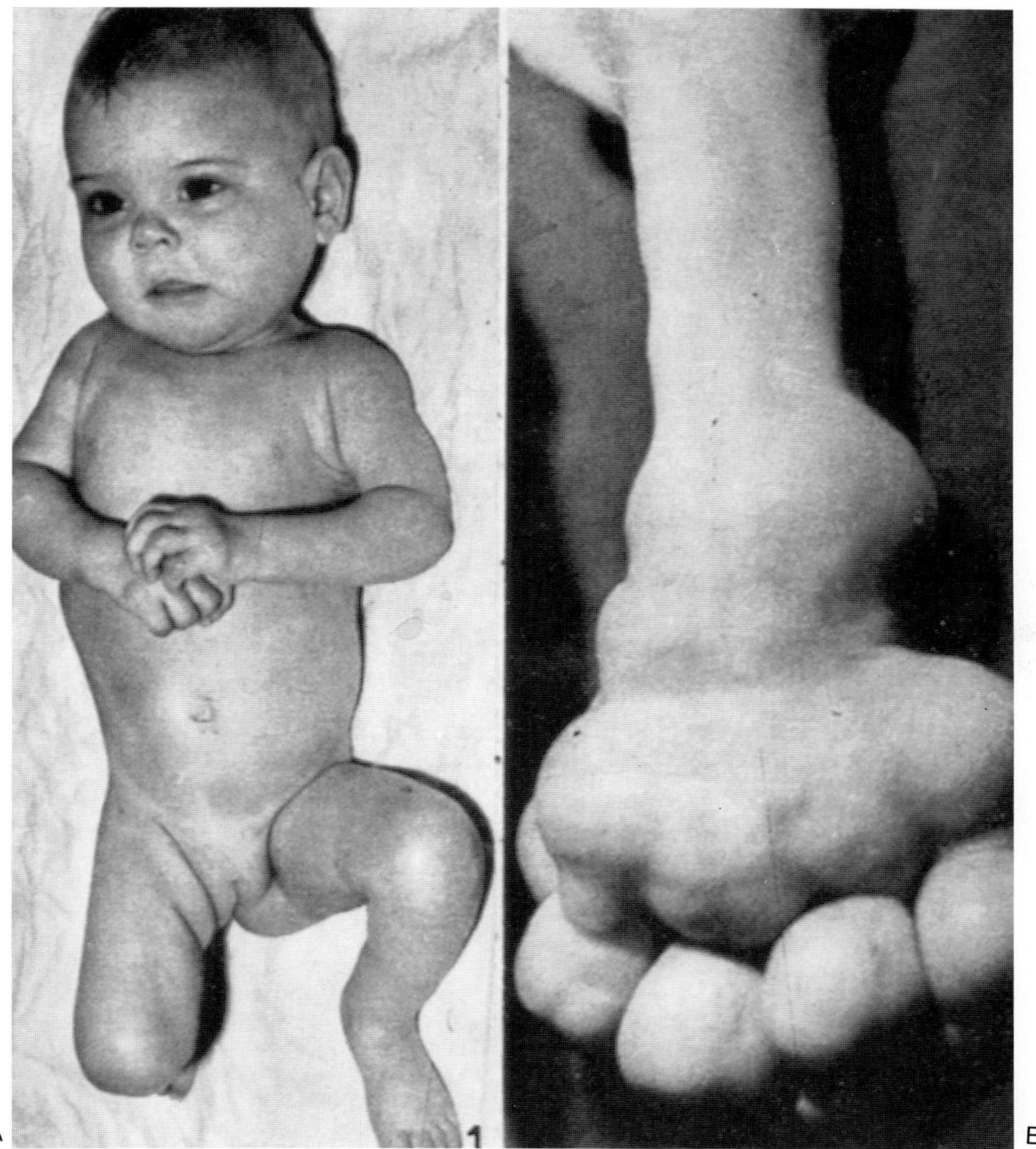

Figure 6.8. **(A)** Infant at 8 months with mild joint swelling over hands. **(B)** Hands at the time of death at age 21 months. (From Dustin et al., 1973.)

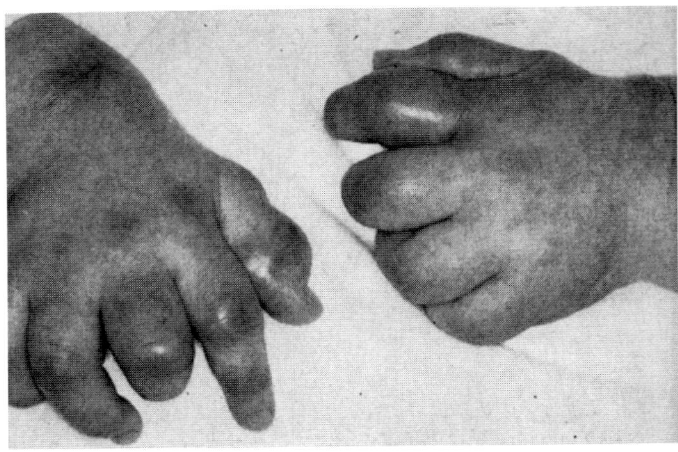

Figure 6.9. Hands with hyperpigmented nodules over joints. (From Abul-Haj et al., 1962.)

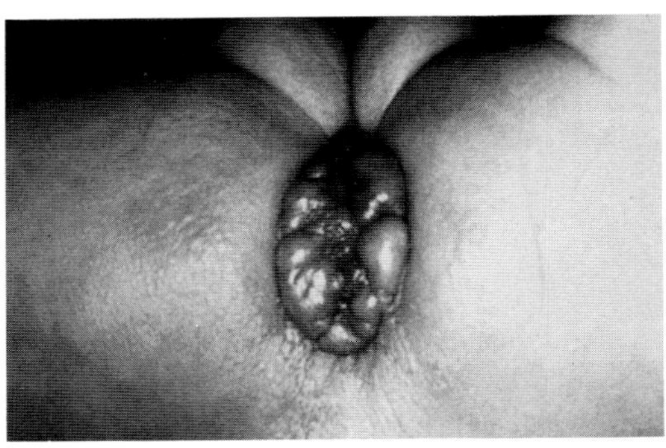

Figure 6.10. Perianal soft tissue masses. (From Chanoki et al., 1989.)

DIFFERENTIAL DIAGNOSIS

Infants with systemic hyalinosis (MIM:228600, 236490) share in common early onset of failure to thrive, joint stiffening, and diffuse nodules in the skin. Acid ceramidase activity is normal in systemic hyalinosis.

Support Group: N.O.R.D.
P.O. Box 8923
New Fairfield, CT
06812
1-800-999-6673

SELECTED BIBLIOGRAPHY

Zappatini-Tommasi, L., Dumontel, C., Guibaud, P., and Girod, C. (1992). Farber disease: an ultrastructural study. *Virchows Arch. A. Pathol. Anat. Histopathol.* **420,** 281–290.
Case report. Bone marrow grafting resulted in improvement of skin, mucosal, joint, and pulmonary symptoms, but neurologic status continued to deteriorate and the patient died. This article reviews the literature and focuses on the ultrastructural features.

PARTIAL LIPODYSTROPHY (MIM:151660, 308980)

(Kobberling-Dunnigan Syndrome; Familial Lipoatrophic Diabetes)

DERMATOLOGIC FEATURES

Major. The term *partial* is misleading, as loss of subcutaneous tissue may be localized or generalized in this heterogeneous group of syndromes that share in common vertical transmission and onset of loss of fat, usually during childhood or puberty. Different patterns of

A
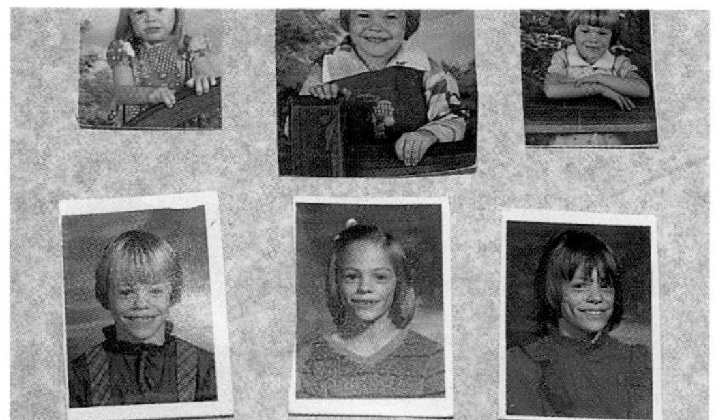

B
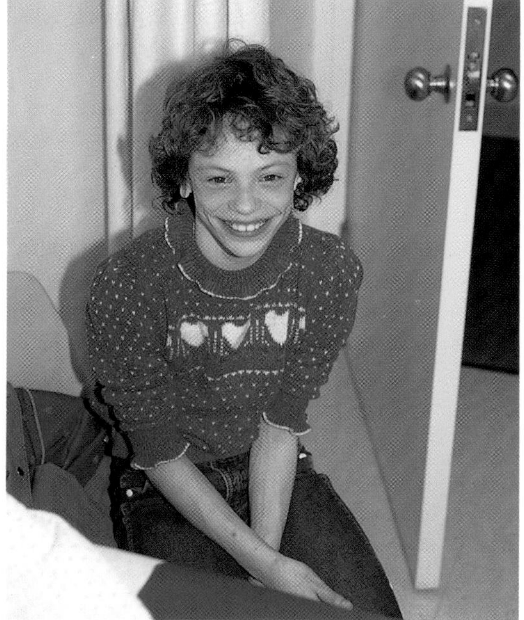

Figure 6.11. **(A)** Gradual loss over time of subcutaneous fat on face. **(B)** Sharply demarcated muscle and bones of face. Prominence of ropy veins on arms at age 10½ years.

involvement have been described, and overlap can be seen within some families. Thus, the specificity of the pattern of subcutaneous loss vis-à-vis allelic heterogeneity is uncertain. The face may be spared, the face and trunk spared, or the face, trunk, and abdomen spared, with loss of fat from, respectively, the trunk and extremities, the extremities, or the extremities and buttocks. Patients do not look emaciated but hardened, with clear definition of muscle groups.

Acanthosis nigricans, brown velvety hyperkeratosis of the skin of the body folds, is common. Eruptive xanthomas, raised yellow papules, and nodules, may appear in early childhood and continue to develop throughout adult life.

MINOR. None.

ASSOCIATED ABNORMALITIES

These conditions appear to be syndromes of insulin resistance, with nonketotic insulin-resistant diabetes developing in childhood and adolescence. Hyperlipidemia is common. Hepatomegaly, presumably due to fatty infiltration of the liver, is reported. In one family, deficiency of C_3 cosegregated with the lipodystrophy.

HISTOPATHOLOGY

LIGHT. Loss of subcutaneous fat, with the dermis abutting the fascia or muscle.

EM. No information.

BASIC DEFECT

Unknown.

TREATMENT

Dietary restriction of fats and carbohydrates was successful in one family, resulting in resolution of xanthomas and improvement in hyperlipidemia and hyperglycemia.

MODE OF INHERITANCE

Questionably autosomal dominant. There have been no instances of male-to-male transmission, and there is a female to male preponderance among affected individuals. In reported pedigrees, none of seven males at risk was affected. Sixteen of 27 females were. The paucity of males at risk was not explained by an increase in pregnancy loss, as might be expected were these X-linked dominant disorders.

PRENATAL DIAGNOSIS

None.

DIFFERENTIAL DIAGNOSIS

In progressive partial lipodystrophy, onset is in childhood or adolescence. Females are almost exclusively involved. The face and trunk are primary sites of involvement. Affected individuals have a bottom-heavy appearance, with preservation or increase of fat in the lower half of the body. Nephropathy, diabetes mellitus, and hyperlipidemia can also develop, but may not. It may be that involvement of the face is a feature that can separate this acquired condition with no risk to offspring from partial lipodystrophy, which has a recurrence risk associated with it. Seip-Berardinelli syndrome (autosomal recessive congenital generalized lipodystrophy, MIM:269700, 272500), usually presents within the first few months of life and is usually more generalized and more severe than partial lipodystrophy, with more severe systemic involvement as well. This is not always true.

Localized atrophy of subcutaneous tissue can occur secondary to trauma and is not genetic. Acquired progressive centrifugal lipodystrophy is marked by the initial appearance of an expanding margin of erythema and progressive loss of subcutaneous tissue from the face and upper trunk.

Familial cervical lipomatosis (MIM:158800) should not be confused with partial lipodystrophy, although in some reports of the latter much is made of the preservation of fat around the neck and face.

Support Group: N.O.R.D.
P.O. Box 8923
New Fairfield, CT 06812
1-800-999-6673

SELECTED BIBLIOGRAPHY

Burn, J., and Baraitser, M. (1986). Partial lipodystrophy with insulin-resistant diabetes and hyperlipidemia (Dunnigan syndrome). *J. Med. Genet.* **23,** 128–130.

This paper nicely demonstrates the marked intrafamilial variability in expression. The one affected male was not more severely involved than the affected females in the family.

Dunnigan, M.G., Cochrane, M.A., Kelly, A., and Scott, J.W. (1974). Familial lipoatrophic diabetes with dominant transmission. A new syndrome. *Q. J. Med.* **43,** 33–48.

Two families with lipoatrophy in which only females were affected. There is a nice discussion of the different types of lipodystrophy. Overlap is evident, and criteria for separating out all the subtypes seem fuzzy.

Kobberling, J., and Dunnigan, M.G. (1986). Familial partial lipodystrophy: two types of an X-linked dominant syndrome, lethal in the hemizygous state. *J. Med. Genet.* **23,** 120–127.

The authors propose X-linkage based on pedigree analysis in which a 1:1:1:0 ratio of affected females to unaffected females to unaffected males to affected males was seen. They offer no hypothesis as to the nature of the lesion presumably causing death in male fetuses, and there are no reports of pregnancy losses. This report pools the two authors' separate experiences.

Power, D.A., Ng, Y.C., and Simpson, J.G. (1990). Familial incidence of C_3 nephritic factor, partial lipodystrophy and membranoproliferative glomerulonephritis. *Q. J. Med.* **75,** 387–398.

One family is described with C_3 deficiency and partial lipodystrophy in a mother and two sons. She and one son also had membranoproliferative glomerulonephritis. The interrelationship of the three features is uncertain. In other reports of inherited C_3 deficiency, no affected members have had partial lipodystrophy.

SEIP-BERARDINELLI SYNDROME (MIM:269700, 272500)

(Congenital Generalized Lipodystrophy)

Includes SHORT Syndrome

DERMATOLOGIC FEATURES

Major. Very soon after birth the affected infant is noted to appear muscular with very little subcutaneous tissue. The face appears haggard. Although the entire body is involved, the abdomen may be protruberant.

Hypertrichosis, of both body and face, is typical, and thick curly scalp hair with low frontal hairline is a feature.

Acanthosis nigricans, with a thickened brown velvety appearance to the skin, develops during childhood in the groins, axillae, and neck and may extend around the mouth and antecubital and popliteal fossae. Although some case reports describe hyperpigmentation alone, I suspect that these authors are observing early alterations of acanthosis nigricans rather than diffuse generalized hyperpigmentation.

Minor. None.

ASSOCIATED ABNORMALITIES

Insulin-resistant diabetes develops in middle to late childhood, as does hyperlipidemia, which is primarily hypertriglyceridemia. Hypertrophic cardiomyopathy with fatty infiltration is described in a significant number of affected individuals who survive into adulthood. Fatty infiltration of the liver leading to cirrhosis and secondary complications such as esophageal varices are a major cause of premature mortality.

Focal osteolysis with cyst formation, primarily involving the long bones, occurs during or after adolescence. There can be absence of fat in the marrow cavity. In childhood, rapid overgrowth with an advanced bone age is typical. Despite this, final height is usually normal or less than normal because early fusion of the epiphyses occurs. Polycystic ovarian disease and clitoromegaly in females and a disproportionately large glans penis in males are common findings. The specificity of renal involvement is less certain. Enlarged kidneys, hydronephrosis, hydroureter, and renal calculi have been noticed in a few patients.

A few individuals have been mentally re-

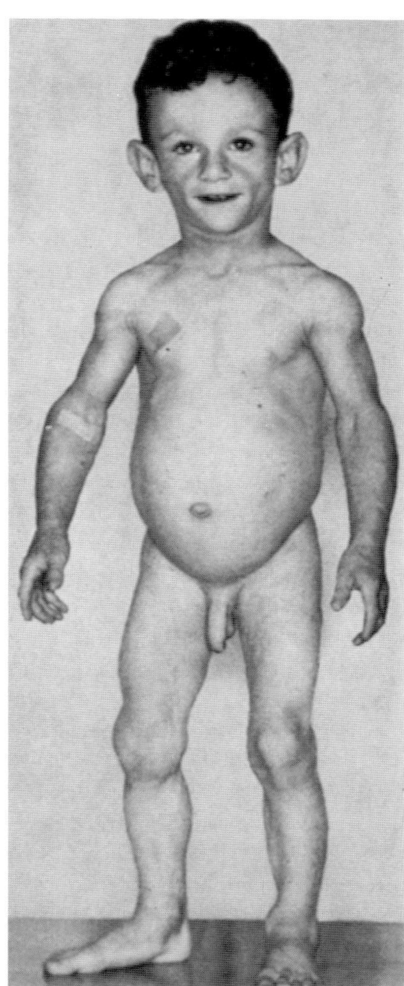

Figure 6.12. Marked definition of muscles due to lack of adipose tissue. Large phallus. (From Seip, 1971.)

tarded, and dilatation of the ventrices has also been noted in a few case reports. These features may be coincidental. Most patients have normal intelligence.

HISTOPATHOLOGY

LIGHT. Decrease to absence of subcutaneous tissue.
EM. No information.

BASIC DEFECT

Unknown. There is a decrease in binding of insulin to receptors.

TREATMENT

None effective for the subcutaneous loss. Dietary management of the diabetes and the hyperlipidemia may result in some improvement.

MODE OF INHERITANCE

Autosomal recessive. There has been recurrence among siblings and consanguinity noted in many parents.

PRENATAL DIAGNOSIS

None.

DIFFERENTIAL DIAGNOSIS

The diencephalic syndrome is an acquired disorder that develops secondary to hypothalamic tumors. There is loss of subcutaneous tissue and premature aging with growth failure. There is no muscular hypertrophy. Children with SHORT syndrome (short stature, hyperextensibility, ocular depression [deepset orbits], Reiger's anomaly, and delayed teething; MIM:151680, 269880) have loss of subcutaneous tissue, particularly of the face, but do not develop acanthosis nigricans and do not have advanced bone age or hypertrichosis. Although the condition was first described in siblings, a similar pattern of anomalies with vertical transmission has also been reported. Premature aging syndromes such as Werner syndrome, progeria, Hallerman-Streiff syndrome, and Cockayne syndrome (MIM:Many) show loss of subcutaneous tissue, but in addition there is loss of dermis, striking facial features, and thinning of hair. These conditions should be easily differentiated from congenital generalized lipodystrophy. In partial lipodystrophy (MIM:151660, 308980) the onset is usually later in childhood and the loss of subcutaneous tissue not generalized. Some overlap cases have been described. Leprechaunism (MIM:246200) is very similar, and infants with it are distinguished primarily by severe intrauterine growth retardation and failure to thrive, earlier onset of insulin resistance, and early death. Children with longstanding dermatomyositis can develop a lipodystrophy-like appearance with hirsutism, loss of subcutaneous tissue, and acanthosis nigricans.

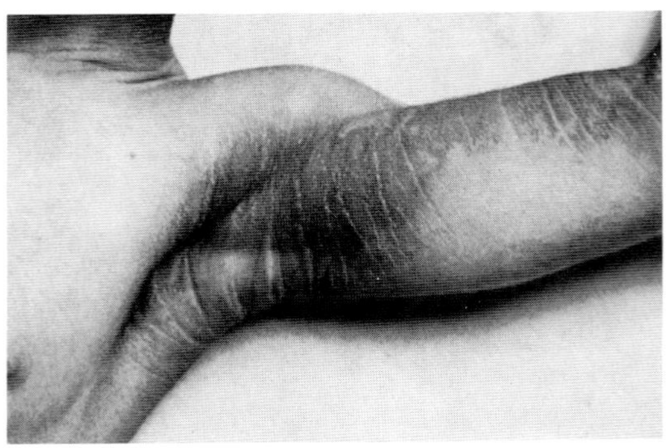

Figure 6.13. Acanthosis nigricans. (From Seip, 1971.)

Support Group: N.O.R.D.
P.O. Box 8923
New Fairfield, CT
06812
1-800-999-6673

SELECTED BIBLIOGRAPHY

Brunzell, J.D., Shankle, S.W., and Bethune, J.E. (1968). Congenital generalized lipodystrophy accompanied by cystic angiomatosis. *Ann. Intern. Med.* **69,** 501–516.

Although the authors describe the bony lesions in lipodystrophy as cystic angiomatosis, subsequent authors have claimed that bone cysts are common in lipodystrophy and not true "cystic angiomatosis," as the latter involves the axial skeleton. The cysts in congenital generalized lipodystrophy involve the long bones, and the cysts are true cysts without a vascular component.

Moller, D.E. (ed.) (1993). *Insulin Resistance.* John Wiley and Sons, New York.

There are chapters discussing treatment (which is not encouraging), recent advances in molecular mechanisms of insulin resistance, and clinical spectrum of the lipodystrophies.

Senior, B., and Gellis, S.S. (1964). The syndromes of total lipodystrophy and of partial lipodystrophy. *Pediatrics* **33,** 593–612.

Ninety-eight references. Puts the confusion into perspective with a detailed review of cases reported up to that time.

VanderVorm, E.R., Kuipers, A., Bonenkamp, J.W., Kleijer, W.J., van Maldergem, L., Herwig, J., and Maassen, J.A. (1993). Patients with lipodystrophic diabetes mellitus of the Seip-Berardinelli type express normal insulin receptors. *Diabetologia* **36,** 172–174.

Fibroblasts from three patients showed normal binding of insulin. The coding regions of both alleles of the insulin receptor gene were sequenced and were normal. The IgF-1 receptor function was also normal.

CHAPTER 7

LYMPHEDEMA

CHOLESTASIS-LYMPHEDEMA SYNDROME (MIM:214900)

(Aagenaes Syndrome; Hereditary Cholestasis Norwegian type)

DERMATOLOGIC FEATURES

MAJOR. Recurrent swelling of the lower extremities begins at infancy in a few patients, later in childhood in most. There is a waxing and waning of the edema, unrelated to the course of the liver disease. The edema is nonpitting.

Icterus secondary to obstructive liver disease develops within the first few weeks of life. The jaundice may gradually resolve in childhood or recur episodically.

MINOR. Pruritis secondary to cholestasis is a common complaint. Typical strawberry hemangiomas were reported in a few cases. It is not clear that this is a true association. Enamel defects with discolored teeth are thought to be secondary to malabsorption and increased bilirubin.

ASSOCIATED ABNORMALITIES

Slowly progressive fibrotic liver disease with a decrease in intrahepatic bile ducts is typical of the disorder. Pale stools are noted shortly after birth. A few patients develop loss of deep tendon reflexes after years of cholestasis. Some

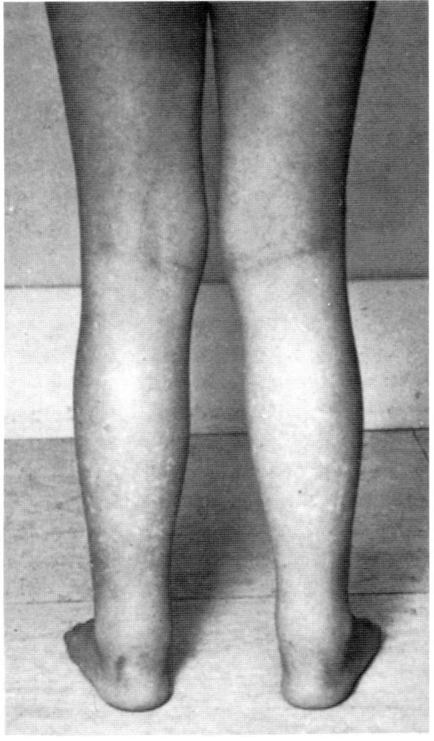

A

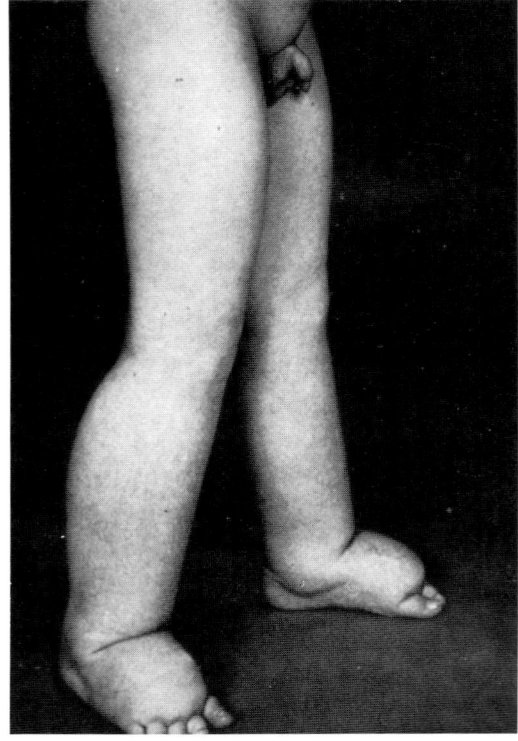

B

Figure 7.1. Mild **(A)** and severe **(B)** lymphedema in siblings. (From Aagenaes, 1974.)

growth failure may occur during childhood, presumably due to malabsorption. Adult height is usually normal.

HISTOPATHOLOGY

LIGHT. No information.
EM. No information.

BASIC DEFECT

Unknown. Lymphangiograms show hypoplastic lymphatics.

TREATMENT

Cholestyramine relieves the itching associated with the increase in bile salts.

MODE OF INHERITANCE

Autosomal recessive.

PRENATAL DIAGNOSIS

None.

DIFFERENTIAL DIAGNOSIS

There are many hereditary causes of cholestasis and jaundice, including Alagille syndrome (arteriohepatic dysplasia, MIM:118450) and α_1-antitrypsin deficiency (MIM:107400), but none of these is associated with edema. Milroy syndrome (MIM:153100) (congenital lymphedema) does not have associated liver disease, nor does Meige syndrome (MIM:153200), with later onset of edema. Both conditions are autosomal dominant. Infants with Noonan syndrome and Turner syndrome can present with neonatal edema. In neither condition is cholestasis a feature.

Support Group: National Lymphedema Network
2211 Post Street, Suite 404
San Francisco, CA 94115
1-415-921-2911

American Liver Foundation
1415 Pompton Avenue
Cedar Grove, NJ 07009
1-201-256-2550

SELECTED BIBLIOGRAPHY

Aagenaes, O., Van der Hagen, C. B., and Refsum, S. (1968). Hereditary recurrent intrahepatic cholestasis from birth. *Arch. Dis. Child.* **43,** 646–657.

A huge, highly inbred Norwegian pedigree, including seven sibships with 16 affected individuals. One instance of possible pseudodominance—an affected mother had an affected child. The father was from the same geographic region but was not known to be related.

Aagenaes, O. (1974). Hereditary recurrent cholestasis with lymphoedema—two new families. *Acta Paediatr. Scand.* **63,** 465–471.

Reports new patient; one was the offspring of first cousins once removed. The patient presented with edema and hypoproteinemia. In the second family, three of seven siblings were affected. They had edema and normal protein. One patient reported previously died of hepatic fibrosis, thus causing the author to temper previous statements regarding a good prognosis in the disorder.

Sharp, H. L., and Krivit, W. (1971). Hereditary lymphedema and obstructive jaundice. *J. Pediatr.* **78,** 491–496.

Report of two sisters. Father, paternal uncle, and paternal grandmother had small lymphangiomas on the feet, and the paternal uncle had resolved capillary hemangiomas. The family is from the same region as, but was not thought to be related to, the Aagenaes kindred. The sisters were subjects of a later report in *J. Pediatr.* **121,** 141–143, 1992. One was treated with spironolactone for edema and failed to progress to menarche. The second sister had normal menarche but became amenorrheic when spironolactone was started. Both appeared to be doing well.

DISTICHIASIS AND LYMPHEDEMA (MIM:153400)

DERMATOLOGIC FEATURES

MAJOR. Edema of the extremities can be present at birth, but usually develops later in life, in the second or third decade. The edema may or may not pit.

Distichiasis, a double row of eyelashes on the upper and lower lids, with the eyelashes growing in toward the corneal surface, is the typical ocular feature. The ectopic eyelashes may be very fine and few in number, and they can be easily overlooked if not suspected.

The features of nuchal webbing, downslanting palpebral fissures, and ptosis are common and suggest that there is prenatal facial edema and cystic hygromas that resolve prior to birth.

MINOR. None.

ASSOCIATED ABNORMALITIES

There can be secondary changes of corneal abrasion, excessive tearing, photophobia, conjunctivitis, and chronic granulation tissue of the eyelids, all due to the mechanical irritation by the extra eyelashes. The lower lids may be pulled down and away from the globe with partial ectropion.

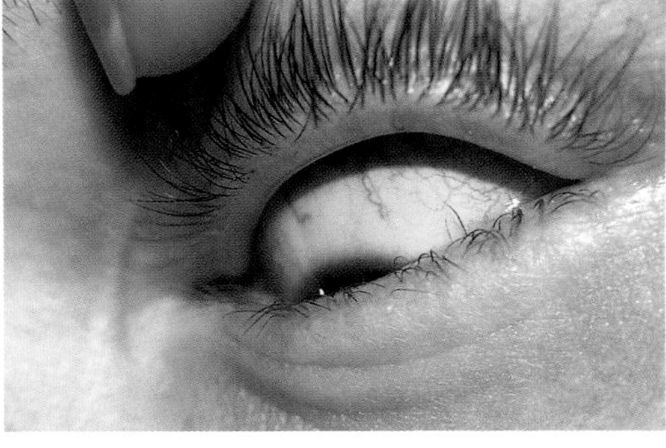

Figure 7.2. Duplication of eyelashes. There are small, fine ectopic lashes on the inner surface of the upper lid.

Vertebral abnormalities and extradural cysts were reported in two families with distichiasis and lymphedema. It is not clear to me that evaluation of the spine in neurologically asymptomatic patients with distichiasis and lymphedema is warranted.

One father–son pair with distichiasis and lymphedema had bifid uvulas. The son also had a submucous cleft of the palate.

HISTOPATHOLOGY

LIGHT. No information.
EM. No information.

BASIC DEFECT

Unknown.

TREATMENT

Epilation or ablation of the aberrant eyelashes may be necessary. Compression stockings, intermittent nighttime use of a compression pump, meticulous hygiene, and prompt use of antibiotics for infection are helpful in the management of the lymphedema. A sudden increase in edema, pain, tenderness, and color change should prompt evaluation for infection. The possibility of malignant change must always be entertained, although this is quite rare.

MODE OF INHERITANCE

Autosomal dominant with high, if not complete, penetrance and variable severity.

PRENATAL DIAGNOSIS

None.

DIFFERENTIAL DIAGNOSIS

The congenital edema of Turner syndrome (gonadal dysgenesis with sex chromosome abnormalities) and Noonan syndrome (MIM:163950) gradually resolves. Both of these conditions can be distinguished either by karyotype or by associated malformations. Patients with Turner syndrome and Noonan syndrome do not have double eyelashes, but the facies of Noonan syndrome and those of distichiasis and lymphedema are otherwise very similar.

The Klippel-Feil anomaly (cervical fusion) (MIM:148900) can give a webbed neck appearance with downslanting palpebral fissures similar to that of distichiasis and lymphedema. Eyelashes are normal in Klippel-Feil syndrome. There is no cervical fusion in distichiasis and lymphedema.

Acquired causes of lymphedema are far more common and, in the absence of a family history, should be searched for vigorously before arriving at the diagnosis of inherited lymphedema.

Distichiasis can be a feature of mandibulofacial dysostosis (MIM:154500), which is readily distinguished by the associated orofacial malformations. Distichiasis can also occur in isolation. Distichiasis is usually not a feature of Meige and Milroy syndromes (hereditary lymphedema, MIM:153100, 153200).

Support Group: National Lymphedema Network
2211 Post Street, Suite 404
San Francisco, CA 94115
1-800-541-3259

SELECTED BIBLIOGRAPHY

Falls, H. F., and Kertesz, E. D. (1964). A new syndrome combining pterygium colli with developmental anomalies of the eyelids and lymphatics of the lower extremities. *Trans. Am. Ophthalmol. Soc.* **62,** 248–275.

A detailed description of a large pedigree with many figures showing the range of severity in facial features, nuchal webbing, and edema among affected siblings.

O'Donnell, B. A., and Collin, J. R. O. (1993). Distichiasis: management with cryotherapy to the posterior lamella. *Br. J. Ophthalmol.* **77,** 289–292.

Twenty-four patients treated by epilation, lid margin cryotherapy, or eyelid splitting cryotherapy to the posterior lamella. The authors favored the last of these three methods. Fifty percent of the patients had a positive family history of distichiasis alone; 30% had a positive family history of lymphedema and distichiasis.

HEREDITARY LYMPHEDEMA (MIM:153100, 153200)

(Hereditary Lymphedema Praecox; Milroy Disease; Nonne-Milroy-Meige Syndrome)

DERMATOLOGIC FEATURES

MAJOR. Congenital, painless, bilateral edema usually involving only the legs is the presenting feature of the form of hereditary lymphedema demarcated by the eponym *Milroy*. Occasionally lymphedema can develop in the arms. The eponym *Meige* has been applied to those individuals in whom the edema develops at or around puberty.

The edema can be pitting or nonpitting, and epidermal changes secondary to longstanding lymphedema can develop. The scrotum can be involved. The degree of edema is variable within families.

MINOR. Malignant angiosarcoma is a recognized risk in chronic lymphedema and has been reported in a few patients with congenital lymphedema. The lesions are marked by red-purple nodules. Almost all of the reports of malignant degeneration that I was able to find occurred in individuals with unilateral limb edema (either an arm or a leg) with no mention of family history. Chronic edema can result in thickening, cracking, and eczematous-like changes of the skin, referred to as *elephantiasis*. It does not invariably develop.

Some patients in families with Milroy disease have been noted to have distichiasis.

Yellow nails are a nonspecific finding associated with lymphedema from a variety of causes, including chylous ascites and pleural effusions. They probably do not define a distinctive subtype of inherited lymphedema (MIM:153300), despite inclusion in McKusick's catalog.

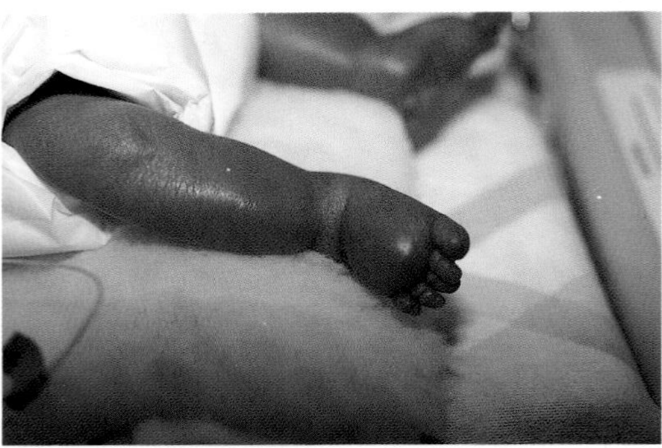

Figure 7.3. Newborn with positive family history, showing edema of legs.

ASSOCIATED ABNORMALITIES

Choanal atresia was reported in one inbred pedigree.

Intestinal lymphangiectasia can occur in association with inherited congenital lymphedema. It appears to be a very rare complication.

One family with Meige (onset in teen years) had bilateral sensorineural hearing loss. One member of this family also had distichiasis.

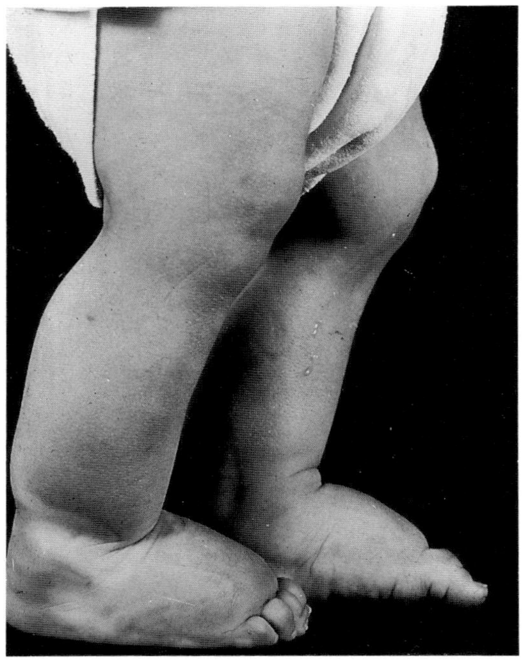

Figure 7.4. Older child, severely involved. (Courtesy of Dr. J. G. Hall, Vancouver, British Columbia.)

HISTOPATHOLOGY

Light. Empty spaces devoid of epithelial lining; homogenization and widening of collagen bundles with extension of strands of collagen into the subcutaneous tissue. Not specific.
EM. No information.

BASIC DEFECT

It is stated that in Milroy syndrome there are abnormal hypoplastic lymphatics and that in later onset lymphedema there are hyperplastic lymphatics. The exact nature of the alterations in lymph channels remains unclear.

TREATMENT

Compression stockings, use of a compression pump, meticulous hygiene, and prompt institution of antibiotics for infection are the mainstays of therapy. While sudden increase in edema, pain, tenderness, and color change should prompt evaluation for infection, the potential for malignant change should always be considered, despite its low likelihood.

MODE OF INHERITANCE

Autosomal dominant; high if not complete penetrance, with variable severity.

PRENATAL DIAGNOSIS

None.

DIFFERENTIAL DIAGNOSIS

The congenital edema of Turner syndrome (gonadal dysgenesis with sex chromosome abnormalities) and the prenatal edema of Noonan syndrome (MIM:163950) resolve, whereas the edema of hereditary lymphedema persists. Both Turner and Noonan syndrome, can be distinguished either by karyotype or by associated malformations.

Acquired causes of lymphedema are far more common and in the absence of a positive family history should be searched for vigorously before arriving at the diagnosis of Meige syndrome. In Klippel-Trenaunay-Weber syndrome (MIM:149000), lymphangiomas and soft tissue hypertrophy/atrophy are usually asymmetric, and there is usually a significant vascular component evident.

Onset of cholestasis in infancy associated with lymphedema developing in childhood is also called Aagenaes syndrome (MIM:214900). Microcephaly with normal intelligence and congenital lymphedema have been reported together in two families, one with male-to-male transmission (MIM:152950).

A mother, three of her four sons, and her daughter had onset of edema in childhood or puberty and presumed cerebral arteriovenous malformations. Two of the boys had pulmonary hypertension (MIM:152900).

The congenital edema reported in association with a neuronal migration defect and cerebellar hypoplasia (MIM:None) resolves over several years. Affected individuals are obviously neurologically compromised from birth. There are numerous central nervous system abnormalities, including pachymicrogyria, hypoplasia of the vermis, and decreased white matter evident on computed tomographic scan.

PEHO syndrome (MIM:260565) is marked by optic atrophy, progressive encephalopathy evident within the first few weeks to months, and hypsarrhythmia, in addition to congenital edema that gradually resolves.

Congenital vein-valve aplasia (MIM:None) is an autosomal dominant disorder in which swelling of the lower extremities occurs with standing and resolves overnight, to recur the next day. The onset of signs is usually at puberty. It is a very rare condition.

An autosomal recessive syndrome of lymphedema, intestinal lymphangiectasia, facial anomalies, and mental retardation was reported in one set of cousins (Hennekens syndrome).

Distichiasis and lymphedema (MIM:153400) is believed to be a distinct genetic disorder. However, there are occasional reports of distichiasis in pedigrees with Milroy or Meige syndrome, and some affected individuals in families with distichiasis and lymphedema have normal eyelashes.

Support Group: National Lymphedema Network
2211 Post Street
Suite 404
San Francisco, CA 94115
1-800-541-3259

SELECTED BIBLIOGRAPHY

Borderon, M. L., and Weiss, M. H. (1991). Choanal atresia and lymphedema. *Ann. Otol. Rhinol. Laryngol.* **100,** 661–664.

A highly inbred Yemenite kindred with congenital choanal atresia and lymphedema of the legs. The pedigree was consistent with autosomal dominant inheritance with reduced penetrance and variable expression, X-linked inheritance, or autosomal recessive inheritance. All affected members are siblings or cousins born to first or second cousins.

Offori, T. W., Platt, C. C., Stephens, M., and Hopkinson, G. B. (1993). Angiosarcoma in congenital hereditary lymphoedema (Milroy's disease)—diagnostic beacons and a review of the literature. *Clin. Exp. Dermatol.* **18,** 174–177.

A grim report of a case and review of the literature. Twelve of 15 patients cited had no family history of edema and onset of lymphedema after infancy. Two of the remaining three patients had edema at birth, but no mention of a positive family history was made in the original report. The prognosis is poor once the tumor has developed.

Pfister, G., Saesseli, B., Hoffmann, U., Geiger, M., and Bollinger, A. (1990). Diameters of lymphatic capillaries in patients with different forms of primary lymphedema. *Lymphology* **23,** 140–144.

A fascinating study that confuses me. By fluorescent lymphography, aplasia of microlymphatics was demonstrated in eight patients with congenital edema, ectasia or enlargement of the lymphatics was demonstrated in four. There is not adequate clinical information to sort out the possible distinguishing clinical features of the two groups, and there was no attempt to study affected family members for specificity of findings. Lymphatics in 12 patients with "sporadic" postpubertal edema were normal in caliber.

Wheeler, E. S., Chan, V., Wassman, R., Rimoin, D. L., and Lesavoy, M. A. (1981). Familial lymphedema praecox: Meige's disease. *Plast. Reconstr. Surg.* **67,** 362–364.

A four generation pedigree with male-to-male transmission. Sensorineural hearing loss in two individuals. There is a clear, short review of the literature.

CHAPTER 8

URTICARIA

All urticarias are marked by the development of wheals—raised, usually itchy, sometimes painful, small papules to large plaques on the skin. Most instances of urticaria are sporadic, but familial occurrence of all types have been reported; usually in only one or two families.

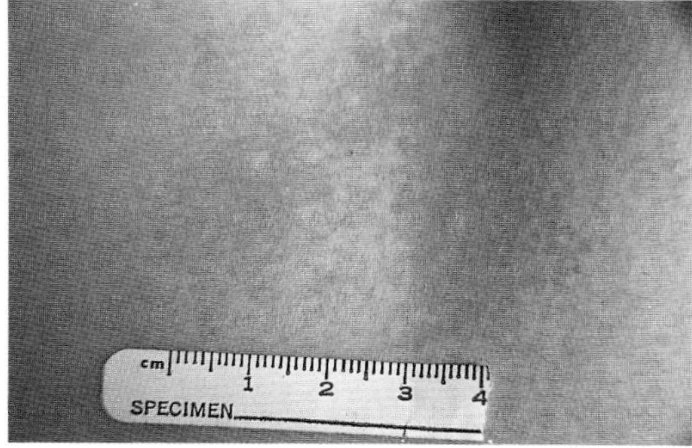

Figure 8.1. Cholinergic urticara with small wheals and large flares. (Courtesy of Division of Dermatology, University of Washington.)

SELECTED BIBLIOGRAPHY

AQUAGENIC URTICARIA (MIM:191850)

Bonnetblanc, J. M., Andrieu-Pfahl, F., Meraud, J. P., and Roux, J. (1979). Familial aquagenic urticaria. *Dermatologica* **158,** 468–470.

Shelley, W. B., and Rawnsley, H. M. (1964). Aquagenic urticaria. Contact sensitivity reaction to water. *JAMA* **189,** 895–898.

In the study of Bonnetblanc et al., (1979) an aunt and niece developed the disorder in childhood. In that of Shelly and Rawnsley (1964) a father and daughter developed hives when the skin came in contact with water, not ice. Inciting contacts included showering, bathing, wet toweling, and perspiration. One family with C_3 deficiency and aquagenic urticaria has been reported.

VIBRATORY ANGIOEDEMA (MIM:193050)

Epstein, P.A., and Kidd, K.K. (1981). Dermodestructive urticaria: an autosomal dominant dermatologic disorder. *Am. J. Med. Genet.* **9,** 307–315.

Hives occurred within 1 to 2 minutes after rubbing or stretching of the skin. These lesions usually resolve within 30 minutes to an hour. Vibratory angioedema may be the same disorder. The authors argue that this phenomenon is not dermographism, as repetitive stimulus, rather than a single stroke, is required to elicit changes.

Patterson, R., Mellies, C. J., Blankenship, M. L., and Pruzansky, J. J. (1972). Vibratory angioedema: a hereditary type of physical hypersensitivity. *J. Allergy Clin. Immunol.* **50,** 174–182.

This is a four generation family with no male-to-male transmission. Urticaria occurred with rubbing, such as toweling dry. The symptoms were present at birth. There was no dermographism.

FAMILIAL DERMOGRAPHISM (MIM:125635)

Jedele, K.B., and Michels, V.V. (1991). Familial dermographism. *Am. J. Med. Genet.* **39,** 201–203.

Four generation family, no male-to-male transmission. Dermographism was the only finding. Suggests that since most people do not complain about dermographism and most doctors do not solicit a family history, familial dermographism may be more common than appreciated.

FAMILIAL LOCALIZED HEAT URTICARIA (MIM:191950)

Michaelsson, G., and Ros, A. M. (1971). Familial localized heat urticaria of delayed type. *Acta Dermatol. Venereol. (Stockh.)* **51,** 279–283.

A similar reaction to heat occurred as in acquired cold urticaria. Direct application of warmth or radiant heat to skin resulted in development of hives approximately 2 hours later. Onset began in late childhood. There was no reaction if the skin was kept wet during sunbathing, but attacks after sauna and use of a hairdryer occurred. The condition seems to require heat, wetness, and moving air, similar to the requirements in familial cold urticaria. Patients complain of burning and itching. Symptoms can last up to 6–10 hours. Biopsy tissue shows edema, vasodilatation, and an inflammatory infiltrate in the upper dermis, with a few degranulated mast cells. There is some symptomatic relief with antihistamines. This pedigree was three generation without any opportunity for male-to-male transmission.

PUPP (MIM:None)

Weiss, R., and Hull, P. (1992). Familial occurrence of pruritic urticarial papules and plaques of pregnancy. *J. Am. Acad. Dermatol.* **26,** 715–717.

Two sisters married to two brothers and a set of identical twin sisters married to a set of identical twin brothers. Each of the females had PUPP in a single pregnancy. PUPP is not generally considered to be genetic.

FAMILIAL COLD URTICARIA (MIM:120180)

(Cold Hypersensitivity)

DERMATOLOGIC FEATURES

Major. Onset of symptoms may be at birth. Lesions are typically raised, red wheals. There may be small purplish macules with a surrounding white halo of vasoconstriction or more generalized erythema. Occasionally, petechiae develop. Lesions may occur anywhere on the skin surface in response to damp cold air and spread to involve covered or protected sites. The hives are often painful rather than pruritic. The development of urticaria may be delayed by several hours after exposure, and the hives themselves may last for hours to several days. The attacks appear to worsen with age.

Minor. Swelling of the lips upon exposure to cold beverages has been described in one patient, but is not a typical finding.

ASSOCIATED ABNORMALITIES

With prolonged exposure to severe cold, the reaction may last upwards of several days, and systemic symptoms of fever, joint pain, and elevated white cell count may occur. Many patients have joint pain, stiffness, and swelling associated with skin changes. Malaise and headache can also occur, similar to the aguey bouts of Muckle-Wells syndrome. In one report, progressive deformity of the fingers occurred; permanent bony changes have not been described in most patients.

HISTOPATHOLOGY

Light. Dilation of vessels, with a perivascular infiltrate composed of neutrophils. More severe lesions show leukocytoclastic vasculitis.

EM. No information.

BASIC DEFECT

Unknown.

TREATMENT

Avoidance of cold wind, prompt warming after exposure. Successful treatment with stanozolol is reported in one family.

MODE OF INHERITANCE

Autosomal dominant. Penetrance may be less than 100%.

PRENATAL DIAGNOSIS

None.

DIFFERENTIAL DIAGNOSIS

In acquired cold contact urticaria, patients make hives in response to cold applied directly to the skin, for example, an ice cube. In familial cold urticaria, the ice cube test response is more often negative; it seems that air movement, as well as decreased air temperature, is required for the generation of hives. Histologic features in acquired cold contact urticaria include edema and a lymphocytic infiltrate in contrast to the polymorphonuclear infiltrate in the dermis associated with familial cold urticaria.

Melkersson-Rosenthal syndrome (MIM: 155900) and hereditary angioedema (MIM: 106100) can cause swelling of the lips. If the history does not differentiate the former from familial cold urticaria, biopsy will. C_1 esterase levels are normal in familial cold urticaria.

The aguey bouts of Muckle-Wells syndrome (MIM:191900) can be mimicked in familial cold urticaria, but cold is not a precipitant in the Muckle-Wells syndrome. One family has been described with a delayed onset reaction to cold of 9 to 18 hours. They were thought to represent a separate disease, but delayed onset of urticaria can occur in familial cold urticaria as well.

Support Group: N.O.R.D.
P.O. Box 8923
New Fairfield, CT
06812
1-800-999-6673

SELECTED BIBLIOGRAPHY

Kile, R.L., and Rusk, H.A. (1940). A case of cold urticaria with an unusual family history. *J.A.M.A.* **114,** 1067–1068.

Four generations with male-to-male transmission. No instances of transmission through unaffected individuals.

Ormerod, A.D., Smart, L., Reid, T.M.S., and Milford-Ward, A. (1993). Familial cold urticaria. Investigation of a family and response to stanozolol. *Arch. Dermatol.* **129,** 343–346.

A five generation pedigree. Five members treated with stanozolol, with good response in four. One unaffected individual transmitted the disease. There are color photographs.

Zip, C.M., Ross, J.B., Greaves, M.W., Scriver, C.R., Mitchell, J.J., and Zoar, S. (1993). Familial cold urticaria. *Clin. Exp. Dermatol.* **18,** 338–341.

Extensive pedigree with many instances of male-to-male transmission. Authors provide a table listing the distinguishing characteristics of familial cold urticaria and acquired cold urticaria, the latter occurring later in life, with shorter duration of symptoms, persistence of itching, and immediate response to physical contact with cold.

HEREDITARY ANGIONEUROTIC EDEMA (MIM:106100)

(C1 Esterase Inhibitor Deficiency; Hereditary Angioedema)

DERMATOLOGIC FEATURES

MAJOR. Recurrent swelling of subcutaneous tissue and mucosa is the hallmark of this condition. Although the onset of attacks may begin in infancy, over 50% of patients first develop problems during the toddler years. The diagnosis of angioneurotic edema is not made until after the age of 30 years in almost 50% of affected individuals, despite the fact that fewer than 1% of patients have their first attack after age 30 years.

Although swelling of the skin, usually of the face (85%) or extremity (96%), can occur, patients do not have true hives or urticaria. The swelling may progress over 1–2 days, but each given area of involvement usually resolves within 72 hours. There is no pitting initially, although as resolution of the edema starts pitting can be induced. There is no itching, usually no overlying erythema, and usually no pain, although a feeling of tightness may occur, both with the edema and as a prodrome to it.

Approximately 25% of patients will experience an annular, serpiginous, or reticulate erythema, preceding attacks by 1–4 days. This rash has variously been described as mottled, erythema multiforme-like, and erythema marginatum.

Attacks can be triggered by emotion, infection, trauma, dental surgery, menstruation, and birth control pills. Symptoms often improve after the menopause and during pregnancy. There is marked variability in severity.

Classically angioneurotic edema is divided into type I and type II. Type I is characterized by decreased levels of C1 esterase inhibitor, decreased function of the inhibitor, and decreased antigen. Individuals with type II have normal levels of C1 esterase inhibitor, with decreased function. From 80% to 85% have type I; 15% have type II.

Minor. Facial lipodystrophy was reported in one patient. It may be a secondary consequence of repeated and longstanding edema, not a primary feature of C1 esterase inhibitor deficiency. Facial lipodystrophy has also been described in four patients with C3 deficiency, glomerular nephritis, and persistent edema.

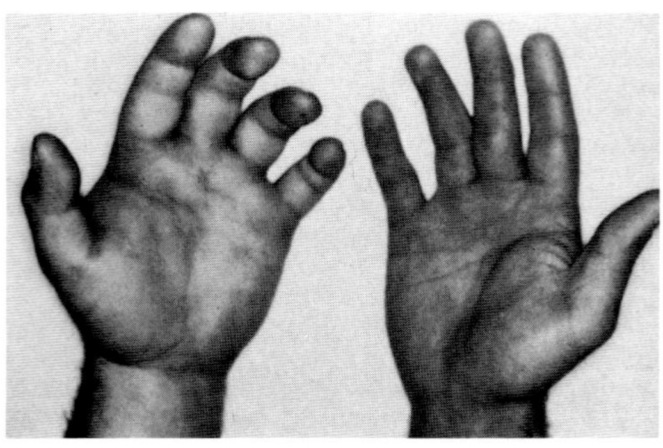

Figure 8.2. Edema of left hand. Right is unaffected. (From Frank et al., 1976.)

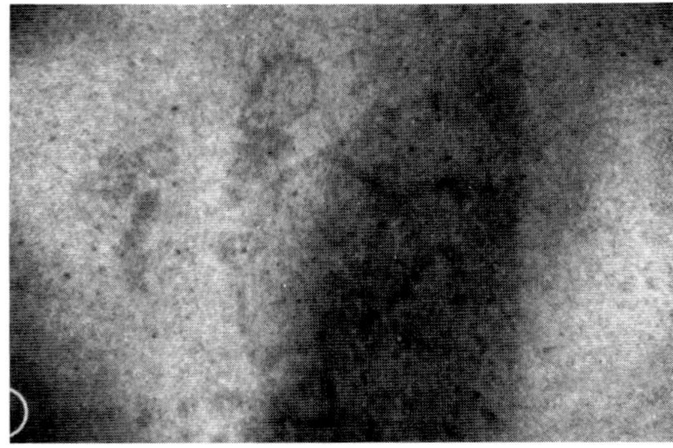

Figure 8.3. Serpiginous expanding lesion of erythema marginatum in patient with hereditary angioneurotic edema. (From Starr and Brasher, 1974.)

ASSOCIATED ABNORMALITIES

Gastrointestinal symptoms occur in 75%–90% of affected individuals. Pain, nausea and vomiting, sensations of distention, and watery diarrhea are typical. Approximately 20% of patients have gastrointestinal symptoms only and do not experience facial swelling or laryngeal involvement.

Oropharyngeal involvement leads to death in over 50% of patients if left untreated. Even with treatment, mortality from airway compromise still occurs because of inadequate or tardy intervention. From 65% to 75% of affected individuals will have laryngeal involvement.

Edema of the bladder, kidneys, lungs, and brain has been reported rarely. Edema of the genitalia has occurred with intercourse. Polycystic or multifollicular ovaries have been described in some affected females.

Collagen vascular diseases, including discoid lupus erythematosus, systemic lupus erythematosus, or systemic erythematosus–like conditions have developed in a few patients with hereditary angioneurotic edema. Involvement of the kidneys with glomerulonephritis has occurred, both within this context and as an isolated complication of hereditary angioneurotic edema. Two of six patients described in the literature developed end-stage renal failure.

HISTOPATHOLOGY

LIGHT. No pathologic changes.
EM. No information.

BASIC DEFECT

Defects in C1 esterase inhibitor are responsible for this condition. Failure to make normal C1 esterase inhibitor results in inability to inhibit the C1r and C1s subunits of C1, kallikrein, plasmin, and factors XI and XII.

TREATMENT

C1 esterase inhibitor concentrate can be administered. From 500 to 1,000 IU IV is recommended for acute attacks; 500 units IU every 2–5 days for prophylaxis.

ϵ-Aminocaproic acid 8 g q4h for acute attacks and 7–12 g/day for prophylaxis is useful. This is the drug of choice for children because of the adrenergic effects of anabolic steroids such as danazol (200 mg q8h for acute attacks, 50–600 mg/day for prophylaxis) or stanozolol 0.5 to 6 mg per day. Both of these anabolic steroids increase C4 and C1 esterase inhibitor synthesis. Occasionally, lower doses on an every other day or every other week basis can provide prophylaxis. In general, therapy is limited to acute attacks and short-term prophylaxis, for example, use prior to exposure to known inciters. Longterm prophylaxis is limited to individuals with severe cases who have recurrent laryngeal involvement.

MODE OF INHERITANCE

Autosomal dominant, allelic heterogeneity between and within subtypes. There appears to be reduced penetrance, and asymptomatic gene carriers have been reported. The gene is mapped to 11q13.

PRENATAL DIAGNOSIS

Possible by mutation analysis.

DIFFERENTIAL DIAGNOSIS

The causes of acute colicky intermittent abdominal pain are legion, and it may be difficult to make the diagnosis of hereditary angioneurotic edema in the absence of facial swelling. The ability to diagnose hereditary angioneurotic edema requires the suspicion of the diagnosis. Complement studies will show a low C4.

Acquired C1 esterase inhibitor deficiency can be distinguished by low C1q levels and is associated with malignancy, most notably B-cell lymphoma, or C1 esterase inhibitor autoantibodies.

Other disorders of the complement pathway may present with angioedema. Patients with these conditions usually have joint pain, true urticaria, and circulating immune complexes.

Support Group: N.O.R.D.
P.O. Box 8923
New Fairfield, CT
06812
1-800-999-6673

SELECTED BIBLIOGRAPHY

Davis, A.E. III, Bissler, J.J., and Cicardi, M. (1993). Mutations in the C1 inhibitor gene that result in hereditary angioneurotic edema. *Behring Inst. Mitt.* **93,** 313–320.

Eighty-five percent of patients with hereditary angioneurotic edema have type I. Of these, 15% are due to duplications or deletions in one or more exons. The article reviews mutations recognized to date, with tables and 45 references. There are many single base substitutions and a possible hot spot for mutations in type II.

Donaldson, V.H., and Evans, R.R. (1963). A biochemical abnormality in hereditary angioneurotic edema. *Am. J. Med.* **35,** 37–44.

These authors demonstrated absence of C1 esterase inhibitor in the skin of affected individuals in three families, both during attacks and while well. They correctly argued that the disease is the result of a primary deficiency and not due to abnormal consumption or destruction of the molecules.

Frank, N.M., Gelfand, J.A., and Atkinson, J.P. (1976). Hereditary angioedema: the clinical syndrome and its management. *Ann. Intern. Med.* **84,** 580–593.

This is an NIH conference report recounting 6 years' experience with 30 patients and 47 affected relatives at the NIH. Patients were symptomatic an average of 21 years prior to diagnosis. Fourteen patients died of complications of the disease. Seven of 30 had a negative family history, but biochemical testing for C1 esterase inhibitor detected abnormalities in parents and siblings of six of these seven. This reference is out of date in regard to mutations and treatment, but it is a very nice clinical review.

Osler, W. (1888). Hereditary angio-neurotic oedema. *Am. J. Med. Sci.* **95,** 362–367.

A beautiful description by the house physician, Dr. Burn, of the proband. Patient had irregular menses, perhaps suggestive of polycystic ovarian disease. There is a detailed family history with at least one obligate carrier expressing no signs. In this case report, the term *urticaria* is used, but it is not clear whether it is being used to describe true hives.

Pan, C. G., Strife, C. F., Ward, M. F., Spitzer, R. E., and McAdams, J. (1992). Longterm follow-up of non-systemic lupus erythematosus glomerulonephritis in patients with hereditary angioedema: report of four cases. *Am. J. Kidney Dis.* **19,** 526–531.

Reviews long-term follow-up of three previously reported cases and one new patient. Contrasts mild outcome in these patients with renal failure reported in two others, remarking on the variability of renal involvement.

Perricone, R., Pasetto, N., DeCarolis, C., Vaquero, E., Noccioli, G., Panerai, A. E., and Fontana, L. (1992). Cystic ovaries in women affected with hereditary angioedema. *Clin. Exp. Immunol.* **90,** 401–404.

The authors found 38% of 13 women to have polycystic ovarian disease, 54% to have multifocal cysts in the ovary. This was compared with 15% and 10%, respectively, of controls. (However, they also quote studies of normal women in which 23% have polycystic ovarian disease.) After 6 months of danazol in six patients, repeat ultrasound evaluation showed normal ovaries.

Robinson, L.C., and Hart, L.L. (1992). Danazol in hereditary angioedema. *Ann. Pharmacother.* **26,** 1251–1252.

Reviews published data on treatment with danazol.

Williamson, D.M. (1979). Reticulate erythema—a prodrome in hereditary angiooedema. *Br. J. Dermatol.* **101,** 549–552.

A patient and mother with hereditary angioneurotic edema had annular erythema. In one, the skin changes preceded the attack. In the other, they appeared to correlate poorly with the onset of attacks.

MELKERSSON-ROSENTHAL SYNDROME (MIM:155900)

DERMATOLOGIC FEATURES

MAJOR. Recurrent painless swelling of the lips, deep folds and grooves in the tongue (lingua plicata), and relapsing peripheral facial palsy form the complete triad of this disorder. The majority of affected individuals do not exhibit all three features. The gums, mucosa, pharynx, and larynx may be involved, in addition to the lips. The swelling is recurrent at first, but most affected individuals end up with permanent distortion of the lips. The usual age of onset is in the third or fourth decade, but the range is from early childhood to old age. All the symptoms can be recurrent or become fixed and may be asymmetric, unilateral, or bilateral.

MINOR. Burning, stinging, and anesthesia are described by a few affected persons. Chapping and redness of the lips occur in a minority.

ASSOCIATED ABNORMALITIES

Migraine-like or cluster headaches are described in about 40% of patients. There are occasional disturbances of taste.

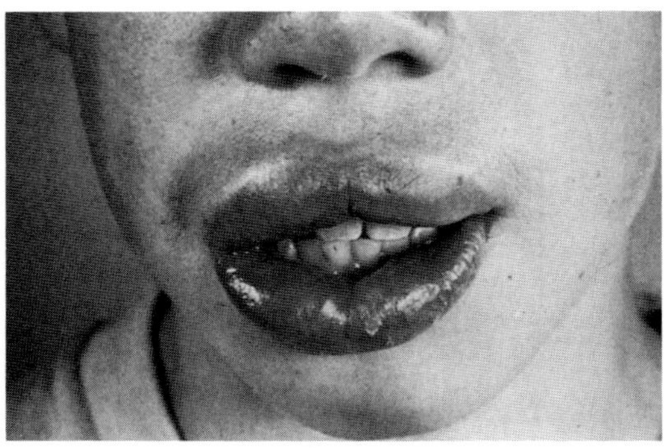

Figure 8.4. Swelling of both lips, with scaling and fissures. (From Zimmer et al., 1992.)

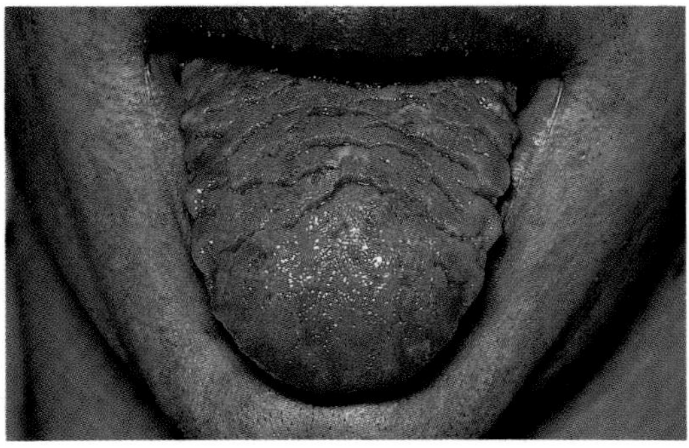

Figure 8.5. Lingua plicata.

HISTOPATHOLOGY

LIGHT. Perivascular tuberculoid granulomas (Meischer's cheilitis granulomatosa) are scattered throughout the involved tissues. Many specimens show only nonspecific inflammation. **EM.** No information.

BASIC DEFECT

Unknown.

TREATMENT

Antihistamines and antibiotics appear to be of little benefit. Intralesional and systemic corticosteroids may be helpful in reducing lip swelling and may improve outcome when used in conjunction with surgical resection. Decompression of the facial nerve has been used to treat longstanding facial palsy.

MODE OF INHERITANCE

Unknown. McMusick lists this condition as an asterisked autosomal dominant, but the evidence is not convincing. Scrotal tongue, which appears to be inherited as an isolated autosomal dominant trait, was the only shared finding in three of seven families.

PRENATAL DIAGNOSIS

None.

DIFFERENTIAL DIAGNOSIS

Lip swelling in angioneurotic edema (MIM: 106100) is usually not red, and extraoral swelling is typical. Normal C1 esterase levels will differentiate Melkersson-Rosenthal syndrome from angioneurotic edema. In Crohn disease (MIM:266600), labial swelling and cobblestoning of the oral mucosa can be seen. Bowel symptoms are not a feature of Melkersson-Rosenthal. History will quickly distinguish trauma, insect bite, and drug-induced gingival hypertrophy from Melkersson-Rosenthal syndrome. Gingival fibromata (MIM:135300) are not associated with swelling of the lips, and again biopsy will differentiate. Individuals with MEN2B (MIM:162300) develop thickening of the lips and tongue because of neuromas. Biopsy will differentiate, as well as the presence of other associated clinical features. Isolated geographic tongue can be sporadic or familial. It is not marked by lip swelling.

Support Group: N.O.R.D.
P.O. Box 8923
New Fairfield, CT
06812
1-800-999-6673

SELECTED BIBLIOGRAPHY

Lygidakis, C., Tsakanikas, C., Ilias, A., and Vassilopoulos, D. (1979). Melkersson-Rosenthal's syndrome in four generations. *Clin. Genet.* **15,** 189–192.

This is the only report in which male-to-male transmission has been claimed to occur. This was a four generation family with seven affected members, one instance of nonpenetrance, and physical examination was limited to evaluation of a mother and a daughter. The supporting evidence for male-to-male transmission is the statement that "from the records and our personal communication with the general practitioner, there was no doubt that all the affected persons had Melkersson-Rosenthal syndrome."

Meisel-Stosiek, M., Hornstein, O. P., and Stosiek, N. (1990). Family study on Melkersson-Rosenthal syndrome. Some hereditary aspects of the disease and review of the literature. *Acta Dermatol. Venereol. (Stockh.)* **70,** 221–226.

The family histories for 42 of 73 unrelated probands were evaluated. No consanguinity was found, and no familial cases of full-blown Melkersson-Rosenthal were seen in 88 first degree and 37 second degree relatives. However, there were 10 families in whom individuals other than the proband had one of the major features of Melkersson-Rosenthal syndrome, or several minor features. For example, lingua plicata occurred in 62% of probands, 36% of first degree relatives, and 5% of second degree relatives. It also occurred in 11% of spouses.

Zimmer, W. M., Rogers, R. S. III, Reeve, C. M., and Sheridan, P. J. (1992). Orofacial manifestations of Melkersson-Rosenthal syndrome. A study of 42 patients and review of 220 cases from the literature. *Oral Surg. Oral Med. Oral Pathol.* **74,** 610–619.

The title says it all.

MUCKLE-WELLS SYNDROME (MIM:191900)

(Urticaria, Deafness, and Amyloid Neuropathy)

DERMATOLOGIC FEATURES

Major. Urticaria, marked by slightly inflamed small to large, sore, painful papules, develops on the trunk and extremities. The lesions are generally not itchy but may be "achey." Onset of symptoms is usually in adolescence. The skin changes may last up to 36 hours, appear to be worsened by heat and exertion, and tempered by cold.

Minor. Dry mouth was reported in one patient to accompany bouts of urticaria. Conjunctivae may be involved and swell.

ASSOCIATED ABNORMALITIES

The deafness is marked by gradual progression of loss of medium- to high-tone frequencies. Onset is usually in the twenties and thirties, but may present earlier in childhood. There appears to be an absence of the organ of Corti and vestibular sensory epithelium, along with atrophy of the cochlear nerve. Amyloid nephropathy with progressive renal failure occurs. Arthralgias, characterized by recurrent bouts of aching joints, chills, and malaise, referred to as "aguey bouts," accompanied by the urticarial rash may begin in infancy or be delayed in onset until adolescence.

Laboratory abnormalities include elevated erythrocyte sedimentation rate, elevated white cell count, hyperglycinemia, and hypergammaglobulinemia.

HISTOPATHOLOGY

Light. No information.
EM. No information.

BASIC DEFECT

Unknown.

TREATMENT

None effective.

MODE OF INHERITANCE

Autosomal dominant with variable expression.

PRENATAL DIAGNOSIS

None.

DIFFERENTIAL DIAGNOSIS

The urticaria of Muckle-Wells syndrome is more painful and less pruritic than acquired urticaria. Individuals with familial cold urticaria (MIM:120180) may have similar aguey bouts with malaise and headache. Cold is not a precipitant in Muckle-Wells syndrome.

Individuals with familial Mediterranean fever (MIM:249100) have similar aguey bouts and also develop amyloid nephropathy. They do not have hearing loss or urticaria.

Familial Mediterranean fever is autosomal recessive.

Support Group: N.O.R.D.
P.O. Box 8923
New Fairfield, CT 06812
1-800-999-6673

SELECTED BIBLIOGRAPHY

Black, J.T. (1969). Amyloidosis, deafness, urticaria, and limb pains: a hereditary syndrome. *Ann. Intern. Med.* **70,** 989–994.

A second family of different ethnic background from that reported by Muckle and Wells (1962).

Muckle, T.J. (1979). The "Muckle-Wells" syndrome. *Br. J. Dermatol.* **100,** 87–92.

Reviews this syndrome. Table of case reports. Uses the term *incomplete penetrance* to describe variable expression. Argues that renal involvement is secondary to inflammation associated with recurrent aguey bouts.

Muckle, T.J., and Wells, M. (1962). Urticaria, deafness, and amyloidosis. A new heredofamilial syndrome. *O. J. Med.* **31,** 235–245.

A four generation family with variable expression. Male-to-male transmission. Loss of libido in young adulthood seemed to be a constant finding. Their pedigrees showed "anticipation," with worsening symptoms and earlier onset in subsequent generations.

URTICARIA PIGMENTOSA (MIM:154800)

(Mastocytosis)

DERMATOLOGIC FEATURES

Major. Mastocytomas, the lesions of urticaria pigmentosa, are usually light brown with an "aura" of pink or yellow. They are flat lesions that may have a small papular component. Ranging in diameter from a few millimeters to centimeters, these patches are marked by irregular and poorly demarcated margins. One may not be able to tell exactly where the lesion stops and the normal skin starts. There may be subtle wrinkling of the skin or increased epidermal markings. When rubbed, the areas urticate (Darier's sign); they turn red and swell and develop into a hive. Lesions that have been rubbed within the last 24–48 hours will not urticate, as the mast cells have not had enough time to regranulate. Vesicles or bullae can occur in the wheal.

Itching can be intense.

Mastocytomas may be isolated (the most common presentation and one that is not genetic) or multiple. Most isolated lesions will develop within the first year of life. They may occur anywhere on the body and tend to spare the face. Multiple lesions usually appear at the same time or within a few days of each other. Thus, an infant who presents initially with an isolated lesion is unlikely to develop multiple sites of involvement later. However, in infants and young children who present initially with multiple lesions, new lesions may continue to appear over several years.

Minor. Affected individuals may have generalized dermographism. This is a more common finding in those who have multiple skin lesions.

ASSOCIATED ABNORMALITIES

Release of histamine by irritation of skin lesions can cause systemic symptoms, including flushing, sweating, hypotension, syncope, diarrhea, and headache.

Although mast cell lesions can occur in bone and liver, this does not occur in familial urticaria pigmentosa.

There have been two case reports of children with Nager syndrome (acrofacial dysostosis, MIM:154400) or a Nager-like syndrome, who have had urticaria pigmentosa.

HISTOPATHOLOGY

Light. Mast cell infiltrates are seen in the dermis. These may extend up to the dermoepidermal junction, or there may be a clear or Grenz zone between the epidermis and the dermal infiltrate. Bullae, when present, may be subepidermal.

EM. Giant granules, with absent or poorly formed lamellae, are seen in the mast cells.

BASIC DEFECT

Unknown.

TREATMENT

None is needed for asymptomatic patients. Lesions gradually lose their tendency to urticate and ultimately, usually by puberty, fade away and become asymptomatic, barely visible, light-colored macules or disappear entirely.

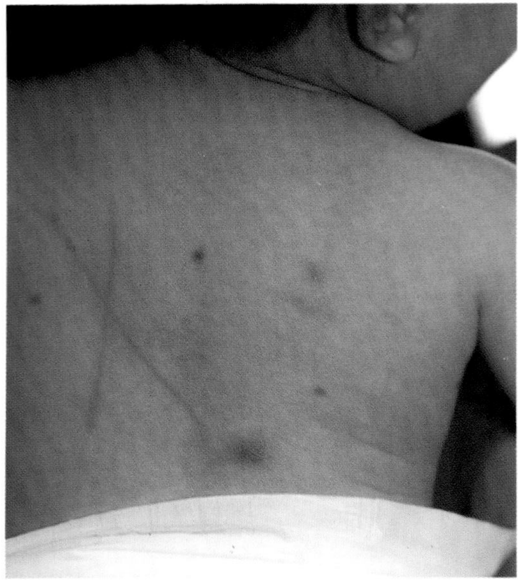

Figure 8.6. Marked dermographism. Brown spots are unrubbed; there is a new hive at 6 o'clock where lesion was rubbed.

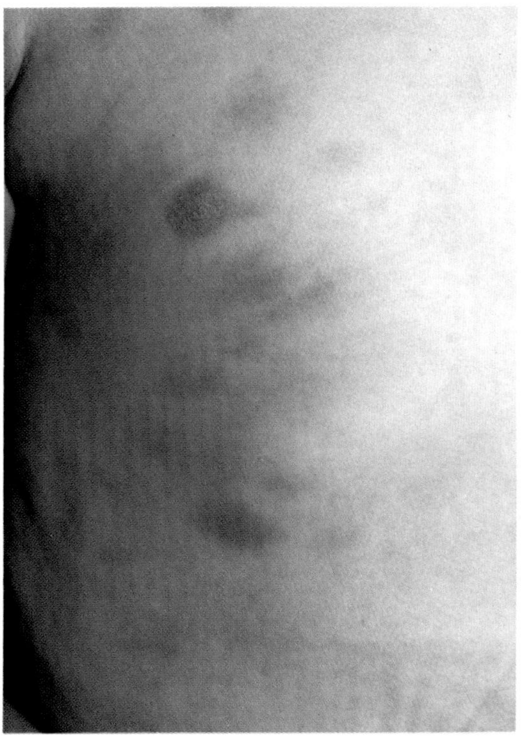

Figure 8.7. Lesions mimicking café-au-lait spots or bruises.

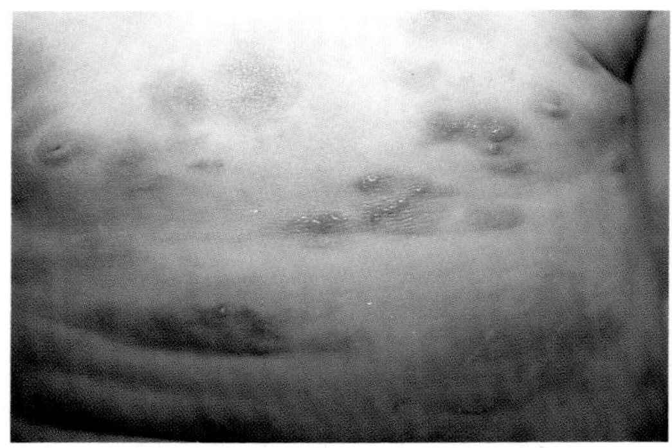

Figure 8.8. Vesicles associated with acute irritation.

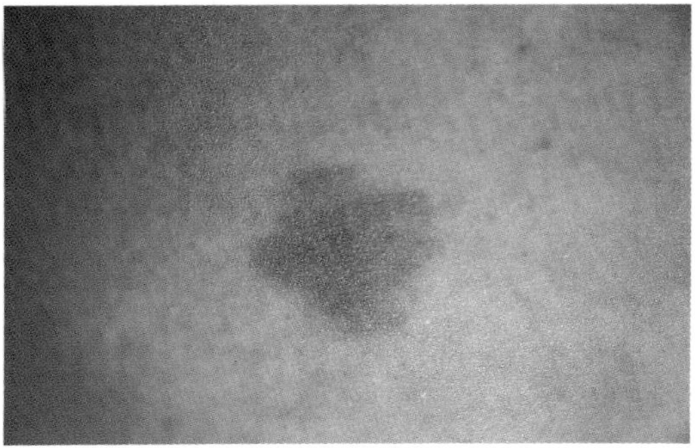

Figure 8.9. Indistinct margins, central faintly palpable element.

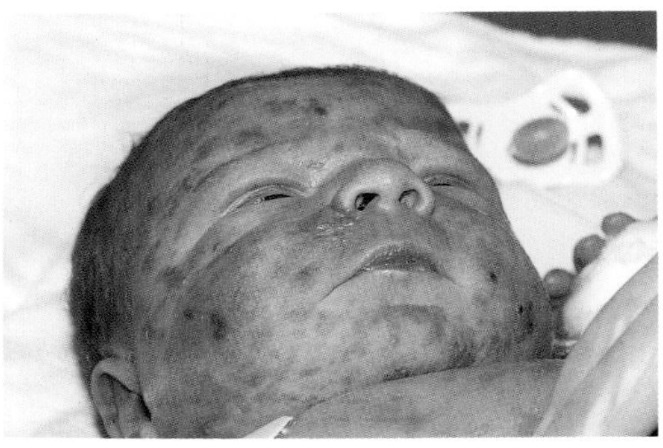

Figure 8.10. Bullous mastocytosis in a newborn.

Avoidance of trauma is wise when possible. Topical steroids may be of some value. Systemic antihistamines and oral Cromolyn may also help to alleviate symptoms. Rarely, excision of symptomatic lesions may be required. There are numerous drugs that are thought to potentiate mast cell release of histamine, and it is generally recommended that their use be avoided in patients with urticaria pigmentosa. The most common of these are aspirin, codeine, and opiates.

MODE OF INHERITANCE

Most cases are sporadic. ?Autosomal dominant. Two of 33 pedigrees reported in the literature showed male-to-male transmission. Eight of 12 sets of identical twins have been concordant for mastocytosis. Pedigrees with bullous mastocytosis, pedigrees with diffuse cutaneous and systemic mastocytosis, and pedigrees with telangiectasia macularis eruptiva perstans in more than one family member have been reported. None of these has occurred with sufficient frequency to make statements about inheritance.

PRENATAL DIAGNOSIS

None.

DIFFERENTIAL DIAGNOSIS

There are other variants of mast cell invasion in the skin, including bullous mastocytosis, diffuse cutaneous mastocytosis, systemic mastocytosis, and telangiectasia macularis eruptiva perstans (TMEP). Bullous mastocytosis is marked by purple nodules and plaques, bullae, and erosions of the skin and generally presents at birth or soon thereafter. In diffuse cutaneous mastocytosis the skin is thickened and may be yellow in color and pebbly in texture. Nodules and tumors may be present. Blistering also occurs. In systemic mastocytosis there is involvement of internal organs with mast cell infiltration. This is almost always an acquired disease of adult life. However, infants with mast cell infiltration of internal organs have been reported, as have newborns with mast cell leukemia. In some, spontaneous resolution has occurred. In TMEP, the skin changes consist of flat vascular lesions that may not urticate.

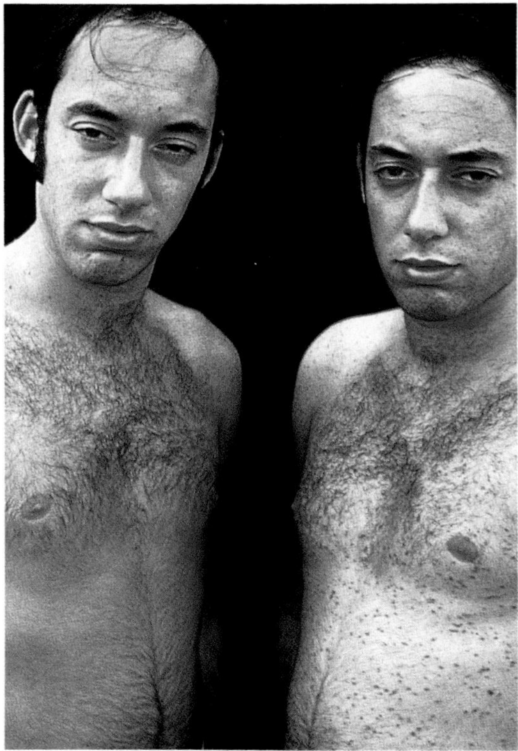

Figure 8.11. Identical twins discordant for mastocytosis. (From Selmanowitz and Orentreich, 1970.)

The diagnosis is most often made by biopsy. The condition is limited to adults. There are very few instances of familial occurrence of these variants.

The patches of urticaria pigmentosa are often mistaken for café-au-lait spots. Café-au-lait spots do not urticate with rubbing, they have sharply defined borders and are easily distinguished from the contiguous normal skin, and they do not have the pink-yellow tinge of the patches of urticaria pigmentosa. The subtle wrinkling and pinpoint papules that can sometimes be seen in mastocytomas are not seen in café-au-lait spots. I see several children each year who have been referred because of concern for neurofibromatosis (MIM:162200) who turn out to have urticaria pigmentosa. When in doubt, the best rule is always to rub the spots. If they are true café-au-lait spots, they will not urticate.

Bullous mastocytosis presents at birth with multiple purple nodules, massive blistering, and denudation, which can be mistaken for epidermolysis bullosa (MIM:Many), congenital leukemia, and staphylococcal scalded skin. With experience, these conditions can be distinguished clinically, but biopsy confirmation is usually warranted.

Support Group: N.O.R.D.
P.O. Box 8923
New Fairfield, CT
06812
1-800-999-6673

SELECTED BIBLIOGRAPHY

Bazex, A., Dupré, A., Christol, B., and Andrieu, H., (1971). Les mastocytoses familiales. Présentation de deux observations. Review générale, intérêt nosologique. *Ann. Dermatol. Syphiligr. (Paris)* **98,** 241–260.

The authors review 30 reports in the literature, one personal communication, and two families of their own. The authors reject the term *urticaria pigmentosa* in favor of *mastocytoses*. They contend that the isolated mastocytoma and widespread cutaneous mastocytosis are the same, based on co-occurrence within families. They believe that inheritance is most likely autosomal dominant, but admit that the data do not support a classic Mendelian mode of transmission.

Clark, D.P., Buescher, L., and Havey, A. (1990). Familial urticaria pigmentosa. *Arch. Intern. Med.* **150,** 1742–1744.

A three generation pedigree with no opportunity for male-to-male transmission. Six females had typical lesions in childhood that disappeared. They then went on to develop TMEP in adult life. Two young children had onset of typical lesions at ages 2 and 3, later than is usual for classic urticaria pigmentosa. This article reviews the literature for familial cases.

Oku, T., Hashizume, H., Yokote, R., Sano, T., and Yamada, M. (1990). The familial occurrence of bullous mastocytosis (diffuse cutaneous mastocytosis). *Arch. Dermatol.* **126,** 1478–1484.

This is an atypical family. The mother developed skin lesions at age 23, after delivery of her first child. This child, at age 5 months, developed widespread cutaneous disease, hyperpigmentation, and thickening of the skin. Two children born to her subsequently were also affected. All the patients improved over time.

Shaw, J.T. (1968). Genetic aspects of urticaria pigmentosa. *Arch. Dermatol.* **97,** 137–138.

Presents 13 pedigrees from the literature and one of his own. States that inheritance is autosomal dominant with decreased penetrance, but the data are not convincing. In four pedigrees, only siblings were affected, four had affected identical twins, three showed mother-to-daughter transmission, two showed female-to-male transmission, one showed male-to-female transmission, but none showed male-to-male transmission.

Touraine, M. A. (1948). Urticaire pigmentaire familiale. *Bull. Soc. Fr. Dermatol. Syphiligr.* **55,** 105–106.

Father, son, and first cousin affected with multiple lesions.

CHAPTER 9

OTHER DISORDERS

ERYTHROMELALGIA (MIM:133020)

(Erythermalgia)

DERMATOLOGIC FEATURES

Much discussion has centered on the correct term for this disorder, with arguments for *erythermalgia* because of the primary importance of heat versus *erythromelalgia* because of the primary importance of swelling. The terms are essentially interchangeable.

MAJOR. Redness, warmth, swelling, and intense pain and burning of the distal extremities with exposure to heat, exercise, and other causes of overheating are typical of this condition. Attacks of heat, redness, and pain may last for minutes to days. In the primary or genetic form of erythromelalgia the onset of symptoms is usually in middle to late childhood in contrast to the later onset of secondary disease.

Initially, the feet and hands are affected. Involvement is always bilateral and may extend proximally. The lower extremities are usually more severely involved than the upper, perhaps due to increased friction and heat with walking and entrapment in footwear.

One author states that toes are spared in primary erythromelalgia; this is not borne out in clinical descriptions or in my own clinical experience.

MINOR. Secondary changes of maceration, ulceration, and tissue damage because of repetitive and prolonged immersion in cold water, application of ice, or self-inflicted trauma in response to pain can occur.

ASSOCIATED ABNORMALITIES

None. The erythromelalgia and nephritis described in one family were both subsequently recognized to be features of Fabry disease, which was segregating in the family.

HISTOPATHOLOGY

LIGHT. No information.
EM. No information.

BASIC DEFECT

Unknown. Defective prostaglandin metabolism has been hypothesized, based on unusual reactions to intradermal injection of PGE and PGE_2 and elevated levels of prostaglandin-like activity in perfusates from the skin of two individuals with nonfamilial primary erythromelalgia. A decrease in peripheral vasoconstrictor tone, coupled with a hypersensitive response to circulating catecholamines, has also been posited.

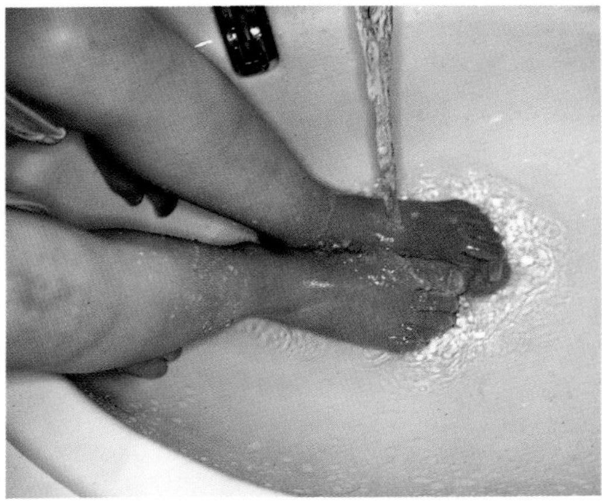

Figure 9.1. Red feet immersed in cold running water for comfort. (Courtesy of Dr. G. Lorette, Tours, France.)

TREATMENT

Cooling of the involved limbs by fanning, immersion in cold water, application of ice packs, and the like is temporarily effective. Success with hypnotherapy has been reported in an 18-year-old female with a 4 week history of symptoms.

Aspirin may relieve symptoms; this is most often successful in secondary erythromelalgia due to thrombocythemia, and is rarely effective in the inherited form of the disorder.

Sympathectomy has resulted in cessation of redness but not in alleviation of pain and is not to be recommended.

MODE OF INHERITANCE

Probable autosomal dominant. One extended pedigree ascertained independently through two probands was the subject of two papers. I have seen an unrelated family with two affected generations. In neither family has male-to-male transmission occurred, but by chance alone there has only been one male at risk who was old enough to be sure of disease status born to an affected male. There is no difference in severity of symptoms between males and females, and affected males have had unaffected daughters, suggesting that X-linked inheritance is unlikely.

One set of two affected siblings with normal parents was reported by Cohen and Samorodin (1982). The majority of "primary" cases with onset in early childhood have had no family history.

PRENATAL DIAGNOSIS

None.

DIFFERENTIAL DIAGNOSIS

Erythromelalgia has been reported as a symptom of Fabry syndrome (MIM:301500). This disorder of α-galactosidase activity should be excluded in any individual presenting with the complaint of erythromelalgia.

Secondary erythromelalgia is associated with myeloproliferative diseases, polycythemia, thrombocytosis, collagen vascular diseases, diabetes, gout, and postviral syndromes. The age of onset in secondary disease is usually later in adult life.

Support Group: N.O.R.D.
P.O. Box 8923
New Fairfield, CT
06812
1-800-999-6673

SELECTED BIBLIOGRAPHY

Cohen, I.J.K., Samorodin, C.S. (1982). Familial erythromelalgia. *Arch. Dermatol.* **118,** 953–954.

An affected brother and sister. Parents were unaffected. No other information given regarding pedigree (e.g. number of siblings, consanguinity).

Drenth, J.P.H., and Michiels, J.J. (1992). Clinical characteristics and pathophysiology of erythromelalgia and erythermalgia. *Am. J. Med.* **93,** 111–112.

Kurzrock, R. and Cohen, P.R. (1992). Reply. *Am. J. Med.,* **93,** 112–114.

The terminologists (Drenth and Michiels, 1992; Kurzrock and Cohen, 1992) duke it out, and in support of their viewpoints give a concise review of clinical features, causes, and linguistic history.

Finley, W.H., Lindsey, J.R., Jr., Fine, J.-D., Dixon, G.A., and Burbank, M.K. (1992). Autosomal dominant erythromelalgia. *Am. J. Med. Genet.* **42,** 310–315.

Nice review of the literature with report of a large kindred originally reported by the senior author in 1966. Despite awareness that Cross' family had Fabry syndrome, not erythromelalgia, the authors still cite this reference as showing reduced penetrance for erythromelalgia.

Kirby, R.L. (1987). Erythromelalgia—not so benign. *Arch. Phys. Med. Rehabil.* **68,** 389.

Thompson, G.H., Hahn, G., and Rang, M.

(1979). Erythromelalgia. *Clin. Orthop.* **144,** 249–254.

A distressing account of a 14-year-old girl, with an affected mother and two affected brothers, who came to bilateral lower leg amputations because of severe infection secondary to self-inflicted tissue damage because of pain. Pain control was finally achieved by intermittent use of a cooling suit. Her brother had bilateral amputations at age 20 for infected ulcerations. He was the subject of the subsequent report by Kirby (1987).

Michiels, J.J., and van Joost, Th. (1988). Primary and secondary erythermalgia, a critical review. *Neth. J. Med.* **33,** 205–208.

Proposes restricting the term *erythromelalgia* to that disease associated with myeloproliferative disorders and using the terms *primary* and *secondary erythermalgia* for the others. Nicely written; clear definition of the symptom complex.

MICHELIN TIRE BABY, (MIM:156610)

DERMATOLOGIC FEATURES

MAJOR. There is no distinct Michelin tire syndrome. Rather than being an entity with a single cause, the phenotype is common to several underlying abnormalities. Folds of thickened skin traversed by circumferential deep grooves can result from underlying smooth muscle hamartomas or an increase in fat, or they can be found in infants with apparently histologically normal skin. The clinical appearance has been compared with the advertising icon of the Michelin Tire Company, a figure composed of multiple overlying inner tubes. On this side of the Atlantic, the Pillsbury doughboy may be a closer reference.

In familial reports, the skin changes seem to disappear over time.

MINOR. One patient was described with stellate scars on the skin.

Hirsutism, either congenital or acquired, has been noted in several case reports.

ASSOCIATED ABNORMALITIES

In one family, an affected son had a median cleft palate and neuroblastoma. His affected father had neither. In a second family, an affected father and an affected child did not share the median cleft palate of a second affected child. Isolated patients have had hemihypertrophy, mental retardation, seizures, clefting, and a variety of facial anomalies.

HISTOPATHOLOGY

LIGHT. The thickening may be due to hamartomas of the skin. Both smooth muscle hamartomas and nevus lipomatosis have been described. In a few cases, the biopsies were read as normal.

EM. No information.

BASIC DEFECT

Unknown.

TREATMENT

None. The creases and folds appear to smooth out over time.

→

Figure 9.2. **(A)** Arm of infant with multiple circumferential rings. Father at age 15 months **(B)** and age 3 years **(C)** with similar rings. (From Kunze and Riehm, 1982.)

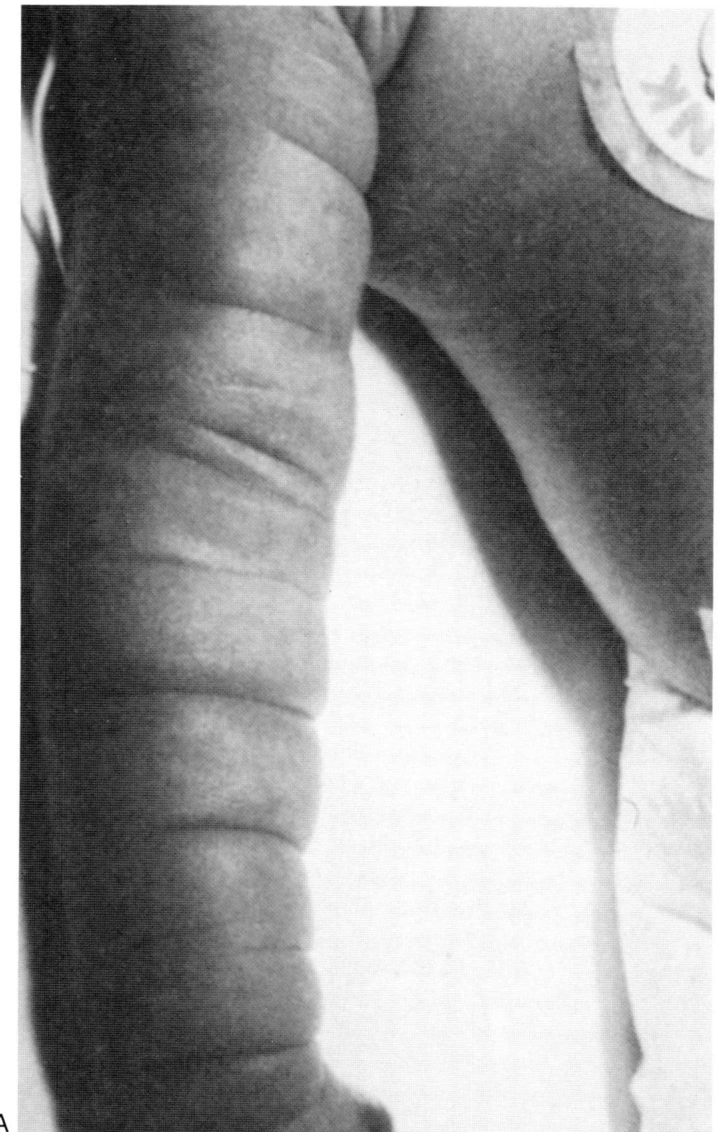

A

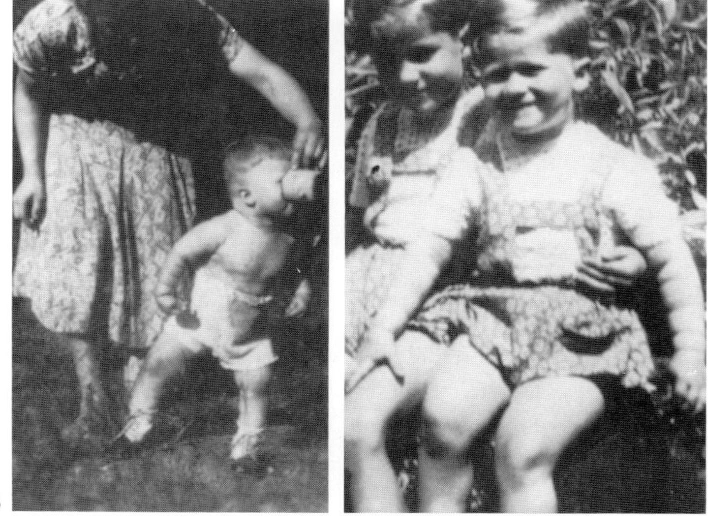

B C

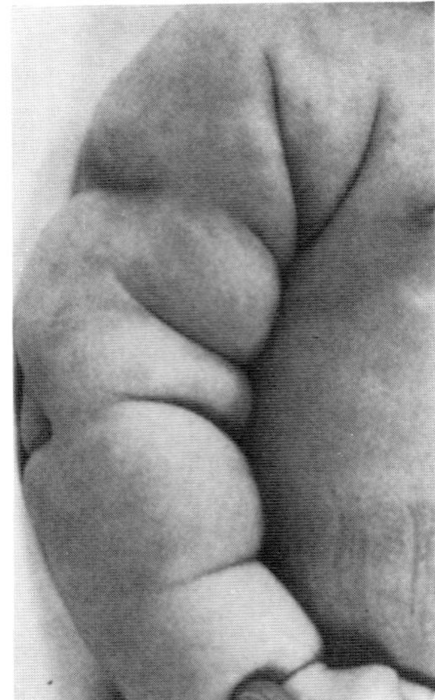
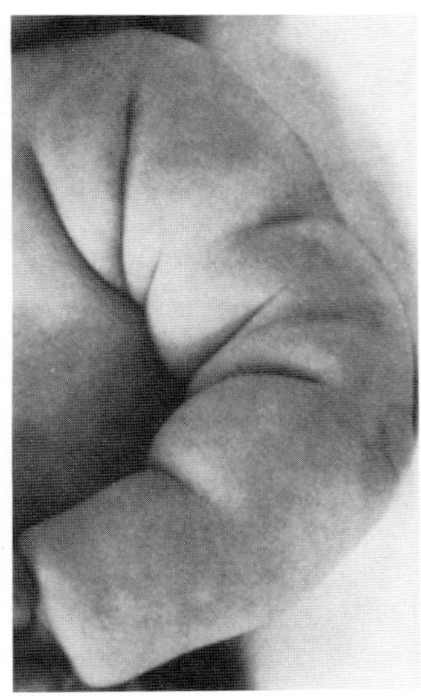

Figure 9.3. Obese infant with multiple creases on both arms. (From Kunze and Riehm, 1982.)

MODE OF INHERITANCE

Autosomal dominant. Male-to-male transmission has been documented. Most cases are sporadic.

PRENATAL DIAGNOSIS

None.

DIFFERENTIAL DIAGNOSIS

Redundant thickened skin was reported in one infant with Laron dwarfism (MIM:262500). In leprechaunism (MIM:246200) there are redundant folds of thin skin due to emaciation. In cutis laxa (MIM:123700, 219100, 304150) the skin is lax and droopy, not full and thickened. Infants with adrenocortical hormone overproduction may have remarkable fullness of the skin, mimicking the changes of Michelin tire syndrome.

Both ainhum (MIM:103400) and amniotic bands (MIM:217100) are distinguished by the presence of constriction bands. The grooves of the Michelin tire baby are not restrictive bands.

Support Group: N.O.R.D.
P.O. Box 8923
New Fairfield, CT
06812
1-800-999-6673

SELECTED BIBLIOGRAPHY

Glover, M.T., Malone, M., and Atherton, D.J. (1989). Michelin-tire baby syndrome resulting from diffuse smooth muscle hamartoma. *Pediatr. Dermatol.* **6,** 329–331.

A clear discussion that proposes and supports the concept that the Michelin tire phenotype results from a variety of causes.

Ross, C.M. (1969). Generalized folded skin with an underlying lipomatous nevus. "The Michelin Tire Baby." *Arch. Dermatol.* **100,** 320–323.

First description. Patient had evidence of abnormal fat on biopsy. Description of the patient is instructive in its bluntness. "She was big, heavy, strong, sturdy, thickset, bad-tempered and ugly."

Schnur, R.E., Herzberg, A.J., Spinner, N.,

Kant, J.A., Magnusson, M., McDonald-McGinn, D., Rehberg, K., Honig, P.J., and Zachai, E.H. (1993). Variability in the Michelin tire syndrome. A child with multiple anomalies, smooth muscle hamartoma, and familial paracentric inversion of chromosome 7q. *J. Am. Acad. Dermatol.* **28,** 364–370.

A detailed case report with tabular review of the literature, giving strong sense that the Michelin tire syndrome is a nonspecific phenotype.

Wallach, D., Sorin, M., and Saurat, J.-H. (1980). Naevus musculaire généralisé avec aspect clinique de "Bébé Michelin." *Ann. Dermatol. Venereol.* **107,** 923–927.

An infant with diffuse folds of skin proved to have smooth muscle hamartomas. Over the years the epidermis became thickened and hirsute. The child was noted to have developmental delay. The initial presentation was identical to Ross' patient (1969).

STIFF SKIN (MIM:184900, 260530)

Includes Parana Stiff Skin; Mucolipidosis II

DERMATOLOGIC FEATURES

MAJOR. There are two variants of stiff skin syndrome described. In one, rock hard skin is present at birth or develops progressively in early childhood. The skin color is unchanged, as are sensation, temperature, and texture. There is no epidermal or dermal atrophy, and involvement is most severe on the buttocks and upper thighs. These changes are relatively mild and do not threaten health.

In the second type of stiff skin (Parana syndrome), onset is in infancy, and progression is rapid and severe. In this group, there is loss of subcutaneous tissue, growth failure, hirsutism, and generalized hyperpigmentation, in addition to hardening of the skin.

MINOR. None.

ASSOCIATED ABNORMALITIES

In the mild form, joint contractures may occur concurrently with the hardening of the skin and may not be progressive, suggesting that the joint involvement may be primary rather than secondary to longstanding restricted movement because of skin tightness. Strength remains normal.

In Parana stiff skin, joint contractures are widespread, severe, and progressive, and pulmonary insufficiency due to restricted chest wall movement can lead to death.

Intellect is unaffected in both conditions.

HISTOPATHOLOGY

LIGHT. Despite severe clinical findings, histopathologic changes are relatively mild, with some increase in staining with Alcian blue and an increase in colloidal iron staining in the dermis.

EM. In some patients studied, no changes in collagen were noted. In fascial biopsy material from patients in one family, aggregated microfibrils and "amianthoid" large collagen fibers were described.

BASIC DEFECT

Unknown. There have been no abnormalities demonstrated in mucopolysaccharide metabolism.

TREATMENT

None. There are no reports of attempts at physical therapy or use of Dilantin (for its anticollagenase activity).

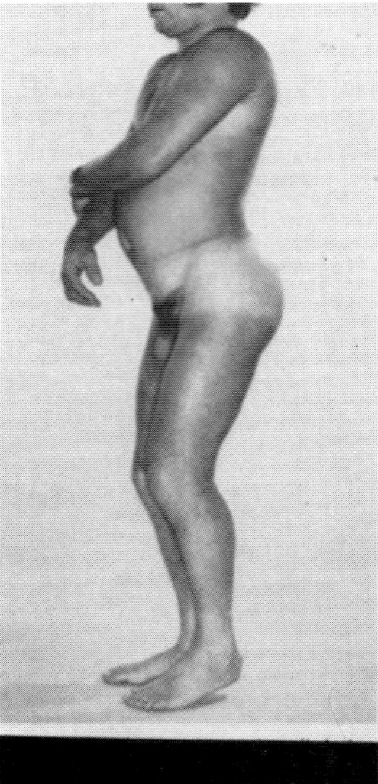
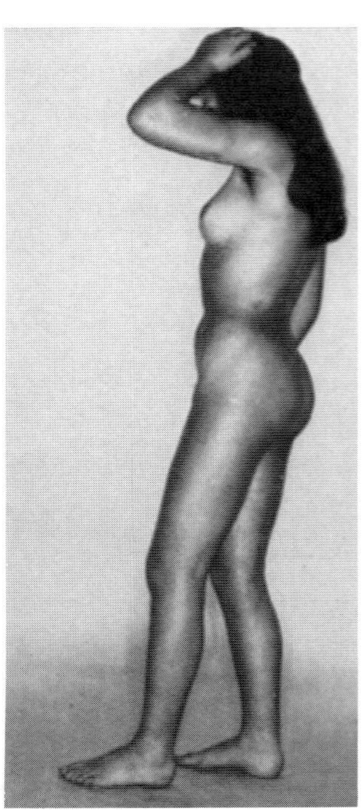

Figure 9.4. Tight skin with joint contractures in siblings. (From Jablonska et al., 1989.)

MODE OF INHERITANCE

The mild form of stiff skin is autosomal dominant. In one family, a mother and two children were affected. However, the father was second cousin to the mother, so pseudodominance was possible. In the mouse, tight skin is autosomal dominant.

The Parana syndrome is autosomal recessive.

PRENATAL DIAGNOSIS

None.

DIFFERENTIAL DIAGNOSIS

In sclerema adultorum, acute progressive woodiness of the skin results from mucopolysaccharide deposition in the dermis. It is most often associated with diabetes mellitus. Onset is considerably later than in familial stiff skin.

Tight, firm, thick skin is a transient feature of mucolipidosis II (I-cell disease, MIM:252500). This feature is striking when present, but its diagnostic importance may not be appreciated. It usually resolves after the first year. The associated abnormalities including developmental delay, abnormal facies, and abnormal excretion of lysosomal enzymes readily distinguish it from stiff skin syndrome.

Focal pebbly thickening of the skin can be seen in the Hurler (MIM:252800), Scheie (MIM:252800), and Hunter (MIM:309900) syndromes, but these are easily differentiated by their associated skeletal and neurologic manifestations and by urine metabolic screening.

In localized scleroderma there are epidermal changes of atrophy, hypo- and hyperpigmentation, and telangiectasias, all absent in stiff skin.

In a family reported with autosomal dominant diffuse lipomatosis (Stevenson et al., 1984), progressive stiffening of the skin of the head, torso, and arms beginning in adult life was described. Skin biopsy showed only lipomas. In addition to the cutaneous change, affected individuals developed renal stones, cardiomyopathy, and deafness.

Support Group: N.O.R.D.
P.O. Box 8923
New Fairfield, CT 06812
1-800-999-6673

SELECTED BIBLIOGRAPHY

Cat, I., Magdalena, N.I.R., Marinoni, L. P., Wong, M. P., Freitas, O.T., Malfi, A., Costa, O., Esteves, L., Giraldi, D. J., and Opitz, J. M. (1974). Parana hard-skin syndrome: study of seven families. *Lancet* **i,** 215–216.

Eight probands, two of whom were siblings, another from a consanguineous mating, all from a small region in southern Parana, Brazil.

Esterly, N. B., and McKusick, V. A. (1971). Stiff skin syndrome. *Pediatrics* **47,** 360–369.

A detailed clinical description of three members of one pedigree and a fourth unrelated patient. They compared the skin to a "piece of marble." Two patients had normal muscle biopsies.

Jablonska, S., Schubert, H., and Kikudu, I. (1989). Congenital fascial dystrophy: stiff skin syndrome—a human counterpart of the tight-skin mouse. *J. Am. Acad. Dermatol.* **21,** 943–950.

Four patients (two of whom were siblings) with stiff skin demonstrated remarkably thickened fascia. Authors suggest two forms of stiff skin: one due to abnormal mucopolysaccharide metabolism and one secondary to abnormal collagen metabolism. One patient had marked hypertrichosis.

Stevenson, R. E., Lucas, T. L., Jr., and Martin, J. B., Jr. (1984) Symmetrical lipomatosis associated with stiff skin and systemic manifestations in four generations. *Proc. Greenwood Genet. Center* **3,** 56–64.

Males and females affected to same degree. Skin described as inelastic and insensitive.

CHAPTER 10

TUMORS/HAMARTOMAS

Any benign or malignant tumor can occur in any individual without a predisposing genetic condition. Multiple occurrences of a benign tumor, however, are more likely to be found only in persons with a genetic disorder or major malformation syndrome. This is true for lipomas, collagenomas, neurofibromas, hemangiomas, glomus tumors, pilomatricomas, and so on. As a general rule, most genetic conditions characterized by multiple benign growths are autosomal dominant in inheritance. Multiple hamartomas can occur in isolation (e.g., lipomas in familial lipomatosis, hemangiomas in familial benign hemangiomatosis) or as a feature of a pleiotropic syndrome (e.g., neurofibromas in neurofibromatosis, pilomatricomas in myotonic dystrophy).

Onset of tumors and, when it occurs, malignant transformation generally occur at a younger age than isolated lesions in individuals without a genetic disorder.

BASAL CELL NEVUS SYNDROME (MIM:109400)

(Nevoid Basal Cell Carcinoma Syndrome; Gorlin Syndrome)

Includes Bazex Syndrome; Rombo Syndrome

DERMATOLOGIC FEATURES

Major. Basal cell nevi may appear in early childhood, although the majority develop in puberty or later. Initially, they are small, skin-colored to light brown translucent papules that can be misdiagnosed clinically as skin tags or nevocytic nevi. They tend to cluster in sun-exposed areas, although they can occur on any skin surface. Although it is stated that the lesions do not become aggressive until after puberty, the histologic features of lesions removed in childhood are typical of basal cell carcinomas and not different from those in adults. Tumors can become locally invasive.

Palmar and plantar pits are reported in about 65% of patients; the prevalence increases with age. These are small depressed areas, which can resemble pitted keratolysis.

Minor. Epidermal cysts and milia also occur in 30%–50% of published patients. Chalazia have been reported occasionally.

ASSOCIATED ABNORMALITIES

Dental: Odontogenic keratocytes, occurring in upwards of 80% of patients, usually become symptomatic after age 10 years, and their occurrence peaks by age 30. The mandible is usually more involved than the maxilla. They may be entirely asymptomatic or may require excision, and they can recur.

Skeletal: Macrocephaly, prominent supraorbital ridging, frontal bossing, and a broad nasal ridge give the classic facies of the disorder, present in more than 65% of patients. Bifid, hypoplastic, and fused ribs occur in 60% of affected individuals. Spina bifida occulta has been described.

CNS: Calcification of the falx cerebri occurs in 85%, bridging of the sella turcica in 60%–80%, and mental retardation in less than 5%–10% of patients with basal cell nevus syndrome. Agenesis of the corpus callosum has been reported, but is rare.

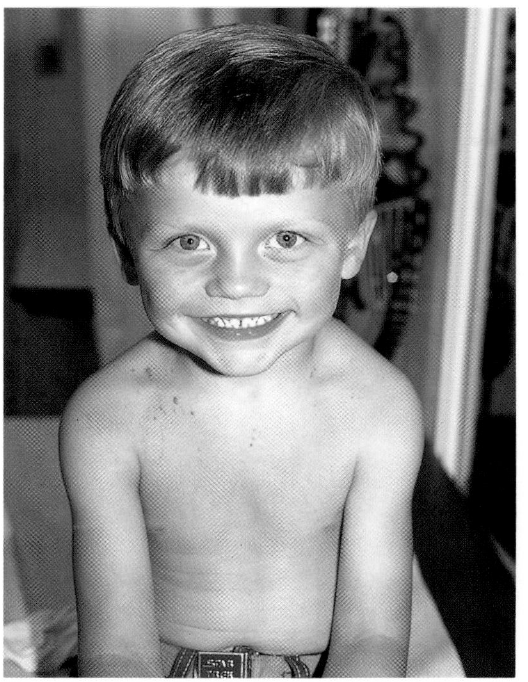

Figure 10.1. Four-year-old with macrocephaly, broad nasal root, and obvious papules on upper chest.

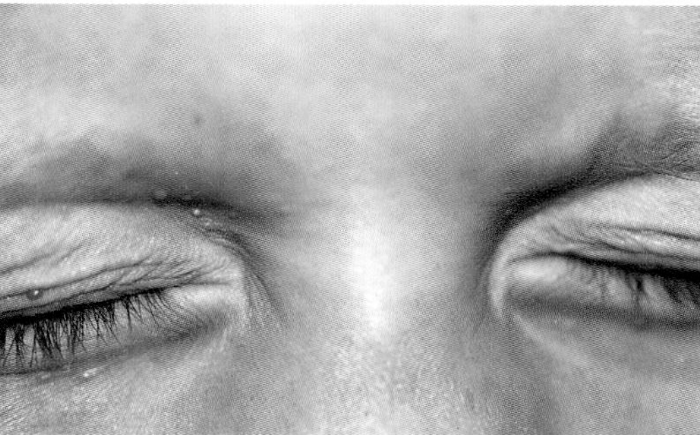

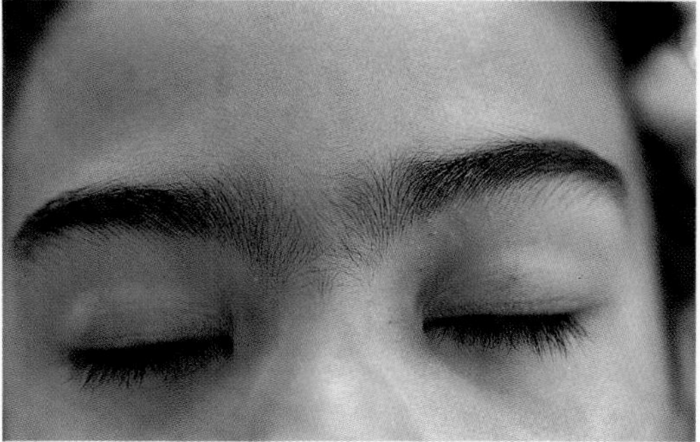

Figure 10.2. Tiny pearly papules on eyelids and in eyebrows in two patients.

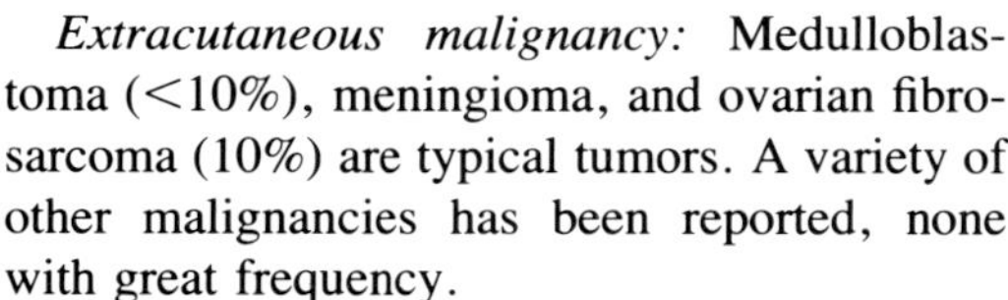

Extracutaneous malignancy: Medulloblastoma (<10%), meningioma, and ovarian fibrosarcoma (10%) are typical tumors. A variety of other malignancies has been reported, none with great frequency.

Ocular: Strabismus (15%–40%), corneal clouding (<10%), coloboma (<10%), and glaucoma (<10%) are the most common findings.

Other: Marfanoid habitus, hypogonadism in the male (<10%), calcified ovarian cysts (25%–50%), cleft lip/palate (5%), and early cardiac fibroma (≤3%) have all been noted.

HISTOPATHOLOGY

LIGHT. The histopathologic features of basal cell nevi are indistinguishable from those of typical basal cell carcinomas. Nests or sheets of basal cells with many mitotic figures are classic findings.

The palmoplantar pits are characterized by acanthosis of the rete ridges, vacuolar changes in the spinous layer, and thinning of the stratum corneum.

EM. The pits show decreased desmosomal attachments, large keratohyaline granules with "white speckles," and abnormally large keratinosomes. Compact clumping of tonofilaments in the periphery of the cytoplasm is seen.

BASIC DEFECT

The basic defect in basal cell nevus syndrome is unknown. In vivo, patients exposed to radiotherapy often develop multiple basal cell tumors in the radiated field within 6 months to 3 years after treatment. Tumors tend to cluster in areas of sun exposure, and affected blacks tend to have later onset of tumors and fewer numbers of them than whites. These findings suggest that a defect in the ability to repair radiation- or ultraviolet-induced damage might play a role in this disorder.

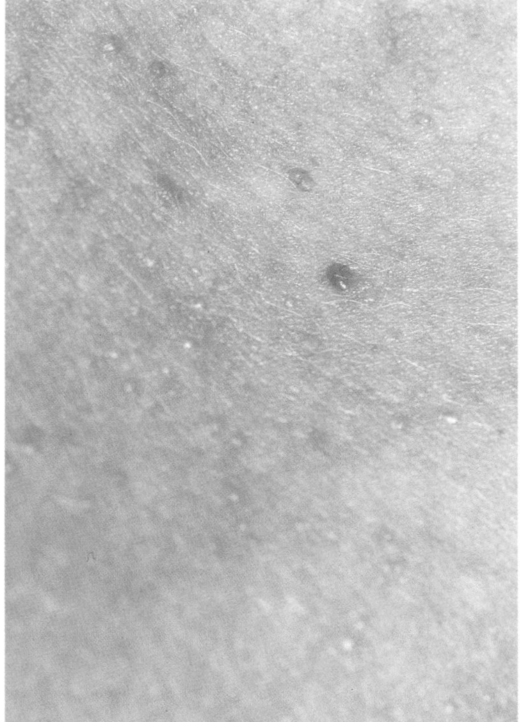

Figure 10.3. Lesions can be extremely subtle, often with specks of pigment in otherwise flesh-colored lesion. Papules may lack the telangiectases of basal cell epitheliomas.

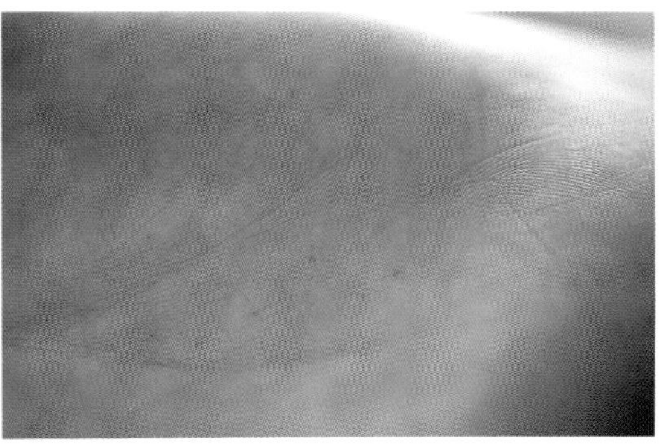

Figure 10.4. Palmar pits can be very subtle.

However, in vitro studies have given conflicting results about increased sensitivity of both leukocytes and fibroblasts from patients with basal cell nevus syndrome to the effects of ionizing radiation (UVB, UVC, x-irradiation), and no consistent findings have been demonstrated.

The candidate gene, *PTC,* in basal cell nevus syndrome is believed to function both in embryogenesis and in tumor suppression. Thus loss of function could result in both the malformations and malignant transformation which occur in this disorder.

TREATMENT

Avoidance of sun exposure is a logical practice for people with basal cell nevus syndrome. The role of sun damage in causing basal cell carcinoma in normal people is undisputed. Blacks with basal cell nevus syndrome have fewer basal cell carcinomas at later ages than do whites, presumably due to photoprotection by melanin. Despite conflicting in vitro studies of the cellular response of basal cell nevus syndrome cells to ultraviolet light, it seems the better part of valor to avoid unnecessary exposure to the "second hit" of sunlight.

Oral retinoids (Accutane) appear to decrease the rate of new tumor formation and perhaps suppress the growth of existing tumors. Colleagues and I studied two patients and were not convinced of any change in tumor occurrence over a 1 year period. Others have noted the difficulty in quantifying improvement because of large numbers of lesions and the episodic nature of tumor development and progression, which has been well documented. Any regimen presumed to suppress new tumor formation needs to be evaluated over long periods. Both the short- and long-term side effects of the retinoids limit their usefulness.

Mohs' chemosurgery is the treatment of choice for large lesions and those showing ulceration or hemorrhage. Electrodessication and curettage is appropriate for smaller lesions, as are cryotherapy, 5-fluoruracil, and topical immunotherapy. Lesions around the eye deserve the attention of both a dermatologist and an ophthalmologist skilled in plastic repair. Systemic administration of a hematoporphyrin dye (which is preferentially taken up by rapidly dividing cells) and subsequent exposure to red light has been tried in three patients with basal

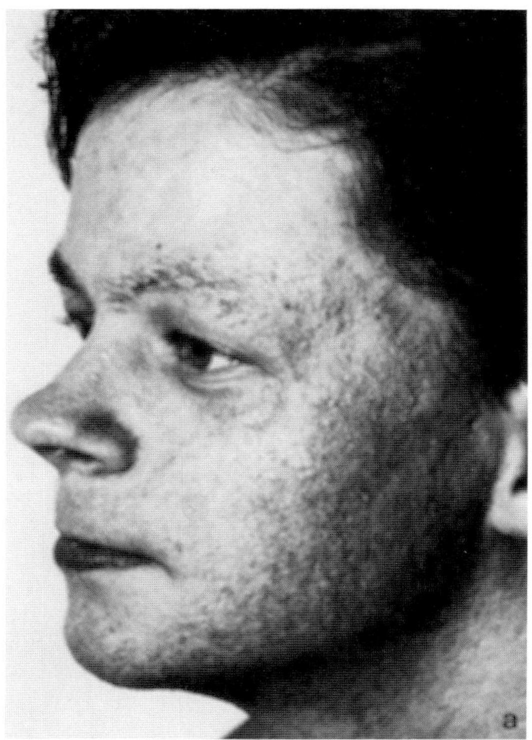

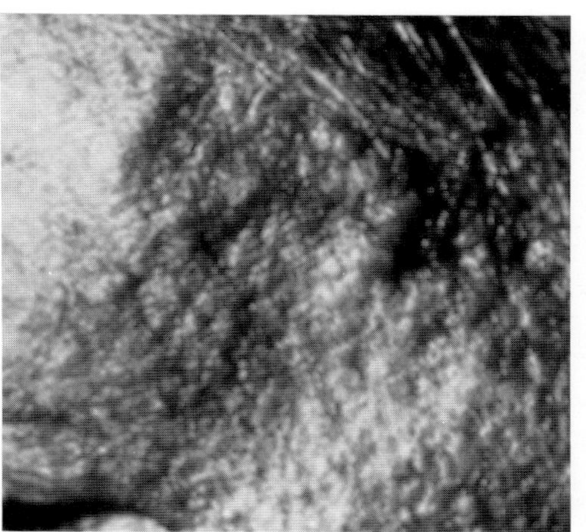

Figure 10.5. **(A)** Rombo syndrome: sparse eyebrows, loss of lower lashes. **(B)** Close-up shows grainy quality of skin and milia. (From Michaëlsson et al., 1981.)

cell nevus syndrome. Eighty percent of 40 tumors resolved completely; 10% of tumors recurred 1 year after treatment, suggesting that results may be temporary. Some lesions that showed clinical ablation had microscopic residua.

Symptomatic jaw cysts require complete enucleation and may recur.

MODE OF INHERITANCE

Autosomal dominant with variable expression. Penetrance is reported to be 100%. From 40% to 60% of cases represent new mutations. A paternal age effect has been found. The gene has been mapped to 9q22.3–q31.

A candidate gene, *PTC,* has been identified in this region. It is homologous to the *patched (ptc)* gene in *Drosophila,* whose function in the fly is integral to normal embryologic development. Preliminary work has shown mutations in *PTC* in sporadic basal cell tumors and in a number of patients with basal cell nevus syndrome.

PRENATAL DIAGNOSIS

Possible now by linkage studies in informative families, potentially by direct mutation analysis if specific mutation identified.

DIFFERENTIAL DIAGNOSIS

Some patients with basal cell nevus syndrome have a marfanoid habitus. I have seen two patients with basal cell nevus syndrome who were misdiagnosed as having Marfan syndrome (MIM:154700). In the latter disorder, none of the skin changes or the rib and calvarial changes are present.

Unilateral linear nevoid basal cell carcinomas with comedones may represent a postzygotic mutation for the basal cell nevus syndrome allele.

Bazex syndrome (MIM:301845) is characterized by basal cell carcinomas of the face, follicular atrophoderma of the hands, feet, and elbows, hypotrichosis with twisting and flattening of hair shafts, and decreased or absent sweating

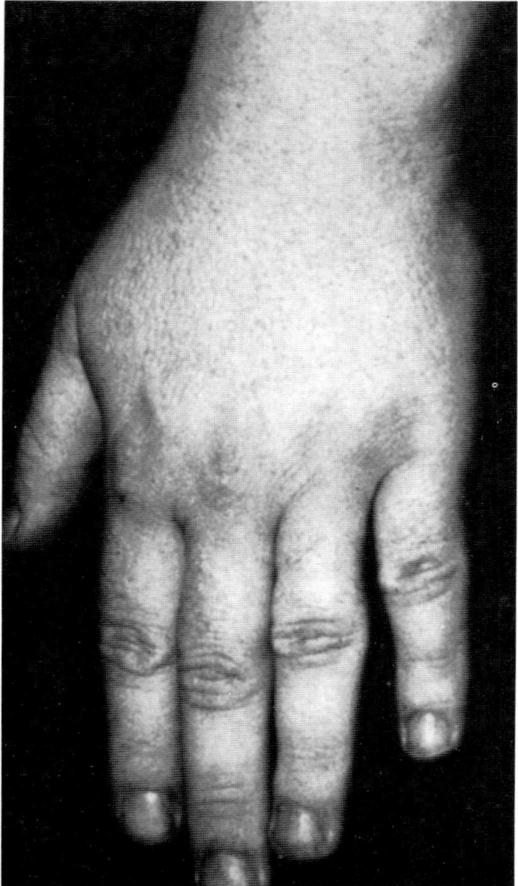

Figure 10.6. Follicular atrophoderma over the back of the hand in Bazex syndrome. (From Gould and Barker, 1978.)

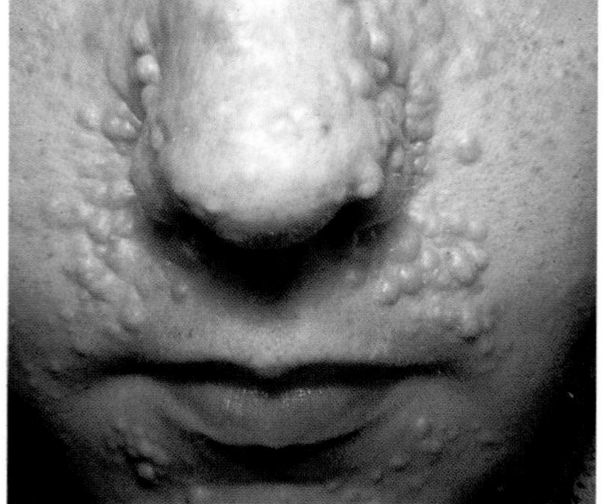

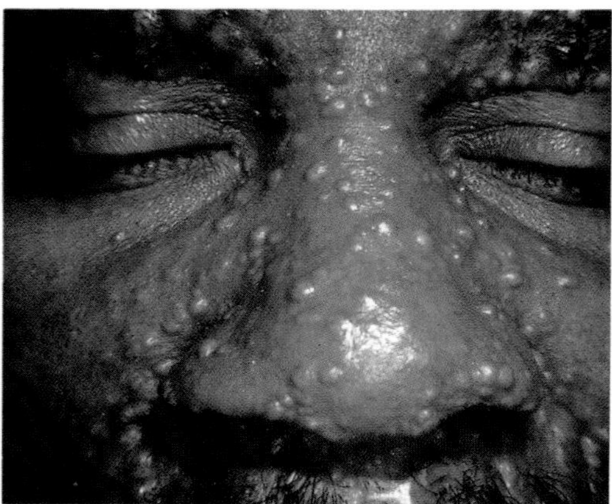

Figure 10.7. (A, B) Multiple trichoepitheliomas. (Courtesy of Division of Dermatology, University of Washington.)

of the face and head. The follicular atrophoderma is present at very young ages without antecedent inflammation. Sweat glands on the forehead appear to be diminished or absent. Eczema is a common complaint in affected individuals. The inheritance pattern of Bazex syndrome is thought to be either X-linked or autosomal dominant. Of 80 individuals in the literature at risk to inherit the condition, 42 have been affected (20 male and 22 female), with equal severity of expression in males and females. Of all males in the published pedigrees, only six were at risk to have inherited the gene from a male. Despite preliminary linkage data suggesting X-linked inheritance, there may be some families with autosomal dominant inheritance. Bazex's name is also appended to a nongenetic disorder of scaling dermatitis associated with laryngopharyngeal structures (acrokeratosis paraneoplastica).

Rombo syndrome (MIM:180730) differs from Bazex syndrome in that the lesions of atrophoderma in Rombo syndrome have later onset; the affected members of the single reported family also had perioral and distal acrocyanosis, no decrease in sweating, and trichoepitheliomas. Male-to-male transmission occurred. It is not clear to me if Rombo syndrome is truly a distinct entity from Bazex syndrome. Both are easily differentiated from basal cell nevus syndrome by the atrophoderma lesions and the absence of skeletal changes and palmoplantar pits.

Support Group: Nevoid Basal Cell Carcinoma Syndrome Support Network (NBCCS Support Network)
3902 Greencastle Ridge Drive, No. 204
Burtonsville, MD 20866
1-800-264-8099

SELECTED BIBLIOGRAPHY

Applegate, L.A., Goldberg, L.H., Ley, R.D., and Ananthaswamy, H.N. (1990). Hypersensitivity of skin fibroblasts from basal cell nevus syndrome patients to killing by ultraviolet B but not by ultraviolet C radiation. *Cancer Res.* **50,** 637–641.

Frentz, G., Munch-Petersen, B., Wulf, H., Niebuhr, E., and da Cunha Bang, F. (1987). The nevoid basal cell carcinoma syndrome: sensitivity to ultraviolet and x-ray irradiation. *J. Am. Acad. Dermatol.* **17,** 637–643.

Little, J.B., Nichols, W.W., Troilo, P., Nagasawa, H., and Strong, L.C. (1989). Radiation sensitivity of cell strains from families with genetic disorders predisposing to radiation-induced cancer. *Cancer Res.* **49,** 4705–4714.

Nagasawa, H., Burke, M.J., Little, F.F., McCone E.F., Chan, G.L., and Little, J.B. (1988). Multiple abnormalities in the ultraviolet light response of cultured fibroblasts derived from patients with the basal cell nevus syndrome. *Teratog. Carcinog. Mutagen.* **8,** 25–33.

Newton, J.A., Black A.K., Arlett, C.F., and Cole, J. (1990). Radiobiological studies in the naevoid basal cell carcinoma syndrome. *Br. J. Dermatol.* **123,** 573–580.

Ringborg, U., Lambert, B., Landegren, J., and Lewensohn, R. (1981). Decreased UV-induced DNA repair synthesis in peripheral leukocytes from patients with the nevoid basal cell carcinoma syndrome. *J. Invest. Dermatol.* **76,** 268–270.

Sharpe, G.R., and Cox, N.H. (1990). Unilateral naevoid basal-cell-carcinoma syndrome—an individually controlled study of fibroblast sensitivity to radiation. *Clin. Exp. Dermatol.* **15,** 352–355.

Applegate et al. (1990), Frentz et al. (1987), Little et al. (1989), Nagasawa et al. (1988), Newton et al. (1990), Ringborg et al. (1981) and Sharpe and Cox (1990) deal with the in vitro responses of leukocytes or fibroblasts from patients with basal cell nevus syndrome to the effects of a variety of insults including UVA, UVB, UVC, and x-ray.

Cristofolini, M., Zumiani, G., Scappini, P., and Piscioli, F. (1984). Aromatic retinoid in chemoprevention of the progression of nevoid basal cell carcinoma syndrome. *J. Dermatol. Surg. Oncol.* **10,** 778–781.

Goldberg, L.H., Hsu, S.H., and Alcalay, J. (1989). Effectiveness of isotretinoin in preventing the appearance of basal cell carcinomas in basal cell nevus syndrome. *J. Am. Acad. Dermatol.* **21,** 144–145.

Hodak, E., Ginzburg, A., David, M., and Sandbank, M. (1987). Etretinate treatment of the nevoid basal cell carcinoma syndrome. *Int. J. Dermatol.* **26,** 606–609.

Peck, G.L., Gross, E.G., Butkus, D., and DiGiovanni, J.J. (1982). Chemoprevention of basal cell carcinoma with isotretinoin. *J. Am. Acad. Dermatol.* **6,** 815–823.

Christofolini et al. (1984), Goldberg et al. (1989), Hodak et al. (1987), and Peck et al. (1987) provide case reports of decreases in basal cell carcinoma formation and growth by oral treatment with isotretinoin. Short- and long-term side effects need to be weighed carefully. Most follow-up periods are short. Goldberg et al. showed a dose effect in identical twins.

Gorlin, R.J. (1987). Nevoid basal cell carcinoma syndrome. *Medicine* **66,** 98–113.

Everything you ever wanted to know about basal cell nevus syndrome is presented in Dr. Gorlin's lucid, detailed, and rational review of this syndrome that bears his name. He prefers the designation *nevoid basal cell carcinoma syndrome.* There are 216 references cited.

Hahn, H., Wicking, C., Zaphiropoulos, P.G., Gailani, M.R., Shanley, S., Chidambaram, A., Vorechovsky, I., Holmberg, E., Unden, A.B., Gillies, S., Negus, K., Smyth, I., Pressman, C., Leffell, D.J., Gerrard, B., Goldstein,

A.M., Dean, M., Toftgard, R., Chenevix-Trench, G., Wainwright, B., Bale, A.E. (1996) Mutations of the human homolog of Drosophila *patched* in the nevoid basal cell carcinoma syndrome. *Cell.* **85,** 841–851.

Johnson, R.L., Rothman, A.L., Xie, J., Goodrich, L.V., Bare, J.W., Bonifas, J.M., Quinn, A.G., Myers, R.M., Cox, D.R., Epstein, E.H. Jr., Scott, M.P. (1996). Human homolog of *patched,* a candidate gene for the basal cell nevus syndrome. *Science.* **272,** 1668–1671.

Both report mutations in *PTC* in sporadic basal cell tumors and in individuals with basal cell nevus syndrome. There appears to be considerable allelic heterogeneity.

Michaelsson, G., Olsson, E., and Westermark, P. (1981). The Rombo syndrome: a familial disorder with vermiculate atrophoderma, milia, hypotrichosis, trichoepitheliomas, basal cell carcinomas and peripheral vasodilation with cyanosis. *Acta Dermatol. Venereol.* **61,** 497–503.

Report of a Swedish family with this perhaps unique autosomal dominant disorder.

Plosila, M., Kiistala, R., and Niemi, K.M. (1981). The Bazex syndrome: follicular atrophoderma with multiple basal cell carcinomas, hypotrichosis and hypohidrosis. *Clin. Exp. Dermatol.* **6,** 31–41.

Histologic evaluation and sweat measurements in a Finnish family with Bazex syndrome. Authors suggest that a primary defect in the follicular apparatus underlies all the lesions of Bazex. Bibliography quite complete for familial reports.

Tse, D.T., Kersten, R.C., and Anderson, R.L. (1984). Hematoporphyrin derivative photoradiation therapy in managing nevoid basal-cell carcinoma syndrome. A preliminary report. *Arch. Ophthalmol.* **102,** 990–994.

Three patients with basal cell nevus syndrome were injected with a hematoporphyrin derivative. The authors appropriately offer this therapy as an adjunct to Mohs' for those patients who have limited tissue reserves for conventional therapy. Disadvantages include expense and the sustained photosensitivity of patients, who must avoid sunlight for a month.

Ullman, S., Sondergaard, J., and Kobayasi, T. (1972). Ultrastructure of palmar and plantar pits in basal cell nevus syndrome. *Acta Dermatol. Venereol.* **52,** 329–336.

Transmission and scanning electron microscopy of palmoplantar pits from two patients with basal cell nevus syndrome.

Vabres, P., Lacombe, D., Rabinowitz, L.G., Aubert, G., Anderson, C.E., Taieb, A., Bonafe, J.-L., and Hors-Cayla, M.-C. (1995). The gene for Bazex-Dupre-Christol syndrome maps to chromosome Xq. *J. Invest. Dermatol.* **105,** 87–91.

Three families with additive lod score of 5.26 for linkage to Xq24–q27 for Bazex.

Viksnins, P., and Berlin, A. (1977). Follicular atrophoderma and basal cell carcinomas. The Bazex syndrome. *Arch. Dermatol.* **113,** 948–951.

Describes a large pedigree of Bazex syndrome, with three affected generations, but no male-to-male transmission. All daughters and no sons of an affected male were affected. The severity of expression did not differ between the sexes.

BATHING TRUNK NEVUS (MIM:137550)

(Giant Congenital Nevocytic Nevus)

Includes Neurocutaneous Melanosis

DERMATOLOGIC FEATURES

MAJOR. The giant congenital nevocytic nevus or bathing trunk nevus can occur in isolation or as part of neurocutaneous melanosis.

The brown, hairy areas may be light tan or pink at birth and gradually darken, or dark at the start. They may become pebbly or verrucous over time. The hairs are usually dark, but may be light and uneven in distribution. Although definitions vary, it is generally accepted that a giant lesion is greater than 20 cm in diameter in the adult. In 65% of patients, the nevus is lumbosacral in distribution. There

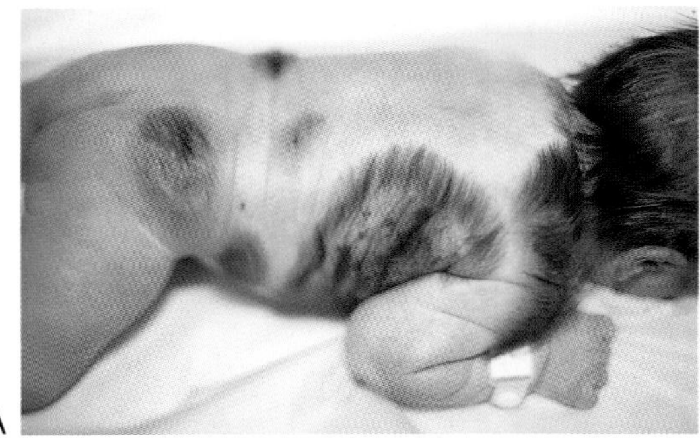

A

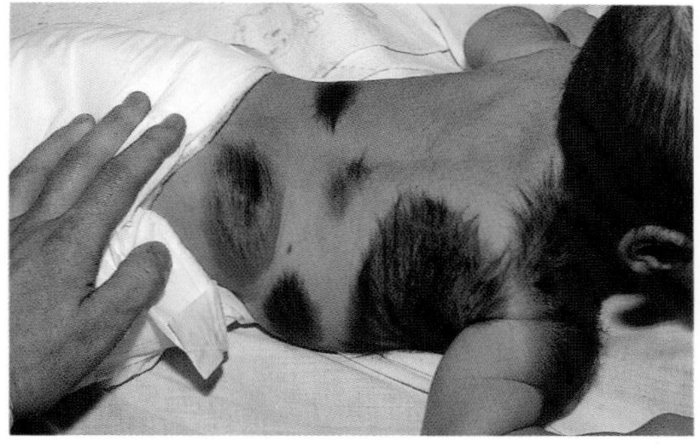

B

Figure 10.8. (A) Newborn. **(B)** At 2 months. Lesions have darkened, and hair growth has increased.

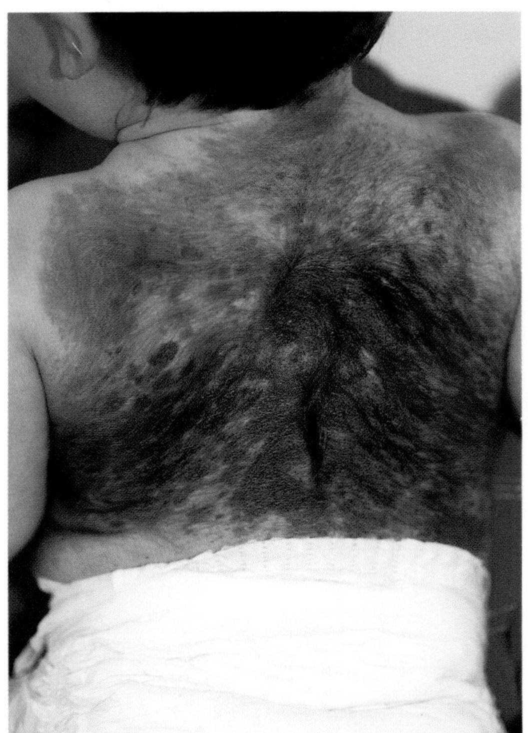

A

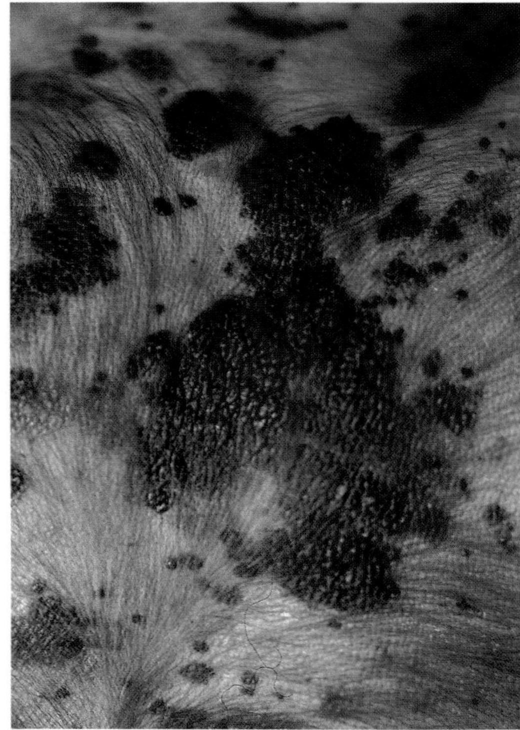

B

Figure 10.9. Marked variegation in pigment and thickness.

may be multiple small satellite lesions as well.

At birth there may be multiple raised pink to purple areas that can mimic or represent true melanoma. These can be mistaken for open neural tube defects when over the midline back or for hemangiomas because of their reddish-purple and moist appearance.

Melanoma develops in 4%–10% of patients. Higher estimates are based on biased series from pathology specimens or surgical clinics. Melanoma may be present at birth or develop later, for the most part before 1 year or after puberty.

MINOR. None.

ASSOCIATED ABNORMALITIES

Neurologic associations include benign or malignant tumors of the leptomeninges (neurocutaneous melanosis). Although central nervous system malignancy has been described in 40%–60% of infants who have leptomeningeal involvement with pigmented melanocytes, this may reflect overreporting in that patients have not been routinely screened for leptomeningeal involvement in the absence of neurologic symptoms. The overall proportion of infants with giant congenital nevocytic nevi who have leptomeningeal involvement is unknown.

Dandy-Walker malformations, seizures, mental retardation, cranial nerve palsies, and neurologic dysfunction can all accompany central nervous system involvement. If present, these signs have grave prognostic implications, with death occurring in over 50% of such patients by age 13 years. In my experience with approximately 20 patients, only 1 has had clinical neurologic complications.

HISTOPATHOLOGY

Light. Nevus cells are present, both in nests and scattered down in single file deep into the lower two-thirds of the dermis and subcutane-

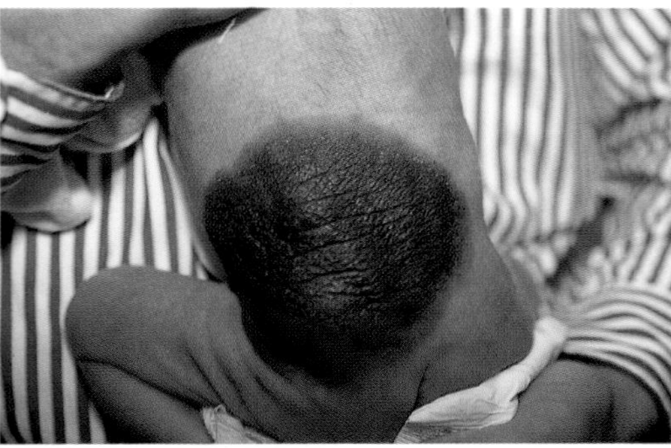

Figure 10.10. Uniformly dark without hair; purple margins are typical.

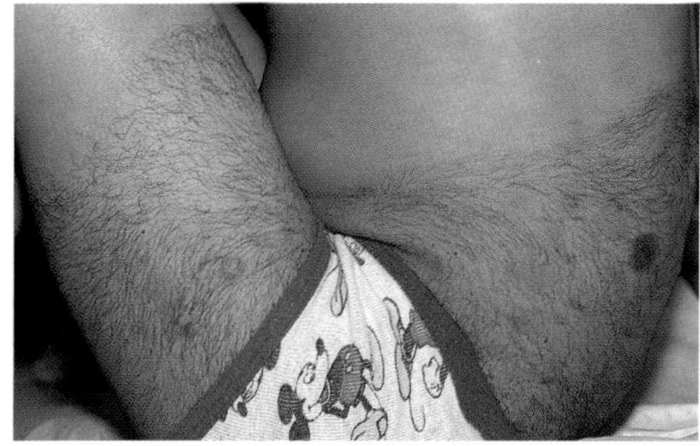

Figure 10.11. Much lighter lesion with hairs; scattered islands of darker and lighter plaques.

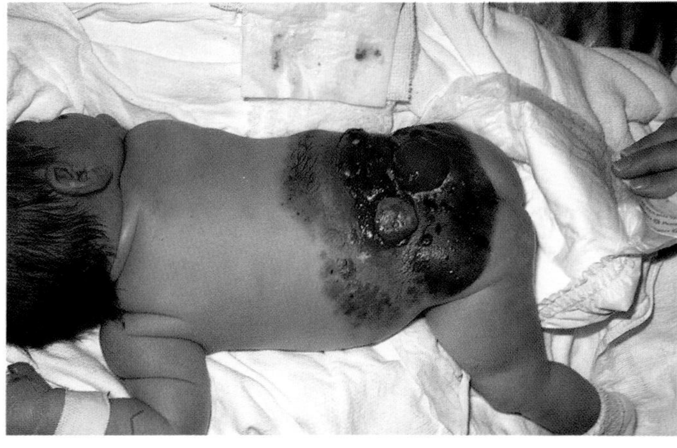

Figure 10.12. Lesion with congenital melanoma. This was resected, and patient was alive at age 5 years without evidence of disease.

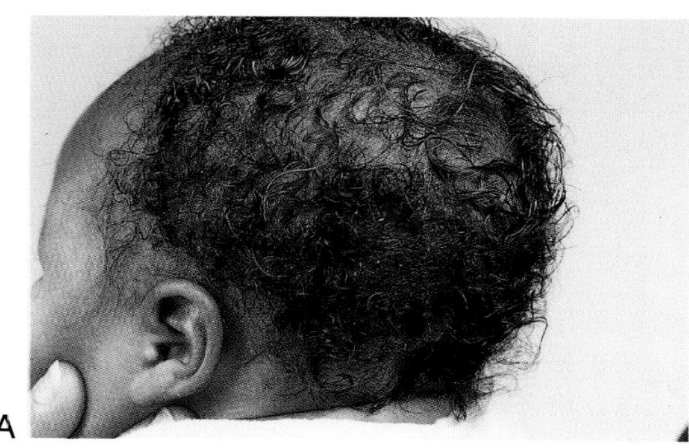

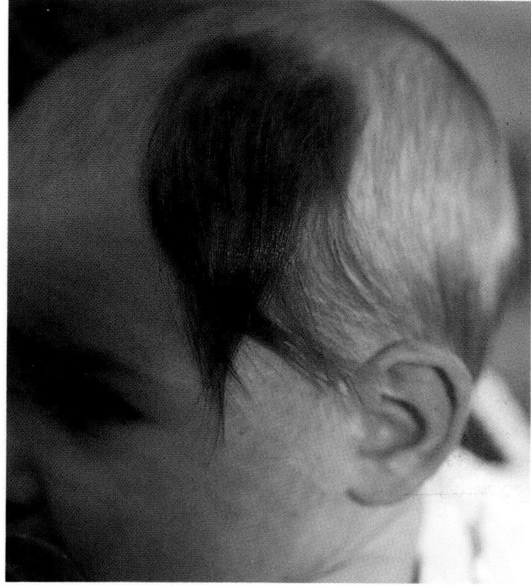

Figure 10.13. (A) Scalp lesion. (B) Much darker hair associated with the nevus.

ous tissue, between collagen bundles, and along appendages, nerves, and blood vessels. Some lesions have a "neural" pattern with neroid tubes and nevic corpuscles, similar to neurofibromas.

EM. No specific diagnostic features.

BASIC DEFECT

Unknown.

TREATMENT

Screening of all infants with giant congenital nevocytic nevi by magnetic resonance imaging with gadolinium contrast to find leptomeningeal involvement has been suggested. In a neurologically intact infant this may have a low yield and questionable prognostic value.

Dermabrasion of these lesions has enjoyed brief popularity, but probably does not result in a lower risk of malignancy and may not give adequate cosmetic results. It may have value in a few specific situations.

Prophylactic and staged excision of these lesions, accompanied by tissue expansion when appropriate, is the treatment of choice. This is not an emergency situation; melanomas are either congenital or develop within the first year and therefore prophylactic removal cannot be done in time; or they do not occur until later childhood and thereafter and there is time for careful planning for removal to ensure the best cosmetic result. Removal of the giant lesion in its entirety with one procedure is almost always impossible. Removal should be planned to give the best cosmetic results. Affected infants should be seen by a plastic surgeon early so that the family can plan and prepare for multiple surgeries, which usually begin at age 3 years or thereafter. Careful skin examination by a dermatologist on a regular basis and immediate removal of areas suspicious for malignancy are mandatory. Although excision is usually aimed at removal of the large lesions, malignant potential may also reside in the scattered smaller lesions. Lifelong skin examination is appropriate.

MODE OF INHERITANCE

Sporadic. There have been a few case reports of multiple small congenital nevocytic nevi in relatives and bathing trunk nevus in a child. In most instances, no family history is elicited.

PRENATAL DIAGNOSIS

None.

DIFFERENTIAL DIAGNOSIS

There is rarely a problem in recognizing the giant lesion. Exophytic fungating areas can be confused with hemangiomas or neural tube defects.

Support Group: Nevus Network
P.O. Box 2057
Arlington, VA 22202-0057
1-703-920-2349

Nevus Registry
Alfred W. Kopf, MD
Department of Dermatology
NYU School of Medicine
562 1st Avenue
New York, NY 10016
1-212-340-5260

SELECTED BIBLIOGRAPHY

Gari, L.M., Rivers, J.K., and Kopf, A.W. (1988). Melanomas arising in large congenital nevocytic nevi: a prospective study. *Pediatr. Dermatol.* **5,** 151–158.

Premature results of a prospective study (mean follow-up time only 53 months) but good review of the literature. Hopefully this cohort will continue to be followed, and a more accurate risk figure for development of melanoma can be developed.

Kadonaga, J.N., and Frieden, I.J. (1991). Neurocutaneous melanosis: definition and review of the literature. *J. Am. Acad. Dermatol.* **24,** 747–755.

Excellent review of this subset of giant congenital nevocytic nevi with central nervous system involvement. Seventy-six references.

Mark, G.J., Mihm, M.C., Liteplo, M.G., Reed, R.J., and Clark, W.H. (1973). Congenital melanocytic nevi of the small and garment type. Clinical, histologic and ultrastructural studies. *Hum. Pathol.* **4,** 395–418.

Compares 60 lesions present at birth to 60 acquired nevi. Describes electron microscopic findings.

COWDEN DISEASE (MIM:158350)

(Multiple Hamartoma Syndrome)

Includes Byars-Jurkiewicz Syndrome

DERMATOLOGIC FEATURES

MAJOR. Cowden disease is characterized by the development of multiple hamartomas.

Keratoses of the face and extremities (acral keratoses) occur in 85%–95% of affected individuals. They are skin colored, perifollicular, and may be smooth or verrucous. They are usually evident by age 20 years.

Papules of the face, which are most often tricholemmomas, are equally common and also develop within the first two decades. These are small, 1–4 mm, flesh-colored bumps that occur around the eyes, nasolabial folds, and mouth and in the preauricular areas.

Oral papillomas are an almost constant finding. They can occur on all mucosal surfaces and tend to be most prominent on the gingiva. They may coalesce to form large plaques. They may be smooth or verrucous. The description of "cobblestoning" of the mucosa has been used. On the lips they are usually rose colored or pearly.

Palmoplantar keratoses also occur. These are papular and do not resemble the pits of the basal cell nevus syndrome.

MINOR. Dermatofibromas can be found in about 50% of affected individuals. Those often appear at an earlier age than isolated dermatofibromas in normal individuals. They can occur anywhere on the body.

Acrochordons on the face, neck, and axillae are a common finding.

Scrotal tongue, oral fibromas, oral lipomas, and angiolipomas are seen in 20%–40% of persons with Cowden syndrome.

Cutaneous malignancies, including melanoma, basal cell carcinoma, and squamous cell carcinoma, have been reported in a minority of patients.

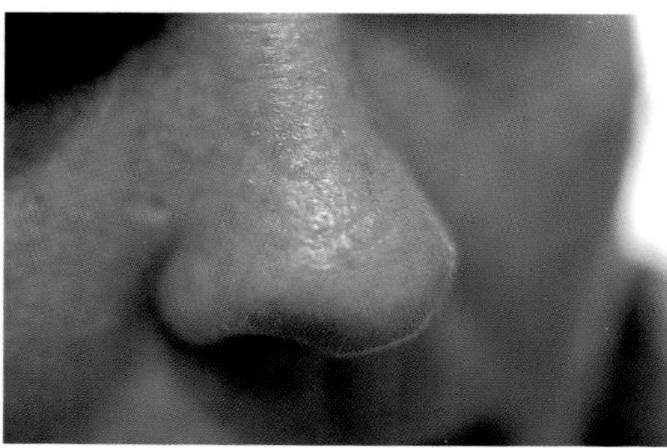

Figure 10.14. Tiny translucent papules on nose.

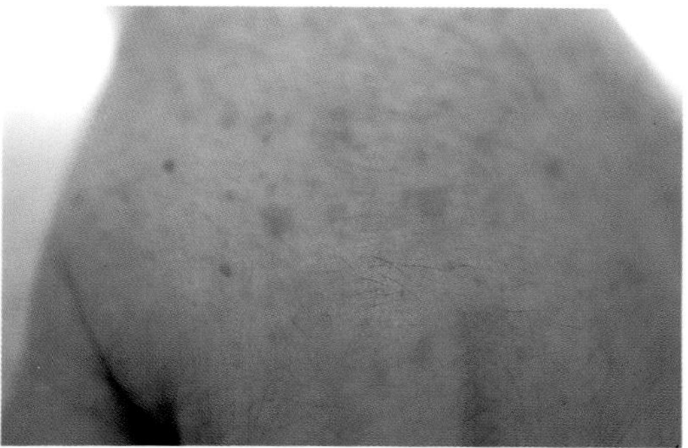

Figure 10.15. Acral keratoses.

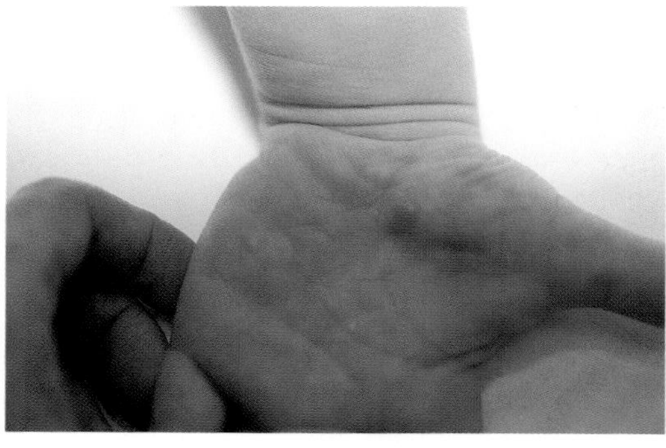

Figure 10.16. Palmar papular keratoses.

ASSOCIATED ABNORMALITIES

No organ seems spared in this disorder. The thyroid diseases associated with Cowden disease include adenomatous goiter, hyperthyroidism, and hypothyroidism. As many as 65% of affected individuals will ultimately develop a goiter. Thyroid carcinoma has been reported in upwards of 5% of patients.

Fibrocystic disease of the breast and follicular adenocarcinoma of the breast in women with Cowden disease are very common. Fibrocystic changes are described in 75% of reported patients. One-third of the females in the literature developed breast cancer. Benign gynecomastia has been mentioned in a few males with Cowden disease.

Gastrointestinal involvement includes multiple hamartomatous polyps in both large and small bowel. Mucosal changes similar to those in the mouth have been seen in the esophagus and duodenum.

Menstrual irregularities, uterine leiomyomas, ovarian cysts, and cervical, uterine, and ovarian cancer occur more often than expected by chance alone.

Bladder cancer, renal cancer, and leukemia have been reported in a single patient each.

Skeletal abnormalities, including macrocephaly, midfacial hypoplasia, scoliosis, bone cysts, and pectus excavatum, are described in about 30% of patients.

Ophthalmologic involvement has been reported in about 15% of cases. There does not appear to be a single specific lesion, and reported abnormalities have ranged from simple myopia to coloboma. Given the variety of findings and the relatively common occurrence of many of them in the general population (e. g., cataracts, myopia), it is possible that these ocular features are associated by chance only.

Peripheral neuromas and neurofibromas are reported in 5% of patients; meningiomas and sensorineural deafness have a similar prevalence. Padberg et al. (1991) have suggested that Lhermite-Duclos disease, a hamartoma of the cerebellum, is a feature of Cowden disease.

HISTOPATHOLOGY

LIGHT. The facial papules are often tricholemmomas arising from the outer root sheath of the hair follicle. Not all lesions show these changes, and multiple biopsies may be necessary.

The keratoses are usually hyperkeratotic papillomas that may or may not have a follicular component and may appear histologically similar to warts.

Lesions in the oral mucosa are fibromas with whorls of relatively acellular fibers. An increase in vascular elements may be seen.

EM. No information.

BASIC DEFECT

Unknown. In one investigation, epidermal growth factor levels in blood and urine were measured and found to be normal.

TREATMENT

Excision or destruction is the only treatment available for the cutaneous lesions.

Careful monitoring for the development of breast and gynecologic malignancy in females, bladder cancer in males, and thyroid and renal cancer in both sexes is mandatory.

MODE OF INHERITANCE

Autosomal dominant with variable and sex-influenced expression. The female predominance in many series may reflect the more frequent ascertainment of women through the development of breast disease.

PRENATAL DIAGNOSIS

None.

DIFFERENTIAL DIAGNOSIS

Basal cell nevus syndrome (MIM:109400) is also characterized by macrocephaly and multiple facial papules. If the distinguishing clinical features of basal cell nevus syndrome (calcification of the falx, bifid ribs, palmoplantar pits) are not present, biopsy of the facial lesions will reveal the correct diagnosis, with basal cell nevi in basal cell nevus syndrome and trichelemmomas in Cowden disease.

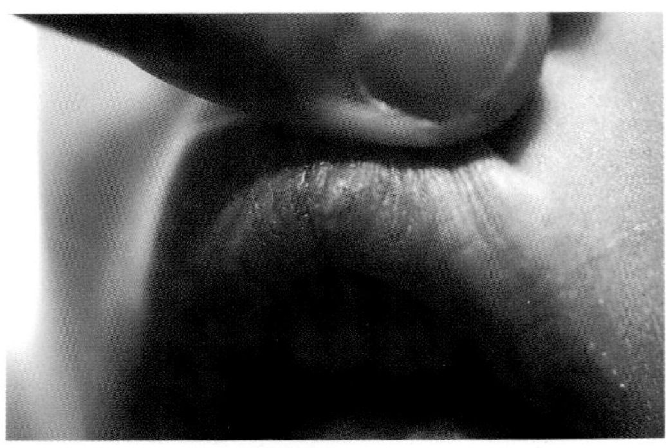
A

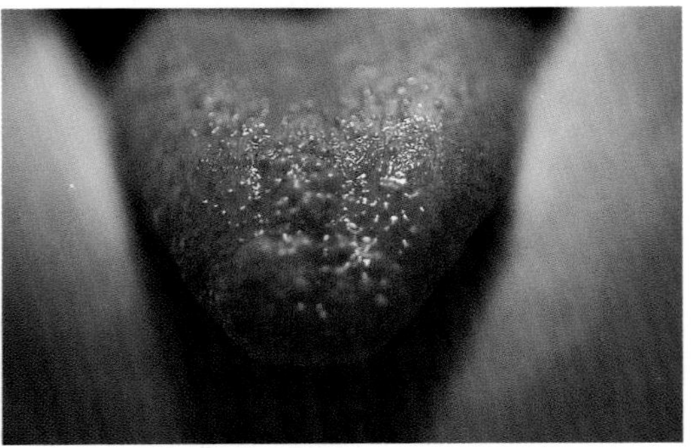
B

Figure 10.17. Papillomas on upper lip **(A)** and tongue **(B)**.

While there is some overlap with neurofibromatosis (MIM:162200), café-au-lait spots, neurofibromas, and optic gliomas have been reported in only a minority of individuals with Cowden disease.

The other familial multiple colonic polyposis syndromes including Gardner syndrome (MIM: 175100), Peutz-Jeghers syndrome (MIM: 175200), and familial polyposis (MIM:175100) can be distinguished by their different cutaneous manifestations and the absence of the typical features of Cowden disease.

The angiofibromas of tuberous sclerosis (MIM:191100) can clinically mimic the tricholemmomas of Cowden disease, especially when the collagenous component predominates and the lesions are more flesh colored and less vascular. The presence of associated cutaneous and systemic findings and/or biopsy will allow for correct diagnosis.

In Byars-Jurkiewicz syndrome, affected individuals have gingival fibromatosis, hypertrichosis, and fibroadenomas of the breast. It is not clear that this is a distinct disorder, but may reflect variable expression of Cowden syndrome.

Support Group: N.O.R.D.
P.O. Box 8923
New Fairfield, CT
06812
1-800-999-6673

SELECTED BIBLIOGRAPHY

Ackerman, A.B. (1978). Tricholemmoma (Letter to the Editor). *Arch. Dermatol.* **114,** 286.

Ackerman suggests that tricholemmomas in general are histopathologically and clinically similar or identical to warts. He states that some of the biopsys specimens described as tricholemmomas by Brownstein et al. (1979) were originally read by Ackerman as warts. To my knowledge, papilloma virus cultures and virus typing have not been attempted or reported with lesions from patients with Cowden disease.

Brownstein, M.H., Mehregan, A.H., Bikowski, J.B., Lupulescu, A., and Patterson, J.C. (1979). The dermatopathology of Cowden's syndrome. *Br. J. Dermatol.* **100,** 667–673.

Of 53 facial lesions from 19 patients, 29 were definite tricholemmomas and 23 were probable. All 14 lesions from oral mucosa were fibromas. Several biopsies were required in some instances to make the diagnosis. The authors believe that multiple tricholemmomas are pathognomonic for and specific to Cowden disease.

Carlson, H.E., Burns, T.W., Davenport, S.L., Luger, A.M., Spence, A., Sparkes, R.S., and Orth, D.N. (1986). Cowden disease: gene marker studies and measurements of epidermal growth factor. *Am. J. Hum. Genet.* **38,** 908–917.

In the single family studied, no linkage with a battery of anonymous probes was detected. Epidermal growth factor levels in saliva, serum, plasma, and urine from affected individuals were normal.

Lloyd, K.M., and Dennis, M. (1963). Cowden's syndrome: a possible new symptom complex with multiple involvement. *Ann. Intern. Med.* **58,** 136–142.

You may search in vain for references to Dr. Cowden. The authors of one of the first reports of the disorder named it after their patient, Rachel Cowden. She later died of breast cancer, as did her mother.

Padberg, G.W., Schot, J.D.L., Vielvoye, J., Bots, T.Th.A.M., and de Beer, F.C. (1991). Lhermite-Duclos disease and Cowden disease: a single phakomatosis. *Ann. Neurol.* **29,** 517–523.

Two unrelated patients from two large pedigrees with Cowden disease presented with hamartomatous lesions in the cerebellum. The authors agree that Lhermite-Duclos is probably not a separate and distinct autosomal dominant disorder but a feature of Cowden syndrome. A previously reported patient with Lhermite-Duclos disease, who had an affected son, died of metastatic breast carcinoma, also suggestive of Cowden disease.

Starink, Th.M., van der Veen, J.P.W., Arwert, F., de Waal, L.P., de Lange, G.G., Gille, J.J.P., and Eriksson, A.W. (1986). The Cowden syndrome: a clinical and genetic study in 21 patients. *Clin. Genet.* **29,** 222–233.

Review of literature and report of findings in four families and three sporadic cases. Excellent table listing features of the disorder. Failed to demonstrate linkage with HLA immunoglobulin haplotypes. Starink has written extensively on Cowden syndrome.

CYLINDROMATOSIS (MIM:123850, 313100)

(Multiple Cylindromas; Spiegler's Tumor; Nevoepithelioma Adenoides [Hoffmann]; Ancell-Spiegler Cylindromas; Epithelioma Adenoides Cysticum; Brooke-Fordyce Tumour; Turban Tumors)
Includes Multiple Trichoepitheliomas

DERMATOLOGIC FEATURES

Major. Multiple lesions are the hallmark of the inherited form of the cylindromas. Papules and nodules develop on the scalp and face, around the ears and neck, usually beginning at puberty and continuing to develop throughout life. They increase in size as well as number with age. Over time they can become progressively disfiguring. These dermal nodules can be pink, red, flesh-colored, or bluish. They are firm and may appear similar to hypertrophic scars or neurofibromas. They range in size from a few millimeters to centimeters in diameter. The face is involved less often than the scalp. The back and the chest are involved least often. There are few or no hair follicles present in the nodules. Necrosis of tumors can occur, and they can become odiferous.

Malignant degeneration, primarily to basal cell epitheliomas, occurs. It is difficult to estimate incidence from the literature, but it may be as high as 10% over a lifetime.

Minor. Trichoepitheliomas are reported in some patients (see Differential Diagnosis). These lesions tend to cluster around the nose.

One family has been reported with multiple milia in addition to trichoepitheliomas and cylindromas.

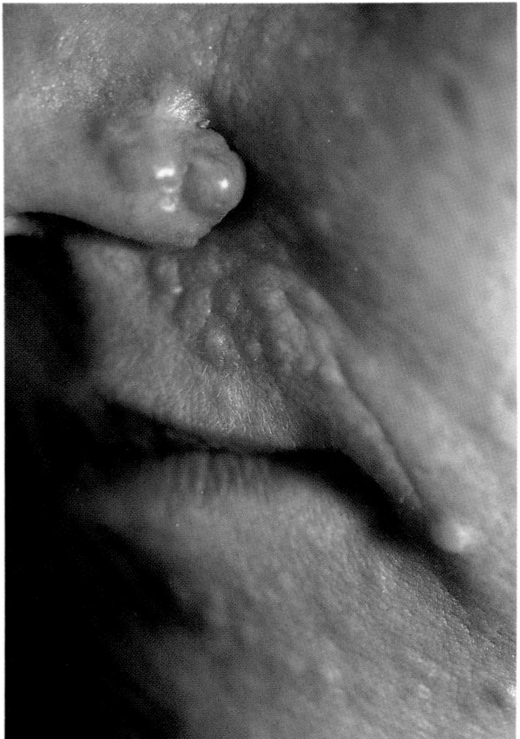

Figure 10.18. Facial lesions around the nostrils and on the cheek and chin.

ASSOCIATED ABNORMALITIES

In one patient with skin involvement, an additional isolated lesion of the lung was found at postmortem.

HISTOPATHOLOGY

Light. Unencapsulated dermal collection of cords and cylinders of basophilic epithelial cells, surrounded by and intercollated with a hyaline membrane. There is hyaline material within the cytoplasm of some cells. The pattern is described as a jigsaw puzzle, with the hyaline membrane separating the pieces.

EM. Two types of cells, one with few desmosomes, abundant heterochromatin, and a small nucleolus with light cytoplasm. The other has dark cytoplasm and an increased number of desmosomes. The hyaline material is granular.

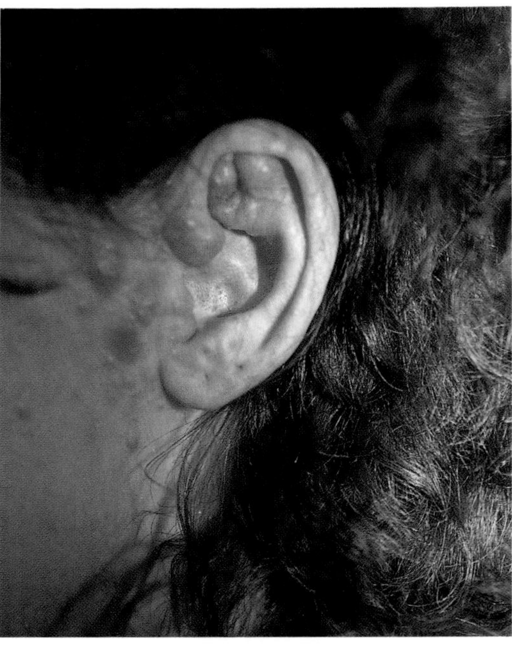

Figure 10.19. Nodules in pinna.

BASIC DEFECT

The origin of cylindromas remains a topic of debate. Some argue for eccrine origin, others

A

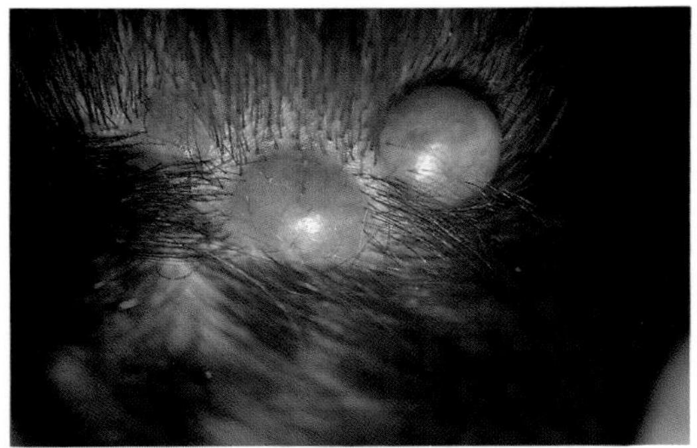

B

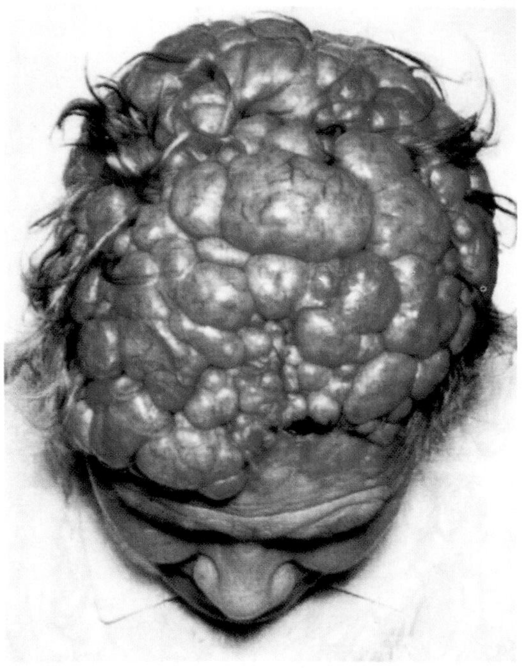

Figure 10.20. Mild **(A)** and severe **(B)** scalp involvement. (B, from Biggs et al., 1995, original courtesy of Dr. M. Stratton.)

for pilar precursors, others for apocrine derivatives.

TREATMENT

Surgical excision. One group recommended electrocoagulation for lesions greater than 1 cm and for multiple scalp lesions to preserve scalp and hair as long as possible. Scalping procedures have been performed for severely involved patients.

MODE OF INHERITANCE

Autosomal dominant. There has been male-to-male transmission. The expression may be more severe in females; this has not been proven. There may be less than 100% penetrance. The gene has been mapped to 16q12–q13.

PRENATAL DIAGNOSIS

None.

DIFFERENTIAL DIAGNOSIS

Multiple syringomas (MIM:186600) can look like trichoepitheliomas and small cylindromas. Histologically they are differentiated by absence of a hyaline capsule.

Hereditary trichoepitheliomas (MIM: 132700) (Brooke-Spiegler syndrome) may be a separate disorder, but some families with cylindromas have had multiple trichoepitheliomas as well, and it is unclear whether this represents a distinct entity versus variability in expression. Desmoplastic trichoepitheliomas (MIM:190345) may also be a distinct entity. The term *cylindroma* has also been used as a synonym for adenoid cystic carcinoma, which is an entirely different tumor and should not be confused with cylindromas of the skin. Some use the adjective *dermal* to define cylindromas involving the skin.

Clinically, the neurofibromas of neurofibromatosis (MIM:162200) could be confused. Café-au-lait spots, axillary freckling, and widespread distribution of lesions are not features of cylindromatosis. If neither history nor associated features lead to the correct diagnosis, biopsy easily distinguishes the lesions of cylindromatosis from other diagnostic considerations, including leukemia cutis, multiple trichoepitheliomas, and neurofibromas.

In basal cell nevus syndrome (MIM:109400), the basal cell nevi are smaller than the turban tumors of cylindromatosis, although initially trichoepitheliomas and basal cell epitheliomas might be confused. Biopsy findings and associated features will quickly differentiate between the two. In the older literature, the term *epithelioma adenoides cysticum* was applied to some cases of basal cell nevus syndrome.

The Rombo syndrome (MIM:180730) is also an autosomal dominant disorder comprised of vermiculate atrophoderma—a lacy pattern of icepick-like scarring of the face, hypotrichosis of the eyebrows, eyelashes, and secondary sexual hairs, distal and perioral cyanotic erythema and trichoepitheliomas, milia, and basal cell epitheliomas. Onset of features is in late childhood, and they are progressive.

Cowden syndrome (MIM:158350) is marked by multiple tricholemmomas, fibrocystic disease of the breast, gastrointestinal polyposis, and malignancy. The tricholemmomas can be distinguished histologically from trichoepitheliomas.

Support Group: SUPORT GROUP
N.O.R.D.
P.O. Box 8923
New Fairfield, CT 06812
1-800-999-6673

SELECTED BIBLIOGRAPHY

Delfino, M., D'Anna, F., Ianniello, S., and Donofrio, V. (1991). Multiple hereditary trichoepithelioma and cylindroma (Brooke-Spiegler syndrome). *Dermatologica* **183,** 150–153.

A mother with trichoepitheliomas and cylindromas, a daughter with trichoepitheliomas, a second affected daughter not examined. The authors suggest that the eponym Brooke-Spiegler be used for those families with multiple adnexal cell hamartomas.

Gaul, L.E. (1953). Heredity of multiple benign cystic epithelioma. *A.M.A. Arch. Dermatol. Syphilol.* **68,** 517–524.

This is a wonderful paper describing a large kindred in Indiana. The photos show multiple small tumors and in one patient a lesion similar to a cylindroma. The author also noted seborrheic dermatitis and milia in affected patients. The biopsy showed milium or trichoepithelioma. The author quietly alludes to the frustration in getting cooperation from family members who often failed their appointments for his study. The trials of clinical research!

Gerretsen, A.L., Beemer, F.A., Deenstra, W., Hennekam, F.A. M., and van Vloten, W.A. (1995). Familial cutaneous cylindromas: investigations in five generations of a family. *J. Am. Acad. Dermatol.* **33,** 199–206.

Extensive pedigree, follow-up to their 1993 report. Thirty affected members of a 237 member pedigree.

Gerretsen, A.L., van der Putte, S.C.J., Deenstra, W., and Van Vloten, W. A. (1993). Cutaneous cylindroma with malignant transformation. *Cancer* **72,** 1618–1623.

Authors suggest that malignant degeneration is much higher in the familial form of this tumor. They present two cases, a brother and a sister, and discuss 26 other cases reported in the literature.

Given, K., Pickrell, K., and Smith, D. (1977). Dermal cylindroma (turban tumor). Case report. *Plast. Reconstr. Surg.* **59:** 582–587.

Vernon, H.J., Olsen, E.A., and Vollmer, R.T. (1988). Autosomal dominant multiple cylindromas associated with solitary lung cylindroma. *J. Am. Acad. Dermatol.* **19:** 397–400.

Given et al. (1977) and Vernon et al. (1988) provide two reports of the same patient with different family history. In the Given et al. report, a sister is said to be affected and the parents unaffected. In the Vernon et al. report, the father and the sister are described as affected. In neither study did the authors examine relatives. The later report did not cite the earlier. A cautionary note to those of us who combine pedigrees to analyze mode of inheritance. Watch out for duplicates, and beware hearsay.

Irwin, L.R., Bainbridge, L.C., Reid, C.A., Piggot, T.A., and Brown, H.G. (1990). Dermal eccrine cylindroma (turban tumor). *Br. J. Plast. Surg.* **43,** 702–705.

An incredible pedigree. It puts to rest any question regarding X-linkage. Of one sibship with 11 members, 3 of 6 females and 2 of 5 males were affected. There is one instance of male-to-male transmission and one normal daughter born to an affected male. They also present a smaller pedigree with transmission to a daughter through an unaffected father whose sister was affected.

Munger, B.L., Graham, J.H., and Helwig, E.B. (1962). Ultrastructure and histochemical characteristics of dermal eccrine cylindroma (turban tumor). *J. Invest. Dermatol.* **39,** 577–595.

Three nodules from one patient were evaluated. There are many micrographs. The authors argue for eccrine origin.

Oikarinen, A., and Peltonen, L. (1985). Basement membrane components and keratin in the dominantly inherited form of cylindroma. *Acta Dermatol. Venereol. (Stockh.)* **65,** 121–125.

The hyaline membrane surrounding the cords of cells stains for type IV collagen, type V collagen, laminin, fibronectin, and proteoglycan. The authors use this to argue the epithelial origin of the tumors. They suggest that the disease could be used to study basement membrane metabolism. Others have shown the presence of both type I and type III collagen in the lesions.

Reynes, M., Puissant, A., Delanoe, J., Noury-Dupperat, G., and Saurat, J.H. (1976). Ultrastructural study of cylindromas (Poncet-Spiegler tumor). *J. Cutan. Pathol.* **3,** 95–101.

The described patient was a member of a four generation pedigree with five affected males. The authors found two cell types, both eccrine in appearance.

Welch, J.P., Wells, R.S., and Kerr, C.B. (1968). Ancell-Spiegler cylindromas (turban tumours) and Brooke-Fordyce trichoepitheliomas: evidence for a single genetic entity. *J. Med. Genet.* **5,** 29–35.

Authors present two large pedigrees and review of the literature. They discuss the overlap between trichoepitheliomas and cylindromas. They did not find evidence for a significant preponderance of affected females.

DYSPLASTIC NEVUS SYNDROME (MIM:155600)

(BK mole syndrome; FAMMM; Familial atypical multiple moles-melanoma; Familial atypical nevus syndrome)

Includes Familial Melanoma

DERMATOLOGIC FEATURES

MAJOR. That there are families with an increased risk for melanoma (with or without dysplastic nevi) is incontrovertible. That there are families with what appears to be an autosomal dominant condition characterized by multiple unusual-appearing moles in widespread distribution (with or without melanoma) is also uncontested. That there is an increased risk for melanoma in individuals with such moles, irrespective of a family history, also seems true. What is currently still poorly understood is the relationship among these—causal or coincidental.

The literature teems with vociferous arguments regarding nomenclature. *Dysplastic nevi* are so named because of their histologic pattern. *Atypical nevi* are so named because of their appearance clinically. The two do not always correspond. Some atypical moles have no dysplastic changes; some moles with dysplasia appear quite uniform clinically.

Classically, the atypical nevus is a fairly large lesion (≥5 mm) with both macular and palpable elements, variegation of pigment (tan, black, red, purple, or pink), and irregular margins. They are usually numerous and may number greater than 100. They usually vary one to the next in appearance. They are widely distributed, often in areas such as the buttocks, which typical moles usually shun. They tend to cluster on the trunk, lower extremities, and scalp. These nevi start to develop in childhood, but often do not assume their atypical appearance until puberty.

Malignancy may develop in a nevus or in normal skin in an individual with many nevi. The risk for melanoma may approach 50%–100% in a person with dysplastic nevi and two or more family members with melanoma. Peripubertal malignancy occurs rarely, prepubertal melanoma almost never. Multiple primary melanomas are common.

MINOR. None.

ASSOCIATED ABNORMALITIES

A few kindreds have been reported with an apparently increased rate of pancreatic carcinoma. There may be an increased risk for intraocular melanoma. The magnitude of the risk for tumors other than melanoma of the skin remains uncertain, and if there is an increased risk it appears to be limited to some families.

HISTOPATHOLOGY

LIGHT. Hotly debated. Melanocytic atypia (cells with hyperchromatic irregular large nuclei) with irregular proliferation at the dermoepidermal junction, architectural atypia, dermal fibrosis, and chronic lymphocytic infiltrate are typical. The rete ridges may be elongated, and there may be telangiectatic vessels.

EM. No information.

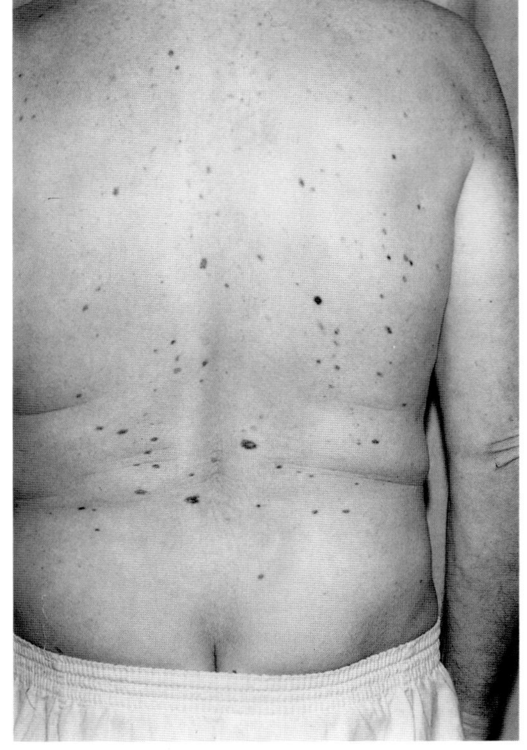

Figure 10.21. Many moles, varying in size and color.

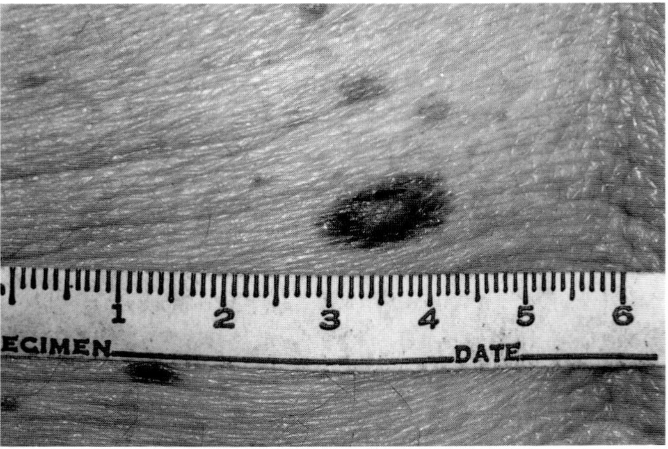

Figure 10.22. Close-up of lesion with macular and papular elements; variegation of pigment and irregular margins.

BASIC DEFECT

Unknown. Some studies suggest chromosomal instability upon exposure of cells to ultraviolet light.

TREATMENT

Good photographs to document size, placement, and appearance of lesions are useful for comparison during monthly self-examination and semiannual dermatologic examinations. Excision of lesions that are changing, rapidly growing, darkening, losing color, or bleeding is always warranted. Despite little compelling evidence that sunscreens reduce the rate of melanoma, given the association of sunlight with nevus formation and the uncertain role of ultraviolet light exposure as causal for melanoma, sunscreen use is still recommended. Sun avoidance and protective clothing are of primary importance. Examination of all first degree relatives should be recommended. Proband recall and historical information regarding relatives is unreliable. Children at risk should be examined initially and then again prior to, during, and after puberty. If they have not developed atypical moles by age 20, they are likely to remain unaffected, but still need to practice routine self-examination.

MODE OF INHERITANCE

Possibly autosomal dominant with variable expression and perhaps with reduced penetrance. Genetic heterogeneity has been inferred from disparate linkage data (some families appear to be linked to 9p21, but not all). The magnitude of the risk to develop malignant melanoma with a positive family history, irrespective of the presence of dysplastic nevi, is uncertain. Within dysplastic nevi families with malignant melanoma, the risk may approach 100% if dysplastic nevi are present in the individual. It is not clear that there is no risk for melanoma to individuals without dysplastic nevi in dysplastic nevus families. Instances of unaffected obligate carriers (no nevi, no melanoma, but affected parent and offspring) have been noted, as well as individuals with melanoma without nevi in dysplastic nevus families.

PRENATAL DIAGNOSIS

None.

DIFFERENTIAL DIAGNOSIS

It is the differentiation between a worrisome lesion and a benign lesion in patients with dysplastic nevi that is problematic, not any confusion between this condition and any other dermatosis.

Support Group: N.O.R.D.
P.O. Box 8923
New Fairfield, CT
06812
1-800-999-6673

SELECTED BIBLIOGRAPHY

Carey, W.P., Jr., Thompson, C.J., Synnestvedt, M., Guerry, D., Halperin, A., Schultz, D., and Elder, D. E. (1994). Dysplastic nevi as a melanoma risk factor in patients with malignant melanoma. *Cancer* **74,** 3118–3125.

Authors evaluated 710 members of 311 melanoma families (those having at least two relatives with melanoma). Rate of melanoma was almost sevenfold greater in family members with dysplastic nevi and a positive history of melanoma than in families with dysplastic nevi alone.

Hussussian, C.J., Struewing, J.P., Goldstein, A.M., Higgins, P.A.T., Ally, D.S., Sheahan, M.D., Clark, W.H., Jr., Tucker, M.A., and Dracopoli, N.C. (1994). Germline p16 mutations in familial melanoma. *Nat. Genet.* **8,** 15–21.

In families with dysplastic nevi and malignant melanoma within pedigrees, individuals with dysplastic nevi only did not have mutations in p16. Those with dysplastic nevi and malignant melanoma or malignant melanoma alone did.

This is a very confusing paper. It suggests to me that even within families where p16 mutations exist, there is another controlling element for the development of dysplastic nevi.

Salmon, J.A., Rivers, J.K., Donald, J.A., Shaw, H.M., McCarthy, W.H., and Kefford, R.F. (1992). Clinical aspects of hereditary melanoma in Australia. *Cytogenet. Cell Genet.* **59,** 170–172.

Eight pedigrees with familial melanoma fell into three groups: no dysplastic nevi, occasional dysplastic nevi, many dysplastic nevi. One of a series of papers in this issue of the journal describing the pedigrees comprising individual laboratory data sets. Statistically analyzes the relationship of moles to melanoma and linkage studies. The authors suggest that 5%–8% of melanomas occur in melanoma families.

Shapiro, P.E. (1992). Making sense of the dysplastic nevus controversy. A unifying perspective. *Am. J. Dermatopathol.* **14,** 350–356.

Two pages of contradictory statements culled from the literature regarding criteria for dysplastic nevi. The author does a nice job summarizing the utility of the concept despite the absence of definitive histopathologic features.

Skolnick, M.H., Cannon-Albright, L.A., and Kamb, A., (1994). Genetic predisposition to melanoma. *Eur. J. Cancer* **30A,** 1991–1995.

The authors argue that the initial linkage reported to 1p was specious and that linkage to 9p21 is clear. The candidate gene, *CDKN2* (aka *MTS1*), may only confer secondary risk. Penetrance appears to be higher in families with detectable *CDKN2* mutations.

Slade, J., Marghoob, A.A., Salopek, T.G., Rigel, D.S., Kopf, A.W., and Bare, R.S. (1995). Atypical mole syndrome: risk factor for cutaneous malignant melanoma and implications for management. *J. Am. Acad. Dermatol.* **32,** 479–494.

There are too many abbreviations (MM, RR, CAMS, AMS, NN, TCE, and so forth) to make for easy reading, but nonetheless the article outlines classification for risk for melanoma based on several factors (Rigel classification) and gives guidelines for management.

EPIDERMAL NEVUS (MIM:163200)

(Linear Epidermal Nevus Syndrome)

DERMATOLOGIC FEATURES

MAJOR. The term *epidermal nevus* has been applied to a spectrum of congenital lesions (although not always recognized at birth and not always developed to full extent) characterized by raised, hyperkeratotic, or verrucous (wart-like) yellow-brown lesions, sometimes with accompanying erythema, usually distributed along the lines of Blaschko. Lesions may have various components of sebaceous elements and keratotic elements and are usually devoid of hairs. When sebaceous elements predominate, the term *nevus sebaceous* (see separate entry) may be used; when hyperkeratosis is the major feature, *epidermal nevus* is the descriptor. It has been suggested that the term *organoid nevus* be used to reflect this overlap, and this may be the most appropriate term for those lesions for which a specific somatic mutation has not been identified.

Epidermal nevi may be small (solitary), widespread but confined to one side of the body (nevus unius lateris) or widespread and bilateral (systematized nevus), and occur in association with other structural abnormalities (epidermal nevus syndrome). These lesions often begin as flat or slightly raised, small, skin-colored to yellow plaques that gradually become more wart-like and darken. On the scalp, the absence of hair is very obvious. These nevi may become papillomatous and resemble an archipelago of brown papules. Lesions may not reach their full extent until late childhood. Extension after adolescence is very rare.

Malignant degeneration is less often reported in epidermal nevi than in sebaceous nevi, but has occurred.

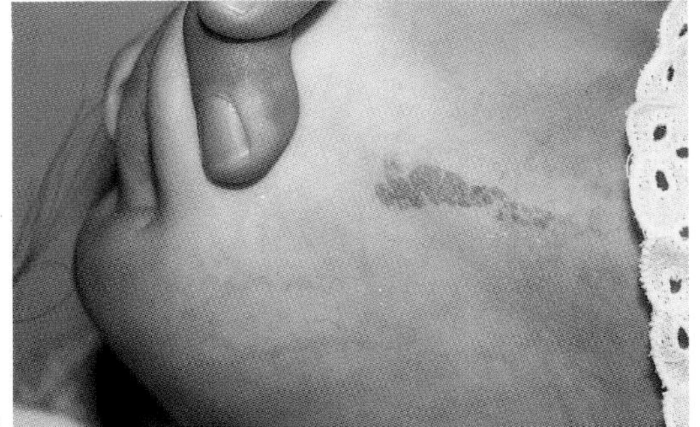

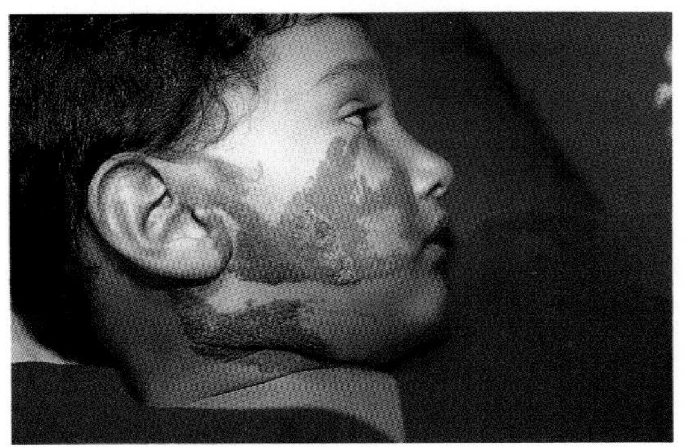

Figure 10.23. **(A)** Small nevus on face. **(B)** Large lesion involving second and third branches of the trigeminal nerve. The hyperkeratosis is not uniform.

MINOR. There may be oral involvement with nevus.

ASSOCIATED ABNORMALITIES

It is difficult to tease out from the literature the range of abnormalities associated with epidermal nevi versus that associated with sebaceous nevi.

Neurologic abnormalities include mental retardation, astrocytoma, cortical blindness, seizures, hemiparesis, quadriplegia, and cranial nerve abnormalities. Structural alterations in the brain are legion and include hemimegalencephaly and polymicrogyria. There appears to be an increased risk for central nervous system involvement if the nevus involves the head or is generalized.

Orthopedic alterations include hemiatrophy, hemihypertrophy, and macrodactyly. Three pa-

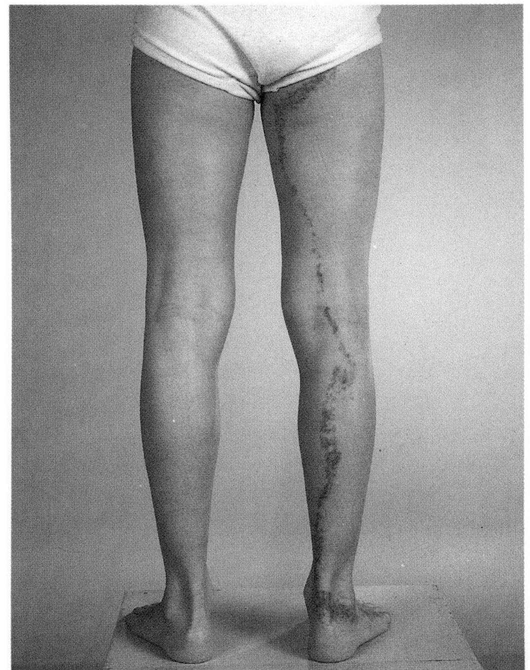

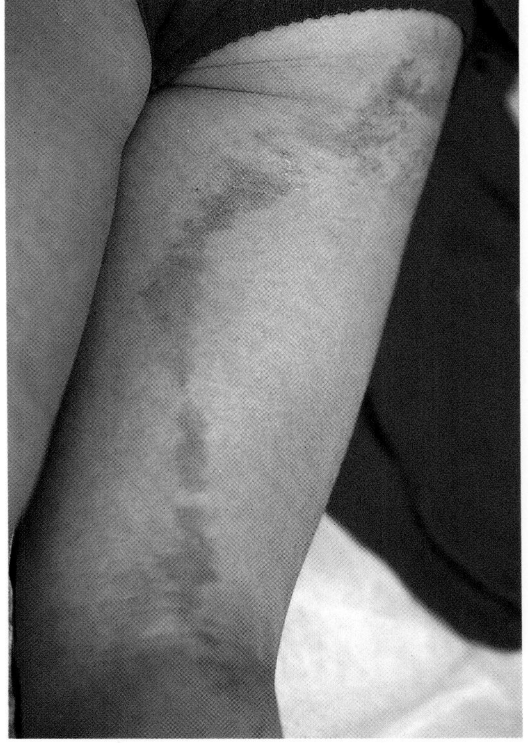

Figure 10.24. **(A)** Linear inflammatory verrucous epidermal nevus. **(B)** Acquired lesion of lichen striatus, clinically very similar.

tients with epidermal nevi have had polyostotic fibrous dysplasia.

Internal malignancies have also been reported. Eye abnormalities are more commonly associated with nevus sebaceous but have also been reported with epidermal nevi and include a variety of structural alterations.

HISTOPATHOLOGY

LIGHT. Hyperkeratosis, acanthosis, papillomatosis, and occasional parakeratosis. The histopathologic features are variable, and some lesions show epidermolytic hyperkeratosis, spongiosis, and vacuolization of basal and suprabasal keratinocytes. Abnormal hair follicles are typical. Histologic features may change with aging. Lesions of ILVEN are associated with an inflammatory infiltrate.

EM. Some lesions demonstrate alterations in keratohyaline granules.

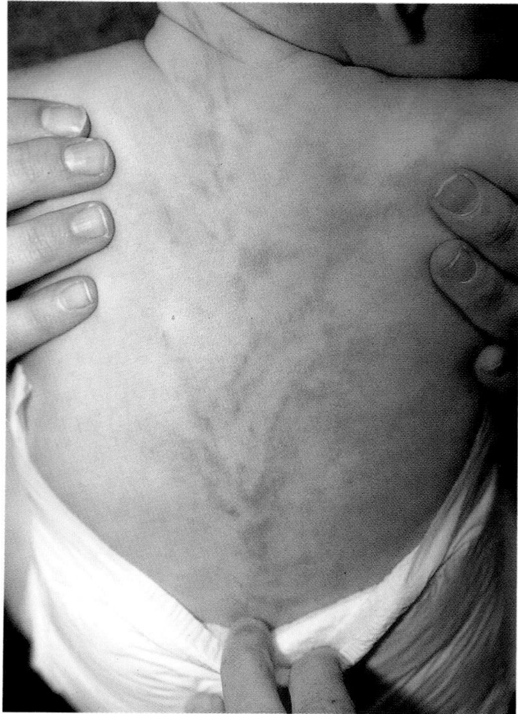

Figure 10.25. Widespread epidermal nevus along the lines of Blaschko. The patient is mosaic for a mutation in K_{10}. (Mutation analysis courtesy of Dr. A. Paller, Chicago, Illinois.)

BASIC DEFECT

In those lesions with epidermolytic hyperkeratosis, somatic mosaicism for mutations in keratin 1 (K_1) or keratin 10 (K_{10}) have been demonstrated. Presumably all forms of organoid nevi have the same causal mechanism, i.e., postzygotic mutation, albeit for different genes or alleles.

TREATMENT

5-Fluorouracil 5% and tretinoin 1% under occlusion bid has been reported by some to result in softening of the nevi. Surgical excision is problematic because there may be recurrence along surgical margins. Spontaneous resolution has been reported on rare occasions.

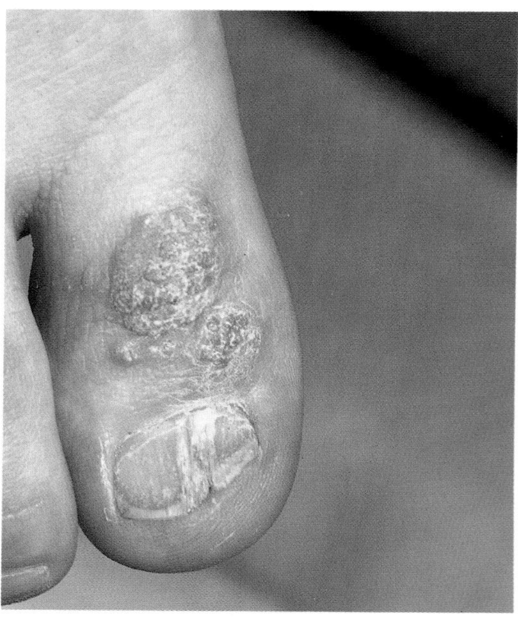

Figure 10.26. Small lesion, with nail dystrophy.

MODE OF INHERITANCE

Sporadic. Some epidermal nevi appear to result from somatic mosaicism for a recognized disorder. In a few instances, individuals with widespread epidermal nevus with epidermolytic hyperkeratosis have had offspring with bullous congenital ichthyosiform erythroderma. There have been rare reports of familial recurrence of localized lesions.

PRENATAL DIAGNOSIS

Potentially possible by molecular techniques for conceptions to individuals with epidermal nevi who are identified to have mosaicism for a specific mutation.

DIFFERENTIAL DIAGNOSIS

Lichen striatus is an acquired, self-limited condition comprised of small, discrete, confluent papules in a distribution along the lines of Blaschko, usually involving an extremity but possibly involving other areas. The papules may be lighter or darker than normal skin. The age of onset usually differentiates this condition clinically from epidermal nevi. Biopsy can confirm the diagnosis but should be unnecessary in most instances.

The lesions of ILVEN (inflammatory linear verrucous epidermal nevus) may be present at birth or may develop much later. They usually involve a limb and are intensely pruritic. There is hyperkeratosis on an erythematous base. Histologically they show chronic psoriasiform or eczematous changes and an inflammatory infiltrate. Laser therapy has been used with some success in inflammatory linear verrucous epidermal nevi.

In unilateral linear Darier-White disease (MIM:124200), lesions are often more waxy and greasy in appearance. Biopsy will show acantholysis and dyskeratosis, the features of Darier disease. The mechanism here is presumably the same as that for the epidermolytic hyperkeratotic epidermal nevus in that there has been a postzygotic mutation for the disorder.

Support Group: F.I.R.S.T.
P.O. Box 20921
Raleigh, NC 27619
1-800-545-3286

SELECTED BIBLIOGRAPHY

Pack, G.T., and Sunderland, D.A. (1941). Naevus unius lateris. *Ann. Surg.* **43,** 341–375.

Presents four cases. One patient who was treated repeatedly with radiation and excision of a lesion on the breast, chest, and thighs subsequently developed "mammary carcinoma" and died at age 23 years. A second patient died of gastric carcinoma without radiation treatment. A third had spontaneous malignant degeneration of the nevus. There is an exhaustive review of earlier reports of nevi, clearly including many different types and extent of organoid nevi. This paper convinced me that the term *nevus unius lateris* is probably not useful.

Paller, A.S., Syder, A.J., Chan, Y.-M., Yu, Q.-C., Hutton, E., Tadini, G., and Fuchs, E. (1994). Genetic and clinical mosaicism in a type of epidermal nevus. *N. Engl. J. Med.* **331,** 1408–1415.

Three patients with widespread and epidermal nevi had offspring with bullous congenital ichthyosiform erythroderma. Mutational analysis showed there to be alterations in K_1 or K_{10}, germline in the offspring, and mosaic in the progenitors. Biopsy specimens from all lesions showed epidermolytic hyperkeratosis.

Rogers, M., McCrossin, I., and Commens, C. (1989). Epidermal nevi and the epidermal nevus syndrome. *J. Am. Acad. Dermatol.* **20,** 476–488.

Rogers, M. (1992). Epidermal nevi and the epidermal nevus syndromes: a review of 233 cases. *Pediatr. Dermatol.* **9,** 342–344.

The term *epidermal nevi* refers to sebaceous nevi (104), keratinocytic nevi (125), and follicular nevi (4). Rogers et al. (1989) review 171 patients in detail. Rogers (1992) added another 102 cases and a discussion of mosaicism.

Solomon, L.M., and Esterly, N.B. (1975). Epidermal and other congenital organoid nevi. *Curr. Probl. Pediatr.* **6(1),** 3–56.

This is an all-time comprehensive review and thoughtful discussion of the overlap among the histologic features of epidrmal/sebaceous/comedonal nevi. The authors prefer the term *organoid nevus* and present cogent arguments for its use. Although I think there is utility in using distinct terms to describe lesions more typical of one or another of these nevi, conceptually I agree that they represent a continuum subsumed within the term *organoid*.

Su, W.P.D. (1982). Histopathologic varieties of epidermal nevus. A study of 160 cases. *Am. J.* Dermatopathol. **4,** 161–170.

This is a Mayo Clinic review. Eight of 167 lesions showed epidermolytic hyperkeratosis. Two of the 167 were porokeratotic, and two showed Darier-like changes. This underscores that clinically similar epidermal nevi may have different histopathologic features.

GARDNER SYNDROME (MIM:175100)

(Intestinal Polyposis With Jaw Cysts)

DERMATOLOGIC FEATURES

MAJOR. From 50% to 60% of patients will develop multiple soft to firm subcutaneous masses. Most will prove to be epidermal cysts; some are fibromas. These lesions commonly appear during childhood and puberty and involve the trunk, scalp, and extremities.

MINOR. Desmoid tumors are proliferations of fibrous and muscle tissue and most often occur at sites of scars. They are reported in about 25% of individuals with Gardner syndrome. The term *desmoid* comes from the band-like appearance of the tissue seen histologically. Fibrous overgrowth in response to surgery can also occur and may also result in intestinal or ureteral obstruction.

Lipomas have been reported in some reviews, but these have not been confirmed histologically.

ASSOCIATED ABNORMALITIES

Osteomas are multiple irregular bony masses that occur most frequently in the mandible. These may result in facial distortion. They can also develop in the maxilla, the skull, and the long bones.

Intestinal polyposis develops during the teen years. Malignant degeneration occurs in 100% of affected colons. The small intestine and duodenum may also have polyps that have malignant potential. The polyps are multiclonal. Periampullary adenocarcinoma has been reported.

Tooth abnormalities include supernumerary teeth and failure of tooth eruption.

Hypertrophy of the retinal pigment epithelium, which appears as dark brown to black patches, can be seen on funduscopic examination. These changes are asymptomatic. Hypertrophy of the retinal pigment epithelium occurring outside the setting of Gardner syndrome is most often unilateral; in Gardner syndrome the findings are bilateral. This change in the retina is believed to be present at birth and may be used as a screening tool for asymptomatic carriers.

Thyroid carcinoma has occurred in patients

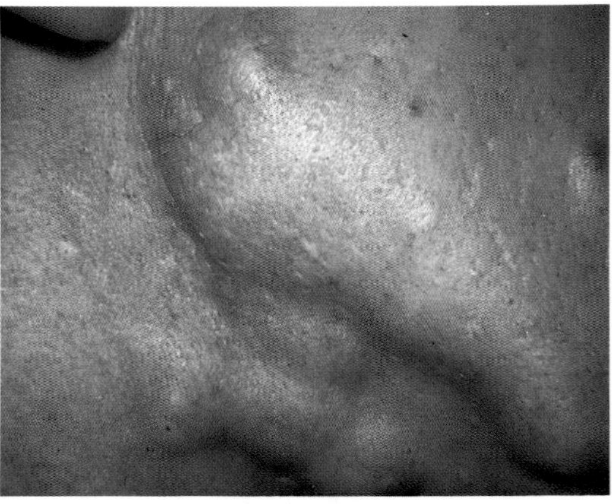

Figure 10.27. Multiple epidermal inclusion cysts on neck. (Courtesy of Dr. J. Halloran, Division of Dermatology, University of Washington.)

with Gardner syndrome and with familial polyposis coli more often than would be expected by chance alone. Hepatoblastoma has been reported in a few patients with Gardner syndrome, as have a host of other malignancies.

HISTOPATHOLOGY

LIGHT. The intestinal lesions are adenomatous polyps.

The epidermal inclusion cysts are lined by epithelial cells. Areas may show features of pilomatricomas with shadow cells that project into the lumen or typical changes of epidermoid cysts or both.

EM. No information.

BASIC DEFECT

Mutations in the gene *APC* have been found. The function of the protein for which it codes is still unknown.

TREATMENT

Screening beginning at age 5 years for polyps. When polyps are present, colectomy is the treatment of choice, with follow-up examinations of other at-risk intestinal sites throughout life.

Sulindac (Clinoral) has been reported to result in regression of colonic polyps in patients with Gardner syndrome. It does not obviate the need for colectomy.

Surgical excision of desmoids is the treatment of choice despite 50% recurrence rate after surgery. Tamoxifen and interferon-α have been reported useful in a few isolated reports.

MODE OF INHERITANCE

Autosomal dominant with 100% penetrance and variable expression. The allelic nature of familial polyposis coli and Gardner syndrome has been proven by mutation analysis. It is still uncertain whether the Gardner syndrome phenotype is associated with specific mutations or if the extra-colonic features are due to factors unrelated to the *APC* mutation. The term familial adenomatous polyposis (FAP) is now considered to apply to both. The gene maps to 5q21-q22.

PRENATAL DIAGNOSIS

Possible by linkage in informative families.

DIFFERENTIAL DIAGNOSIS

Multiple intestinal polyps and skin findings are also a feature of Peutz-Jeghers syndrome, (MIM:175200), which is distinguished by the presence of multiple lentigines and a low risk for malignant degeneration of the intestinal polyps. Patients with Turcot syndrome (MIM: 276300) and Cowden syndrome (MIM:158350) in which central nervous system tumors, especially medulloblastomas, are found, may also have intestinal polyposis. The skin changes of acrokeratoses and facial papules in these two conditions are distinctive.

Multiple epidermal cysts (MIM:131600) can occur as an isolated dominant condition. Bony overgrowth of the jaw occurs in cherubism (MIM:118400), and odontogenic cysts of the jaw occur in the basal cell nevus syndrome (MIM:109400). Again, the associated abnormalities easily distinguish all of these disorders.

Intestinal polyps are reported in the Bannayan-Riley-Ruvalcaba syndrome (MIM: 153480). This disorder can be distinguished from Gardner syndrome by the presence of penile pigmentation and macrocephaly. These patients lack the epidermoid cysts and bony changes of Gardner syndrome. Birt-Hogg-Dubé (MIM:135150) is a rare autosomal dominant disorder with perifollicular fibromas, acrochordons, and trichodiscomas. A few patients have had a few colonic polyps.

Support Group: Familial Gastrointestinal Registry
600 University Avenue, No. 1157

Toronto, Ontario,
Canada M5G 1X5
1-416-586-8334

Intestinal Multiple
Polyposis and
Colorectal Cancer
(IMPACC)
P.O. Box 11
Conyngham, PA 18219
1-717-788-3712

SELECTED BIBLIOGRAPHY

Gardner, E.J. (1972). Discovery of the Gardner syndrome. *Birth Defects* **8(2),** 48–51.

This review of the history of the discovery and evaluation of the Utah kindred first reported by the author is an interesting read. The bibliography cites his prior publications.

Giardello, F.M., Hamilton, S.R., Krush, A.J., Piantadosi, S., Hylind, L.M., Celano, P., Booker, S.V., Robinson, C.R., and Offerhaus, G.J. (1993). Treatment of colonic and rectal adenomas with Sulindac in familial adenomatous polyposis. *N. Engl. J. Med.* **328,** 1313–1316.

A double-blind placebo-controlled study of 22 patients with 150 mg of Sulindac bid for 9 months. During the 9 months of treatment, polyps decreased in number and size in the treatment group; after 3 months of no treatment, slow regrowth was seen. Responses were reported as percent of change from baseline, and number of polyps at baseline was two times greater in the placebo group. The authors concluded that the drug probably is useful, but does not replace colectomy.

Groden, J., Thliveris, A., Samovitz, W., Carlson, M., Gelbert, L., Albertson, H., Joslyn, G., Stevens, J., Spirio, L., Robertson, M., Sargeant, L., Krapcho, K., Wolff, E., Burt, R., Hughes, J.P., Warrington, J., McPherson, J., Wasmuth, J., Le Paslier, D., Abderrahim, H., Cohen, D., Leppert, M., and White, R. (1991). Identification and characterization of the familial adenomatous polyposis gene. *Cell* **66,** 589–600.

The authors found two patients with stop codon mutations and two with deletions leading to frameshift mutations in patients with familial adenomatous polyposis. One individual transmitted the gene to two of his three offspring. Confirmation that these offspring also have the disorder is absent.

Krush, A.J., Traboulsi, E.I., Offerhaus, J.A., Maumanee, I.H., Yardley, J.H., and Levin, L.S. (1988). Hepatoblastoma, pigmented ocular fundus lesions and jaw lesions in Gardner syndrome. *Am. J. Med. Genet.* **29,** 323–332.

Report of five cases of infants and children with hepatoblastoma and a family history of Gardner syndrome. The authors recommend evaluating first degree relatives of children with hepatoblastoma for signs of Gardner syndrome.

Rongioletti, F., Hazini, R., Gianotti, G., and Rebora, A. (1989). Fibrofolliculomas, tricodiscomas and acrochordons (Birt-Hogg-Dubé) associated with intestinal polyposis. *Clin. Exp. Dermatol.* **14,** 72–74.

An individual with Birt-Hogg-Dubé disease who had a few colonic polyps. Authors propose the polyps are part of the disorder.

Shields, J.A., Shields, C.L., Shah, P.G., Pastore, D.J., and Imperiale, S.M. Jr. (1992). Lack of association among typical congenital hypertrophy of the retinal pigment epithelium, adenomatous polyposis and Gardner syndrome. *Ophthalmology* **99,** 1709–1713.

One hundred thirty-two individuals with congenital hypertrophy of the retinal pigment epithelium were evaluated. None had intestinal polyposis by history. The authors detail the differences in appearance between isolated congenital hypertrophy of the retinal pigment epithelium and that associated with familial adenomatous polyposis.

Traboulsi, E.I., Krush, A.J., Gardner, E.J., Booker, S.V., Offerhaus, G.J.A., Yardley, J.H., Hamilton, S.R., Luk, G.D., Giardiello, F.M., Welsh, S.B., Hughes, J.P., and Maumanee, I.H. (1987). Prevalence and importance of pigmented ocular fundus lesions in Gardner's syndrome. *N. Engl. J. Med.* **316,** 661–667.

One hundred thirty-four family members (41 affected, 43 at 50% risk, 30 second degree or greater relatives, and 20 spouses) from 16 families with Gardner syndrome were examined for retinal pigmentation, as were an additional 22 controls. Five percent of controls had bilateral pigment changes; one-third of these were unilateral. Eighty percent of affected individuals had bilateral lesions; 12% had unilateral lesions. The authors concluded that in at-risk individuals, large pigmented lesions were diagnostic, but one or two small peripheral lesions were not.

HEREDITARY KERATOACANTHOMAS (MIM:132800)

(Ferguson-Smith Syndrome; Molluscum Sebaceum; Self-healing Squamous Epitheliomas)
Includes Muir-Torre Syndrome

DERMATOLOGIC FEATURES

MAJOR. Starting as red macules, rapidly growing nodules develop on any skin surface, especially the face, ears, scalp, forearms, and legs. The lesions appear and grow over 1–2 months and then resolve over 4–6 months. Most lesions develop central ulceration or crust with rolled borders and undermining of the edges. As these regress and spontaneously heal, they leave crater-like scars on the face and neck. Flatter, finer scars occur on the extremities. Onset has been reported as early as the teen years and as late as the mid-fifties, with the median age of onset in the twenties. The rate of spontaneous resolution may decrease with age.

Open comedones are described as "common" in these patients. No affected individual has died from cutaneous malignancy.

MINOR. Rarely, lesions can develop on the mucosal surfaces. Itching of lesions was described in one sibling pair.

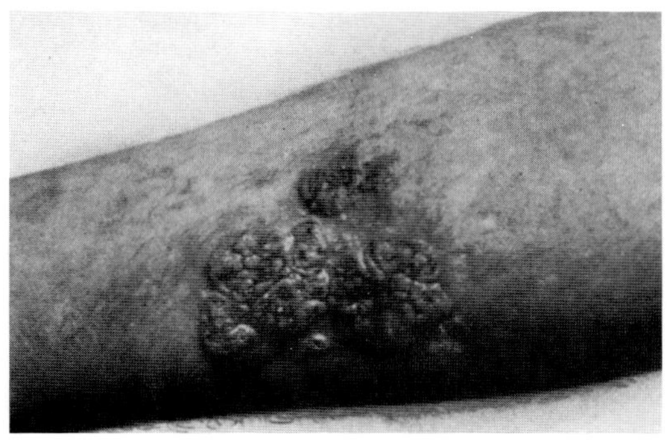

Figure 10.28. Active lesions in plaque on arm. (From Ferguson Smith, 1934.)

ASSOCIATED ABNORMALITIES

None.

HISTOPATHOLOGY

LIGHT. Well-differentiated squamous cell carcinoma with few mitoses, fully keratinized nests of cells, necrosis, invaginations with kera-

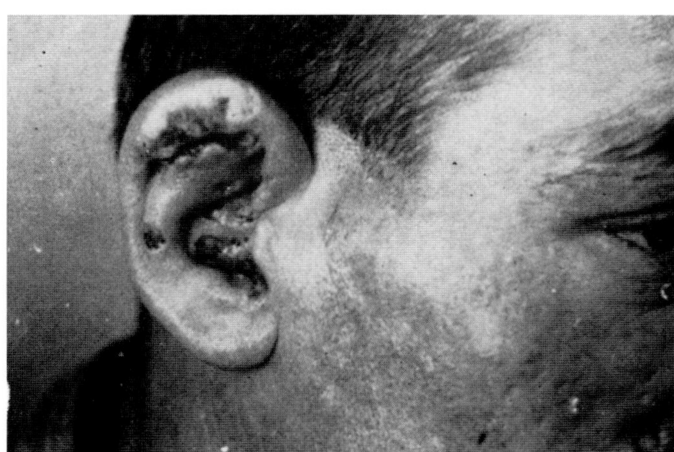

Figure 10.29. Lesions on pinnae in various stages. Scars on cheeks at sites of previous nodules. (From Charteris, 1951.)

tin plugs, and columnar epithelial infiltrates can be seen in the dermis.

EM. No evidence for viral particles has been shown.

BASIC DEFECT

Unknown. Sites of predilection support the role of sun exposure.

TREATMENT

Natural resolution or excision. Tumors are said to recur rarely after surgical removal, but excision may cause more scarring than natural resolution. Radiation therapy is to be avoided on the supposition that these patients may be more likely to develop malignancy, despite lack of spontaneous malignant degeneration. Unless the correct diagnosis can be established by history, biopsy and treatment for squamous cell carcinoma are obligatory, as it is impossible to distinguish between these self-healing lesions and squamous cell carcinoma. Thus, most patients with this condition will undergo several rounds of treatment before correct diagnosis is established.

MODE OF INHERITANCE

Autosomal dominant. The gene has been mapped to 9q22–q31.

PRENATAL DIAGNOSIS

None.

DIFFERENTIAL DIAGNOSIS

The multiplicity of lesions helps to distinguish the keratoacanthomas of this disorder from acquired squamous cell carcinoma, wart, and keratoacanthoma. Individuals with atrophoderma vermiculatum (MIM:209700) and healed lesions of acne vulgaris have similar scarring

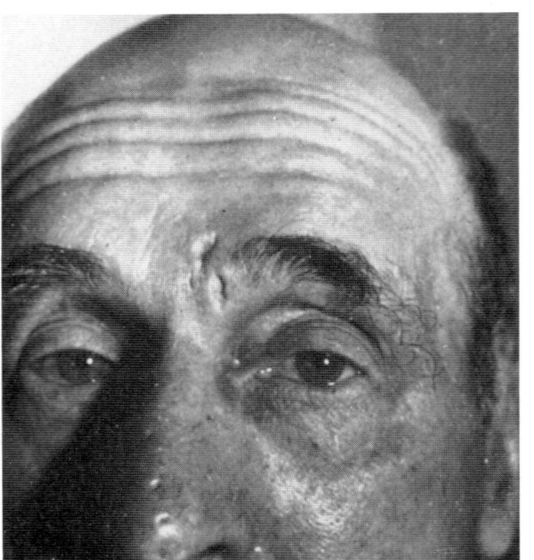

A

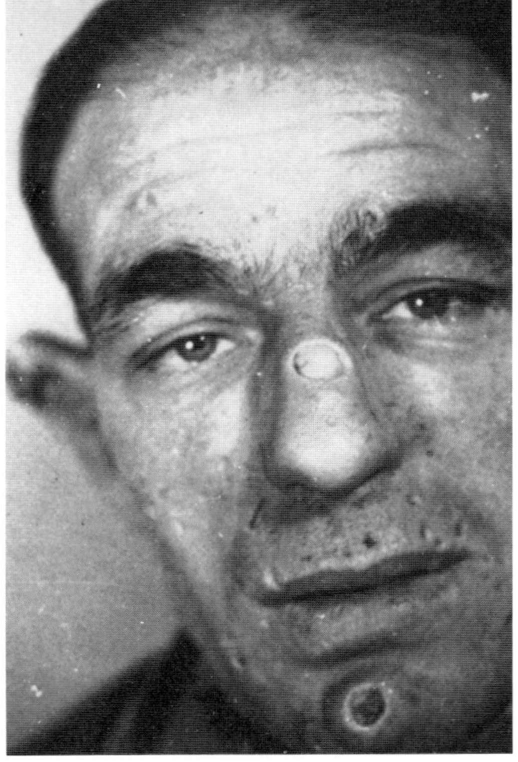

B

Figure 10.30. Scars from self healing **(A)** versus scars from surgical excision **(B).** (From Charteris, 1951.)

and comedones of the face, but do not have involvement elsewhere, do not have spontaneous healing, and do not show squamous cell carcinoma changes on biopsy.

There are occasional descriptions of multiple self-healing keratoacanthomas appearing in injured skin in otherwise normal individuals. In Muir-Torre syndrome (MIM:158320) multiple keratoacanthomas develop in association with internal malignancies, usually of the gastrointestinal tract. The age of onset is usually in late adult life. Spontaneous healing of the skin lesions is not described. Other skin tumor types, including basal cell epitheliomas, sebaceous carcinomas, and sebaceous adenomas, have also been reported in Muir-Torre, and the condition has been described in some members of a subset of "cancer families."

Support Group: N.O.R.D.
P.O. Box 8923
New Fairfield, CT
06812
1-800-999-6673

SELECTED BIBLIOGRAPHY

Currie, A.R., and Ferguson Smith, J. (1952). Multiple primary spontaneous-healing squamous cell carcinomata of the skin. *J. Pathol. Bacteriol.* **64,** 827–839.

In follow-up of original patients reported in 1951, the authors found an additional affected first cousin related through an unaffected parent. There are extensive histologic plates.

Ferguson-Smith, M.A., Wallace, D.C., James, Z.H., and Renwick, J.H. (1971). Multiple self-healing squamous epithelioma. *Birth Defects* **XII(8),** 157–163.

Ferguson Smith's son, Ferguson-Smith, acquired a hyphen and described 11 families with 62 individuals, including both of the original Ferguson Smith (no hyphen) pedigrees. At least one instance of an unaffected gene carrier, a healthy 57-year-old woman with an affected daughter, brother, and nephews.

Goudie, D.R., Yuille, M.A.R., Leversha, M.A., Furlong, R.A., Carter, N.P., Lush, M.J., Affara, N.A., and Ferguson-Smith, M.A. (1993). Multiple self-healing squamous epitheliomata (*ESSI*) mapped to chromosome 9q22–q31 in families with common ancestry. *Nat. Genet.* **3,** 165–169.

Linkage analysis in 13 families, all from west central Scotland. Gave a lod score of 9.02 at a recombination fraction of 0.03 for a region on 9q.

Hall, N.R., Williams, M.A.T., Murday, V.A., Newton, J.A., and Bishop, D.T. (1994). Muir-Torre syndrome: a variant of the cancer family syndrome. *J. Med. Genet.* **31,** 627–631.

The phenotype of Muir-Torre—the occurrence of multiple cutaneous tumors coupled with internal malignancy—appears to be an inconstant feature in some cancer families. Of 15 family members with cancer, one had actinic keratoses, one had multiple basal cell carcinomas and sebaceous epithelioma, and one had multiple sebaceous adenomas and keratoacanthoses. Twelve had no significant skin changes.

Haydey, R.P., Reed, M.L., Dzubow, L.M., and Shupack, J.L. (1980). Treatment of keratoacanthomas with oral 13-cis-retinoic acid. *N. Engl. J. Med.* **303,** 560–562.

Case report of an atypical patient with persistent, nonhealing, debilitating keratoacanthomas who responded to oral retinoids. In their introductory paragraph, the authors state that familial keratoacanthomas fail to resolve spontaneously and recur rapidly after excision, neither of which statement is supported by the literature.

Schwartz, R.A., Flieger, D.N., and Sared, N.K. (1980). The Torre syndrome with gastrointestinal polyposis. *Arch. Dermatol.* **116,** 312–314.

Case report of an elderly male with adenocarcinoma of the bowel in the setting of colonic polyposis. Authors review other cases and propose a possible association. They allude to a familial risk for Torre syndrome.

INFANTILE MYOFIBROMATOSIS (MIM:228550)

(Congenital Generalized Fibromatosis)

DERMATOLOGIC FEATURES

Major. Infantile myofibromatosis is divided into three categories: solitary, multicentric, and multicentric with visceral involvement. All three can be seen recurring in families.

The conditions are marked by the development of firm, discrete, sometimes flesh colored but usually more purplish nodules that develop in the skin, underlying muscle, or subcutaneous tissue. They range in size from half to several centimeters in diameter and may number from a few to a hundred.

One half of reported cases involve isolated lesions. They are usually benign with a good prognosis and spontaneous resolution. A third of reported cases have multicentric lesions without visceral involvement. These also show spontaneous resolution and a low rate of recurrence after surgical resection. The term *multiple myofibromatosis* is used by some to indicate disease limited to the skin only, reserving the term *generalized* for those with visceral involvement. The remaining one-sixth of patients have multiple lesions with visceral involvement, and the course in these patients can be fatal.

Minor. None.

ASSOCIATED ABNORMALITIES

Visceral involvement is the leading cause of death. Both the cardiopulmonary system and the gastrointestinal tract can be involved. One patient developed obstruction of the bile duct by a myofibroma.

Involvement of the skeleton with lytic areas in the metaphyses of the long bones is a feature of the systemic disease. These lesions are often symmetric. The flat bones—pelvis, ribs and scapulae—may also be involved. No organ is invariably spared in this condition. There are rare reports of myofibromas developing in the brain.

Death is usually due to secondary consequences: pneumonia or respiratory obstruction. Spontaneous resolution of visceral involvement has been reported.

HISTOPATHOLOGY

Light. Plump and spindle-shaped cells grouped in bundles or fascicles at the periphery of lesions surround areas of necrosis and calcification with immature spindle cells. There is an increased number of mitoses and an increase in the number of vessels.

EM. There is a fibroblastic-like appearance of the cells with irregular nuclei; there are bundles of myofilaments within which focal densities appear.

BASIC DEFECT

Unknown.

TREATMENT

Spontaneous resolution is typical of solitary and multicentric lesions. Surgical excision is sometimes required for rapidly growing, locally destructive lesions or those that are obstructive. The value of chemotherapy in visceral disease is uncertain.

MODE OF INHERITANCE

Uncertain. The disorder is rare, and familial occurrences are even rarer. Affected cousins, half-siblings, and parent–offspring pairs have all been reported.

A 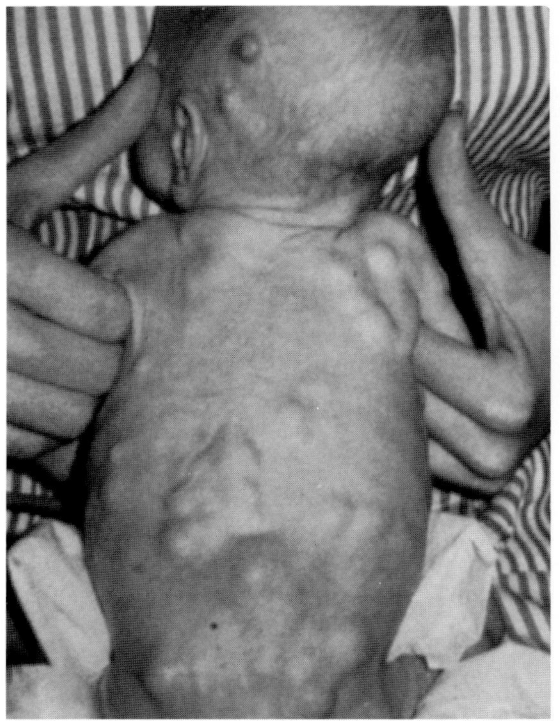

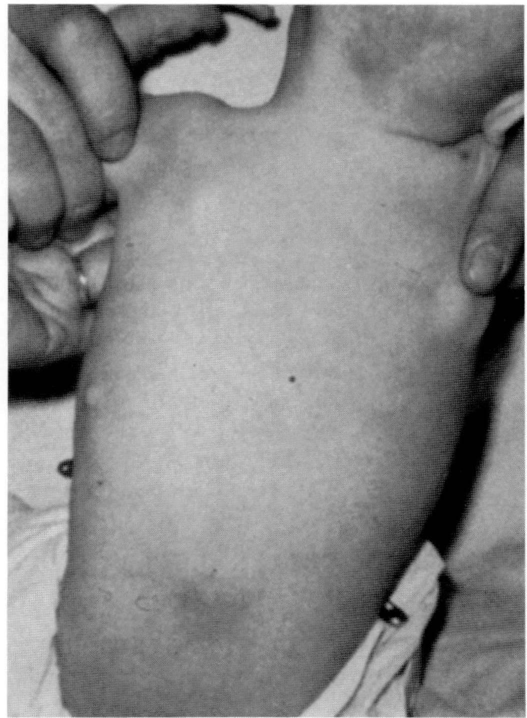 B

Figure 10.31. **(A)** At age 1 month multiple nodules are evident. **(B)** Almost complete regression by 1 year. (From Schaffzin et al., 1972.)

PRENATAL DIAGNOSIS

No information.

DIFFERENTIAL DIAGNOSIS

The nodules themselves may be mistaken for deep hemangiomas or cutaneous malignancy, other infiltrative lesions, fibrous hamartomas, hyaline fibromatosis, and neurofibromas. Biopsy will differentiate. Histologically, lesions in the generalized form of the disorder can be confused with fibrosarcomas.

Support Group: N.O.R.D.
P.O. Box 8923
New Fairfield, CT 06812
1-800-999-6673

SELECTED BIBLIOGRAPHY

Bracko, M., Cindro, L., and Gouloh, R. (1992). Familial occurrence of infantile myofibromatosis. *Cancer* **69,** 1294–1299.

Two brothers presented at birth. New lesions appeared throughout childhood. The authors review 10 pedigrees to date, two with two or more involved generations, seven with affected siblings or cousins, one with affected half-siblings. No pedigree showed male-to-male transmission. In some families just skin was involved; in some, skin and bone; in some, skin, bone, and viscera. There was also variability within families. This reference includes all previous familial reports except for that of Nasr et al. (1986).

Goldberg, N.S., Bauer, B.S., Kraus, H., Crussi, F.G., and Esterly, N.B. (1988). Infantile myofibromatosis: a review of clinical pathology with perspectives in new treatment choices. *Pediatr. Dermatol.* **5,** 37–46.

A useful table of the fibromatoses of childhood.

Jennings, T.A., Duray, P.H., Collins, F.S., Sabetta, J., and Enzinger, F.M. (1984). Infantile myofibromatosis. Evidence for an autosomal-dominant disorder. *Am. J. Surg. Pathol.* **8,** 529–538.

A father with a congenital lesion removed from the neck at day 6 developed a new lesion under the tongue at age 25 years. His newborn daughter manifested multiple skin and bony tumors.

Nasr, A.M., Blodi, F.C., Lindahl, S., and Jenkins, J. (1986). Congenital generalized multicentric myofibromatosis with orbital involvement. *Am. J. Ophthalmol.* **102,** 779–787.

The focus of the paper is on surgical management. The familial occurrence of this condition was noted in passing. Three first cousins were affected in a Saudi Arabian family. There was no mention of consanguinity.

Venenci, P.Y., Bigel, P., Desgruelles, C., Lortat-Jacob, S., Dufier, J.L., and Saurat, J.H. (1987). Infantile myofibromatosis. Report of two cases in one family. *Br. J. Dermatol.* **117,** 255–259.

Bone and skin involvement with spontaneous resolution in two siblings. Three other siblings were normal. There was no consanguinity.

MULTIPLE ENDOCRINE NEOPLASIA TYPES 2A/2B (MIM:162300, 171400)

(MEN IIa/IIb; MEN III; Froboese Syndrome)

There are three syndromes that are identified by the term *multiple endocrine neoplasia* (MEN). MEN 1 has no skin findings. MEN 2A (medullary thyroid carcinoma, parathyroid hyperplasia, and pheochromocytoma) is also usually without skin manifestations, although some pedigrees with cutaneous amyloidosis have been discussed. MEN 2B or MEN 3 is characterized by multiple neuromas of the mucosae in addition to medullary thyroid carcinoma and pheochromocytoma without parathyroid disease.

DERMATOLOGIC FEATURES

Major. The mucosal neuromas typically develop within the first year of life and result in a thickened, blubbery, or irregular appearance to the lips. The oral mucosa, tongue, eyelids and conjunctiva may also be involved. The lesions are shiny, yellow to flesh-colored papules and nodules.

Minor. Localized pruritis of the upper back is a symptom associated with the cutaneous amyloidosis reported in a subset of families with MEN 2A. The area may be raised, thickened, pigmented, and scaly. These may be secondary changes due to chronic scratching. At least two patients with MEN 2B have been described with perioral or periocular lentigines, freckles, or hyperpigmentation. In one of these it appeared to be the consequence of thyroid disease, as the skin changes disappeared after thyroidectomy.

One patient in one report had multiple café-au-lait spots. Other individuals have been reported to have one or two.

ASSOCIATED ABNORMALITIES

A marfanoid appearance with asthenic habitus, pectus excavatum, scoliosis, and muscle wasting is typical of individuals with MEN 2B. Pes cavus, rather than pes planus, is often described and is likely due to peroneal muscle weakness. Generalized hypotonia and distal muscle wasting and weakness with abnormal electromyographic and nerve conduction velocity studies are common. The symptoms and signs may go

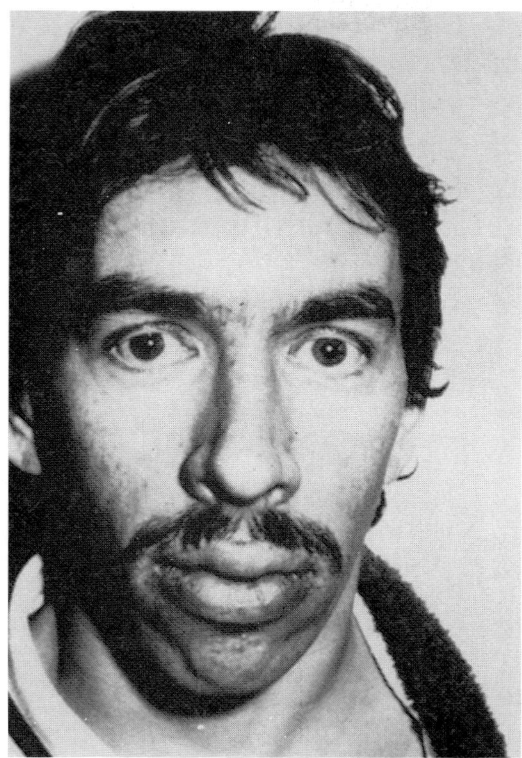

Figure 10.32. Full lips and elongated slender face. (From Fryns and Chrzanowska, 1988.)

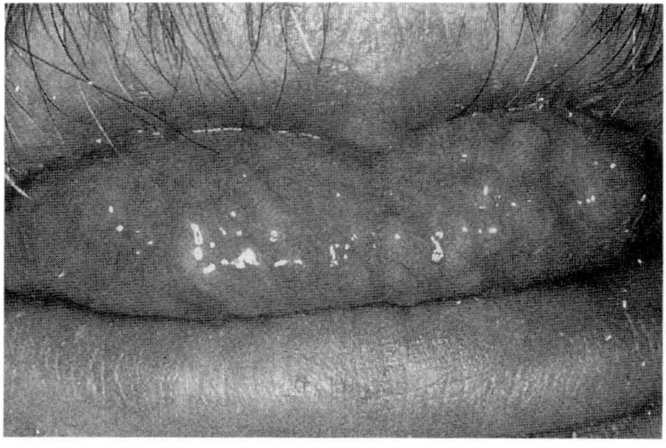

Figure 10.33. Neuromas on tongue. (From Kirk et al., 1991.)

unrecognized by the physician because of mild degree unless specifically sought.

Ganglioneuromas of the gastrointestinal tract are typical, if not universal, and gastrointestinal symptoms of colic, cramping, and bowel irregularities are common in childhood.

Focal or general hyperplasia of the C cells of the thyroid precedes development of medullary thyroid carcinoma and may be present in very early childhood. Medullary thyroid carcinoma is the most common tumor of both MEN 2A and MEN 2B. Malignant degeneration has been reported in childhood; tumors may be bilateral and multifocal.

Pheochromocytomas occur in about 50% of patients with MEN 2A; they develop in more than 50% of patients with MEN 2B. Again, these are bilateral and multifocal.

Hyperparathyroidism develops in about 25% of MEN 2A patients; it is not a feature of MEN-2B.

Medullated corneal nerves are an asymptomatic feature of MEN 2B. Delay of puberty may be a feature in both males and females; the basis for this is unknown.

HISTOPATHOLOGY

LIGHT. The neuromas are plexiform, comprised of unencapsulated nerve fibers with axonal proliferation, surrounded by a thickened perineurium. There is no increase in connective tissue stroma.

EM. No information.

BASIC DEFECT

Mutations in the *RET* oncogene, a protein tyrosine kinase gene.

TREATMENT

The only effective treatment for the neuromas if they interfere with oral function is excision. Screening for thyroid carcinoma by regular calcitonin levels is advocated by some, but the risk of metastasis is very high once evidence of thyroid disease has developed. Therefore, some advocate prophylactic thyroidectomy in childhood, once the clinical diagnosis of MEN 2A or 2B has been made on the basis of phenotype. Screening for pheochromocytomas is recommended; however, each method (e.g., measurement of urinary catecholamines, radioisotope screening) has its proponents.

MODE OF INHERITANCE

Autosomal dominant. MEN 2A and 2B are allelic. The gene maps to the centromeric region of chromosome 10, at 10q11.2.

PRENATAL DIAGNOSIS

Possible by linkage studies with informative markers or by direct mutational analysis.

DIFFERENTIAL DIAGNOSIS

Neurofibromatosis (MIM:162200) can be confused with MEN 2B, as café-au-lait spots have been described in patients with the latter and the mucosal neuromas have the histologic appearance of plexiform neuromas. The orofacial swelling of Melkersson-Rosenthal syndrome (MIM:155900) can be confused clinically. Biopsy should differentiate. Any patient with multiple mucosal neuromas should be screened for MEN 2B. Bowel symptoms often result in the misdiagnosis of Hirschprung disease (MIM:249200), Crohn disease (MIM:266600), and ulcerative colitis (MIM:191390). Rectal biopsy will lead to the correct diagnosis.

Individuals with Marfan syndrome (MIM:154700) do not have mucosal neuromas. Patients with MEN 2B lack the cardiovascular and ocular complications of Marfan syndrome, although they share the asthenic habitus.

The oral changes of Cowden syndrome (MIM:158350) can appear similar; the presence of other cutaneous findings and biopsy, if necessary, will differentiate between the two. Isolated cutaneous lichen amyloidosis (MIM: 105250) can be inherited as an autosomal dominant trait. Whether the skin changes reported in some pedigrees with MEN 2A are due to coinheritance of the genes for two conditions or to a single causal mutation remains uncertain.

Support Group: N.O.R.D.
P.O. Box 8923
New Fairfield, CT 06812
1-800-999-6673

SELECTED BIBLIOGRAPHY

Laimore, T.C., Howe, J.R., Korte, J.A., Dilley, W.G., Aine, L., Aine, E., Wells, S.A., Jr., and Donis-Keller, H. (1991). Familial medullary thyroid carcinoma and multiple endocrine neoplasia type 2B map to the same region of chromosome 10 as multiple endocrine neoplasia type 2A. *Genomics* **9,** 181–192.

Studies in two large kindreds with medullary thyroid carcinoma and six kindreds with MEN 2B showed linkage to the same centromeric region of 10q as MEN 2A. There is a well-written discussion regarding whether alleles versus contiguous genes versus epigenetic factors are responsible for the different manifestations of the disorders.

The Third International Workshop on Multiple Endocrine Neoplasia Type 2 Syndromes (1989). *Henry Ford Hospital Med. J.* **37,** 98–224.

The entire issue is devoted to the MEN syndromes. The workshop recommended the preferred designations MEN 2, MEN 2A, and MEN 2B to denote the disorders and MEN2A and MEN2B to designate the gene(s). Two papers within this collection recommend screening for MEN 2A in all patients with hereditary cutaneous amyloidosis.

Van Heyningen, V. (1994). One gene—four syndromes. *Nature* **367,** 319–320.

Hofstra, R.M.W., Landsvater, R.M., Ceccherini, I., Stulp, R.P., Stelwagen, T., Luo, Y., Pasini, B., Hoppener, J.W.M., van Amstel, H.K.P., Romeo, G., Lips, C.J.M., and Buys, C.H.C.M. (1994). A mutation in the *RET* proto-oncogene associated with multiple endocrine neoplasia type 2B and sporadic medullary thyroid carcinoma. *Nature* **367,** 375–376.

Romeo, G., Ronchetto, P., Luo, Y., Barone, V., Seri, M., Ceccherini, I., Pasini, B., Bocciardi, R., Lerone, M., Kaariainen, H., and Martucciello, G. (1994). Point mutations affecting the tyrosine kinase domain of the *RET* proto-oncogene in Hirschprung's disease. *Nature* **367,** 377–378.

Êdery, P., Lyonnet, S., Mulligan, L.M., Pelet, A., Dow, E., Abel, L., Holder, S., Nihoul-Fekete, C., Ponder, B.A.J., and Munnich, A. (1994). Mutations of the *RET* proto-oncogene in Hirschprung's disease. *Nature* **367,** 378–380.

Van Heyningen (1994) gives a clear editorial and review of disorders caused by specific mutations in the *RET* proto-oncogene. Hofstra et al. (1994), Romeo et al. (1994), and Edery et al. (1994) provide papers identifying mutations responsible for MEN 2B, sporadic medullary thyroid carcinoma, and Hirschprung disease.

MULTIPLE LEIOMYOMATOSIS (MIM:150800)

DERMATOLOGIC FEATURES

MAJOR. Leiomyomas of the skin are discrete firm papules and nodules that are fixed to the overlying epidermis and move freely over deeper structures. Lesions may present at birth or may not develop until the teen years. They gradually increase in size and number over the lifetime and may coalesce to form plaques. They may be widespread and bilateral, distributed in a dermatomal pattern, or unilateral. The overlying skin is pink or red or purple-brown and may have superficial telangiectases.

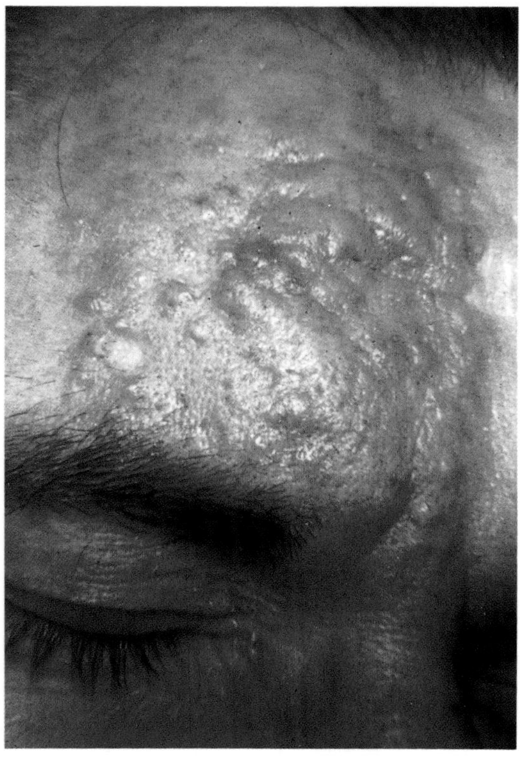

Figure 10.34. Infiltrated plaque on forehead. (Courtesy of Dr. J. Halloran, Division of Dermatology, University of Washington.)

The lesions are spontaneously painful. Pain is often precipitated by cold. Malignant degeneration of cutaneous lesions has not been reported.

MINOR. In some patients pain may be associated with transient color change in the leiomyomas—redenning or darkening.

ASSOCIATED ABNORMALITIES

Multiple leiomyomata of the uterus have been reported in several affected females. Isolated uterine involvement occurred in the mother of several children with cutaneous involvement with and without uterine involvement.

In two patients, uterine leiomyosarcoma developed.

HISTOPATHOLOGY

LIGHT. The epidermis may be normal or thinned or acanthotic. There is a clear area of

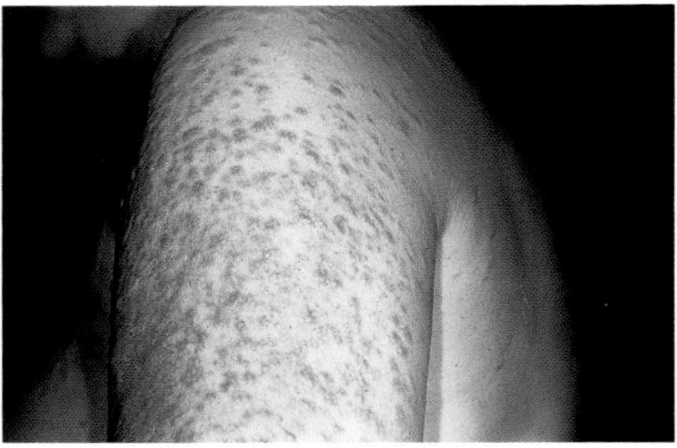

Figure 10.35. Multiple tiny papules. (Courtesy of Dr. W. Baker, Division of Dermatology, University of Washington.)

uninvolved dermis at the dermal junction, below which irregular bundles of spindle-shaped smooth muscle cells interdigitate with collagen bundles.

EM. No information for genetic form specifically. The smooth muscle cells appear normal in leiomyomas.

BASIC DEFECT

Unknown.

TREATMENT

Recurrence after surgical extirpation is the rule.

MODE OF INHERITANCE

Autosomal dominant. Male-to-male transmission has been reported.

PRENATAL DIAGNOSIS

None.

DIFFERENTIAL DIAGNOSIS

Alport syndrome has been associated with esophageal leiomyomas and vulvar leiomyomas (MIM:106801) but not with cutaneous lesions. Any adnexal tumor such as a neurofibroma, epidermal cyst, dermatofibroma, or angiofibroma can appear clinically similar. Spontaneous pain is a hallmark of leiomyomas and is not seen with these other tumors. A biopsy may be necessary for the correct diagnosis.

Support Group: N.O.R.D.
P.O. Box 8923
New Fairfield, CT 06812
1-800-999-6673

SELECTED BIBLIOGRAPHY

Fisher, W.C., and Helwig, E.B. (1963). Leiomyomas of the skin. *Arch. Dermatol.* **88,** 510–520.

Reviews series of slides sent to the Armed Forces Institute of Pathology. Most cases were not correctly diagnosed prior to biopsy. There are seven families represented. In one of the families, all of three affected siblings had lesions limited to the right side, arguing against segmental or postzygotic mutation as a cause for unilateral involvement.

Joliffe, D.S. (1978). Multiple cutaneous leiomyomata. *Clin. Exp. Dermatol.* **3,** 89–92.

Two female patients with cutaneous and uterine leiomyomas; one had two affected sisters. The author comments that with a 10%–25% prevalence of uterine leiomyomas in women over 40 years, the co-occurrence of skin and uterine lesions may be coincidental. He did not explore family histories beyond what was offered, so one cannot use this report to invoke autosomal recessive or X-linked dominant inheritance.

Reed, W.B., Walker, R., and Horowitz, R. (1973). Cutaneous leiomyomata with uterine leiomyomata. *Arch. Dermatol. Venereol. (Stockh.)* **53,** 409–416.

Reviews the literature. Points out the risks for malignant degeneration of uterine lesions. States that the onset of uterine tumors is earlier in the hereditary condition than in the general population.

PILOMATRICOMA (MIM:132600)

(Pilomatrixoma; Calcifying Epithelioma of Malherbe)

DERMATOLOGIC FEATURES

MAJOR. Pilomatricomas are small, firm dermal nodules ranging in size from that of a pea to 1–2 cm in diameter and 0.5 to 1 cm in thickness. Giant lesions have been described. The nodules have sharply demarcated and often irregular margins. They may appear yellow or bluish. Upon stretching of the skin, pinpoint nodularity may be appreciated. The nodules are attached to the overlying skin and move freely over the subcutaneous tissue. They are usually, but not always, painless. Occasionally they can rupture and extrude material.

Isolated lesions are not rare in children and can develop throughout childhood. Antecedent trauma is described in about 30% of instances. Sites of predilection are around the ears, in the eyebrows, on the upper arms, and chest.

Multiple lesions occur in 2%–3.5% of reported series. Multiple lesions have been described in sporadic cases, in association with myotonic dystrophy, and in a few families without clinical evidence of myotonic dystrophy.

MINOR. None.

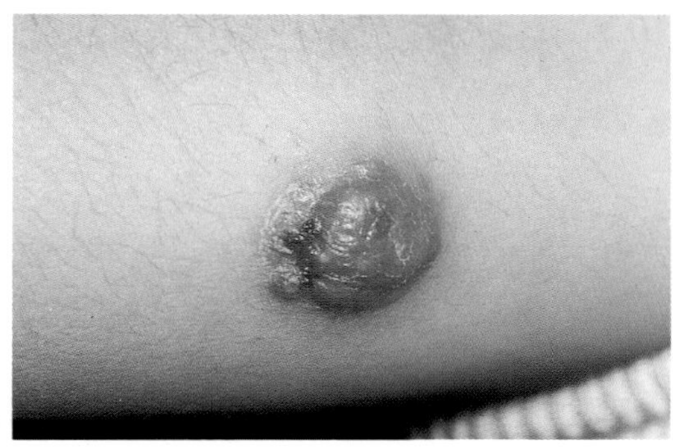

Figure 10.36. **(A)** Pinkish nodule. **(B)** Pilomatricoma extruding material. (Courtesy of Division of Dermatology, University of Washington.)

ASSOCIATED ABNORMALITIES

Some individuals with myotonic dystrophy will have multiple pilomatricomas.

HISTOPATHOLOGY

LIGHT. Irregular islands of epithelial cells are separated by fibrous tissue. The islands are composed of basophilic cells and shadow cells that have lost their nuclei. Calcium deposits occur in about 75% of lesions, frank ossification in 15%–20%. Foreign body giant cells are often seen adjacent to the shadow cells. Presumably the basophilic cells are immature hair matrix cells.

EM. α-Keratin strands are seen in cells; hairlike structures are found as well, suggesting derivation from hair matrix cells.

BASIC DEFECT

The tumor arises from hair matrix cells. The cause is unknown.

TREATMENT

Surgical excision. Although most lesions are benign and stabilize, some continue to grow, and, extremely rarely, malignant degeneration with metastasis has occurred.

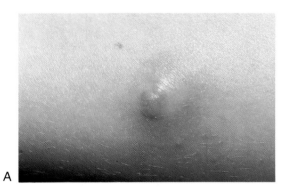

MODE OF INHERITANCE

Isolated lesions are sporadic. Multiple lesions, not in association with myotonic dystrophy, may be autosomal dominant. Three sets of siblings; one father–daughter pair; one father, his two daughters, his brother and sister; one mother–daughter pair; and one sibling pair with possibly two affected paternal aunts and an uncle have been described. There have been no instances of male-to-male transmission.

PRENATAL DIAGNOSIS

None.

DIFFERENTIAL DIAGNOSIS

Signs and symptoms of myotonic dystrophy (Steinert disease, MIM:160900) should be sought in any patient with more than one pilomatricoma and in any individual with a family history of pilomatricoma. The cysts of Gardner syndrome (familial polyposis coli, MIM: 175100) can occasionally show histologic features similar to pilomatricomas. The associated features of osteomas, tooth abnormalities, and intestinal polyposis should lead to the correct diagnosis if biopsy of the lesion does not.

Any calcified lesion may appear clinically similar to a pilomatricoma, including epidermal inclusion cysts, lymph nodes, hematomas, and hemangiomas. Lesions in the eyebrow may be confused clinically with dermoids. Dermoids tend to be more fixed to the underlying tissue and have a smooth surface when the epidermis is stretched. They usually have normal skin color and regular smooth margins.

Support Group: N.O.R.D.
P.O. Box 8923
New Fairfield, CT
06812
1-800-999-6673

Muscular Dystrophy
Association
3300 East Sunrise Drive
Tucson, AZ 85718-3208
1-602-529-2000

SELECTED BIBLIOGRAPHY

Cambiaghi, S., Ermacora, E., Brusasco, A., Canzi, L., and Caputo, R. (1994). Multiple pilomatricomas in Rubenstein-Taybi syndrome: a case report. *Pediatr. Dermatol.* **11,** 21–25.

A single patient with multiple lesions. No other instances of this association in the literature.

Harper, P.S. (1972). Calcifying epithelioma of Malherbe—association with myotonic muscular dystrophy. *Arch. Dermatol.* **106,** 41–44.

Seven of 167 patients with myotonic dystrophy had pilomatricomas. The tumors were multiple in four of these. One sibling pair [previously reported in *Birth Defects* **7(8),** 1971] and one mother–son pair. Other relatives in these pedigrees with myotonic dystrophy did not have pilomatricomas. Of 18 relatives in these families who did not have myotonic dystrophy, none had pilomatricomas when examined by Harper.

Hills, R.J., and Ive, F.A. (1992). Familial multiple pilomatrixomas (Letter). *Br. J. Dermatol.* **127,** 194–195.

This mother and daughter pair with no clinical evidence of myotonic dystrophy presented with multiple pilomatrixomas. The lesions in the mother were asymptomatic. In the daughter they were painful and discharged yellowish material.

Mohlenbeck, F.W. (1973). Pilomatrixoma (calcifying epithelioma). A statistical study. *Arch. Dermatol.* **108,** 532–534.

Reviews 170 cases of his own and 1,399 from the literature for age at appearance, site, and incidence among biopsied lesions.

PROTEUS SYNDROME (MIM:176920)

(Partial Gigantism with Macrodactyly, Hemihypertrophy, and Connective Tissue Nevi)
Includes Bannayan-Riley-Ruvalcaba Syndrome

DERMATOLOGIC FEATURES

MAJOR. Proteus syndrome is a disorder marked by a variety of hamartomas. Overgrowth of soft tissues with deep and superficial lipomatosis is extremely common, along with asymmetric bony overgrowth. Hemihypertrophy and macrodactyly are progressive; the latter is a hallmark of the disorder. These changes may be present at birth or develop within the first few years of life.

The soft tissue enlargement of the hands and feet is composed of fatty tissue. Cerebriform thickening of the soles is common and, when examined histologically, has proven to be a connective tissue nevus, which can also occur elsewhere on the skin.

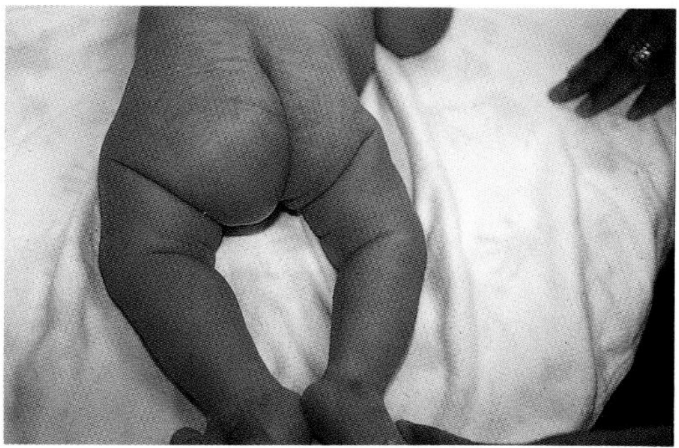

Figure 10.37. Large mass in left buttocks.

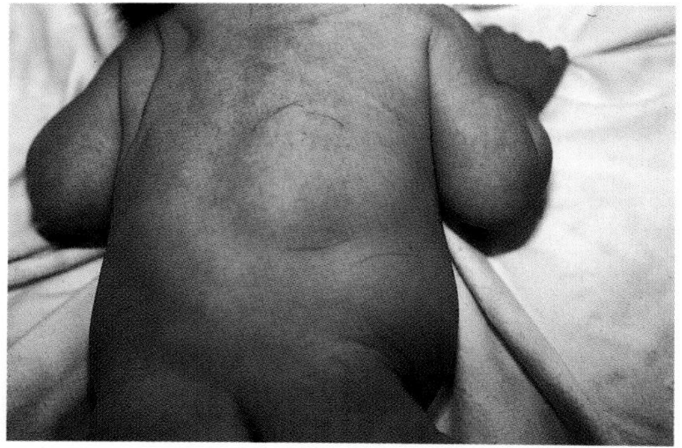

Figure 10.38. Soft tissue masses evident on right back.

Hyperpigmentation in a diffuse, linear, or patchy distribution is common to many reports. In some, there appears to be epidermal thickening with verrucous changes typical of an epidermal or organoid nevus.

Muscular atrophy and loss of subcutaneous tissue are common in the "unaffected" areas of the body.

MINOR. Lymphangiomas and angiomas can occur anywhere and may progress, stabilize, or regress during life.

Extraosseus calcification occurs commonly in the soft tissues of the overgrown fingers and toes.

ASSOCIATION ABNORMALITIES

Ocular: The eye findings are as protean as other manifestations of this disorder. Epibulbar masses have been noted in several patients. Histopathology of a mass from one patient demonstrated a fibrous hamartoma.

Strabismus and amblyopia, nystagmus, high myopia, and optic disc pallor have been reported in more than one instance. Heterochromia iridis has occurred. Ocular involvement is often asymmetric, with the more severe eye findings on the same side of the body as the more marked overgrowth.

Skeletal: Asymmetric bony overgrowth with leg length discrepancy is common. Any bone can be involved. Overgrowth of individual phalanges, metacarpals, and metatarsals is frequent. This is referred to as *partial gigantism of the hands and/or feet* in many reports. Genu valgum and scoliosis are reported in most patients. Bossing of the cranial vault has been described in many patients. While sometimes frontal, it can occur elsewhere in the skull and may be secondary to fat deposition in the diploie of the cranial bones. Osteomas, endondromas, and osteochondromas are also seen.

Intelligence: Ranges from normal to severely retarded.

Pulmonary: Cystic malformations in the lung have been documented in a few patients.

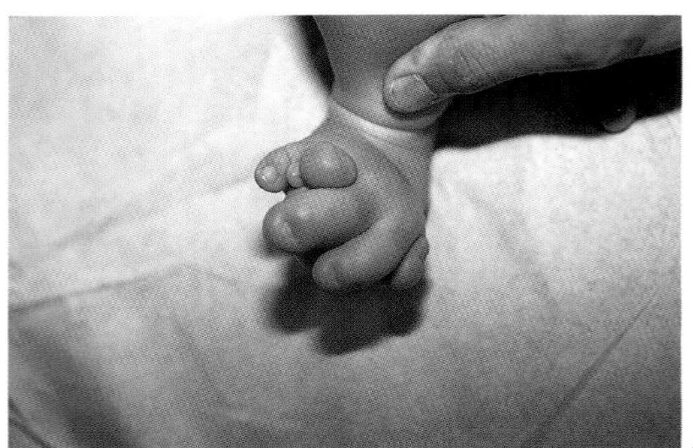

A

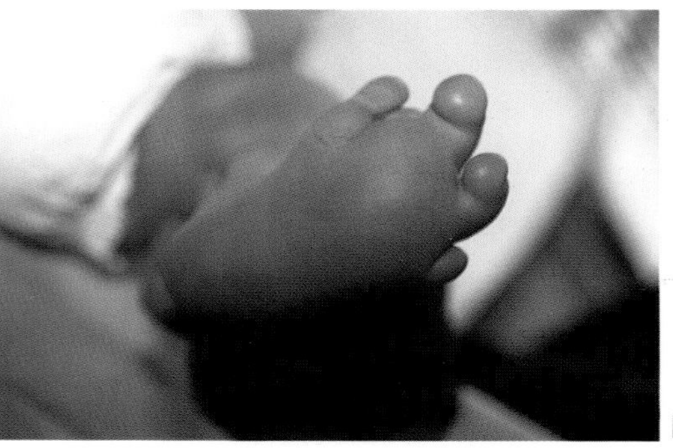

B

Figure 10.39. **(A, B)** Malformed left foot.

HISTOPATHOLOGY

LIGHT. The findings are those of the specific hamartoma and include changes consistent with lipomas, angiolipomas, and hemangiomas. The changes in the skull result from fatty deposition in the spongy matter between the inner and outer table of the skull.

EM. Electron microscopy of a linear nevus from one individual showed extensive vacuolization at the melanocyte–keratinocyte margins and aggregation of densely packed granules in the intracellular spaces.

BASIC DEFECT

Unknown. Just as the manifestations of the Proteus syndrome are multiple, so may be the causes. The clinical features are quite variable, and it is reasonable to believe that there is not a single unifying cause for all cases. A variety of genetic or acquired alterations in factors controlling growth may lead to the common features of asymmetric soft tissue and bony overgrowth.

TREATMENT

Surgical excision, including amputation of involved digits or limbs and life-threatening or crippling tumors may be necessary. Orthopedic management of bony complications and careful ophthalmologic evaluation and management need to be individualized.

MODE OF INHERITANCE

All cases have been sporadic. New mutation for an autosomal dominant disorder has been suggested. Somatic mutation for a lethal autosomal dominant condition seems a likely causal mechanism and might explain the asymmetric distribution of findings. Extensive karyotyping of multiple tissues to look for chromosomal mosaicism has not been done.

PRENATAL DIAGNOSIS

None.

DIFFERENTIAL DIAGNOSIS

Maffucci syndrome (MIM:166000): There is clearly overlap between Maffucci and Proteus syndromes, and some patients reported as one may, in fact, represent the other. Lipomas are not features of Maffucci syndrome, which is characterized by enchondromatosis and hemangiomatosis, and are an invariable feature of Proteus syndrome.

Neurofibromatosis (MIM:162200): The café-au-lait spots of neurofibromatosis are reported in Proteus syndrome, but axillary freckling is not. Cerebriform cutaneous neurofibromas look clinically similar to the cerebriform tumors of Proteus. A positive family history for neurofibromatosis would rule out Proteus syndrome; the presence of other features of Proteus syndrome would eliminate the diagnosis of neurofibromatosis. Biopsy and histopathology of soft tissue changes should discriminate between a neurofibroma and a lipoma or organoid nevus.

Klippel-Trenaunay-Weber syndrome (MIM: 149000): The bony and soft tissue overgrowths of Klippel-Trenaunay-Weber syndrome are associated with hemangiomas and lymphangiomas. There may be considerable overlap with the Proteus syndrome. Lipomatosis is not a feature of Klippel-Trenaunay-Weber syndrome.

Encephalocraniocutaneous syndrome: This differs from Proteus syndrome in that the hamartomas in it are lipomatous only. Intracranial and scleral involvement are typical. Some authors believe that this disorder and Proteus syndrome are both part of the spectrum of a single disorder.

Bannayan-Riley-Ruvalcaba syndrome (macrocephaly, multiple lipomas, and hemangiomas, MIM:153480): This syndrome is extremely rare. Reported patients have not had progressive macrodactyly, bossing of the skull, or soft tissue changes on the palms and soles. They share in common with Proteus syndrome subcutaneous hamartomas and organoid nevi. Affected males often have brown macules on the glans and shaft of the penis. Mental retardation has been described in 50% of reported patients. Intestinal hamartomas are typical, as is a lipid storage myopathy.

Support Group: Neurofibromatosis, Inc. (NF, Inc.)
8855 Annapolis Road, No. 110
Lanham, MO 20706-2924
1-301-577-8984

SELECTED BIBLIOGRAPHY

Burke, J.P., Bowell, R., and O'Doherty, N. (1988). Proteus syndrome: ocular complications. *J. Pediatr. Ophthalmol. Strabismus* **25,** 99–102.

Reviews the literature on eye findings in Proteus syndrome along with a case of their own.

Clark, R.D., Donnai, D., Rogers, J., Cooper, J., and Baraitser, M. (1987). Proteus syndrome: an expanded phenotype. *Am. J. Med. Genet.* **27,** 99–117.

These authors report 11 new cases of Proteus syndrome in detail. They emphasize the changing nature of the disorder, with the development of different features over time in individual patients.

Cremin, B.J., Viljoen, D.L., Wynchank, S., and Beighton, P. (1987). The Proteus syndrome: the magnetic resonance and radiological features. *Pediatr. Radiol.* **17,** 486–488.

These authors suggest that magnetic resonance imaging is useful in the evaluation of the mesodermal soft tissue (lipomas, fibromas) malformations of Proteus.

Happle, R. (1986). Cutaneous manifestation of lethal genes. *Hum. Genet.* **72,** 280.

A letter to the editor that puts forth the hypothesis that mosaicism for lethal genes is a mechanism common to disorders that express along the lines of Blaschko in the skin.

Hotamisigil, G.S., and Ertogan, F. (1990). The Proteus syndrome: association with nephrogenic diabetes insipidus. *Clin. Genet.* **38,** 139–144.

Single case report of female with Proteus and nephrogenic diabetes insipidus. Presents a table reviewing clinical features in 49 patients reported in the literature.

Viljoen, D.L., Nelson, N.M., de Jong, G., and Beighton, P. (1987). Proteus syndrome in Southern Africa: natural history and clinical manifestations in six individuals. *Am. J. Med. Genet.* **27,** 87–97.

Description of six patients and very clear detailed discussion of differential diagnosis.

Wiedemann, H.-R., Burgio, G.R., Aldenhoff, P., Kunze, J., Kaufmann, H.J., and Schirg, E. (1983). The Proteus syndrome. *Eur. J. Pediatr.* **140,** 5–12.

First coined the term *Proteus,* after the Greek god who was able to change shape. Reports four cases in detail.

SEBACEOUS NEVUS SYNDROME (MIM:163200)

(Linear Nevus Sebaceous; Solomon's Epidermal Nevus; Schimmelpenning-Feuerstein-Mims; Nevus Sebaceous of Jadassohn)

Includes Encephalocraniocutaneous Lipomatosis

DERMATOLOGIC FEATURES

MAJOR. Typical lesions are yellow and may appear waxy. They are devoid of hairs and have a slightly irregular surface. Sebaceous nevi may be any size. When widespread, they are usually distributed along the lines of Blaschko. Solitary lesions may be oval or linear. Over time, the surface often becomes more erose and thickened and may become papillomatous and bumpy. There is a risk for both benign and malignant transformation, which generally occurs after puberty. The risk is approximately 10%. Benign syringocystadenoma papilliferum is the most common tumor that develops. Basal cell carcinoma, squamous cell carcinoma, keratoacanthoma, sebaceous carcinoma, eccrine porocarcinoma, and apocrine carcinoma have all been described.

MINOR. There are a few case reports in which multiple hemangiomas accompany the sebaceous nevus.

ASSOCIATED ABNORMALITIES

As with epidermal nevi, there are usually no abnormalities associated with isolated small lesions. The more widespread a lesion is, the more likely it is to be associated with other malformations and to represent a global hamartomatous disorder. When lesions involve the face and, in particular, the forehead, the risk

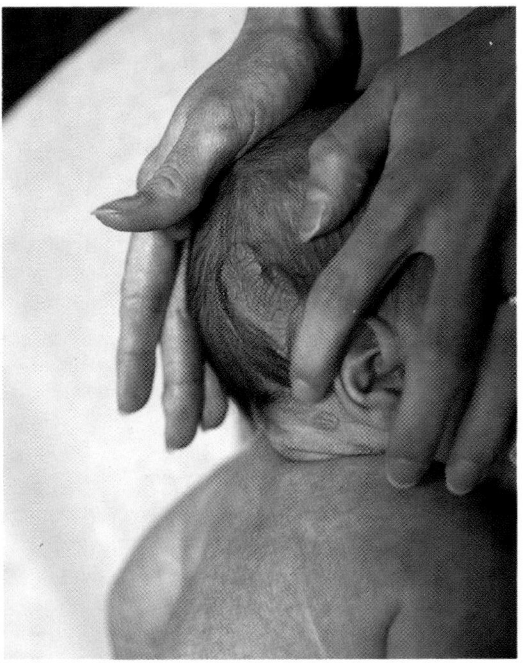

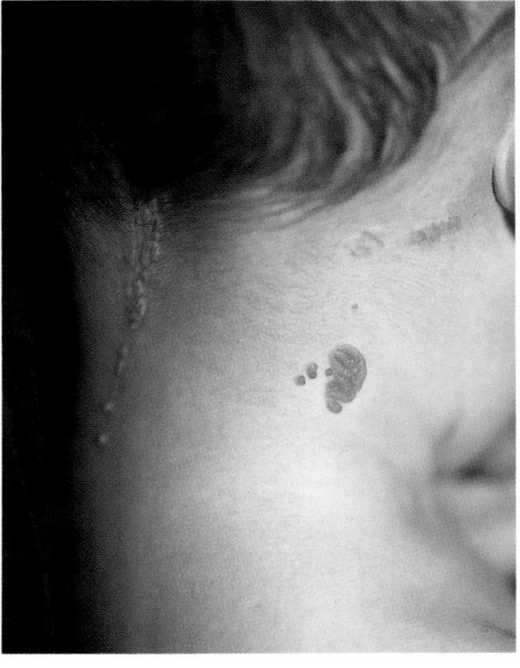

A B

Figure 10.40. **(A)** Cerebriform lesion on scalp; satellite lesions on neck. **(B)** Extension down onto nape. Lesions vary in color.

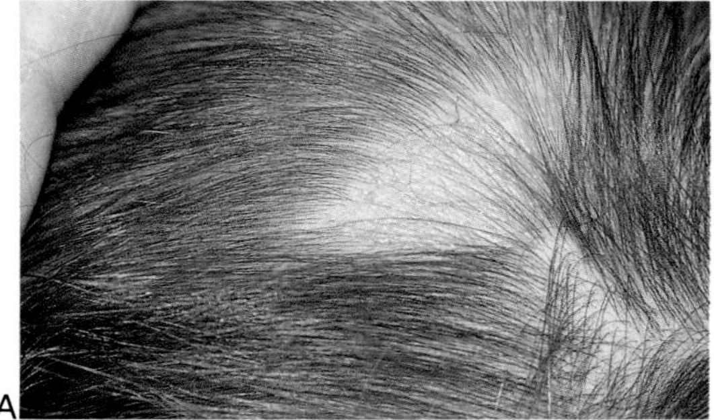

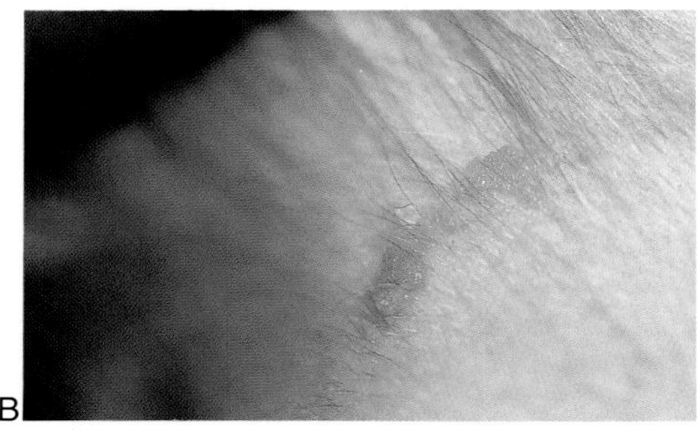

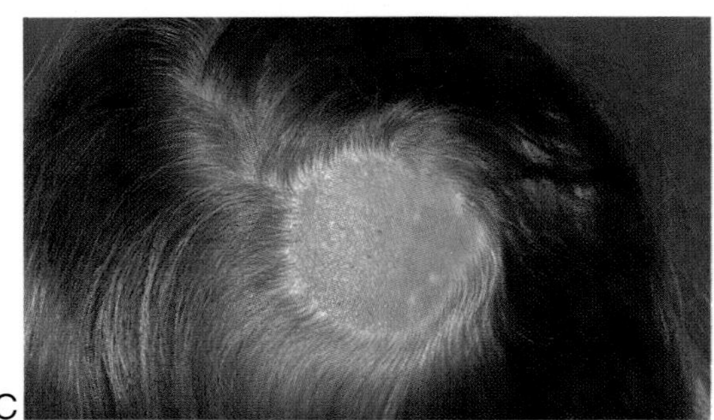

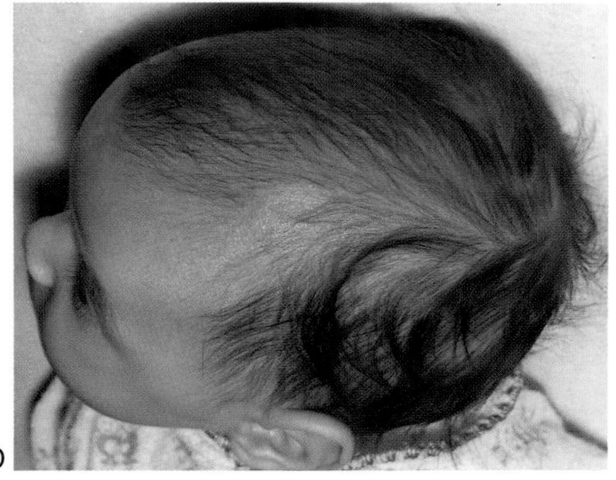

Figure 10.41. **(A)** Flat, typical yellow grainy appearance. **(B)** Raised lesion. **(C)** Leathery patch. **(D)** Lanceolate lesion coming down onto forehead. This infant was developmentally normal.

for associated central nervous system abnormalities is very high. Of almost 40 case reports in the literature in which facial involvement was present, only 5 had normal intellect. The central nervous system abnormalities include mental retardation, seizures, and structural malformations. Unilateral megalencephaly has been reported several times. There are a handful of case reports in which affected individuals have structural brain malformations and cerebral atrophy with normal intellect and no seizures. It is important to recognize that solitary sebaceous nevi are quite common on the scalp, and they are, in general, not associated with underlying central nervous system problems. It is those that involve the face that are problematic. Ocular abnormalities are common in the nevus sebaceous syndrome, and there are a host of abnormalities described. Lipodermoids of the lid and conjunctivae are typical. There may be colobomas. Ptosis has also been described. There may be intrascleral hamartomatous bone or cartilage development.

There are several reports of children with extensive lesions who developed rickets due to a defect in renal tubular reabsorption of phosphate and deficiency of 1,25-$(OH)_2$ vitamin D. Individual case reports describe a plethora of unique malformations.

HISTOPATHOLOGY

Light. The epidermis is papillomatous with buds of basaloid cells. There are mature sebaceous glands with venting to the surface. Typically there are absent or abnormal, incompletely formed hair follicles. Histologic features change with time and maturation of the lesions. **EM.** No information.

BASIC DEFECT

Unknown.

TREATMENT

Surgical excision is the treatment of choice for small lesions to address the risk for malignant degeneration. There may be recurrence along the margins. Laser ablation has been attempted, but only short-term follow-up information is available.

MODE OF INHERITANCE

Sporadic. It has been posited that these lesions are the result of somatic mutations for an otherwise lethal autosomal dominant gene. There have been only three reports of familial recurrence of isolated lesions without associated abnormalities. One mother–daughter pair and one grandfather–mother–granddaughter pedigree have been reported with lesions on the vertex of the scalp. There is a third report of two maternal half-brothers with isolated lesions born to an unaffected mother.

PRENATAL DIAGNOSIS

None.

DIFFERENTIAL DIAGNOSIS

In encephalocraniocutaneous lipomatosis, ipsilateral epibulbar choristomas, connective tissue nevi of the eyelid, and lipomas of the scalp, face, and central nervous system occur together. There is usually an area of alopecia in the scalp, often with no change in the appearance of the underlying skin. Hemifacial microsomia may also occur. Mental retardation is typical. Various structural central nervous system malformations, in addition to lipomas, are seen. In two case reports, sebaceous nevi were also described. The lipomas and the connective tissue nevi may be the differentiating feature between the linear sebaceous nevus syndrome and encephalocraniocutaneous lipomatosis, or they may represent different points along a continuum.

Isolated lesions on the scalp can be mistaken for aplasia cutis congenita (MIM:Many). Plaque-like molluscum contagiosum in HIV-positive patients can give a similar appearance. A Tzanck smear or biopsy will differentiate between the two. Warts and xanthomas might sometimes be confused. In general, sebaceous nevi are readily recognized.

Support Group: N.O.R.D.
P.O. Box 8923
New Fairfield, CT
06812
1-800-999-6673

SELECTED BIBLIOGRAPHY

Cavenagh, E.C., Hart, B.L., and Rose, D. (1993). Association of linear sebaceous nevus syndrome and unilateral megalencephaly. *A.J.N.R.* **14,** 405–408.

Case report. Reviews literature and states that 26 of 36 patients with central nervous system symptoms who underwent magnetic resonance imaging and computed tomographic scanning had evidence for megalencephaly. Both epidermal nevus syndrome and linear nevus sebaceous syndrome patients were included.

Jones, E.W., and Heyl, T. (1970). Naevus sebaceous. A report of 140 cases with special regard to the development of secondary malignant tumors. *Br. J. Dermatol.* **82,** 99–117.

Included both sebaceous and epidermal nevi. Twenty-seven developed syringocystadenoma papilliferum; nine developed basal cell epitheliomas, but only three of these showed signs of aggressive growth. There was one squamous cell epithelioma, three syringomas, two apocrine cystadenomas, and two osteomata. There were 14 lesions that showed basaloid hamartomatous proliferation.

Mehregan, A.H., and Pinkus, H. (1965). Life history of organoid nevi. *Arch. Dermatol.* **91,** 574–588.

These authors describe 150 cases of organoid nevi. They clearly demonstrate the overlap of features between epidermal nevi and sebaceous nevi. They discuss the life cycle of the lesions and Jadassohn's work. The appellation *of Jadassohn* is not useful, and there is no difference inherent in the terms *nevus sebaceous* and *nevus sebaceous of Jadassohn.* Authors use the term *nevus sebaceous of Jadassohn* interchangeably with *organoid nevi.*

TUMORAL CALCINOSIS (MIM:114120, 211900)

(Calcinosis Cutis Circumscripta)

DERMATOLOGIC FEATURES

MAJOR. Usually painless, large, firm, irregular subcutaneous nodules develop in midchildhood through adult life. They occur primarily over the joints, buttocks, and hips. Growth of lesions may arrest spontaneously after puberty or continue.

MINOR. Gingivitis and perleche are described in some patients. A preceding asymptomatic erythematous rash in early childhood was noted in one report.

ASSOCIATED ABNORMALITIES

Hoarse voice.

HISTOPATHOLOGY

LIGHT. Deposits of calcium apatite with occasional foreign body giant cells. There are fibrous septae separating the deposits.

EM. No information.

BASIC DEFECT

Unknown. Hyperphosphatemia is often found, but the underlying cause remains elusive.

TREATMENT

None is consistently effective. Recurrence after surgical excision is common.

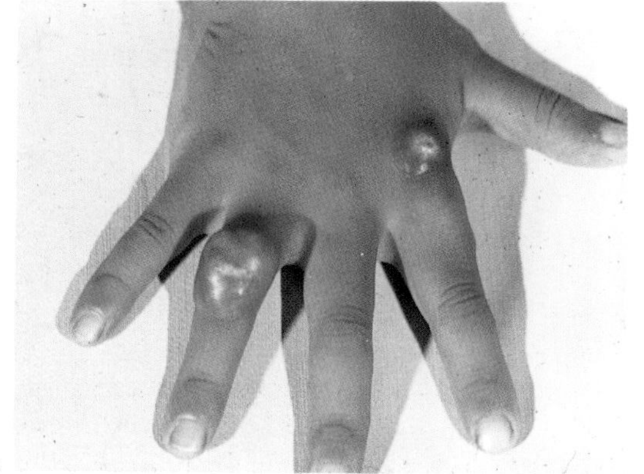

A

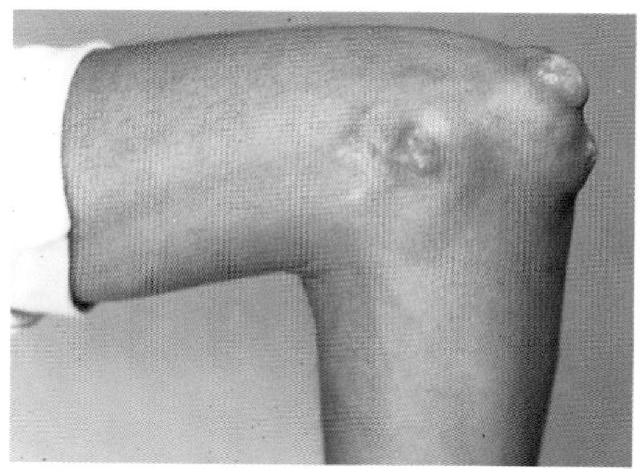

B

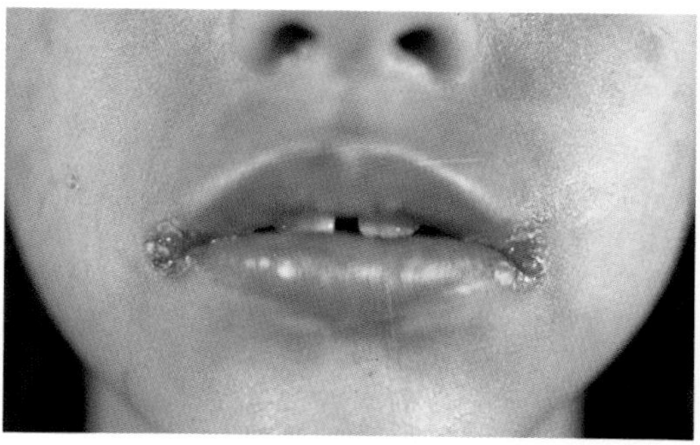

C

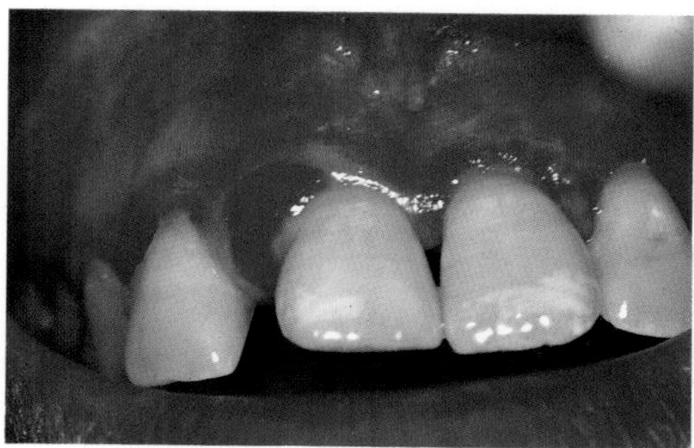

D

Figure 10.42. Nodules on hands **(A)**; elbow **(B)**; perleche **(C)**; and gingivitis **(D)**. (From Metzker, A., et al., 1988. Originals courtesy of Dr. A. Metzger, Israel.)

MODE OF INHERITANCE

Most are sporadic. Autosomal recessive inheritance in many families. One pedigree suggested autosomal dominant inheritance (see Lyles et al., 1985)

PRENATAL DIAGNOSIS

None.

DIFFERENTIAL DIAGNOSIS

Calcinosis cutis can occur in association with pseudopseudohypoparathyroidism (Albright hereditary osteodystrophy, MIM:103580, 203330, 300800); has been reported rarely in Rothmund-Thomson syndrome (MIM:268400), hereditary sclerosing poikiloderma (Weary syndrome, MIM:173700), scleroderma (MIM: 181750), CREST syndrome (MIM:181750), dermatomyositis, Raynaud disease (MIM: 179600), and hypervitaminosis D. It is a rare complication of pseudoxanthoma elasticum (MIM:177850, 177860, 264800, 264810). COPS syndrome is marked by poikiloderma and exuberant calcinosis cutis.

Support Group: N.O.R.D.
P.O. Box 8923
New Fairfield, CT 06812
1-800-999-6673

SELECTED BIBLIOGRAPHY

Lyles, K.W., Burkes, E.J., Ellis, G.J., Lucas, K.J., Dolan, E.A., and Drezner, M.K. (1985). Genetic transmission of tumoral calcinosis: autosomal dominant with variable clinical expressivity. *J. Clin. Endocrinol. Metab.* **60,** 1093–1096.

Authors claim autosomal dominant inheritance, but this may be a different disease from classic tumoral calcinosis. In this family, hypoplastic teeth with bulbous roots and pulp stones were found in three of nine affected individuals, calcinosis cutis occurred in only four of nine affected individuals, and 1,25$(OH)_2$ vitamin D levels were elevated in all. There was no description given of the skin lesions beyond "tumorous and calcific deposits" and no information regarding number, age of onset, distribution, and so forth.

Metzker, A., Eisenstein, B., Oren, J., and Samuel, R. (1988). Tumoral calcinosis revisited—common and uncommon features. Report of ten cases and review. *Eur. J. Pediatr.* **147,** 128–132.

Two consanguineous pedigrees. Notes persistent red vasculitic-like rash with no evidence of vasculitis on pathology. Twenty-six references.

Pursley, T.V., Prince, M.J., Chausmer, A.B., and Raimer, S.S. (1979). Cutaneous manifestations of tumoral calcinosis. *Arch. Dermatol.* **115,** 1100–1102.

Seven of 15 siblings were affected. The proband failed to respond to dietary management of phosphate depletion and topical steroid therapy.

CHAPTER 11

METABOLIC DISORDERS

PORPHYRIAS

Among the porphyrias, there are three that usually come to diagnosis by virtue of their skin changes and two others in which skin findings play a role. In only one, acute intermittent porphyria, is the skin entirely unaffected.

The enzymatic pathway of heme biosynthesis is well worked out, and the enzymatic defects are known for these disorders. Correct diagnosis depends on clinical assessment and on the typical pattern of excretion of porphyrins in blood, urine, and stool. The names of the disorders reflect their historical distinction into those with primary hematologic, hepatic, and cutaneous involvement. They are also classified into acute and nonacute; those with abdominal and neuropsychiatric features are acute. As with most genetic disorders, allelic heterogeneity is proving to be the rule, and compound heterozygosity will probably come to explain the "reduced" penetrance of porphyria cutanea tarda and erythropoietic protoporphyria.

Photosensitivity in the porphyrias occurs because of porphyrin deposition into the skin or because of direct production of porphyrins by keratinocytes and fibroblasts. Ultraviolet light is absorbed by the porphyrin molecules, which become "excited" and transfer their "energy" to the skin cells, resulting in phototoxicity. Many factors, including complement and lysosomal enzymes, play roles, and the precise mechanisms of the destructive effects of these molecules on the skin remain to be proven. Maximum skin reactivity to light in the porphyrias is in the 400–410 nm range, a wavelength not blocked by glass or by the epidermis.

Direct enzymatic or molecular diagnosis may become the method of choice as more laboratories offer these services. Initial screening for the porphyrias using stool, blood, and urine will still play a role. I have always been confused about which porphyrins are elevated in which excreta or body fluid and offer Table 11.1 as a quick guide to the patterns of each of the disorders with skin manifestation. I must note that in reviewing numerous references, the excretion patterns detailed for each disorder varied somewhat among authors as to the specific porphyrin excreted, the relative proportions of the porphyrin excreted, and the changes during acute and quiescent phases. It is im-

Table 11.1. Porphyrin Excretion Patterns

	Blood	*Urine*	*Stool*
Congenital erythropoietic porphyria	Uro > copro > proto	Uro >>>>> copro	Copro
Erythropoietic protoporphyria	Proto	—	Proto
Hereditary coproporphyria	−/+ Copro (RBCs)	Copro > ALA/PBG/uro	Copro > uro/proto
Porphyria cutanea tarda	—	Uro >>> copro	Isocopro
Variegate porphyria	PBG	PBG/ALA/uro/copro	Proto > copro
Hepatic erythropoietic porphyria	Proto (RBC)	Uro >>> copro	Isocopro

ALA, δ-aminolevulinic synthase; copro, coproporphyria; PBG, porphobilinogen; proto, coproprotoporphyrin; uro, uroporphyrin.

portant to remember the meaning of the term *screening test*. These are not definitive diagnostic tests.

Brown eggs from chickens result from increased uterine content of protoporphyrin.

SELECTED BIBLIOGRAPHY

Disler, P.B., and Moore, M.R. (1985). Porphyria. *Clin. Dermatol.* **3 (2).**

Moore, M.R., McColl, K.E.L., Rimington, C., and Goldberg, A. (1987). *Disorders of Porphyrin Metabolism*. Plenum Medical, New York.

Both Disler et al. (1985) and Moore et al. (1987) are readable reviews with detailed information on basic mechanisms, diagnosis, and treatment of porphyrias.

Epstein, J.H., Tuffanelli, D.L., and Epstein, W.L. (1973). Cutaneous changes in the porphyrias: a microscopic study. *Arch. Dermatol.* **107,** 689–698.

Fluorescent microscopic and electron microscopic studies of 22 patients with active porphyria tarda, five with erythropoietic protoporphyria, two with variegate porphyria and one with hereditary coproporphyria, and 10 with quiescent porphyria cutanea tarda. Biopsy changes were similar in all patients, with minor variations.

CONGENITAL ERYTHROPOIETIC PORPHYRIA (MIM:263700)

(Gunther Disease)

DERMATOLOGIC FEATURES

MAJOR. This is an extremely rare condition. I have seen it once in a Yupik child.

There is a broad range of severity in congenital erythropoietic porphyria, likely to be correlated with specific mutations. Some affected individuals showed signs at birth; others do not develop typical features until later. Usually there is marked photosensitivity during the first few years of life as exposure to sunlight occurs. Exposed skin blisters and develops erosions, which ulcerate and heal with scarring. The fluid in the vesicles will fluoresce with Wood's lamp.

Mutilation of the nasal tip, ears, fingertips, and eyelids develops over time in many. Others with the same enzyme deficiency have little permanent skin damage.

Hirsutism develops in involved areas, characterized by fine, dark lanugo hairs. The skin may also lichenify, and hyperpigmentation is common.

MINOR. Dystrophic nails have been described. Scarring alopecia can occur with repeated blistering of the scalp.

ASSOCIATED ABNORMALITIES

The characteristics secondary to hemolysis include splenomegaly, jaundice, anemia, and an elevated reticulocyte count. Affected newborns have presented with anemia, hepatosplenomegaly, and jaundice and have been diagnosed prior to the development of skin changes, suggesting that exposure to light is not the only precipitant.

The teeth are discolored, pink or reddish-brown (erythrodontia), and show red fluorescence under Wood's lamp. This is thought to be due to porphyrin binding to calcium phosphate. The deciduous teeth are involved, again indicating that the disease is active in utero.

Porphyrin also binds to bones, and osteoporosis and fractures are complications that can develop in childhood. Swollen-appearing joints with limited range of motion develop, along with acroosteolysis of the distal phalanges. Ectopic calcification of soft tissue has also been described.

The urine is pink or reddish-brown, and this may be the first noticeable sign of the disorder.

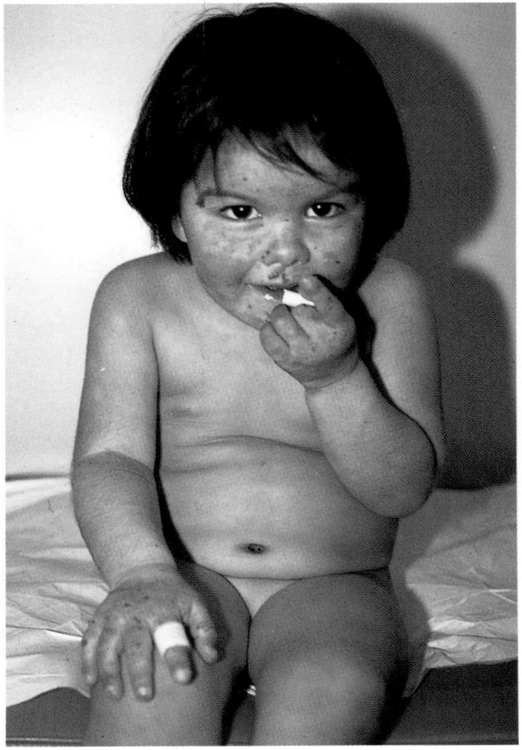

Figure 11.1. Crust and erosions on face and hands; very hirsute arms. (Courtesy of Dr. C. R. Scott, Seattle, Washington.)

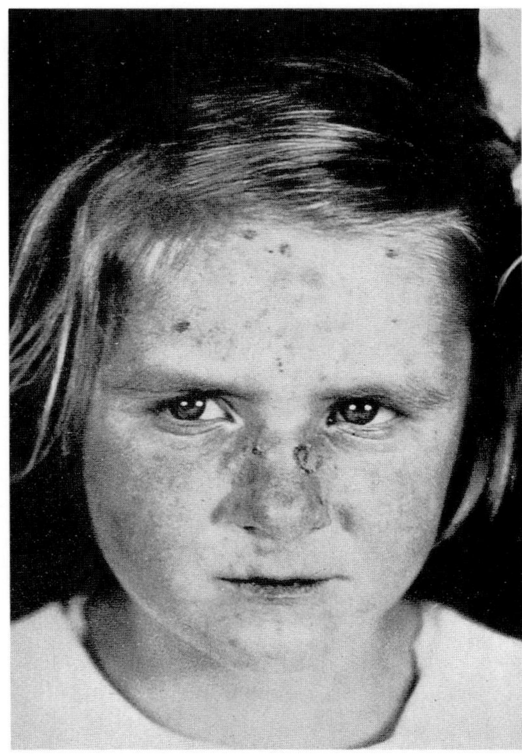

Figure 11.2. Older patient with erosions, scarring, and increased hairiness at temples and lateral aspects of eyebrows. (From Vannotti, 1954.)

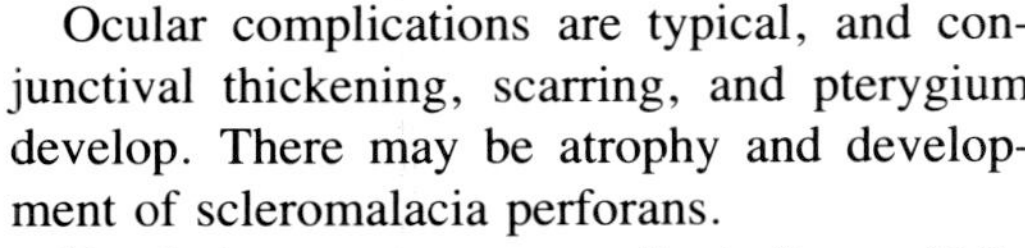

Ocular complications are typical, and conjunctival thickening, scarring, and pterygium develop. There may be atrophy and development of scleromalacia perforans.

Death is premature, usually before middle age, usually caused by repeated hemolytic crises, cirrhosis, and renal failure.

HISTOPATHOLOGY

LIGHT. Deposition of hyalin in the walls of the capillaries of the upper dermis and in the basement membrane zone. Bullae are subepidermal. Atrophy, dermal fibrosis, and loss of adnexae can be seen in later stages.

EM. Redundant rings of basement membrane around dermal blood vessels. Filamentous and amorphous material in upper dermis.

BASIC DEFECT

Defects in uroporphyrinogen III cosynthetase (URO-synthase) activity due to a variety of mutations. Cows can get Gunther disease and also demonstrate allelic heterogeneity. The first reports were from South African herds, but affected Danish and English cows have also been described.

TREATMENT

None effective. Hematin administration and hypertransfusion give modest and short-term benefit. Splenectomy improves red blood cell life span, but clinical improvement is limited. Bone marrow transplantation in one patient resulted in improvement in the disease, but the

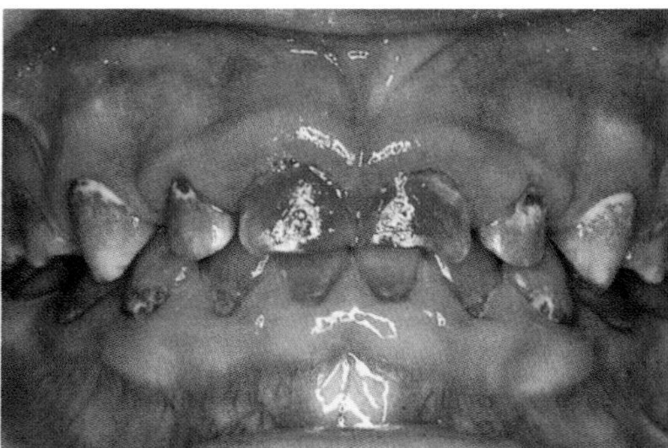

Figure 11.3. Teeth with marked discoloration. (From Fayle and Pollard, 1994.)

patient died of cytomegalic virus infection 8 months later. Avoidance of sun exposure is important. β-carotene has minimal benefit. Barrier sunscreens may be of use. Photoprotective yellow lenses may decrease the eye damage.

Several authors describe a need for psychiatric support in dealing with disfigurement.

MODE OF INHERITANCE

Autosomal recessive. Heterogeneous based on molecular studies, and compound heterozygosity has been demonstrated.

PRENATAL DIAGNOSIS

Enzymatic assay of amniocytes has been successful. Presumably molecular diagnosis is possible.

DIFFERENTIAL DIAGNOSIS

The demonstration of elevated uroporphyrin in red blood cells, plasma, and urine is definitive. Upon clinical presentation alone, other diagnostic considerations include the following.

Polymorphous light eruption (MIM:174770): This is rare in infancy and is usually marked by more eczematous-like skin changes with red papules and small vesicles. Although clinical phototesting to different wavelengths of light can distinguish this from congenital erythropoietic porphyria, it seems cruel when painless evaluation for fluorescence of red blood cells will diagnose congenital erythropoietic porphyria.

Erythropoietic protoporphyria (MIM: 177080): This usually has later onset with more severe symptoms and milder signs. The porphyrin excretion pattern will distinguish between these two conditions. There are no tooth changes or urine color changes in erythropoietic protoporphyria.

Epidermolysis bullosa (MIM:Many): Although patients with epidermolysis bullosa share blistering in common with Gunther disease, the disorders are readily distinguished by other clinical features.

Scleroderma: There are some similarities with congenital erythropoietic porphyria in joint restriction, cutaneous atrophy, and calcinosis cutis, but the age of onset and lack of associated photosensitivity in scleroderma should make quick work of distinguishing the two conditions.

Homozygous porphyria cutanea tarda (hepatoerythropoietic porphyria): presents with similar features. The pattern of excretion of porphyrins is different.

Poikiloderma of Kindler-Weary (MIM: 173650): This shares blistering and atrophy with congenital erythropoietic porphyria. Patients with Kindler-Weary do not excrete porphyrins in the urine, have no staining of the teeth, and usually do not have such severe scarring.

Support Group: Iron Overload Diseases Association, Inc.
433 Westwind Drive
North Palm Beach, FL 33408
1-407-840-8512

American Porphyria Foundation
P.O. Box 22712
Houston, TX 77027
1-713-266-9617

SELECTED BIBLIOGRAPHY

Boulechfar, S., Dasilva, V., Deybach, J.-C., Nordmann, Y., Grandchamp, B., and Verneuil, H.de. (1992). Heterogeneity of mutations in the uroporphyrinogen III synthase gene in congenital erythropoietic porphyria. *Hum. Genet.* **88,** 320–324.

A total of seven families (two from prior publications) with four different point mutations, one deletion and one insertion, based on mRNA studies. Summarizes mutations reported in the literature. C73R appears to be a relative hot spot.

Cripps, D.J. (1986). Porphyria: genetic and acquired. *I.A.R.C. Sci.Publ.* **77,** 549–566.

A brief summary chapter with a precis for each disorder, including screening tests, porphyrin excretion pattern, and enzyme defects.

Hift, R.J., Meissner, P.N., and Kirsch, R.E. (1993). The effect of oral activated charcoal on the course of congenital erythropoietic porphyria. *Br. J. Dermatol.* **129,** 14–17.

A follow-up of two earlier anecdotal reports of clinical response to activated charcoal. The authors report initial improvement, but subsequent failure with treatment in one patient.

Illis, L. (1964). On porphyria and the aetiology of werwolves. *Proc. Natl. Acad. Sci. U.S.A.* **57,** 23–26.

The author argues that hirsutism, scarring, and photomutilation, along with preference for nocturnal activity in individuals with porphyria, might account for the development of the werwolf legends.

Pain, R.W., Welch, F.W., Woodroffe, A.J., Handley, D.A., and Lockwood, W. H. (1975). Erythropoietic uroporphyria of Gunther first presenting at 58 years with positive family studies. *Br. Med. J.* **iii,** 621–623.

A 58-year-old man presented with a 3 month history of blistering and hirsutism. His teeth were normal in color, his urine was discolored, and his spleen and liver were normal. Porphyrin excretion was consistent with the diagnosis of Gunther disease. Five asymptomatic relatives also had a urine excretion pattern consistent with the diagnosis of Gunther disease. The authors suggest that the patient was a manifesting heterozygote. This may be the situation for the few case reports of late onset of congenital erythropoietic porphyria.

Townsend-Coles, W.F., and Barnes, H.D. (1957). Erythropoietic (congenital) porphyria. Two cases in Sudanese siblings. *Lancet* **ii,** 271–273.

Murphy, G.M., Hawk, J.L.M., Nicholson, D.C., and Magnus, I.A. (1987). Congenital erythropoietic porphyria (Gunther's disease). *Clin. Exp. Dermatol.* **12,** 61–65.

Initial report (Townsend and Barnes, 1957) and 30 year follow-up (Murphy et al., 1987) of two siblings in whom severity was considerably different, suggesting that the clinical variation may not be entirely attributable to different molecular lesions (unless both were differing compound heterozygotes).

Warner, C.A., Yoo, H.-W., Roberts, A.G., and Desnick, R.J. (1992). Congenital erythropoietic porphyria: identification and expression of exonic mutations in the uroporphyrinogen III synthase gene. *J. Clin. Invest.* **89,** 693–700.

Twenty-one patients. The authors attempt genotype–phenotype correlations, with homozygosity for *C73R* alleles conferring marked severity.

ERYTHROPOIETIC PROTOPORPHYRIA (MIM:177000)

(Erythrohepatic Protoporphyria; EPP)

DERMATOLOGIC FEATURES

Major. Acute photosensitivity with burning and intense itching usually presents early in childhood. In some individuals, onset of symptoms is delayed until early adolescence. Symptoms occur within a few minutes to a few hours of sun exposure. Redness and swelling can occur, usually after repeated attacks, but early on there may be no clinical signs, and the correct diagnosis may be missed.

Late changes include thickening of the skin

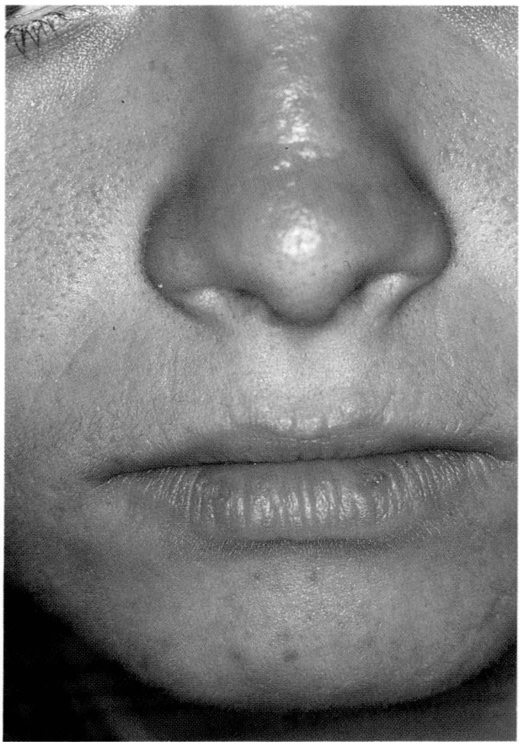

Figure 11.4. Thickening of skin on cheeks and nose. (Courtesy of Division of Dermatology, University of Washington.)

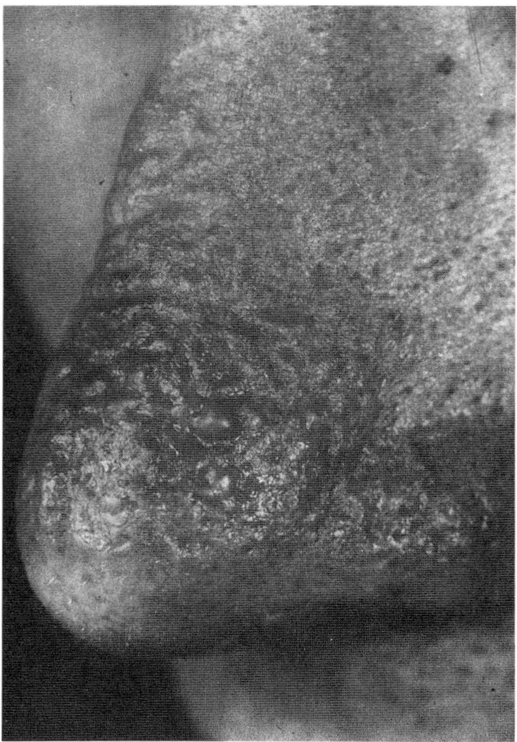

Figure 11.5. Thickened orange peel-like changes in disease of longstanding duration. (From Moore et al., 1987.)

with a waxy or leathery-like pseudosclerodermatous appearance, described as similar to colloid milium. These changes tend to be relatively mild. Superficial, shallow, chicken pox-like, or linear scars and pits appear on the face, and pseudorrhagades—linear creases around the mouth—may develop. These can also involve the lips themselves.

Minor. Petechiae and vesicles have been described in some individuals.

ASSOCIATED ABNORMALITIES

Anemia is found in about 25% of affected individuals and is usually mild.

Abnormalities in liver function tests develop in about 30% of patients. Progressive liver failure is rare, usually occurring after the age of 30 years. Estimates of its occurrence range from 1% to 4% of affected individuals. There have been several case reports of individuals with erythropoietic protoporphyria in whom the correct diagnosis was not suspected until liver disease developed. The cause of the liver disease remains unknown. Once jaundice develops, progression to end stage liver failure is inevitable.

Urine porphyrin is normal; plasma, stool, and erythrocyte protoporphyrins are elevated. Gallstones develop in about 30%.

HISTOPATHOLOGY

Light. Epidermal hyperkeratosis, acanthosis, and thickening of blood vessel walls are typical features. Deposition of IgA and mucopolysaccharides around blood vessels in the superficial dermis can be seen.

EM. *Acute lesions:* Swollen endothelial cells

of the dermal vessels with cell lysis and degranulation of mast cells. *Chronic lesions:* Variable findings from no change to necrosis of basal cells, replication of the basement membrane of upper dermal capillaries, and hyalin deposition.

BASIC DEFECT

Defects in the mitochondrial enzyme ferrochelatase.

TREATMENT

Oral β-carotene is the treatment of choice. Adult doses range from 120 to 180 mg/day to achieve serum levels of 6–8 mg/l (400–800 μg/dl). Sunscreens have limited usefulness but nonetheless should be used.

In patients resistant to β-carotene, transfusion treatment with packed red blood cells has been moderately successful. This treatment is not without risk and is not considered to be standard therapy. Plasmapheresis has also been mentioned as effective.

Although not entirely reliable, liver functions should be monitored in all individuals. Should these rise, then liver biopsy is indicated. Some patients will develop liver failure without any prior indication. Treatment with cholestyramine, activated charcoal, and bile salts may postpone, but probably does not prevent, development of liver failure.

MODE OF INHERITANCE

Autosomal dominant with reduced penetrance and marked allelic heterogeneity. It may require compound heterozygosity for clinical expression of the disorder. Recurrence risk to clinically affected individuals to have clinically affected offspring is much lower than 50%. In the mouse, erythropoietic protoporphyria is a recessive condition with no clinical expression in heterozygotes. The gene for ferrochelatase maps to the long arm of chromosome 18.

PRENATAL DIAGNOSIS

Not performed. Presumably possible by molecular techniques.

DIFFERENTIAL DIAGNOSIS

Porphyria cutanea tarda (MIM:176100) is usually later in onset. Patients with porphyria cutania tarda often do not recognize the association of the symptoms with sun exposure. There is more cutaneous change and usually absence of pain and burning. In polymorphic light eruption (MIM:174770) symptoms usually develop hours, not minutes, after sun exposure. Itching may be more prominent than burning and stinging. Scarring is rare. Red blood cell protoporphyrin levels are normal. Gunther disease (CEP, MIM:263700) is much more severe, of earlier onset, and distinguished by elevated levels of urine porphyrins.

Erythropoietic protoporphyria has been misdiagnosed as hydroa aestivale and solar urticaria. It is appropriate to screen patients for erythropoietic protoporphyria when these diagnoses are being considered. The waxy-like skin changes of erythropoietic protoporphyria are somewhat similar to the skin changes of lipoid proteinosis (MIM:247100), but the absence of associated photosensitivity, the presence of mucosal involvement, and involvement of nonsun-exposed skin in lipoid proteinosis are distinctive.

While psychogenic dermatitis or dermatitis artifactua are sometimes considered in the differential diagnosis of erythropoietic protoporphyria, these disorders are rare in children. The direct association of symptoms with sun exposure should trigger measurement of red blood cell protophorphyrins to exclude factitial disease.

Support Group: Iron Overload Diseases Association, Inc.
433 Westwind Drive
North Palm Beach, FL 33408
1-407-840-8512

American Porphyria Foundation

P.O. Box 22712
Houston, TX 77027
1-713-266-9617

SELECTED BIBLIOGRAPHY

Bickers, D.R. (1987). The dermatologic manifestations of human porphyria. *Ann. N.Y. Acad. Sci.* **514,** 261–267.

Review of the dermatologic manifestations of porphyria cutanea tarda and erythropoietic protoporphyria, with a concise historical accounting of the recognition of the diseases and a review of pathophysiology.

De Leo, V.A., Poh-Fitzpatrick, M., Mathews-Roth, M., and Harber, L.C. (1976). Erythropoietic protoporphyria. 10 years experience. *Am. J. Med.* **60,** 8–22.

Thirty-two patients: 97% had burning, 80% itching, 94% edema, 64% erythema. Only 28% had scarring. The tolerance for sun exposure and the severity of symptoms and signs varied widely. One hundred seventeen references.

Mathews-Roth, M.M. (1986). Beta-carotene therapy for erythropoietic protoporphyria and other photosensitivity diseases. *Biochimie* **68,** 875–884.

Gives dosing schedule: 1–4 years, 60–80 mg/day; 5–8 years, 90–120 mg/day; 9–12 years, 120–150 mg/day; 13–15 years, 150–180 mg/day; > 16 years, 180 mg/day. Administer the dose for 4–6 weeks and avoid increasing sun exposure until the carotenemic skin tone develops. Then exposure can be gradually increased to tolerance. Treatment does not result in complete sun tolerance. The dose can be increased to a maximum of 300 mg/day, with blood levels of 800 ng/dl. If there is no improvement after 3 months, the drug will not be helpful and should be discontinued.

Nordmann, Y. (1992). Erythropoietic protoporphyria and hepatic complications. *J. Hepatol.* **16,** 4–6.

States that approximately 1% of patients with erythropoietic protoporphyria will develop fatal liver disease. Summarizes experience and states that once jaundice develops the course is invariably fatal, short of liver transplantation.

Rufener, E.A. (1987). Erythropoietic protoporphyria: a study of its psychosocial aspects. *Br. J. Dermatol.* **116,** 703–708.

Twelve individuals answered a questionnaire and were interviewed, giving fascinating results. The statistical analysis of the questionnaire suggested that the impact of the disease was minimal. However, in interviews, the degree of distress and the alienation attributed to the disorder were marked. Most patients no longer consulted physicians for symptoms, and most were averse to trying new treatments.

Sarkany, R.P.E. (1995). The molecular genetics of erythropoietic protoporphyria. *Curr. Opin. Dermatol.* 219–224.

Todd, D.J. (1994) Erythropoietic protoporphyria. *Br. J. Dermatol.* **131,** 751–766.

Sarkany (1995) and Todd (1994) provide superb reviews of the current state of knowledge. Todd's paper lists 223 references.

Went, L.N., and Klasen, E.C. (1984). Genetic aspects of erythropoietic protoporphyria. *Ann. Hum. Genet.* **48,** 105–117.

Ninety-one families in the Netherlands. Forty-six singleton cases, 23 with two or more affected individuals within sibships, 22 pedigrees with more complex involvement. Fluorescence of red blood cells followed classic autosomal dominant inheritance pattern; symptomatic offspring had markedly higher percentage of fluorescent cells than asymptomatic parents. The authors postulate a three allele system.

HEREDITARY COPROPORPHYRIA (MIM:121300)

(HCP; CP)

DERMATOLOGIC FEATURES

Major. This is a rare form of porphyria. Acute photosensitivity develops in about 30% of patients and is similar to the pattern of porphyria cutanea tarda, with development of blisters and vesicles. The onset is usually in adult life. Skin changes rarely occur in the absence of acute systemic attacks.

Minor. None.

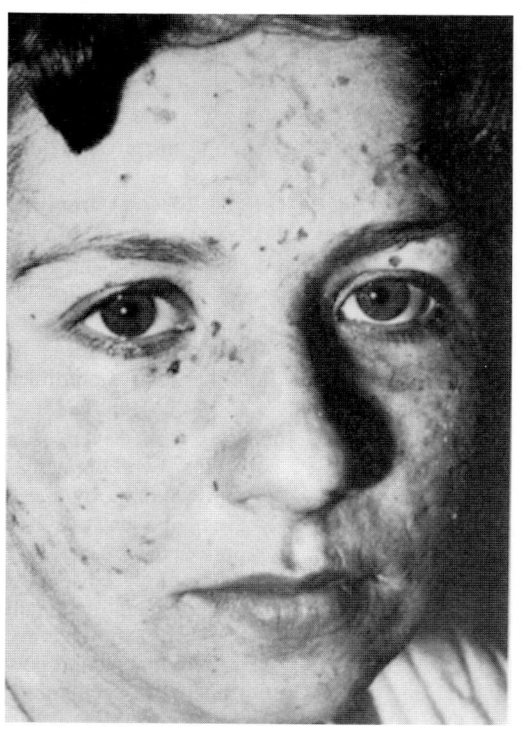
A

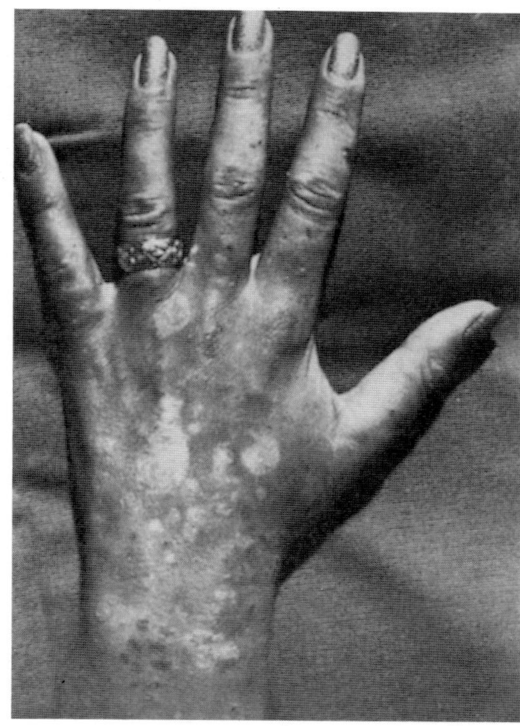
B

Figure 11.6. Typical superficial erosions, crusts and scars on face **(A)** and hands **(B)**. (From Hunter et al., 1971.)

ASSOCIATED ABNORMALITIES

Acute abdominal pain and vomiting, with or without neuropsychiatric attacks, are common and can be precipitated by drugs that increase the activity of hepatic cytochrome P450 (e.g., griseofulvin, barbiturates, phenytoin).

HISTOPATHOLOGY

LIGHT. Described in only one patient. Changes are similar to those in the other porphyrias.
EM. No information.

BASIC DEFECT

Defect in coprophryinogen oxidase.

TREATMENT

Avoidance of precipitating drugs. Affected individuals should wear a medical alert bracelet. Screening of relatives at risk is warranted. During attacks, hematin or high carbohydrate/ protein feeding is helpful.

MODE OF INHERITANCE

Autosomal dominant, with as few as 20%–30% of gene carriers experiencing attacks.

PRENATAL DIAGNOSIS

None.

DIFFERENTIAL DIAGNOSIS

The clinical features are very similar to those of variegate porphyria (MIM:176200); skin lesions are less common in hereditary coproporphyria and tend to occur in those patients with concomitant liver disease. The systemic complaints are similar to those of acute intermittent porphyria (MIM:176000).

Support Group: American Porphyria Foundation
P.O. Box 22712
Houston, TX 77027
1-713-266-9617

SELECTED BIBLIOGRAPHY

Brodie, M.J., Thompson, G.G., Moore, M.R., Beattie, A.D., and Goldberg, A. (1977). Hereditary coproporphyria. Demonstration of the abnormalities in haem biosynthesis in peripheral blood. *Q. J. Med.* **182,** 229–241.

Eight of 20 individuals with the enzyme defect were symptomatic. The authors reviewed 111 cases from the literature of which 35 were symptomatic. Thirty percent of these had skin signs. Over 50% of the acute attacks were precipitated by drug exposure.

Goldberg, A., Rimington, C., and Lockhead, A.C. (1967). Hereditary coproporphyria. *Lancet* **i,** 632–636.

Ten cases of their own and 20 cases from the literature. The case details are instructive in the list of psychiatric diagnoses and treatments given to patients prior to arriving at the correct diagnosis.

Grandchamp, B., Phung, N., and Nordmann, Y. (1977). Homozygous case of hereditary coproporphyria. *Lancet* **ii,** 1348–1349.

An affected homozygote in whom severe skin changes of hypertrichosis and hyperpigmentation on the hands and face developed by age 4 years. Enzymatic activity in the patient was 2%. The first cousin parents both had 50% activity. The patient had one acute systemic episode at age 10 and was well until she became pregnant at age 20 years. She also had short stature, similar to the first case of hereditary coproporphyria reported, who may also have been homozygous.

PORPHYRIA CUTANEA TARDA (MIM:176100)

(Type II PCT)

Includes Hepatic Erythropoietic Porphyria (HEP)

DERMATOLOGIC FEATURES

MAJOR. The skin of sun-exposed areas (ears, hands, forearms, face) is fragile and develops vesicles and bullae with minor trauma. The blisters denude, and the superficial erosions heal with scarring and/or milia. Hypertrichosis, particularly on the temples, forehead, and around the eyes, is typical. The hairs are fine and dark. Hyperpigmentation can be mild or severe, is usually patchy and mottled, and may the sole presenting complaint. The hands and the face are most often involved. In women whose legs are exposed to sunlight, the legs and the feet may also be involved. Patients usually do not complain of photosensitivity and may not recognize the role that sunlight plays in their skin changes.

Hepatic erythropoietic porphyria is most likely the homozygous form of porphyria cutanea tarda. Homozygotes present with severe photosensitivity as neonates, go on to develop all the cutaneous signs of congenital erythropoietic porphyria, but lack erythrodontia, are not anemic, and they do not develop splenomegaly or liver disease.

MINOR. Long-term changes include scarring alopecia. Sclerodermatous-like skin changes are reported in approximately 20% of patients. There may be loss of nail plates. Less than 10% of patients develop ectopic calcinosis cutis.

ASSOCIATED ABNORMALITIES

Acquired porphyria cutanea tarda is very common and associated with liver disease due to ethanol abuse or estrogen use. Liver disease may be a concomitant of the disorder, as in erythropoietic protoporphyria, or a primary causal factor in provoking symptoms.

Keratoconjunctivitis, pinguecula, and pterygia are frequent ocular findings. Pinguecula are brown or yellow nodules that develop on the bulbar conjunctiva and have been described in 60% of patients with porphyria cutanea tarda examined for them. Pterygia occur in approximately 10%, and both are believed to result from actinic damage to the conjunctiva.

A

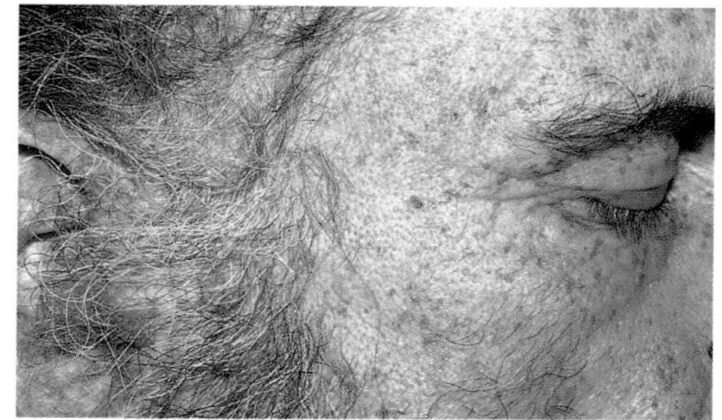

B

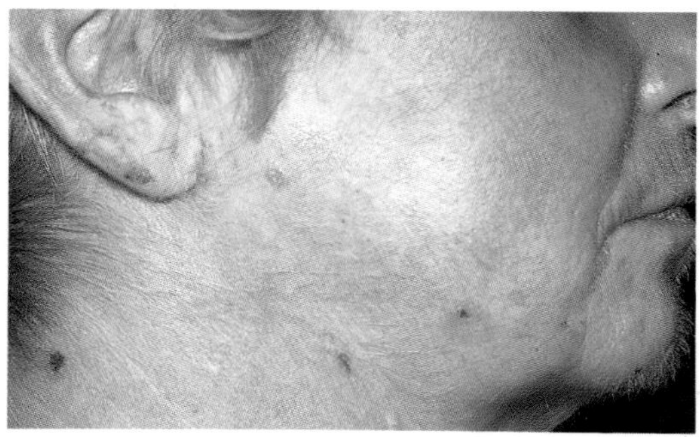

Figure 11.7. **(A)** Hairiness over zygoma; subtle atrophic scarring lateral to the eyebrow. **(B)** Hirsutism in a female with crusted erosions. (Courtesy of Division of Dermatology, University of Washington.)

HISTOPATHOLOGY

Light. Subepidermal bullae with "festooning" of dermal papillae into the blister cavity. The changes are consistent with solar damage. Patchy IgG deposition in dermal vessels and at the dermoepidermal junction is seen. There is little inflammatory infiltrate. The sclerodermatous lesions show sclerodermatous changes.

EM. Reduplication of the basal lamina small vessels in the upper dermis.

BASIC DEFECT

Reduction in uroporphyrinogen decarboxylase activity in all tissues. In acquired disease, the enzyme activity in the liver is decreased but is normal in all other tissues.

TREATMENT

Low-dose chloroquine (3 mg/kg/week in children).

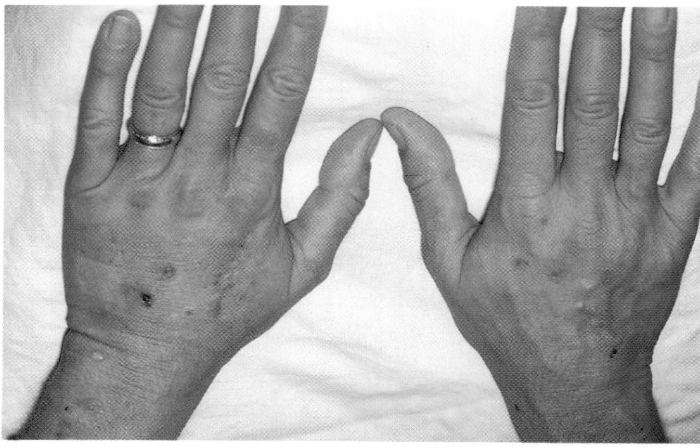

Figure 11.8. Typical erosions, scars, and blisters on backs of hands. (Courtesy of Division of Dermatology, University of Washington.)

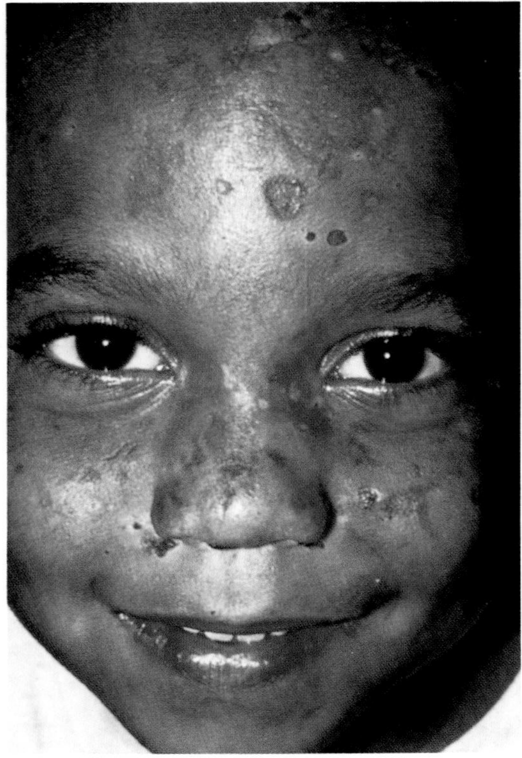

A

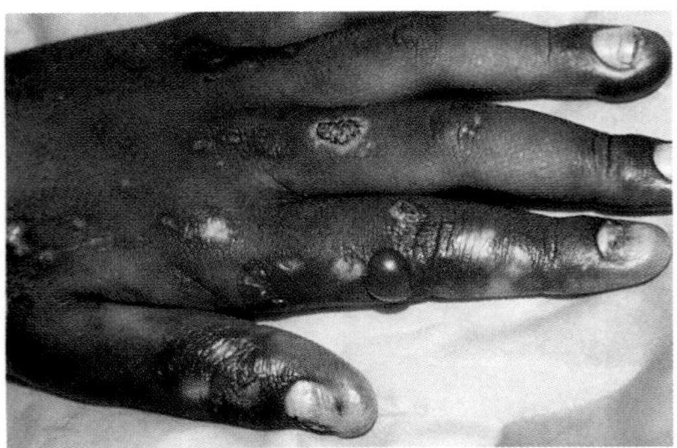

B

Figure 11.9. Face **(A)** and hands **(B)** of child with HEP. Marked scarring. (From Parsons et al., 1994.)

Phlebotomy to bring the hemoglobin level down to 11–12 g/dl.

Elimination of environmental triggers such as alcohol or estrogen.

MODE OF INHERITANCE

Autosomal dominant. Most heterozygotes are asymptomatic. Homozygotes have severe disease. The gene maps to 1p34.

PRENATAL DIAGNOSIS

None.

DIFFERENTIAL DIAGNOSIS

To discriminate between the acquired and genetic forms, red blood cell activity of the enzyme should be measured. It is normal in the acquired form. In the porphyria cutanea tarda-like syndrome associated with chronic renal dialysis, there is no abnormal excretion of porphyrins. Nalidixic acid, tetracycline, Dapsone, and Naproxen are among the drugs that can induce porphyria cutanea-like skin changes.

Variegate porphyria (MIM:176200) can be clinically indistinguishable from porphyria cutanea tarda in individuals who have primary skin involvement rather than systemic complaints. The porphyrin excretion pattern will distinguish between the two disorders. The plasma of patients with variegate porphyria fluoresces at 626 nm. Plasma from individuals with porphyria cutanea tarda does not.

With hereditary coproporphyria (MIM: 121300), the systemic symptoms of abdominal pain and neurologic abnormalities overshadow the cutaneous features.

In epidermolysis bullosa acquisita, blisters are not limited to sun-exposed areas, and generalized skin fragility is the rule.

Support Group: Iron Overload Diseases Association, Inc. (IOD)
433 Westwind Drive
North Palm Beach, FL 33408
1-407-840-8512

American Porphyria Foundation (APF)
P.O. Box 22712
Houston, TX 77027
1-713-266-9617

SELECTED BIBLIOGRAPHY

Egbert, B.M., LeBoit, P.E., McCalmont, T., Hu, C.-H., and Austin, C. (1993). Caterpillar bodies: distinctive basement membrane-containing structures in blisters of porphyria. *Am. J. Dermatopathol.* **15,** 199–202.

In almost all patients with porphyria cutanea tarda and pseudo-porphyria cutanea tarda, linear pink-staining bodies that contain type IV collagen and laminin are found in the basal and suprabasal epidermal cells of the blister roof. They are not specific for porphyria cutanea tarda and are found in approximately 10% of patients with other bullous diseases; they were also seen in one patient with erythropoietic protoporphyria.

Elder, G.H. (1990). The cutaneous porphyrias. *Semin. Dermatol.* **9,** 63–69.

Nice succinct review of the porphyrias of interest to dermatologists.

Roberts, A.G., Elder, G.H., De Salamanca, R.E., Herrero, C., Lecha, M., and Mascaro, J.M. (1995). A mutation (G281E) of the human uroporphyrinogen decarboxylase gene causes both hepatoerythropoietic porphyria and overt familial porphyria cutanea tarda: biochemical and genetic studies on Spanish patients. *J. Invest. Dermatol.* **104,** 500–502.

Four of five Spanish patients with hepatoerythropoietic porphyria were homozygous for the same mutation; one was a compound heterozygote. One heterozygote carrier of the mutation had overt porphyria cutanea tarda. Discussion of confusion that still exists regarding relationship between these disorders.

VARIEGATE PORPHYRIA (MIM:176200)

DERMATOLOGIC FEATURES

Major. The skin in sun-exposed areas is fragile, blisters with little or no trauma, and develops erosions. Scarring is a common late feature of the disorder.

As in porphyria cutanea tarda, milia, hyperpigmentation, and hypertrichosis can develop. As in erythropoietic protoporphyria, pseudosclerodermatous changes also develop. Although approximately 80% of patients have cutaneous involvement, only about 50% present first with skin involvement alone. The skin changes are usually present after puberty and develop between the ages of 20 and 40 years in most patients. Typically acute photosensitivity develops late and usually is accompanied by liver disease.

Homozygosity for variegate porphyria has been reported. Affected individuals have developmental delay, growth retardation, seizures, and marked photosensitivity and present within the first few months of life. Carrier parents have been asymptomatic.

Minor. None.

ASSOCIATED ABNORMALITIES

Acute abdominal pain and acute neuropsychiatric symptoms, identical with those of acute intermittent porphyria, can occur with or without cutaneous involvement. The abdominal pain is colicky. Constipation is common, diarrhea is uncommon. Nausea, anxiety, headaches, confusion, seizures, abnormal behavior, coma, peripheral neuropathy, and bulbar palsy can all occur. Approximately 40% of patients have abdominal or central nervous system involvement along with skin involvement. Approximately 20% have systemic symptoms without skin involvement. Acute attacks usually do not begin until after puberty.

Although cholelithiasis is not a prominent feature of variegate porphyria, it occurs in these patients more often than would be expected by chance alone.

Autonomic dysfunction with hypertension and tachycardia is also reported.

Mortality due to the disease is most commonly precipitated by exacerbating drug exposure and results from respiratory failure.

HISTOPATHOLOGY

Light. Subepidermal blisters with mucopolysaccharide deposition around blood vessels.
EM. Reduplication of the basement membranes of small blood vessels in the dermis. Fibrillar material is deposited in the perivascular spaces and extends through the epidermis in threads, not clumps.

BASIC DEFECT

Deficiency of protoporphyrinogen oxidase activity.

TREATMENT

Avoidance of precipitating agents, e.g., certain drugs, alcohol, birth control pills, and fasting. Hematin infusion during acute states with rehydration and restoration of electrolyte balance.

MODE OF INHERITANCE

Autosomal dominant with higher penetrance than demonstrated in other porphyrias. The disorder is most common in South Africa, and a founder effect has been suggested. Close linkage to the α_1-antitrypsin locus on chromosome 14.

PRENATAL DIAGNOSIS

None.

DIFFERENTIAL DIAGNOSIS

Porphyria cutanea tarda (MIM:176100), acute intermittent porphyria (MIM:176000), and hereditary coproporphyria (MIM:121300) are distinguished by their porphyrin excretion patterns in urine and stool. In variegate porphyria, between attacks the urine excretion of porphyrins is normal. However, fecal protoporphyrin levels remain elevated.

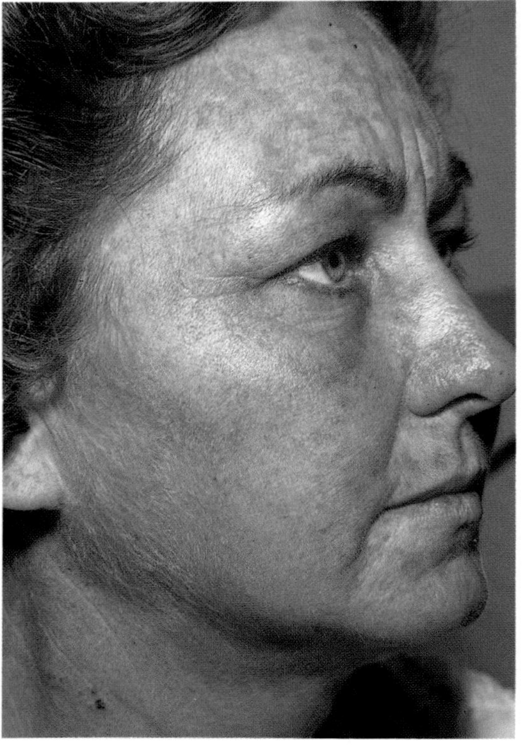

Figure 11.10. Mild facial hirsutism and scattered telangiectases. (Courtesy of Division of Dermatology, Seattle, Washington.)

An extensive menu of disorders from colitis to pancreatitis to esophageal dysfunction is usually entertained in the differential diagnosis of the acute attacks of variegate porphyria.

Support Group: American Porphyria Foundation (APF)
P.O. Box 22712
Houston, TX 77027
1-713-266-9617

SELECTED BIBLIOGRAPHY

Eales, L., Day, R.S., and Blekkenhorst, G.H. (1980). The clinical and biochemical features of variegate porphyria: an analysis of 300 cases studied at Groote Schuur Hospital, Capetown. *Int. J. Biochem.* **12,** 837–853.
This disease is most common in the South Afri-

can Caucasian and Colored populations. The authors bemoan the inability to trace the Dutch founders and progenitors because of the "dastardly attack by the Luftwaffe which razed central Rotterdam." A detailed review of a huge population with very good clinical descriptions.

Hift, R.J., Meissner, P.N., Todd, G., Kirby, P., Bilsland, D., Collins, P., Ferguson, J., and Moore, M.R. (1993). Homozygous variegate porphyria: an evolving clinical syndrome. *Postgrad. Med. J.* **69,** 781–786.

Two patients and a tabular review of the literature.

Macalpine, I., Hunter, R., and Rimington, C. (1968). Porphyria in the royal houses of Stuart, Hanover and Prussia. A follow-up study of George 3d's illness. *Br. Med. J.* **1,** 7–18.

The authors did a yeoman's job of tracing the pedigree both forward and back. They found two living descendants of George III and, by testing them, made the retrospective diagnosis of variegate porphyria in him.

MUCOPOLYSACCHARIDOSES

HUNTER SYNDROME (MIM:309900)

(MPS-IIA; MPS-IIB)

DERMATOLOGIC FEATURES

Major. Hunter syndrome is the only mucopolysaccharidosis that is associated with distinctive skin lesions beyond the generalized coarsening of features and hirsutism associated with storage diseases.

Flesh-colored to whitish small papules develop over the scapulae, usually at some time during the toddler years. They increase in number with time. Lesions may coalesce to form linear ridges and plaques. Involvement gradually extends to the shoulders, upper arms, upper chest, and lateral thighs. The nape of the neck may also show changes. Occasionally, spontaneous involution can occur.

Minor. The skin in general may appear thickened. Eyebrows, eyelashes, and scalp hair are luxurious. The tongue becomes progressively thickened, as do the gums.

ASSOCIATED ABNORMALITIES

Central nervous system anomalies include progressive mental retardation in most affected boys. Recognition of delays usually occurs by the second year of life. Progressive behavioral changes develop in the preschool years. Hyperactivity, oppositional behavior, aggression, and "exuberance" are common. There is a plateauing of skills, and gradual degeneration follows in the severe form of the disorder. In the more mild variants of Hunter syndrome, affected individuals may have normal intelligence.

Both progressive conductive and sensorineural hearing loss occur. Mucoid otorrhea is frequent.

Skeletal changes include macrocrania, short stature, gibbous deformity, kyphosis, and thickening and stiffening of the small and large joints. The hands become progressively clawed, the joints fixed in flexion. Radiologic changes include a J-shaped sella turcica and vertebral beaking, as well as broadening of the phalanges and the generalized changes of dysostosis multiplex.

The facies are characterized by thickened features and protruberant tongue and lips.

Hepatosplenomegaly is the rule, and abdominal and inguinal hernias are common. Intractable diarrhea is a complaint in many affected individuals. The cause for this is unclear.

A hoarse voice and recurrent upper airway

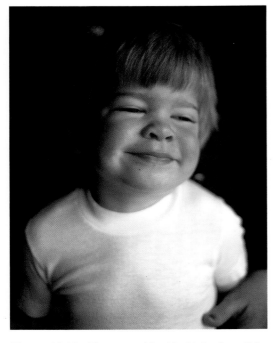

Figure 11.11. Five-year-old with thickening of facial features and luxuriant head of hair.

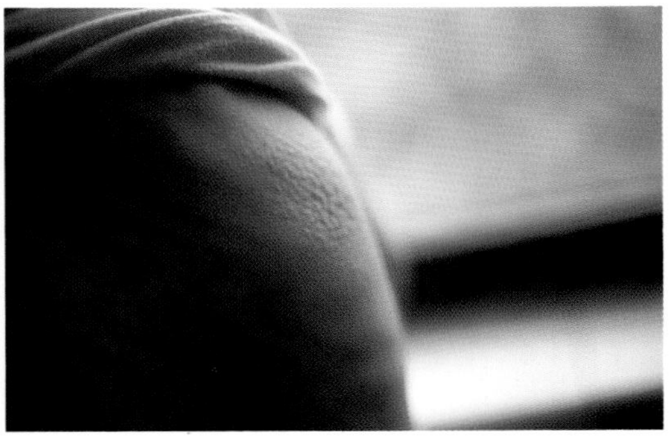

Figure 11.12. Cobblestoned plaque over scapula.

obstruction due to storage in mucosa are typical. Affected individuals have recurrent upper respiratory tract infections, adenoidal and tonsillar hypertrophy, and nasal congestion. Supraglottic swelling may result in sleep apnea.

Progressive cardiomyopathy and valvular disease is often the cause of death, which occurs within the first and second decades in the more severe variants.

Corneal clouding in Hunter syndrome is very rare. Progressive visual loss can occur, and increased retinal pigment degeneration has been described.

HISTOPATHOLOGY

Light. Increased amounts of mucinous material (glycosaminoglycans) in the reticular dermis that stain positively with Alcian blue separate the collagen bundles. Metachromatic granules are present in the fibrolasts.
EM. No information.

BASIC DEFECT

Mutations in iduronate-2 sulfatase (IDS), a lysosomal enzyme, result in intracellular storage of glycosaminoglycans, both dermatan sulfate and heparan sulfate.

TREATMENT

Supportive. Bone marrow transplantation has not been proven to be curative.

MODE OF INHERITANCE

X-linked recessive. Large and small deletions and point mutations have been found in the gene, mapped to Xq28.

PRENATAL DIAGNOSIS

DNA based. Carrier detection is also possible by molecular techniques.

DIFFERENTIAL DIAGNOSIS

The individual skin changes are similar to connective tissue nevi. If the color is slightly yellow, then they may be confused with xanthomas. The general cobblestone appearance can mimic the changes of pseudoxanthoma elasticum (MIM:177850, 264800) and lipoid proteinosis (MIM:247100). The associated clinical features of Hunter syndrome should lead easily to the correct diagnosis.

Support Group: National MPS Society, Inc.
17 Kraemer Street
Hicksville, NY 11801
1-516-931-6338

SELECTED BIBLIOGRAPHY

Bergstrom, S.K., Quinn, J.J., Greenstein, R., and Ascensas, J. (1994). Longterm followup of a patient transplanted for Hunter's disease type IIB: a case report and literature review. *Bone Marrow Transplant.* **14,** 653–681.

In this report of bone marrow transplantation in an 18-year-old with mild disease, the skin lesions resolved within a few months. The remainder of his manifestations also improved. His brother, the donor, had been treated successfully for acute lymphocytic leukemia 6 years before. At the time of transplant, the rearranged TCR-γ gene associated with his tumor was not detectable in marrow cells. There is a table reviewing results in six cases to date.

DiFerrante, N., and Nichols, B.L. (1972). A case of the Hunter syndrome in progeny. *Johns Hopkins Med. J.* **130,** 325–328.

A male with presumably a mild form of Hunter syndrome had a carrier daughter and two affected grandsons. There are wonderful family photos.

Froissart, R., Blond, J.-L., Maire, I., Guibaud, P., Hopwood, J.J., Mathieu, M., and Bozon, D. (1993). Hunter syndrome: gene deletions and rearrangements. *Hum. Mutat.* **2,** 138–140.

Analyzed 36 patients. Genotype–phenotype correlations are not exact, although complete deletion of the gene appears to always result in a severe phenotype.

Prystowsky, S.D., Maumenee, I.H., Freeman, R.G., Herndon, J.H., Jr., and Harrod, M.J. (1977). A cutaneous marker in Hunter syndrome. A report of four cases. *Arch. Dermatol.* **113,** 602–605.

Photos, clinical description, and review of nine previously described cases.

Sasaki, C.T., Ruiz, R., Kirchner, J.A., Gaito, R., Jr., and Seshi, B. (1987). Hunter's syndrome: a study in airway obstruction. *Laryngoscope.* **97,** 280–285.

Dismal review of five cases. Describes progression of signs and symptoms based on anatomy of involvement. States that surgical procedures in older (>15 years) patients require tracheostomy, as the airway changes prevent successful intubation.

Young, I.D., and Harper, P.S. (1982). Mild form of Hunter's syndrome: clinical delineation based on 31 cases. *Arch. Dis. Child.* **57,** 828–836.

Young, I.D., Harper, P.S., Newcombe, R.G., and Ancher, I.M. (1982). A clinical and genetic study of Hunter's syndrome. 2. Differences between the mild and severe forms. *J. Med. Genet.* **19,** 408–411.

Features of 52 severely and 31 mildly affected patients are reviewed succinctly. More details about the mild cases are provided by Young and Harper (1982).

OTHER METABOLIC DISORDERS

ACRODERMATITIS ENTEROPATHICA (MIM:201100)

DERMATOLOGIC FEATURES

MAJOR. Although the initial lesions of acrodermatitis enteropathica are blisters occurring soon after breast feeding is reduced or stopped, most clinical descriptions do not mention blisters or note them only as a minor feature. The blisters rapidly become pustular, and a weeping, oozing, red, eczematous rash occurs around the mouth, genitals, anus and distal extremities. Scaling is a late feature. Lesions heal without scarring.

Softening of the nail plate and swelling of the paronychial soft tissue is common. There may be nail dystrophy.

The hair is invariably affected, and total alopecia is common. Residual hairs are thin, brittle, and fragile and may show trichorrhexis nodosa.

Minor. Glossitis and stomatitis may occur.

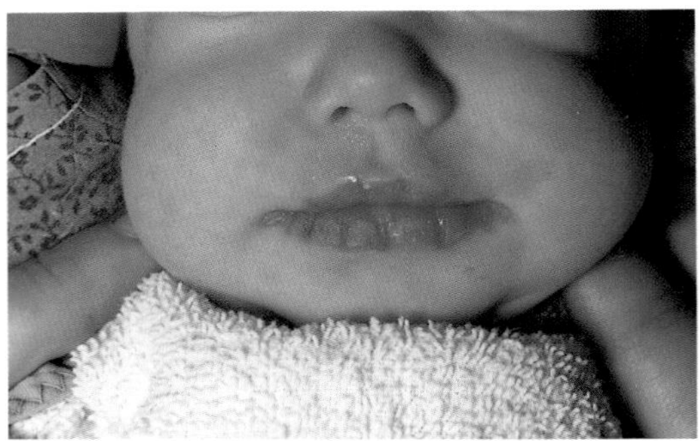

Figure 11.13. Early fissures at angles of mouth; cracking lips.

ASSOCIATED ABNORMALITIES

Neurologic abnormalities are typical of acrodermatitis enteropathica, with progressive ataxia, depression, irritability, and lethargy. These changes are reversible with zinc therapy, and permanent neurologic damage is uncommon in treated patients.

Growth retardation and failure to thrive are seen. Diarrhea is typical and associated with lactose intolerance. Recurrent infections are typical; *Candida albicans* and *Staphylococcus aureus* are common pathogens. Zinc deficiency results in impairment of monocyte and neutrophil function and depression of IgA and IgG, and both humoral and cellular immunity are adversely affected. The thymus is often hypoplastic or absent.

Many patients have eye involvement with blepharitis, keratitis, and conjunctivitis.

Hypogonadism has been reported but may be a secondary phenomenon of malnutrition rather than directly related to zinc deficiency.

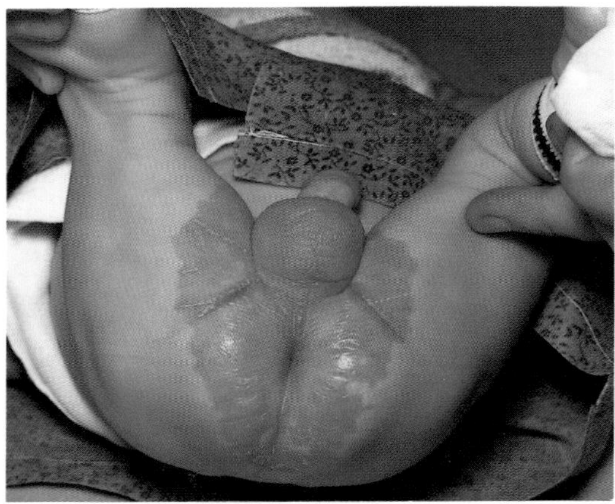

Figure 11.14. Shiny erosions around perineum.

HISTOPATHOLOGY

Light. In early lesions, there is pallor in the upper epidermis with clear cells that have empty or hazy cytoplasm, followed by psoriasiform changes. Diffuse parakeratosis overlies these areas and becomes more generalized with time. Occasional subcorneal vesicles can be found. Dermal vessels are dilated and tortuous. These findings are nonspecific.

EM. EM features are described primarily for jejeunal mucosa, and none is diagnostic. One report of EM of a skin biopsy in one patient described abnormal accumulation of lipid droplets in the cytoplasm, intracellular edema, and loss of normal intracellular architecture in the spinous cells. Basal cells were normal.

BASIC DEFECT

There is an abnormality, as yet undefined, in the intestinal absorption of zinc. Zinc is essential for the function of at least 90 enzymes, including DNA and RNA polymerases, carbonic anhydrase, and retinol dehydrogenase.

Breastfed infants do not manifest the disorder, as human breast milk contains high levels of low-molecular-weight zinc ligands that bind

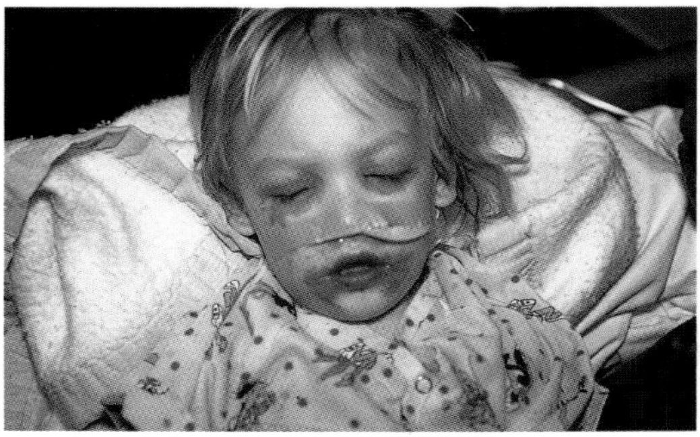

Figure 11.15. Severe perioral and periorbital involvement.

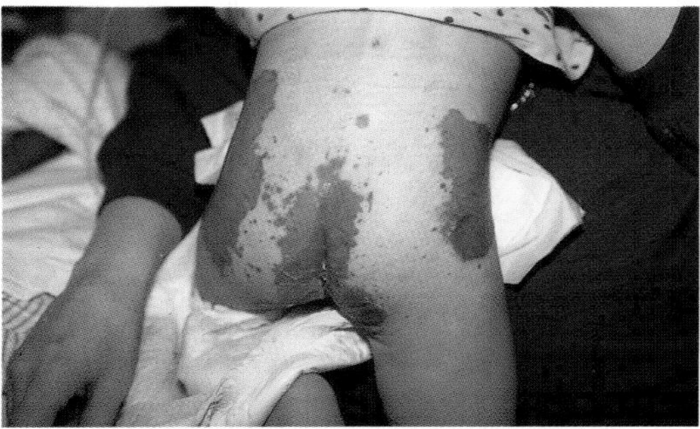

Figure 11.16. Same patient as in Fig. 11.15, with involvement of buttocks and flanks.

to zinc and facilitate its uptake from the small intestine.

There is an animal model for inherited acrodermatitis enteropathica. A-46 in Holstein-Freisian cattle is a lethal recessive condition characterized by similar skin involvement, infection, and death. It reverses promptly with zinc therapy.

Milk from the *lm/lm* mouse causes zinc deficiency and an acrodermatitis enteropathica phenocopy in mouse pups to whom it is fed, irrespective of the genotype of the recipient pup. The milk appears to be deficient in zinc because of a defect in transport of the metal from maternal serum to milk.

TREATMENT

Di-iodohydroxy quiniline (diodoquin) was the mainstay of therapy for 25 years until Moynahan (1974) administered oral zinc to patients and reversed the disease. From 35 to 100 mg of elemental zinc (50mg/220 mg zinc sulfate heptahydrate) daily in divided doses is the usual treatment. Doses may need to be adjusted, and zinc requirements may decrease after puberty. If improvement occurs, some authors suggest a withdrawal period to document relapse and confirm the diagnosis, as transient acrodermatitis enteropathica has been reported.

MODE OF INHERITANCE

Autosomal recessive. Carrier detection is not reliable, as the range of zinc levels in normals is too great.

PRENATAL DIAGNOSIS

Not attempted. For a treatable disease that responds without sequelae irrespective of the timing of institution of treatment, prenatal diagnosis is probably not appropriate. There is some suggestion that zinc deficiency in untreated acrodermatitis enteropathica patients during pregnancy may be teratogenic. There is no evidence for adverse outcome of pregnancy in treated patients.

DIFFERENTIAL DIAGNOSIS

Dietary insufficiency of zinc results in a phenocopy that is indistinguishable from the autosomal recessive form of the disease. The acquired disease is much more common, especially in Third World countries.

Blisters are a more persistent and major feature of epidermolysis bullosa (MIM:Many); erosions are more prominent in acrodermatitis enteropathica. There are no eczematous changes in the epidermolyses bullosa, and the hair is usually normal. The distribution of lesions is different. Electron microscopy will allow for correct diagnosis.

Candida diaper dermatitis can initially be confused with acrodermatitis enteropathica. While secondary yeast overgrowth is common in acrodermatitis enteropathica, the timing of onset of signs and the specific and widespread distribution of acrodermatitis enteropathica lesions should suggest the correct diagnosis.

Bullous congenital ichthyosiform erythroderma (MIM:113800) is usually congenital in onset. Acrodermatitis enteropathica appears later in infancy. Acrodermatitis enteropathica does not have the large bullae of congenital ichthyosiform erythroderma, and the hyperkeratosis of acrodermatitis enteropathica is later in onset and less severe. Generalized erythroderma is not typical of acrodermatitis enteropathica.

Familial pemphigus (Hailey-Hailey disease, MIM:169600) presents with intertriginous blistering without the eczematous features of acrodermatitis enteropathica. It rarely presents in infancy. Hair is normal in familial pemphigus.

Necrolytic migratory erythema is most often associated with glucagonoma and has not been reported in infancy. Clinically and histologically it is otherwise similar to acrodermatitis enteropathica.

The skin lesions of chronic mucocutaneous candidiasis (MIM:114580, 212050, 240300) can mimic those of acrodermatitis enteropathica. Demonstration of hyphae in skin scrapings may help distinguish the two. Oral involvement with *Candida* is not part of acrodermatitis enteropathica.

Although the perioral lesions and nail changes of mucoepithelial dysplasia (gap junction disease, Witkop syndrome, MIM:158310) are similar to those of acrodermatitis enteropathica and alopecia is seen in both conditions, the histopathology and electron microscopic findings are distinct.

The diagnosis of acrodermatitis enteropathica is clinical. Serum zinc levels may be abnormally low, but can be in the normal range. If the diagnosis is suspected, an empiric trial of 35–100 mg/day of elemental zinc is warranted.

Support Group: N.O.R.D
PO Box 8923
New Fairfield, Ct 06812
1-800-999-6673

SELECTED BIBLIOGRAPHY

Aggett, P.J. (1983). Acrodermatitis enteropathica. *J. Inherit. Metab. Dis.* **6,** 39–43.

Review of the role of zinc metabolism in acrodermatitis enteropathica. Sixty-nine references.

Danbolt, N., and Closs, K. (1942). Akrodermatitis enteropathica. *Acta Dermatol. Venereol.* **23,** 127–169.

Describes two children with a pustular dermatosis that the authors termed *acrodermatitis enteropathica,* believing that an intestinal abnormality of some kind resulted in a metabolic disturbance and the clinical syndrome. The article is in German with English and French summaries.

Gonzalez, J.R., Botet, M.V., and Sanchez, J.L. (1982). The histopathology of acrodermatitis enteropathica. *Am J. Dermatopathol.* **4,** 303–311.

Describes the histopathology in 12 cases of acrodermatitis enteropathica. Excellent clinical color photos. Well written and covers clinical presentation of disease well. States that pallor in upper epidermis is fairly diagnostic, although not specific.

Moynahan, E.J. (1974). Acrodermatitis enteropathica: a lethal inherited human zinc-deficiency disorder (Letter to the Editor). *Lancet.* **ii,** 399–400.

Follow-up of initial reported case and seven other patients with acrodermatitis enteropathica who responded to zinc replacement therapy.

ALKAPTONURIA (MIM:203500)

(Homogentisic Acid Oxidase Deficiency; Ochronosis)

DERMATOLOGIC FEATURES

Major. The deposition of polymers of homogentisic acid in cartilage and dermis and excreta results in blue-black pigmentation of the earwax, urine, cartilage of the ear and tip of the nose, sclerae, bones, skin of the axillae, around the areolae, and at the ends of the fin-

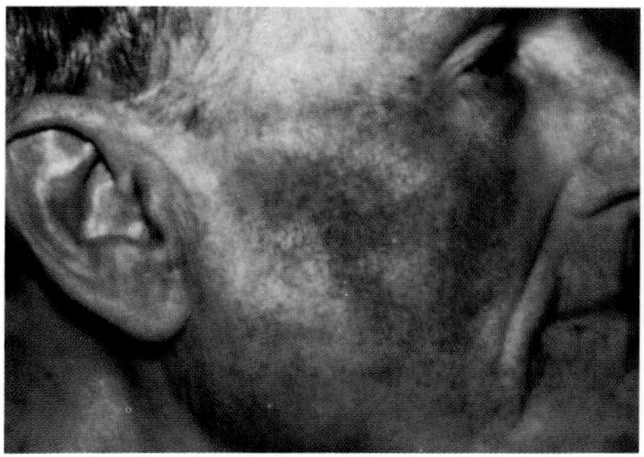
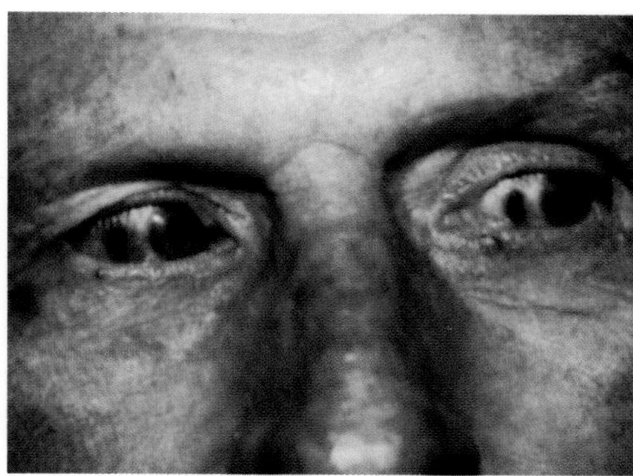

Figure 11.17. Black pigment in ear, on cheeks, sclerae, and over nasal bridge. (From Albers et al., 1992.)

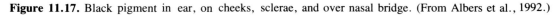

gers. The pigment changes are progressive and develop in adult life. By age 50 years almost all patients will have these clinical findings. Pigmentation of earwax and urine are usually the only signs of alkaptonuria in children.

The staining of the axillae, genital region, and cheeks is presumably due to increased homogentisic acid secretion in sweat glands and in the sweat. Where the skin over cartilage is thin (nose, pinnae, small joints, extensor tendons of the hands) it appears darker. The fingernails may also be bluish-gray.

Patients may complain of the ears being stiff and painful.

Minor. None.

ASSOCIATED ABNORMALITIES

Arthritis is the major deleterious aspect of ochronosis. It is progressive, involves all the joints, and usually begins in the thirties. The mechanism by which deposition of homogentisic acid in the bones and cartilage causes arthritis is not understood. The term *ochronosis* refers to the bony involvement of alkaptonuria. Males usually have more problems than females. Calcification of the intravertebral discs results in a clinical picture similar to that of ankylosing spondylitis. The small joints are usually spared.

The urine contains homogentisic acid, and standing urine turns dark over time because of oxidation. Renal stones can occur in both females and males. Stones in the prostate develop in almost all affected males and may be symptomatic.

Conductive hearing loss may result from ochronosis of the ossicles. Tinnitus is common. The tympanic membranes may appear blue. Cardiac involvement includes high blood pressure and cardiac murmurs. The heart valves show a bluish color, as do the endocardium and the intima of the aorta. Functional cardiac disease is rare. Pigment can develop in any part of the eyeball and lids, including the cornea, conjunctiva, sclera, tarsal plates, and eyelid skin.

HISTOPATHOLOGY

Light. Intracellular deposition of fine granular pigment occurs in the sweat glands and along the basement membrane. There are clumps of pigment in the dermis, on collagen fibers, and accompanying degeneration of elastic fibers. Macrophages can be seen.

EM. Cross sections of collagen bundles show homogeneous large, electron dense aggregates. Similar ochronotic pigment is found in macrophages and in elastic fibers.

BASIC DEFECT

Defective or absent homogentisic acid oxidase results in accumulation of homogentisic acid, a degradation product of tyrosine. Homogentisic acid oxidizes and converts to quinone derivatives, which make the color.

TREATMENT

Large doses of vitamin C have been proposed as a means to help delay or prevent arthritis. Vitamin C prevents oxidation of homogentisic acid to benzoquinone acetic acid, which is the molecule that binds to connective tissue. There are no long-term clinical studies of efficacy.

MODE OF INHERITANCE

Autosomal recessive. The gene, *(HGO)*, maps to 3q2. It has been cloned and mutations have been identified in individuals with alkaptonuria. The disorder occurs with increased frequency among Slovaks (one per 19,000) and in the Dominican Republic.

PRENATAL DIAGNOSIS

None.

DIFFERENTIAL DIAGNOSIS

Exogenous causes of ochronosis include chronic application of phenyl or carbolic acid to ulcers and industrial exposure to quinones.

Support Group: The National Arthritis Foundation
1314 Spring Street NW
Atlanta, GA 30309
1-404-872-7100.

SELECTED BIBLIOGRAPHY

Garrod, A.E. (1902). The incidence of alkaptonuria: a study in chemical individuality. *Lancet* **ii,** 1616–1620.

Proposed the autosomal recessive mode of inheritance for alkaptonuria but did not recognize morbidity associated with the condition. He considered it to be a "sport" or "alternative mode of metabolism."

O'Brien, W.M., LaDu, B.N., and Bunim, J.J. (1963). Biochemical, pathologic, and clinical aspects of alcaptonuria, ochronosis and ochronotic arthropathy. *Am. J. Med.* **34,** 813–838.

A review with great historical detail and delineation of both clinical features and biochemical defects. Reviews the genetics and shows that pedigrees purporting autosomal dominant inheritance were inbred and probably reflect pseudodominance. They show that the male-to-female preponderance of propositi was a result of bias of ascertainment. The ratio of males to females is 1:1 when all cases are examined. "The diagnosis of alcaptonuria and ochronosis poses no difficulty; it needs only to be thought of to be made." Three hundred fifty-three references.

Pollak, M.R., Chou, Y.-H.W., Cerda, J.J., Steinmann, N.B., LaDu, B.N., Seidman, J.G., and Seidman, C.E. (1993). Homozygosity mapping of the gene for alkaptonuria to 3q2. *Nat. Genet.* **5,** 201–204.

McKusick, V.A. (1994). Alkaptonuria tracked down to chromosome 3 (Editorial). *Genomics* **19,** 3–4.

Janocha, S., Wolz, W., Srsen, S., Srsnova, K., Montagutelli, X., Guenet, J.-L., Grimm, T., Kress, W., and Muller, C.K. (1994). The human gene for alkaptonuria (*AKU*) maps to chromosome 3q. *Genomics* **19,** 5–8.

Montagutelli, X., Lalouette, A., Coude, M., Kamoun, P., Forest, M., and Guenet, J.-L. (1994). *Aku,* a mutation of the mouse homologous to human alkaptonuria maps to chromosome 16. *Genomics* **19,** 9–11.

The articles of Pollak et al. (1993), McKusick (1994), Janocha et al. (1994), and Montagutelli et al. (1994) demonstrate that the gene maps to the long arm of chromosome 3 in humans and in the homologous region on 16 in the mouse. Mice with alkaptonuria were discovered by noticing black wood shavings in their cages. Mapping in the humans was based on a Slovak population. Janocha et al. (1994) has a nice table of signs and symptoms that develop with aging. The mouse does not develop staining of connective tissue.

Stenn, F.F., Milgram, J.W., Lee, S.L., Weigand, R.J., and Veis, A. (1977). Biochemical identification of homogentisic acid pigment in an ochronotic Egyptian mummy. *Science* **197,** 566–568.

Harwa (so much for patient confidentiality) died in approximately 1500 BC. He suffered from arthritis manifested by articular narrowing in the hips and knees. Biopsy of his bones revealed black pigment bands consistent with ochronosis. The authors argue that the frequent finding of black pigment in Egyptian mummies is due to the high frequency of alkaptonuria and not to artifact from mummification.

BIOTINIDASE DEFICIENCY (MIM:253260)

(Multiple Carboxylase Deficiency Late Onset)

DERMATOLOGIC FEATURES

MAJOR. The rash of biotinidase deficiency usually develops in midinfancy and is variously described as eczematous, seborrheic, erythematous, patchy, scaly, and nonspecific. There appears to be nothing to distinguish it from the common papulosquamous disorders of infancy such as eczema and seborrheic dermatitis. More than 50% of patients will have skin findings; in 25% it is the presenting sign.

Thinning of the hair, sparse hair, poor hair growth, and hair loss occur in more than 50% of affected individuals.

MINOR. Thrush is a common complication.

ASSOCIATED ABNORMALITIES

Biotinidase deficiency occurs in about 1 in 40,000 liveborn children. The signs of the condition are usually not present at birth, and most states have neonatal screening programs.

Neurologic problems associated with biotinidase deficiency include developmental delay; hypotonia, most marked in the lower extremities and trunk; ataxia, which may be intermittent or progressive; and seizures. Infantile spasms and myoclonic seizures are typical and respond poorly to anticonvulsants.

Hearing loss occurs in more than 50% of patients and is not improved with biotin treatment.

Laryngeal stridor has been described in several reports. Respiratory difficulties occur in 25%–50% of patients and are unresponsive to standard measures such as oxygen and bronchodilators. These problems do resolve with biotin administration. There is an intermittent metabolic acidosis.

Eye findings include keratoconjunctivitis, blepharitis, optic atrophy, and motility disturbances.

HISTOPATHOLOGY

LIGHT. No information.
EM. No information.

BASIC DEFECT

There is an inability to cleave biotin from other compounds (e.g., carboxylases). Thus affected individuals cannot recycle the vitamin biotin.

TREATMENT

Biotin supplementation promptly reverses skin and hair changes, the respiratory problems, and the metabolic disturbance. The standard dose is 15–20 mg/day PO.

MODE OF INHERITANCE

Autosomal recessive. The gene has been mapped to 3p25.

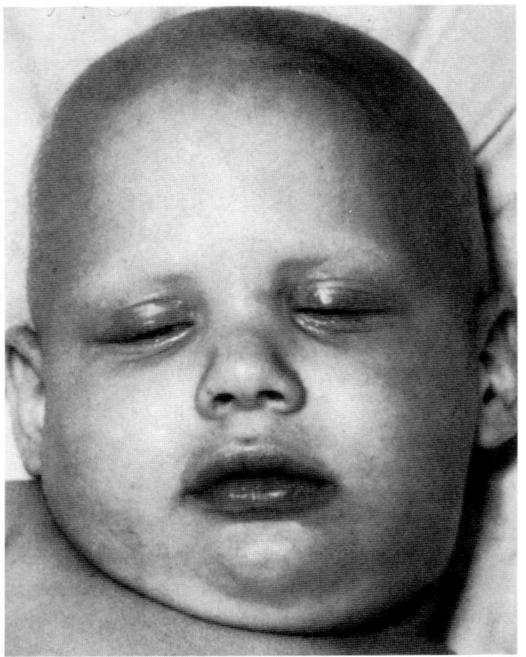

A

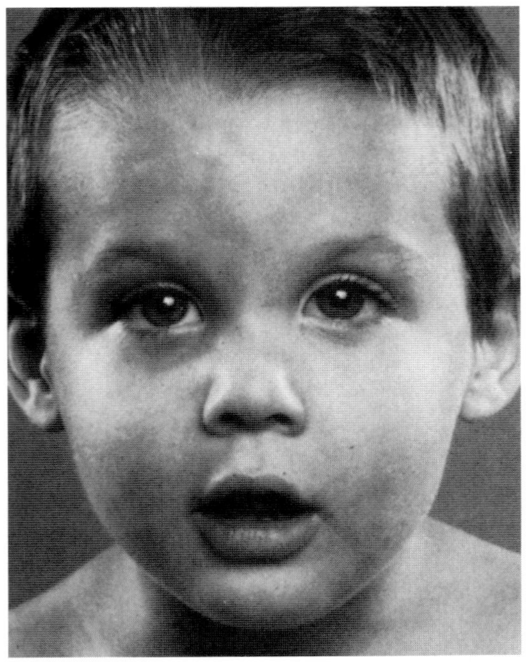

B

Figure 11.18. **(A)** Untreated girl at 2 years 9 months with alopecia and perioral and periorbital dermatitis. **(B)** After 4 months of biotin treatment, regrowth of scalp hair, eyelashes, and eyebrows. (From Thoene et al., 1981.)

PRENATAL DIAGNOSIS

Possible using cultured amniotic fluid or chorionic villi cells.

DIFFERENTIAL DIAGNOSIS

The co-occurrence of an eczematous dermatitis and neurologic symptoms should prompt consideration of biotinidase deficiency. Similar skin changes are seen in common childhood dermatoses and in association with a variety of metabolic and immunologic defects. The correct diagnosis depends on recognition of the associated features and appropriate laboratory investigation.

Neonatal biotinidase deficiency is also referred to as *holocarboxylase synthase deficiency* (MIM:253270). Neonates usually present with neurologic complications, which lead to diagnosis prior to development of skin rash. This is in contrast to late onset disease. In acrodermatitis enteropathica (MIM:201100), the skin changes are usually more erosive, localized to groin, around the mouth, and distal extremities, and affected infants usually do not have seizures or eye changes.

Iatrogenic biotin deficiency can result from chronic hemodialysis, bizarre diets, long-term administration of anticonvulsants, or total parenteral nutrition.

Support Group: Association for Neuro-Metabolic Disorders
5223 Brookfield Lane
Sylvania, OH 43560-1809
1-419-885-1497

SELECTED BIBLIOGRAPHY

Cole, H., Weremowicz, S., Morton, C.C., and Wolf, B. (1994). Localization of serum biotinidase (*BTD*) to human chromosome 3 in band p25. *Genomics* **22,** 662–663.

The cDNA for this gene was cloned and hybridized to this region on 3.

Sweetman, L., and Nyhan, W.L. (1986). Inheritable biotin-treatable disorders and associated phenomena. *Annu. Rev. Nutr.* **6,** 317–343.

This review chapter suggests that hair loss and rash are due to a deficiency of acetyl coA carboxylase, which is required for fatty acid synthesis, because defects in the other three carboxylases do not cause hair loss or skin changes.

Wastell, H.J., Bartlett, K., Dale, G., and Shein, A. (1988). Biotinidase deficiency: a survey of 10 cases. *Arch. Dis. Child.* **63,** 1244–1249.

Age at onset ranged from 1 1/2 months to 1 1/2 years. Four of nine affected patients had dermatitis. Seven of nine had alopecia, seven of nine had recurrent respiratory infections, and six of nine ataxia. Five had hearing loss that did not improve with treatment. Three had visual findings, and one, who was diagnosed earliest, had intellectual problems. There is a detailed review of all the cases.

Wolf, B., and Heard, G.S. (1991). Biotinidase deficiency. *Adv. Pediatr.* **38,** 1–21.

Summarizes clinical information in 33 reports in the literature, as well as their own patients, for a total of 83 cases.

FAMILIAL CUTANEOUS AMYLOIDOSIS (MIM:105250, 204950, 301220)

(Familial Primary Cutaneous Amyloidosis; Familial Lichen Amyloidosis)

Includes Partington Syndrome; X-Linked Cutaneous Amyloidosis;

X-Linked Reticulate Pigmentary Disorder

DERMATOLOGIC FEATURES

MAJOR. The cutaneous amyloidoses are classified by distribution (macular, biphasic, lichenoid), associated disease, type of amyloid protein, and other features. It is not evident to me that these distinctions have much applicability to the minority of patients with inherited cutaneous amyloidosis, as the clinical features can vary, even within families, and the derivation of the amyloid protein is uncertain.

In the autosomal dominant forms of cutaneous amyloidosis, diffuse brown macules and patches develop on the upper back and over the shins. The arms and thighs may also be involved. Itching is common, and secondary changes of lichenification may occur. Hyperkeratotic yellow-brown papules are described in a number of patients. Whether these are primary or secondary to repeated excoriation is unclear. A salt-and-pepper appearance of the skin with both hyperpigmented and hypopigmented areas has also been noted. The onset of the color change may be in early childhood or delayed until after puberty.

In an X-linked form of cutaneous amyloidosis, manifesting carrier females show distribution of pigment along the lines of Blaschko, while males have generalized reticulate hyperpigmentation. In autosomal dominant forms, distribution is more diffuse or patchy.

MINOR. Palmoplantar hyperkeratosis in males with the X-linked form has been described. Blonde, unruly hair with a frontal upsweep was described in two of six affected males with the X-linked form.

ASSOCIATED ABNORMALITIES

In one family with X-linked disease, symptoms of failure to thrive, recurrent pulmonary infections, and severe neonatal colitis may have been a consequence of the disorder or the result of an unrelated X-linked condition or due to unrecognized cystic fibrosis. At autopsy, one 50-year-old was found to have pulmonary fibrosis with no evidence of amyloid deposition except in the skin. Corneal dystrophy was

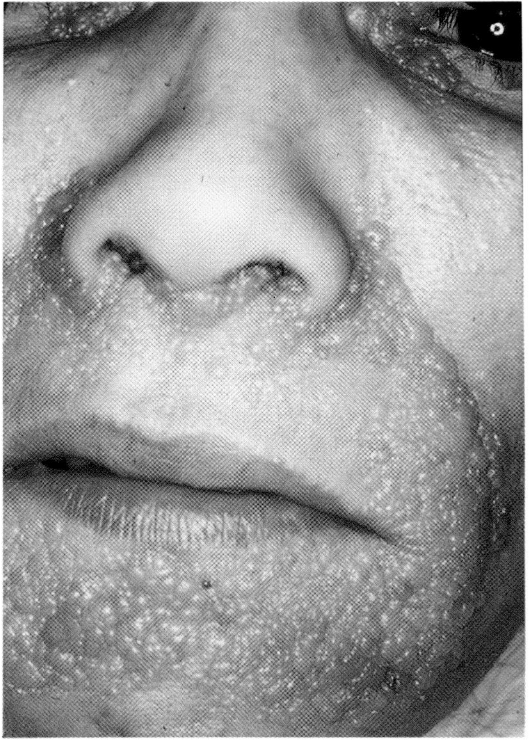

Figure 11.19. Plaque of coalesced papules in lichen amyloidosis. (Courtesy of Division of Dermatology, University of Washington.)

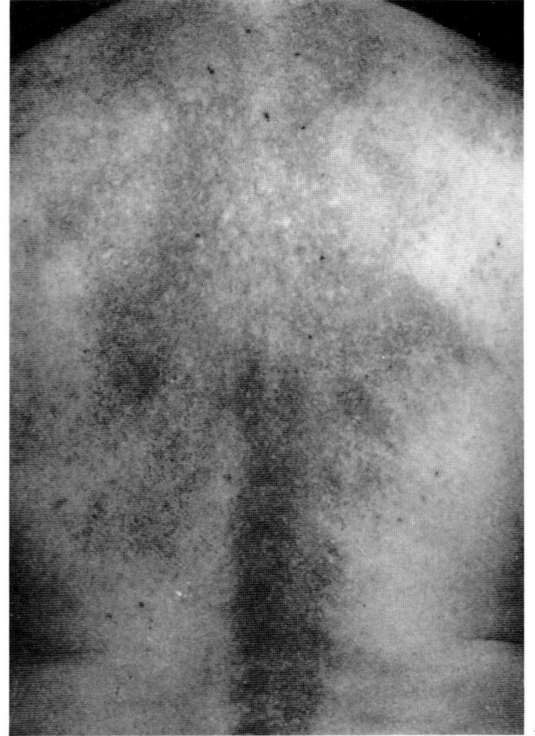

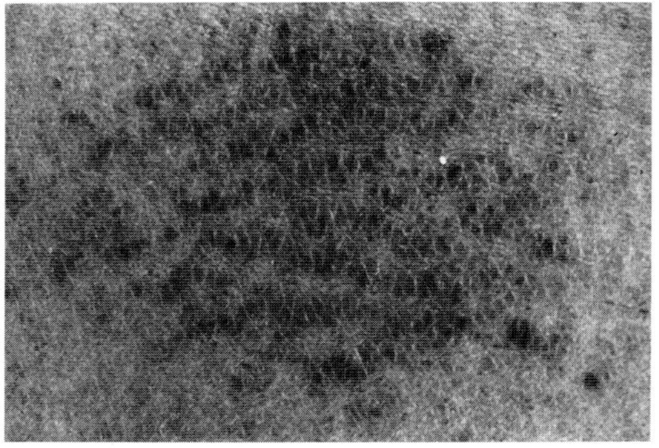

Figure 11.20. **(A)** Pigment changes in affected male. **(B)** Close-up shows stippled appearance. (From Black and Wilson Jones, 1971.)

found in three of the six affected males in this family.

HISTOPATHOLOGY

LIGHT. Amyloid deposition in the papillary dermis with an increase in melanin and hyperkeratosis. The amyloid deposits stain with Congo red.

EM. The amyloid deposits appear as ovoid bodies filled with fibrillar material.

BASIC DEFECT

Unknown. The amyloid in cutaneous amyloidosis is thought to derive from filamentous degeneration of keratinocytes, in concert with dermal proteins.

TREATMENT

Two cases of sporadic primary cutaneous amyloidosis were treated successfully with etretinate. These individuals sustained prolonged remission of pruritis and had clearing of amyloid from the skin.

MODE OF INHERITANCE

Autosomal dominant, questionable autosomal recessive, and X-linked recessive.

It is unclear if the autosomal dominant form is genetically heterogeneous or only clinically heterogeneous. There are no distinct patterns of skin findings that can distinguish among the subtypes, if they truly exist.

There has only been one family reported in which only siblings were affected. These individuals had bullae and amyloid deposition in the skin. The parents were not evaluated.

The X-linked form has been tentatively linked to Xp21–p22.

PRENATAL DIAGNOSIS

None.

DIFFERENTIAL DIAGNOSIS

There are three inherited amyloidoses whose major clinical features are neurologic and cardiac. For the most part, there are no overt cutaneous changes in these disorders, although there may be histologic evidence of amyloid deposition in the skin.

Secondary deposition of amyloid in the skin and in other organs is a consequence of many disorders, all readily distinguished by their other clinical features (e.g., familial Mediterranean fever, MIM:134610, 249100; multiple myeloma; chronic inflammatory disease). In most instances there are no clinically obvious changes in the skin, despite histopathologic evidence of amyloid deposition. In a minority, dermatologic findings have included petechiae, purpura, sclerodermatous-like changes, alopecia, waxy papules in the body folds, bullae, and tumors or nodules—quite distinct from the cutaneous features of familial primary cutaneous amyloidosis. Pruritis is common in all these disorders.

Localized amyloidosis of the skin is almost always sporadic, and most individuals with cutaneous amyloid will probably fall into this group.

Muckle-Wells syndrome (MIM:191900) is an autosomal dominant disorder characterized by hives, fever, deafness, and systemic amyloidosis.

Cutaneous amyloidosis was reported in one patient with Alagille syndrome (MIM:118450), one patient with Fanconi anemia (MIM:227650), and several families with familial medullary thyroid carcinoma (MIM:155240) or MEN 2A (MIM:171400). In one family with the last disorder, the plaques of lichen amyloidosis were not invariably present. Therefore, they are not a reliable identifier of gene carriers. Amyloid deposition in females with the X-linked form of familial primary cutaneous amyloidosis can mimic the pigment distribution of incontinentia pigmenti (MIM:308310). The absence of blistering and verrucous stages, coupled with typical histologic features, should allow for correct diagnosis.

Support Group: N.O.R.D.
P.O. Box 8923
New Fairfield, CT 06812
1-800-999-6673

SELECTED BIBLIOGRAPHY

Dahlback, K., and Sakai, L. (1990). Immunohistochemical studies on fibrillin in amyloidosis, lichen ruber planus, and porphyria. *Acta Dermatol. Venereol. (Stockh.)* **70,** 275–280.

In skin from three patients with macular amyloidosis, the amyloid deposits stained with antibodies to fibrillin. In three biopsies specimens from patients with lichen amyloidosis and from one with secondary cutaneous amyloidosis, no significant staining was seen. The authors suggest fibrillin may be involved in the pathogenesis of primary cutaneous amyloidosis. There is no mention of positive family histories in any of these patients.

Gagel, R.F., Levy, M.L., Donovan, D.T., Alford, B.R., Wheeler, T., and Tschen, J.A. (1989). Multiple endocrine neoplasia type 2a associated with cutaneous lichen amyloidosis. *Ann. Intern. Med.* **111,** 802–886.

Three of five family members affected with MEN 2A had single plaques on the upper back that developed at or after 18 years of age and slowly progressed. Itching was intense. The authors suggest screening families with lichen amyloidosis for MEN 2A.

Sagher, F., and Shanon, J. (1963). Amyloidosis cutis. Familial occurrence in three generations. *Arch. Dermatol.* **87,** 171–175.

Three individuals in three generations shared an isolated congenital asymptomatic "nevus" of confluent papules on the back. On biopsy these showed amyloid. This appears to be a unique disorder.

CHAPTER 12

PREMATURE AGING

COCKAYNE SYNDROME (MIM:216400, 216410)

(Cockayne Syndrome-A and Cockayne Syndrome-B, Cockayne Syndrome-I and Cockayne Syndrome-II)

DERMATOLOGIC FEATURES

MAJOR. The Cockayne syndrome has been divided into three subtypes. CS-I (CS-A) presents in childhood. CS-II (CS-B) presents at birth or infancy and has a worse prognosis with an earlier demise. CS-III (CS-C) is identical to xeroderma pigmentosa subgroup B and will not be further discussed here. The degree of skin changes is quite variable, both within the groups and between the groups. The descriptions of skin findings in most case reports of Cockayne syndrome are fairly cursory. Patients typically have gradual thinning of the skin with loss of subcutaneous tissue and an increase in telangiectases. The skin is described as dry and rough. Thinning of the hair is typical. There appears to be marked photosensitivity with mild, if any, pigment changes, and marked facial erythema with sun exposure.

MINOR. Anhidrosis or hypohidrosis can develop, but hyperthermia as a result of a decreased ability to sweat has not been a problem. Erythema of the hands and feet has been described, and, despite the redness, they are described as being cold.

ASSOCIATED ABNORMALITIES

The typical facial appearance of the patients includes a pinched look and a beaked nose. This appearance develops gradually over time.

Retinal pigment degeneration, corneal opacities, cataracts (which appear to correlate with poorer outcome and earlier death), and nystagmus are described. Vision appears to be relatively well preserved despite retinal pigment changes. Optic atrophy and miotic pupils have also been noted.

Progressive mental retardation and microcephaly, progressive ataxia, tremors, and cogwheeling, as well as progressive sensorineural hearing loss, are the neurologic features of the disorder. On magnetic resonance imaging and computed tomographic scan, calcifications within the cerebrum, cerebellum, and basal ganglia are seen. There is white matter atrophy with patchy demyelinization in both the central and peripheral nervous systems.

There is progressive growth failure with failure to thrive, and all patients have short stature.

The skeletal changes, in addition to short stature, include relatively large hands and feet, limited range of motion of the joints with kyphosis, a thickened calvarium evident on x-ray, vertebral body alterations, sclerotic epiphyses of the fingers, and osteoporosis.

Hypogonadism has been described in about 30% of the males. Irregular menses and "underdeveloped" breasts have been described in some females.

Renal changes seen on biopsy include thickened glomerular basement membranes, hyalinization and atrophy of the tubules and glomeruli, and renal fibrosis. Arteriosclerotic changes and hypertension have also been described.

Dental caries are often mentioned and may be due to poor hygiene. The jaw opening is often restricted, and good oral toilet is difficult.

Cachexia, pneumonia, and progressive neurologic deterioration usually lead to death, the median age of which is 12–13 years.

HISTOPATHOLOGY

Light. No information.
EM. No information.

BASIC DEFECT

There is an increase in ultraviolet sensitivity of cells in culture. The cells seem to be deficient in the repair of actively transcribed genes. There appear to be three complementation groups.

TREATMENT

None specific.

MODE OF INHERITANCE

Autosomal recessive.

PRENATAL DIAGNOSIS

Cultured amniocytes exposed to ultraviolet light fail to recover normal RNA synthesis.

DIFFERENTIAL DIAGNOSIS

Unlike those with xeroderma pigmentosa (MIM:278700), patients with Cockayne syndrome do not develop skin cancer. There have been case reports of individuals with features of both diseases. Excision repair studies are probably indicated in patients in whom Cockayne syndrome is suspected to rule out the possibility of xeroderma pigmentosa. Patients with Cockayne syndrome have been misdiagnosed as having cerebral palsy. Neurologic regression is an important clue to differentiate Cockayne syndrome from this broader category. The magnetic resonance imaging changes of Cockayne syndrome can distinguish it from Bloom syndrome (MIM:210900). The skin of patients with Bloom syndrome is also characterized by marked hypopigmentation and hyper-

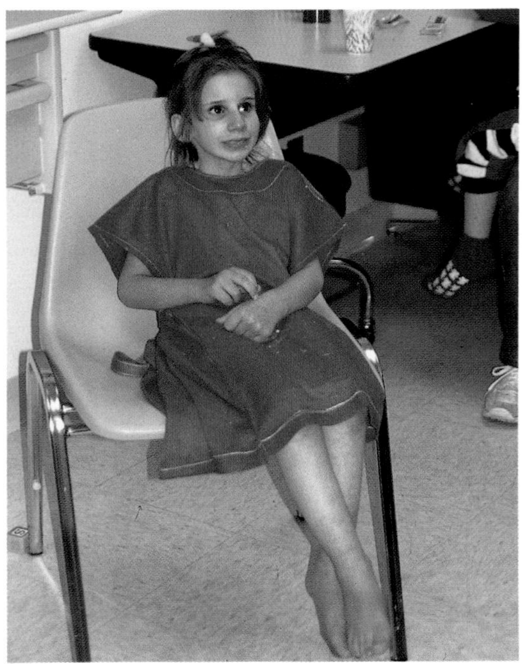

Figure 12.1. Affected 9-year-old with height at the 50th percentile for a 3-year-old, weight at 50th percentile for a 2-year-old, and head circumference of a 3-month-old.

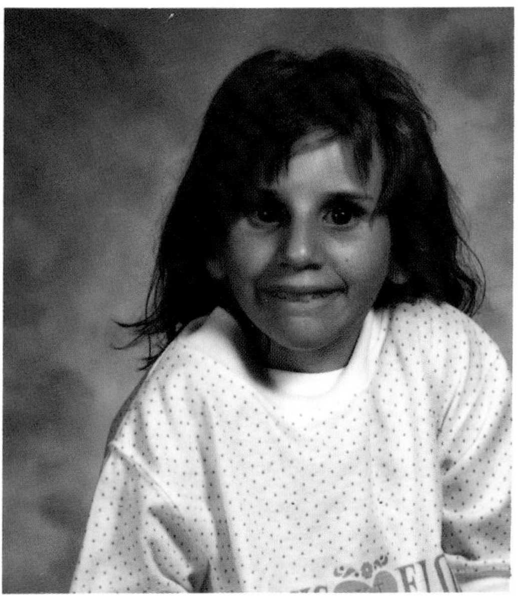

Figure 12.2. Close-up showing pinched facial appearance.

pigmentation, which is not a typical feature of Cockayne syndrome. COFS (cerebro-oculo-facial-skeletal) syndrome (MIM:214150) shares in common with CS-II facial changes evident at birth, plus arthrogryposis and growth failure. UVA sensitivity studies have not been performed in infants diagnosed with COFS syndrome. Thus, whether they are the same or distinct conditions is still uncertain. CAMFAK, or CAMAK (MIM:212540), is a term used to describe an entity similar to CS-II, and it may be the same condition. PIBIDS syndrome (MIM:278720) shares many features in common with Cockayne syndrome. Ichthyosis and trichothiodystrophy distinguish it. Among the disorders of premature aging, progeria (MIM:176670) is marked by much more severe wasting and growth failure. Children with progeria do not have the neurologic features of Cockayne syndrome. Seckel syndrome (MIM: 210600), or bird-headed dwarfism, shares in common with Cockayne syndrome failure to thrive and neurologic abnormalities, but has no skin changes associated with it.

Support Group: Share and Care Cockayne Syndrome Network
P.O. Box 552
Stanleytown, VA 24168-0552
1-703-629-2369

SELECTED BIBLIOGRAPHY

Cockayne, E.A. (1936). Dwarfism with retinal atrophy and deafness. *Arch. Dis. Child.* **11,** 1–8.

Cockayne, E.A. (1946). Dwarfism with retinal atrophy and deafness. *Arch. Dis. Child.* **46,** 52–54.

Two siblings. Describes dry, red, scaly rash on the face, ears, backs of hands, wrists, and legs. Beautiful color plates of the eye changes. Approaches syndrome identification from the feature of retinitis pigmentosa and concludes that the syndrome is distinct. Ten years of natural history are reported in the follow-up paper.

Hirooka, M., Hirota, M., and Kamada, M. (1988). Renal lesions in Cockayne syndrome. *Pediatr. Nephrol.* **2,** 239–243.

Report of two siblings. Reviews literature to date of renal findings in Cockayne syndrome, which are quite varied.

Lehmann, A.R., Francis, A.J., and Giannelli, F. (1985). Prenatal diagnosis of Cockayne's syndrome. *Lancet* **i,** 486–488.

Two fetuses at risk. The authors measured RNA synthesis after UVA radiation of amniocyte cell cultures for 3–4 days. Both true-positive and true-negative results obtained.

Nance, M.A., and Berry, S.A. (1992). Cockayne syndrome: review of 140 cases. *Am. J. Med. Genet.* **42,** 68–84.

One hundred forty-three references. Extensive review of the literature. Tables are somewhat confusing and do not always agree with the text (e.g., "all patients with Cockayne syndrome are mentally retarded" with no listing of mental retardation as a neurologic manifestation in the table). This problem can be overcome by careful reading. Clear discussion of the differential diagnosis based on presentation.

Patton, M.A., Giannelli, F., Frances, A.J., Baraitser, M., Harding, B., and Williams, A.J. (1989). Early onset Cockayne's syndrome: case reports with neuropathological and fibroblast studies. *J. Med. Genet.* **26,** 154–159.

Presents two patients and discusses similarities with COFS syndrome. Recounts evidence to support and refute arguments for the separation of these two disorders.

Venema, J., Mullenders, L.H.F., Natarajan, A.T., van Zeeland, A.A., and Mayne, L.V. (1990). The genetic defect in Cockayne syndrome is associated with the defect in repair of UV-induced DNA damage in transcriptionally active DNA. *Proc. Natl. Acad. Sci. U.S.A.* **87,** 4707–4711.

Two cell lines in Cockayne syndrome patients in complementation groups A and B showed decreased ability to repair pyrimidine dimers in transcriptionally active DNA formed after ultraviolet irradiation. Authors suggest this defect correlates with neurologic involvement, as it is seen in xeroderma pigmentosum type D and type A, both of which have mental retardation, as does Cockayne syndrome. This defect is not seen in xeroderma pigmentosum type C, in which intellectual ability is normal.

Weeda, G., Van Ham, R.C.A., Vermeulen,

W., Bootsma, D., Van Der Eb, A.J., and Hoeijimakers, J.H.J. (1990). A presumed DNA helicase encoded by ERCC-3 is involved in human repair disorders xeroderma pigmentosum and Cockayne's syndrome. *Cell* **62,** 777–791.

A mutation in *XPBC/ERCC-3* was found in a patient and a heterozygous mother. However, because only the single mutant allele was expressed in the patient, the authors postulated that the paternal allele must contain a mutation resulting in reduced or absent mRNA production. They could not confirm this hypothesis, because they could not get cells from the father.

DE BARSY SYNDROME (MIM:219150)

(Cutis Laxa, Corneal Clouding and Mental Retardation; Progeroid Syndrome of de Barsy)

DERMATOLOGIC FEATURES

MAJOR. The "aged" appearance of infants with de Barsy syndrome is based on the thin skin of the face and pinched midface with lack of subcutaneous tissue and on the wrinkled appearance of the skin elsewhere. These changes are not progressive. The vascular pattern of the skin is prominent. There have been only about a dozen case reports, and I am not convinced that all have had the same disorder.

MINOR. The sparse hair is an inconstant feature.

ASSOCIATED ABNORMALITIES

Intrauterine growth retardation is common, and poor postnatal growth is universal. There is a progressive choreoathetosis and stable, severe mental retardation. The joints may be lax with multiple dislocations, but the hands are typically held in an unusual fisted pattern. The facies are marked by large-appearing deep-set eyes, relatively large ears, and a pinched or beaked nose. Ocular involvement includes cataracts, strabismus, and myopia.

HISTOPATHOLOGY

LIGHT. There is a variable decrease in the amount of elastic fibers with thin, short fibers. Not all case reports have demonstrated this finding.

EM. There is variability in collagen bundle size, with a decrease in the amorphous component of elastin and an increase in the microfibrillar component of elastin.

BASIC DEFECT

Unknown.

TREATMENT

None.

MODE OF INHERITANCE

Uncertain. Although two sibships with several affected members have been described, the reported clinical features of these patients do not convince me that the diagnosis of de Barsy syndrome in them is correct.

PRENATAL DIAGNOSIS

None.

DIFFERENTIAL DIAGNOSIS

Infants with cutis laxa have similar wrinkled skin; progeroid, thin, pinched facies are usually not seen. Rather, infants with cutis laxa (MIM:123700, 219100, 304150) have a hound

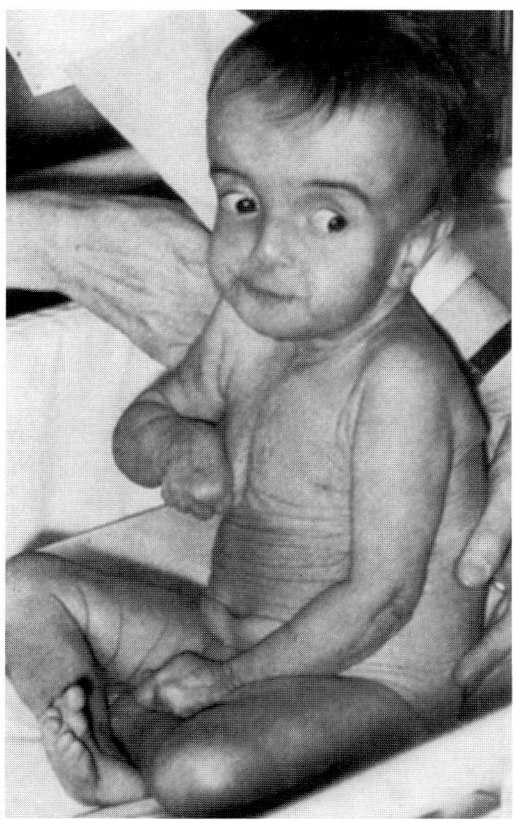

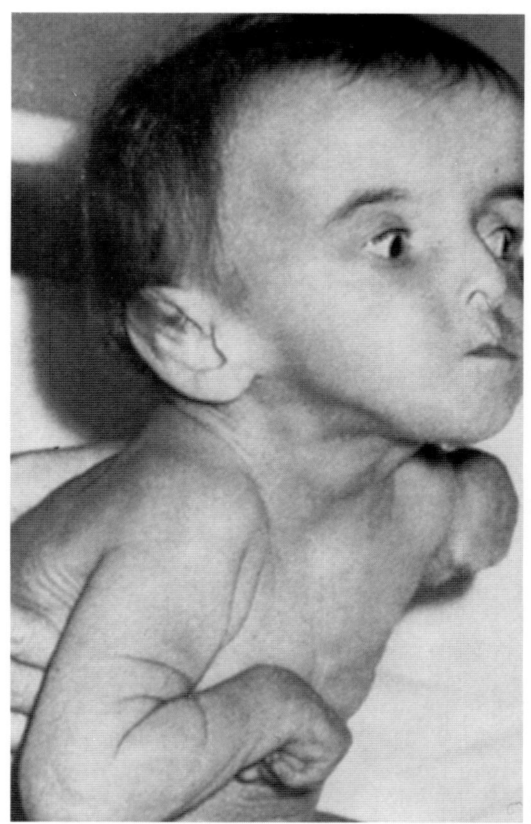

Figure 12.3. **(A, B)** Lax skin with many wrinkles. Facies marked by thin hair, frontal bossing, hypertelorism, abnormal ears, and pinched nose. (From de Barsy et al., 1968.)

dog or loose-jowled appearance. Children with progeria (Hutchinson-Gilford, MIM:176670) and Cockayne syndrome (MIM:216400) have a similar facial appearance. In these conditions, however, the abnormal facies are usually not present at birth, but develop later in infancy. They usually do not have wrinkled skin, and athetosis is not typical.

Wiedemann-Rautenstrauch syndrome (MIM: 264090) is very similar to de Barsy. Both conditions have carried the descriptor *neonatal progeroid syndrome*. Natal teeth are common to Weidemann-Rautenstrauch syndrome. Athetosis seems to be specific to de Barsy syndrome.

Support Group: N.O.R.D.
P.O. Box 8923
New Fairfield, CT 06812
1-800-999-6673

SELECTED BIBLIOGRAPHY

de Barsy, A.M., Moens, E., and Dierckx, L. (1966). Dwarfism, oligophrenia, and degeneration of the elastic tissue in skin and cornea: a new syndrome? *Helv. Paediatr. Acta* **23,** 305–313.

The authors describe their patient as having cutis laxa with thin, wrinkled, translucent skin. She also had progressive choreoathetosis. Abnormal short elastic fibers reduced in number were seen on biopsy. They thought that the patient's ocular findings, which included degeneration of Bowman's membrane and corneal scarring, distinguished her from other cases of cutis laxa.

Karnes, P.S., Shamban, A.T., Olsen, D.R., Fazio, M.J., and Falk, R.E. (1992). de Barsy syndrome: report of a case, literature review, and elastin gene expression in studies of skin. *Am. J. Med. Genet.* **42,** 29–34.

Case description. Tables compare de Barsy syndrome with other disorders and convince me of the significant overlap among them. The authors demonstrated a decrease in the steady-state levels of mRNA for elastin in fibroblast cultures, the significance of which remains unexplained.

Kunze, J., Majewski, F., Montgomery, Ph., Hockey, H., Karkut, I., and Riebel, Th. (1985). De Barsy syndrome—an autosomal recessive progeroid syndrome. *Eur. J. Pediatr.* **144,** 348–354.

Unfortunately, the pedigree with four affected siblings and the pedigree with three appear to have different disorders, neither of which is compellingly similar to de Barsy, based on review of the photographs. The wrinkly skin appeared limited to the hands and feet and overlarge joints. The facies do not give the same pinched appearance, and there is no hypotrichosis. To use this report to argue for the autosomal recessive inheritance of the de Barsy syndrome seems somewhat risky.

HALLERMANN-STREIFF SYNDROME (MIM:234100)

(François Dyscephalic Syndrome; Oculomandibulodyscephaly; Oculomandibulofacial Syndrome)

DERMATOLOGIC FEATURES

MAJOR. Rarely diagnosed on the basis of skin changes, nonetheless this disorder of premature aging has marked skin abnormalities. The skin of the face is atrophic, thin, and taut appearing. Telangiectases are common. In photographs, the atrophic characteristics of the skin are not as striking as the bony craniofacial alterations. There is generalized hypotrichosis of the scalp, which may also involve the eyebrows and eyelashes and secondary sexual hairs. The hairs are fine and usually light colored.

MINOR. Mild xerosis to frank ichthyosis has been noted in some case descriptions.

ASSOCIATED ABNORMALITIES

The term *dyscephaly* refers to the abnormal shape of the head and face. Wormian bones are seen in infancy. The term *bird-headed dwarfism* is also often used. The cranium may be small as well as altered in shape.

The face is characterized by a pinched beaked nose and extraordinary retrognathia. The mouth is marked by an everted lower lip. One-third of affected individuals are small at birth, and there is proportionate short stature in 50%–65% of patients. Although final adult height is reported to be 152 cm for females and 155–157 cm for males, numerous case descriptions of adult women give heights of 145 cm or so. I am uncertain of the validity of the taller heights alluded to in reviews.

Ophthalmologic features include microphthalmia and/or congenital cataracts in 90% of patients. Cataracts are always bilateral. A host of other ocular abnormalities has been noted in a minority of patients.

Dental anomalies are seen in 80% of patients and include absence of teeth, natal teeth, malformed teeth, enamel hypoplasia, and supernumerary teeth.

Estimates of the proportion of patients with mental retardation range from 15% to 30%, and the degree of intellectual handicap varies greatly. Obstructive sleep apnea has been the focus of several case reports, and a few patients have had upper airway obstruction because of a narrow trachea. At least three pregnancies have been reported in affected females and have resulted in normal outcomes.

HISTOPATHOLOGY

LIGHT. Decrease in mucopolysaccharides; alterations in both collagen and elastin, which appear to be nonspecific.

EM. No information.

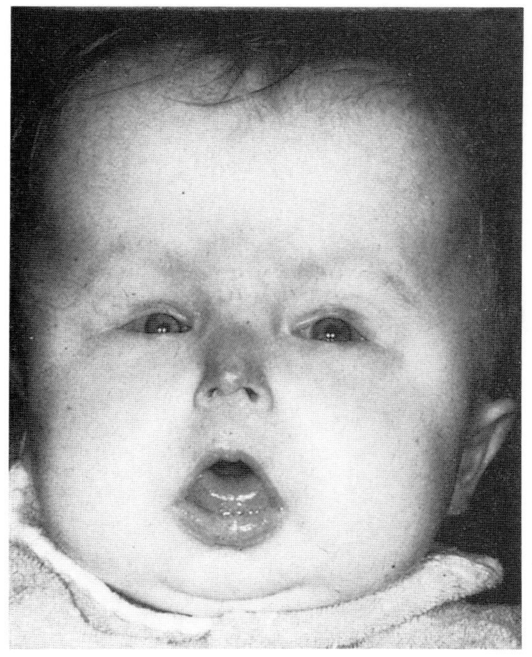
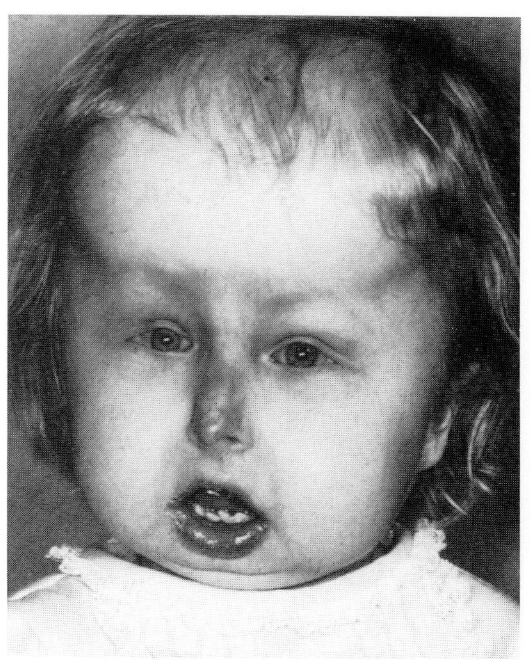

Figure 12.4. Same patient at ages 1 year **(A)** and 3½ years **(B)** sparse hair, beaked nose and small mouth. (From Cohen, 1991.)

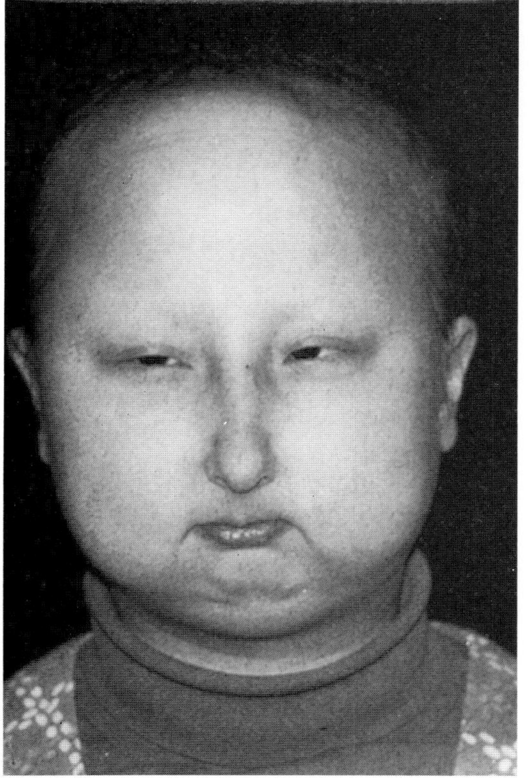
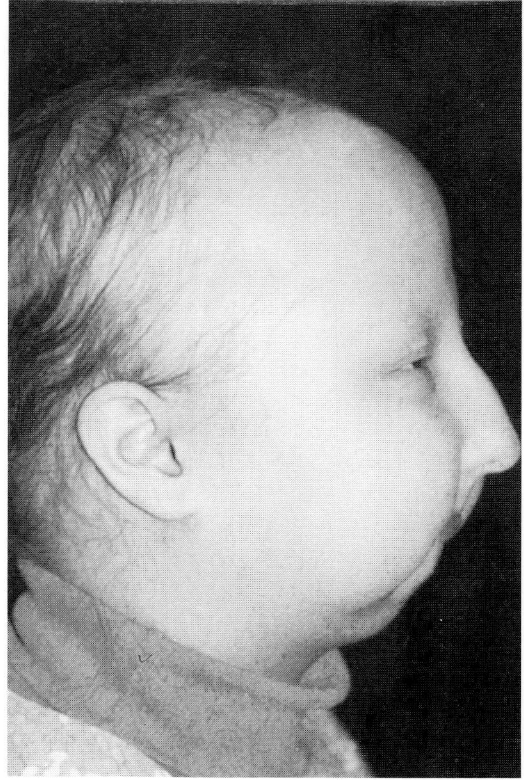

Figure 12.5. (A, B) Small palpebral fissures, beaked nose, hypotrichosis, and marked micrognathia. (From Cohen, 1991.)

BASIC DEFECT

Unknown.

TREATMENT

Craniofacial reconstruction, orthodontia, and cataract extraction are all part of management. Attention to the risk of obstructive airway involvement is important.

MODE OF INHERITANCE

Appears to be sporadic

PRENATAL DIAGNOSIS

None.

DIFFERENTIAL DIAGNOSIS

Rothmund-Thomson syndrome (poikiloderma congenitale, MIM:268400) and Bloom syndrome (MIM:210900) share facial telangiectases and skin atrophy with Hallermann-Streiff syndrome, but the facies of Hallermann-Streiff syndrome are distinctive. Children with progeria (MIM:176670) do not have the eye changes of Hallermann-Streiff syndrome or the marked micrognathia. Wiedemann-Rautenstrauch syndrome (MIM:264090) and Seckel syndrome (MIM:210600) may have a somewhat similar facial appearance, but do not show the eye findings of Hallermann-Streiff syndrome. Children with Seckel syndrome do not have cutaneous atrophy.

Support Group: N.O.R.D.
P.O. Box 8923
New Fairfield, CT
06812
1-800-999-6673

Little People of
America.
P.O. Box 9897
Washington, D.C.
20016
1-800-243-9273

SELECTED BIBLIOGRAPHY

Cohen, M.M., Jr. (1991). Hallermann-Streiff syndrome—a review. *Am. J. Med. Genet.* **41,** 488–499.

Nice discourse critiquing the evidence for familial transmission. Many tables listing clinical features. The author is interested in receiving information about cases and asks that they be reported to him. This is the lead article of a symposium on Hallermann-Streiff syndrome that appears in this edition of the journal. Seventy-six references.

Dinwiddie, R., Gewitz, M., and Taylor, J.F.N. (1978). Cardiac defects in the Hallermann-Streiff syndrome. *J. Pediatr.* **92,** 77–78.

Beware. They report three patients with Hallermann-Streiff syndrome and congenital heart disease. They extrapolate to an incidence of congenital heart disease of 4.8% based on their three patients and a total of 60 patients with Hallermann-Streiff syndrome in the literature. There is no bibliographic confirmation of the source of the 60 cases. The 4.8% figure has entered into legend and is repeatedly cited without alteration, even now, when over 150 cases have been logged.

François, J. (1982). François' dyscephalic syndrome. *Birth Defects* **XVIII(6),** 595–619.

In describing possible modes of inheritance, François states that the fact that patients resemble each other as closely as brothers and sisters "favors a genetic explanation." This review of the literature has several tables and many references.

HUTCHINSON-GILFORD PROGERIA (MIM:176670)

Includes Wiedemann-Rautenstrauch Syndrome; Carbohydrate Deficient Glycoprotein Syndrome; Mandibuloacral Dysplasia

Disorders of premature aging share in common cutaneous changes including loss of subcutaneous tissue, graying and thinning of the hair, and prominence of the vascular pattern of the skin. They are separated by specific systemic features (e.g., atherosclerosis) and age of onset and rate of progression. In addition to well-delineated syndromes there are numerous isolated case reports of "unique" patients who give the appearance of premature aging. Despite its rarity (1 in 8,000,000 births), the phenotype of Hutchinson-Gilford progeria is familiar to most practitioners because it is so striking.

DERMATOLOGIC FEATURES

MAJOR. Loss of subcutaneous tissue occurs everywhere with the exception of the suprapubic fat pad, which is preserved. The skin appears thin with a prominent venous pattern. The epidermis may look taut and shiny, giving a sclerodermatous appearance. Thick, inelastic skin on the lower extremities has been described in some children. One patient of mine presented with soft, lipomatous-like lesions on his buttocks and lower extremities, rather than stiff skin. These clinical features usually develop between 6 months and 1 year. When present at birth, they may indicate the Wiedemann-Rautenstrauch syndrome.

Pigmentary changes develop over time, may be patchy, and occur primarily in sun-exposed areas. Both guttate hypermelanosis and hypomelanosis can occur.

The hair may be normal early on, but gradually thins, becomes wispy, and loses its color. Within the first 2 years alopecia may become complete. Any hairs that remain are fine, white, or blonde. There is an absence of secondary sexual hairs; eyelashes and eyebrows are often absent.

MINOR. A bluish tinge around the mouth and the nasolabial folds referred to as *midfacial cyanosis* is often described. This may reflect a decrease in the thickness of the dermis with visual prominence of the underlying vascular network. Sweating may be decreased. Nail changes can occur. The nails may be thinned, short, and small. Hypoplastic or absent nipples have been described in a minority of patients.

ASSOCIATED ABNORMALITIES

Abnormal facies with a glyphic nasal tip are classic. The nose becomes sharp and sculpted with loss of the softer tissue of the nares. The

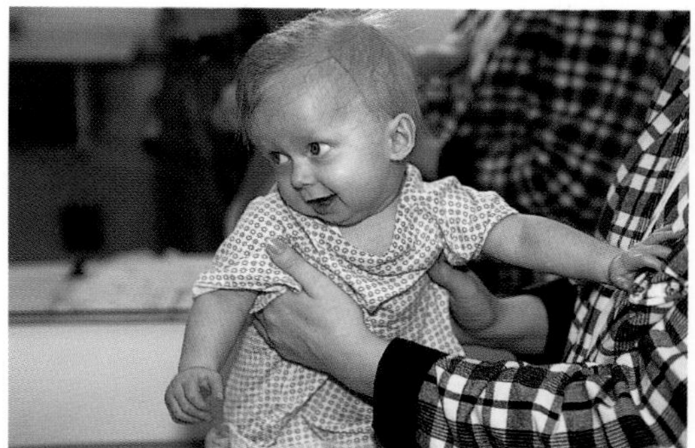

A

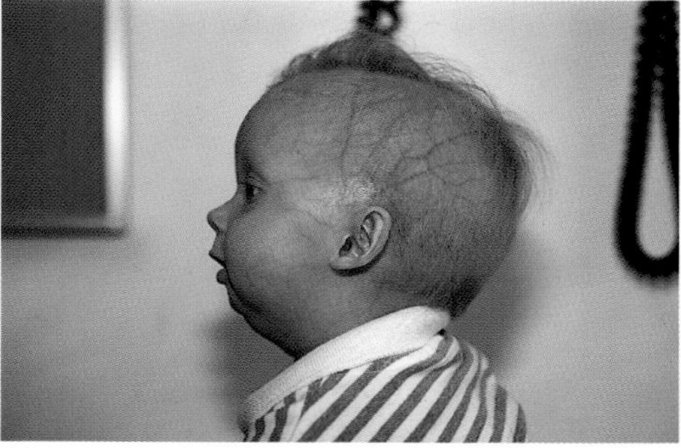

B

Figure 12.6. (A, B) Thinning of hair, prominent venous pattern, frontal bossing, and full cheeks with micrognathia in an 8 month old.

nasal cartilage becomes visible. Micrognathia and prominent eyes with hypoplastic inferior orbital ridges are typical, and the terms *bird-like* or *plucked bird appearance* are used. Absence of the earlobes, commented on in many reports, is an acquired feature. The lobes gradually atrophy, possibly due to loss of subcutaneous tissue.

Growth failure is usually evident by 3–12 months of age with a fall-off in height and weight. The head circumference is preserved. Short stature persists into adult life, and patients show very little in the way of weight gain. Growth failure is often the reason for initial evaluation of infants, and it is an invariable finding in children with progeria.

Failure to develop secondary sexual characteristics is typical. There has been one successful pregnancy reported in a patient who had onset of typical progeric features in late childhood; she thus may represent a different syndrome.

Skeletal changes early on include loss of the distal tufts of the phalanges with acroosteolysis. Osteoporosis and resorption of the distal ends of the clavicles occur somewhat later. The cranium is large relative to the face. There is limited range of motion at the knees, and other joints may become stiff. The anterior fontanelle often remains open. Coxa valga generally occurs by age 2, and affected children have a wide-based gait. Aseptic necrosis of the hips is also reported.

Intelligence is normal. The voice is thin and high pitched.

Dentition may be delayed. The teeth may be abnormal in structure and in number. The secondary teeth are usually more severely involved than the primary teeth.

Death comes early to children with progeria. The median age is in the early teens. The cause of death is usually myocardial infarction occurring secondary to atherosclerosis. Widespread atherosclerotic disease is the rule. Angina and strokes are common. In addition to atherosclerosis, myocardial fibrosis can develop.

Insulin resistance by biochemical testing is common, but frank hyperglycemia and diabetes occur rarely.

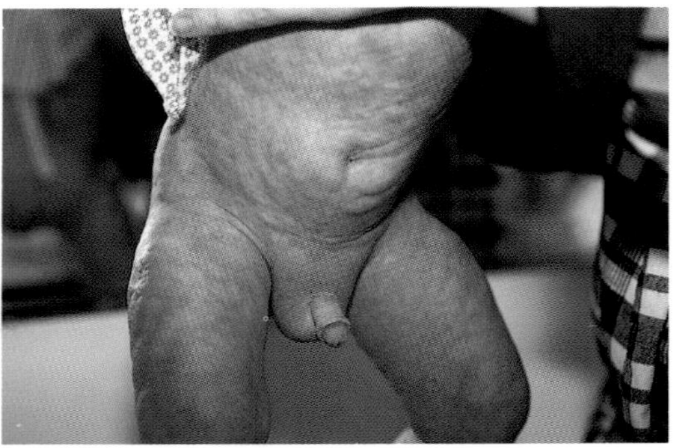

Figure 12.7. Marbled appearance of the skin. The nodules are soft, and the skin has a pebbly texture.

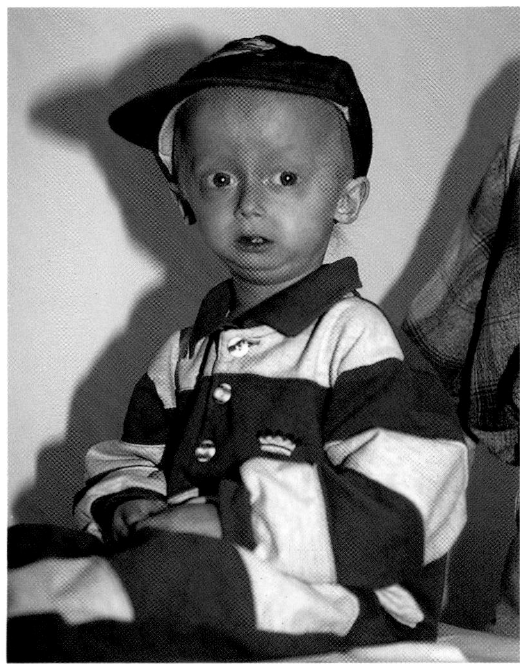

Figure 12.8. Same patient at 31 months with progressive changes.

HISTOPATHOLOGY

Light. In the sclerodermatous-like skin there is a decrease in sebaceous glands and hair follicles with normal sweat glands, prominent arrector pilorum muscles, and a decrease of subcutaneous fat. There is an increase in melanin in the basal keratinocytes. The epidermis may be normal or hyperkeratotic. In the dermis, there is a normal to increased number of blood vessels with thickened walls. There is disorganization, thickening, and hyalinization of collagen fiber bundles.

EM. No information.

BASIC DEFECT

Unknown. Many abnormalities in cell culture have been reported, including decreased insulin receptor gene expression, increased type IV collagen mRNA, increased amounts of fibronectin, decreased repair after ultraviolet light radiation, decreased cell lifespan, decreased response to epidermal growth factor, and so forth. An increased excretion of hyaluronic acid in the urine has been demonstrated. Total glycosaminoglycans in the urine are normal, but the proportion of hyaluronic acid is increased.

TREATMENT

None effective. Physical therapy and occupational therapy may help to maintain range of motion of the joints. Dietary management may be necessary for hyperlipidemia. One patient had coronary artery bypass surgery performed at age 14 years. One year follow-up showed significant relief of symptoms of angina, but central nervous system symptoms due to impaired blood flow continued to worsen.

MODE OF INHERITANCE

Uncertain. In support of autosomal dominant inheritance is an increase in the mean paternal age and very few recurrences in sibships. In support of autosomal recessive inheritance is one inbred pedigree with two generations of involved siblings. The few recurrences within sibships could be the result of autosomal recessive inheritance or gonadal mosaicism.

PRENATAL DIAGNOSIS

None.

DIFFERENTIAL DIAGNOSIS

In Rothmund-Thomson syndrome (MIM: 268400) photosensitivity, telangiectases, and poikilodermatous skin changes are marked. Failure to thrive is less obvious. In Cockayne syndrome (MIM:216400), photosensitivity is a major feature, as are progressive neurologic symptoms, including ataxia, mental retardation, and spasticity.

Mandibuloacral dysplasia (MIM:248370) has been compared with progeria but is quite readily distinguished. It is an autosomal recessive disorder. Affected individuals have a normal lifespan. Onset of signs occurs in midchildhood with mild hair and skin changes, mild to moderate short stature, and marked micrognathia, with failure of the mandible to grow. Radiographic changes are similar to those of progeria, with resorption of the distal tufts of the phalanges and the clavicles.

The skin changes of scleroderma are similar in appearance, but the age of onset and lack of associated systemic features differentiate it from progeria.

In Wiedemann-Rautenstrauch syndrome (neonatal pseudohydrocephalic progeroid syndrome, MIM:264090), the changes are present at birth. Affected infants often have natal teeth. They share the same skin changes and joint limitation with progeria. They retain paradoxical cushions of subcutaneous fat between the finger joints, in the lumbar region, and in the armpits. Mental retardation is more typical in these infants. Photographs of affected infants show a fairly prominent jaw with a small mouth. This condition is believed to be autosomal recessive.

Fat pads or pseudolipomas on the labia and buttocks, which disappear during childhood, are a feature of carbohydrate-deficient glycoprotein syndrome (MIM:212065). Failure to thrive, mental retardation, and ataxia, along with retinal pigmentary degeneration, are cardinal features.

Support Group: International Progeria Registry
NY State Institute for Basic Research

1050 Forest Hill Road
Staten Island, NY
10314
1-718-494-5333

SELECTED BIBLIOGRAPHY

Brown, W.T. (1990). Genetic diseases of premature aging as models of senescence. *Annu. Rev. Gerontol. Geriatr.* **10,** 23–42.

Reviews progeria, Werner, Down, and Cockayne syndromes. Argues for new dominant mutations as a cause for progeria. Reviews research.

Castineyra, G., Panal, M., Lopez Presas, H., Goldschmidt, E., and Sanchez, J.M. (1992). Two sibs with Wiedemann-Rautenstrauch syndrome: possibilities of prenatal diagnosis by ultrasound. *J. Med. Genet.* **29,** 434–436.

On ultrasound performed for other reasons, intrauterine growth retardation was noted at 20 weeks. The pregnancy resulted in a female with progeric features and natal teeth. During a subsequent pregnancy, ultrasound at 12 and 16 weeks was normal; at 20 weeks there was a decrease in head circumference and abdominal diameter. This was confirmed at 25 weeks. Termination at 28 weeks showed an affected male fetus. Femoral lengths were normal in both fetuses. Authors suggest that it is possible to diagnose the condition by ultrasound on the basis of the pattern of growth failure.

DeBusk, F.L. (1972). The Hutchinson-Gilford progeria syndrome. Report of 4 cases and review of the literature. *J. Pediatr.* **80,** 697–724.

Historical review. Extraordinary photographs. Detailed review of clinical features with a nice presentation of information regarding mode of inheritance to date.

Gilford, H. (1904). Progeria: a form of senilism. *Practitioner* **73,** 188–217.

A long, beautifully detailed discursive with follow-up of Hutchinson's original patient who died at age 17 years. In addition, observations in life and of a postmortem examination of a patient of Gilford's who died at age 18 years. There is a description of the patient's skin as "withered and juiceless." The thymus was enlarged at age 18. In the discussion, Gilford mentions an American child who died at age 8 months of senile decay, a wizened, hirsute infant. Perhaps this was the first case of leprechaunism? He also describes a woman of 41 whose brother was also affected, both with milder changes. This most likely represents Werner syndrome.

Hamer, L., Kaplan, F., and Fallon, M. (1988). The musculoskeletal manifestations of progeria. A literature review. *Orthopedics* **11,** 763–769.

No primary data but a clear and detailed review of the literature regarding the bone and muscle features of progeria.

Mulvihill, J.J., and Smith, D.W. (1975) Another disorder with prenatal shortness of stature and premature aging. *Birth Defects* **XI(2),** 368–371.

Bird-like facies, multiple nevi, high-pitched voice, sparse hair, hypogonadism, microcephaly with low IQ, and sensorineural hearing loss.

Rudin, C., Thommen, L., Fliegel, C., Steinmann, B., and Bühler, U. (1988). The neonatal pseudo-hydrocephalic progeroid syndrome (Wiedemann-Rautenstrauch). *Eur. J. Pediatr.* **147,** 433–438.

Reviews five previous case reports and presents a patient of their own and a clear discussion of the differential diagnosis.

Tenconi, R., Miotti, F., Miotti, A., Audino, G., Ferro, R., and Clementi, M. (1986). Another Italian family with mandibuloacral dysplasia: why does it seem more frequent in Italy? *Am. J. Med. Genet.* **24,** 357–364.

Three siblings and a review of eight families reported in the literature.

WERNER SYNDROME (MIM:277700)

(Progeria of the Adult)

Includes Flynn-Aird Syndrome

DERMATOLOGIC FEATURES

Major. In the second and third decades, signs of "premature aging" develop. These have been appreciated in individuals as young as 13 years or delayed until the sixth decade.

The hair thins and grays and loses its luster, and progressive balding ensues. The eyebrows and eyelashes may be affected.

There is loss of subcutaneous tissue with binding down of the skin; sclerodermatous-like alterations with thinned, taut, shiny skin and telangiectases are typical. Ulcerations occur, and calcinosis cutis is described in about 30% of patients. Patchy hyperpigmentation and hypopigmentation are typical.

Loss of muscle mass and loss of subcutaneous tissue accompany the epidermal and dermal atrophy.

Hyperkeratoses develop over bony prominences and on the soles. These may ulcerate and are slow to heal.

Minor. Axillary and pubic hair may be absent or sparse.

ASSOCIATED ABNORMALITIES

Early atherosclerosis—at 25 to 40 years of age—is a major cause of death, the mean age of which is in the forties. Calcification of the heart valves and within blood vessels is severe.

Cataracts develop in the third and fourth decades and may be of any type. Glaucoma occurs in a significant proportion of patients.

Growth arrest at puberty is typical, and short stature (146 cm for females, 157 cm for males) is a constant finding. Hypogonadism in males and irregular menses and premature menopause in females are the norm. Although fertility appears to be reduced, affected males and females have reproduced.

The voice is typically high pitched, and the facies are marked by beaking of the nose, similar to the other progerias.

The extremities are very thin, and the trunk appears relatively stocky.

Osteoporosis develops, most severely in the legs. Arthritis and joint destruction result in significant disability in the middle years.

Two-fifths of reported patients develop diabetes mellitus.

A variety of malignancies, the other leading cause of mortality, occurs in these patients. Many types of sarcomas and carcinomas, as well as benign tumors—adenomas, myomas, meningiomas—are reported. Cutaneous malignancy has not been noted. The risk for malignancy is hard to quantify but may approach 10%–15%.

HISTOPATHOLOGY

Light. Epidermal atrophy with dropout of appendageal structures, loss of subcutaneous fat, and mild hyperkeratosis with occasional perivascular and periappendageal lymphocytic infiltrate.

There is mild dermal fibrosis with hyalinization, similar to scleroderma.

EM. Interstitial calcification around collagen fibrils was described in one patient.

BASIC DEFECT

Unknown. Fibroblasts have decreased lifespan in culture—20 or so doublings versus about 60 in normal individuals. The gene for Werner syndrome is believed to code for a DNA helicase. Thus alterations in its protein product could disrupt any of the steps of DNA replication that require unwinding.

TREATMENT

None specific to Werner syndrome.

A

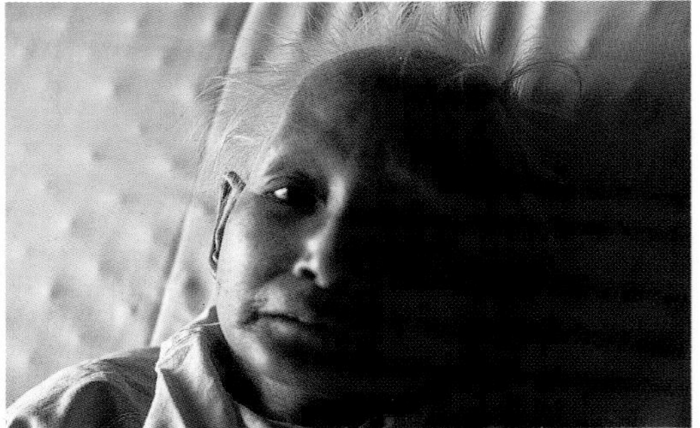

B

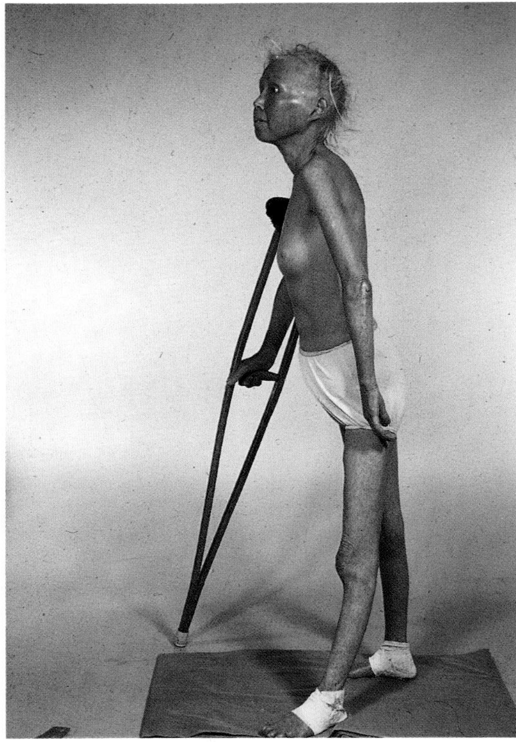

Figure 12.9. **(A)** Patient in her late forties. **(B)** Sister also in her late forties. (B, courtesy of Dr. G. Martin, Seattle, Washington.)

MODE OF INHERITANCE

Autosomal recessive based on reports of affected siblings and offspring born to consanguineous couples. The gene (*WRN*) has been mapped to 8p12, identified and sequenced. There is allelic heterogeneity, with four different mutations found in five families studied to date.

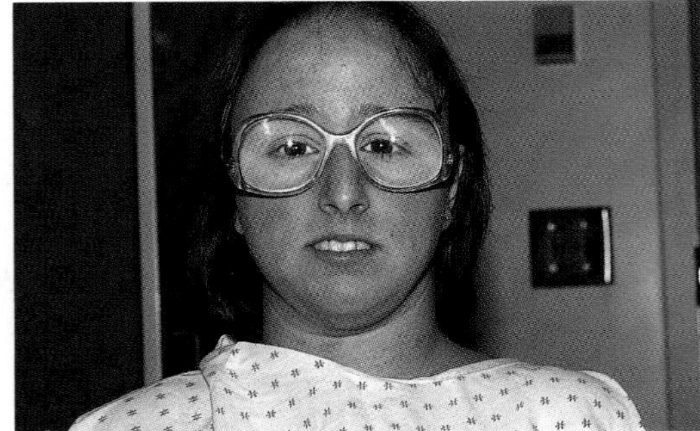

Figure 12.10. Patient with myocardial infarction at age 26 years, with thinning of scalp hair and beaked nose.

PRENATAL DIAGNOSIS

Presumably possible using molecular techniques in families where the mutation has been identified.

DIFFERENTIAL DIAGNOSIS

In the absence of cataracts, or if their presence is overlooked, a misdiagnosis of scleroderma might be made. Graying of the hair, short stature, and hypogonadism are not typical of scleroderma. Involvement of the fingertips is more typical of scleroderma than of Werner syndrome. Rothmund-Thomson syndrome (poikiloderma congenitale, MIM:264800) presents in early childhood. These patients share in common with Werner syndrome short stature, cataracts, and telangiectases, but in Rothmund-Thomson syndrome these features have earlier onset, and patients with Rothmund-Thomson syndrome lack the sclerodermatous-like changes of the skin. Patients with Hutchinson-Gilford syndrome (MIM:176670) present in early childhood and infancy; patients with Werner syndrome present later. In the Japanese, a rare, presumably autosomal recessive disorder of progressive loss of fat in the face and extremities, joint contractures, mental retardation, and a recurrent erythema nodosum-like rash, progressive weakness, hepatomegaly, macroglossia, and calcifications of the basal ganglia, all with onset in the first two decades, has been reported.

Flynn-Aird syndrome (MIM:136300) shares in common with Werner syndrome sclerodermatous-like changes of the skin, gradual neurologic problems, and bony changes. In Flynn-Aird syndrome, progressive sensorineural deafness is the first feature, and there appears to be significantly greater nervous system involvement with atypical epilepsy, expressive aphasia, numbness and paresthesias of the skin, and ataxia.

Support Group: International Progeria Registry
NY State Institute for Basic Research
1050 Forest Hill Road
Staten Island, NY 10314
1-718-494-5333

SELECTED BIBLIOGRAPHY

Epstein, C.J., Martin, G.M., Schultz, A.L., and Motulsky, A.G. (1966). Werner's syndrome. *Medicine* **45,** 177–221.

Describes one family of their own, one of whose members I was privileged to examine in 1977. This article reviews the previous literature in detail regarding age of onset of various signs and symptoms and gives pedigree analysis. Raises question about premature canities in heterozygous siblings.

Flynn, P., and Aird, B. (1965). A neuroectodermal syndrome of dominant inheritance. *J. Neurol. Sci.* **2,** 161–182.

In the second decade, nerve deafness develops, followed by ataxia, muscle wasting, stiff joints, and neuritic pain. Intellectual testing is normal, but intellectual function appears to be impaired. Atypical epilepsy with intermittent expressive aphasia, blurring of vision, and numbness and paresthesias of the skin develop. Retinitis pigmentosa, cataracts, severe myopia, and blindness occur. Osteoporosis, cystic bony changes and dental caries are also features. Atrophy of the skin and subcutaneous tissue similar to that of scleroderma is characteristic, and ulceration with poor healing is common. Skin biopsy shows atrophy. Life expectancy does not appear to be significantly reduced. In this report, one patient is described as being deeply tanned. One questions whether Flynn-Aird syndrome might be an adrenoleukodystrophy.

Goto, M., Rubenstein, M., Weber, J., Woods, K., and Drayna, D. (1992). Genetic linkage of Werner's syndrome to five markers on chromosome 8. *Nature* **355,** 735–738.

In 21 Japanese families, a shotgun approach with a palette of markers across the autosomes proved successful. Subsequent studies refined linkage to 8p12.

Hoepffner, H.-J., Dreyer, M., Reimers, U., Schmidt-Preuss, U., Koepp, H.-P., and Rüdiger, H.W. (1989). A new familial syndrome with impaired function of three related peptide growth factors. *Hum. Genet.* **83,** 209–216.

Three brothers with normal stature, joint contractures, lipodystrophy, and bird-like facies. It seems very different from Werner syndrome in description and photographs. Fibroblasts show normal replication, unlike Werner syndrome.

Ruprecht, K.W. (1989). Ophthalmological aspects in patients with Werner's syndrome. *Arch. Gerontol. Geriatr.* **9,** 263–270.

In 10 of 18 eyes operated on for cataracts, wound dehiscence occurred. The author suggests techniques to reduce the likelihood of bad outcome. He posits that poor results may be due to inadequate healing because of reduced potential for fibroblasts to divide.

Thweatt, R., and Goldstein, S. (1993). Werner syndrome and biological ageing: A molecular genetic hypothesis. *Bioassays* **15,** 421–426.

Reviews experimental information to date, 56 references. The authors propose a mutation in a gene for a *trans*-acting protein that ultimately results in inappropriate inhibition of DNA synthesis, causing cell senescence.

Yu, C.-E., Oshima, J., Fu, Y.-H., Wijsman, E.M., Hisama, F., Alisch, R., Matthews, S., Nakura, J., Miki, T., Ouais, S., Martin, G.M., Mulligan, J., Schellenberg, G.D. (1996). Positional cloning of the Werner's syndrome gene. *Science.* **272,** 258–262.

One Japanese and one Caucasian family shared the same mutations. Three others (2 Japanese, 1 Syrian) had three distinct alterations in the *WRN* gene. The predicted protein is similar to known DNA helicases. George Martin persevered successfully!

CHAPTER 13

PHOTOSENSITIVITY

BLOOM SYNDROME (MIM:210900)

(Congenital Telangiectatic Erythema and Stunted Growth)

DERMATOLOGIC FEATURES

MAJOR. Telangiectases and erythema of the face in a butterfly distribution similar to that of lupus erythematosus develop in infancy after exposure to sunlight. The forearms and hands may also be involved. These changes are exacerbated by continued sun exposure. The telangiectases may lessen with time, although atrophy and hyper- and hypopigmentation usually follow

The diagnosis should be suspected in any young child with growth failure and lupus-like facial rash.

Multiple café-au-lait spots have been described in more than 50% of patients. I am unable, from the descriptions in these reports, to determine if these are part of the hypo/hyperpigmentation process or represent true café-au-lait spots.

MINOR. Acanthosis nigricans, possibly associated with diabetes mellitus and hirsutism, has been mentioned in case reports. A single case of Bloom syndrome has been described to have coarse, ichthyotic skin. Loss of eyelashes can occur.

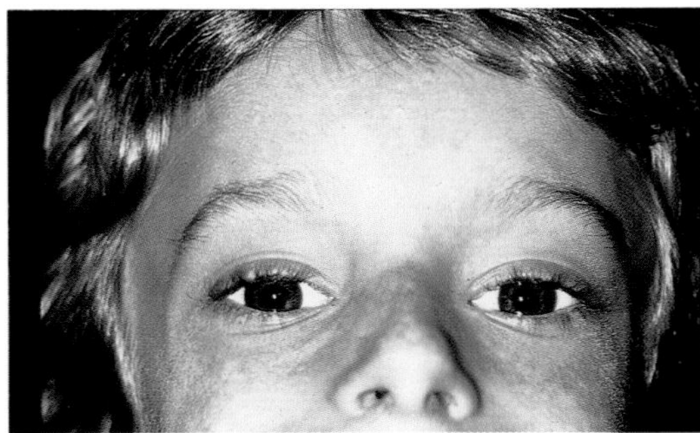

Figure 13.1. Subtle facial erythema across cheeks and across bridge of nose.

ASSOCIATED ABNORMALITIES

Immunodeficiency: Childhood is marked by repeated infections. Severe chronic lung disease appears to be a significant complication in the teen years, ostensibly secondary to repeated infections and bronchiectasis. Most patients have abnormally low levels of one or more of IgA, IgG, and IgM.

Increased risk of malignancy: Malignancy has occurred in almost 50% of patients in the Bloom Syndrome Registry. The variety of tumors is great; skin cancers in unusual, nonsunexposed areas; cancer of the breast, colon, tongue, larynx, and cervix; leukemia; and Wilms tumor lead the list. Multiple primaries have occurred in at least 5% of patients, and the age of onset of tumors is extremely young, consistent with the "two-hit" theory of carcinogenesis.

Infertility/hypogonadism: Males with Bloom syndrome have small testes and no sperm production. The cause of this is unknown. Although a few affected females have reproduced, fertility in women with Bloom syndrome also seems reduced. Despite the abnormalities in gamete production, pubertal development is usually normal, suggesting that some gonadal function is unimpaired.

Growth Failure: This is of prenatal onset and persists after birth. Head size is also small, although intelligence is usually normal. The facies are characteristically small and sharp featured.

Diabetes mellitus has been reported in 10% of patients.

Survival to age 40 years is rare.

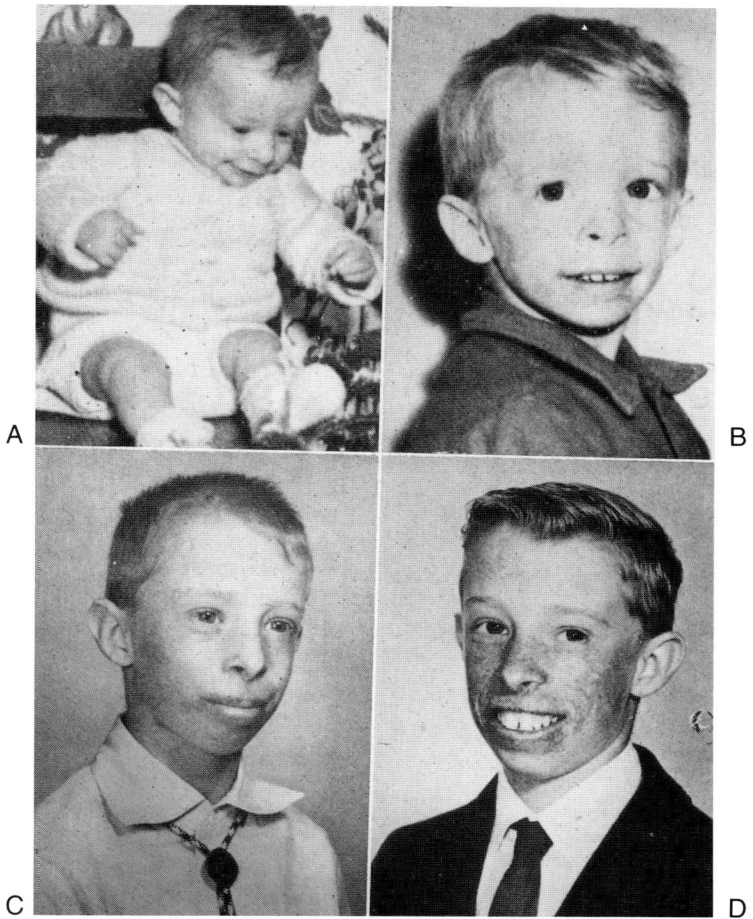

Figure 13.2. Patient at ages 6 months **(A),** 5 years **(B),** 11 years **(C),** and 14 years **(D),** showing progressive telangiectases. Typical sculptured nasal tip evident. (From German, 1969.)

HISTOPATHOLOGY

Light. Increased numbers of dilated capillaries with a hyperplastic endothelium are found. The atrophic changes are nonspecific. The histology of Bloom syndrome is not diagnosis.
EM. No information.

BASIC DEFECT

Absence of a DNA helicase is posited based on identification of homozygosity for loss of function alleles for the causative gene. Cells from Bloom syndrome patients show increased chromosome breakage and a 5- to 10-fold increase in sister chromatid exchange (breaks and reanastomoses of the two homologous strands of a single chromosome).

TREATMENT

Treatment is limited to avoidance of sun exposure, use of sunscreens, and appropriate therapy for associated malignancies.

MODE OF INHERITANCE

Autosomal recessive. Although the disorder has been reported most often among Ashkenazi Jews, it has occurred in many other disparate ethnic groups, usually in offspring of consanguineous matings. Heterozygotes do not demonstrate increased sister chromatid exchange. The gene, *BLM,* maps to 15q26.1.

PRENATAL DIAGNOSIS

Theoretically possible by assay of sister chromatid exchange in chorionic villi or amniocytes. With identification of mutations, direct DNA studies are possible.

DIFFERENTIAL DIAGNOSIS

Rothmund-Thomson syndrome (MIM:268400): The skin changes of Rothmund-Thomson syndrome are similar, but the facies are different, with a small saddle nose rather than the beakish nose of Bloom syndrome. The cataracts, radial ray abnormalities, alopecia, and tooth abnormalities of Rothmund-Thomson syndrome may also help to distinguish between the disorders.

Gunther disease (congenital erythropoietic porphyria, MIM:263700): The photosensitivity of congenital erythropoietic porphyria usually appears somewhat later, in the first few years of childhood. There is no prenatal growth deficiency. Splenomegaly and staining of teeth are not seen in Bloom syndrome. Porphyrin screening should allow for correct diagnosis.

Xeroderma pigmentosa (MIM:278700–278810): The hyperpigmented, hypopigmented, and xerotic lesions of the xeroderma pigmentosa disorders may help distinguish them from Bloom syndrome. Multiple skin cancers in sun-exposed areas are more typical of xeroderma pigmentosa than Bloom syndrome. Although telangiectases are seen in xeroderma pigmentosa, a "butterfly" distribution of these is not. Growth failure may or may not be seen. Differentiation between the two disorders may depend on the laboratory (i.e., increase in sister chromatid exchange versus defects in DNA excision repair).

Systemic lupus erythematosus (MIM: 152700): Systemic lupus erythematosus rarely occurs in infancy. The atrophy and poikiloderma of Bloom syndrome are quite different. Prenatal growth failure does not occur in systemic lupus erythematosus.

Polymorphic light eruption (MIM:174770): Individuals with polymorphic light eruption have no associated growth failure and a normal head circumference.

Cockayne syndrome (MIM:216400–216410): The features of premature aging are much more global in Cockayne syndrome than in Bloom syndrome, and the skin changes are later in onset.

If the diagnosis of Bloom syndrome is suspected, appropriate cytogenetic studies looking for increased sister chromatid exchange should be performed.

Support Group: Bloom Syndrome Registry
c/o James German, MD
310 East 67th Street
New York, NY 10021

National Foundation for Jewish Genetic Disease
250 Park Avenue, Suite 1000
New York, NY 10017
212-371-1030

SELECTED BIBLIOGRAPHY

Bloom, D. (1966). The syndrome of congenital telangiectatic erythema and stunted growth. *J. Pediatr.* **68,** 103–113.

Longitudinal natural history study of three original cases and four new cases.

Chan, J.Y., Becker, F.F., German, J., and Ray, J.H. (1987). Altered DNA ligase I activity in Bloom's syndrome cells. *Nature* **325,** 357–359.

Willis, A.E., and Lindahl, T. (1987). DNA ligase I deficiency in Bloom's syndrome. *Nature* **325,** 355–357.

Chan et al. and Willis and Lindahl (1987) each report an abnormality in one of two DNA ligases involved in semiconservative DNA replication in patients with Bloom syndrome.

Ellis, N.A., Groden, J., Ye, T.-Z., Straughen, J., Lennon, D.J., Ciocci, S., Proytcheva, M., and German, J. (1995). The Bloom's syndrome gene product is homologous to RecQ helicases. *Cell* **83,** 655–666.

Authors hypothesize that absence of DNA helicase destabilizes other enzymes involved in DNA replication and repair.

German, J., and Passarge, E. (1989). Report from the Registry for 1987. *Clin. Genet.* **35,** 57–69.

Information on 130 patients in the International Bloom Syndrome Registry.

HARTNUP DISORDER (MIM:234500)

DERMATOLOGIC FEATURES

MAJOR. Most individuals with the defective amino acid transport of Hartnup disorder will not be symptomatic. Among those who are, there is an acute photosensitivity, marked by acute inflammation and blistering. Irregular hyperpigmentation and hypopigmentation, along with dry, scaling, red skin are typical and similar to the rash of pellagra. These scaly red thickened plaques and patches develop on the sun-exposed skin of the face, hands, neck, and legs. The rash is usually asymptomatic, although it can be itchy. The rash can develop in infancy or may be delayed in onset. There is extreme variability in severity.

MINOR. Mucosal involvement with inflammation of the tongue, lips, and angular stomatitis and atrophic glossitis have been described. Vulvar and vaginal mucosa may also be affected.

The hair may be thin and break easily.

ASSOCIATED ABNORMALITIES

Malnutrition secondary to a defect in gastrointestinal transport of neutral amino acids, especially tryptophan, and abnormal renal excretion of the same can occur. There may be a generalized renal amino aciduria. Chronic diarrhea and failure to thrive are common. Whether short stature is primary or due to growth delay and inadequate calories is unclear.

Neurologic symptoms may occur at the same time as skin changes or develop subsequent to the skin lesions. Cerebellar ataxia is often intermittent and is the primary neurologic finding. Nystagmus, ptosis, diplopia, increased reflexes, and pyramidal signs have been reported in a few patients. It is unclear if mental retardation is a related or coincidental finding. Episodic psychotic features and disordered thought processes are described in some patients, often occurring in conjunction with ataxia.

HISTOPATHOLOGY

LIGHT. Not diagnostic. Orthohyperkeratosis and thickened granular layer.

EM. Tightly packed tonofilaments with globular keratohyaline granules.

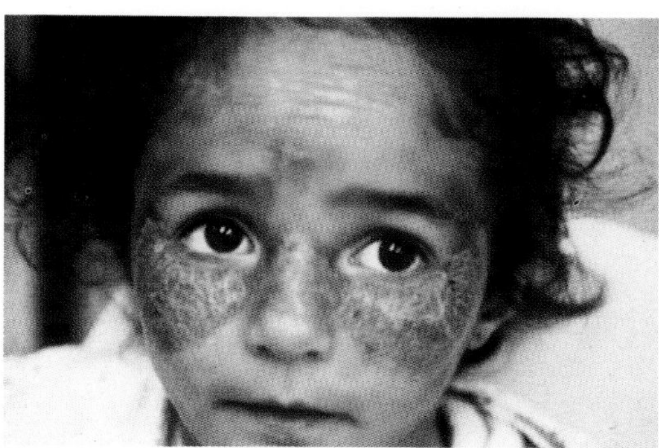

Figure 13.3. Scaling, crusted dermatitis in a butterfly distribution. (From Galadari et al., 1993.)

BASIC DEFECT

There is a defect in renal and intestinal neutral amino acid transport.

TREATMENT

Nicotinamide (50–300 mg/day by mouth) clears the skin findings and may help the neurologic symptoms. The basis for its effectiveness is unclear.

MODE OF INHERITANCE

Autosomal recessive for the disorder, but expression of the disease is multifactorial and appears to depend on external factors such as diet.

PRENATAL DIAGNOSIS

None. Maternal disease is not detrimental to the fetus.

DIFFERENTIAL DIAGNOSIS

For the eczema, limitation of involvement to sun-exposed areas and associated neurologic abnormalities may point the way to the correct diagnosis of Hartnup disorder. A dietary history should quickly exclude the diagnosis of pellagra.

Support Group: N.O.R.D.
P.O. Box 8923
New Fairfield, CT 06812
1-800-999-6673

SELECTED BIBLIOGRAPHY

Levy, H.L. (1995). Hartnup disorder. In *The Metabolic Basis of Inherited Disease*. Scriver, C.R., Beaudet, A.L., Sly W.S., and Valle, D. (eds.). McGraw-Hill, New York, 7th ed., pp. 3629–3642.

This is an excellent chapter. Hartnup disorder truly belonged to Hartnup. He was a 12-year-old with a tentative diagnosis of pellagra who had a 19-year-old sister with similar findings. The latter had been treated for pellagra. Two other siblings showed similar abnormalities of amino acid excretion in urine, but were essentially asymptomatic. The author emphasizes that most patients have no problems. He graciously acknowledges the contribution of the author of the chapter in the 4th edition, Dr. Jepson, now deceased. There are 130 references.

Scriver, C.R., Mahon, B., Levy, H.L., Clow, C.L., Reade, T.M., Kronick, J., Lemieux, B., and Laberge, C. (1987). The Hartnup phenotype: Mendelian transport disorder, multifactorial disease. *Am. J. Hum. Genet.* **40,** 401–412.

Authors suggest that the amino acid transport defect is the result of a single gene alteration but that expression of the disorder depends on multiple other factors. Nineteen of 21 individuals presumably homozygous for the abnormal gene had essentially no clinical problems.

Wilcken, B., Yu, J.S., and Brown, D.A. (1977). Natural history of Hartnup disease. *Arch. Dis. Child.* **52,** 38–40.

Twelve probands, and 3 of the 15 siblings detected by routine urine screening. They were followed for up to 8 years. The authors estimate a frequency of 1 in 33,000 in Australia. Six of the patients were treated. None developed a rash. One in the treatment group developed sun sensitivity when the medications were stopped. This resolved when treatment was reinstituted.

KINDLER SYNDROME (MIM:173650)

(Kindler-Weary Hereditary Acrokeratotic Poikiloderma; Brain Syndrome)

Includes Hereditary Sclerosing Poikiloderma; Mendes da Costa–Hereditary Bullous Dystrophy, Macular Type

DERMATOLOGIC FEATURES

MAJOR. Poikiloderma—reticular telangiectases, hypopigmentation, and hyperpigmentation with epidermal atrophy—begins in early childhood. It is most marked in sun-exposed areas. There is fine cigarette paper-like wrinkling of the skin over the hands and elsewhere.

Photosensitivity is variable and decreases with age.

Blisters on the hands and feet in response to little or no trauma begin in infancy and improve in adult life. This may be the only symptom for the first few years and may falsely lead to the diagnosis of epidermolysis bullosa.

Palmoplantar hyperkeratosis is generally mild and occurs in about 65% of individuals. Acrokeratoses resembling flat warts and punctate keratoses on the palms and soles were described by Weary et al. (1971)

MINOR. Gingivitis and/or leukokeratosis in a few reports.

Mild onychodystrophy with ridging, grooving, and atrophy. Blisters can occasionally occur in the oral mucosa. Several case reports of esophageal, urethral, rectal, and/or conjunctival scarring. Eczema, dermatitis, and xerosis described in a number of patients. One patient was described with squamous cell carcinoma of the skin and a transitional cell bladder carcinoma.

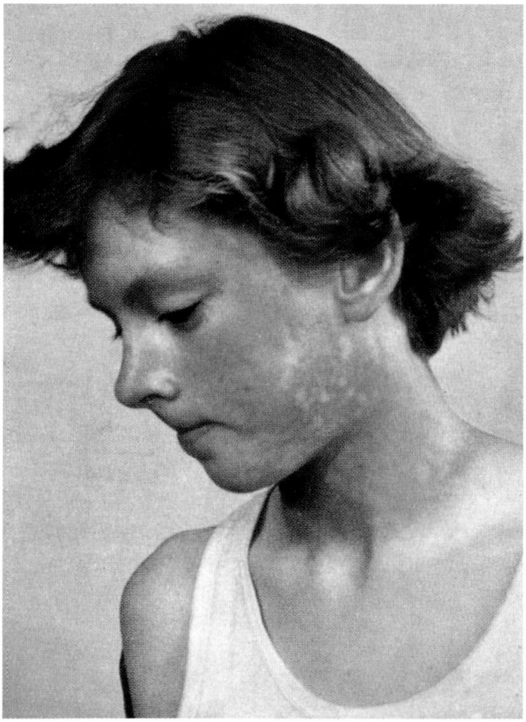

Figure 13.4. Telangiectases on face and neck with pigment changes. (From Kindler, 1954.)

ASSOCIATED ABNORMALITIES

Dental caries have been noted in a number of case reports.

HISTOPATHOLOGY

LIGHT. Nonspecific epidermal atrophy, dermal edema, incontinence of pigment with or without cytoid bodies, with or without a decrease in elastic fibers.

EM. Level of cleavage of the blisters is uncertain; intradermal, junctional, and dermal cleavage planes were all described in single biopsies from single individuals. In others the level of the split appeared to be intraepidermal.

BASIC DEFECT

Unknown.

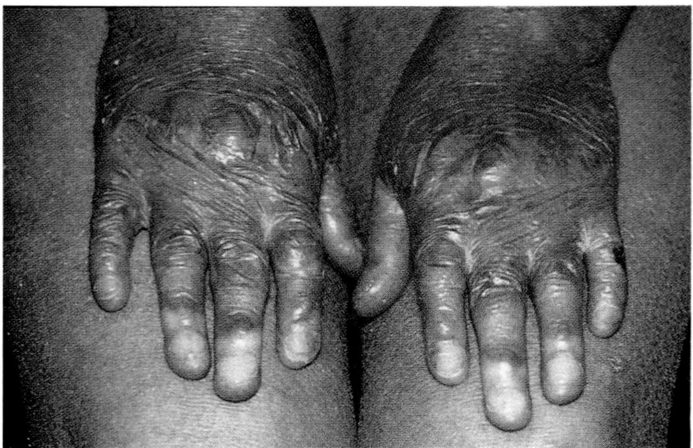

Figure 13.5. Cigarette paper scarring on hands; cutaneous fusion up to the PIP joints. (From Forman et al., 1989.)

TREATMENT

None, beyond standard emollient and blister care.

MODE OF INHERITANCE

Autosomal dominant (?Weary), autosomal recessive (?Kindler). The disorders are similar clinically and differ only in the reported mode of inheritance. It is impossible in a sporadic case to determine in which group it belongs.

PRENATAL DIAGNOSIS

None.

DIFFERENTIAL DIAGNOSIS

Epidermolysis bullosa with mottled hyperpigmentation (MIM:131960) is strikingly similar. Lack of telangiectases in epidermolysis bullosa may differentiate the two, but I believe that they are identical.

Dyskeratosis congenita (MIM:224230, 305000) is marked by leukokeratosis. The skin changes are more hyperpigmented, but telangiectases are also described. Some cases of Kindler syndrome have been noted to have leukokeratosis.

Mendes da Costa syndrome (hereditary bullous dystrophy, macular type, MIM:302000) is X-linked and marked by microcephaly, short stature, mild mental retardation, and conical fingers, in addition to skin changes similar to those in Kindler syndrome. It has been described in a Dutch family and in a family from Italy. Linkage to Xq27.3–28 has been suggested.

Hereditary sclerosing poikiloderma (MIM: 173700, also described by Weary et al., 1969) lacks bullae, photosensitivity, telangiectases, atrophy, and acrokeratoses. Although described as poikilodermatous, the skin changes are marked by hyper- and hypopigmentation, without telangiectases or atrophy. The fibrous bands of sclerosing poikiloderma are not found in acrokeratotic poikiloderma. Calcinosis cutis was reported in one patient.

Rothmund-Thomson syndrome (MIM: 268400) shares skin changes in common with Kindler-Weary, but has, in addition, short stature, cataracts, and other manifestations.

In the xeroderma pigmentosa disorders (MIM:278700–278800) photosensitivity results in pigment changes and atrophy. Acral blistering is atypical, and palmoplantar hyperkeratosis does not occur.

Cutaneous amyloidoses (MIM:105250,

204900, 301220) can give a poikilodermatous appearance to the skin, but the onset is much later in adult life. A biopsy should differentiate.

Support Group: D.E.B.R.A.
40 Rector Street, 8th Floor
New York, NY 10006
1-212-693-6610

SELECTED BIBLIOGRAPHY

Bruckner-Tuderman, L., Vogel, A., Ruegger, S., Odermatt, B., Tonz, O., and Schnyder, U.W. (1989). Epidermolysis bullosa simplex with mottled hyperpigmentation. *J. Am. Acad. Dermatol.* **21,** 425–432.

Striking similarity to Kindler syndrome, with cigarette paper changes, acral blistering improving with age, photosensitivity, gingivitis, and nail dystrophy. Color change was noted to be more hyperpigmented than telangiectatic, but hypopigmentation consistent with poikiloderma also described. Involvement tended to be more truncal and on the extremities, sparing the face.

Forman, A.B., Prendiville, J.S., Esterly, N.B., Hebert, A.A., Duvic, M., Horiguchi, Y., and Fine, J.-D. (1989). Kindler syndrome: report of two cases and review of the literature. *Pediatr. Dermatol.* **6,** 91–101.

Good review of the differential diagnosis of poikilodermatous syndromes.

Hachem-Zadeh, S., and Garfunkel, A.A. (1985). Kindler syndrome in two related Kurdish families. *Am. J. Med. Genet.* **20,** 43–48.

Two sibships of cousins; clear review of the literature.

Larrègue, M., Prigent, F., Lorette, G., Canuel, C., and Ramdenee, P. (1981). Acrokeratose poikilodermique bulleuse et héréditaire de Weary-Kindler. *Ann. Dermatol. Venereol.* **108,** 69–76.

Report of an affected father and son with excellent review of familial data in the literature. Discussion also notes rather liberal use of the term *poikiloderma* and inability to differentiate Weary syndrome clinically from Kindler syndrome.

Weary, P.E., Hsu, Y.T., Richardson, D.R., Caravati, C.M., and Wood, B.T. (1969). Hereditary sclerosing poikiloderma. Report of two families with an unusual and distinctive genodermatosis. *Arch. Dermatol.* **100,** 413–422.

Generalized mottling with hypo- and hyperpigmentation and firm hyperkeratotic reticular or parallel sclerotic bands in axillae and antecubital and popliteal fossae develop in adolescent and adult life. Palms and soles are waxy and tight. Presumed autosomal dominant inheritance, but no opportunity for male-to-male transmission in the pedigree. By description, skin changes are not truly poikilodermatous, as no atrophy and no telangiectases were noted.

Weary, P.E., Manley, W.F., Jr., and Graham, G.F. (1971). Hereditary acrokeratotic poikiloderma. *Arch. Dermatol.* **103,** 409–422.

Ten family members in three generations with male-to-male transmission. Color photos.

Wijker, M., Ligtenberg, M.J.L., Schoute, F., Defesche, J.C., Pals, G., Bolhuis, P.A., Ropers, H.H., Hulsebos, T.J.M., Menko, F.H., van Oost, B.A., Lungarotti, M.S., and Arwert, F. (1995). The gene for hereditary bullous dystrophy, X-linked macular type, maps to the Xq27.3-qter region. *Am. J. Hum. Genet.* **56,** 1096–1100.

Although only one Dutch pedigree initially described, a second Italian family was found. The genetic relationship (i.e. ancestors in common), if any, between the two families, is under investigation.

POLYMORPHOUS LIGHT ERUPTION (MIM:174770)

(PMLE; Familial Actinic Prurigo)

DERMATOLOGIC FEATURES

MAJOR. The term *polymorphous* refers to the protean nature of the skin changes associated with photosensitivity in this condition. Small and large papules, vesicles, eczematous or edematous plaques, prurigo nodules, and even target-like lesions can occur. Typically, skin changes develop on sun-exposed skin in childhood (compared with later onset in acquired polymorphous light eruption). Seventy-five percent of patients have developed signs by age 18 years. In general, the rash begins in the spring and gradually diminishes toward fall. This "hardening" phenomenon is not understood. The symptoms then recur in the subsequent spring. After years, the rash may persist throughout the seasons without significant winter remission. Lesions usually resolve, but with longstanding disease scarring is common, although it may occur with slightly less frequency among affected Native Americans.

Pruritus is a major complaint.

The infraorbital area, upper eyelids, upper philtrum, forehead, and the skin under the chin and that of the anterior neck are often spared because they are in shadow. The tops of the hands and arms are also usually involved. Cheleitis of the lower lip is common in the hereditary form in Native Americans.

MINOR. Blistering of the helices of the ears may occur. When skin changes are limited to the ears without more generalized rash, it is sometimes referred to as juvenile spring eruption, which also has been reported to occur in families and may reflect variable expression rather than a distinct disorder.

ASSOCIATED ABNORMALITIES

Tearing and itching of the eyes can be initiated by sun exposure. Conjunctivitis may develop, and there have been reports of pterygia formation with chronic eye involvement.

HISTOPATHOLOGY

LIGHT. Edema and spongiosis with acanthosis and parakeratosis are seen in the small papular and eczematous lesions. The large papules show edema with mild liquefaction of the basal layer. Both small and large papules share a dense perivascular lymphocytic infiltrate in the upper and middle dermis, along with edema.

EM. No information.

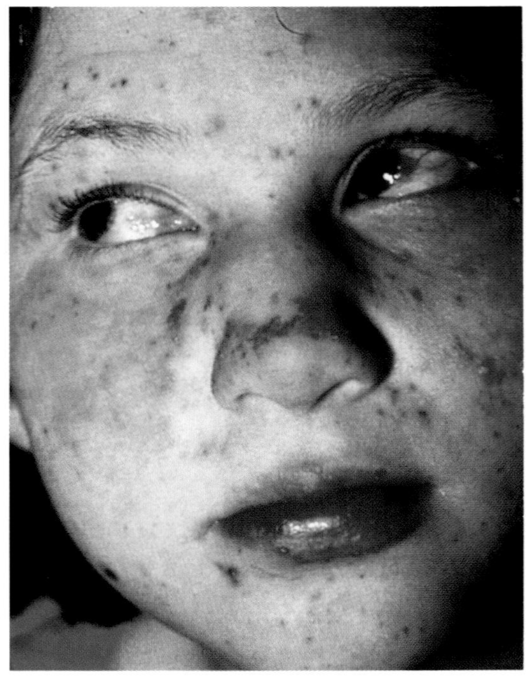

Figure 13.6. Lips, conjunctivae, and skin with lesions. (Draelos and Hansen, 1986.)

BASIC DEFECT

Unknown.

TREATMENT

Avoidance of sun exposure. Antimalarials have met with some success. Intermittent use of systemic corticosteroids has been suggested. PUVA therapy starting in the spring may decrease severity of symptoms. β-carotene may be helpful in some, along with use of broad-spectrum (UVA and UVB) sunscreens. Thalidomide has also been used. Antibiotics may be necessary to treat secondary infection.

MODE OF INHERITANCE

Uncertain. Among North and Central American natives, 30%–75% of cases have a positive

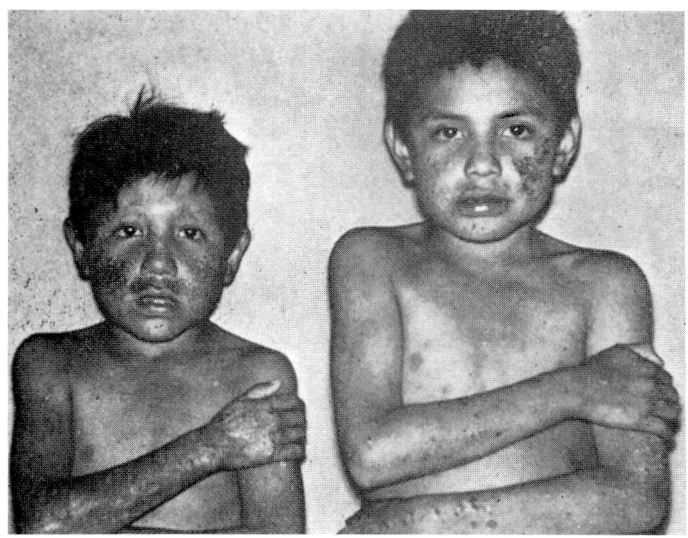

Figure 13.7. Brothers with facial and forearm involvement. (From Birt and Davis, 1975.)

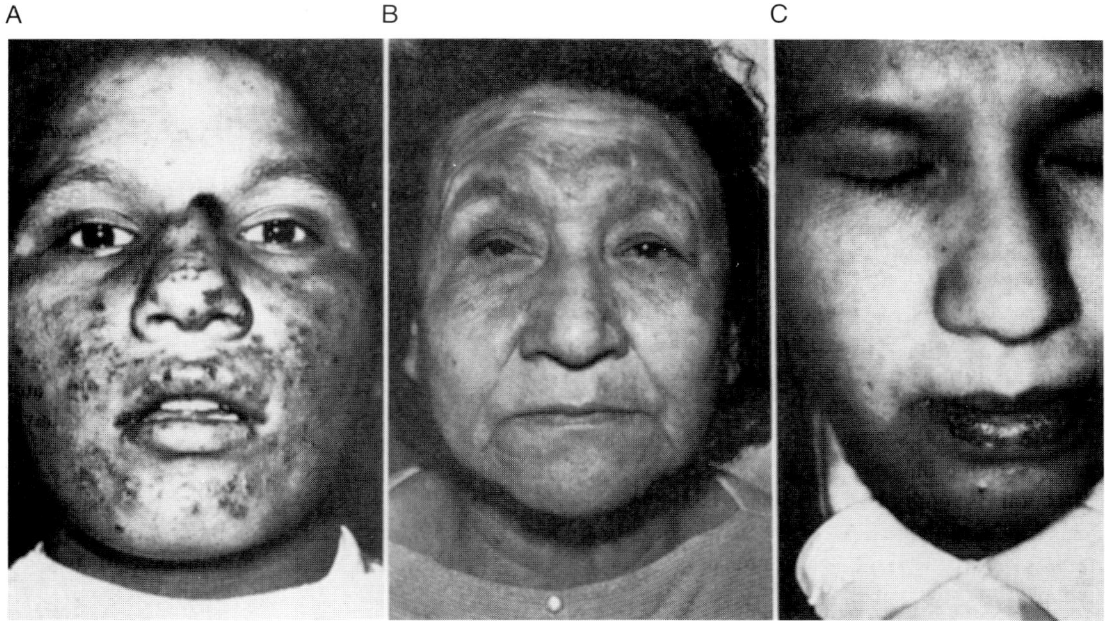

Figure 13.8. (**A**) Crusted papules. (**B**) Plaques. (**C**) Cheilitis. (From Birt and Davis, 1975.)

family history. Among the Native American tribal groups, Chippewa, Navajo, Cree, and Columbian Indians seem to be most commonly affected. In the Finns, 56% of patients have other affected family members.

PRENATAL DIAGNOSIS

None.

DIFFERENTIAL DIAGNOSIS

Itchy, raised, eczematous patches are common to many dermatologic disorders. Atopic dermatitis, in contrast to polymorphous light eruption, is not limited to sun-exposed areas. Airborne contact dermatitis usually involves the eyelids, chin, and philtrum, areas that are protected from sun contact and usually not involved in polymorphous light eruption. Contact dermatitis looks the same, but history should differentiate it from polymorphous light eruption. Allergic photocontact dermatitis can appear identical; history and phototesting may be helpful. In the nodular form of polymorphous light eruption, discoid and systemic lupus erythematosus pose diagnostic confusion. The lack of scalp involvement, the absence of follicular plugging and atrophy, and the absence of telangiectases are useful clinical clues suggestive of polymorphous light eruption. Erythropoietic protoporphyria (MIM:177000) can mimic polymorphous light eruption. Porphyrin screening and fluorescent scanning of red blood cells can determine the correct diagnosis. Secondary infection is common in polymorphous light eruption, and there is a risk of misdiagnosis of recurrent impetigo with failure to recognize the underlying photosensitivity.

Support Group: N.O.R.D.
P.O. Box 8923
New Fairfield, CT
06812
1-800-999-6673

SELECTED BIBLIOGRAPHY

Berth-Jones, J., Norris, P.G., Graham-Brown, R.A.C., Burns, D.A., Hutchinson, P.E., Adams, J., and Hawk, J.L.M. (1991). Juvenile spring eruption of the ears; a probable variant of polymorphous light eruption. *Br. J. Dermatol.* **124,** 375–378.

Of 18 cases, 5 had no family history. In one family, two brothers had classic polymorphous light eruption, while their father and two other brothers had ear involvement only.

Birt, A.R., and Davis, R.A. (1975). Hereditary polymorphous light eruption of American Indians. *Int. J. Dermatol.* **14,** 105–111.

Reviews and updates original publication of 1968. Discusses distribution of certain ethnic groups with distribution of disease. They treated with oral trimethylpsoralen without extra exposure to ultraviolet light and with 0.1% betamethasone valerate with good results, inducing remission in some patients.

Draelos, Z.K., and Hansen, R.C. (1986). Polymorphic light eruption in pediatric patients with American Indian ancestry. *Pediatr. Dermatol.* **3,** 384–389.

Nice discussion of treatment options.

Jansen, C.T. (1978). Heredity of chronic polymorphous light eruptions. *Arch. Dermatol.* **114,** 188–190.

All patients in Finland. Among those with vesiculopapular lesions, 26 had a positive family history. Ten of 16 with prurigo nodules had a positive family history, 2 of 11 with an eczematous morphology did also. Four of 10 with macronodular disease and 9 of 12 with other types of skin lesions had positive family histories. Interestingly, of 15 familial cases that the authors attempted to confirm, one proved to have a different disease. (This suggests that the reliability of these data is questionable.) Fifty-six percent of patients gave a family history of affected individuals in multiple generations, and there was male-to-male transmission in some.

Van Praag, M.C.G., Boom, B.W., and Vermeer, B.J. (1994). Diagnosis and treatment of polymorphous light eruption. *Int. J. Dermatol.* **33,** 233–239.

Discusses the differential diagnosis of photosensitivity, with tables highlighting the differences in history, histopathology, and morphology. Does not emphasize genetic aspects.

ROTHMUND-THOMSON SYNDROME (MIM:268400)

(Hereditary Poikiloderma Congenitale)

Includes COPS Syndrome

DERMATOLOGIC FEATURES

MAJOR. Facial telangiectases with atrophy and hypopigmentation develop in early infancy and progress. Blotchy hyperpigmentation may also develop. Occasionally blisters can occur. The extensor aspects of the extremities, backs of hands, legs, and buttocks are involved with truncal and flexural sparing. Progression usually stops in late childhood.

There is thinning or alopecia of scalp, facial, body, and secondary sexual hairs. Absent or sparse eyebrows and eyelashes are most common.

MINOR. Diffuse hyperkeratotic lesions have been described in approximately 30%, as has photosensitivity. Variable nail dystrophy is noted in about 25% of patients. Calcinosis cutis is an uncommon finding. Squamous cell carcinoma of the skin has been described.

ASSOCIATED ABNORMALITIES

Short stature is reported in 50%–65% of individuals. Skeletal malformations include radial ray defects, small hands and feet, absent patel-

A

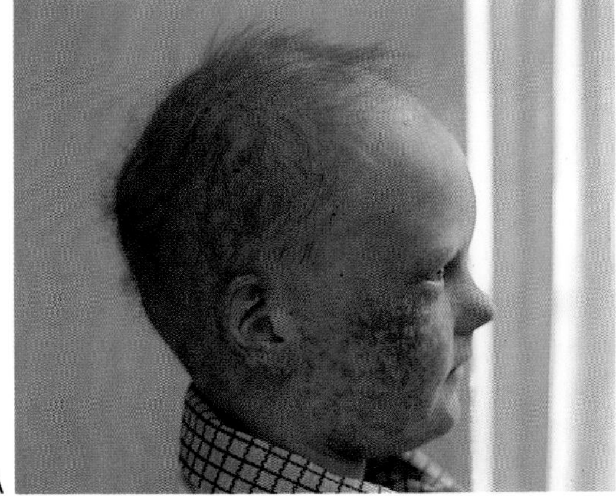

B

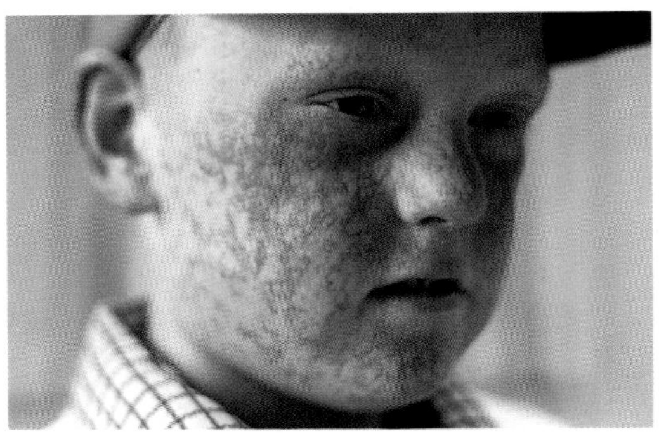

Figure 13.9. **(A)** Marked vascular changes and sparse hair. **(B)** Atrophic nature of skin changes is evident.

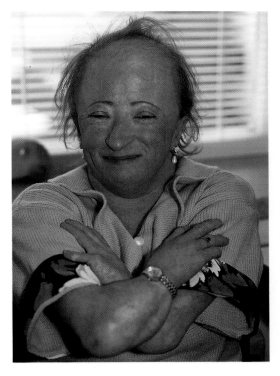

Figure 13.10. Thirty-eight year old with progressive hair loss and radial ray defects.

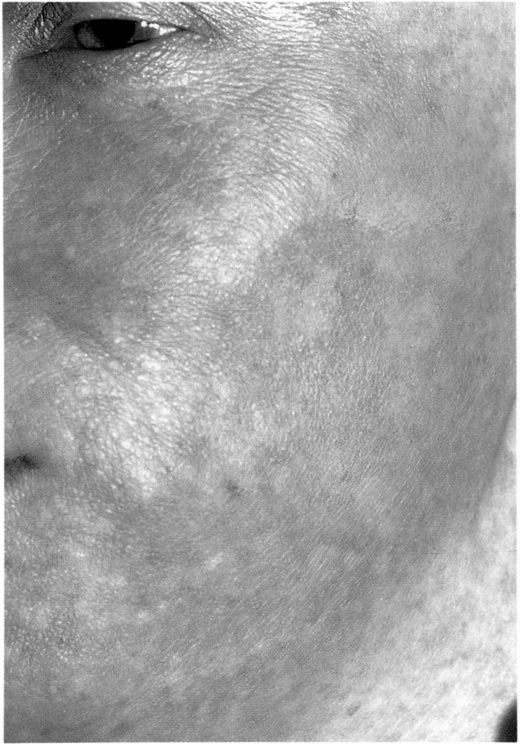

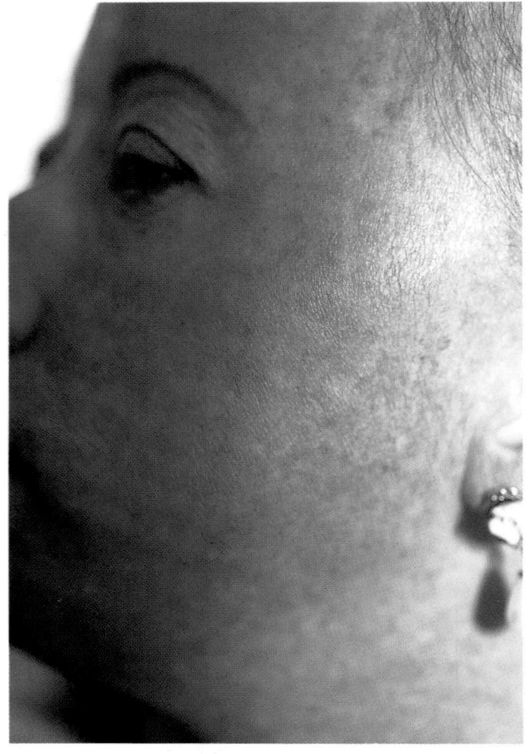

Figure 13.11. Age 27 (**A**) and age 38 (**B**) showing mild atrophy, marked vascular and pigment changes and little progression in severity over time. Eyebrows and eyelashes are absent.

lae and osteoporosis. Osteogenic sarcoma has been reported in nine patients and appears to be a real and specific association.

Hypogonadism and infertility are described in approximately 25%. There have been some successful pregnancies to affected women.

Juvenile cataracts are reported in approximately 50% of patients. Mental retardation occurs in less than 10% of patients. Most have normal intelligence.

Hypodontia occurs in approximately 40% of patients. Facial changes, including triangular facies, frontal bossing, hypertelorism, and prominent and flattened nose are described in a minority of patients.

HISTOPATHOLOGY

LIGHT. Mild epidermal atrophy, perivascular lymphocytic infiltrate, telangiectasias, and fragmentation of elastic fibers.
EM. No information.

BASIC DEFECT

Unknown. A variety of chromosomal alterations have been reported in a minority of patients.

TREATMENT

Laser for facial telangiectases.

MODE OF INHERITANCE

Autosomal recessive.

PRENATAL DIAGNOSIS

None.

DIFFERENTIAL DIAGNOSIS

Fanconi syndrome (MIM:227650, 227660), Bloom syndrome (MIM:210900), and ataxia telangiectasia (MIM:208900) share facial telangiectases but not poikilodermatous (atrophic) alterations. Kindler syndrome (MIM:173650) is marked by bullae, which are a minor feature in Rothmund-Thomson syndrome. In dyskeratosis congenita (MIM:224230, 305000) there is usually later onset of the skin changes. Leukokeratosis is not a prominent feature of Rothmund-Thomson syndrome.

COPS syndrome (calcinosis cutis, osteoma cutis, poikiloderma, and skeletal abnormalities) is marked by metaphyseal bone changes similar to rickets and exuberant calcinosis cutis, which is a rare complication of Rothmund-Thomson syndrome.

Support Group: N.O.R.D.
P.O. Box 8923
New Fairfield, CT 06812
1-800-999-6673

SELECTED BIBLIOGRAPHY

Berg, E., Chuang, T.-Y., and Cripps, D. (1987). Rothmund-Thomson syndrome. A case report, photo testing, and literature review. *J. Am. Acad. Dermatol.* **17,** 332–338.

A table with manifestations reported in earlier reviews, representing a putative total of 107 patients. Moss (1989) points out that there are many duplicate reports, which brings the total of patients to less than 100.

Hallman, N., and Patiala, R. (1951). Congenital poikiloderma atrophicans vasculare in a mother and her son. *Acta Dermatol. Venereol.* **31,** 401–406.

A mother and son with poikiloderma, thin atrophic skin over the hands. Joint contractures present in the mother. Hands and feet are described as small in both, but with no measurements given. Palmoplantar keratoderma present in the son. This is the only case of vertical transmission of putative Rothmund-Thomson syndrome.

Moss, C. (1989). Duplicate reporting of patients with Rothmund-Thomson syndrome. (Letter) *J. Am. Acad. Dermatol.* **21,** 816–817.

Moss points out that bias toward an impression of more severe phenotype is a likely consequence of duplicate reporting of patients.

Oranje, A.P., de Muinck Keizer-Schrama, S.M.P.F., Vuzevski, V.D., and Meradji, M. (1991). Calcinosis cutis, osteoma cutis, poikiloderma and skeletal abnormalities (COPS syndrome)—a new entity? *Eur. J. Pediatr.* **150,** 343–346.

Single case report. Poikiloderma preceded calcinosis, both present by 1 year of age.

Starr, D.G., McClure, J.P., and Connor, J.M. (1985). Non-dermatological complications and genetic aspects of the Rothmund-Thomson syndrome. *Clin. Genet.* **27,** 102–104.

Twenty-five of 73 siblings at risk also affected. One mother–son pair (see Hallman and Patiala, 1951). Consanguinity present in 16% of families. Frequency of clinical features differs in their tables from those in other reports.

Vennos, E.M., Collins, M., and James, W.D. (1992). Rothmund-Thomson syndrome: review of the world literature. *J. Am. Acad. Dermatol.* **27,** 750–762.

Well written and detailed with 150 references. Wonderful photographs. Extensive table with differential diagnosis.

XERODERMA PIGMENTOSUM (MIM:194400, 133510.0001, 278700–278800)

Includes All Complementation Groups; DeSanctis-Cacchione Syndrome

DERMATOLOGIC FEATURES

Major. The skin changes of xeroderma pigmentosum usually present in early childhood, during the toddler years in 50%, by kindergarten in 75%, and in almost all patients by adulthood. Patients give a history of easy sunburning, acute photosensitivity, and unusual

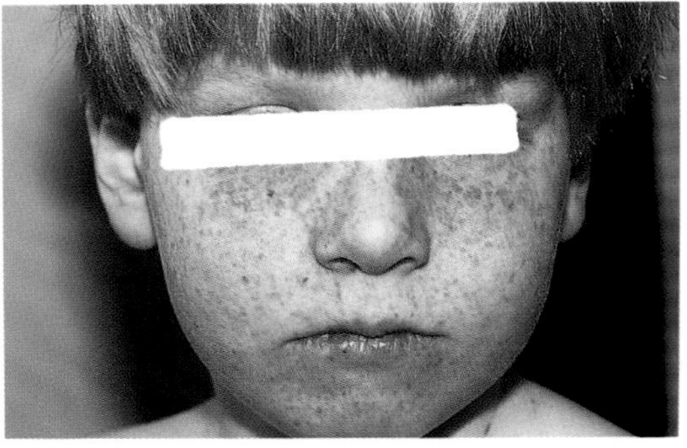

A

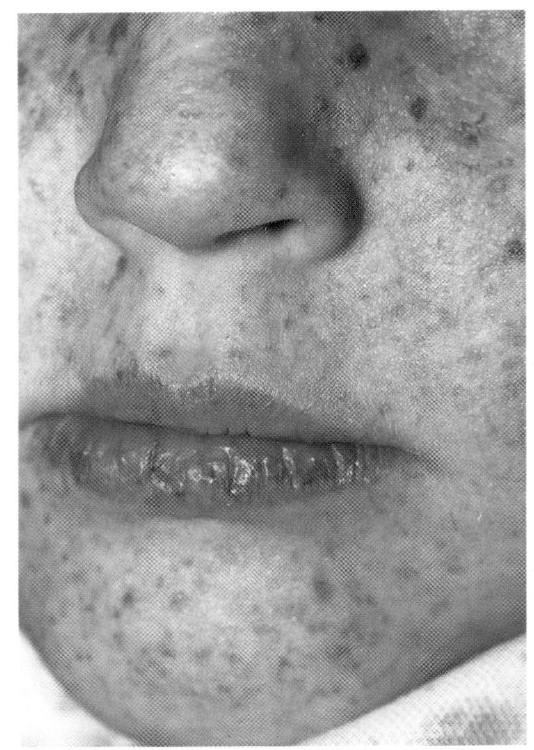

B

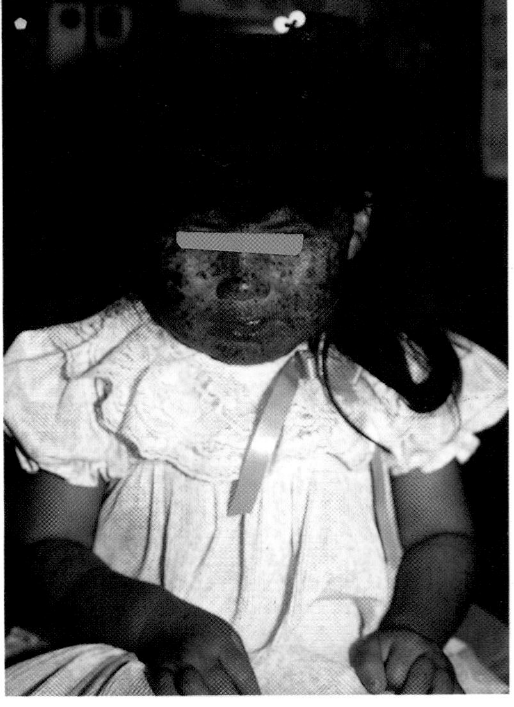

C

Figure 13.12. (A–C) Three children with actinic pigment change and telangiectases. Child in C is more severely involved. (B, from Sybert and Holbrook, 1987; C, courtesy of Dr. R. Wagner, Freeland, Washington.)

freckling and xerosis of the face, backs of the hands, and forearms. The correct diagnosis is often not made initially. Progressive changes of premature aging with thinning of the epidermis, dermal elastosis and wrinkling, marked splotchy hyperpigmentation with irregular tan to dark brown macules (solar lentigines), hypopigmentation, and actinic keratoses develop. These changes are all those associated with excessive sun exposure in normal individuals.

Cutaneous malignancy is invariable. Actinic keratoses, basal cell epithelioma, squamous cell carcinoma, and melanoma, in order of decreasing frequency, are reported. Approximately 5% of patients develop melanoma. Onset of malignancy can be as early as age 2 years. The mean age at which the first cutaneous malignancy develops is 8 years.

Progressive disfigurement due to repeated surgeries is an almost invariable outcome.

MINOR. Malignancies of the tip of the tongue have been reported rarely.

ASSOCIATED ABNORMALITIES

There are complementation groups A through G. Only three patients have been reported with XP-B. XP-F appears primarily in the Japanese and is associated with mild disease. Growth retardation and progressive mental retardation is typical of XP-A (De Sanctis-Cacchione syn-

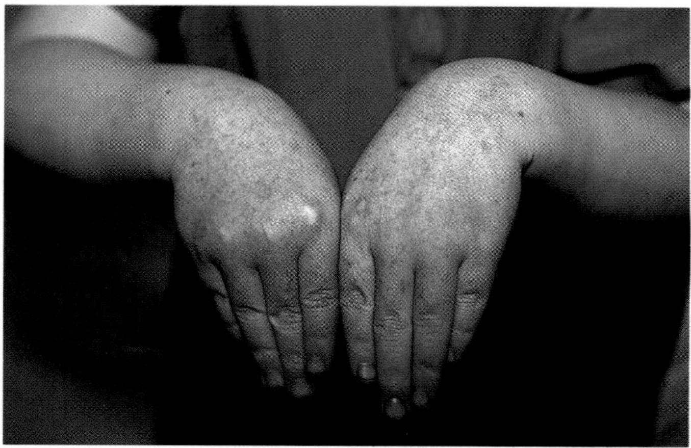

Figure 13.13. Tops of hands showing actinic damage in child.

drome). In addition, children with XP-A have microcephaly, quadriparesis, ataxia, choreoathetosis, and progressive sensorineural hearing loss. In XP-D mental retardation may develop in the second decade.

Individuals with XP-F, XP-E, and variant XP usually have normal neurologic status, as do some patients with XP-A and most, but not all, with XP-C. One adult with XP-C who survived into her forties began exhibiting sensorineural hearing loss, atrophy, and gait abnormalities, suggesting that neurologic involvement may be part of the syndrome if patients survive long enough.

No part of the exposed globe is spared. Photophobia is common. Abnormal melanin deposition along the eyelid margins, tumor formation, scarring, and blepharitis are typical. Conjunctival telangiectases and atrophy with secondary conjunctivitis and conjunctival malignancies occur. Corneal opacification, keratitis, and neovascularization and tumor have also been described.

HISTOPATHOLOGY

LIGHT. Nondiagnostic. The changes are those of solar damage or of cutaneous malignancy.
EM. Pigmented lesions show an increase in number and pleomorphism of melanosomes, and giant melanosomes can be found in melanocytes and keratinocytes.

BASIC DEFECT

Abnormalities in DNA excision repair enzymes have been demonstrated. The cells are unable to excise DNA dimers that are formed in the skin cells by exposure to ultraviolet light. They differ in their rates of repair. In variant xeroderma pigmentosum repair excision is normal. In XP-B, the defect is in *ERCC3;* in XP-D, *ERCC2;* in XP-G, *ERCC5;* in XP-C, *XPCC;* and in XP-A, the defect is in *XPAC*.

TREATMENT

Avoidance of exposure to both UVA and UVB light. This includes light from the sun and from artificial sources. Light from incandescent bulbs is usually tolerated, but unshielded fluorescent lights and sunlamps are problematic. Protective glasses are also important to prevent eye changes. Special glass or UVA-blocking film for car windows and home windows is appropriate. Occlusive clothing, such as that made by Solumbra, or leather and denim is advised. Broad-spectrum sunscreens are mandatory. Careful skin examinations with appropriate surgical management are vital. Currently, an experimental protocol for topical treatment with liposomes containing DNA repair enzymes is underway.

Oral isotretinoin showed some promise in decreasing the formation of tumors, but after cessation of the drug rebound occurred. Side effects of the medication at 2 mg/kg/day were severe. The results of a protocol using 0.5 mg/kg/day have not been published to date. In a few reports of individuals with milder variant disease, etretinate appeared to be useful. I would not recommend its use in children at this time.

MODE OF INHERITANCE

Autosomal recessive. One study suggested an increased risk of skin cancer in heterozygotes. However, this increased risk appeared to cluster primarily within four families so that generalization to all carriers is uncertain. One study demonstrated an increase in mental retardation and microcephaly in relatives of patients with xeroderma pigmentosum, but did not address the contribution of the consanguinity in these families to these features. *XPAC* is mapped to 9q34.1, *XPCC* to 3p25, *ERCC3* to 2q21, *ERCC2* to 19q13.2-q13.3, *ERCC5* to 13q33,.

PRENATAL DIAGNOSIS

Measurement of ultraviolet light–induced DNA dimer excision repair in amniotic fluid cells.

DIFFERENTIAL DIAGNOSIS

PIBIDS (MIM:278730) (trichothiodystrophy with photosensitivity) is allelic to XP-D, yet patients do not develop cutaneous tumors despite photosensitivity, and children with XP-D do not have trichothiodystrophy. In ataxia telangiectasia (MIM:208900), patients can present with telangiectases similar to those seen in xeroderma pigmentosum and with neurologic findings similar to those found in the XP-D group. However, patients with ataxia telangiectasia do not have abnormal freckling and have no history of sun sensitivity.

Cockayne syndrome (MIM:216400) is also marked by defective nucleotide excision repair, short stature, and photosensitivity, but affected individuals usually do not have the xerosis and pigmentary changes of xeroderma pigmentosum. Microcephaly, a beaked nose, severe dwarfing, and loss of subcutaneous tissue without development of skin cancers is typical of Cockayne syndrome. Retinal atrophy and progressive deafness are also limited to Cockayne syndrome. Calcification of the basal ganglia is seen in Cockayne syndrome, as are joint contractures, and these are not part of xeroderma pigmentosum. There are extremely rare case reports of overlap individuals designated with XP-B, in addition, a few patients with XP-F and XP-C with features of Cockayne syndrome have been described.

In hereditary polymorphic light eruption (MIM:174770), there can be similar skin changes, but there is no defect in excision repair. Patients with this disorder may be somewhat less photosensitive than those with xeroderma pigmentosum and have their symptoms primarily in the spring and summer. Associated malignancies at an early age have not been noted.

Erythropoietic protoporphyria (MIM:177000) is marked by burning, pain, and fewer cutaneous findings. Gunther disease (congenital erythropoietic porphyria, MIM:263700) shows similar skin changes, but blistering is more prominent than pigment change. Porphyrin screening is appropriate in any patient suspected to have xeroderma pigmentosa. Rothmund-Thomson syndrome (MIM:268400) shares in common with xeroderma pigmentosa telangiectases and poikiloderma, although it lacks the propensity for malignancy.

Support Group: The Xeroderma Pigmentosa Registry
UMDNJ-New Jersey Medical School
Dept. of Dermatology
Rm H576
Medical Science Building
185 South Orange Avenue
Newark, NJ 07103
1-201-982-6255

Share and Care
Cockayne Syndrome
Network
PO Box 552
Stanleytown, VA
24168-0552
1-703-629-2369

SELECTED BIBLIOGRAPHY

Bech-Thomsen, N., Wulf, H.C., and Ullman, S. (1991). Xeroderma pigmentosum lesions related to ultraviolet transmittance by clothes. *J. Am. Acad. Dermatol.* **24,** 365–368.

A neat study. Faced with one patient with a fair amount of skin damage in clothing-protected areas, the authors measured UVB transmittance of her clothing and correlated milder damage on her buttocks with greater protection by denim. This is a nice example of quantifying common sense.

Bootsma, D. (1993). The genetic defect in DNA repair deficiency syndromes. EACR—Muhlbock Memorial Lecture. *Eur. J. Cancer* **29A,** 1482–1488.

Well-written, concise review with table listing complementation groups and their shared and distinctive features. Presents current understanding of the basic defects in terms accessible to clinicians.

Imray, F.P., Hockey, A., Relf, W., Ramsay, R.G., and Kidson, C. (1986). Sensitivity to ultraviolet radiation in a dominantly inherited form of xeroderma pigmentosum. *J. Med. Genet.* **23,** 72–78.

Anderson, T.E., and Begg, M. (1950). Xeroderma pigmentosum of mild type. *Br. J. Dermatol. Syphilol.* **62,** 402–407.

One Australian family with autosomal dominant sun sensitivity and abnormal freckling. Minimal occurrence of malignancy. The family had excision repair rates similar to those seen in XP-E (40%–60% of normal), but complementation studies with XP-E were not done.

Kraemer, K.H., Lee, M.M., and Scotto, J. (1987). Xeroderma pigmentosum. Cutaneous, ocular and neurologic abnormalities in 830 published cases. *Arch. Dermatol.* **123,** 241–250.

A massive literature review. Thirty percent of patients were dead by age 40 years. Forty percent had eye involvement, 5% had melanoma, and 18% had neurologic abnormalities. There was no correlation with complementation groups, so it is difficult to apply likelihoods of each of these problems occurring in a single individual. Many tables, including one with reports of rare associations such as internal malignancy and immune defects.

Mimaki, T., Itoh, N., Abe, J., Tagawa, T., Sato, K., Yabuuchi, H., and Takebe, H. (1986). Neurological manifestations in xeroderma pigmentosum. *Ann. Neurol.* **20,** 70–75.

Even with a single complementation group, here xeroderma pigmentosum XP-A, which is frequent among Japanese, variability in expression is the rule and the typical clinical features, such as short stature, microcephaly, and mental retardation, had delayed and variable onset.

Parshad, R., Sanford, K.K., Kraemer, K.H., Jones, G.M., and Tarone, R.E. (1990). Carrier detection in xeroderma pigmentosum. *J. Clin. Invest.* **85,** 135–138.

In a blinded study, lymphocytes and fibroblasts from eight obligate carriers showed a twofold higher rate of chromatid damage 2–3 hours after x-irradiation. The authors suggest that the test may be useful in families with known xeroderma pigmentosum to detect heterozygote carrier siblings. This does not make much sense to me, as carrier testing of the sibling's spouse would not be reliable.

Thielmann, H.W., Popanda, O., Edler, L., and Jung, E.G. (1991). Clinical symptoms and DNA repair characteristics of xeroderma pigmentosum: patients from Germany. *Cancer Res.* **51,** 3456–3470.

Among 61 xeroderma pigmentosum patients in Germany, three were group A, 26 C, 16 D, 3 E, 2 F, and 11 were variant. Groups C, D, and variant patients developed basal cell carcinoma, squamous cell carcinoma, and melanoma. Those in groups A, E, and F did not. The authors were struck with the preponderance of melanomas that occurred in type D, but the percentages of patients with XP-D and XP-C who developed melanoma were 62% and 46% respectively—not too dissimilar, given the small number of patients. These findings are interesting in that they suggest that it is problems with specific types of excision repair that give rise to one or another type of cutaneous malignancy.

CHAPTER 14

IMMUNE DEFICIENCY DISEASES

CHEDIAK-HIGASHI DISEASE (MIM:214500)

(Chediak-Higashi-Steinbrinck Disease, Beguez-Cesar-Chediak Disease)

Includes Griscelli syndrome (MIM:214450)

DERMATOLOGIC FEATURES

Major. Patients with Chediak-Higashi have "dilute" pigmentation—they are lighter in color than their familial and racial background would predict. There may be a grayish tone to the skin. Perhaps 10%–15% of patients do not have pigment changes.

The hair is often silvery or steely gray. Even when the hair color is blonde to dark brown, there may still be a silvery glint to it. Eye color is usually normal.

Patients can freckle and have pigmented moles despite their generalized decrease in pigment. Dyschromia with patchy pigmentation in sun-exposed areas has also been described.

Minor. Severe sunburn has been described in some patients. Scarring secondary to recurrent pyoderma can occur.

ASSOCIATED ABNORMALITIES

Visual disturbances are occasionally reported. Nystagmus is not an invariable finding.

Increased susceptibility to common bacterial infections (e.g., *Staphylococcus aureus*, β-hemolytic *Streptococcus*) is thought to be due to defective degranulation of leukocytes. This feature presents early in childhood. Otitis, pyoderma, and pneumonias are common.

Chediak-Higashi disease is marked by a rapid, progressive, explosive downhill course, also called the *accelerated phase*, characterized by lymphoproliferative disease with lymphadenopathy, hepatosplenomegaly, pancytopenia, recurrent fever, and death. This is said to occur in 85% of patients. Death usually occurs before age 10 years and often before age 5. There have been some long-term survivors. Hepatosplenomegaly may develop within the first few years, prior to the accelerated phase.

Neurologic symptoms are primarily that of a progressive neuropathy and include clumsiness, abnormal gait, and paresthesias. Patients with these neurologic signs tend to be much older, in their teens, twenties, and thirties. Young children may die before they can exhibit neurologic involvement, or patients with neurologic disease may have a distinct disorder. There are a few patients who have had mental retardation. Most of these are the products of consanguineous matings, so there may be a separate reason for the mental retardation unrelated to the Chediak-Higashi disease.

HISTOPATHOLOGY

Light. Cytoplasmic large granules are seen in all cells that produce granules. Histiocytic and lymphohistiocytic infiltrates of all organs occur in the accelerated phase. There may be a decrease in the number of melanocytes.

EM. Large electron-dense lysosomal granules are present in dermal fibroblasts. Giant clumped melanosomes are found in melanocytes, with decreased numbers of melanosomes in keratinocytes.

BASIC DEFECT

Unknown. There is a decrease in leukocyte chemotaxis and a defect in natural killer cells. Cats have what appears to be a homologous disease.

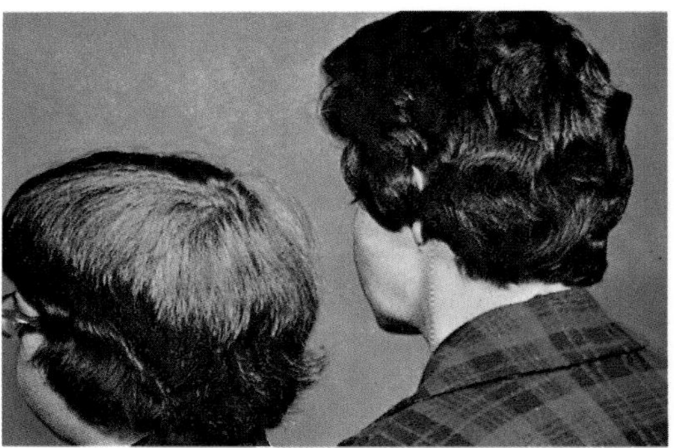

Figure 14.1. Mother and daughter; silver sheen of daughter's hair is evident. (From Windhorst et al., 1968.)

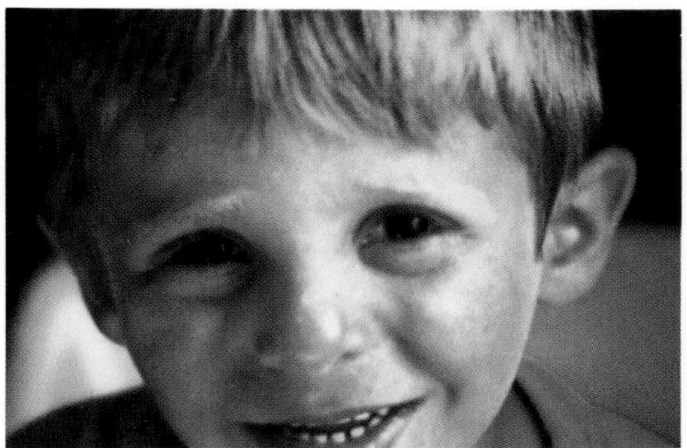

Figure 14.2. Silver-gray hair of scalp, eyebrows, eyelashes, and facial down in Griscelli syndrome. (From Hurvitz et al., 1993.)

TREATMENT

Careful management of bouts of infection and photoprotection are important. Treatment of the lymphoproliferative stage is limited to a choice between antimetabolites and bone marrow transplant.

MODE OF INHERITANCE

Autosomal recessive. Heterozygote detection is probably not reliable.

PRENATAL DIAGNOSIS

Successful prenatal diagnosis has been performed in cats by screening amniotic fluid cells for giant lysosomes and by looking at blood for enlarged granules in leukocytes. In humans, electron microscopic analysis of fetal blood from affected fetuses shows typical inclusions in neutrophils. Scalp biopsies of fetuses at risk demonstrated abnormal giant melanin granules in the hairs of affected Chediak-Higashi fetuses.

DIFFERENTIAL DIAGNOSIS

Griscelli syndrome (MIM:214450) shares in common with Chediak-Higashi diffuse hypopigmentation and recurrent infections. Affected individuals have silvery hair, hypotonia, and motor retardation. Hematologic features of Griscelli syndrome include thrombocytopenia, neutropenia, and recurrent anemia. In contrast to Chediak-Higashi, granulocytes are normal but there is impaired natural killer cell function. Delayed hypersensitivity responses are absent and there is a decrease in IgA and IgG. There is an increased number of mature melanosomes within melanocytes, and these are not aggregated in clumps. The pigment in the hair, however, is clumped. Prenatal diagnosis of Griselli syndrome has been performed using this feature as a marker in fetal scalp biopsies. Patients with Menkes disease (MIM:309400) may have silvery hair. They also have pili torti, a structural hair defect not seen in Chediak-Higashi syndrome. Neurologic symptoms are typical in Menkes disease and present early. In general, the giant peroxidase-positive granules seen in leukocytes are pathognomonic of Chediak-Higashi disease. However, they have been occasionally reported in patients with acquired leukemia.

Support Group: N.O.R.D.
P.O. Box 8923
New Fairfield, CT
06812
1-800-999-6673

SELECTED BIBLIOGRAPHY

Bejaoui, M., Veber, F., Girault, D., Gaud, C., Blanche, S., Griscelli, C., and Fischer, A.

(1989). Phase accélerée de la maladie de Chediak-Higashi. *Arch. Fr. Pediatr.* **46,** 733–736.

Eighteen accelerated phases in 11 patients. In seven, remission was achieved with etoposide, prednisone, and intrathecal methotrexate. Relapse occurred in all. Bone marrow transplant was successful in three, lethal in one. The authors note that there was an increase in triglycerides in a majority of patients. They give their treatment protocol.

Blume, R.S., and Wolff, S.M. (1972). The Chediak-Higashi syndrome: studies in four patients and a review of the literature. *Medicine* **51,** 247–280.

A review of 59 cases reported to date of publication. They discussed four patients in detail. One hundred seventeen references.

Klein, C., Philippe, N., LeDeist, F., Fraitag, S., Prost, C., Durandy, A., Fischer, A., and Griscelli, C. (1994) Partial albinism with immunodeficiency (Griscelli syndrome). *J. Pediatr.* **125,** 886–895.

Seven patients in whom no cutaneous pigment changes were seen, only silvery hair. Large pigment granules present in hair shafts. Skin biopsy showed accumulation of melanosomes in melanocytes, with decrease in transfer to keratinocytes. One of three children who underwent bone marrow transplantation survives.

Misra, V.P., King, R.H.M., Harding, A.E., Muddle, J.R., and Thomas, P.K. (1991). Peripheral neuropathy in the Chediak-Higashi syndrome. *Acta Neuropathol. (Berl.)* **81,** 354–358.

A brother and sister with progressive peripheral neuropathy are described. These patients had a course very atypical of Chediak-Higashi disease. One was age 33 and one was age 29. The authors reviewed the previous literature and state that the neuropathy is the result of axonal problems, not the result of demyelinization.

Peron, C.M., and Kaplan, J. (1993). Complementation analysis of Chediak-Higashi syndrome. The same gene may be responsible for the defect in all patients and species. *Somatic Cell Mol. Genet.* **19,** 459–463.

Neat study. Fusion of wild-type fibroblasts with Chediak-Higashi cells corrected defect in all species. They used beige mice and Aleutian mink. There was cross-species wild-type/affected correction as well. However, beige mouse–human Chediak-Higashi cell hybrids did not correct, suggesting that these are allelic defects.

Sato, A. (1955). Chediak and Higashi's disease: probable identity of "a new leucocytal anomaly (Chediak) "and" congenital gigantism of peroxidase granules (Higashi)." *Tokushima J. Exp. Med.* **6,** 201–210.

This paper is transcribed from a speech. Sato put together a case report of Higashi's with one of Chediak's and felt that both patients had the same disease. A delightful read, and I would vote for the eponym of Sato syndrome myself.

CHRONIC GRANULOMATOUS DISEASE (MIM:233700, 306400)

DERMATOLOGIC FEATURES

MAJOR. Recurrent suppurative skin infections characterized by furunculosis and perirectal abscesses are primary features in chronic granulomatous disease. Cervical and inguinal lymphadenitis is typical, and draining abscesses overlying involved nodes are common. Signs usually present within the first year, and 80% will manifest by age 2. Almost 50% of affected individuals will present first with dermatitis. This "dermatitis" is often pustular and vesicular rather than eczematous. It is often periorificial and impetiginized. It may involve the scalp and appear seborrheic-like.

Causative infective organisms are *Staphylococcus aureus, Aspergillus, Pseudomonas,* and *Serratia marcescens.* Catalase-positive organisms predominate as infectious agents.

Paronychia occur frequently.

MINOR. Sweet syndrome (acute febrile neutrophilic dermatitis) characterized by red, raised plaques and nodules with ulcerating centers was reported in one infant with chronic granulomatous disease.

Approximately 30% of female carriers of chronic granulomatous disease experience skin changes consistent with discoid lupus erythematosus. These skin changes are marked by scaling erythematous plaques, atrophy, and hypopigmentation developing in sun-exposed areas. Immunofluorescence is negative, and histopathology shows some changes consistent with discoid lupus erythematosus.

Some patients develop gingivitis.

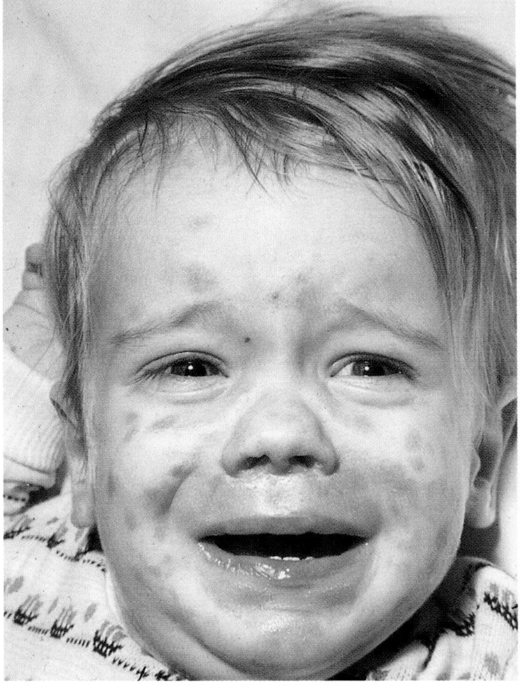

Figure 14.3. Seborrheic-like, eczematous facial rash. (Courtesy of Dr. H. Ochs, Seattle, Washington.)

ASSOCIATED ABNORMALITIES

Lymphadenopathy, hepatosplenomegaly, failure to thrive, chronic diarrhea, and anemia are common features.

Recurrent suppurative internal infections, pneumonia with lung abscesses, osteomyelitis, and liver abscesses are most common. Osteomyelitis occurs in up to 30% of patients. Hematogenous or local spread can result in infection in virtually any organ.

In general, affected individuals have hypergammaglobulinemia.

Chronic granulomas can develop in the bladder and stomach and may cause obstructive symptoms.

Survival has improved with earlier recognition of the condition and prophylactic antibiotic treatment. Approximately 30%–50% of affected individuals succumb to the disease by age 10 years.

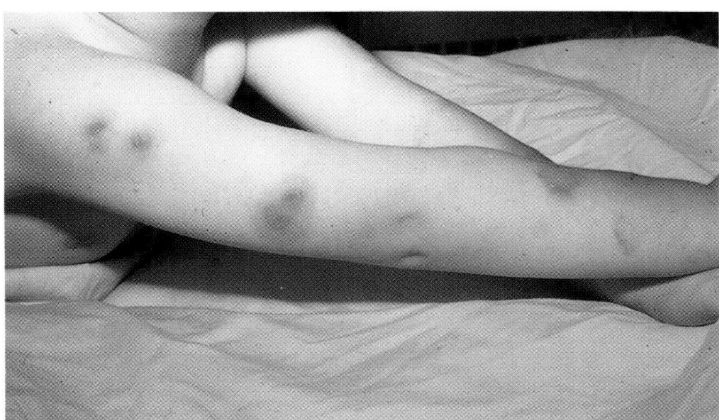

Figure 14.4. Lesions of serratia marcessens. (Courtesy of Dr. H. Ochs, Seattle, Washington.)

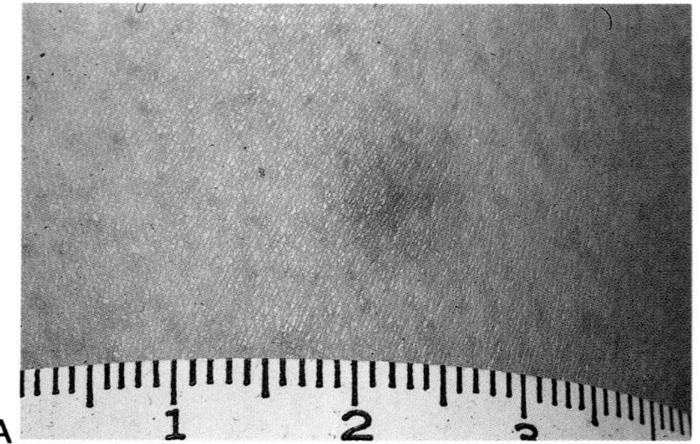

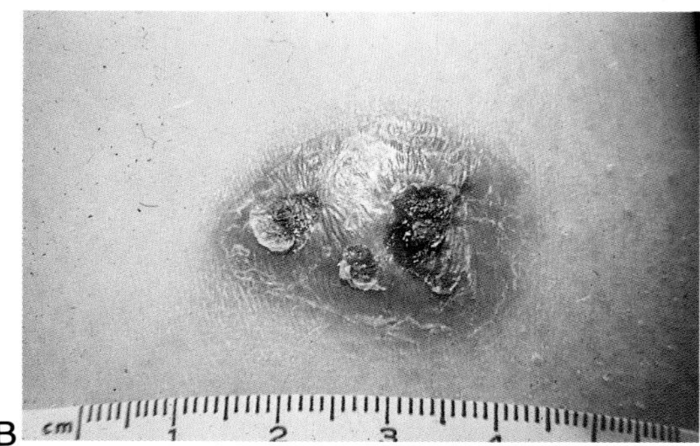

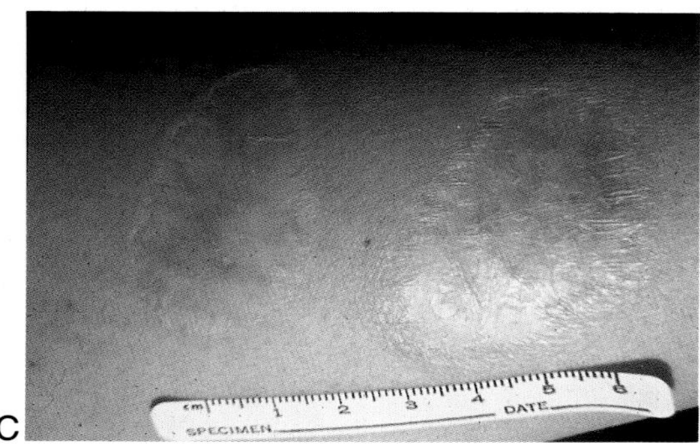

Figure 14.5. (A–C) Lesions in stages of evolution and healing with scarring. (Courtesy of Dr. H. Ochs, Seattle, Washington.)

HISTOPATHOLOGY

LIGHT. The granulomatous reactions are composed of epithelioid histiocytes, lymphocytes, plasma cells, and multinucleated Langerhans-type giant cells. There may be central caseation. Pigment-laden histiocytes with foamy cytoplasm, coupled with typical clinical features, are pathognomonic.
EM. No information.

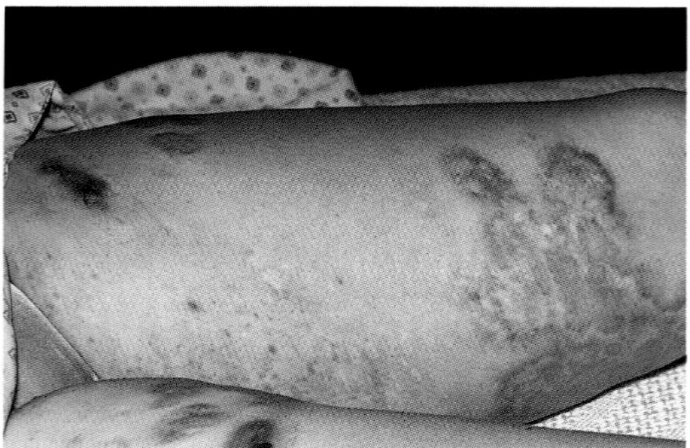

Figure 14.6. Old scars and active disease in adult. (Courtesy of Dr. H. Ochs, Seattle, Washington.)

BASIC DEFECT

Mutations in any of the four components of cytochrome b 588 coded for by genes on the X chromosome and at autosomal loci result in defective NADPH oxidase so that phagocytic cells cannot produce superoxide anions necessary for bacteriocidal and fungicidal activity.

TREATMENT

Prophylactic antibiotics. Treatment primarily with trimethoprim-sulfamethoxazole helps to reduce the occurrence of infection. Human interferon-γ injections appear to decrease the frequency and severity of infections.

MODE OF INHERITANCE

Approximately 65% are X-linked recessive; the gene is located at Xp21.1. Thirty-five percent are autosomal recessive with loci at 1q25, 16q24, and 7q11.23. There is both allelic and locus heterogeneity, and many specific mutations have now been identified.

PRENATAL DIAGNOSIS

Possible by NADPH oxidase activity of fetal blood, by linkage studies, or by direct mutational analysis if the mutation is known.

DIFFERENTIAL DIAGNOSIS

Many immunodeficiency diseases present with cutaneous infection in infancy. The nature of the infecting organism may help to point to the correct diagnosis. The NBT test will different chronic granulomatous disease from other diseases such as leukocyte adhesion deficiency syndrome (MIM:116920) or Job syndrome (MIM:243700). The NBT test demonstrates the failure of the white cells of chronic granulomatous disease patients to turn NBT blue. Job syndrome and Wiskott-Aldrich syndrome (MIM:301000) present more commonly with chronic eczema, chronic granulomatous disease with suppurative nodules.

Severe atopic dermatitis in association with recurrent infections should prompt an evaluation for underlying immune defects. If the patient has recurrent abscesses, chronic granulomatous disease is highly suspect.

Support Group: The Immunodeficiency Foundation
25 West Chesapeake Avenue, Suite 206
Towson, MD 21204-4820
1-800-296-4433

SELECTED BIBLIOGRAPHY

Curnette, J.T. (1993). Chronic granulomatous disease: the solving of a clinical riddle at the molecular level. *Clin. Immunol. Immunopathol.* **67,** S2–S15.

Review with tabular presentation of clinical features. Nicely summarizes sites of infection: "occur most commonly in those organs in contact with the outside world—the lungs, gastrointestinal tract, and skin, as well as the lymph nodes that drain those structures."

Fischer, A., Segal, A.W., Seger, R., and Weening, R.S. (1993). The management of chronic granulomatous disease. *Eur. J. Pediatr.* **152,** 896–899.

Reviews current treatment based on their experience with over 100 patients. Does not discuss current research and gene replacement therapy, which is actively being investigated.

Forehand, J.R., and Johnston, R.B., Jr. (1994). Chronic granulomatous disease: newly defined molecular abnormalities explain disease variability and normal phagocytic physiology. *Curr. Opin. Pediatr.* **6,** 668–675.

Concise and superficial review with clear explanation of mechanisms of defects in NADPH oxidase activity. Sixty-seven references.

Quie, P.G. (1993). Chronic granulomatous disease of childhood. A saga of discovery and understanding. *Pediatr. Infect. Dis. J.* **12,** 395–398.

The author had made the original observation of the decreased bacteriocidal activity of polymorphonuclear cells in chronic granulomatous disease. Here he reviews the voyage of discovery, which underscores the importance of collegial interactions and hallway brainstorming.

Sillevis Smith, J.H., Weening, R.S., Krieg, S.R., and Bos, J.D. (1990). Discoid lupus erythematosus-like lesions in carriers of X-linked chronic granulomatous disease. *Br. J. Dermatol.* **122,** 643–650.

Fifteen of 16 carriers responded to a questionnaire. Seventy percent had recurrent aphthous stomatitis, and 65% had recurrent skin rash, which appeared to be provoked by sunlight in more than 50%. Twenty percent had Raynaud phenomenon, and a similar proportion had recurrent skin infection.

Windhorst, D.B., and Good, R.A. (1971). Dermatologic manifestations of fatal granulomatous disease of childhood. *Arch. Dermatol.* **103,** 351–356.

This is the only detailed description of the skin changes in chronic granulomatous disease that I could find. Most other reports use the catch-all term of *dermatitis* without any further description. The "dermatitis" is not typically generalized and eczematous, but rather localized and scrofulous.

EPIDERMODYSPLASIA VERRUCIFORMIS (MIM:226400, 305350)

DERMATOLOGIC FEATURES

MAJOR. The classic lesions of epidermodysplasia verruciformis consist of disseminated, usually skin-colored, flat wart-like papules on the backs of the hands, tops of the feet, extremities, face, and trunk. The palms and soles are usually spared. These lesions may be whitish or pink and almost flat. They may be discrete or confluent. Onset has been reported at birth and as late as age 40 years, but usually occurs in the first and second decades, with 80% of cases occurring prior to age 20.

Also typical are a widespread eruption of red to reddish-brown or achromic plaques and a pityriasis versicolor-like eruption of scaly patches that are widely disseminated. Both types of lesions may show the Koebner phenomenon, and the first occurrence of lesions has been reported after sunburn.

Malignant transformation of lesions to squamous cell carcinoma occurs in 30%–50% of reported cases, particularly in sun-exposed areas of the body. These malignancies are almost always microinvasive and nonmetastasizing. Human papilloma virus (HPV) types 5, 8 and 14 are found in the primary malignancies. Although malignant degeneration in individuals of African descent with epidermodysplasia verruciformis is purportedly extremely rare, in the only series addressing this question, the mean age of 12 patients was 20.9 years, with only two individuals older than 25, and most patients were lost to follow-up. Thus, the development of malignancy may have been missed. At least one case report of malignant change in a Congolese native has been published.

MINOR. Common warts and condyloma acuminata can also be found; the latter may be limited to individuals with acquired immunodeficiency.

Pigmented papillomatous seborrhea-like growths on the forehead have been described. An eccrine poroma was found in one patient. The mucous membranes of the mouth are generally not involved.

ASSOCIATED ABNORMALITIES

The term *epidermodysplasia verruciformis* has been applied to the clinical phenomenon of widespread HPV infection in the setting of known causes of immunoincompetence, as if it were a unitary phenomenon. Epidermodysplasia verruciformis can be seen in association with HIV infection and systemic lupus erythematosus and after immunosuppressive treatment for malignancy. In most instances of familial epidermodysplasia verruciformis, no specific immune defect has been demonstrated, although a variety of alterations in cell-mediated immunity have been found.

Mental retardation has been described in several case reports, but the descriptions are usually very limited, and in most cases intelligence is either normal or not discussed. The occurrence of mental retardation may be related more to the effect of the consanguinity present in the families than to epidermodysplasia verruciformis.

HISTOPATHOLOGY

LIGHT. The epidermis is populated by large, clear, dysplastic cells in clumps or nests with homogeneous, finely granular cytoplasm, especially in the spinous and granular layers. Within the nuclei there are clear spaces (intranuclear vacuoles) that are pathognomonic. Patchy keratosis may also be seen. There are prominent keratohyaline granules in the dysplastic cells of the stratum granulosum.

EM. The pityriasis versicolor-like lesions show cells with clear cytoplasm with few tonofilament bundles and a paucity of keratohyaline granules. HPV particles are seen in the cells.

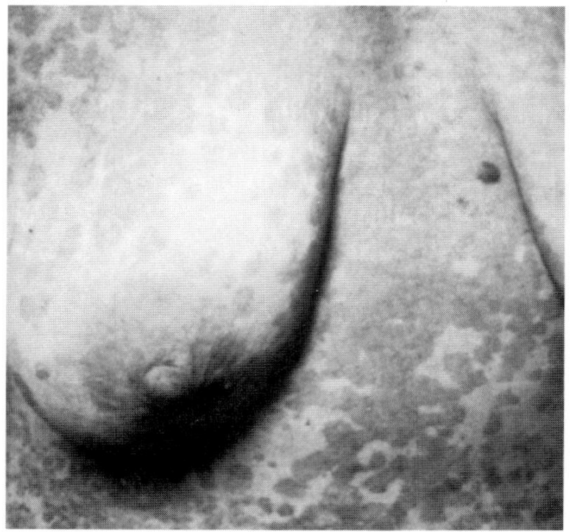

Figure 14.7. Pityriasis versicolor-like lesions. (From Lutzner and Blanchet-Bardon, 1985.)

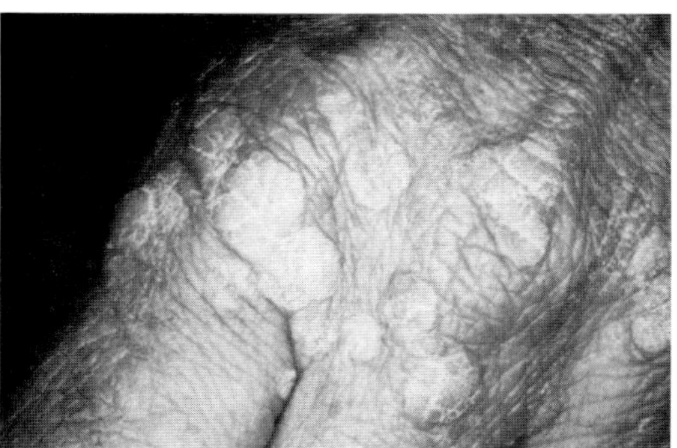

Figure 14.8. Wart-like papules over the back of the hand. (From Lutzner and Blanchet-Bardon, 1985.)

BASIC DEFECT

There appears to be an inability of the skin to resist infection by HPV subtypes that are not typical of warts in the general population (5, 8, 9, 12, 14, 15, 17, 19–25). Infection with typical HPV subtypes (2, 3, 10) also occurs.

Defects demonstrated in one or more, but never consistently in all, patients with epidermodysplasia verruciformis include anergy to DNCB sensitization; increase in TGF-β1 and TNF-α; defective natural cell-mediated cytotoxicity; increased activity of natural killer cell activity in four of six patients (all four had malignancy, the two with normal activity had no malignancies); and defect of T-cell response to HPV-infected keratinocytes.

TREATMENT

A variety of therapies have been tried with mixed success. Etretinate treatment has resulted in improvement but not clearing of warts in some patients and no response in others. Relapse occurs with cessation of treatment. Jablonska (1986) has suggested that etretinate is helpful for HPV type 3 infections but not type 5 infections. 5-FU has also been used.

Skin cancer surveillance, use of photoprotection, and avoidance of radiation are reasonable measures to take.

In the family with probable X-linked epidermodysplasia verruciformis, treatment with injections of transfer factor resulted in improvement. In another patient with immunodeficiency, the lesions improved, but did not disappear, after bone marrow transplant.

MODE OF INHERITANCE

Unclear, but autosomal recessive inheritance is likely. Among case reports consanguinity is common (greater than 30%), and affected sibships have been reported 10 times.

Of four reports often cited as describing possible autosomal dominant inheritance, two are from one family (Jablonska et al., 1979) in which the HPV virotypes are atypical for epidermodysplasia verruciformis. In a third, the patient had no family history, and in the fourth the patient did not have epidermodysplasia verruciformis.

In one pedigree with possible X-linked inheritance of epidermodysplasia verruciformis (which was the subject of two separate reports in the literature), a grandfather and four grandsons born to healthy daughters were affected. They were shown to have severely depressed levels of suppressor T cells, a finding not theretofore reported. This family may represent a specific X-linked immune defect with secondary HPV infection.

In the absence of a known cause for immunoincompetence, recurrence risks are likely to be 25% to siblings.

The statement is made in the literature that epidermodysplasia verruciformis was "considered a genodermatosis until human papilloma virus was demonstrated by electron microscopy." I think that there is still a genodermatosis(es) characterized by HPV infection and clinical epidermodysplasia verruciformis, whose underlying cause is sure to be inherited immune defects, as well as phenocopies due to acquired immune surveillance failure.

PRENATAL DIAGNOSIS

None.

DIFFERENTIAL DIAGNOSIS

Acrokeratosis verruciformis of Hopf (AKH) (MIM:101900): The distribution of wart-like lesions on the hands and feet in this condition is different than that of epidermodysplasia verruciformis, which is far more generalized. The pityriasis versicolor-like rash of epidermodysplasia verruciformis is not seen in AKH. The palmar hyperkeratoses of AKH are not a feature of epidermodysplasia verruciformis. Viral particles and parakeratosis are not seen in AKH.

Darier-White disease (MIM:124200): The greasy appearance to the scaling of Darier-White disease is not typical of epidermodysplasia verruciformis. Neither malignant degeneration nor the pityriasis versicolor-like changes of epidermodysplasia verruciformis are seen in Darier-White. Histologically the disorders can be distinguished.

Epidermal nevus: The distribution of epidermal nevi is usually along the lines of Blaschko. There are not the pityriasis versicolor-like changes or individual flat plane wart-like lesions. The texture is usually more hyperkeratotic or velvety in nevi, and lesions show no evidence for koebnerization.

Acquired epidermodysplasia verruciformis: The development of widespread warts in an immunocompromised individual (e.g., AIDS, status postchemotherapy) should not trigger concern for genetic risk.

Plane warts due to typical HPV subtypes differ histologically with a basket weave stratum corneum, empty perinuclear space surrounded by a rim of condensed tonofilaments, and keratohyaline granules. HPV typing may help to distinguish patients at risk for malignancy.

Support Group: N.O.R.D.
P.O. Box 8923
New Fairfield, CT 06812
1-800-999-6673

SELECTED BIBLIOGRAPHY

Jablonska, S., Obalek, S., Wolska, H. (1986). Follow-up of patients with epidermodysplasia verruciformis treated with etretinate. (Letter) *Dermatologica* **173,** 196–199.

Response in three patients. Remission in one, improvement in another while on treatment, but recurrence after cessation of medication, improvement in third. Warts were concurrently treated by scraping.

Jablonska, S., and Orth, G. (1985). Epidermodysplasia verruciformis. *Clin. Dermatol.* **3,** 83–96.

Detailed review with 54 references. Discussion includes both familial and acquired epidermodysplasia verruciformis without distinguishing or contrasting between them. There are excellent photographs.

Jablonska, S., Orth, G., Jarzabek-Chorzelska, M., Glinski, W., Obalek, S., Rzesa, G., Croissant, O., and Favre, M. (1979). Twenty-one years of follow-up studies of familial epidermodysplasia verruciformis. *Dermatologica* **158,** 309–327.

A two generation family is reported, but they have some features atypical of epidermodysplasia verruciformis, including infection with HPV types 3 and 4 only and regression of warts after two pregnancies in one individual. This family has been the subject of several reports.

Lutzner, M.A. (1978). Epidermodysplasia verruciformis, an autosomal recessive disease characterized by viral warts and skin cancer.

A model for viral oncogenesis. *Bull. Cancer (Paris)* **65,** 169–182.

Review of the literature with 132 references from American, European, and Asian journals.

Rajagopalan, K., Loo, D.S.C., Tay, C.H., Chin, K.N., and Tan, K.K. (1972). Familial epidermodysplasia verruciformis of Lewandowsky and Lutz. *Arch. Dermatol.* **105,** 73–78.

Six of seven female siblings at risk (the unaffected girl died at 1 month of age) and none of four males in the sibship born to first cousins had epidermodysplasia verruciformis. The authors suggest that epidermodysplasia verruciformis may be a sex-limited trait, but the findings in this family may simply reflect the higher number of females at risk.

Ross, C.M. (1971). On the fundamental identity of epidermodysplasia verruciformis, acrokeratosis verruciformis, and disseminated plane warts. *Br. J. Dermatol.* **85(suppl 7),** 102–109.

This paper is a classic example of the problems posed by overlapping disorders with fuzzy borders. Ross presents two patients, one in whom the diagnosis of epidermodysplasia verruciformis is made. This patient had limited disease, starting at age 18 years, on the scalp after bacterial infection. Lesions were clinically plane warts, and this was confirmed by electron microscopic demonstration of viral particles. Thus, Ross argues, disseminated plane warts and epidermodysplasia verruciformis are the same. Others would argue that the patient only had the former, not the latter, disorder. The second patient, given the diagnosis of AKH by Ross, had widespread lesions typical of epidermodysplasia verruciformis, including the pityriasis versicolor-like changes, with onset at age 36 years. There were multiple typical papules on the body surface. The palms and fingers were covered by dark brown depressed macules and hyperpigmentation of the dermal ridges. The toenails were dystrophic with subungual debris. No fungal studies were done. The palm lesions showed hyperkeratosis. Biopsy from the papules showed viral particles. Ross chooses to interpret these findings as showing that epidermodysplasia verruciformis is the same as AKH, but perhaps the diagnosis of AKH is inappropriate and this patient had epidermodysplasia verruciformis alone. The clinical appearance of the palm lesions was atypical for AKH, and the toenail changes could have been acquired. It is difficult to claim unity among diseases when the diagnosis is not firm.

Sezary, A., and Levy-Coblentz, G. (1933). Naevi verruciformes. *Bull. Fr. Soc. Dermatol. Syphilol.* **40,** 220–223.

A delightful passage in this case report explains why their patient, seen for complaints of eczema, had not sought medical help for her "epidermal nevus": It never gave her any troubling symptoms, many other family members had the same thing, it had not changed since infancy, and, because most of the lesions were not readily seen, her ability to charm, flirt, and/or seduce ("la coquetterie") was minimally affected (translation mine). This case is cited in reviews as epidermodysplasia verruciformis affecting two generations with a putatively affected father and two of his offspring. However, the authors clearly stated that this disorder is distinct and suggested the term *verrucous nevus.*

FAMILIAL MUCOCUTANEOUS CANDIDIASIS (MIM:114580, 212050)

Includes Familial Mucocutaneous Candidiasis and Polyendocrinopathy (MIM:240300)

DERMATOLOGIC FEATURES

MAJOR. Familial mucocutaneous candidiasis is not a single disease but can result from a variety of immune defects that hamper resistance to fungal infections. Candidal diaper rash and oral thrush are the typical first presentations. Onset of thrush in familial mucocutaneous candidiasis is usually within the first year, and almost always occurs by age 5. The oral mucosa is often red with whitish plaques. Nail involvement usually appears in later childhood. The nails are thickened and discolored with subungual debris. Marked hyperkeratosis of skin lesions is a feature of chronic localized candidiasis. In widespread chronic disease the groin, hands, face, and scalp are usually involved, and hyperkeratosis is mild.

MINOR. Other cutaneous fungal and bacterial infections may also occur.

ASSOCIATED ABNORMALITIES

A variety of defects in cell-mediated immunity can be associated. In a subset of families, susceptibility to candidal infection is accompanied by polyendocrinopathy including the adrenal glands and parathyroids, less often the thyroid and ovaries. The endocrinopathies usually develop in childhood after onset of the candidiasis and may go unrecognized for a number of years. Vitiligo and alopecia totalis occur with increased frequency in these patients, as does diabetes mellitus.

Iron deficiency anemia occurs more often than expected by chance alone.

Systemic infection with a wide range of bacterial, mycobacterial, and other fungal organisms can occur. Systemic candidiasis is rare.

HISTOPATHOLOGY

LIGHT. *Candida* organisms seen.

EM. No information.

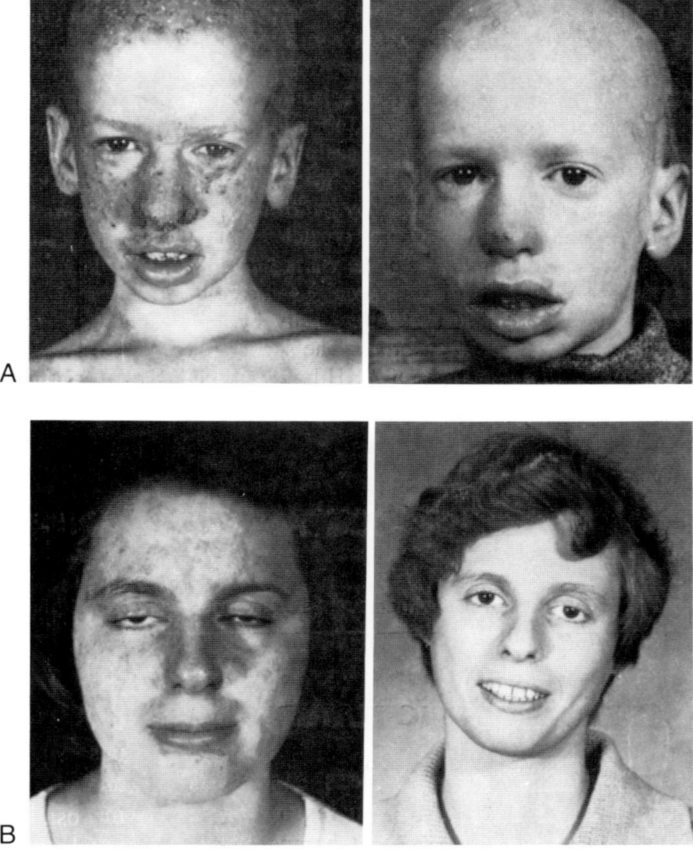

Figure 14.9. (A, B) Patients before and during topical clotrimazole treatment. (From Pazin, 1979.)

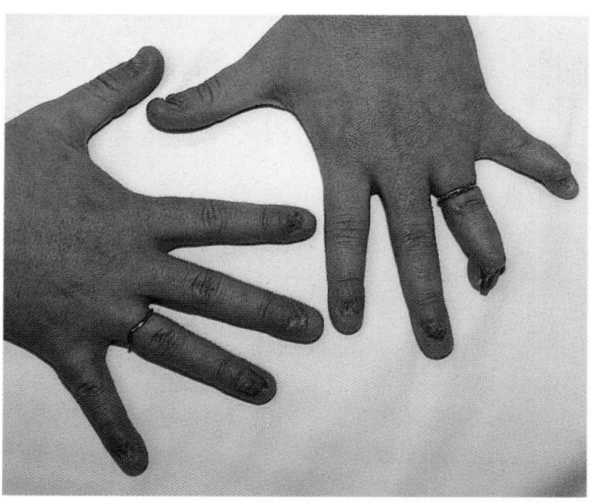

Figure 14.10. Hands and nails of patient with marked nail dystrophy and periungual swelling.

BASIC DEFECT

Except where specific immune defect is recognized, the cause is unknown.

TREATMENT

Ketoconazole is effective, but relapse occurs if treatment is stopped. One patient whose infections were refractory to ketoconazole responded to itraconazole.

In chronic mucocutaneous candidiasis with polyendocrinopathy, successful treatment of the hormone disorder does not ameliorate the skin infection. In chronic mucocutaneous candidiasis with iron deficiency, parenteral iron replacement results in clearing or improvement in the candidiasis.

MODE OF INHERITANCE

Autosomal recessive: Affected cousins, consanguinity, and affected sibships all reported.

?Autosomal dominant; see references.

PRENATAL DIAGNOSIS

None.

DIFFERENTIAL DIAGNOSIS

Candidiasis can accompany any immune deficiency and has been associated with thymic aplasiab (Nezelof syndrome, MIM:242700), Swiss-type agammaglobulinemia (MIM: 202500), and, rarely, with DiGeorge syndrome (MIM:188400). Individuals with hyper-IgE syndrome (MIM:147060, 243700) may also suffer from chronic candidal infections. Chronic candidiasis limited to the oral mucosa has no recognized genetic component, nor does the candidiasis associated with development of thymoma. Mucoepithelial dysplasia (gap junction disease, MIM:158310) is clinically very similar. Affected individuals have keratitis and photophobia, which is not part of chronic mucocutaneous candidiasis. Electron microscopic findings should discriminate.

Support Group: N.O.R.D.
P.O. Box 8923
New Fairfield, CT
06812
1-800-999-6673

SELECTED BIBLIOGRAPHY

Canales, L., Middlemas, R.O., III, Louro, J.M., and South, M.A. (1969). Immunological observations in chronic mucocutaneous candidiasis. *Lancet* **ii,** 567–571.

Male proband with severe disease, by history had mildly affected sister and niece. Could be X-linked, autosomal dominant, or inaccurate diagnosis in unexamined relatives.

Herrod, H.G. (1990). Chronic mucocutaneous candidiasis in childhood and complications of non-*candida* infection. A report of the Pediatric Immunodeficiency Collaborative Study Group. *J. Pediatr.* **116,** 377–382.

A mixed bag of 43 patients, some with polyendocrinopathy. Rate of recurrent severe infection from non-*Candida* organisms was 80%. Seven patients died.

Kroll, J.J., Einbinder, J.M., and Merz, W.G. (1973). Mucocutaneous candidiasis in a mother and son. *Arch. Dermatol.* **108,** 259–262.

Onset in the mother at age 16 years. She had keratitis and marked scalp involvement with alopecia; her 3-year-old son also had hypothyroidism. Autosomal dominant inheritance of familial mucocutaneous candidiasis with polyendocrinopathy, or perhaps unrecognized gap junction disease.

Mobacken, H., and Moberg, S. (1986). Ketoconazole treatment of 13 patients with chronic mucocutaneous candidiasis. A prospective three-year trial. *Dermatologica* **173,** 229–236.
The group included two twins and one father–son pair and six patients with polyendocrinopathy. Oral treatment with ketoconazole cleared cutaneous *Candida* over several months (it took longer for the nails). Two long-term remissions were achieved.

Sams, W.M., Jr., Jorizzo, J.L., Snyderman, R., Jegasothy, B. V., Ward, F.E., Weiner, M., Wilson, J.G., Yount, W.J., and Dillard, S.B. (1979). Chronic mucocutaneous candidiasis. Immunological studies of three generations of a single family. *Am. J. Med.* **67,** 948–959.
This is a confusing family. Nine affected family members, no male-to-male transmission. Two of nine had candidiasis and normal lymphocyte transformation (LTF), one had no skin infection with abnormal LTF, and six had both candidiasis and abnormal LTF. Six of nine had enamel dysplasia. Curiously, while the text states that the spouse of the proband was normal, the table indicates that he developed hypoadrenalism at age 9. All four of their children had either clinical disease or laboratory evidence of abnormal LTF. Typographical error or pseudodominance for a recessive disorder.

JOB SYNDROME (MIM:147060, 243700)

(Quie-Hill Syndrome; Buckley Syndrome; Job Disease; Hyper-IgE Syndrome)

An atopic dermatitis-like picture with recurrent infection and elevated IgE is common to many immune defects, some of which are not well defined. This heterogeneity is reflected in the case reports of Job syndrome. Some occasionally reported associated features may be unrecognized diagnostic discriminators rather than variable expression of a single gene defect. Although McKusick lists *hyper-IgE* as dominant and *Job syndrome* as recessive, the two terms have been used interchangeably in the literature.

DERMATOLOGIC FEATURES

MAJOR. Severe eczema with variable redness, scaling, and oozing develops soon after birth. Lichenification and pruritus are common. Sites of predilection include the face and extensors. Subcutaneous staphylococcal abscesses with no evidence of inflammation (cold abscesses) are typical and usually develop after 6 months of age.

Mucocutaneous candidiasis often occurs; vulvar and oral mucosa and nails may all be involved.

Gingivitis is noted in more than 50% of cases.

MINOR. Hidradenitis suppurativa occurs in some.

ASSOCIATED ABNORMALITIES

Infections of other organs including the eye, lung, ear, sinuses, bone, and lymphatics are typical.

Elevated levels of IgE, usually in the many thousands, is the hallmark of the disorder. T-cell defects, B-cell defects, and eosinophilia are variable, and, although a chemotactic defect in circulating neutrophils is thought to be typical of the disorder, it is not present in all cases. Other atopic diseases, hay fever, asthma, and allergies are conspicuously absent.

Coarse facies with a broad nasal bridge, prominent nose, and "irregular" jaws and cheeks are described in some patients. It is not clear whether these result from recurrent cutaneous and subcutaneous bacterial and candidal infection and chronic lichenification or represent primary facial structural abnormali-

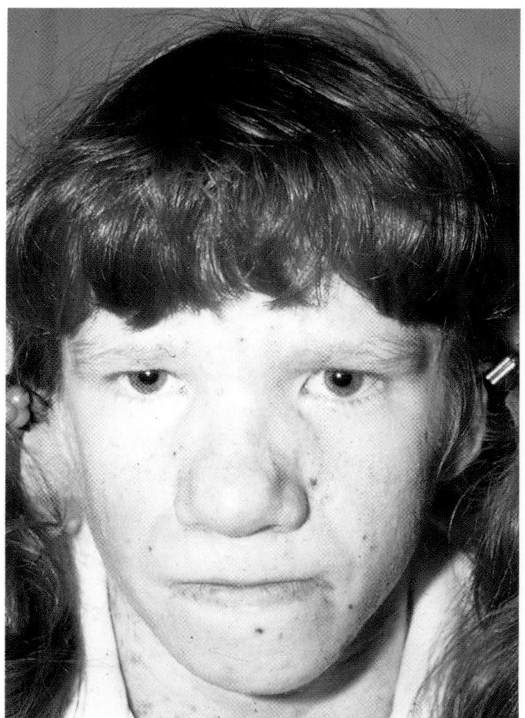

Figure 14.11. Coarse, facial features with thickening of skin. (Courtesy of Dr. H. Ochs, Seattle, Washington.)

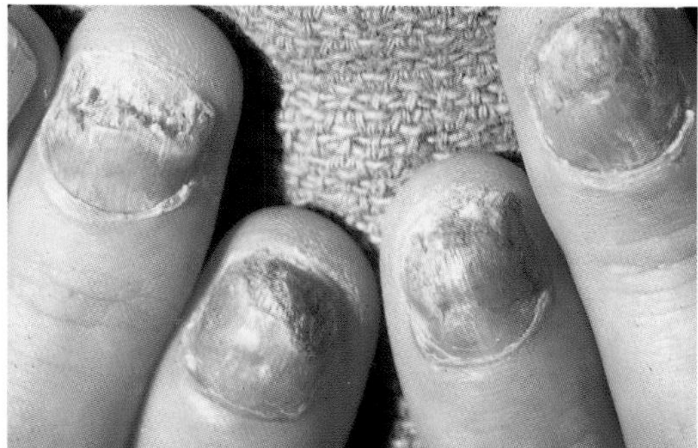

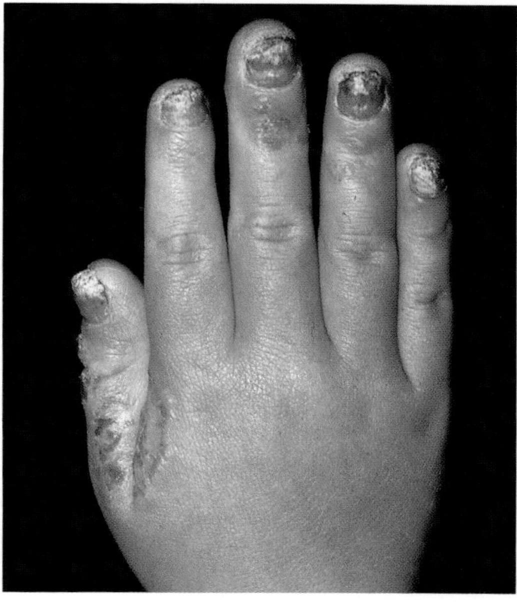

Figure 14.12. (A, B) Typical nail changes and hand dermatitis. (Courtesy of Dr. H. Ochs, Seattle, Washington.)

ties. Craniosynostosis has been described in four patients.

Growth retardation, presumably secondary to chronic illness, is typical. Reduced bone mass and fractures are reported in some patients. Chronic keratoconjunctivitis with corneal ulceration has been described.

HISTOPATHOLOGY

LIGHT. Not diagnostic.
EM. No information.

BASIC DEFECT

Unknown.

TREATMENT

Parenteral antibiotics, incision and drainage of abscesses, and topical skin care with prophylactic oral antibiotics are standard therapy. Intravenous gammaglobulin and plasmaphoresis remain experimental.

MODE OF INHERITANCE

Uncertain. Most cases are sporadic. Both vertical and horizontal transmission have been reported, with one father–son affected pair.

PRENATAL DIAGNOSIS

None.

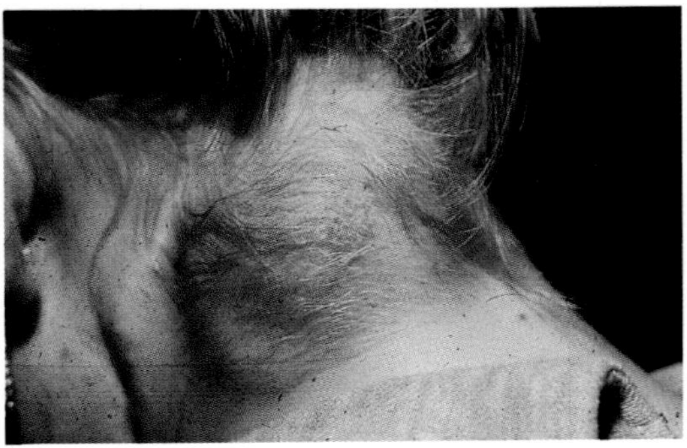

Figure 14.13. Abscess. (Courtesy of Dr. H. Ochs, Seattle, Washington.)

DIFFERENTIAL DIAGNOSIS

Severe atopic dermatitis can be associated with a host of immune defects, and an elevated IgE level is not uncommon in chronic atopics without an underlying immune defect. While impetiginization in atopic dermatitis is common, abscesses are not. Onset of skin changes in atopic dermatitis is often later than the eczema of Job syndrome, and distribution of the latter tends to be extensor rather than flexural. Nonetheless, differentiation between severe atopic dermatitis and Job syndrome may be difficult and arbitrary.

Patients with Wiskott-Aldrich syndrome (MIM:301000) may also have elevated IgE levels. Skin changes in chronic granulomatous disease (MIM:233690, 233700, 306400) can be similar.

Patients with mucocutaneous candidiasis and keratoconjunctivitis could be confused with Job syndrome, as can individuals with mucoepithelial dysplasia (MIM:158310). Electron microscopy should distinguish among them.

Support Group: N.O.R.D.
P.O. Box 8923
New Fairfield, CT 06812
1-800-999-6673

SELECTED BIBLIOGRAPHY

Donabedian, H., and Gallin, J.I. (1983). The hyperimmunoglobulin E recurrent-infection (Job's) syndrome. A review of the NIH experience. *Medicine* **62,** 195–208.

A report of 13 patients.

Hill, H.R. (1982). The syndrome of hyperimmunoglobulin E and recurrent infections. *Am. J. Dis. Child.* **136,** 767–770.

Very interesting review of the laboratory investigation into the initial delineation of Job syndrome. The technical conundrums and uncertainty involved are revealed.

Leung, D.Y.M., and Geha, R.S. (1988). Clinical and immunological aspects of the hyperimmunoglobulin E syndrome. *Hematol. Oncol. Clin. North Am.* **2,** 81–100.

Comprehensive review of over 100 patients referred to them. Only nine fit the hyper-IgE criteria. The rest had other primary immunodeficiencies or severe atopic dermatitis and superficial staphylococcal infections.

Ring, J., and Landthaler, M. (1989). Hyper IgE syndromes. *Curr. Probl. Dermatol.* **18,** 79–88.

These authors define Buckley syndrome as marked by a paucity of skin findings. However, Buckley's patients are described as having chronic skin rashes. I am therefore unsure that their classification scheme is legitimate.

MUCOEPITHELIAL DYSPLASIA (MIM:158310)

(Gap Junction Disease)

DERMATOLOGIC FEATURES

This is an extremely rare disorder with three families and one sporadic case reported.

Major. Inflammation of all mucous membranes, simulating candidiasis, begins in early to middle childhood. The mucosa are fiery red and thickened. The skin is dry and rough with

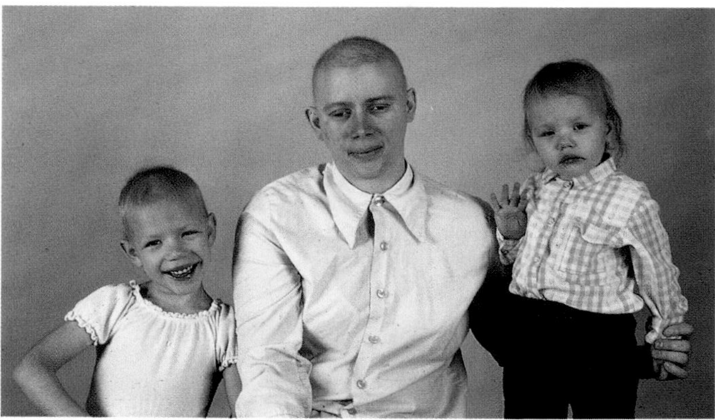

Figure 14.14. Mother and two affected daughters. (From Okamoto et al., 1977.)

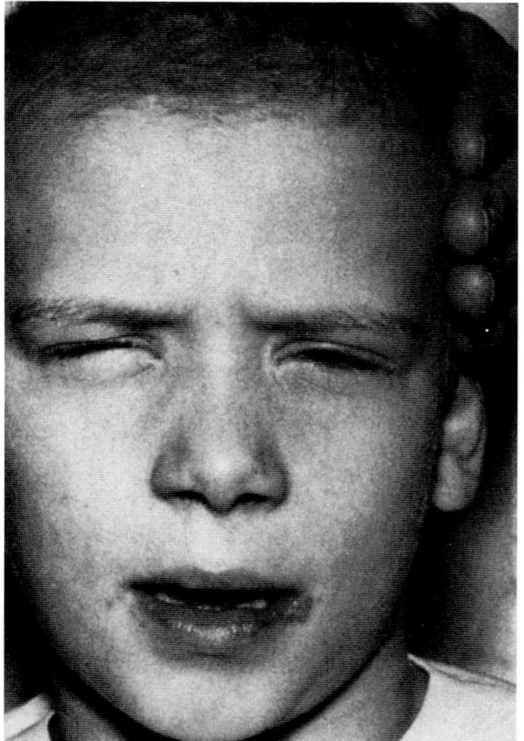

Figure 14.15. Close-up showing perleche. Patient is photophobic secondary to keratitis. (From Okamoto et al., 1977.)

keratosis pilaris. The scalp hair initially is thin and dry and scanty and may fall out permanently in childhood. Pubic and axillary hair may be absent. Alopecia can be recurrent or permanent.

Minor. Nails can be dystrophic, thickened, thinned, or clubbed in the presence of lung disease.

Vaginal Pap smears are typically abnormal.

ASSOCIATED ABNORMALITIES

Chronic keratoconjunctivitis with neovascularization of the cornea leading to blindness is preceded by photophobia and excess tearing. Cataracts have also been described.

Recurrent upper respiratory tract infections with rhinorrhea are typical. No specific underlying immune defect has been demonstrated. Perhaps the mechanical defenses of the mucosa are impaired. Recurrent pneumonias with secondary changes result in fibrocystic lung disease and recurrent pneumothoraces.

Eosinophilia is a variable finding.

HISTOPATHOLOGY

Light. In mucosa there is a decrease in number of epithelial cells with lack of normal maturation and presence of dyskeratosis. The skin shows hyperkeratotic plugs in the follicles, with moderate perifollicular inflammatory infiltrate. **EM.** Mucosal fibroblasts are filled with dilated rough endoplasmic reticulum, a decrease in desmosomes with absence of tonofilament attachments, and keratohyaline granules. "Undulating" bands of desmosome-like and gap

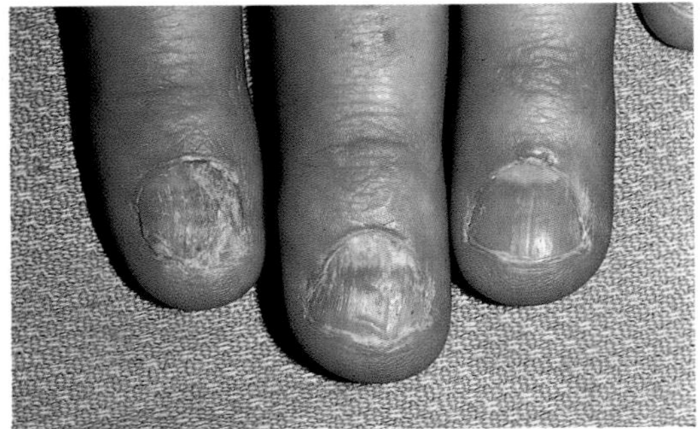

Figure 14.16. Nail changes. (From Okamoto et al., 1977.)

junction-like material are present in the cytoplasm.

BASIC DEFECT

Unknown. Although genes for gap junction proteins have been found, there is no information regarding their role in this disorder.

TREATMENT

Corneal transplants have failed.

MODE OF INHERITANCE

Autosomal dominant.

PRENATAL DIAGNOSIS

None.

DIFFERENTIAL DIAGNOSIS

Misdiagnosis of familial mucocutaneous candidiasis (MIM:114580, 212050) is possible. Cultures are generally negative in mucoepithelial dysplasia. The ultrastructural findings should confirm the diagnosis. Misdiagnosis of an ectodermal dysplasia, type unspecified or unknown, is a possibility.

Support Group: N.O.R.D.
P.O. Box 8923
New Fairfield, CT
06812
1-800-999-6673

SELECTED BIBLIOGRAPHY

Okamoto, G.A., Hall, J.G., Ochs, H., Jackson, C., Rodaway, K., and Chandler, J. (1977). New syndrome of chronic mucocutaneous candidiasis. *Birth Defects* **XIII(3B),** 117–125.

In retrospect, this family most likely had gap junction disease. I have seen this family, and, on multiple occasions, cultures for *Candida* were negative.

Urban, M.D., Schosser, R., Spohn, W., Wentling, W.O., and Robinow, M. (1991). New clinical aspects of hereditary mucoepithelial dysplasia. *Am. J. Med. Genet.* **39,** 338–341.

Autosomal dominant pedigree with more mild eye and lung involvement. Shared some electron microscopic features with gap junction disease, but not all.

Witkop, C.J., Jr., White, J.G., King, R.A., Dahl, M.V., Young, W.G., and Sauk, J.J., Jr. (1979). Hereditary mucoepithelial dysplasia: a disease apparently of desmosome and gap junction formation. *Am. J. Hum. Genet.* **31,** 414–427.

A large pedigree with extensive evaluation of electron microscopic features.

WISKOTT-ALDRICH SYNDROME (MIM:301000)

DERMATOLOGIC FEATURES

Major. Eczematous changes of lichenified, red, scaling, weeping plaques and patches on the cheeks, hands, trunk, and extremities clinically indistinguishable from atopic dermatitis develop within the first 6 months of life. Itching and secondary infection with typical staphylococcal and streptococcal impetigo is common. Petechiae and purpura also develop, secondary to thrombocytopenia.

Minor. As in any patient with atopic disease, eczema herpeticum (widespread herpes simplex) and molluscum contagiosum can occur.

Extensive warts have also been described in some patients.

ASSOCIATED ABNORMALITIES

Immune defects include elevated IgA and IgE and decreased IgM levels. There is a progressive deterioration of immune function with a decrease in the number of suppressor T cells and impaired helper T cells. Recurrent infections, especially pneumonias, otitis media, and skin abscesses due to encapsulated organisms such as meningococci, pneumococci, and *Haemophilus influenzae* account for more than 50% of the deaths. Although patients are initially more susceptible to bacterial infections, as cell-mediated immunity wanes, viral and fungal diseases increase.

Decreases in platelet size, number, and function result in bleeding. Melena, hematemesis, and epistaxis are common. Intracranial hemorrhages are responsible for another 25% of deaths.

Allergies, typically to cow's milk, eggs, and medications, are common. Autoimmune diseases, including hemolytic anemia, a JRA-like syndrome, autoimmune thrombocytopenia, glomerulonephritis or nephrotic syndrome, and interstitial nephritis, are common. Renal involvement is often progressive.

Malignancy is common. Non-Hodgkin lymphoma with brainstem and spinal cord involvement and leukemia are the typical tumors. Twenty-five percent of the deaths in Wiskott-Aldrich syndrome are attributable to these disorders.

The median age of death is between 6.5 and 8 years of age.

HISTOPATHOLOGY

Light. The features are identical to atopic dermatitis. The presence of extravasated red blood cells in the papillary and/or reticular dermis in the absence of inflammatory reaction around

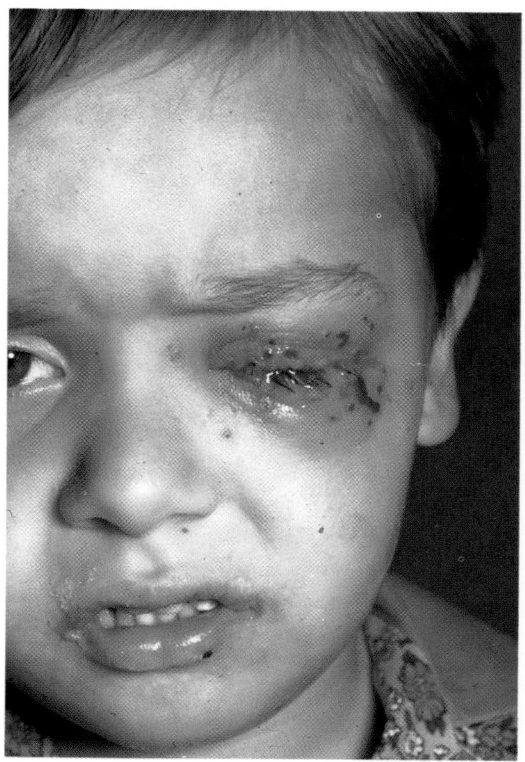

Figure 14.17. Herpetic infection. (Courtesy of Dr. H. Ochs, Seattle, Washington.)

vessels may differentiate Wiskott-Aldrich syndrome from atopic dermatitis.

EM. No information.

BASIC DEFECT

Unknown. There has been recent identification of the causative gene *WASP*.

TREATMENT

Bone marrow transplantation. Other treatment, including prophylactic antibiotics and immunoglobulin transfusions, are of limited utility. Splenectomy may be necessary to control the thrombocytopenia, but raises the risk for infection.

MODE OF INHERITANCE

X-linked recessive. The gene maps to Xp11.2. Carrier detection is possible by detection of a skewed X inactivation pattern. There is nonrandom inactivation of the X bearing the abnormal gene in all hemopoietic cells. The test is not 100% reliable.

PRENATAL DIAGNOSIS

Currently possible by linkage studies. With identification of the gene, direct DNA testing is likely to become available.

DIFFERENTIAL DIAGNOSIS

Atopic dermatitis clinically mimics the skin changes of Wiskott-Aldrich syndrome. There is lack of responsiveness to standard treatment in Wiskott-Aldrich syndrome, and the presence of other infections should raise suspicion of the diagnosis. In any infant with severe unresponsive atopic dermatitis, evaluation of platelet size and function is reasonable to rule out Wiskott-Aldrich syndrome.

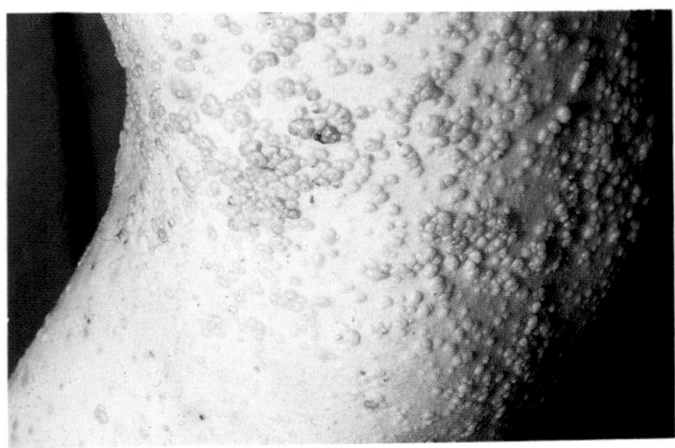

Figure 14.18. Widespread molluscum contagiosum. (Courtesy of Dr. H. Ochs, Seattle, Washington.)

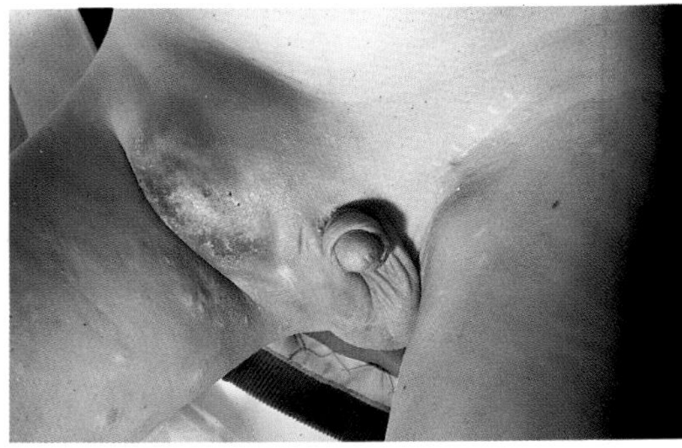

Figure 14.19. Huge inguinal abscess. Extensive scarring from previous infections. (Courtesy of Dr. H. Ochs, Seattle, Washington.)

Patients with hyper IgE or Job syndrome (MIM:243700) have similar eczematous changes and suffer from recurrent staphylococcal abscesses. Their platelets are normal and their IgE levels are extremely high.

Other immune defects (MIM:Many) can present with eczematous-like skin changes. The platelet abnormality of Wiskott-Aldrich syndrome appears to be specific to it.

The gene for X-linked thrombocytopenia appears to be allelic to the Wiskott-Aldrich gene, and some patients with the former disorder show mild manifestations (e.g., eczema, susceptibility to infection) of Wiskott-Aldrich syndrome.

Support Group: Immune Deficiency Foundation (IDF)

25 West Chesapeake
Avenue, Suite 206
Towson MD 21204-
4820
1-800-296-4433.

SELECTED BIBLIOGRAPHY

Aldrich, R.A., Steinberg, A.G., and Campbell, D.C. (1954). Pedigree demonstrating a sex-linked recessive condition characterized by draining ears, eczematoid dermatitis and bloody diarrhea. *Pediatrics* **13,** 133–139.

Beautiful pedigree analysis; 16 affected males in three generations. Discussion of the diploid 48 chromosome complement of humans does not interfere with the authors' understanding of Mendelian inheritance.

Derry, J.M., Ochs, H.D., and Francke, U. (1994). Isolation of a novel gene mutated in Wiskott-Aldrich syndrome. *Cell* **78,** 635–644.

Identified a cDNA sequence expressed in lymphoblastic and megakaryocytic cell lineages that was altered in four affected males (two unrelated and one uncle–nephew pair). They termed the gene *WASP* (Wiskott-Aldrich syndrome protein). They identified three independent mutations in exon 2.

Kolluri, R., Shehabeldin, A., Peacocke, M., Lamhonwah, A.-M., Teichert-Kuliszewska, K., Weissman, S.M., and Siminovitch, K.A. (1995). Identification of *WASP* mutations in patients with Wiskott-Aldrich syndrome and isolated thrombocytopenia reveals allelic heterogeneity at the *WAS* locus. *Hum. Mol. Genet.* **4,** 1119–1126.

Found mutations in 22 males from 19 families with either Wiskott-Aldrich syndrome or isolated thrombocytopenia. No phenotype–genotype correlations were recognized. Identical mutations resulted in both mild and severe disease.

Lorenz, P., Bollmann, R., Hinkel, G.K., Mackler, M., Siegert, G., Stamminger, G., Wendisch, J., and Ziemer, S. (1991). False-negative prenatal exclusion of Wiskott-Aldrich syndrome by measurement of fetal platelet count and size. *Prenat. Diagn.* **11,** 819–825.

Fetal blood sampling at 22 weeks showed platelet number and size both at the lower range of normal. The pregnancy resulted in an affected male. Presumably two pregnancies at risk with normal platelet parameters resulted in normal children. The authors cautioned that DNA studies are the only reliable method of prenatal diagnosis.

Perry, G.S., Spector, B.D., Schuman, L.M., Mandel, J.S., Anderson, E., McHugh, R.B., Hanson, M.R., Fahlstrom, S.M., Krivit, W., and Kersey, J.H. (1980). The Wiskott-Aldrich syndrome in the United States and Canada (1892–1979). *J. Pediatr.* **97,** 72–78.

Patients identified through a subset of a registry for immunodeficiency and malignancy. A total of 301 cases reviewed.

Sullivan, K.E., Mullen, C.A., Blaese, R.M., and Winkelstein, J.A. (1994). A multiinstitutional survey of the Wiskott-Aldrich syndrome. *J. Pediatr.* **125,** 876–885.

Results of a mailed survey to physicians. Results obtained for 154 patients. All patients had thrombocytopenia and immune defects. Thirty percent had the full triad with eczema, small platelets, and laboratory-defined immunodeficiency. The average age of diagnosis was 21 months (10 months in the presence of a positive family history, 24 months without). Eighty-one percent of patients had eczema at some point in the course of their disease. Reviews treatment.

Appendix A: Glossary

PRIMARY LESIONS

abscess: a pus-filled accumulation deep in the dermis or subcutaneous tissue

bulla: lesion larger than 1 cm, serous-fluid filled, superficial, and elevated

comedo(nes): papule(s) with central white or black plug of keratinous material within the pilosebaceous unit

cyst: a sac that contains liquid or semisolid material. Similar to a nodule but somewhat resilient to touch

macule: a flat, discolored (red, white, brown, blue) spot, nonpalpable, usually <1 cm in diameter

milia: white papules with no follicular orifice or pore

nodule: a mass >0.5 cm to <1 cm diameter that can be palpated and/or elevates the skin. Defined by level at which it is formed, e.g., dermal, subcutaneous. Usually deeper and larger than a papule

papule: a raised solid, superficial bump, usually less than 0.5–1 cm. May be single, grouped, or confluent

patch: a flat discolored area, nonpalpable, >1–2 cm in diameter

petechia: pinpoint hemorrhage into the epidermis

plaque: a raised superficial area usually 1–2 cm may be comprised of confluent papules or nodules

purpura: circumscribed deposit of blood or blood pigments in the skin, >1 cm

pustule: pus-filled, small, <1 cm, superficial elevated lesion. May be sterile or contain bacteria

tumor: a mass larger than a nodule. May be superficial or deep

vesicle: serous-fluid filled, small, <1 cm, superficial, elevated lesion

wheal: irregular in shape, raised, evanescent lesion caused by tissue edema

SECONDARY CHANGES

atrophy: loss of substance. May be superficial, deep, or both. Marked by textural and color changes

crust: dried exudate (serum, pus, blood) overlying a primary lesion

erosion: superficial loss of tissue, usually heals without scarring. An open base of a blister is an erosion

excoriation: breaks in the epidermis caused by scratches

fissure: linear breaks in the skin, with sharp, defined walls

lichenification: thickening of the epidermis with exaggeration of skin markings

scale: desquamating accumulation of thickened stratum corneum

scar: replacement of normal epidermis with connective tissue

ulcer: irregular, deep erosion, often heals with scarring

DISTRIBUTION

annular: in rings or circles

dermatomal: along lines defined by the dermatomes

flexural: antecubital, popliteal fossae, volar wrists, anterior ankles

follicular: around hair follicles—intervening skin is clear

generalized: involves most skin surfaces; mucosa may or may not be affected

intertriginous: in the folds (axillae, groins, under neck)

koebnerization (isomorphic phenomenon): distribution of lesions at sites of trauma, e.g., within excoriations

linear: along lines, often trauma induced (see koebnerization)

lines of Blaschko: pattern of lines on the skin similar, but not identical, to dermatomes, along which many congenital skin lesions are distributed, e.g., incontinentia pigmenti, organoid nevi. May reflect migration pattern of cells during embryogenesis.

photosensitive: sun-exposed areas are face and tops of ears, (with sparing of infraorbital area; subnasal tip, philtrum, and forehead areas protected by hair) nape of neck, backs of hands, arms, upper chest, back, and shins in women. Clothing-covered areas (buttocks, groins, breasts) spared

seborrheic: in scalp, along hairline, eyebrows, eyelid margins, sternum

DESCRIPTIVE

eczematous: early on, red, weeping, raised, pruritic, vesicular, crusted lesions. Later stages marked by lichenification, scaling, erythema, and hyperpigmentation

guttate: droplet, "raindrop," "teardrop" distribution

nevus: a relatively stable malformation or hamartoma of the skin. May be present at birth. Presumably directed by genetic factors, sometimes with additive environmental effect (e.g., sun exposure and acquired nevocytic nevi)

papulosquamous: raised scaling lesions (e.g., psoriasis, seborrhea, lichen planus)

vascular: results from proliferation, dilation, or malformation of any blood vessel and further differentiated by type of vessel (capillary, arteriovenous malformation, venous, arterial). Distinct from hemorrhage, petechiae, or purpura, in which leakage of blood into skin is cause and which will not blanch with pressure (diascopy)

verrucous: wart-like, irregular surface

Appendix B: Differential Diagnosis by Skin Sign

The skin signs are set out in the following categories:

A. Primary signs

1. Macules
2. Patches
3. Papules
4. Nodules
5. Plaques
6. Cysts
7. Tumors
8. Vesicles/bullae
9. Absence
10. Scars
11. Erosions
12. Abscesses
13. Ulcers
14. Wheals

B. Vascular lesions

1. Angiokeratoma
2. Erythema
3. Port wine stain
4. Telangiectases
5. Vascular mottling/cutis marmorata
6. Venous/mixed/cavernous

C. Specific lesions

1. Acanthosis nigricans
2. Acrochordons
3. Ankyloblepharon filiforme adnatum
4. Calcinosis cutis/osteoma cutis
5. Comedones
6. Connective tissue nevi
7. Cutis verticis gyrata
8. Dermatofibroma
9. Elastosis perforans serpiginosa
10. Follicular atrophoderma
11. Freckles/lentigines
12. Granulomas
13. Juvenile xanthogranuloma
14. Keratoacanthoma
15. Knuckle pads
16. Lipomas
17. Milia
18. Neurofibromas
19. Nevocytic nevi
20. Organoid nevi
21. Pilomatricomas
22. Porokeratoses
23. Steatocystoma multiplex
24. Syringoma
25. Trichoepithelioma
26. Trichlemmoma
27. Warts
28. Xanthoma/xanthelasma

D. Disease processes

1. Acne
2. Atrophy/thinning
3. Collodion membrane
4. Constriction bands
5. Discoid/systemic lupus erythematosus
6. Eczema/seborrheic dermatitis
7. Edema/lymphedema
8. Erythroderma
9. Fragility
10. Hypertrophy/thickening
11. Keratosis pilaris
12. Lax/hyperelastic skin
13. Lipodystrophy
14. Malignancy-cutaneous
15. Malignancy-noncutaneous
16. Photosensitivity
17. Poikiloderma
18. Premature aging
19. Pruritis
20. Scleroderma
21. Tight skin
22. Urticaria

E. Regional involvement

1. Abnormal dermatoglyphics
2. Localized absence

3. Mucosal involvement
4. Palmo/plantar
5. Scalp

F. Pigment abnormalities

1. Albinism
2. Patchy depigmentation/hypopigmentation
3. Hyperpigmentation
4. Jaundice

G. Ichthyosis/Scaling

1. Generalized
2. Xerosis
3. Patterned/localized/migratory

H. Hair

1. Absence/alopecia
2. Thin/sparse
3. Coarse
4. Hair shaft abnormality
5. Curly
6. Male pattern baldness
7. Hirsutism/hypertrichosis
8. Decrease/absence hair color
9. Eyelashes/eyebrows

I. Nails

1. Absence/hypoplasia/loss
2. Hypertrophic
3. Thin/koilonychia
4. Leukonychia
5. Clubbing
6. Paronychia
7. Other

J. Sweat Glands

1. Hypohidrosis
2. Hyperhidrosis

PRIMARY SIGNS

MACULES

Brown

Bannayan-Riley-Ruvalcaba syndrome (penile lentigines), 525
Centrofacial lentiginosis (lentigines), 279
Familial cutaneous amyloidosis, 555–58
Familial multiple café-au-lait spots, 292–98
Fanconi syndrome, 267–70
LEOPARD syndrome (lentigines), 277–80
McCune-Albright syndrome (café-au-lait), 283–87
Multiple endocrine neoplasia 2A/2B (café-au-lait, freckles), 516–19
NAME/Carney/LAMB complex (lentigines, ephelides), 289–92
Neurofibromatosis (café-au-lait, axillary freckling), 292–98
Peutz-Jeghers syndrome (lentigines), 300–3
Proteus syndrome (café-au-lait), 523–25
Schimke immuno-osseous dysplasia (small café-au-lait), 296
Universal melanosis (palms, soles), 303–5
Urticaria pigmentosa (mast cell inclusions), 471–75
Watson syndrome (café-au-lait), 296
Xeroderma pigmentosa (solar lentigines), 587–91

White

Epidermolysis bullosa junctional inversa (albostriate spots), 144–47
Hereditary palmoplantar keratoderma punctate (guttate hypopigmentation), 63–66
Tuberous sclerosis (ash leaf spots, guttate hypopigmentation), 409–14

PATCHES

Blue/Black

Alkaptonuria, 550–53
Nevus phakomatosis pigmentovascularis (Mongolian spots), 298–300

Brown

Bloom syndrome (patchy hyperpigmentation, café-au-lait), 574–77
Epidermodysplasia verruciformis (tinea versicolor-like), 598–601
Familial cutaneous amyloidosis, 555–58
Hypomelanosis of Ito (along the lines of Blaschko), 318–22
Incontinentia pigmenti (swirly, along lines of Blaschko), 273–77
LEOPARD syndrome ("café-noir"), 277–80

Red

White

PAPULES

Flesh Colored /White

Hyperkeratotic

Yellow

Papules, Other

NAME/Carney/LAMB complex (blue nevi), 289–92

NODULES

Flesh Colored/White

Buschke-Ollendorf syndrome (connective tissue nevi), 340–41
Congenital generalized fibromatosis, 514–16
Cowden syndrome, 494–97
Cylindromatosis, 497–501
François syndrome (white, waxy), 424–26
Gardner syndrome (fibromas), 508–10
Infantile myofibromatosis, 514–16
Multiple leiomyomatosis, 519–20
Multiple pilomatricoma, 521–22
Multiple syringomas, 229–31
Myotonic dystrophy (pilomatricoma), 521–22
Pachyonychia congenita (steatocystoma multiplex), 222–26
Steatocystoma multiplex, 238–40
Systemic hyalinosis (perianal, subcutaneous), 433–37

Hyperkeratotic

Hereditary keratoacanthomas, 511–13
Kyrle/Flegel disease (hyperkeratoses), 99–101

Red/Blue

Blue rubber bleb nevus syndrome, 369–72
Hereditary glomus tumors, 380–83
Maffucci syndrome, 392–95

Yellow

Alagille syndrome (eruptive xanthomas), 457, 557
Bannayan-Riley-Ruvalcaba syndrome (lipomas), 525
Cerebrotendinous xanthomatosis (xanthomas), 438–40
Encephalocraniocutaneous lipomatosis (lipomas), 528
Familial multiple lipomatosis (lipomas), 441–43
Proteus syndrome (lipomas), 523–25

Other

Albright hereditary osteodystrophy (osteoma cutis), 415–17
Ehlers-Danlos types I and II (spheroids), 343–45
Fibrodysplasia ossificans progressiva (osteoma cutis), 445–48
Hereditary angiolipomatosis, 441–43
Lipogranulomatosis (histocytic), 448–50
McCune-Albright syndrome (myxomas), 283–87
NAME/Carney/LAMB complex (neurofibromas, myxoid tumors), 289–92
Neurofibromatosis (neurofibromas), 292–98
Urticaria pigmentosa (mast cell inclusions), 471–75

PLAQUES

Flesh Colored/White

Buschke-Ollendorff syndrome (connective tissue nevi), 340–41
Hunter syndrome (flesh, yellow), 545–47
Tuberous sclerosis (shagreen patches, connective tissue nevi), 409–14
Hereditary palmoplantar keratosis Vohwinkel (starfish hyperkeratoses), 71–73

Hyperkeratotic

Darier-White disease (verrucous), 88–92
Epidermal nevus (verrucous, hyperkeratotic), 504–8
Erythrokeratodermia variabilis (hyperkeratotic), 40–43
Incontinentia pigmenti (verrucous, stage II), 273–77
Werner syndrome (calcinosis cutis), 571–73

Brown

Acanthosis nigricans (brown, velvety), 85–87
Bathing trunk nevus, 490–94

Yellow

Cerebrotendinous xanthomatosis, 438–40
Lipoid proteinosis, 426–29
Pseudoxanthoma elasticum, 362–65
Sebaceous nevus, 526–28

Other

Epidermodysplasia verruciformis (reddish-brown to white), 598–601
Hartnup disorder (scaly, red), 577–78

CYSTS

TUMORS

VESICLES/BULLAE

ABSENCE

SCARS

EROSIONS

ABSCESSES

ULCERS

WHEALS

VASCULAR LESIONS

ANGIOKERATOMA

ERYTHEMA

PORT WINE STAIN

Sturge-Weber syndrome, 396–99
Wyburn-Mason syndrome, 398

TELANGIECTASES

Angioma serpiginosum, 379, 387
Ataxia telangiectasia, 366–69
Bloom syndrome, 574–77
Cockayne syndrome, 559–62
COPS syndrome, 587
Cutis marmorata telangiectatica congenita, 372–77
Dowling-Degos disease, 262–64
Focal dermal hypoplasia, 405–9
Hallermann-Streiff syndrome, 564–66
Hereditary benign essential telangiectasia, 386
Hereditary hemorrhagic telangiectasia, 383–88
Kindler syndrome, 579–81
Rothmund-Thomson syndrome, 585–87
Telangiectatica macularis eruptiva perstans, 471–75
Unilateral nevoid telangiectasia, 386
Werner syndrome, 571–73

VASCULAR MOTTLING/CUTIS MARMORATA

Aplasia cutis congenita, 399–404
Cutis marmorata telangiectatica congenita, 372–77
Diffuse cortical meningeal angiomatosis of Divry and Van Bogaert, 398
Familial dysautonomia, 421–24
Menkes disease, 195–98

VENOUS/MIXED/CAVERNOUS

Bannayan-Riley-Ruvalcaba syndrome, 525
Blue rubber bleb nevus syndrome, 369–72
Cutis marmorata telangiectatica congenita, 372–77
Diffuse hemangiomatosis, 391
Familial cavernous angiomas, 398
Hereditary glomus tumors, 380–83
Klippel-Trenaunay-Weber syndrome, 388–92
Maffucci syndrome, 392–95
Proteus syndrome (angiolipomas, lymphangiomas, angiomas), 523–25

SPECIFIC LESIONS

ACANTHOSIS NIGRICANS

Acanthosis nigricans, 85–87
Beare-Stevenson syndrome, 419–20
Bloom syndrome (rare), 574–77
Costello syndrome, 352–55
Crouzon syndrome, 85–87
Familial insulin resistance, 85–87
Ichthyosis with hypogonadism, 114–15
Leprechaunism, 176–77
Partial lipodystrophy, 450–52
Polycystic ovarian disease, 180–82
Prader-Willi syndrome, 86
Rabson-Mendenhall syndrome, 177
Seip-Berardinelli syndrome, 453–55

ACROCHORDONS

Birt-Hogg-Dubé syndrome, 509
Costello syndrome, 352–55
Cowden syndrome, 494–97

ANKYLOBLEPHARON FILIFORME ADNATUM

AEC syndrome, 241–44
CHANDS, 193–95
Lethal popliteal pterygium syndrome, 430–33
Popliteal pterygium syndrome (facio-genito-popliteal syndrome), 430–33

CALCINOSIS CUTIS/OSTEOMA CUTIS

Albright hereditary osteodystrophy, 415–17
COPS syndrome, 587
Fibrodysplasia ossificans progressiva, 445–48
Hereditary sclerosing poikiloderma, 580
Multiple pilomatricoma, 521–22
Porphyria cutanea tarda, 540–43
Proteus syndrome, 523–25
Pseudoxanthoma elasticum (rare), 362–65

Rothmund-Thomson syndrome (rare), 585–87
Tumoral calcinosis, 529–30
Werner syndrome, 571–73

COMEDONES

Atrophoderma vermiculatum, 102–4
Dowling-Degos disease, 262–64
Familial dyskeratotic comedones, 233–35
Hereditary keratoacanthomas, 511–13

CONNECTIVE TISSUE NEVI

Buschke-Ollendorff syndrome, 340–41
Proteus syndrome, 523–25
Tuberous sclerosis, 409–14

CUTIS VERTICIS GYRATA

Beare-Stevenson syndrome, 419–20
Cutis verticis gyrata, 417–21
Pachydermoperiostosis, 420

DERMATOFIBROMA

Cowden syndrome, 494–97

ELASTOSIS PERFORANS SERPIGNOSA

Down syndrome, 346
Ehlers-Danlos type IV, 345–47
Elastosis perforans serpiginosa, 362–65
Marfan syndrome, 365
Pseudoxanthoma elasticum, 362–65

FOLLICULAR ATROPHODERMA

Bazex syndrome, 487–88
Chondrodysplasia punctata, 108–13
Focal dermal hypoplasia, 405–9
Ulerythema ophryogenes, 102–4

FRECKLES/LENTIGINES

Bannayan-Riley Ruvalcaba syndrome (penile lentigines), 525
Centrofacial lentiginosis, 279
LEOPARD syndrome, 277–80
Multiple endocrine neoplasia 2B, 516–19
NAME/Carney/LAMB complex, 289–92
Neurofibromatosis (axillary, inguinal), 292–98
Nevus phakomatosis pigmentovascularis, 298–300
Partial unilateral lentiginosis, 279–80
Peutz-Jeghers syndrome, 300–3
Schimke immunoosseous dysplasia, 296
Xeroderma pigmentosum (solar lentigines), 587–91

GRANULOMAS

Blau syndrome, 426
Chronic granulomatous disease, 594–97

JUVENILE XANTHOGRANULOMA

Neurofibromatosis, 292–98

KERATOACANTHOMA

Dowling-Degos disease, 262–64
Hereditary keratoacanthomas, 511–13
Muir-Torre syndrome, 513

KNUCKLE PADS

Acrokeratoelastoidosis, 49–50
Dupuytren contracture, 97–99
Ehlers-Danlos type I, 343–45
Hereditary palmoplantar keratoderma with leukonychia, 98
Knuckle pads, 97–99

LIPOMAS

Bannayan-Riley-Ruvalcaba syndrome, 525
Carbohydrate-deficient glycoprotein syndrome, 569
Familial multiple lipomatosis, 441–43
Familial symmetric lipomatosis, 443–45
Proteus syndrome, 523–25

MILIA

Absence of dermatoglyphics, 83–85
Basal cell nevus syndrome, 484–90
Cylindromatosis, 497–501

NEUROFIBROMAS

NEVOCYTIC NEVI

ORGANOID NEVI

PILOMATRICOMAS

POROKERATOSES

STEATOCYSTOMA MULTIPLEX

SYRINGOMA

TRICHOEPITHELIOMA

TRICHOLEMMOMA

WARTS

XANTHOMA/XANTHELASMA

DISEASE PROCESSES

ACNE

ATROPHY/THINNING (see also poikiloderma)

COLLODION MEMBRANE

CONSTRICTION BANDS

DISCOID LUPUS/SYSTEMIC LUPUS ERYTHEMATOSUS

ECZEMA/SEBORRHEIC DERMATITIS

EDEMA/LYMPHEDEMA

ERYTHRODERMA

Nonbullous congenital ichthyosiform erythroderma, 27–30
Pityriasis rubra pilaris, 43–46

FRAGILITY

Dermatosparaxis, 341–43
Ehlers-Danlos types I and II, 343–45
Ehlers-Danlos type IV, 345–47
Epidermolysis bullosa syndromes, all forms, 129–160
Porphyrias, all forms, 531–45

HYPERTROPHY/THICKENING

Beare-Stevenson syndrome, 419–20
Cutis verticus gyrata (forehead, scalp), 417–21
GAPO syndrome (face), 251–53
Melkersson-Rosenthal syndrome (lips), 468–70
Michelin tire baby, 478–81
Multiple endocrine neoplasia 2B (lips), 516–19
Pachydermoperiostosis, 420
Systemic hyalinosis, 433–37
Urticaria pigmentosa, 471–75

KERATOSIS PILARIS

Atrophoderma vermiculatum, 102–4
Buschke-Ollendorff syndrome, 340–41
Cardio-facio-cutaneous syndrome, 104
Erythromelanosis follicularis faciei et colli, 102–4
Hereditary palmoplantar keratoderma Howel-Evans, 58–60
Ichthyosis vulgaris, 21–23
Mucoepithelial dysplasia, 606–8
Noonan syndrome, 102–4
Onychotrichodysplasia with neutropenia, 220–21
Ulerythema ophryogenes, 102–4

LAX/HYPERELASTIC SKIN

Barber-Say syndrome, 175
Beare-Stevenson syndrome, 419–20
Costello syndrome, 352–55
Cutis laxa, 255–61
de Barsy syndrome, 562–64
Dermatosparaxis, 341–43
Ehlers-Danlos types I, II, and III, 343–45
Ehlers-Danlos type type VIII, 349–50
Leprechaunism (loose, excessive wrinkling), 176–77
Neonatal Marfan syndrome, 360
Pseudoxanthoma elasticum (late), 362–65
SCARF, 355–61
Tricho-rhino-phalangeal syndrome type II, 201–4
Wrinkly skin, 355–61

LIPODYSTROPHY

Carbohydrate-deficient glycoprotein syndrome, 569
Hereditary angioneurotic edema (rare), 465–68
Hutchinson-Gilford progeria, 567–70
Leprechaunism, 176–77
Partial lipodystrophy, 450–52
Proteus syndrome, 523–25
Seip-Berardinelli syndrome, 453–55
SHORT syndrome, 454
Stiff skin, 481–83
Trichothiodystrophy (IBIDS), 205–8
Wiedemann-Rautenstrauch syndrome, 569

MALIGNANCY, CUTANEOUS

Acrokeratosis verruciformis, 50–53
Basal cell nevus syndrome, 484–90
Bazex syndrome, 487–88
Bathing trunk nevus, 490–94
Cowden syndrome, 494–97
Cylindromatosis, 497–501
Darier-White disease (rare), 88–92
Dyskeratosis congenita, 264–67
Dysplastic nevus syndrome, 501–4
Epidermal nevus syndrome (rare), 504–8
Epidermodysplasia verruciformis, 598–61
Epidermolysis bullosa dystrophica dominant, 148–51
Epidermolysis bullosa dystrophica recessive Hallopeau Siemens, 151–56
François syndrome, 424–26
Hereditary keratoacanthomas, 511–13

KID syndrome, 115–18
Kyrle/Flegel disease, 99–101
Muir-Torre syndrome, 513
Rombo syndrome, 487–89
Rothmund-Thomson syndrome, 585–87
Scleroatrophic and keratotic dermatosis of the limbs, 78–80
Sebaceous nevus, 526–28
Xeroderma pigmentosum, 587–91

MALIGNANCY, NONCUTANEOUS

Ataxia telangiectasia, 366–69
Basal cell nevus syndrome, 484–90
Bloom syndrome, 574–77
Cowden syndrome, 494–97
Dyskeratosis congenita, 264–67
Fanconi syndrome, 267–70
Gardner syndrome, 508–10
Hereditary palmoplantar hyperkeratosis Howel-Evans, 58–60
Maffucci syndrome, 392–95
McCune-Albright syndrome, 283–87
Multiple endocrine neoplasia 2A/2B, 516–19
Multiple leiomyomatosis, 519–20
Neurofibromatosis, 292–98
Peutz-Jeghers syndrome, 300–3
Rothmund-Thomson syndrome, 585–87
Wiskott-Aldrich syndrome, 609–11

PHOTOSENSITIVITY

Bloom syndrome, 574–77
Cockayne syndrome, 559–62
Congenital erythropoietic porphyria, 532–35
Erythropoietic protoporphyria, 535–38
Hartnup disorder, 577–78
Hepatic erythropoietic porphyria, 540–43
Hereditary coproporphyria, 538–40
Kindler syndrome, 579–81
Polymorphous light eruption, 581–84
Porphyria cutanea tarda, 540–43
Rothmund-Thomson syndrome, 585–87
Trichothiodystrophy (PIBIDS), 205–8
Variegate porphyria, 543–45
Xeroderma pigmentosum, 587–91

POIKILODERMA

Ataxia telangiectasia, 366–69
Bloom syndrome, 574–77
COPS syndrome, 587
Dyskeratosis congenita, 264–67
Hereditary sclerosing poikiloderma, 580
Kindler syndrome, 579–81
Mendes da Costa syndrome, 579–81
Rothmund-Thomson syndrome, 585–87
Xeroderma pigmentosum, 587–91

PREMATURE AGING

Cockayne syndrome, 559–62
de Barsy syndrome, 562–64
Dyskeratosis congenita, 264–67
Ehlers-Danlos type IV, 345–47
Flynn-Aird syndrome, 571–73
Hallermann-Streiff syndrome, 564–66
Hutchinson-Gilford progeria, 567–70
Mandibuloacral dysplasia (mild), 569
Rothmund-Thomson syndrome, 585–87
Trichothiodystrophy (IBIDS), 205–8
Weidemann-Rautenstrauch syndrome, 567–70
Werner syndrome, 571–73

PRURITUS

Cholestasis and lymphedema, 456–57
Continuous peeling skin, 10–12
Darier-White disease, 88–92
Epidermolysis bullosa dystrophica pretibial, 156–58
Epidermolysis bullosa simplex Dowling-Meara, 131–34
Erythrokeratodermia variabilis, 40–43
Erythropoietic protoporphyria, 535–38
Familial cutaneous amyloidosis, 555–58
Hailey-Hailey disease, 160–62
Multiple endocrine neoplasia 2B (with amyloidosis), 516–19
Netherton syndrome, 31–34
Polymorphous light eruption, 581–84
Pruritic urticarial papules and plaques of pregnancy, 464
Pseudoxanthoma elasticum (occasional), 362–65
Sjögren-Larsson syndrome, 126–28
Urticaria pigmentosa, 471–75

SCLERODERMA

Erythropoietic protoporphyria (pseudosclerodermatous), 535–38

Hutchinson-Gilford progeria (early), 567–70
Porphyria cutanea tarda, 540–43
Variegate porphyria (pseudoscleromatous), 543–45
Werner syndrome, 571–73

TIGHT SKIN

Collodion membrane, 23–26
Lamellar exfoliation of the newborn, 23–26
Mucolipidosis II, 481–83
Neu-Laxova syndrome, 118–20
Restrictive dermopathy, 34–37
Stiff skin, 481–83

URTICARIA

Aquagenic urticaria, 463
Dermo-destructive urticaria, 463
Familial cold urticaria, 464–65
Familial localized heat urticaria, 463–64
Hereditary angioneurotic edema, 465–68
Muckle-Wells syndrome, 470–71
Netherton syndrome, 31–34
Pruritic urticarial papules and plaques of pregnancy, 464
Vibratory angioedema, 463

REGIONAL INVOLVEMENT

ABNORMAL DERMATOGLYPHICS

Absence of dermatoglyphics, 83–85
Anonychia with flexural pigmentation, 218
Epidermolysis bullosa junctional progressiva, 144–47
Hypohidrotic ectodermal dysplasia, 254–57
KID syndrome, 115–18
Naegeli syndrome, 287–89
Scleroatrophic and keratotic dermatosis of the limbs, 78–80

LOCALIZED ABSENCE

4 p−, 399–404
Amniotic bands, 337–40
Aplasia cutis congenita, 399–404
Epidermolysis bullosa dystrophica, all forms, 148–58
Epidermolysis bullosa junctional, all forms, 140–47
Focal dermal hypoplasia, 405–9
Johansson-Blizzard syndrome, 401
Microphthalmia with linear skin defects, 405–9
Scalp-ear-nipple syndrome, 399–401
Trisomy 13, 399–404

MUCOSAL INVOLVEMENT

Acrodermatitis enteropathica (erosions), 547–50
Byars-Jurkiewicz syndrome (fibromatosis), 494–97
Chronic granulomatous disease (gingivitis), 594–97
Clouston syndrome (leukoplakia), 244–47
Cowden syndrome (oral papillomas), 494–97
Cross syndrome (gingival fibromatosis), 316–18
Darier-White disease (white papules), 88–92
Dyskeratosis congenita (leukoplakia), 264–67
Ehlers-Danlos type VIII (periodontitis), 349–50
Fabry syndrome (angiokeratoma), 377–80
Familial mucocutaneous candidiasis, 601–4
François syndrome (gingival hypertrophy), 424–26
Gingival fibromatosis and hypertrichosis, 169–71
Hartnup disorder (gingivitis, stomatitis), 577–78
Hemochromatosis (hyperpigmentation), 271–73
Hereditary hemorrhagic telangiectasia (telangiectasia, epistaxis), 383–88
Hereditary palmoplantar keratoderma Howel-Evans (leukoplakia), 58–60
Hereditary palmoplantar keratoderma Olmsted (leukoplakia), 60–63
Hystrix-like ichthyosis with deafness (leukoplakia), 20
Job syndrome (candidiasis), 604–6
KID (leukokeratosis and scrotal tongue), 115–18
Kindler syndrome (gingivitis, leukokeratosis), 579–81

Laband syndrome (gingival hypertrophy), 468–70
Melkersson-Rosenthal syndrome (lingua plicata), 468–70
Mucoepithelial dysplasia (mucositis), 606–8
Multiple endocrine neoplasia 2B (neuromas), 516–19
Pachyonychia congenita (leukoplakia), 222–26
Papillon-Lefèvre (periodontitis), 75–78
Porokeratosis palmaris plantaris et disseminata (porokeratosis), 81–83
Pseudoxanthoma elasticum (cobblestoning), 362–65
Rutherfurd syndrome (gingival hypertrophy), 171
Systemic hyalinosis (gingival hypertrophy), 433–37
Tumoral calcinosis (gingivitis, pèrleche), 529–30
Winchester syndrome (gingival hypertrophy), 433–37

PALMO/PLANTAR

Erythema

Cockayne syndrome, 559–62
Erythromelalgia, 476–78
Hemochromatosis, 271–73

Hyperkeratosis

Acrokeratoelastoidosis, 49–50
Acrokeratosis verruciformis (punctate), 50–53
Bullous congenital ichthyosiform erythroderma, 5–10
Clouston syndrome, 244–47
Cowden syndrome (papules), 494–97
Darier-White disease, 88–92
Dyskeratosis congenita, 264–67
Epidermolysis bullosa junctional generalized atrophic benign, 143–47
Epidermolysis bullosa simplex, 131–40
Erythokeratodermia variabilis (occasional), 40–43
Familial cutaneous amyloidosis (X-linked), 555–58
Hereditary painful callosities (calluses), 92–94
Hereditary palmoplantar keratoderma with deafness, 54–55
Hereditary palmoplantar keratoderma with leukonychia, deafness, 97–99
Hereditary palmoplantar keratoderma epidermolytic hyperkeratosis, 56–58
Hereditary palmoplantar keratoderma Greither, 68–70
Hereditary palmoplantar keratoderma Howel-Evans, 58–60
Hereditary palmoplantar keratoderma Olmsted, 60–63
Hereditary palmoplantar keratoderma punctate, 63–66
Hereditary palmoplantar keratoderma striata, 66–67
Hereditary palmoplantar keratoderma Unna-Thost, 68–70
Hereditary palmoplantar keratoderma Vohwinkel, 71–73
Hereditary papulotranslucent acrokeratoderma, 49–50
Hereditary sclerosing poikiloderma, 580
Kindler syndrome, 579–81
Knuckle pads, 97–99
Mal de Meleda, 73–75
Naegeli syndrome, 287–89
Pachyonychia congenita, 222–26
Papillon-Lefèvre, 75–78
Pityriasis rubra pilaris, 43–46
Progressive systemic erythrokeratoderma, 46–49
Richner-Hanhart syndrome, 124–26
Scleroatrophic and keratotic dermatosis of the limbs, 78–80

Pits

Basal cell nevus syndrome, 484–90
Darier-White disease, 88–92
Mutliple syringomas, 229–31

Other

Anonychia with flexural pigmentation (peeling), 218
Epidermolysis bullosa dystrophica Hallopeau-Siemens (fusion), 151–56
Epidermolysis bullosa junctional progressiva (thinning, fusion), 144–47

SCALP

PIGMENT ABNORMALITIES

ALBINISM

PATCHY DEPIGMENTATION/ HYPOPIGMENTATION

HYPERPIGMENTATION

Generalized

Localized/Patterned/Patchy

JAUNDICE

ICHTHYOSIS/SCALING

GENERALIZED

XEROSIS

PATTERNED/LOCALIZED/MIGRATORY (see also palmo/plantar hyperkeratosis)

HAIR

ABSENCE/ALOPECIA

Congenital Nonscarring

Congenital Scarring

Acquired Nonscarring

Lipoid proteinosis, 426–29
Male pattern baldness, 165–67
Marie Unna syndrome, 167–68
Mucoepithelial dysplasia, 606–8
Rapp-Hodgkin syndrome, 257–60

Acquired Scarring

Clouston syndrome, 244–47
Congenital erythropoietic porphyria, 532–35
Epidermolysis bullosa junctional generalized atrophic benign, 143–47
Incontinentia pigmenti, 273–77
Porphyria cutanea tarda, 540–43

THIN/SPARSE

Acrodermatitis enteropathica, 547–50
Bazex syndrome, 487–88
Biotinidase deficiency, 553–55
Cartilage-hair hypoplasia, 220–21
Clouston syndrome, 244–47
Cockayne syndrome, 559–62
Coffin-Siris syndrome, 246
Costello syndrome, 352–55
de Barsy syndrome (occasional), 562–64
Dyskeratosis congenita, 264–67
EEC syndrome, 247–49
Fibrodysplasia ossificans progressiva (progressive loss), 445–48
Hallermann-Streiff syndrome, 564–66
Hartnup disorder, 577–78
Hemochromatosis (progressive loss), 271–73
Hutchinson-Gilford progeria, 567–70
Hypohidrotic ectodermal dysplasia, 254–57
Hypotrichosis with light colored hair and facial milia, 168
Kallin syndrome, 134–40
Loose anagen hair, 163–65
Menkes disease, 195–98
Onychotrichodysplasia and neutropenia (thin or congenital alopecia), 220–21
Oral-facial-digital syndrome type I, 235–38
Pachyonychia congenita, 222–26
Rapp-Hodgkin syndrome, 257–60
Rothmund-Thomson syndrome, 585–87
Trichodental syndrome, 198–201
Tricho-rhino-phalangeal type I, 201–4
Tricho-rhino-phalangeal type II, 201–4
Trichothiodystrophy, 205–8
Werner syndrome, 571–73

COARSE

AEC syndrome, 241–44
Anonychia with flexural pigmentation, 218
Clouston syndrome, 244–47
Rapp-Hodgkin syndrome, 257–60
Trichodentosseus syndrome, 198–201
Woolly hair, 193–95

HAIR SHAFT ABNORMALITY

Bjornstad syndrome (pili torti), 186–88
Marie Unna syndrome (various), 167–69
Menkes disease (pili torti), 195–98
Monilethrix, 182–84
Netherton syndrome (trichorrhexis invaginata), 31–34
Pachyonychia congenita (pili torti), 222–26
Pili annulati, 185–86
Pili torti, 186–88
Pili trianguli et canaliculi, 188–90
Pseudomonilethrix, 182–84
Rapp-Hodgkin syndrome (various), 257–60
Trichorrhexis invaginata, 190–91
Trichorrhexis nodosa, 191–93
Trichothiodystrophy, 205–8

CURLY

Cardio-facio-cutaneous syndrome, 104
CHANDS, 193–95
Costello syndrome, 352–55
Hereditary palmoplantar keratoderma striata, 66–67
Noonan syndrome, 193–95
Seip-Berardinelli syndrome, 453–55
Trichodentosseus syndrome, 198–201
Woolly hair, 193–95

MALE PATTERN BALDNESS

Male pattern baldness, 165–67
Polycystic ovarian disease, 180–82
Tricho-rhino-phalangeal type I, 201–4
Tricho-rhino-phalangeal type II, 201–4

HIRSUTISM/HYPERTRICHOSIS

Ambras syndrome, 172–75
Barber-Say syndrome, 172–75
Byars-Jurkieviez syndrome, 494–97

DECREASE/ABSENCE HAIR COLOR

EYELASHES/EYEBROWS

NAILS

ABSENCE/HYPOPLASIA/LOSS

Congenital

ACQUIRED

Dyskeratosis congenita, 264–67
Epidermolysis bullosa dystrophica, all forms, 148–58
Epidermolysis bullosa junctional, all forms, 140–47
Familial dystrophic shedding of the nails, 211–12
Porphyria cutanea tarda, 540–43
Scleroatrophic and keratotic dermatosis of the limbs, 78–80
Transient bullous dermatolysis of the newborn, 158–60
Twenty nail dystrophy, 214–16

HYPERTROPHIC

AEC syndrome, 241–44
CHILD syndrome, 105–8
Clouston syndrome, 244–47
Congenital erythropoietic porphyria (occasional), 532–35
EEC syndrome, 247–49
Epidermolysis bullosa dystrophica dominant, all forms, 148–58
Epidermolysis bullosa junctional, all forms, 140–47
Epidermolysis bullosa simplex, all forms, 131–40
Familial mucocutaneous candidiasis, 601–4
GAPO syndrome, 251–53
LOGIC syndrome, 144, 148
Mucoepithelial dysplasia, 606–8
Pachyonychia congenita, 222–26
Pityriasis rubra pilaris, 43–46
Rabson-Mendenhall syndrome, 177
Rapp-Hodgkin syndrome, 257–60

THIN/KOILONYCHIA

Acrokeratosis verruciformis (thin, friable), 50–53
Cardio-facio-cutaneous syndrome, 104
Costello syndrome, 352–55
Hemochromatosis (acquired), 271–73
Hereditary palmoplantar keratoderma with deafness, 54–55
Hutchinson-Gilford progeria, 567–70
Kindler syndrome (mild changes), 579–81
Onychotrichodysplasia with neutropenia, 220–21
Tooth and nail syndrome, 260–61
Tricho-rhino-phalangeal type I, 201–4
Tricho-rhino-phalangeal type II, 201–4
Twenty nail dystrophy, 214–16
Universal melanosis (occasional), 303–5

LEUKONYCHIA

Acrokeratosis verruciformis, 50–53
Darier-White disease (white bands), 88–92
Hailey-Hailey disease (white bands), 160–62
Hemochromatosis, 271–73
Hereditary palmoplantar keratoderma with deafness, 54–55
Leukonychia, 213–14
Leukonychia, deafness, enamel hypoplasia, 214
Leukonychia, sebaceous cysts, renal calculi, 213–14

CLUBBING

Pachydermoperiostosis, 420

PARONYCHIA

Acrodermatitis enteropathica, 547–50
Chronic granulomatous disease, 594–97
Familial mucocutaneous candidiasis, 601–4

OTHER

Alkaptonuria (bluish grey), 550–53
Congenital malalignment of great toenails, 210–11
Darier-White disease (red/white streaks, notching), 88–92
Dyskeratosis congenita (ridging, splitting, pterygia), 264–67
Hereditary palmoplantar keratoderma Olmstead (variable), 60–63
Hereditary palmoplanta keratoderma punctate (variable), 63–66
Hereditary palmoplantar keratoderma Vohwinkel (variable), 71–73
Incontinentia pigmenti (variable), 273–77
Keratosis follicularis spinulosa decalvans (high cuticles), 94–97
Naegeli syndrome (variable), 287–89
Onychogryphosis, 225
Papillon-Lefèvre (occasional-splits, grooves, pits), 75–78

Rothmund-Thomson syndrome (variable), 585–87
Trichothiodystrophy (variable), 205–8
Tuberous sclerosis (periungual fibromas), 409–14

SWEAT GLANDS

HYPOHIDROSIS

AEC syndrome (mild), 241–44
Bazex syndrome (head, face), 487–88
Fabry syndrome (acquired), 377–80
Hereditary sensory and autonomic neuropathy type IV, 423
Hypohidrotic ectodermal dysplasia, 254–57
Lamellar ichthyosis (occasional), 27–30
Naegeli syndrome, 287–89
Pachydermoperiostosis (palmar/plantar), 420
Passarge syndrome, 256
Rapp-Hodgkin syndrome (mild), 257–60
Scleroatrophic and keratotic dermatosis of the limbs (palms/soles), 78–80

HYPERHIDROSIS

Acrokeratoelastoidosis (palmoplantar), 49–50
Blue rubber bleb nevus syndrome (localized), 369–72
Böök syndrome, 229
Charcot-Marie-Tooth disease, 229
Dyskeratosis congenita (palmoplantar), 264–67
Familial dysautonomia, 421–24
Hereditary glomus tumors (localized), 380–83
Hereditary palmoplantar keratoderma
Olmsted, 60–63
Hyperhidrosis, 228–29
Klippel-Trenaunay-Weber syndrome (localized), 388–92
Maffucci syndrome (localized), 392–95
Mal de Meleda (palmoplantar), 73–75
Nail-patella syndrome (rare), 216–20
Pachyonychia congenita (palmoplantar), 222–26
Richner-Hanhart syndrome (palmoplantar), 124–26

Figure Credits

2.1 Sybert, V.P., and Holbrook, K.A. (1987). Prenatal diagnosis and screening. *Dermatol. Clin.* **5,** 17–41.

2.2 ibid.

2.8 Abdel-Hafez, K., Safer, A.M., Selim, M.M., and Rehak, A. (1983). Familial continual skin peeling. *Dermatologica* **166,** 23–31. Copyright S. Karger A.G., Basel.

2.10 Dale, B.A., Holbrook, K.A., Fleckman, P., Kimball, J.R., Brumbaugh, S., and Sybert, V.P. (1990). Heterogeneity in harlequin ichthyosis, an inborn error of epidermal keratinization: Variable morphology and structural protein expression and a defect in lamellar granules. *J. Invest. Dermatol.* **94,** 6–18.

2.12 Steijlen, P.M., van Dooren-Greebe, R.J., Happle, R., and Van de Kerkhof, P.C. (1991). Ichthyosis bullosa of Siemens responds well to low-dosage oral retinoids. *Br. J. Dermatol.* **125,** 469–471. Copyright Blackwell Science Ltd.

2.13 Steijlen, P.M., Perret, C.M., Schuurmans-Stekhoven, J.H., Ruiter, D.J., and Happle, R. (1990). Ichthyosis bullosa of Siemens: Further delineation of the phenotype. *Arch. Dermatol. Res.* **282,** Fig. 4.5, p. 2. Copyright Springer-Verlag.

2.14 Curth, H.O., and Macklin, M.T. (1954). The genetic basis of various types of ichthyosis in a family group. *Am. J. Hum. Genet.* **6,** 371–382. University of Chicago Press. Copyright American Society of Human Genetics.

2.27 Traupe, H. (1989). *The Ichthyoses: A Guide to Clinical Diagnosis, Genetic Counseling and Therapy.* Fig. 61A, B, p. 170. Copyright Springer-Verlag, New York.

2.28 Judge, M.R., Morgan, G., and Harper, J.I. (1994). A clinical and immunological study of Netherton's syndrome. *Br. J. Dermatol.* **131,** 615–621.

2.29A Holbrook, K.A., Dale, B.A., Witt, D.R., Hayden, M.R., and Toriello, H.V. (1987). Arrested epidermal morphogenesis in three newborn infants with a fatal genetic disorder (restrictive dermopathy). *J. Invest. Dermatol.* **88,** 330–339. Reprinted by permission of Blackwell Science, Inc.

2.29B Witt, D.R., Hayden, M.R., Holbrook, K.A., Dale, B.A., Baldwin, V.J., and Taylor, G.P. (1986). Restrictive dermopathy: a newly recognized autosomal recessive skin dysplasia. *Am. J. Med. Genet.* **24,** 631–648. Copyright Alan R. Liss, Inc. Reprinted by permission of John Wiley and Sons, Inc.

2.38 Dupertuis, M.C., Laroche, L., Huault, M.C., and Blanchet-Bardon, C. (1991). Érythrokératodermie progressive et symétrique de Darier-Gottron. *Ann. Dermatol. Venereol.* **118,** 775–778.

2.39 ibid.

2.40 Dowd, P.M., Harman, R.R., and Black, M.M. (1983). Focal acral hyperkeratosis. *Br. J. Dermatol.* **109,** 97–103. Copyright Blackwell Science Ltd.

2.41 ibid.

2.43 Sybert, V.P., Dale, B.A., and Holbrook, K.A. (1988). Palmar-plantar keratoderma. A clinical, ultrastructural, and biochemical study. *J. Am. Acad. Dermatol.* **18,** 75–86.

2.44 Bititci, O.O. (1975). Familial hereditary, progressive sensori-neural hearing loss with keratosis palmaris and plantaris. *J. Laryngol. Otol.* **89,** 1143–1146.

2.46 O'Mahony, M.Y., Ellis, J.P., Hellier, M., Mann, R., and Huddy, P. Familial tylosis and carcinoma of the oesophagus. *J. R. Soc. Med.* **77,** 514–517.

2.47 ibid.

2.48 Lucker, G.P.H., and Steijlen, P.M. (1994). The Olmsted syndrome: Mutilating palmoplantar and periorificial keratoderma. *J. Am. Acad. Dermatol.* **31,** 508–509.

2.49 Atherton, D.J., Sutton, C., and Jones, B.M. (1990). Mutilating palmoplantar keratoderma with periorificial keratotic plaques (Olmsted's syndrome). *Br. J. Dermatol.* **122,** 245–252. Copyright Blackwell Science Ltd.

2.50 Osman, Y., Daly, T.J., and Don, P.C. (1992). Spiny keratoderma of the palms and soles. *J. Am. Acad. Dermatol.* **26,** 879–881.

2.51 Žmegač, Z.J., and Sarajlič, M.V. (1964). A rare form of an inheritable palmar and plantar keratosis. *Dermatologica* **130,** 40–52. Copyright S. Karger A.G., Basel

2.53 Baes, H., De Beukelaar, L., and Wachters, D. (1969). Keratoderma palmo-plantaris varians. *Ann. Dermatol. Syphiligr. Paris* **96,** 45–50.

2.56 Gibbs, R.C., and Frank, S.B. (1966). Keratoma hereditaria mutilans (Vohwinkel). Differentiating features of conditions with constriction of digits. *Arch. Dermatol.* **94,** 619–625. Copyright American Medical Association.

2.57 Franceschetti, A.T., Reinhart, V., and

Schnyder, U.W. (1972). La maladie de Meleda. *J. Genet. Hum.* **20,** 267–296.

2.58 ibid.

2.62 Delaporte, E., N'guyen-Mailfer, C., Janin, A., Savary, J.B., Vasseur, F., Feingold, N., Piette, F., and Bergoend, H. (1995). Keratoderma with scleroatrophy of the extremities or sclerotylosis (Huriez syndrome): A reappraisal. *Br. J. Dermatol.* **133,** 409–416. Copyright Blackwell Science Ltd.

2.63 ibid.

2.66 Baird, H.W. III (1964). Kindred showing congenital absence of the dermal ridges (fingerprints) and associated anomalies. *J. Pediatr.* **64,** 621–631.

2.67 ibid.

2.78 van Osch, L.D., Oranje, A.P., Keukens, F.M., van Voorst-Vader, P.C., and Veldman, E. (1992). Keratosis follicularis spinulosa decalvans: A family study of seven male cases and six female carriers. *J. Med. Genet.* **29,** 36–40.

2.79 ibid.

2.80 ibid.

2.82 Ramer, J.C., Vasily, D.B., and Ladda, R.L. (1994). Familial leuconychia, knuckle pads, hearing loss, and palmoplantar hyperkeratosis: An additional family with Bart-Pumphrey syndrome. *J. Med. Genet.* **31,** 68–71.

2.83 Cunningham, S.R., Walsh, M., Matthews, R., Fulton, R., and Burrows, D. (1987). Kyrle's disease. *J. Am. Acad. Dermatol.* **16,** 117–123.

2.84 Tidman, M.J., Price, M.L., and MacDonald, D.M. (1987). Lamellar bodies in hyperkeratosis lenticularis perstans. *J. Cutan. Pathol.* **14,** 207–211. Copyright Munksgaard International Publishers, Ltd., Copenhagen.

2.88 Happle, R., Koch, H., and Lenz, W. (1980). The CHILD syndrome. Congenital hemidysplasia with ichthyosiform erythroderma and limb defects. *Eur. J. Pediatr.* **134,** 27–33. Fig. 3a–c, p. 28. Copyright Springer-Verlag.

2.89 Hashimoto, K., Topper, S., Sharata, H., and Edwards, M. (1995). CHILD syndrome: Analysis of abnormal keratinization and ultrastructure. *Pediatr. Dermatol.* **12,** 116–129. Reprinted by permission of Blackwell Science, Inc.

2.96 Langer, K., Konrad, K., and Wolff, K. (1990). Keratitis, ichthyosis and deafness (KID) syndrome: Report of three cases and a review of the literature. *Br. J. Dermatol.* **122,** 689–697. Copyright Blackwell Science Ltd.

2.98 Nazzaro, V., Blanchet-Bardon, C., Lorette, G., and Civatte, J. (1990). Familial occurrence of KID (keratitis, ichthyosis, deafness) syndrome. Case reports of a mother and daughter. *J. Am. Acad. Dermatol.* **23,** 385–388.

2.99 Ejeckam, G.G., Wadhwa, J.K., Williams, J.P., and Lacson, A.G. (1986). Neu-Laxova syndrome: Report of two cases. *Pediatr. Pathol.* **5,** 295–306.

2.101 Venencie, P.Y., Pauwels, C., Rekik, A., Mielot, F., Hadchouel, M., and Odievre, M. (1993). Ichtyose avec accumulation de lipides neutres. Syndrome de Dorfman-Chanarin. A propos d'une observation familiale. *Ann. Dermatol. Venereol.* **120,** 758–760.

2.102 ibid.

2.103 Refsum, S., Salomonsen, L., and Skatvedt, M. (1949). Heredopathia atactica polyneuritiformis in children. A preliminary communication. *J. Pediatr.* **35,** 335–343.

2.104 Davies, M.G., Marks, R., Dykes, P.J., and Reynolds, D. (1977). Epidermal abnormalities in Refsum's disease. *Br. J. Dermatol.* **97,** 401–406. Copyright Blackwell Science Ltd.

2.105 Fraser, N.G., MacDonald, J., Griffiths, W.A., and McPhie, J.L. (1987). Tyrosinaemia type II (Richner-Hanhart syndrome)—report of two cases treated with etretinate. *Clin. Exp. Dermatol.* **12,** 440–443. Copyright Blackwell Science Ltd.

2.132 Hashimoto, K., Burk, J.D., Bale, G.F., Eto, H., Hashimoto, A., Kameyama, K., Kanzaki, T., and Nishiyama, S. (1989). Transient bullous dermolysis of the newborn: Two additional cases. *J. Am. Acad. Dermatol.* **21,** 708–713.

3.5 Macías-Flores, M.A., García Cruz, D., Rivera, H., Escobar-Luján, M., Melendrez-Vega, A., Rivas-Campos, D., Rodríguez-Collazo, R., Moreno-Arellano, I., and Cantú, J.M. (1984). A new form of hypertrichosis inherited as an X-linked dominant trait. *Hum. Genet.* **66,** 66–70. Fig. 2,3, p. 67. Copyright Springer-Verlag.

3.6 Santana, S.M., Alvarez, F.P., Frías, J.L., and Martínez-Frias, M.L. (1993). Hypertrichosis, atrophic skin, ectropion, and macrostomia (Barber-Say syndrome): Report of a new case. *Am. J. Med. Genet.* **47,** 20–23.

3.8 Reed, O.M., Mellette, J.R., Jr., and Fitzpatrick, J.E. (1989). Familial cervical hypertrichosis with underlying kyphoscoliosis. *J. Am. Acad. Dermatol.* **20,** 1069–1072.

3.9 Reprinted by permission of the publisher from

Rudolph, R.I. Hairy elbows. *Cutis* **36,** 69. Copyright 1985 by Excerpta Medica Inc.

3.12 Reprinted by permission of the publisher from Price, V.H. Office diagnosis of structural hair anomalies. *Cutis* **15,** 231–240. Copyright 1975 by Excerpta Medica Inc.

3.13 Juon, M. (1942). Eine Beobachtung familiären Auftretens von Pili anulati. *Dermatologica* **86,** 117–122. Copyright S. Karger A.G., Basel.

3.14 ibid.

3.20 Traupe, H. (1989). *The Ichthyoses: A Guide to Clinical Diagnosis, Genetic Counseling and Therapy*. Springer-Verlag, New York, p. 170, Fig. 61A, B.

3.21 Porter, P.S. The genetics of human hair growth. In Bergsma, D. (Ed.). *The Clinical Delineation of Birth Defects*. Baltimore: Williams and Wilkins Company for the National Foundation-March of Dimes. *BD:OAS* **VII(8),** 1971, 69–85, with permission of the copyright holder.

3.25 Sybert, V.P., and Holbrook, K.A. (1987). Prenatal diagnosis and screening. *Dermatol. Clin.* **5,** 17–41.

3.27 Lichtenstein, J., Warson, R., Jorgenson, R., Dorst, J.P., and McKusick, V.A. (1972). The tricho-dento-osseous (TDO) syndrome. *Am. J. Hum. Genet.* **24,** 569–582. University of Chicago Press. Copyright American Society Human Genetics.

3.28 Quattromani, F., Shapiro, S.D., Young, R.S., Jorgenson, R.J., Parker, J.W., Blumhardt, R., and Reece, R.R. (1983). Clinical heterogeneity in the tricho-dento-osseous syndrome. *Hum. Genet.* **64,** 116–121. Fig. 3a,b, p. 118. Copyright Springer-Verlag.

3.31 Happle, R., Traupe, H., Grobe, H., and Bonsmann, G. (1984). The Tay syndrome (congenital ichthyosis with trichothiodystrophy). *Eur. J. Pediatr.* **141,** 147–152. Fig. 1a–d, p. 150. Copyright Springer-Verlag.

3.32 Happle, R., Traupe, H., Grobe, H., and Bonsmann, G. (1984). The Tay syndrome (congenital ichthyosis with trichothiodystrophy). *Eur. J. Pediatr.* **141,** 147–152. Fig. 2a–f, p. 151. Copyright Springer-Verlag.

3.36 Reprinted by permission of the publisher from Martin, S., and Rudolph, A.H. Familial dystrophic periodic shedding of the nails. *Cutis* **25,** 622–623. Copyright 1980 by Excerpta Medica Inc.

3.40 Verhage, J., Habbema, L., Vrensen, G.F., Roord, J.J., and Bleeker-Wagemakers, E.M. (1987). A patient with onychotrichodysplasia, neutropenia and normal intelligence. *Clin. Genet.* **31,** 374–380. Copyright Munksgaard International Publishers, Ltd., Copenhagen.

3.41 ibid.

3.42 ibid.

3.52 Yesudian, P., and Thambiah, A. (1975). Familial syringoma. *Dermatologica* **150,** 32–35. Copyright S. Karger A.G., Basel.

3.53B Piepkorn, M.W., Clark, L., and Lombardi, D.L. (1981). A kindred with congenital vellus hair cysts. *J. Am. Acad. Dermatol.* **5,** 661–665.

3.56 Gorlin, R.J., and Psaume, J. (1962). Orodigitofacial dysostosis—a new syndrome. A study of 22 cases. *J. Pediatr.* **61,** 520–530.

3.57 ibid.

3.58 ibid.

3.60 Magid, M.L., Wentzell, J.M., and Roenigk, H.H, Jr., (1989). Multiple cystic lesions. *Arch. Dermatol.* **126,** 101, 104. Copyright American Medical Association.

3.62 Vanderhooft, S.L., Stephan, M.J., and Sybert, V.P. (1993). Severe skin erosions and scalp infections in AEC syndrome. *Pediatr. Dermatol.* **10,** 334–340.

3.64 ibid.

3.65 ibid.

3.66 ibid.

3.75A Jensen, N.E. (1971). Congenital ectodermal dysplasia of the face. *Br. J. Dermatol.* **84,** 410–416.

3.75B Kowalski, D.C., and Fenske, N.A. (1992). The focal facial dermal dysplasias: Report of a kindred and a proposed new classification. *J. Am. Acad. Dermatol.* **27,** 575–582.

3.77A,B A. Tipton, R.E., and Gorlin, R.J. (1984). Growth retardation, alopecia, pseudo-anodontia, and optic atrophy—the GAPO syndrome: Report of a patient and review of the literature. *Am. J. Med. Genet.* **19,** 209–216. Copyright Wiley-Liss, Inc. Reprinted by permission of Wiley-Liss, Inc., a division of John Wiley and Sons, Inc. B. Original figure courtesy of J.J. Pindborg.

3.80 Sybert, V.P. (1989). Hypohidrotic ectodermal dysplasia: Argument against an autosomal recessive form clinically indistinguishable from X-linked hypohidrotic ectodermal dysplasia (Christ-Siemens-Touraine syndrome). *Pediatr. Dermatol.* **6,** 76–81.

3.81 The Executive and Scientific Advisory Boards of the National Foundation for Ectodermal Dysplasias, Mascoutah, Illinois (1989). Scaling skin in the neonate: A clue to the early diagnosis of X-linked hypohidrotic ectodermal dysplasia (Christ-Siemens-Touraine syndrome). *J. Pediatr.* **114,** 600–602.

3.82 Schroeder, H.W., Jr., and Sybert, V.P. (1987). Rapp-Hodgkin ectodermal dysplasia. *J. Pediatr.* **110,** 72–75.

3.83 ibid.

4.1 Crovato, F., Desirello, G., and Rebora, A. (1983). Is Dowling-Degos disease the same disease as Kitamura's reticulate acropigmentation? *Br. J. Dermatol.* **109,** 105–110. Copyright Blackwell Science Ltd.

4.2 Crovato, F., Nazzari, G., and Rebora, A. (1983). Dowling-Degos disease (reticulate pigmented anomaly of the flexures) is an autosomal dominant condition. *Br. J. Dermatol.* **108,** 473–476. Copyright Blackwell Science Ltd.

4.9 Held, J.L., Yankiver, B., and Kohn, S.R. (1993). Hyperpigmentation and secondary hemochromatosis: A novel treatment with extracorporeal chelation. *J. Am. Acad. Dermatol.* **28,** 253–254.

4.10A Sybert, V.P., and Holbrook, K.A. (1987). Prenatal diagnosis and screening. *Dermatol. Clin.* **5,** 17–41.

4.10B–D Francis, J.S., and Sybert, V.P. (1995). Update on incontinentia pigmenti. *Curr. Opin. Dermatol.,* 55–60.

4.13 ibid.

4.14 ibid.

4.17B Ting, H.C., and Ng, S.C. (1983). The leopard (multiple lentigines) syndrome: A case report. *Med. J. Malaysia* **38,** 98–101.

4.23 Itin, P.H., Lautenschlager, S., Meyer, R., Mevorah, B., and Rufli, T. (1993). Natural history of the Naegeli-Franceschetti-Jadassohn syndrome and further delineation of its clinical manifestations. *J. Am. Acad. Dermatol.* **28,** 942–950.

4.24 ibid.

4.25 ibid.

4.26 Carney, J.A., Gordon, H., Carpenter, P.C., Shenoy, B.V., and Go, V.L. (1985). The complex of myxomas, spotty pigmentation, and endocrine overactivity. *Medicine Baltimore* **64,** 270–283.

4.27 Atherton, D.J., Pitcher, D.W., Wells, R.S., and MacDonald, D.M. (1980). A syndrome of various cutaneous pigmented lesions, myxoid neurofibromata and atrial myxoma: The NAME syndrome. *Br. J. Dermatol.* **103,** 421–429.

4.28 Koopman, R.J., and Happle, R. (1991). Autosomal dominant transmission of the NAME syndrome (nevi, atrial myxoma, mucinosis of the skin and endocrine overactivity). *Hum. Genet.* **86,** 300–304. Fig. 2, p. 301. Copyright Springer-Verlag.

4.38 Kint, A., Oomen, C., Geerts, M.L., and Breuillard, F. (1987). Mélanose diffuse congénitale. *Ann. Dermatol. Venereol.* **114,** 11–16.

4.39 Shiloh, Y., Litvak, G., Ziv, Y., Lehner, T., Sandkuyl, L., Hildesheimer, M., Buchris, V., Cremers, F.P., Szabo, P., White, B.N., Holden, J.J.A., and Ott, J. (1990). Genetic mapping of X-linked albinism-deafness syndrome (ADFN) to Xq26.3–q27.1. *Am. J. Hum. Genet.* **47,** 20–27. University of Chicago Press. Copyright American Society of Human Genetics. Original figure courtesy of Dr. Kalman Fried.

4.40 Witkop, C.J., Jr. (1985). Inherited disorders of pigmentation. *Clin. Dermatol.* **3,** 70–134. Reprinted by permission of the publisher. Copyright Elsevier Science, Inc.

4.42 Walsh, R.J. (1971). A distinctive pigment of the skin in New Guinea indigenes. *Ann. Hum. Genet.* **34,** 379–388.

4.43 Nance, W.E., Jackson, C.E., and Witkop, C.J., Jr. (1970). Amish albinism: A distinctive autosomal recessive phenotype. *Am. J. Hum. Genet.* **22,** 579–586. University of Chicago Press. Copyright American Society of Human Genetics.

4.44 Fryns, J.P., Dereymaeker, A.M., Heremans, G., Marien, J., van Hauwaert, J., Turner, G., Hockey, A., and van den Berghe, H. (1988). Oculocerebral syndrome with hypopigmentation (Cross syndrome). Report of two siblings born to consanguineous parents. *Clin. Genet.* **34,** 81–84. Copyright Munksgaard International Publishers, Ltd., Copenhagen.

4.45 ibid.

4.46 Sybert, V.P., Pagon, R.A., Donlan, M., and Bradley, C.M. (1990). Pigmentary abnormalities and mosaicism for chromosomal aberration: Association with clinical features similar to hypomelanosis of Ito. *J. Pediatr.* **116,** 581–586.

5.3 Weinstein, H. (1913). A description of ainhum as seen on the Canal Zone, with report of interesting cases occurring in one family. *South Med. J.* **6,** 651–656.

5.8A Petty, E.M., Seashore, M.R., Braverman, I.M., Spiesel, S.Z., Smith, L.T., and Milstone, L.M. (1993). Dermatosparaxis in children. A case report and review of the newly recognized phenotype. *Arch. Dermatol.* **129,** 1310–1315.

5.20 Nelson, D.L., and King, R.A. (1981).

Ehlers-Danlos syndrome type VIII. *J. Am. Acad. Dermatol.* **5,** 297–303.

5.21 Mehregan, A.H. (1970). Transepithelial elimination. *Curr. Probl. Dermatol.* **3,** 124–147. Copyright S. Karger A.G., Basel.

5.22 ibid.

5.23 Davies, S.J., and Hughes, H.E. (1994). Costello syndrome: Natural history and differential diagnosis of cutis laxa. *J. Med. Genet.* **31,** 486–489.

5.24 Costa, T., Eichenfield, L.F., and Krafchik, B.R. (1994). What syndrome is this? Costello syndrome. *Pediatr. Dermatol.* **11,** 277–279. Reprinted by permission of Blackwell Science, Inc.

5.25 ibid.

5.26A Philip A.G.S. (1978). Cutis laxa with intrauterine growth retardation and hip dislocation in a male. *J. Pediatr.* **93,** 150–151.

5.28 Ledoux-Corbusier, M. (1983). Cutis laxa, congenital form with pulmonary emphysema: An ultrastructural study. *J. Cutan. Pathol.* **10,** 340–349. Copyright Munksgaard International Publishers Ltd., Copenhagen.

5.29 Koppe, R., Kaplan, P., Hunter, A., and MacMurray, B. (1989). Ambiguous genitalia associated with skeletal abnormalities, cutis laxa, craniostenosis, psychomotor retardation, and facial abnormalities (SCARF syndrome). *Am. J. Med. Genet.* **34,** 305–312.

5.30 ibid.

5.31A,B Hurvitz, S.A., Baumgarten, A., and Goodman, R.M. (1990). The wrinkly skin syndrome: A report of a case and review of the literature. *Clin. Genet.* **38,** 307–313. Copyright Munksgaard International Publishers Ltd., Copenhagen.

5.34 van Joost, T., Vuzevski, V.D., ten Kate, F.J., Stolz, E., and Heule, F. (1988). Elastosis perforans serpiginosa: Clinical, histomorphological and immunological studies. *J. Cutan. Pathol.* **15,** 92–97. Copyright Munksgaard International Publishers, Ltd., Copenhagen.

5.44 Sybert, V.P., and Holbrook, K.A. (1987). Prenatal diagnosis and screening. *Dermatol. Clin.* **5,** 17–41.

5.59 Sybert, V.P. (1985). Aplasia cutis congenita: A report of 12 new families and review of the literature. *Pediatr. Dermatol.* **3,** 1–14. Blackwell Scientific Publ. Ltd.

5.60 ibid.

5.61 ibid.

5.62 ibid.

5.63 ibid.

5.73A Oikarinen, A., Palatsi, R., Kylmaniemi, M., Keski-Oja, J., Risteli, J., and Kallioinen, M. (1994). Pachydermoperiostosis: Analysis of the connective tissue abnormality in one family. *J. Am. Acad. Dermatol.* **31,** 947–953.

5.75 Beare, J.M., Dodge, J.A., and Nevin, N.C. (1969). Cutis gyratum, acanthosis nigricans and other congenital anomalies. A new syndrome. *Br. J. Dermatol.* **81,** 241–247. Copyright Blackwell Science Ltd.

5.76 Axelrod, F.B., Nachtigal, R., Dancis, J., (1974). Familial dysautonomia: Diagnosis, pathogenesis and management. *Adv. Pediatr.* **21,** 75–96.

5.77 Ruiz-Maldonado, R., Tamayo, L., and Velazquez, E. (1977). Dystrophie dermo-chondro-corneene familiale (syndrome de François). *Ann. Dermatol. Venereol.* **104,** 475–478.

5.82 Hall, J.G., Reed, S.D., and Greene, G. (1982). The distal arthrogryposes: Delineation of new entities—review and nosologic discussion. *Am. J. Med. Genet.* **11,** 185–239.

5.83A ibid.

5.84 ibid.

5.85 Glover, M.T., Lake, B.D., and Atherton, D.J. (1992). Clinical, histologic, and ultrastructural findings in two cases of infantile systemic hyalinosis. *Pediatr. Dermatol.* **9,** 255–258. Reprinted by permission of Blackwell Science Ltd.

5.87 Hollister, D.W., Rimoin, D.L., Lachman, R.S., Cohen, A.H., Reed, W.B., and Westin, G.W. (1974). The Winchester syndrome: A nonlysosomal connective tissue disease. *J. Pediatr.* **84,** 701–709.

6.1 Bacchi, O., Stefanucci, S., Brustenghi, P.L., Pagliacci, A., and Bellanti, G.M. (1992). Cerebrotendinous xanthomatosis. Case report. *Ital. J. Neurol. Sci.* **13,** 511–515.

6.6 Reprinted by permission of the publisher from Pereyo, N. Fibrodysplasia ossificans progressiva. *Cutis* **17,** 376, 381. Copyright 1976 by Excerpta Medica Inc.

6.8 Dustin, P., Tondeur, M., Jonniaux, G., Vamos-Hurwitz, E., and Pelc, S. (1973). La maladie de Farber. Etude anatomo- clinique et ultrastructurale. *Bull. Acad. Méd. Belg.* **128,** 733–762.

6.9 Abul-Haj, S.K., Martz, D.G., Douglas, W.F., and Geppert, L.J. (1962). Farber's disease. Report of a case with observations on its histogenesis and notes on the nature of the stored material. *J. Pediatr.* **61,** 221–232.

6.10 Chanoki, M., Ishii, M., Fukai, K., Kobayashi, H., Hamada, T., Murakami, K., and Tanaka, A. (1989). Farber's lipogranulomatosis in siblings: Light and electron microscopic studies. *Br. J. Dermatol.* **121,** 779–785. Copyright Blackwell Science Ltd.

6.12 Seip, M. (1971). Generalized lipodystrophy. *Ergeb. Inn. Med. Kinderheilkd.* **31,** 59–95. Fig. 1, p. 68. Copyright Springer-Verlag.

6.13 op. cit. Fig. 2, p. 71. Copyright Springer-Verlag.

7.1 Aagenaes, O. (1974). Hereditary recurrent cholestasis with lymphoedema—two new families. *Acta Paediatr. Scand.* **63,** 465–471.

8.2 Frank, M.M., Gelfand, J.A., and Atkinson, J.P. (1976). Hereditary angioedema: The clinical syndrome and its management. *Ann. Intern. Med.* **84,** 580–593. Reproduced with permission.

8.3 Starr, J.C., and Brasher, G.W. (1974). Erythema marginatum preceding hereditary angioedema. *J. Allergy Clin. Immunol.* **53,** 352–355.

8.4 Zimmer, W.M., Rogers, R.S.III, Reeve, C.M., and Sheridan, P.J. (1992). Orofacial manifestations of Melkersson-Rosenthal syndrome. A study of 42 patients and review of 220 cases from the literature. *Oral Surg. Oral Med. Oral Pathol.* **74,** 610–619.

8.11 Selmanowitz, V.J., and Orentreich, N. (1970). Mastocytosis. A clinical genetic evaluation. *J. Hered.* **61,** 91–94. By permission of Oxford University Press.

9.2 Kunze, J., and Riehm, H. (1982). A new genetic disorder: Autosomal-dominant multiple benign ring-shaped skin creases. *Eur. J. Pediatr.* **138,** 301–303.

9.3 ibid.

9.4 Jablonska, S., Schubert, H., and Kikuchi, I. (1989). Congenital fascial dystrophy: Stiff skin syndrome—a human counterpart of the tight-skin mouse. *J. Am. Acad. Dermatol.* **21,** 943–950.

10.5A,B Michaelsson, G., Olsson, E., and Westermark, P. (1981). The Rombo syndrome: A familial disorder with vermiculate atrophoderma, milia, hypotrichosis, trichoepitheliomas, basal cell carcinomas and peripheral vasodilation with cyanosis. *Acta Derm. Venereol.* **61,** 497–503.

10.6 Gould, D.J., and Barker, D.J. (1978). Follicular atrophoderma with multiple basal cell carcinomas (Bazex). *Br. J. Dermatol.* **99,** 431–435. Copyright Blackwell Science Ltd.

10.20 Biggs, P.J., Wooster, R., Ford, D., Chapman, P., Mangion, J., Quirk, Y., Easton, D.F., Burn, J., and Stratton, M.R. (1995). Familial cylindromatosis (turban tumour syndrome) gene localised to chromosome 16q12–q13: Evidence for its role as a tumour suppressor gene. *Nat. Genet.* **11,** 441–443.

10.28 Ferguson Smith, J., (1934). A case of multiple primary squamous-celled carcinomata of the skin in a young man with spontaneous healing. *Br. J. Dermatol. Syphil.* **46,** 267–272. Copyright Blackwell Science Ltd.

10.29 Charteris, A.A. (1951). Self-healing epithelioma of the skin. *Am. J. Roentgenol. Rad. Ther.* **65,** 459–464.

10.30 ibid.

10.31 Schaffzin, E.A., Chung, S.M., and Kaye, R. (1972). Congenital generalized fibromatosis with complete spontaneous regression. A case report. *J. Bone Joint Surg. Am.* **54,** 657–662.

10.32 Fryns, J.P., and Chrzanowska, K. (1988). Mucosal neuromata syndrome (MEN type IIB (III)). *J. Med. Genet.* **25,** 703–706.

10.33 Kirk, J.F., Flowers, F.P., Ramos-Caro, F.A., and Browder, J.F. (1991). Multiple endocrine neoplasia type III: Case report and review. *Pediatr. Dermatol.* **8,** 124–128. Reprinted by permission of Blackwell Scientific Publications, Inc.

10.42 Metzker, A., Eisenstein, B., Oren, J., and Samuel, R. (1988). Tumoral calcinosis revisited—common and uncommon features. Report of ten cases and review. *Eur. J. Pediatr.* **147,** 128–132. Fig. 3-7, p. 130. Copyright Springer-Verlag.

11.2 Vanotti, A. (1954). *Porphyrins; Their Biological and Chemical Importance.* Hilgers and Watts, London.

11.3 Fayle, S.A., and Pollard, M.A. (1994). Congenital erythropoietic porphyria—oral manifestations and dental treatment in childhood: A case report. *Quintessence Int.* **25,** 551–554. Copyright Quintessence Publishing.

11.5 Moore, M.R., McColl, K.E.L., Rimington, C., and Goldberg, A. (1987). *Disorders of Porphyrin Metabolism.* Plenum Medical Book Co., New York, p. 203. Original attributed to I.A. Magnus.

11.6 Hunter, J.A.A., Khan, S.A., Hope, E., Beattie, A.D., Beveridge, G.W., Smith, A.W., and Goldberg, A. (1971). Hereditary coproporphyria. Photosensitivity, jaundice and neuropsychiatric manifestations associated with pregnancy. *Br. J. Dermatol.* **84,** 301–310. Copyright Blackwell Science Ltd.

11.9 Parsons, J.L., Sahn, E.E., Holden, K.R.,

and Pai, G.S. (1994). Neurologic disease in a child with hepatoerythropoietic porphyria. *Pediatr. Dermatol.* **11,** 216–221. Reprinted by permission of Blackwell Science Ltd.

11.17 Albers, S.E., Brozena, S.J., Glass, L.F., and Fenske, N.A. (1992). Alkaptonuria and ochronosis: Case report and review. *J. Am. Acad. Dermatol.* **27,** 609–614.

11.18 Thoene, J., Baker, H., Yoshino, M., and Sweetman, L. (1981). Biotin-responsive carboxylase deficiency associated with subnormal plasma and urinary biotin. *N. Engl. J. Med.* **304,** 817–820.

11.20 Black, M.M., and Wilson Jones, E. (1971). Macular amyloidosis. A study of 21 cases with special reference to the role of the epidermis in its histogenesis. *Br. J. Dermatol.* **84,** 199–209. Blackwell Scientific Publications Ltd.

12.3 de Barsy, A.M., Moens, E., and Dierckx, L. (1968). Dwarfism, oligophrenia and degeneration of the elastic tissue in skin and cornea. A new syndrome? *Helv. Paediatr. Acta* **23,** 305–313.

12.4 Cohen, M.M., Jr. (1991). Hallermann-Streiff syndrome: A review. *Am. J. Med. Genet.* **41,** 488–499. Copyright Wiley-Liss, Inc. Reprinted by permission of Wiley-Liss, Inc., a division of John Wiley and Sons, Inc. Original courtesy of Dr. R. Gorlin.

12.5 ibid.

13.2 German, J. (1969). Bloom's syndrome. I. Genetical and clinical observations in the first twenty-seven patients. (1969). *Am. J. Hum. Genet.* **21,** 196–227. University of Chicago Press. Copyright American Society of Human Genetics.

13.3 Galadari, E., Hadi, S., and Sabarinathan, K. (1993). Hartnup disease. *Int. J. Dermatol.* **32,** 904.

13.4 Kindler, T. (1954). Congenital poikiloderma with traumatic bulla formation and progressive cutaneous atrophy. A case report. *Br. J. Dermatol.* **66,** 104–111. Copyright Blackwell Science Ltd.

13.5 Forman, A.B., Prendiville, J.S., Esterly, N.B., Hebert, A.A., Duvic, M., Horiguchi, Y., and Fine, J.D. (1989). Kindler syndrome: Report of two cases and review of the literature. *Pediatr. Dermatol.* **6,** 91–101. Reprinted by permission of Blackwell Science Ltd.

13.6 Draelos, Z.K., and Hansen, R.C. (1986). Polymorphic light eruption in pediatric patients with American Indian ancestry. *Pediatr. Dermatol.* **3,** 384–389. Reprinted by permission of Blackwell Science Ltd.

13.7 Birt, A.R., and Davis, R.A. (1975). Hereditary polymorphic light eruption of American Indians. *Int. J. Dermatol.* **14,** 105–111.

13.8 ibid.

13.12B Sybert, V.P., and Holbrook, K.A. (1987). Prenatal diagnosis and screening. *Dermatol. Clin.* **5,** 17–41.

14.1 Windhorst, D.B., Zelickson, A.S., and Good, R.A. (1968). A human pigmentary dilution based on a heritable subcellular structural defect—the Chediak-Higashi syndrome. *J. Invest. Dermatol.* **50,** 9–18. Reprinted by permission of Blackwell Science, Inc.

14.2 Hurvitz, H., Gillis, R., Klaus, S., Klar, A., Gross-Kieselstein, F., and Okon, E. (1993). A kindred with Griscelli disease: Spectrum of neurological involvement. *Eur. J. Pediatr.* **152,** 402–405. Fig. 2, p. 403. Copyright Springer-Verlag.

14.7 Lutzner, M.A., and Blanchet-Bardon, C. (1985). Epidermodysplasia verruciformis. *Curr. Probl. Dermatol.* **13,** 164–185.

14.8 ibid.

14.9 Pazin, G.J., Nagel, J.E., Friday, G.A., and Fireman, P. (1979). Topical clotrimazole treatment of chronic mucocutaneous candidiasis. *J. Pediatr.* **94,** 322–324.

14.14 Okamoto, G.A., Hall, J.G., Ochs, H., Jackson, C., Rodaway, K., and Chandler, J. New syndrome of chronic mucocutaneous candidiasis. In Bergsma, D. & Lowry, R.B. (Eds.). *New Syndromes.* New York: Alan R. Liss for The National Foundation—March of Dimes. *BD:OAS* **XIII(3B),** 1977, 117–125, with permission of the copyright holder.

14.15 ibid.

14.16 ibid.

Index

Page numbers in italics refer to listings in the differential diagnosis section of other disorders.